Foundations of Adult Health Nursing

Third Edition

DEDICATIONS

Lois White:
To my beloved husband, John, who is on his last great adventure and learning experience.

Gena Duncan:
To my husband, who gives me unconditional love and brings balance, calmness, and excitement to my life.
To Lois White, who modeled the role of an author and committed much of her life to this textbook.
To Wendy Baumle, for her hard work and dedication in developing this textbook. Thanks.
To future nurses who are caring and competent.

Wendy Baumle:
This book is dedicated to my beloved family—Patrick, Taylor, Madeline, Blair, Connor, Janet, and Robert—for their love and support, to Juliet Steiner for inspiring me and for making a difference in my life, to Gena Duncan for her guidance and friendship, and to my friends, colleagues, and students for their support and valuable insight into today's nursing education.

Foundations of Adult Health Nursing

Third Edition

Lois White, RN, PhD
Former Chairperson and Professor Department of Vocational Nurse Education, Del Mar College, Corpus Christi, Texas

Gena Duncan, RN, MSEd, MSN
Former Associate Professor of Nursing, Ivy Tech Community College, Fort Wayne, Indiana

Wendy Baumle, RN, MSN
James A. Rhodes State College, School of Nursing, Lima, Ohio

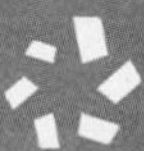

CENGAGE Learning™

Australia • Brazil • Japan • Korea • Mexico • Singapore • Spain • United Kingdom • United States

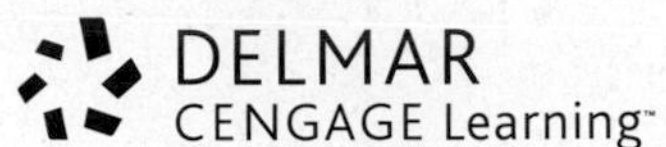

Foundations of Adult Health Nursing, Third Edition
Lois White, RN, PhD, Gena Duncan, RN, MSEd, MSN, and Wendy Baumle, RN, MSN

Vice President, Career and Professional Editorial: Dave Garza

Director of Learning Solutions: Matt Kane

Executive Editor: Steven Helba

Managing Editor: Marah Bellegarde

Senior Product Manager: Juliet Steiner

Editorial Assistant: Meghan E. Orvis

Vice President, Career and Professional Marketing: Jennifer Ann Baker

Marketing Director: Wendy Mapstone

Senior Marketing Manager: Michele McTighe

Marketing Coordinator: Scott Chrysler

Production Director: Carolyn Miller

Production Manager: Andrew Crouth

Senior Content Project Manager: James Zayicek

Senior Art Director: Jack Pendleton

Technology Project Manager: Mary Colleen Liburdi

Production Technology Analyst: Patricia Allen

Production Technology Analyst: Ben Knapp

Library of Congress Control Number: 2010920751
ISBN-13: 978-1-4283-1775-8
ISBN-10: 1-4283-1775-9

Delmar
5 Maxwell Drive
Clifton Park, NY 12065-2919
USA

Cengage Learning is a leading provider of customized learning solutions with office locations around the globe, including Singapore, the United Kingdom, Australia, Mexico, Brazil, and Japan. Locate your local office at: **international.cengage.com/region**

Cengage Learning products are represented in Canada by Nelson Education, Ltd.

To learn more about Delmar, visit **www.cengage.com/delmar**

Purchase any of our products at your local college store or at our preferred online store **www.CengageBrain.com**

Printed in the United States of America
1 2 3 4 5 6 7 12 11 10

CONTENTS

CHAPTER 3: ONCOLOGY / 44

UNIT 2

Nursing Care of the Client: Oxygenation and Perfusion / 69

CHAPTER 4: RESPIRATORY SYSTEM / 70

CHAPTER 5: CARDIOVASCULAR SYSTEM / 119

CHAPTER 6: HEMATOLOGIC AND LYMPHATIC SYSTEMS / 163

UNIT 3

Nursing Care of the Client: Digestion and Elimination / 195

CHAPTER 7: GASTROINTESTINAL SYSTEM / 196

CHAPTER 8: URINARY SYSTEM / 238

UNIT 4

Nursing Care of the Client: Mobility, Coordination, and Regulation / 275

CHAPTER 9: MUSCULOSKELETAL SYSTEM / 276

CHAPTER 12: ENDOCRINE SYSTEM / 388

UNIT 5

Nursing Care of the Client: Reproductive and Sexual Health / 429

CHAPTER 13: REPRODUCTIVE SYSTEM / 430

CHAPTER 14: SEXUALLY TRANSMITTED INFECTIONS / 481

UNIT 6

Nursing Care of the Client: Body Defenses / 499

CHAPTER 15: INTEGUMENTARY SYSTEM / 500

CHAPTER 16: IMMUNE SYSTEM / 543

UNIT 7

Nursing Care of the Client: Physical and Mental Integrity / 581

CHAPTER 17: MENTAL ILLNESS / 582

UNIT 8

Nursing Care of the Client: Older Adult / 645

CHAPTER 19: THE OLDER ADULT / 646

UNIT 9

Nursing Care of the Client: Health Care in the Community / 677

CHAPTER 20: AMBULATORY, RESTORATIVE, AND PALLIATIVE CARE IN COMMUNITY SETTINGS / 678

CHAPTER 22: INTEGRATION / 725

CONTRIBUTORS

Carol A. Fetters Andersen, RN, MSN
Director of Mental Health Services
St. Anthony Regional Hospital and Nursing Home
Carroll, IA
Chapter 19, The Older Adult

Carma Andrus, RN, MN,CNS
Dauterive Primary Care Clinic
St. Martinville, LA
Chapter 11, Sensory System

Diane R. Behrens, RNCS, MA, MSEd
Instructor
University of Saint Francis
Fort Wayne, IN
Chaptere 16, Immune System

Gyl A. Burkhard, RN, BSN, MS
Instructor
OCM BOCES
Syracuse, NY
Chapter 8, Urinary System

Diana L. Case, RN, MA, FNP
Neighborhood Health Clinic
Fort Wayne, IN
Chapter 2, Surgery

Janice Eilerman, MSN, RN
Rhodes State College
Lima, OH
Chapter 15: Integumentary System

Mary Elias, RNC, BSN, CCE
Instructor
Practical Nursing Program
Ivy Tech State College
Fort Wayne, IN
Chapter 13, Reproductive System

Michael A. Fiedler, CRNA, MS
Assistant Professor
Applied Health Sciences
University of Alabama at Birmingham
Birmingham, AL
Chapter 1, Anesthesia

Nancy Fieldhouse, RNBC, MSN
Ivy Tech Community College Northeast
Fort Wayne, IN
Chapter 20, Ambulatory, Restorative, and Palliative Care in Community Settings

Lynn Franck, MS, RN
Assistant Professor
Rhodes State College
Lima, OH
Chapter 12: Endocrine System

Norma Fujise, RN, C, MS
School of Nursing
University of Hawaii
Honoloulu, HI
Chapter 15, Integumentary System

Cathy Greer, RN, MS
Instructor
Lutheran College of Health Professions
Fort Wayne, IN
Chapter 2, Surgery

Margaret L. Griffin, RN, BSN, MS
Instructor
Luthern College of Health Professions
Fort Wayne, IN
Chapter 15, Integumentary System

Beverly F. Hidebrand, RN, BSN, MS
Former Health Occupations Coordinator
Washington, Saratoga, Warren, Hamilton, & Essex Counties BOCES
Saratoga, NY
Chapter 8, Urinary System

Janet Leah Joost, RN, BSN
Instructor
Front Range Community College
Boulder, CO
Chapter 4, Respiratory System

Janet E. Keith, RN, MSEd
Instructor Practical Nursing Program
Ivy Tech State College
Fort Wayne, IN
Chapter 9, Musculoskeletal System

Vicki L. Khouli, RN, BSN, MA, IBCLC
Instructor
Practical Nursing Program
Ivy Tech State College
Fort Wayne, IN
Chapter 14, Sexually Transmitted Infections

Celinda Kay Leach, RN, BS, MPH
Program Chair
Practical Nursing Program
Ivy Tech State College
Bloomington, IN
Chapter 3, Oncology

Sandra Liming, RN, MN
Nursing Instructor
North Seattle Community College
North Seattle, WA
Chapter 13, Reproductive System

Patricia Lokken, MSN, FNP-C
Family Nurse Practitioner
Blearwater Health Services
Bagley, MN
Chapter 20, Ambulatory, Restorative, and Palliative Care in Community Settings

Cheryl McGaffic, RN, PhD
Clinical Instructor
College of Nursing
The University of Arizona
Tucson, AZ
Chapter 16, Immune System

Robin Theresa McKenzie, RN, MSN, CCRN
Assistant Chairman
Navy Medical Center
San Diego, CA
Chapter 11, Sensory System

David K. Miller, RNC, BSN, MSEd
ICU/Medical-Surgical Manager
W. S. Major Hospital
Shelbyville, IN
Chapter 16, Immune System

Joan Fritsch Needham, RNC, MS
Director of Education
DeKalb County Nursing Home
DeKalb, IL
Chapter 19, The Older Adult

Raymond Phillips, RN, MS, CCRN
Clinical Nurse Specialist
Staff Development Coordinator
U.S. Naval Hospital
Rota, Spain
Chapter 11, Sensory System

Susan Reinhart, RN, MS
Assistant Professor
Department of Registered Nurse Education
Del Mar College
Corpus Christi, TX
Chapter 17, Mental Illness

Kathy Rockwell, RN, BSN, MA, MSN, PNP
Professor
Department of RN Education
Del Mar College Corpus Christi, TX
and
Supervisor, Surgical Services
94th General Hospital
Seagoville, TX
Chapter 21, Responding to Emergencies

Martha Ann Rust, RN, BSN, MSN
Instructor
Lutheran College of Health Professions
Fort Wayne, IN
Chapter 10, Neurological System

Mary Kay Schultz, RN, MSN, ANP
Instructor
Department of Nursing
Regis University
Denver, CO
Chapter 12, Endocrine System

Leslee R. Sinn, RN, BSN
Instructor
Front Range Community College
Boulder, CO
Chapter 7, Gastrointestinal System

Russlyn A. St. John, RN, MSN
Associate Professor & Coordinator Practical Nursing
St. Charles Community College
St. Peters, MO
Chapter 12, Endocrine System

Patricia Tutor, PhD
Riverside Community College
Riverside, CA
Chapter 7: Gastrointestinal System

Donna Jean White, RN, MS
Rhodes State College
Lima, OH
Chapter 19: The Older Adult

Lorrie Wong, RN, MS
School of Nursing
University of Hawaii
Honolulu HI
Chapter 15, Integumentary System

REVIEWERS

Charlene Bell, RN, MSN, NCSN
Instructor
Associate Degree Nursing Program
Southwest Texas Junior College
Uvalde, TX

Donna Burleson, RN, MS
Chair of Nursing Department
Cisco Junior College
Abilene, TX

Dotty Cales, RN
Instructor
North Coast Medical Training Academy
Kent, OH

Carolyn Du, BSN, MSN, NP, CDe
Director of Education
Pacific College
Costa Mesa, CA

Jennifer Einhorn, RN, MS
Nursing Instructor
Chamberlain College of Nursing
Addison, IL

Patricia Fennessy, RN, MSN
Education Consultant
Connecticut Technical High School System
Middletown, CT

Carol Greulich, CS, RN, MSN
Assistant Professor
University of Saint Francis
Fort Wayne, IN

Helena L. Jermalovic, RN, MSN
Assistant Professor
University of Alaska
Anchorage, AK

Sharon Knarr, RN
Clinical Instructor
LPN Program
Northcoast Medical Training Academy
Kent, OH

Christine Levandowski, RN, BSN, MSN
Director of Nursing
Baker College
Auburn Hills, MI

Wendy Maleki, RN, MS
Director
Vocational Nursing Program
American Career College
Ontario, CA

Katherine C. Pellerin, RN, BS, MS
Department Head, LPN Program
Norwich Technical High School
Norwich, CT

Jennifer Ponto, RN, BSN
Faculty
Vocational Nursing Program
South Plains College
Levelland, TX

Cheryl Pratt, RN, MA, CNAA
Regional Dean of Nursing
Rasmussen College
Mankato, MN

Cherie R. Rebar, RN, MSN, MBA, FNP
Chair, Associate Professor, Nursing Program
Kettering College of Medical Arts
Kettering, OH

Timm Reed, RRT, RN, BS, MSN, MBA
Assistant Professor
University of Saint Francis
Fort Wayne, IN

Patricia Schrull, RN, MSN, MBA, MEd, CNE
Director, Practical Nursing Program
Lorain County Community College
Elyria, OH

Laura Spinelli
Keiser Career College
Miami Lakes, FL

Frances S. Stoner, RN, BSN, PHN
Instructor, NCLEX Coordinator
American Career College
Anaheim, CA

Tina Terpening
Associate Nursing Faculty
University of Phoenix, Southern California Campus

Lori Theodore, RN, BSN
Orlando Tech
Orlando, FL

Kimberly Valich, RN, MSN
Nursing Faculty, Department Chairperson
South Suburban College
South Holland, IL

Sarah Elizabeth Youth Whitaker, DNS, RN
Nursing Program Director
Computer Career Center
El Paso, TX

Shawn White, RN, BSN
Clinical Coordinator, Nursing Instructor
Griffin Technical College
Griffin, GA

Christina R. Wilson, RN, BAN, PHN
Faculty, Practical Nursing Program
Anoka Technical College
Anoka, MN

MARKET REVIEWERS AND CLASS TEST PARTICIPANTS

Deborah Ain
Nursing Professor
College of Southern Nevada
Las Vegas, NV

Mary Ann Ambrose, MSN, FNP
Program Director
Cuesta Community College Vocational Nursing Program
Paso Robles, CA

Jennie Applegate, RN, BSN
Practical Nursing Instructor
Keiser Career College
Greenacres, FL

Charlotte A. Armstrong, RN, BSN
Instructor
Northcoast Medical Training Academy
Kent, OH

Camille Baldwin
High Tech Central
Fort Myers, FL

Priscilla Burks, RN, BSN
Practical Nursing Instructor
Hinds Community College
Pearl, MS

Virginia Chacon
Colorado Technical University
Pueblo, CO

Sherri Comfort, RN
Practical Nursing Instructor Department Chair
Holmes Community College
Goodman, MS

Brandy Coward, BNS, MA
Director of Nursing
Angeles Institute
Lakewood, CA

Scott Coward, RN
Campus Director
Angeles Institute
Lakewood, CA

Jennifer Decker
Clinical Instructor
College of Eastern Utah
Price, UT

C. Kay Devereux
Professor
Department Chair, Vocational Nurse Education
Tyler Junior College
Tyler, TX

Carolyn Du, BSN, MSN, NP, CDe
Director of Education
Pacific College
Costa Mesa, CA

Laura R. Durbin, RN, BSN, CHPN
Instructor
West Kentucky Community and Technical College
Paducah, KY

Robin Ellis, BSN, MS
Nursing Faculty
Provo College
Provo, UT

Suzanne D. Fox, RN
Practical Nursing Instructor
Arkansas State University Technical Center
Marked Tree, AR

Judie Fritz, RN, MSN
Instructor
Keiser Career College
Miami Lakes, FL

Edith Gerdes, RN, MSN, BHCA
Associate Professor of Nursing
Ivy Tech Community College
South Bend, IN

Juanita Hamilton-Gonzalez
Professor
Coordinator – Practical Nursing Program
City University of New York – Medgar Evers
Brooklyn, NY

Jane Harper
Assistant Professor
Southeast Kentucky Community & Technical College
Pineville, KY

Angie Headley
Nursing Instructor
Swainsboro Technical College
Swainsboro, GA

Lillie Hill
Clinical Coordinator/Instructor
Practical Nursing
Durham Technical Community College
Durham, NC

Michelle Hopper
Sanford-Brown College
St. Peters, MO

Karla Huntsman, RN, MSN
Instructor
Nursing Program
AmeriTech College
Draper, UT

Connie M. Hyde, RN, BSN
Practical Nursing Instructor
Louisiana Technical College
Lafayette, LA

Denise Isackila
Instructor
North Coast Medical Training Academy
Kent, OH

Kimball Johnson, RN, MS
Nursing Professor
College of Eastern Utah
Price, UT

Sandy Kamhoot, BSN
Faculty
Santa Fe College
Gainesville, FL

Juanita Kaness, MSN, RN, CRNP
Nursing Program Coordinator
Lehigh Carbon Community College
Schnecksville, PA

Mary E. Kilbourn-Huey, MSN
Assistant Professor
Maysville Community and Technical College
Maysville, KY

Gloria D. Kline, RN
Practical Nursing Instructor
Hinds Community College
Vicksburg, MS

Christine Levandowski, RN, BSN, MSN
Director of Nursing
Baker College
Auburn Hills, MI

Mary Luckett, RN, MS
Professor Vocational Nursing
Level 1 Coordinator
Houston Community College
Coleman College for Health Sciences
Houston, TX

Wendy Maleki, RN, MS
Director
Vocational Nursing Program
American Career College
Ontario, CA

Luzviminda A. Malihan
Assistant Professor
Hostos Community College
Bronx, NY

Vanessa Norwood McGregor, RN, BSN, MBA
Practical Nursing Instructor
West Kentucky Community and Technical College
Paducah, KY

Kristie Oles, RN, MSN
Practical Nursing Chair
Brown Mackie College
North Canton, OH

Beverly Pacas
Department Head/Instructor
Practical Nursing
Louisiana Technical College
Baton Rouge, LA

Debra Perry, RN, MSN
Instructor
Lorain County Community College
Elyria, OH

Cheryl Pratt, RN, MA, CNAA
Regional Dean of Nursing
Rasmussen College
Mankato, MN

Charlotte Prewitt, RN, BSN
Practical Nursing Instructor
Meridian Technology Center
Stillwater, OK

Stephanie Price
Faculty, Practical Nursing
Holmes Community College
Goodman, MS

Patricia Schrull, RN, MSN, MBA, MEd, CNE
Director, Practical Nursing Program
Lorain County Community College
Elyria, OH

Margi J. Schutlz, RN, MSN, PhD
Director, Nursing Division
GateWay Community College
Phoenix, AZ

Sherie A. Shupe, RN, MSN
Director of Nursing
Computer Career Center
Las Cruces, NM

Sherri Smith, RN
Chairwoman
Arkansas State University Technical Center
Jonesboro, AR

Cheryl Smith, RN, BSN
Practical Nursing Instructor
Colorado Technical University
North Kansas City, MO

Laura Spinelli
Keiser Career College
Miami Lakes, FL

Jennifer Teerlink, RN, MSN
Nursing Faculty
Provo College
Provo, UT

Dana L. Trowell, RN, BSN
LPN Program Director
Dalton State College
Dalton, GA

Racheal Vargas, LVN
Clinical Liaison
Medical Assisting/Vocational Nursing
Lake College
Reading, CA

Sarah Elizabeth Youth Whitaker, DNS, RN
Nursing Program Director
Computer Career Center
El Paso, TX

Shawn White, RN, BSN
Clinical Coordinator, Nursing Instructor
Griffin Technical College
Griffin, GA

Sharon Wilson
Program Director/Instructor, Practical Nursing
Durham Technical Community College
Durham, NC

Vladmir Yarosh, LVN, BS
Program Coordinator —Vocational Nurse Program
Gurnick Academy of Medical Arts
San Mateo, CA

DiAnn Zimmerman
Director, Instructor
Dakota County Technical College
Rosemount, MN

PREFACE

Foundations of Adult Health Nursing, third edition, covers the common medical/surgical conditions generally encountered by Practical/Vocational nurses. An anatomy and physiology review is provided at the beginning of each body system chapter. Each condition is presented and is followed by medical-surgical management topics—including pharmacological, dietary, activity aspects, and nursing management. The nursing process is presented in great detail and incorporates the current NANDA-I diagnoses and NIC/NOC references. As well, it identifies subjective and objective data with health history questions, possible nursing diagnoses, goals/outcomes, interventions, and evaluation. Each chapter contains a sample care plan. The student is provided with opportunities to demonstrate knowledge and develop critical thinking skills by completing the Case Studies included in many of the chapters. New client case studies have been added throughout. The student has the opportunity to assess knowledge and critical thinking of essential nursing concepts by answering NCLEX®-style review questions at the end of each chapter.

Although a systems approach is presented, the concept of holistic care is fundamental to this text. Throughout the book, boxes highlight special topics regarding critical thinking questions, memory tricks, life span development, client teaching, cultural considerations, professional tips, community/home health care, safety, and infection control.

Health care settings are changing, multifaceted, challenging, and rewarding. Critical thinking and sound nursing judgments are essential in the present health care environment. Practical/Vocational nursing students confront and adapt to changes in technology, information, and resources by building a solid foundation of accurate, essential information. A firm knowledge base also allows nurses to meet the changing needs of clients. This text was written to equip the LPN/VN with current knowledge, basic problem-solving and critical thinking skills to successfully pass the NCLEX®-PN exam and meet the demanding challenges of today's health care.

ORGANIZATION

Foundations of Adult Health Nursing, third edition, consists of 22 chapters grouped into 10 units.

- **Unit 1:** ESSENTIAL CONCEPTS—discusses the various types of anesthesia and the nursing care required for each. Surgery describes the perioperative care of clients. The Oncology chapter covers the various types of cancer, the usual treatments, and the nursing care required.
- **Unit 2:** NURSING CARE OF THE CLIENT: OXYGENATION AND PERFUSION— includes the respiratory system, cardiovascular system, and hematological and lymphatic systems.
- **Unit 3:** NURSING CARE OF THE CLIENT: DIGESTION AND ELIMINATION— discusses the gastrointestinal system and urinary system.
- **Unit 4:** NURSING CARE OF THE CLIENT: MOBILITY, COORDINATION, AND REGULATION—covers the musculoskeletal system, neurological system, sensory system, and endocrine system.
- **Unit 5:** NURSING CARE OF THE CLIENT: REPRODUCTIVE AND SEXUAL HEALTH—includes the male and female reproductive systems and sexually transmitted infections.
- **Unit 6:** NURSING CARE OF THE CLIENT: BODY DEFENSES—discusses the integumentary system and the immune system.
- **Unit 7:** NURSING CARE OF THE CLIENT: PHYSICAL AND MENTAL INTEGRITY— addresses substance abuse and the care of clients with common mental illnesses. *Substance Abuse* describes substances which are commonly abused, the signs and symptoms of abuse, and treatments available.
- **Unit 8:** NURSING CARE OF THE CLIENT: OLDER ADULT—explains nursing care for the older adult. Physiological changes of aging are presented for each body system.

- **Unit 9:** NURSING CARE OF THE CLIENT: HEALTH CARE IN THE COMMUNITY— defines the role of the nurse in ambulatory, restorative, and palliative care in community settings. Discusses appropriate client assessments and nursing interventions in each health care setting.
- **Unit 10:** APPLICATIONS—describes how nursing knowledge is applied in emergencies. Specific information is provided for common emergencies. A number of scenarios describing clients with multisystem problems assist students to see the integration of the body.

FEATURES

Each chapter includes a variety of learning aids designed to help the reader further a basic understanding of key concepts. Each chapter opens with a **Making the Connection** box that guides the reader to other key chapters related to the current chapter. This highlights the integration of the text material. Procedures used for the care of clients with medical/surgical disorders are identified as appropriate. **Learning Objectives** are presented at the beginning of each chapter as well. These help students focus their study and use their time efficiently. A listing of **Key Terms** is provided to identify the terms the student should know or learn for a better understanding of the subject matter. These are typeset in color and defined at first use in the chapter. Each medical/surgical chapter has a brief review of anatomy and physiology to review the organs and functions of the system being discussed.

The content of each chapter is presented in nursing process format. Where appropriate, a **Sample Nursing Care Plan** is provided in the chapter. These serve as models for students to refer to as they create their own care plans based on case studies. **Case Studies** are presented at the conclusion of most chapters. These call for students to draw upon their knowledge base and synthesize information to develop their own solutions to realistic cases. **Nursing Diagnoses, Planning/Outcomes, and Interventions** are presented in a convenient table format for quick reference.

A bulleted **Summary** list and multiple-choice **NCLEX®-style Review Questions** at the end of each chapter assist the student in remembering and using the material presented. **References/Suggested Readings** allow the student to find the source of the material presented and also to find additional information concerning topics covered. **Resources** are also listed and provide names and internet addresses of organizations specializing in a specific area of health care.

Boxes used throughout the text emphasize key points and provide specific types of information. The boxes are:

- **Critical Thinking**: encourages the student to use the knowledge gained to think critically about a situation.
- **Memory Trick**: provides an easy-to-remember saying or mnemonic to assist the student in remembering important information presented.
- **Life Span Considerations**: provides information related to the care of specific age groups during the life span.
- **Client Teaching**: identifies specific items that the client should know related to the various disorders.
- **Cultural Considerations**: shares beliefs, manners, and ways of providing care, communication, and relationships of various cultural and ethnic groups as a way to provide holistic care.
- **Professional Tip**: offers tips and technical hints for the nurse to ensure quality care.
- **Safety:** emphasizes the importance of and ways to maintain safe care.
- **Community/Home Health Care**: describes factors to consider when providing care in the community or in a client's home, and adaptation in care that may be necessary.
- **Drug Icon**: highlights pharmacological treatments and interventions that may be appropriate for certain conditions and disorders.
- **Collaborative Care**: mentions members of the care team and their roles in providing comprehensive care to clients.
- **Infection Control**: indicates reminders of methods to prevent the spread of infections.

The back matter includes a **Glossary of Terms**. The appendices include **NANDA-I Nursing Diagnoses**; **Recommended Childhood, Adolescent, and Adult Immunization Schedules**; **Abbreviations, Acronyms and Symbols**; and **English/Spanish Words and Phrases. Standard Precautions** are found on the inside back cover.

NEW TO THIS EDITION

Added one new chapter:

- **Chapter 20,** *Ambulatory, Restorative, and Palliative Care in Community Settings* defines the role of the nurse, explains the legal issues when providing nursing care, and discusses appropriate client assessments and nursing interventions in each health care setting.

Extensively updated chapters:

- **Chapter 2,** *Surgery,* now contains additional robotic and minimally invasive surgeries.
- **Chapter 5,** *Cardiovascular System,* has improved anatomy and physiology and assessment sections, explanations of cutting-edge diagnostic tests, and extensively updated content on implantable cardioverter-defibrillator, pacemaker, cardiac valve management, angina, minimally invasive surgery, ventricular assist device, and pharmacological care.
- **Chapter 22,** *Integration,* includes more in-depth case studies to use as appropriate throughout the educational experience.

Updated content within chapters:

- Updates to **Chapter 3**, *Oncology*, include sections on photodynamic therapy, hormone therapy, and targeted cancer therapy, and a table on cancer screening guidelines.
- Updates to **Chapter 6**, *Hematologic* and *Lymphatic Systems*, include a critical thinking activity for students to visually compare the different anemias, pertinent drugs used in system disease conditions, and a section on Hodgkin's disease and nodular lymphocyte predominance Hodgkin's disease.
- A new section to help the student understand issues in caring for clients with obesity.
- Content added to **Chapter 9**, *Musculoskeletal System*, include guidelines for assessing muscle strength, external fixation, and an explanation of the bone mineral density test and medications for osteoporosis. The sections on

cast care, traction, and total hip replacement have also received extensive updates.

- Updates to **Chapter 10**, *Neurological System*, include intrathecal chemotherapy, chemotherapy disk-shaped wafers, Stroke Risk Scorecard, diet therapy, positron emission tomography scanning and ablation procedures for Parkinson's disease; sniff test to diagnose Alzheimer's disease, Parkinson's disease, and other neurodegenerative disorders.
- New sections in **Chapter 21**, *Responding to Emergencies*, discuss disaster triage, mass casualty incidents, and poisoning and drug overdoses.

Other additions:

- Added case studies to all chapters as offering a mixture of critical thinking and nursing process questions.
- Added Concept Maps to several chapters so the student can link facts with real life clinical practice.
- Added Concept Care Maps to chapters as appropriate for visual picture of the nursing process.
- Increased number of challenging and applicable critical thinking questions.
- Updated cultural considerations and cultural content included throughout the text.
- Added Adult Immunization Schedule along with Childhood and Adolescent Immunization Schedules.
- Added objective and subjective assessment guidelines to medical-surgical chapters for student use in clinical settings.
- Cited research articles in understandable manner for easy application of evidence-based practice.
- Added current NANDA-I diagnoses according to North American Nursing Diagnosis Association International (2010) NANDA-I *Nursing Diagnoses: Definitions and Classification (NANDA Nursing Diagnosis)*.
- Added new NCLEX®-style review questions at the end of chapters to help students challenge their understanding of content while gaining practice with this important question style.
- Added memory tricks for ease of student recall of pertinent information.
- Numerous new photos and illustrations for improved presentation of concepts.
- New, free, StudyWARE™ CD-ROM provides interactive games, animations, videos, heart and lung sounds, and much more to augment the learning experience and support mastery of concepts.

EXTENSIVE TEACHING/ LEARNING PACKAGE

The complete supplements package for *Foundations of Adult Health Nursing*, third edition, was developed to achieve two goals:

1. To assist students in learning the information and procedures presented in the text.
2. To assist instructors in planning and implementing their programs for the most efficient use of time and other resources.

INSTRUCTOR RESOURCES

Foundations of Adult Health Nursing Instructor's Resource, third edition

ISBN-10: 1-428-31780-5
ISBN-13: 978-1-428-31780-2

The Instructor's Resource has four components to assist the instructor and enhance classroom activities and discussion.

Instructor's Guide

- **Instructional Approaches**: Ideas and concepts to help educators manage different presentation methods. Suggestions for approaching topics with rich discussion topics and lecture ideas are provided.
- **Student Learning Activities:** Ideas for activities such as classroom discussions, role play, and individual assignments designed to encourage critical thinking as students engage with the concepts presented in the text.
- **Resources:** Additional books, videos, and resources for use in developing and implementing your curriculum.
- **Web Activities:** Suggestions for student learning experiences online, including specific websites and accompanying activities.
- **Suggested Responses to the Case Study:** Case studies located throughout the book challenge student critical thinking with questions about nursing care. Suggested responses are included.
- **Answers to Review Questions:** Answers and rationales for all end-of-chapter NCLEX®-style questions are provided.

Computerized Testbank

- Includes a rich bank of questions that test students on retention and application of material in the text.
- Many questions are now presented in NCLEX® style, with each question providing the answer and rationale, as well as cognitive levels.
- Allows the instructor to mix questions from each of the didactic chapters to customize tests.

Instructor Slides Created in PowerPoint

- A robust offering of instructor slides created in PowerPoint outlines the concepts from text in order to assist the instructor with lectures.
- Ideas presented stimulate discussion and critical thinking.

Image Library

A searchable Image Library provides more than 800 illustrations and photographs that can be incorporated into lectures, class materials, or electronic presentations.

STUDENT RESOURCES

Foundations of Adult Health Nursing Study Guide, third edition

ISBN-10: 1-4283-1785-6
ISBN-13: 978-1-4283-1785-7

A valuable companion to the core book, this student resource provides additional review of all 22 chapters of *Foundations of*

Adult Health Nursing, third edition, with Key Terms matching review questions, Abbreviation Review Exercises, Self-Assessment Questions, and other Review Exercises and Activities. Answers to questions are provided at the back of the book making this an excellent resource for self-study and review.

Foundations of Nursing Online Companion

ISBN-10: 1-4283-1779-1
ISBN-13: 978-1-4283-1779-6

The Online Companion gives online access to all the components in the Instructor's Resource as well as additional tools to reinforce the content in each chapter and enhance classroom teaching. Multimedia animations, Concept Care Map Model, and Physical Assessment Guide are just some of the many resources found on this robust site. To access the site for *Foundations of Nursing,* third edition, simply point your browser to http://www.delmar.cengage.com/companions. Select the nursing discipline and then select *Foundations of Nursing,* third edition.

CL eBook to Accompany *Foundations of Adult Health Nursing,* third edition

Printed access code ISBN-10: 1-4354-8788-5
Printed access code ISBN-13: 978-1-4354-8788-8
Instant access code ISBN-10: 1-4354-8787-7
Instant access code ISBN-13: 978-1-4354-8787-1

Foundations of Nursing WebTutor Advantage on Blackboard

ISBN-10: 1-4283-1781-3
ISBN-13: 978-1-4283-1781-9

Foundations of Nursing WebTutor Advantage on WebCT

ISBN-10: 1-4283-1782-1
ISBN-13: 978-1-4283-1782-6

- A complete online environment that supplements the course provided in both Blackboard and WebCT format.
- Includes chapter overviews, chapter outlines, and competencies.
- Useful classroom management tools include chats and calendars, as well as instructor resources such as the instructor slides created in PowerPoint.
- Multimedia offering includes video clips and 3D animation.
- Comprehensive Audio Glossary with all terms and definitions from this text in downloadable audio format.

ABOUT THE AUTHORS

Lois Elain Wacker White earned a diploma in nursing from Memorial Hospital School of Nursing, Springfield, Illinois; an Associate degree in Science from Del Mar College, Corpus Christi, Texas; a Bachelor of Science in Nursing from Texas A & I University—Corpus Christi, Corpus Christi, Texas; a Master of Science in Education from Corpus Christi State University, Corpus Christi, Texas; and a Doctor of Philosophy degree in Education Administration—Community College from the University of Texas, Austin, Texas.

She has taught at Del Mar College, Corpus Christi, Texas, in both the Associate Degree Nursing program and the Vocational Nursing program. For 14 years, she was also chairperson of the Department of Vocational Nurse Education. Dr. White has taught fundamentals of nursing, mental health/mental illness, medical-surgical nursing, and maternal/pediatric nursing. Her professional career has also included 15 years of clinical practice.

Dr. White has served on the Nursing Education Advisory Committee of the Board of Nurse Examiners for the State of Texas and the Board of Vocational Nurse Examiners, which developed competencies expected of graduates for each level of nursing.

Gena Duncan has worked as an RN for 36 years in the clinical, community health, and educational arenas. This has equipped Mrs. Duncan with a wide range of nursing experiences and varied skills to meet the educational needs of today's students. She has an MSEd and MSN.

During her professional career, Mrs. Duncan served as a staff nurse, an assistant head nurse of a medical-surgical unit, a continuing education instructor, an associate professor in an LPN program, and director of an Associate degree nursing program. She has taught LPN, ADN, BSN, and MSN nursing students. As a faculty member, she taught many nursing courses and served on a statewide curriculum committee for a state college. As director of an Associate degree nursing program, she was instrumental in starting and obtaining state board approval of an LPN-RN nursing program.

Her master's research thesis was entitled "An Investigation of Learning Styles of Practical and Baccalaureate Students." The results of the study are published in the *Journal of Nursing Education*. She has coauthored two textbooks, a medical-surgical textbook and a transitions text for LPN to RN students. She has been an active member of Sigma Theta Tau.

Wendy Baumle is currently a nursing instructor at James A. Rhodes State College in Ohio. She has spent 19 years as a clinician, educator, school district health coordinator, and academician. Mrs. Baumle has taught fundamentals of nursing, medical-surgical nursing, pediatrics, obstetrics, pharmacology, anatomy and physiology, and ethics in health care in practical nursing and associate nursing degree programs. She has previously taught at Lutheran College, Fort Wayne, Indiana, at Northwest State Community College, Archbold, Ohio, and at James. A. Rhodes State College in Lima, Ohio. Mrs. Baumle earned her Bachelor of Science degree in Nursing from The University of Toledo, Toledo, Ohio, and her Master's degree in Nursing from The Medical College of Ohio, Toledo, Ohio. Mrs. Baumle is a member of a number of professional nursing organizations, including Sigma Theta Tau, the American Nurses Association, the National League for Nursing, and the Ohio Nurses Association.

ACKNOWLEDGMENTS

Many people must work together to produce any textbook, but a comprehensive book such as this requires even more people with various areas of expertise. We would like to thank the contributors for their time and effort to share their knowledge gained through years of experience in both the clinical and academic settings. Debra Thorson, RN, MS, nursing instructor at Northwest Technical College at Bemidji, Minnesota, contributed content to Chapter 21, Responding to Emergencies.

To the reviewers, we thank you for your time spent critically reading the manuscript, and for your expertise and valuable suggestions that have added to this text.

We would like to acknowledge and sincerely thank the entire team at Delmar Cengage Learning who has worked to make this textbook a reality. Juliet Steiner, senior product manager, receives a special thank you. She has kept us on track and provided guidance with humor, enthusiasm, sensitivity, and expertise. We extend a special thank you to Steve Helba, executive editor, for his vision for this text, calm demeanor, and patience. Other members on the team—Marah Bellegarde, managing editor; James Zayicek, senior content product manager; Jack Pendleton, senior art director; and Meghan Orvis, editorial assistant, have all worked diligently for the completion of this textbook. Thank you to all.

HOW TO USE THIS TEXT

This text is designed with you, the reader, in mind. Special elements and feature boxes appear throughout the text to guide you in reading and to assist you in learning the material. Following are suggestions for how you can use these features to increase your understanding and mastery of the content.

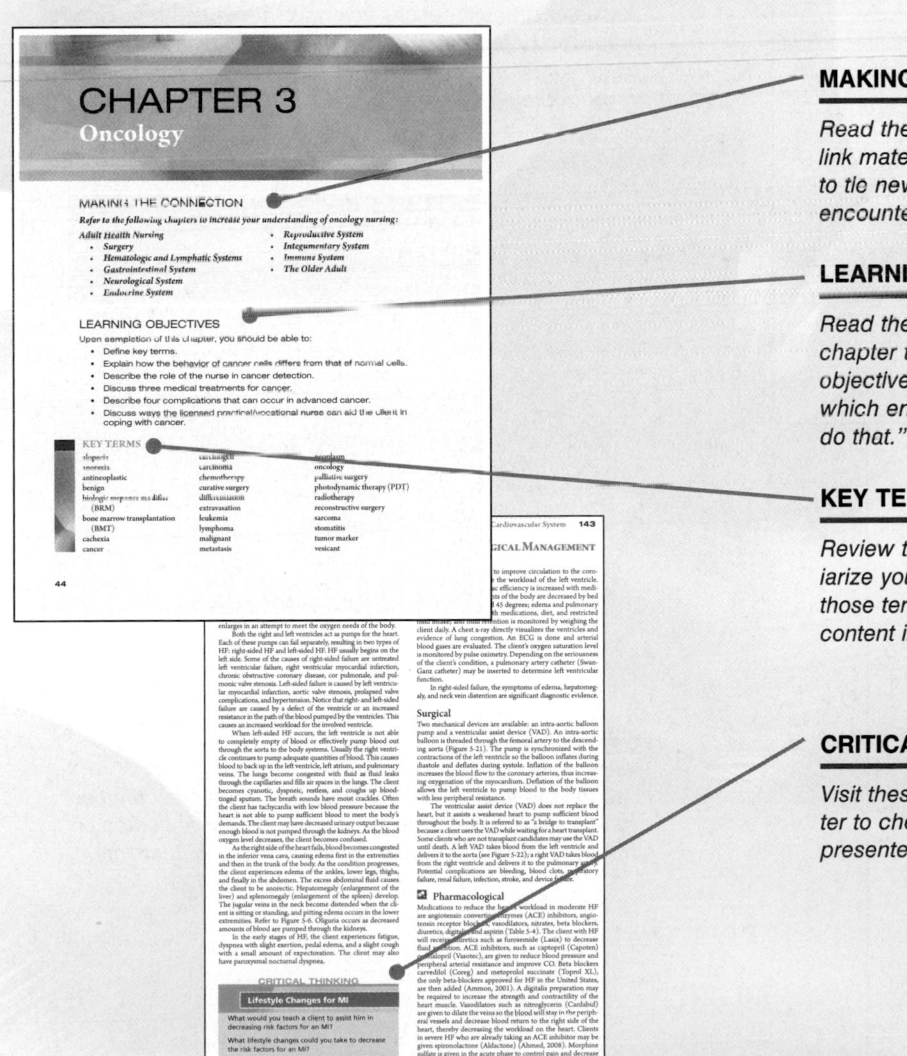

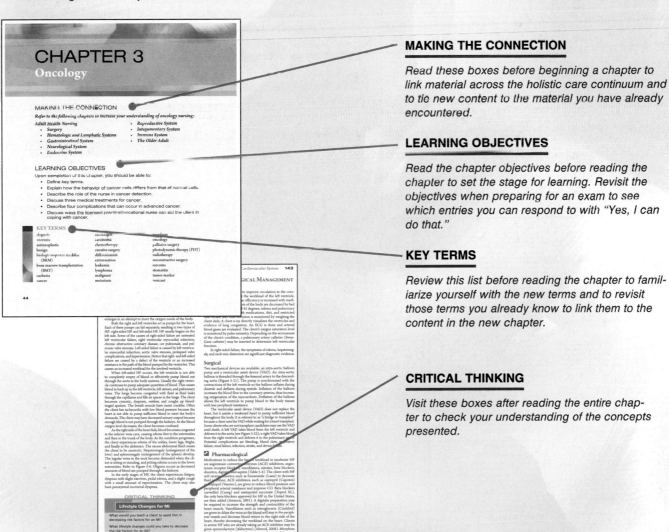

MAKING THE CONNECTION

Read these boxes before beginning a chapter to link material across the holistic care continuum and to tie new content to the material you have already encountered.

LEARNING OBJECTIVES

Read the chapter objectives before reading the chapter to set the stage for learning. Revisit the objectives when preparing for an exam to see which entries you can respond to with "Yes, I can do that."

KEY TERMS

Review this list before reading the chapter to familiarize yourself with the new terms and to revisit those terms you already know to link them to the content in the new chapter.

CRITICAL THINKING

Visit these boxes after reading the entire chapter to check your understanding of the concepts presented.

HOW TO USE THIS TEXT (Continued)

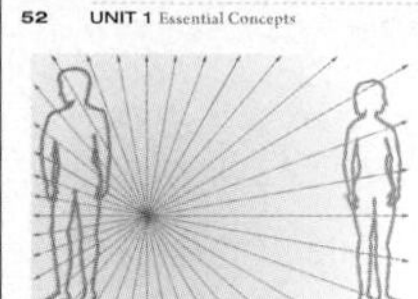

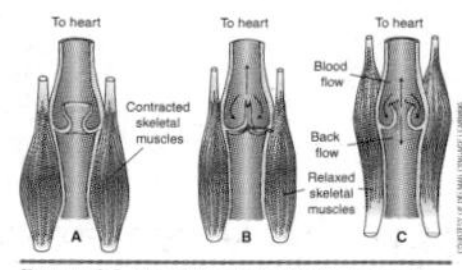

PROFESSIONAL TIP

Use these boxes to increase your professional competence and confidence, and to expand your knowledge base.

COMMUNITY/HOME HEALTH CARE

Read these boxes before making a home visit to a client with a given disorder.

CULTURAL CONSIDERATIONS

Test your sensitivity to cultural and ethnic diversity by scanning these boxes and using the guidelines and suggestions in your practice. You may also want to ask yourself what biases or preconceptions you have about different cultural practices before reading a chapter and then read these boxes for information that may help you be more sensitive in your nursing care and approach to clients.

MEMORY TRICK

Use the mnemonic devices provided in the new Memory Trick feature to help you remember the correct steps or proper order of information when working with clients.

HOW TO USE THIS TEXT (Continued)

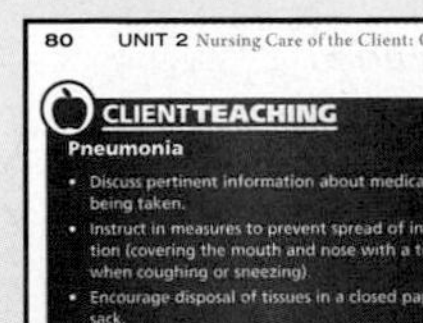

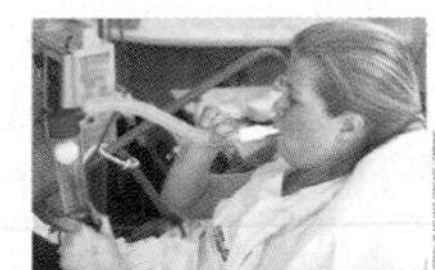

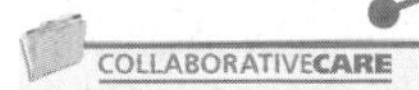

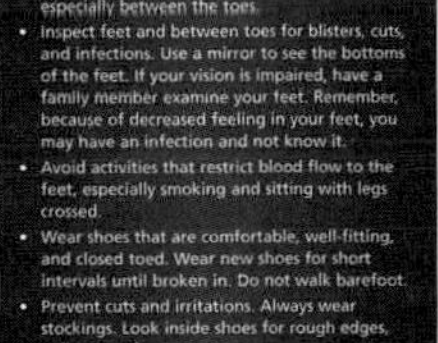

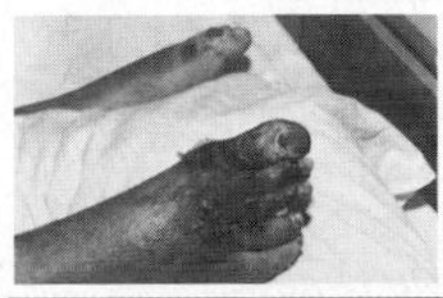

DRUG ICONS

These symbols draw attention to information relating to the pharmacological management available for certain disorders. Review these sections to understand the pharmacological treatments appropriate for your clients' conditions.

COLLABORATIVE CARE

These boxes explain which other health care professionals may be involved in the comprehensive care offered to clients. Review these boxes and ask yourself if you understand how your role as a nurse will complement the care provided by others on the health care team.

INFECTION CONTROL

When reading a chapter, stop and pay attention to these features and ask yourself, "Had I thought of that? Do I practice these precautions?"

CLIENT TEACHING

Read these boxes to gain insight into client learning needs related to the specific disorder or condition. You may want to make your own index cards or electronic notes listing these teaching guidelines to use when you are working with clients.

LIFE SPAN CONSIDERATIONS

Use these boxes to increase your awareness of variations in care based on client age; this will help you deliver more effective and appropriate care.

HOW TO USE THIS TEXT (Continued)

CHAPTER 10 Neurological System 327

EPILEPSY/SEIZURE DISORDER

Epilepsy is a disorder of cerebral function in which the client experiences sudden attacks of altered consciousness, motor activity, or sensory phenomenon. Convulsive seizures are the most common type. Most recurrent seizure patterns are caused by epilepsy. Most clinicians and authors use the term "seizure disorder" for epilepsy or seizures (Hickey, 2008).

A seizure is initiated by an electrical disturbance in the neurons, which, in turn, causes an aberrant discharge of electrical activity from any part of the cerebral cortex and possibly from other areas of the brain (Samuels, 2004). This electrical discharge may cause involuntary episodes of loss of consciousness, excessive muscular movement or loss of muscle tone, and changes in behavior, mood, sensation, and/or perception (Smeltzer, Bare, Hinkle, & Cheever, 2008).

The etiology of the electrical disturbance may be birth trauma, hypoxia, infection, tumor, alcohol toxicity, drugs, drug withdrawal, carbon monoxide or lead poisoning, vascular abnormalities such as CVA, hypoglycemia electrolyte imbalance, or fever. Often, the cause is idiopathic, or unknown.

Seizures are classified as generalized or partial. In generalized seizures, the entire brain is affected simultaneously, causing bilateral, symmetrical reactions. Generalized seizures are classified as tonic and/or clonic (grand mal), absence (petit mal), or myoclonic.

Tonic–clonic seizures involve rigid tonic contractions of muscles and loss of postural control followed by a clonic stage of intermittent contraction and relaxation. Incontinence of stool or urine is common. Absence seizures involve loss of conscious activity without the muscular involvement of tonic–clonic seizures. Myoclonic seizures are very mild, sudden, involuntary contractions of a muscle group or rapid, forceful movements. They usually occur in the trunk or extremities and involve no loss of consciousness.

Partial seizures initiate in a focal point in the brain and involve the function of those specific neurons. Partial seizures are either simple or complex. In simple partial seizures, the area affected may be a hand, a finger, the ability to talk, or a sense such as smell. Consciousness is not lost.

Complex partial seizures generally involve loss of consciousness and produce cognitive, affective, psychosensory, or psychomotor symptoms. The client performs inappropriate purposive behaviors, called **automatisms**, or mechanical, repetitive motor behaviors performed unconsciously, such as lip-smacking. Auras, peculiar sensations that precede a seizure, may take the form of a taste, smell, sight, or sound; dizziness; or a "funny" feeling. After the seizure, the client typically cannot remember the episode.

Diagnostic testing to determine the type of seizure activity includes an EEG to identify abnormal electrical activity and/or the focal point of the seizure. Sleep and video EEGs document changes in electrical activity of the brain. CT scans identify or rule out lesions, degenerative changes, or vascular abnormalities.

MEDICAL–SURGICAL MANAGEMENT

Surgical

Surgical intervention is indicated for a very small percentage of clients; those for whom pharmacological treatment has not been effective and when the focal points are identified. Microsurgery is used to irradiate focal points of abnormal electrical discharge caused by tumor, vascular abnormality, or abscess.

Pharmacological

The primary method of controlling seizure activity is pharmacological. Seizure activity is controlled with an anticonvulsant agent or a combination of anticonvulsants in 75% of clients (Hickey, 2008). Phenytoin (Dilantin), phenobarbital (Phenobarbital), carbamazepine (Tegretol), valproic acid (Depakene), and primidone (Mysoline) are often used. Anticonvulsant agents are started one at a time in gradually increasing doses. The client's blood level is monitored for therapeutic range, and the client is assessed for side effects of the drug and signs of drug toxicity, such as drowsiness, dizziness, gastric distress, rash, blood dyscrasias, and ataxia.

The goal is to obtain seizure control with minimal side effects. Any anticonvulsant is gradually discontinued. Abrupt

SAFETY

Precautions During a Seizure

If the client is in bed:

- Be sure the side rails are up.
- Put padding (blankets) on the side rails to prevent injury.

If the client is out of bed:

- Carefully ease the client to the floor.
- Move nearby objects so that the client will not be injured.
- Place a soft item beneath the client's head.

Whether the client is in or out of bed:

SAFETY

Pause while reading to consider these elements and quiz yourself: "Do I take steps such as these to ensure my own and the client's safety? Do I follow these guidelines in every practice encounter?"

CHAPTER 6 Hematologic and Lymphatic Systems 175

SAMPLE NURSING CARE PLAN (Continued)

EVALUATION

Circulation in lower extremities has improved as manifested by prompt capillary refill and strong pedal and popliteal pulses. Extremities are warm to touch.

NURSING DIAGNOSIS 3 *Deficient Knowledge* related to prescribed treatment regimen as evidenced by a lack of rest and working long hours

Nursing Outcomes Classification (NOC)	Nursing Interventions Classification (NIC)
Knowledge: Energy Conservation	*Self-Modification Assistance*
Knowledge: Treatment Regimen	*Teaching: Individual*

PLANNING/OUTCOMES	NURSING INTERVENTIONS	RATIONALE
R.T. will relate the prescribed treatment regimen before discharge.	Teach R.T. the pathophysiology related to sickle cell disease.	Improves compliance with the medical regimen.
	Encourage R.T. to take medications as ordered.	Improves circulation and postpones sickle cell crisis situations.
	Explain the importance of avoiding stressful situations and the symptoms of infection.	These situations increase oxygen demands.
	Explain the importance of adequate rest on a routine basis.	Allows adequate oxygenation and reduces stress.

EVALUATION

R.T. states his RBCs have Hgb S rather than Hgb A, and a lack of oxygen causes his RBCs to sickle. Sickling is caused by fatigue, lack of oral fluids, emotional and physical stress, infection, exposure to cold and anesthesia. He knows the purpose and side effects of each medication and the times he is to take them. R.T. states he is to avoid high altitudes. R.T. states that he will try to routinely have enough rest.

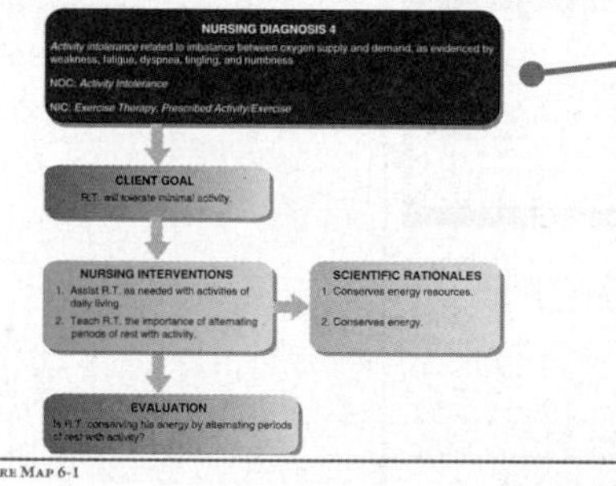
NURSING DIAGNOSIS 4
Activity intolerance related to imbalance between oxygen supply and demand, as evidenced by weakness, fatigue, dyspnea, tingling, and numbness
NOC: Activity Intolerance
NIC: Exercise Therapy, Prescribed Activity/Exercise
CLIENT GOAL
R.T. will tolerate minimal activity.
NURSING INTERVENTIONS
1. Assist R.T. as needed with activities of daily living
2. Teach R.T. the importance of alternating periods of rest with activity.
SCIENTIFIC RATIONALES
1. Conserves energy resources.
2. Conserves energy.
EVALUATION
Is R.T. conserving his energy by alternating periods of rest with activity?

CONCEPT CARE MAP 6-1

SAMPLE NURSING CARE PLAN

Use this feature to test your understanding and application of the content presented. Ask yourself: "Would I have come up with the same nursing diagnoses? Are these the interventions that I would have proposed? What other interventions would be appropriate?"

CONCEPT CARE MAPS

Review these graphical tools to help incorporate the interrelatedness of nursing concepts in preparation for clinical practice.

234 UNIT 3 Nursing Care of the Client: Digestion and

continue using it in the hospital. The nurse assesses pain regularly, monitors PCA use, and obtains appropriate orders to manage pain (Sammons, 2002). If an NG tube is in place, the nurse does not reposition the NG tube as the movement may damage the suture line. The client takes sips of water and, if tolerated, slowly progresses to eating very small portions of pureed food or juices. The nurse teaches diet modifications and exercise to assist the client in controlling weight. Weight loss is a lifetime challenge.

caused by eating simple sugars. It is a benign problem that possibly can be modified by decreasing the ingestion of simple sugar.

CASE STUDY

R.J. is a 52-year-old woman admitted to the hospital with acute abdominal pain. R.J. complains of right upper quadrant pain radiating to the back. She has had previous episodes, usually occurring about 2 hours after eating. This episode, however, is not resolving. R.J. also complains of nausea. Her vital signs are BP 152/88 mm Hg, pulse 92 beats/min, and respirations 24 breaths/min and shallow. R.J. is a slightly obese female who states she has recently been dieting to lose weight. Laboratory analysis includes a CBC with slightly elevated WBCs, elevated bilirubin, and elevated alkaline phosphatase. An IV is started, and R.J. is given meperidine (Demerol) IM for pain. R.J. has been made NPO. An ultrasound of the gallbladder is ordered.

The following questions will guide your development of a nursing care plan for this case study.

1. List subjective and objective data a nurse would want to obtain about R.J.
2. List risk factors other than those R.J. has that would put a client at risk for developing cholecystitis.
3. List two nursing diagnoses and goals for R.J.
4. The ERCP is successful in removing the CBD stone. The decision is made to perform a laparoscopic cholecystectomy. What teaching will R.J. need?
5. Why is meperidine (Demerol) the medication of choice for pain control?
6. List at least three successful outcomes for R.J.

SUMMARY

- The gastrointestinal system is a complex system composed of the digestive tract as well as accessory organs.
- Disorders of the GI tract affect the breakdown and absorption of nutrients, breakdown of wastes and by-products, and the lifestyle of the individual.
- Because the liver is responsible for so many functions in the body, disorders of the liver can affect other systems significantly.
- Peptic ulcers may be either gastric or duodenal. *H. pylori* is a common cause of ulcers and can be treated with antibiotics.
- Diverticulosis is a commonly occurring disorder in the United States and is believed to be caused by a low-fiber diet.
- Inflammatory bowel disease includes both Crohn's disease and ulcerative colitis. IBD can lead to nutritional imbalances, bowel obstructions, alterations in the structure of the intestine, and affected lifestyle.
- Bowel obstructions have multiple causes and can lead to electrolyte imbalances, dehydration, and possibly sepsis.
- Viral hepatitis is a concern for health care professionals at risk for exposure. Standard precautions must be used to prevent the transmission of the virus.
- Colorectal cancer is one of the most preventable forms of cancer if routine screenings are performed.

REVIEW QUESTIONS

1. A client with a bleeding esophageal varix:
   1. should be encouraged to vomit the blood to decrease abdominal distention and pressure.
   2. should have an NG tube placed to suction blood from the stomach
   4. will not need follow-up once the bleeding has stopped.
2. A client with a perforated duodenal ulcer:
   1. requires an EGD to repair the perforation.

CASE STUDY

Read over these boxes within the text. Draw on the knowledge you have gained and synthesize information to develop your own educated responses to the case study challenges.

SUMMARY

Carefully read the bulleted list to review key concepts discussed. This is an excellent resource when studying or preparing for exams.

REVIEW QUESTIONS

Test your knowledge and understanding by answering the NCLEX®-style review questions with each chapter. These are an excellent way to test your mastery of the concepts covered in the chapter, and a good opportunity to become familiar with answering NCLEX®-style review questions.

HOW TO USE STUDYWARE™ TO ACCOMPANY *FOUNDATIONS OF ADULT HEALTH NURSING*, THIRD EDITION

Minimum System Requirements

- Operating systems: Microsoft Windows XP w/SP 2, Windows Vista w/ SP 1, Windows 7
- Processor: Minimum required by Operating System
- Memory: Minimum required by Operating System
- Hard Drive Space: 500 MB
- Screen resolution: 1024 × 768 pixels
- CD-ROM drive
- Sound card and listening device required for audio features
- Flash Player 10. The Adobe Flash Player is free, and can be downloaded from http://www.adobe.com/products/flashplayer/

Set-Up Instructions

1. Insert disc into CD-ROM drive. The StudyWARE™ installation program should start automatically. If it does not, go to step 2.
2. From My Computer, double-click the icon for the CD drive.
3. Double-click the *setup.exe* file to start the program.

Technical Support

Telephone: 1-800-648-7450
8:30 A.M.-6:30 P.M. Eastern Time
E-mail: delmar.help@cengage.com

StudyWARE™ is a trademark used herein under license.

Microsoft® and Windows® are registered trademarks of the Microsoft Corporation.

Pentium® is a registered trademark of the Intel Corporation.

Getting Started

The StudyWARE™ software helps you learn terms and concepts in *Foundations of Adult Health Nursing*, third edition. As you study each chapter in the text, be sure to explore the activities in the corresponding chapter in the software. Use StudyWARE™ as your own private tutor to help you learn the material in your *Foundations of Adult Health Nursing*, third edition textbook.

Getting started is easy! Install the software by following the installation instructions provided above. When you open the software, enter your first and last name so the software can store your quiz results. Then choose a chapter or section from the menu to take a quiz or explore media and activities.

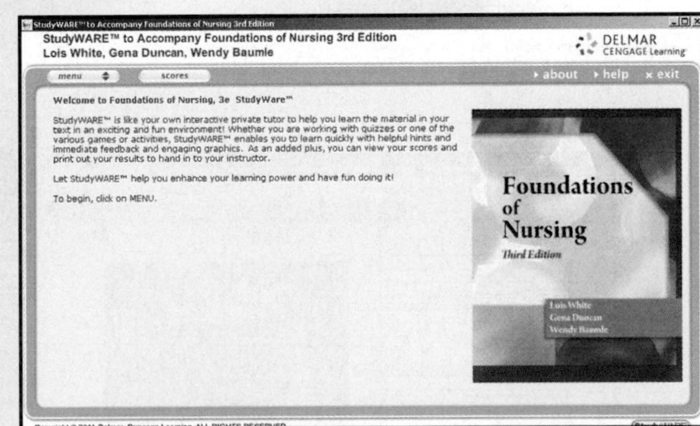

HOW TO USE STUDYWARE™ (Continued)

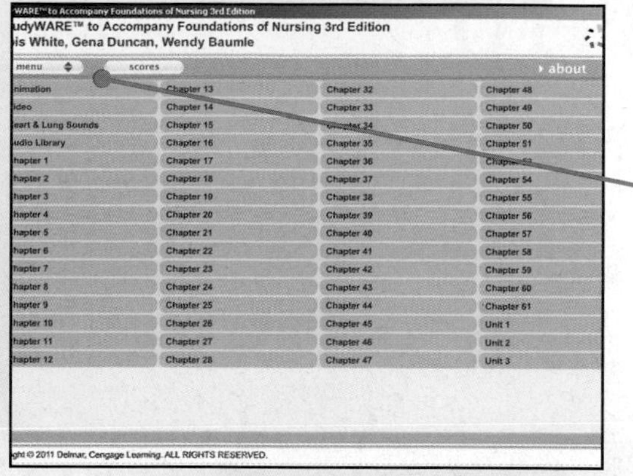

MENU

You can access the menu from wherever you are in the program. The menu includes Animations, Video, Heart & Lung Sounds, Chapter Activities for all didactic chapters, and NCLEX®-style Quizzes for each major unit. You can also access your scores from the button to the right of the main menu button.

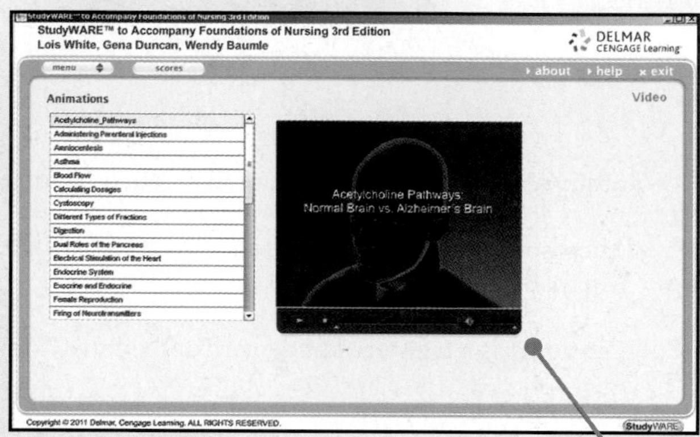

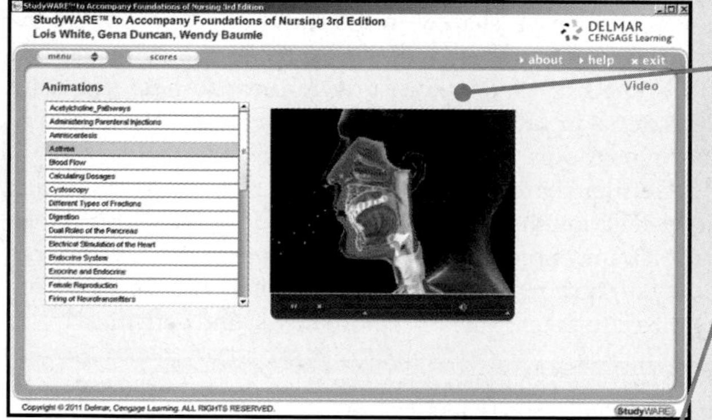

ANIMATION

This section on your StudyWARE™ CD-ROM provides 35 multimedia animations of biological, anatomical, and pharmacological processes. These animations visually explain some of the more difficult concepts and are an engaging resource to support your understanding.

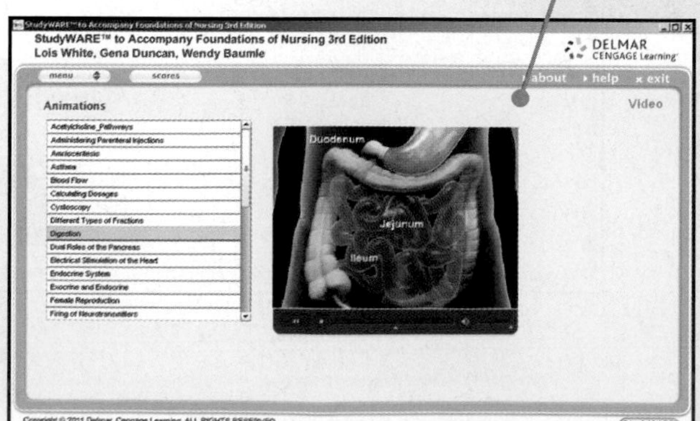

HOW TO USE STUDYWARE™ (Continued)

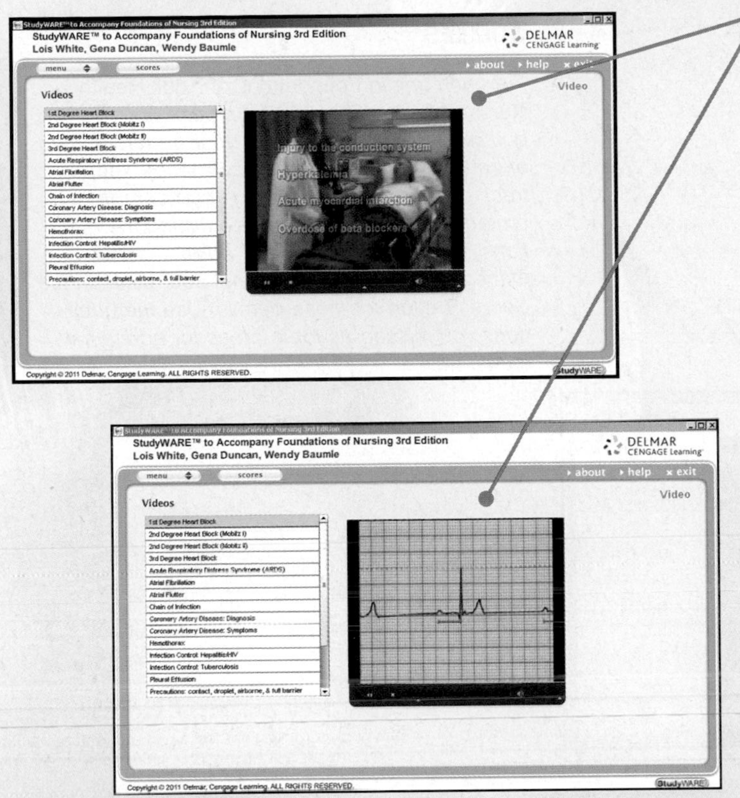

VIDEO

A selection of 20 high quality video clips on topics ranging from infection control to the cardiovascular and respiratory systems has been provided. Click on the clip you would like to view, then click on the play button on the media viewer in the center of the screen. These video clips, many of which were developed by Concept Media, are a wonderful resource to help visualize difficult processes and skills.

HEART & LUNG SOUNDS

This searchable multimedia program provides a comprehensive library of audio files for different heart and lung sounds that will be encountered by nurses. Sounds can be viewed according to category or specific sounds can be found by using the alphabetical term search function. In addition to hearing the sounds, related information about etiology and auscultation is provided.

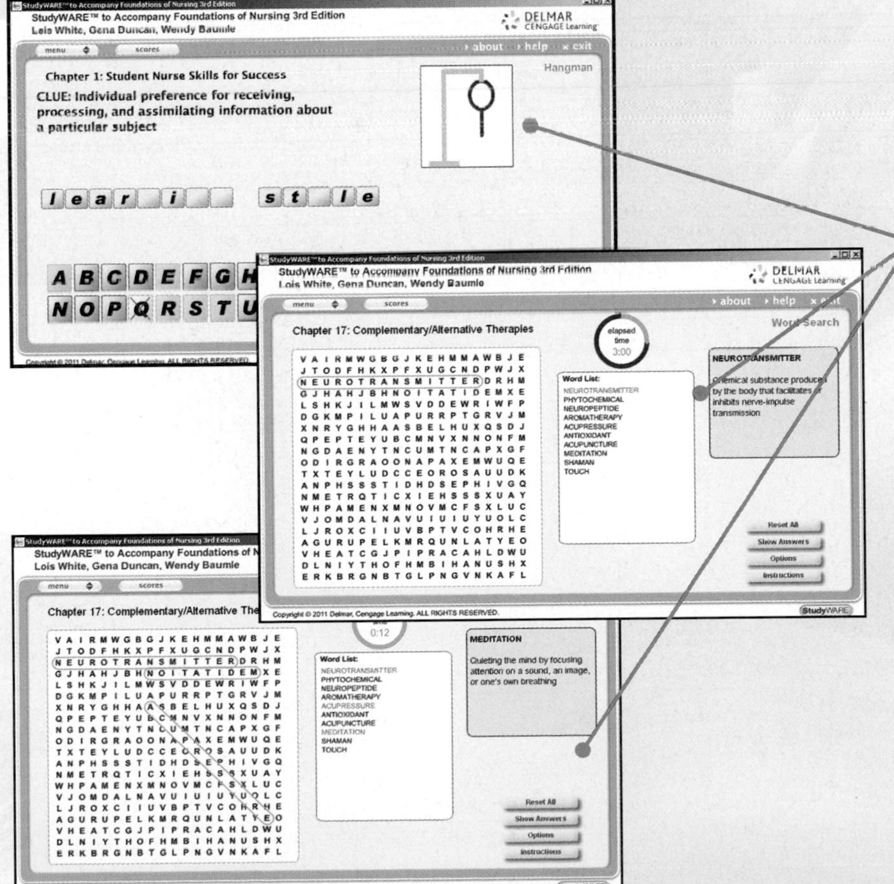

CHAPTER ACTIVITIES

For each chapter from Foundations of Adult Health Nursing, *third edition, games and activities are provided to help you master the glossary terms in a fun and interesting way. Concentration is a memory game that asks you to flip cards to match definitions with their terms. Flash Cards allow you to test your knowledge of a term by reading the term, thinking about the definition, then checking the actual definition. Hangman follows the traditional hangman game format and can be played by one or two players, challenging you to fill in the blanks for a term before the puzzle is completed. Crossword Puzzles provide definitions of key terms as clues so you can fill in the appropriate term and clear the board.*

HOW TO USE STUDYWARE™ (Continued)

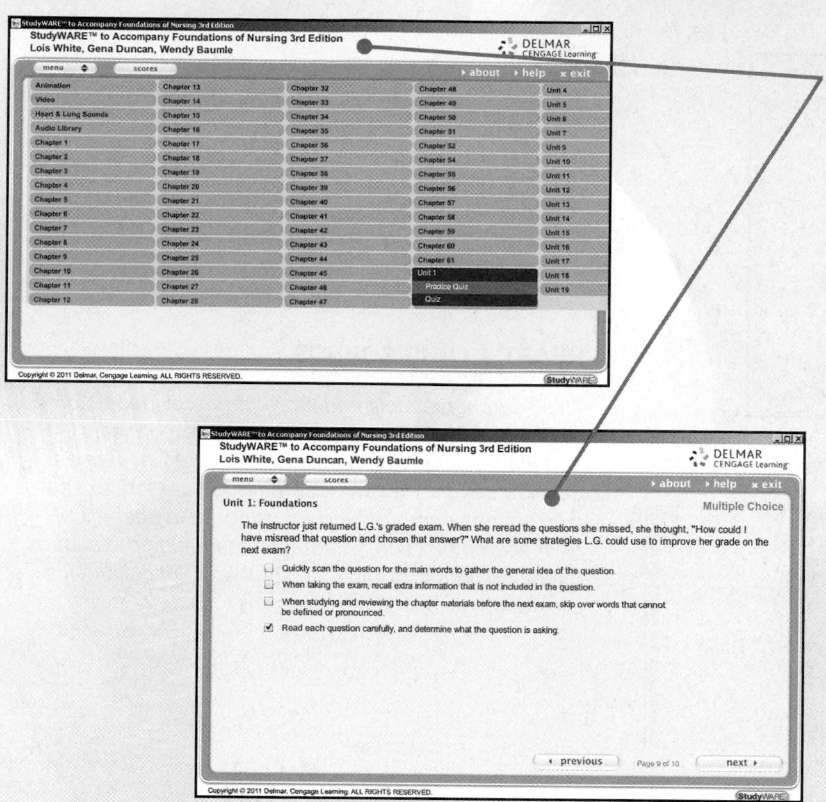

QUIZZES

For each unit in Foundations of Adult Health Nursing, *third edition, both practice and live quizzes are provided to test your understanding of critical concepts. The quiz program keeps track of your answers and a report can be generated at the end of the quiz outlining the questions, your answers, and the correct answers. Once the quiz has been completed, click on the Scores button for these details. Use the questions you missed as topic areas for additional study.*

UNIT 1 Essential Concepts

CHAPTER 1
Anesthesia

MAKING THE CONNECTION

Refer to the following chapters to increase your understanding of anesthesia:

Adult Health Nursing

- ***Surgery***

LEARNING OBJECTIVES

Upon completion of this chapter, you should be able to:

- Define key terms.
- Describe the difference between regional and general anesthesia.
- Identify the purposes of sedation.
- Describe the effects of sedation or general anesthesia on memory and cognitive function.
- Discuss the types of monitoring necessary to ensure client safety during sedation.
- Describe the signs and symptoms and risks of oversedation.
- Discuss the dangers involved in aspiration of gastric contents and how gastric aspiration is prevented during anesthesia.
- List the medications that are typically given on the day of surgery.
- List and describe the different types of regional anesthesia.
- Describe the risks involved with regional and general anesthesia.
- Discuss the residual effects of anesthesia on the client.
- List three methods of postoperative pain management and explain briefly how each is administered.

KEY TERMS

amnesia
analgesia
anesthesia
anesthesiologist
anesthetist
capnography
general anesthesia
orthostatic hypotension
regional anesthesia
sedation
synergism

INTRODUCTION

Anesthesia refers to the absence of normal sensation. **Analgesia** refers to pain relief without producing anesthesia. The delivery of general anesthesia to prevent pain during surgery began in the United States in the 1800s. When surgeons began using anesthesia routinely, they soon realized the need for someone trained in its administration and turned to the nurses with whom they worked daily. Early nurse anesthetists were trained on the job by the surgeons with whom they worked.

Anesthesia is now a specialty of both nursing and medicine. Experienced registered nurses (RNs) with a baccalaureate degree can become certified registered nurse anesthetists (CRNAs) after completing two or more years of graduate education in nurse anesthesia. In November 2001, the Centers for Medicare and Medicaid Services (CMS) published an anesthesia care rule stating a governor could notify CMS of the desire to opt out of the federal physician supervision requirement for nurse anesthetists administering anesthesia to Medicare clients (AANA, 2000). Since then, 13 states have opted out of the supervision rule (AANA, 2005).

Today there are more than 37,000 CRNAs who administer more than 30 million anesthetics in the United States each year and are the only anesthesia providers in two-thirds of all the U.S. rural hospitals (AANA, 2009). CRNAs often work in groups with anesthesiologists.

An **anesthesiologist** is a licensed physician educated and skilled in the delivery of anesthesia who also adds to the knowledge of anesthesia through research or other scholarly pursuits. An **anesthetist** is a qualified RN, dentist, or physician who administers anesthetics.

Before administering an anesthetic, the anesthesia provider assesses the client's health status, discusses the risks and benefits of anesthesia with the client, and plans an anesthetic appropriate for the client and the surgical procedure. Surgical nurses prepare clients to talk with their anesthesia providers by encouraging them to ask any questions they have about anesthesia and the care they will receive.

The use of anesthesia is essential to the health and well-being of clients undergoing surgery. Although anesthesia prevents any sensation of pain, it also temporarily eliminates or diminishes the client's ability to control many essential physiologic functions such as respiration, heart rate, and temperature regulation. In addition to ensuring adequate levels of anesthesia throughout a surgical procedure, the anesthesia provider monitors and, when necessary, controls physiologic functions such as respiratory rate and blood pressure. Before the end of the surgery, the anesthesia provider administers appropriate medications to ensure that the client is comfortable when emerging from the anesthetic. Pain may be relieved with local anesthetic infiltration, opioid analgesics, or nonopioid analgesics.

PREANESTHETIC PREPARATION

Preparing a client for anesthesia and surgery is a cooperative effort involving the surgeon, the anesthesia provider, and the nursing staff who cares for the client both before and after surgery (Figure 1-1). The client may undergo general (total body) anesthesia, where the control of body functions is temporarily lost; regional anesthesia, where a region of the body is made insensible to pain; or local anesthesia, where only a small area of the body is made insensible to pain.

CRITICAL THINKING

Physical Assessment and Anesthesia

What is the relevance of physical assessment and anesthesia?

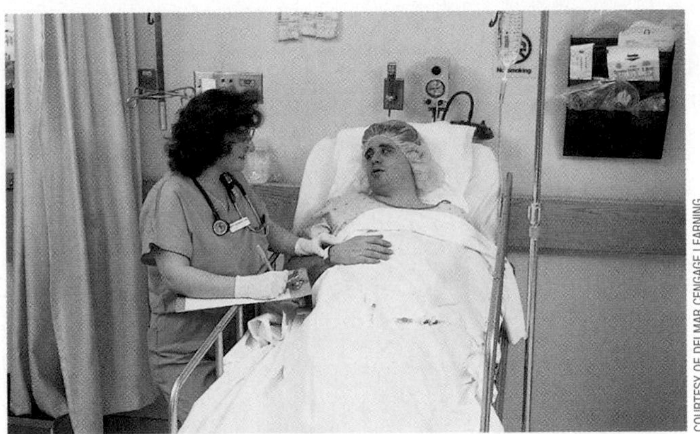

FIGURE 1-1 A nurse prepares a client for anesthesia and surgery.

ORAL INTAKE

Normally, only air should enter the trachea and lungs. The body prevents foreign material from entering the trachea by coughing forcefully when something other than air enters or by tightly closing the vocal cords to prevent entry of the foreign substance. Anyone who has ever drank something and had it go down the trachea knows how uncomfortable it is and how hard the body works to cough up the foreign substance.

General anesthesia removes a person's ability to guard the airway by coughing or closing the vocal cords. Passive regurgitation of stomach contents into the back of the throat can occur at any time during the delivery of general anesthesia. Aspiration of gastric contents into the lungs can cause significant illness or death. An important step in preventing aspiration of gastric contents is ensuring that the stomach is as empty as possible. In the past, adults have been instructed not to eat or drink anything for at least 8 hours before surgery and usually nothing past midnight the night before surgery. More recent information, however, strongly indicates that adults need not go without clear liquids for 8 or more hours before surgery; 2 hours are sufficient (ASA, 1999; ASA, 2007). In fact, the amount of liquid in a person's stomach at the time of surgery may actually be decreased if water is taken a couple of hours

LIFE SPAN CONSIDERATIONS

Anesthesia for Pediatric Clients

- Have a parent present when the anesthesiologist examines the child and performs the preoperative assessment.
- Explain the procedure at the child's level of understanding, such as "This mask will help you go to sleep for a while."
- Allow the child to play with a mask.

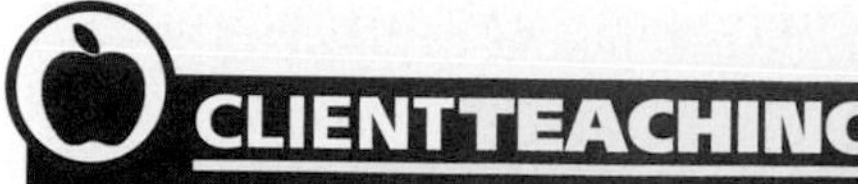

CLIENT TEACHING

Oral Intake Before Surgery

- Clearly explain to clients those things that they will or will not be allowed to eat or drink before surgery.
- Emphasize the need to exactly follow the instructions related to the time at which eating or drinking must cease before surgery.
- Discuss taking usual medications with doctor before surgery.

before surgery. Some anesthesia providers still prefer that their clients not have anything to eat or drink for at least 8 hours before surgery; others may allow water up to 2 hours before.

Preoperative Medication

Most scheduled medications that a person receives while in the hospital or takes at home every day are continued until the time of surgery. Give oral medications with just enough water to swallow them, even when a client is having surgery first thing in the morning. The anesthesia provider usually writes orders specifying how the morning medication should be managed. Diabetic drugs and cardiovascular medications such as antihypertensives and heart medications are especially important for the client to receive.

Exceptions to the practice of continuing scheduled medications before surgery include administration of drugs such as insulin and oral antihyperglycemics, nonsteroidal anti-inflammatory drugs (NSAIDs) such as aspirin, and anticoagulants such as heparin or warfarin (Coumadin). Because food is withheld, giving insulin or oral antihyperglycemic drugs is likely to result in a dangerously low blood sugar level. The way insulin and glucose administration is handled depends on the severity of the client's disease and the preference of the physician and anesthesia provider. Anticoagulants and NSAIDs affect clotting. With some types of surgery, the bleeding caused by aspirin-like drugs or low-dose heparin is more likely. In some cases, no NSAIDs are allowed for 10 days to 2 weeks before surgery. In other circumstances, they are taken right up until surgery. Low-dose heparin or heparinoids may be given preoperatively to prevent postoperative thromboembolism, but higher doses of heparin and any dose of Coumadin is stopped before surgery to allow coagulation times to return to within normal ranges. Coumadin is usually stopped a week to 10 days before surgery and heparin within a few hours of surgery. Health care providers may order laboratory work the morning of surgery if the client takes anticoagulants to check the INR or PT for Coumadin and APTT or PTT levels for heparin.

LIFE SPAN CONSIDERATIONS

Fasting: Infants and Small Children

Infants and small children have a high metabolic need and tolerate only short periods of fasting, 4 hours or less.

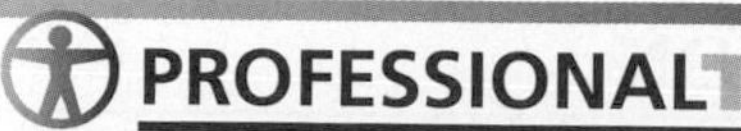

PROFESSIONAL TIP

Preanesthetic Care

- Health care providers explain the risks and benefits of anesthesia and the surgical procedure and have the client sign consent forms before they administer any preoperative medications. The client must be alert to sign consent forms.
- Complete the preoperative checklist.
- Make sure all preoperative orders are executed, especially those for blood tests, preoperative medications, and blood from the blood bank.
- Check, verify, and document the presence or absence of drug allergies for each client.
- Administer regular daily oral medications with a small sip of water as ordered.
- Remind the client of the importance of following instructions regarding any eating or drinking restrictions.
- Administer preoperative medications at the ordered time. Timing can be crucial to achieving the desired effect at the correct time.
- If the client responds abnormally to the preoperative medication, notify the anesthesia department immediately.
- Be sure the client's chart is complete when it goes to the operating room with the client. Recent diagnostic test results are especially important to include; otherwise, surgery may be delayed while these results are sought.
- Make sure the client's consents are in order and included in the chart when the client is transported to surgery.

Additional medications may be ordered to prepare the client for surgery or anesthesia. Surgeons often order prophylactic antibiotics. The anesthesia provider may order a sedative to help the client sleep the night before surgery or to ease the client's anxiety while waiting for surgery. Opioids like morphine or meperidine (Demerol) also are used for pain relief or to ease the induction of anesthesia. Atropine may be given to decrease oral secretions and prevent aspiration. Some anesthesia providers prefer to give preoperative medications in the operating room to precisely control the medication's effect on the client. This is especially true for very sick clients.

Consent

Consent for anesthesia is usually obtained on the same form as is surgical consent, or a separate anesthesia consent form may be used instead of or in addition to the combined consent. In either case, for informed consent to be obtained, the anesthetic must be discussed with the client by someone with expert knowledge of anesthesia, usually an anesthesia provider or the surgeon.

SEDATION

Sedation refers to a reduction of stress, excitement, or irritability and involves some degree of central nervous system (CNS) depression. Sedation is used to decrease awareness of events, relieve anxiety, control the physiologic changes that often accompany anxiety, and ease the induction of general anesthesia. This is welcome news to many clients who fear local or regional anesthesia because they do not want to be awake and see and hear anything during surgery or a diagnostic procedure.

Different sedatives given in combination have a greater effect on the client than does any one of the sedatives given alone. This phenomenon is called **synergism**. The synergistic effect that occurs when different sedative drugs are administered together makes respiratory depression and unconsciousness more likely. In general, benzodiazepines (diazepam [Valium] and midazolam hydrochloride [Versed]) are better sedatives than are opioids (morphine and fentanyl citrate [Sublimaze]). If a client's anxiety is caused by pain, an opioid is a better choice of sedative because the opioid relieves the pain that caused the anxiety.

Sedative medications are administered based on the client's physical condition, weight, mental state, and the procedure being performed, with close observation of the effects of the drugs on the client.

The amount of sedation required by a client for comfort is always balanced with the amount of stimulation experienced as a result of pain or anxiety. Sedation and general anesthesia both involve CNS depression; thus sedation and anesthesia exist on a continuum. As sedation becomes deeper and deeper, it eventually becomes general anesthesia. Sometimes, the line between sedation and general anesthesia is very difficult to distinguish. When sedation becomes general anesthesia, all of the risks of general anesthesia are present, including airway obstruction, respiratory arrest, and aspiration of gastric contents. For this reason, all but the lightest sedation should be administered by an anesthetist or another provider skilled and experienced in airway assessment, protection, and management, as well as assessment of oxygenation and ventilation.

Sedation and Monitoring

Sedation is often used to alleviate client anxiety and discomfort during procedures performed under local anesthesia. Properly administered, local anesthetic injection blocks the painful stimulus of small incisions and minor surgical procedures; however, local anesthetic administration can cause significant discomfort because of edema and tissue irritation caused by the acidity of the local anesthetic solution. Most clients are uncomfortable knowing they are undergoing surgery and prefer to be less alert during the procedure. Procedural sedation (also known as moderate sedation and conscious sedation), decreases the client's perception of these physical and mental discomforts.

During local anesthesia and sedation, the client must remain conscious and in control of his own airway and breathing reflexes. Oversedation is likely to result in airway obstruction and places the client at risk for aspiration of gastric contents. Because sedatives are CNS depressants and, thus, respiratory depressants, give supplemental oxygen to clients during sedation. Monitoring during sedation is done through observation by an individual knowledgeable and experienced in the assessment of respiratory volume and airway patency.

The Joint Commission standards for monitoring clients undergoing procedural sedation require that the BP be measured at frequent and regular intervals and the heart rate and oxygenation be continually monitored by pulse oximetry. They also require the continual monitoring of respiratory rate and pulmonary ventilation. Cardiac rhythm for clients with significant cardiovascular disease or predisposition to dysrhythmias is monitored with an EKG (Joint Commission, 2009).

One method of monitoring pulmonary ventilation is **capnography** that measures a client's carbon dioxide concentration. The capnogram displays the CO_2 level as a waveform (Srinivasa & Kodali, 2008). The individual monitoring the client's breathing and vital signs is devoted to that task to the exclusion of any other duties.

Residual Effects of Sedation

Sedation usually persists beyond the duration of the surgical procedure. The length of time it takes to recover from sedation depends on the health of the client, the properties of the drugs used, other drugs the client may be taking, and the amount of sedative drugs administered.

Amnesia (the inability to remember things) produced by sedatives is commonly found even in clients who appear to be completely recovered. Such clients will probably not remember any instructions given to them during or soon after the procedure. Given that minor procedures and surgery are commonly performed on an outpatient basis, some clients may be discharged before regaining the ability to remember verbal instructions. All instructions should thus be given in writing and explained to the person responsible for taking the client home. Some facilities put the discharge instructions on a CD-ROM, DVD, or video for the client to take home and review.

If heavy sedation was used or the procedure ends suddenly, the client may remain significantly sedated after the procedure is over because the CNS stimulation ended while the CNS depressant effect of the sedative remains. The client is closely monitored until the effects of the sedative medications wear off enough for the client to wake and become oriented.

REGIONAL ANESTHESIA

In **regional anesthesia** a region of the body is temporarily rendered insensible to pain by injection of a local anesthetic. Local anesthetics are a class of drugs that temporarily block the transmission of small electrical impulses through nerves (Table 1-1). The duration of anesthesia produced by a local anesthetic depends on the drug used, the amount injected, and into which part of the body the drug is injected. The amount of insulation surrounding a nerve fiber, the anatomic location of the fiber, and the diameter of the fiber all influence the ease with which nerve impulses are blocked by local anesthetics.

Types of Regional Anesthesia

There are three types of regional anesthesia: local anesthesia, nerve blocks, and spinal and epidural blocks.

Local Anesthesia

Clinically, the use of local anesthetics to block nerves is identified by different names depending on the amount of local anesthetic used and where it is injected. When a small

TABLE 1-1 Drugs Used For Sedation And Anesthesia

Local anesthetics	chloroprocaine (Nesacaine) procaine (Novocain) tetracaine (Pontocaine) bupi vacaine (Marcaine) dibucaine (Nupercaine, Nupercainal) lidocaine (Xylocaine) prilocaine (Citanest)
General anesthetics	enflurane (Ethrane) halothane (Fluothane) isoflurane (Forane)
Intravenous anesthetics	methohexital sodium (Brevital) thiopental sodium (Pentothal) diazepam (Valium) midazolam hydrochloride (Versed) fentanyl citrate (Sublimaze)
Adjuncts to anesthesia	succinylcholine chloride (Anectine, Quelicin, Sucostrin) tubocurarine chloride (Tubocurarin)

Adapted from *Pharmacology for Nurses: A Pathophysiologic Approach*, by M. Adams, L. Holland, and P. Bostwick, 2008, Upper Saddle River, NJ: Pearson Prentice Hall.

amount of local anesthetic drug is injected either into the skin and subcutaneous tissues around a cut or at the site of a needle puncture for a central line placement, it is called local anesthesia. The anesthetic is not aimed at a specific nerve; rather it anesthetizes all small superficial nerves in the target area. Local anesthesia is most commonly performed using lidocaine (Xylocaine) and lasts approximately 1 hour. Serious side effects of lidocaine (Xylocaine) are convulsions, respiratory depression, and dysrhythmias leading to cardiac arrest. Lidocaine with preservatives or epinephrine are used only for local anesthesia and never given for dysrhythmias (Adams, Holland, & Bostwick, 2008). Occasionally, for some types of plastic surgery, this type of anesthesia is used over a large area of the body. In this case, longer-acting local anesthetics are used. Because very small amounts of local anesthetics are generally used, the risk of local anesthetic toxicity is also small.

▼ SAFETY ▼

Preventing Choking and Aspiration

To prevent choking and aspiration after the use of an oral anesthetic solution (e.g., viscous lidocaine) or spray, fluids and foods must be withheld until the gag reflex returns.

Topical anesthesia, achieved with direct application of a local anesthetic to tissue, is desired in some situations (e.g., before insertion of an IV). The anesthetic takes the form of an ointment, lotion, solution, or spray.

Nerve Blocks

When a local anesthetic is injected more deeply into the body and/or is directed at a specific nerve or nerves, it is called a *nerve block*. Nerve blocks are often called by the name of the specific nerve or nerves they block. Examples include an ulnar nerve block in the arm or a brachial plexus block of all the nerves in the arm. Nerve blocks are often performed using lidocaine (Xylocaine), mepivacaine (Carbocaine), or bupivacaine (Marcaine) and may last from 1 to 12 hours.

Spinal and Epidural Blocks

Blocks also are identified according to where the local anesthetic is injected. One example is an *epidural block*, for which local anesthetic is injected into the epidural space near the spinal cord to anesthetize several spinal nerves at once. With spinal blocks (also called subarachnoid blocks), the local anesthetic is injected into the cerebrospinal fluid (CSF), where it can bathe uninsulated spinal nerves as they exit the spinal cord to the periphery of the body (Figure 1-2).

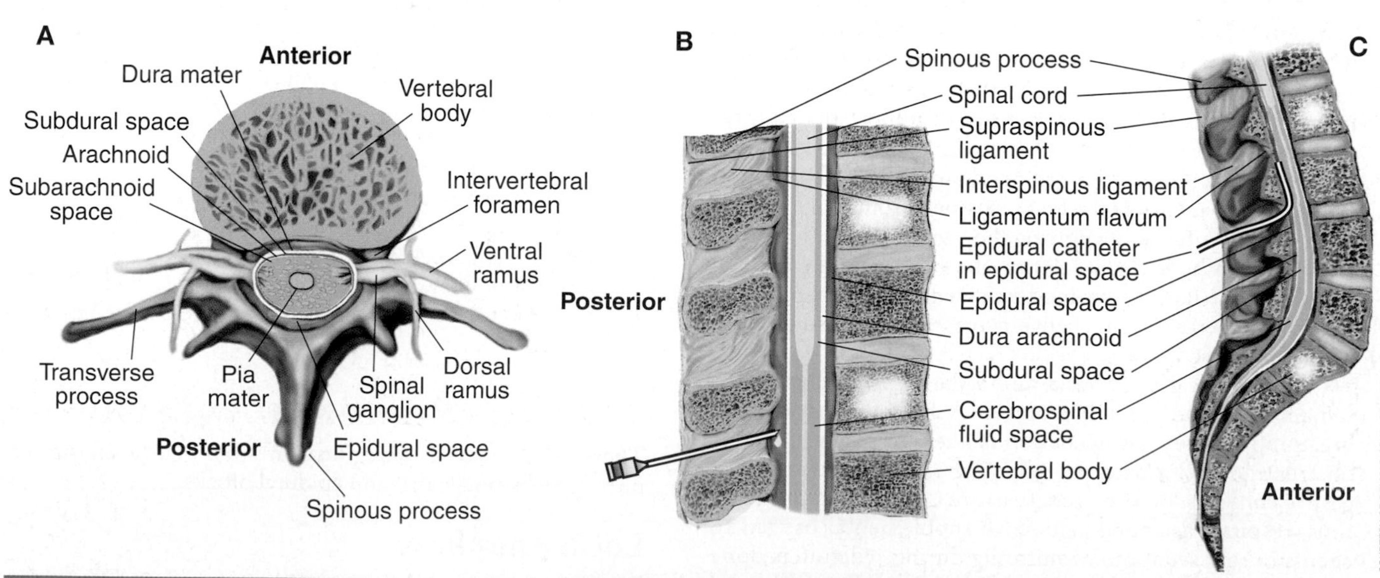

FIGURE 1-2 *A*, **Cross-Sectional Anatomy of the Spine;** *B*, **Side View of Spinal Anatomy with the Tip of an Epidural Needle Placed in the Epidural Space;** *C*, **Side View of Spinal Anatomy with the Tip of an Epidural Catheter Placed in the Epidural Space**

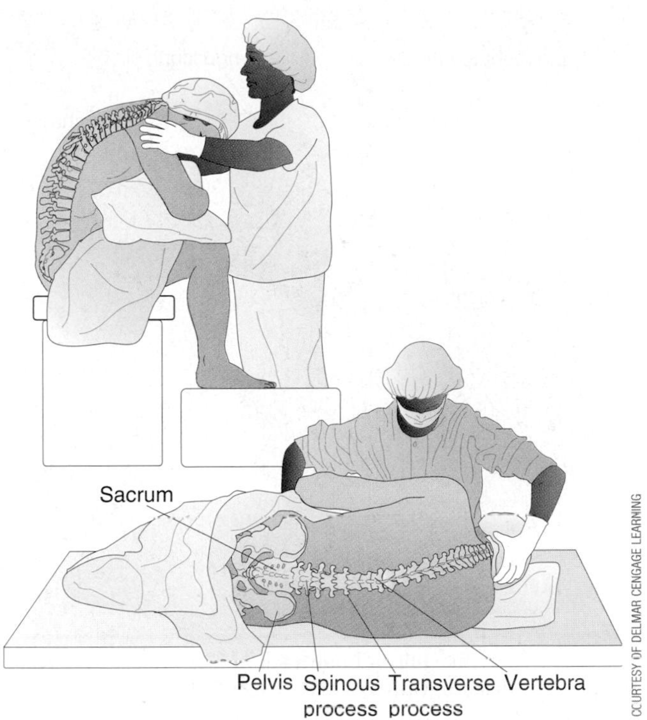

FIGURE 1-3 Correct positions for performing a spinal block or inserting an epidural catheter into the lumbar area. The assistance of trained personnel is crucial to the proper positioning, reassurance, and safety of the client.

Spinal and epidural blocks are generally used to anesthetize a significant area of the body. They are capable of safely producing anesthesia sufficient for surgery in the abdomen, pelvis, perineum, or lower extremities. When an epidural block is performed, a catheter is usually inserted into the epidural space, making it possible to inject additional doses of drug. The client must either be sitting in a bent-over position or lying on the side with head and knees as close together as possible (Figure 1-3). Either position separates the vertebra, making insertion of the needle or catheter possible. Epidural blocks have an added advantage in that by varying the way the anesthetic is used, the block can produce analgesia (pain relief without producing anesthesia), complete anesthesia, and even profound muscular relaxation (needed for some types of surgery). This allows epidural anesthesia to be used not only for surgical procedures, but also for analgesia during labor and for postoperative pain relief.

Spinal blocks are most often performed using lidocaine (Xylocaine) or bupivacaine (Marcaine) and last from 1 to 3 hours. Epidural blocks are most commonly performed using bupivacaine (Marcaine), and the block can be continued as long as local anesthetic is injected through the catheter into the epidural space.

Opioids such as morphine and fentanyl citrate (Sublimaze) may be added to the local anesthetic in either of these blocks to intensify the analgesic or anesthetic effect, or to provide postoperative pain relief after the block has worn off.

One type of complication is peculiar to spinal and epidural regional anesthetics. When CSF leaks out through a hole made in the dural membrane during performance of a subarachnoid block or an accidental dural puncture during the attempted performance of an epidural block, a postdural puncture headache (PDPH) may result. The headache is caused by the loss of CSF from around the brain. The headache is relieved by lying down and returns when the individual sits up or stands. Pain commonly occurs in both the front and the back of the head and is sometimes accompanied by neck and shoulder stiffness. Photophobia or double vision may be present with severe headache. The onset of the headache is usually not immediate and may take 1 to 2 days to become bothersome. Treatment involves adequate hydration to allow the normal production of CSF; analgesics; and bed rest in a supine position. One treatment for significant or persistent PDPH is a procedure called an epidural blood patch, which involves injecting 15 to 20 mL of the client's own blood into the epidural space. Once the blood clots, it plugs the hole in the dural membrane. Another treatment involves connecting an IV infusion to the epidural catheter to replace the lost CSF and treat the headache.

Residual Effects of Regional Anesthesia

All anesthetics wear off as the drug responsible for causing the anesthesia is removed, metabolized, and eliminated. Some effects wear off faster than others. The client may be wide awake and able to carry on a conversation but have residual effects that are not detected by casual observation. Motor, sensory and sympathetic residual block effects are common.

Residual Motor Block

A motor block is a temporary condition caused when local anesthetic blocks nerves that carry instructions to skeletal muscles telling them to contract. Motor block results in the inability to move a body part and is usually the last effect to develop and the first to wear off. It results only when the regional block is very dense and complete.

A complete motor block results in a temporary paralysis, with the client being incapable of moving the blocked part despite tremendous effort. With a complete motor block, there is usually no function in any other type of nerve in the same area. A client with a complete motor block of any part of the body would not likely be released from the recovery area. Clients experiencing residual (incomplete) motor block may be released from recovery. A client who has had any type of block involving the legs is not allowed to get out of bed without assistance until it is demonstrated that a complete recovery of motor strength in the legs is regained. Even a small amount of residual motor block greatly increases the possibility that a client will fall.

As a regional block begins to wear off, motor function begins to return first, sensation begins to return next, and sympathetic nervous function returns last. Motor function and sensation is detected easily by asking the client to move the blocked part or by touching the skin and asking the client whether it feels normal. The return of sympathetic function is more difficult to detect. Orthostatic hypotension may occur even after motor and sensory functions have completely returned and the regional block appears to have worn off. To prevent fainting, the nurse assists the client in getting out of bed until she is able to do so without any dizziness or significant decrease in blood pressure.

Residual Sensory Block

Normal sensation may not have returned completely upon client discharge from the recovery area. As the regional block wears off, sensation returns gradually. As sensation begins to return, the client experiences a "pins-and-needles" feeling in an arm or leg that has been blocked and may feel touch or pressure before recovering complete sensation. Until complete recovery of normal sensation, any blocked areas are frequently checked and carefully protected, as the client may be unaware that a finger or hand, for example, is being pinched or denied blood supply.

Residual Sympathetic Block

The last nerve fibers to recover as a local anesthetic wears off are those responsible for carrying instructions to the muscles that surround blood vessels. When these sympathetic nerves are blocked, veins and arteries dilate, lowering the blood pressure. The venous system has a large capacity, and venous dilation results in the pooling of a large amount of blood. This decreases the amount of blood that returns to the heart, and the blood pressure falls. The amount of blood that pools is greatest in parts of the body that are farthest below the level of the heart. Even in a client who has had a spinal or epidural block and is lying supine, a significant amount of venous pooling occurs, resulting in lower-than-normal blood pressure. If the same client is allowed to sit up, even more venous pooling will occur, less blood will return to the heart, and blood pressure will fall substantially. This phenomenon of having a large drop in blood pressure when sitting up or standing is called **orthostatic hypotension.** *Orthostatic* signifies that it involves body position, and hypotension means low blood pressure. Clients who have had a spinal or epidural block are more likely to have orthostatic hypotension the higher in the spinal column the level of their block.

GENERAL ANESTHESIA

General anesthesia involves unconsciousness, complete insensibility to pain, amnesia, motionlessness, and muscle relaxation. With general anesthesia, the body also loses the ability to control many important functions, including the abilities to maintain an airway, control vital functions such as breathing and heart rate, and regulate temperature. These functions are controlled by the anesthesia provider during administration of general anesthesia.

General anesthesia involves four overlapping stages: induction (going to sleep), maintenance, emergence (waking up), and recovery.

Induction and Airway Management

The induction of general anesthesia is a short but critical period during which the client is rendered unconscious, vital functions are controlled, and enough anesthetic drug is introduced into the body to keep the client asleep during surgery. In adults, drugs are usually injected into an IV line to quickly produce unconsciousness, and additional anesthetic is then inhaled (Table 1-1).

LIFE SPAN CONSIDERATIONS

Induction of Anesthesia in Small Children

Inhalation of an anesthetic vapor is used first, then an IV line is started and additional IV drugs are administered.

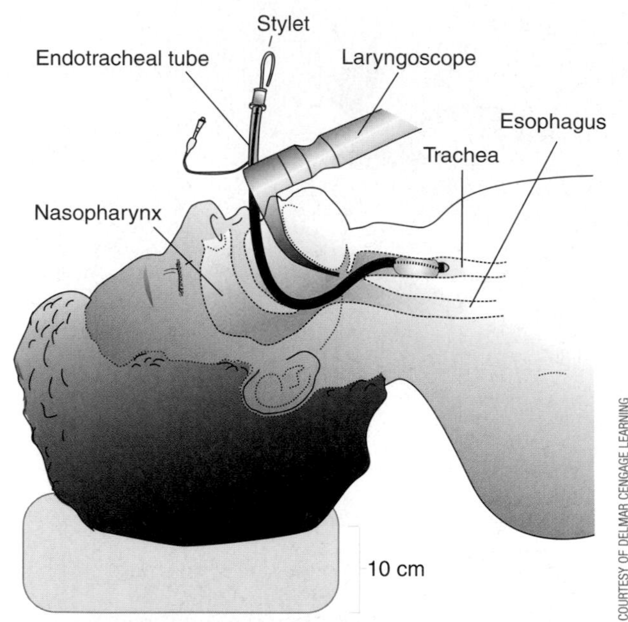

FIGURE 1-4 Placing an Endotracheal Tube in the Trachea with Direct Visualization by Laryngoscopy

Immediately after the induction of general anesthesia, the anesthesia provider secures the airway using a cuffed endotracheal tube (ETT) (Figure 1-4). An ETT provides a breathing passage from outside the client to within the client's trachea.

Maintenance

General anesthesia is maintained with some combination of IV and inhaled drugs. Figure 1-5 shows a client connected to an anesthesia machine by a breathing circuit.

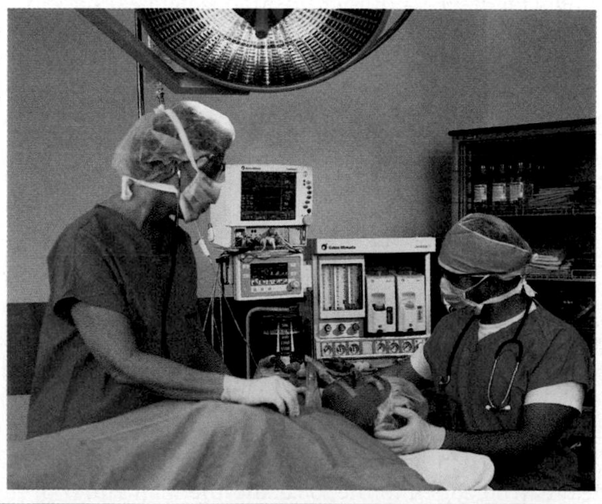

FIGURE 1-5 A typical anesthesia machine is a complex equipment set. This machine has anesthetic vaporizers and flowmeters to deliver oxygen, nitrous oxide, and air. It also supports a ventilator and equipment to monitor ventilation, oxygen content of inspired gas, client oxygen saturation, blood pressure, heart rate, and respiration. (Pictured above is the Datex-Ohmeda Aestiva/5 Anesthesia Delivery System equipped with a Cardiocap/5 Monitor.) (*Reprinted with permission of Datex-Ohmeda, Inc.*)

Skeletal Muscle Relaxation

Some types of surgery require complete relaxation of skeletal muscles. In these cases, the anesthesia provider administers a skeletal muscle relaxant such as pancuronium bromide (Pavulon) or vecuronium bromide (Norcuron) to completely paralyze the client. These types of drugs prevent clients from breathing on their own, requiring the anesthesia provider to ventilate clients during surgery. Paralysis is eliminated before emergence from anesthesia so the client can breathe independently again.

Inadequate reversal of paralysis presents as anything from total skeletal muscle paralysis to the inability of the client to cough and clear the airway. If the client is having difficulty breathing, basic life support is provided until the arrival of an anesthesia provider.

EMERGENCE

Emergence from general anesthesia occurs when anesthetic drugs are allowed to wear off. The anesthesia provider carefully controls the timing and amount of anesthetic drug given in order for the client to emerge from general anesthesia at the desired time. The initial phase of emergence is usually quite quick, allowing the client to awaken enough to respond to verbal directions and maintain an airway. After this time, the client's breathing tube usually is removed, and the client is taken to the postanesthesia care unit (recovery room). If, for some reason, the client is left on a ventilator and with a breathing tube in place, the anesthesia provider takes the client to an intensive care unit asleep instead of waking the client up from the anesthetic.

RECOVERY

Recovery from general anesthesia is not complete simply because the client has regained consciousness. The client may not remember what has happened for minutes or even hours after receiving an anesthetic. The ability to think clearly often takes longer to return, with some residual thinking difficulty persisting for several days or even weeks. Inhalation anesthetics are eliminated from the body through the lungs, and very small amounts of anesthetic are still being exhaled for several weeks. Many anesthetic drugs are stored in body fat and released back into the bloodstream very slowly after anesthetic administration has ended. The speed of this release depends on the amount of anesthetic given during the surgery, the length of the surgery, and how deeply the client is breathing.

LIFE SPAN CONSIDERATIONS

Oxygenation and Ventilation in the Elderly Client

- Impaired mobility allows secretions to pool in the lungs. Therefore, elderly clients must be monitored more closely, and secretions suctioned.
- Most anesthetic agents cause decreased respiratory rate and decreased tidal volume, putting elderly clients at greater risk for hypoventilation.

Oxygenation and Ventilation

Almost all anesthetics are respiratory depressants. Benzodiazepines, opioids, and inhalation anesthetic agents have significant respiratory depressant effects. Any one of these drugs may be used in a dose that causes apnea, or lack of respirations for more than 10 seconds, during a general anesthesia. When used in combination their effect on respiration is at least additive. When the rate or depth of respirations decrease, the elimination of carbon dioxide is retarded, and carbon dioxide builds up in the blood and in the lungs. Oxygen saturation is monitored by pulse oximetry. Even small amounts of supplemental oxygen given to a client whose rate or depth of breathing is decreased adds significantly to the amount of oxygen in the bloodstream. This is the most important reason that oxygen is given to even healthy clients when they are recovering from general anesthesia.

Heart Rate and Blood Pressure

Few direct effects on heart rate (HR) and blood pressure (BP) regulation are seen during recovery from general anesthesia. Some anesthetic techniques that are heavily based on opioids, such as fentanyl citrate (Sublimaze) or sufentanil citrate (Sufenta), can cause a slow HR, but as long as BP is maintained, no specific treatment is necessary. Although most general anesthetics are myocardial depressants, the depressive effects of current agents are mild, especially after anesthetic administration is ended.

Most HR and BP changes seen during recovery result from factors related indirectly to the anesthetic. Both HR and BP increase as a result of sympathetic stimulation. Pain, hypoxia, and fear can all result in sympathetic stimulation with an increase in HR and BP. Discovering and addressing the source of the client's fear often reduces the anxiety. When the causes of sympathetic stimulation are addressed, HR and BP should normalize.

Temperature Regulation and Shivering

With general anesthesia, the body loses its natural ability to regulate temperature. General anesthetic agents dilate the blood vessels close to the surface of the body, exposing the client's warm blood to the cool exterior. During anesthetization, the client is mostly uncovered in a cold operating room, and the body's surgical area is cleaned with cold solutions. After this is done, the client's insulating covering (skin and subcutaneous fat) is cut open to expose the warm interior of the body and allow its heat to escape. Room temperature intravenous (IV) fluids are infused into the veins, and the client breathes cool gases. Surgical clients lose a great amount of heat at a time when the body is least able to respond to warm the tissues. Hypothermia adds to the CNS depression resulting from any residual anesthetics. Surface warming with a forced-air warming blanket is an effective way to increase the temperature of a client intraoperatively and when recovering from general anesthesia; warm cloth blankets also maintain body warmth. Figure 1-6 shows use of a forced-air warming blanket.

All potent inhalation agents are associated with shivering during emergence from general anesthesia when the blood level of the anesthetic agent is very low. The cause of the shivering is not clear but does not appear to be related to the client's body temperature. (Of course, postoperative clients

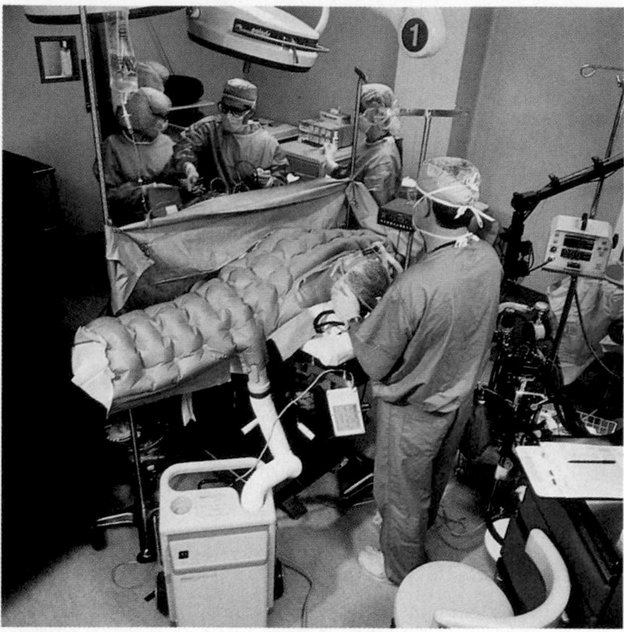

FIGURE 1-6 A forced-air warming blanket applied to the upper abdomen, chest, and arms or lower torso of a client during surgery. The unit on the floor to the left of the anesthesia provider (foreground) is the heating unit, which contains a fan that pushes warm air through the hose and into the blanket, much like a furnace pushes warm air through heating ducts and into a house. Warm air exits hundreds of pinholes on the surface of the blanket and next to the client. (*Courtesy of Mallinckrodt Medical, Inc.*)

also shiver when they are cold.) The key to eliminating shivering postoperatively is to ensure client warmth and encourage deep breathing so that the anesthetic is eliminated as quickly as possible.

Fluid Balance

Surgical procedures and the injuries that necessitate them have major effects on the body's distribution of fluid. Appropriate care during anesthesia sometimes necessitates the delivery of a large volume of IV fluid. This IV fluid does not stay in the vascular system long, moving out of the vascular space to replace losses from the interstitial and intracellular spaces.

Trauma, whether caused by an accidental injury or a surgical incision, results in fluid losses or shifts in three general areas as follows: direct blood loss, evaporation through the surgical wound, and fluid shifts. Large volumes of fluid are lost to the air through the surgical wound, especially during abdominal procedures. A major abdominal procedure, for example, can result in the loss of up to 10 mL/kg/hour of fluid by evaporation.

CRITICAL THINKING

Client Monitoring After Anesthesia

Why must clients be monitored very closely after receiving an anesthetic?

POSTOPERATIVE PAIN MANAGEMENT

Pain has many causes. Postoperative pain results from tissue injury, release of local and hormonal substances, inflammation, mental outlook, and, perhaps, neural hyperexcitability related to excessive noxious input. As such, baseline postoperative pain, pain from pressure placed on an incision, and pain from client movement each respond best to different pain-relieving strategies.

The amount of medication needed to relieve pain depends on the intensity and type of pain, the size of the client, and the client's age. The opioid dose for an elderly client is started at 25–50% of the usual adult dose and then slowly increased by 25–50% increments until the client reports a mild pain level (McDonald, 2006). The opioid of choice for elderly is morphine with hydromorphone hydrochloride (Dilaudid) as the second choice (McDonald, 2006). Monitor the elderly closely for opioid toxicity on a pain scale they understand.

PATIENT-CONTROLLED ANALGESIA

Patient-controlled analgesia (PCA) allows clients to self-administer pain medication by pushing a button when they experience pain. After an IV catheter is in place, a client-controlled analgesia pump is connected "piggyback" to the IV line. The pump is programmed to deliver a predetermined dose of morphine, hydromorphone hydrochloride (Dilaudid), or fentanyl citrate (Sublimaze) when the client pushes a button. It will not, however, deliver unlimited amounts. A set time must pass between each successive dose, and when the total dose of opioid delivered in any hour reaches a preset limit, the pump will not deliver any more medicine until the next hour. This is referred to as lockout.

Properly programmed, PCA allows the client a great deal of control over when pain medicine is received, which is likely to help decrease anxiety. Patient-controlled analgesia also results in a shorter interval between the need for pain medicine and its administration, better pain relief than that obtained with intermittent IM injections, and a reduction in nursing time necessary for the delivery of pain medicine. It does not, however, decrease the need for client assessment of pain while the PCA machine is in use.

REGIONAL ANALGESIA

Regional analgesia and anesthesia have many applications in the relief of postoperative pain. Regional anesthetics do not cease working when the surgery ends and provide pain relief for a variable period of time afterward. The duration of postoperative pain relief can be extended by continuing the infusion of pain medication into the epidural space or by adding opioids to either epidural or spinal anesthetics.

Local Anesthetics

Local anesthetics, either alone or in combination with opioids, are administered into the epidural space at low concentrations that do not cause complete anesthesia. This type of pain relief is most commonly used for women in labor who receive epidural analgesia. Local anesthetic in low concentrations is

CLIENT TEACHING

Patient-Controlled Analgesia (PCA)

- Only the client should push the button to administer more analgesic.
- The client should not ask visitors to push the button.

a powerful analgesic. If local anesthetic is administered in a way to relieve pain in the lower extremities, clients are usually confined to bed, because even dilute concentrations of local anesthetic may affect the strength of leg muscles enough to increase the risk of falling. Clients receiving analgesia via an epidural block are watched carefully to ensure that they do not develop pressure necrosis in the blocked areas.

Opioids

The spinal cord has receptors for opioids, and when opioids are added to a spinal or epidural anesthetic, they provide pain relief even after the anesthetic block has worn off. Morphine added to a spinal or epidural anesthetic provides hours of postoperative pain relief, often enough so that no other pain medication is needed; it may even provide better pain relief than do IM injections or intravenous PCA. Opioids are added to spinal or epidural anesthetics as a single dose or be infused into the epidural space postoperatively. Although spinal and epidural morphine provide excellent pain relief, they may also produce significant respiratory depression. Fortunately, the respiratory depression after spinal or epidural morphine administration is rarely rapid in onset. Respiratory depression is very rare with properly dosed epidural or spinal fentanyl citrate (Sublimaze). With current client selection and dosing protocols, life-threatening respiratory depression is a rare event. When it does occur, it can be detected long before it causes harm, by observing the client frequently, noting respiratory rate and depth, and periodically measuring oxygen saturation by pulse oximetry.

PROFESSIONAL TIP

Postanesthetic Care

- Immediately report to the anesthesia provider or surgeon any client breathing difficulty or a respiratory rate of 12 breaths per minute or less.
- Immediately report to the surgeon or the anesthesia department a fall in the client's BP or increase in HR.
- Verify client's ability to stand or walk with normal motor strength and coordination and without any dizziness before allowing the client to get up without assistance.
- Do not allow clients to rub their eyes. Clients who are still drowsy may try to rub out protective eye moisturizer and, in the process, cause painful corneal abrasions.
- Observe clients immediately and hourly for bladder distention. Both regional and general anesthesia can sometimes cause temporary urinary retention.
- If clients have an epidural catheter for postoperative pain management, ensure that they change positions from time to time to prevent pressure necrosis. Do not allow the lateral aspect of the leg to rest on the side rails.
- Report to the anesthesia department as soon as possible any headache that gets worse when the client sits up or stands.
- Before giving discharge instructions, verify that the client's ability to remember instructions has returned. Always share discharge instructions with the individual responsible for taking the client home and provide the client with a written copy of the instructions.

SUMMARY

- In addition to ensuring an adequate level of anesthesia throughout a surgical procedure, the anesthesia provider monitors and controls physiologic functions.
- Some anesthesia providers prefer that clients not have anything to eat or drink for at least 8 hours before surgery. Others allow water up to 2 hours before surgery.
- Most scheduled medications that a client takes every day are continued up to and including the morning of surgery.
- Sedation depresses brain activity, decreasing awareness, reducing anxiety, and easing the induction of general anesthesia.
- Oversedation results in respiratory depression, which can cause airway obstruction, and places the client at risk for aspiration of gastric contents.
- Regional anesthesia by the injection of a local anesthetic temporarily renders a "region" of the body insensible to pain.
- General anesthesia produces unconsciousness, complete insensibility to pain, amnesia, motionlessness, and muscle relaxation.
- A person is unlikely to remember what has happened for minutes to hours after sedation or a general anesthetic.
- Intravenous patient-controlled analgesia (PCA) allows clients to self-administer pain medication by pushing a button on the PCA machine. Limits are programmed into the machine to prevent overdose.
- Local anesthetics, alone or in combination with opioids, can be injected into the epidural space at low concentrations to provide postoperative analgesia.
- Spinal and epidural morphine can produce dangerous respiratory depression. This can be detected by frequent observations of the client's respiratory rate and depth and by periodic measurement of oxygen saturation via pulse oximetry.

CASE STUDY

C.P. is in the recovery room after outpatient surgery. She received a general anesthetic and is now awake, breathing deeply, and talking to the staff. She has received morphine sulfate intravenously and is quite comfortable. Before being discharged home from the surgery center, C.P. rests in an easy chair in the transitional recovery area. The nurse taking care of her notices that she asks questions about things that have already been discussed and has even asked one question three times.

The following questions will guide your development of a nursing care plan for the case study.

1. After making these observations, what nursing diagnoses and goals might the nurse identify for C.P.?
2. List nursing interventions in caring for C.P.
3. Identify teaching approaches.

REVIEW QUESTIONS

1. Clients are at risk for aspiration of gastric contents into the lungs when receiving a general anesthetic because:
   1. general anesthesia causes stomach distention.
   2. general anesthesia eliminates protective airway reflexes.
   3. gastric peristalsis is reversed during general anesthesia.
   4. vomiting normally occurs during general anesthesia.
2. The most dangerous result of oversedation is:
   1. lack of response to verbal directions.
   2. longer recovery time and resultant delayed discharge.
   3. prolonged amnesia.
   4. inability to breathe adequately.
3. What is a sign that a client has a postdural puncture headache following a spinal or epidural regional block?
   1. The headache subsides after intake of plenty of liquids.
   2. The headache begins after the surgical procedure.
   3. The headache worsens when the client sits up or stands.
   4. The client is confused in addition to having a headache.
4. After cessation of a general anesthetic, how long might it be before the client can think as clearly as before the client received the anesthetic?
   1. Before being discharged from the recovery room.
   2. Within 2 hours.
   3. Six hours.
   4. Several days.
5. What effect might a spinal or epidural anesthetic block still have after normal sensation and motor function have returned?
   1. Decrease in pulse rate when the client is lying in bed.
   2. Decrease in blood pressure when the client stands up.
   3. Inhibition of protective airway reflexes.
   4. Sore muscles.
6. A client returned from surgery and has a PCA for pain. The main purpose of the PCA is:
   1. the client controls pain medication administration.
   2. so the nurse does not have to stop caring for another client to administer medication to the client in pain.
   3. better pain relief for the client than intermittent IM injections.
   4. less time needed to assess the client's pain level.
7. A client is given fentanyl citrate (Sublimaze) with a spinal anesthetic for pain relief. To adequately assess the client for respiratory depression the nurse: (Select all that apply.)
   1. notes respiratory rate and depth.
   2. observes the color the mucous membranes.
   3. measures oxygen saturation with a pulse oximeter on a regular basis.
   4. monitors the client's ventilation by capnography.
   5. checks apical and peripheral pulses.
   6. observes symmetry of chest wall movements and use of accessory muscles.
8. A client had a regional anesthesia. During postoperative care, the nurse assesses for residual effects of the anesthesia by: (Select all that apply.)
   1. asking the client questions and listening to his responses.
   2. asking the client to move an area blocked by the anesthesia.
   3. touching the client's legs and asking if the touch feels normal.
   4. assisting the client to a sitting position and asking if she is dizzy.
   5. assessing the client's mental alertness.
   6. assessing the motor strength in her legs.

9. A client has a nonunion fracture of the fifth phalange and is having a nerve block as the anesthesia. What client statement indicates to the nurse that more teaching is needed about the anesthesia and scheduled procedure?
   1. I may be awake but sleepy throughout the surgery.
   2. I will not be able to move my lower arm during surgery.
   3. I will not have any painful feeling in my lower arm or hand during surgery.
   4. I will be unconscious and put to sleep prior to and during the surgery.

10. The main priority of the anesthesia provider during a general anesthetic is monitoring the:
    1. blood pressure at frequent intervals.
    2. oxygenation by pulse oximetry.
    3. respiratory rate and pulmonary ventilation.
    4. cardiac rhythm by an EKG.

REFERENCES/SUGGESTED READINGS

Adams, M., Holland, L., & Bostwick, P. (2008). *Pharmacology for nurses: A pathophysiologic approach*. Upper Saddle River, N.J.: Pearson Prentice Hall.

American Association of Nurse Anesthetists (AANA). (2001). Administration puts politics before patients; Implements cumbersome anesthesia care rule. Retrieved on April 2, 2009 at http://www.aana.com/Advocacy.aspx?ucNavMenu_TSMenuTargetID=49&ucNavMenu_TSMenuTargetType=4&ucNavMenu_TSMenuID=6&id=2575&terms=administration+puts+politics+before+patients%3a+implements+cumbersome+anesthesia+care+rule

American Association of Nurse Anesthetists (AANA). (2002). New Hampshire becomes fifth state to opt out of federal anesthesia requirement. Retrieved on April 2, 2009 at http://www.aana.com/news.aspx?ucNavMenu_TSMenuTargetID=171&ucNavMenu_TSMenuTargetType=4&ucNavMenu_TSMenuID=6&id=690&terms=opt+out

American Association of Nurse Anesthetists (AANA). (2005). *Governor Rounds removes physician supervision for South Dakota CRNAs*. Retrieved on March 31, 2009 at http://www.aana.com/news.aspx?ucNavMenu_TSMenuTargetID=62&ucNavMenu_TSMenuTargetType=4&ucNavMenu_TSMenuID=6&id=854&terms=opt+out

American Association of Nurse Anesthetists (AANA). (2008). Education of nurse anesthetists in the United States–At a glance. Retrievedon March 31, 2009 at http://www.aana.com/BecomingCRNA.aspx?ucNavMenu_TSMenuTargetID=18&ucNavMenu_TSMenuTargetType=4&ucNavMenu_TSMenuID=6&id=1018

American Association of Nurse Anesthetists (AANA). (2009). Qualifications and capabilities of the certified registered nurse anesthetist. Retrieved on March 31, 2009 at http://www.aana.com/BecomingCRNA.aspx?ucNavMenu_TSMenuTargetID=102&ucNavMenu_TSMenuTargetType=4&ucNavMenu_TSMenuID=6&id=112

American Society of Anesthesiologists (ASA). (1999). 1998 House of delegates passes two new practice guidelines. Retrieved on March 31, 2009 at http://www.asahq.org/Newsletters/1999/02_99/1998_0299.html

American Society of Anesthesiologists (ASA). (2007). Revised guidelines issued for anesthesia, pain relief during labor and delivery. Retrieved on March 31, 2009 at http://www.asahq.org/news/asanews040207.htm

Berkowitz, C. (1997). Epidural pain control—Your job, too. *RN*, 60(8), 22–27.

Carroll, P. (2002). Procedural sedation: Capnography's heightened role. *RN*, 65(10), 54–62.

Clinical News. (1999). "NPO after midnight" outdated? *AJN*, 99(2), 18.

Connolly, M. (1999). Postdural puncture headache. *AJN*, 99(11), 48–49.

Crenshaw, J. (1999). New guidelines for preoperative fasting. *AJN*, 99(4), 49.

Joint Commission. (2009). Standards for operative or other high-risk procedures and/or the administration of moderate or deep sedation or anesthesia. Retrieved on April 1, 2009 at http://www.jointcommission.org/NR/rdonlyres/6530941D-98AD-4AC7-8944-9DDE1116E503/0/OBS_Standards_Sampler_2007_final.pdf

Joint Commission Resources. Joint Commission on Accreditation of Healthcare Organizations. (2000). New definitions, revised standards address the continuum of sedation and anesthesia. *Joint Commission Perspectives*, 20(4), 10.

Kodali, B. (2008). Capnograms during procedural sedation. Retrieved on April 1, 2009 at http://www.capnography.com/new/index.php?option=com_contetn&view=article&id+245&

Kost, M. (1999). Conscious sedation: Guarding your patient against complications. *Nursing99*, 29(4), 34–39.

Kreger, C. (2001). Spinal anesthesia and analgesia. *Nursing2001*, 31(6), 36–41.

McDonald, D. (2006). Postoperative pain management for the aging patient. *Geriatrics Aging*, 9(6), 395-398.

Messinger, J., Hoffman, L., O'Donnell, J., & Dunworth, B. (1999). Getting conscious sedation right. *AJN, 99*(12), 44–49.

O'Donnell, T., Bragg, K., & Sell, S. (2003). Procedural sedation: Safely navigating the twilight zone. *Nursing2003*, 33(4), 36–41, 44.

Pasero, C., & McCaffery, M. (1999). Providing epidural analgesia. *Nursing99, 29*(8), 34–39.

Scott, J., & Stanski, D. (1987). Decreased fentanyl and alfentanil dose requirements with age: A simultaneous pharmacokinetic and pharmacodynamic evaluation. *Journal of Pharmacology and Experimental Therapeutics*, 240, 159–166.

Srinivasa, V., & Kodali, B. (2008). Applications of capnography. Retrieved on November 6, 2009 at http://www.capnography.com/outside/sedation.htm

Wong, D. (2003). Topical local anesthetics. *AJN*, 103(6), 42–45.

Woomer, J., & Berkheimer, D. (2003). Using capnography to monitor ventilation. *Nursing2003*, 33(4), 42–43.

RESOURCES

American Association of Nurse Anesthetists, http://www.aana.com

American Society of Anesthesiologists, http://www.asahq.org

American Society of Peri Anesthesia Nurses, http://www.aspan.org

American Society of Regional Anesthesia and Pain Medicine, http://www.asra.com

Anesthesia Patient Safety Foundation, http://www.gasnet.org/societies/apsf/

Foundation for Anesthesia Education and Research, http://www.faer.org

Society for Education in Anesthesia, http://www.seahq.org

CHAPTER 2
Surgery

MAKING THE CONNECTION

Refer to the following chapters to increase your understanding of perioperative nursing:

Adult Health Nursing

- ***Anesthesia***
- ***Respiratory System***
- ***Cardiovascular System***
- ***Musculoskeletal System***
- ***Integumentary System***

LEARNING OBJECTIVES

Upon completion of this chapter, you should be able to:

- Define key terms.
- List risk factors in a preoperative nursing assessment.
- List information in a general teaching plan for a preoperative client.
- Identify common nursing care for the preoperative, intraoperative, and postoperative phases.
- Describe the principles of asepsis and their application to nursing practice.
- Discuss nursing interventions to prevent or treat postoperative complications.
- Identify information needed by the postoperative client before discharge.
- Discuss the physiologic changes of aging that affect the elderly client's response to surgery.
- Plan care for a postoperative client.

KEY TERMS

Aldrete Score
ambulatory surgery
asepsis
aseptic technique
circulating nurse
dehiscence
evisceration
first assistant
informed consent
intraoperative phase
perioperative
postoperative phase
preoperative phase
scrub nurse
sterile
sterile conscience
sterile field
surgery

INTRODUCTION

Surgery refers to the treatment of injury, disease, or deformity through invasive operative methods. Surgery is a unique experience, with no two clients responding alike to similar operations. Even the same client may respond differently to two separate surgical situations or to the same surgery performed at a later time. Surgery is a major stressor for every client. To a client, there is no such thing as minor surgery; anxiety and fear are normal. Surgery, even when planned well in advance, is a stressor that produces both psychological (anxiety, fear) and physiologic (neuroendocrine) stress reactions. Surgery is a stressful experience because it involves entry into the human body.

Surgeries are classified as minor (presenting little risk to life) or major (possibly involving risk to life) and are performed for a variety of reasons. Table 2-1 lists indications for surgery.

The term **perioperative** encompasses the preoperative (before surgery), intraoperative (during surgery), and postoperative (after surgery) phases of surgery. Each phase refers to a particular time during the surgical experience, and each requires a wide range of specific nursing behaviors and functions. Perioperative nursing has one continuous goal: to provide a standard of excellence in the care of the client before, during, and after surgery. Nursing activities are geared to meet the client's psychosocial needs as well as immediate physical needs.

Individuals face surgery with their own values. Each client has specific expectations of the surgical experience and distinct hopes for the outcome of the surgery. The nurse takes an active part in the entire perioperative process to ensure quality and continuity of client care.

PREOPERATIVE PHASE

The **preoperative phase** is that time during the surgical experience that begins with the client's decision to have surgery and ends with the transfer of the client to the operating table.

The outcome of surgical treatment is tremendously enhanced by accurate preoperative nursing assessment and careful preoperative preparation. The client must be assessed by the nurse both physiologically and psychologically. Assessment of the client involves the integration of factors relating to the client's illness, physical condition, related medical conditions, and current surgical diagnosis. Regardless of how minor the surgical procedure, a thorough health history is essential and available to the perioperative team throughout the client's surgical experience.

The psychological well-being of the client has an impact on the surgical outcome. The surgical client is at risk for anxiety related to the surgical experience and the outcome of surgery. Fear and anxiety are normal responses to the stress of surgery and affect the client's ability to cope with the proposed plan of care. Because individuals differ in their perceptions of the meaning of surgery, the degree of anxiety and fear experienced varies. If fear and anxiety become excessive, however, these emotions interfere with recovery by magnifying the normal physiologic stress response. By assessing and being aware of the fears and anxieties of the surgical client, the nurse provides support and information so that stress does not become overwhelming. The most common fears related to surgery are:

- Fear of the unknown
- Fear of pain and discomfort
- Fear of mutilation and disfigurement
- Fear of anesthesia
- Fear of disruption of life patterns
  - Separation from family/significant others
  - Sexuality
  - Financial
  - Permanent/temporary limitations
- Fear of death/not waking up
- Fear of not being in control

Fear of the unknown is the most prevalent fear before surgery and is the fear the nurse can most easily allay through client education and preoperative teaching.

PREOPERATIVE PHYSIOLOGIC ASSESSMENT

Physiologic assessment includes a physical examination and a review of the client's laboratory values and diagnostic studies. Laboratory and diagnostic studies are divided into those that are routine and those that are performed specifically to evaluate the client's primary disease process or coexisting condition. The common preoperative laboratory tests include:

TABLE 2-1 Indications for Surgery

TYPE OF SURGERY	PURPOSE	EXAMPLE
Diagnostic	Determine cause of symptoms	Biopsy Exploratory laparotomy
Curative	Remove a diseased body part or replace a body part to restore function	Cholecystectomy Total knee arthroplasty
Palliative	Relieve symptoms without curing disease	Tumor resection associated with cancer
Restorative	Strengthen a weakened area	Herniorrhaphy
Cosmetic	Improve appearance Change shape	Face lift Mammoplasty

- Hemoglobin and hematocrit (Hgb and Hct)
- White blood cell (WBC) count
- Blood typing and cross matching (screening)
- Serum electrolytes
- Prothrombin time (PT), International Normalized Ratio (INR), and partial thromboplastin time (PTT)
- Bilirubin
- Liver enzymes: alanine aminotransferase (ALT) and aspartate aminotransferase (AST)
- Urinalysis
- Blood urea nitrogen (BUN) and creatinine

Although it is common practice to obtain a chest x-ray for many clients admitted to the hospital, this study is increasingly omitted for healthy children and healthy adults younger than age 40 years in whom the physical examination is normal and there is no reason to suspect pulmonary or cardiac disease. Additional radiographic or fluoroscopic examinations, sonograms, radioisotopic scans, magnetic resonance imaging, and computerized tomography scans provide useful information about the nature of the disease process and its anatomic location and extent. Any organ that is undergoing major surgery is adequately evaluated with these techniques before the operation.

Electrocardiograms (ECGs) are routinely performed in middle-age and elderly clients undergoing surgery because of the prevalence of ischemic heart disease in these age groups. It is also of value to have a baseline study for comparison in case subsequent ECGs are needed.

Preoperative testing is completed several days before the date of surgery. The type and amount of screening depends on the age and condition of the client, the nature of the surgery, and the surgeon's preference. Surgeons (doctors who perform surgery) are coming under increasing economic pressure to minimize routine testing procedures. The current trend is based on cost versus benefits, moving away from extensive testing in the absence of indicative/warranting data from the health history and physical examination.

The nurse's role in preoperative testing is to ensure that the ordered tests are performed, that the results are placed in the client's chart, and that abnormal results are reported to the physician immediately.

The physiologic nursing assessment is completed before surgery. Preoperative assessment takes place in the surgeon's office, in the hospital during hospitalization, or in the hospital or ambulatory surgery unit on the day of surgery. The nurse collects client health data by interviewing the client, the family, significant others, and health-care providers. Data collection also is accomplished through review of the client's records, assessment, and/or consultation. Assessment is essential to establishing nursing diagnoses and predicting outcomes (Association of periOperative Registered Nurses [AORN], 2002b). When performing the nursing assessment, the nurse screens the client for risks that may contribute to complications in the perioperative period. The nurse's role in the preoperative phase ensures client safety, understanding, and compliance with health care treatment. The variables affecting surgical status are age, medications, nutrition, fluid and electrolytes, and various body systems.

Age

Surgery is performed on individuals of any age, although persons at both extremes of age (infants and elders) are at greater risk for complications. Infants easily become dehydrated or fluid overloaded with resultant electrolyte imbalances. Because their metabolic rate is two to three times that of adults, infants can receive formula up to 6 hours before surgery, and breastfed infants can be nursed up to 4 hours before surgery. Infants may then have clear liquids for up to 2 hours before surgery.

Body temperature regulation and the renal, immune, and respiratory systems are different in infants than in adults. Renal function in the infant is comparatively less efficient because of a lower glomerular filtration rate and less efficient renal tubular function (Phillips, 2007). This leads to retention of anesthesia and medications and to fluid overload. Because of a comparatively larger ratio of body surface area to body mass, infants are also more prone to hypothermia when placed in a cool environment or when large areas of their body surface is exposed. Furthermore, an immature immune system renders the infant more susceptible to infections. Because of a smaller and less developed anatomic structure and enlarged tongue and lymphoid tissue, the infant is also more prone to respiratory obstruction. The nursing process and nursing care is tailored to meet the unique needs of the infant client.

Elderly clients experience many physiologic changes associated with aging and are more likely to have degenerative disease in many organs. Elders are more likely to become dehydrated and are thus less able to adapt to fluid loss during surgery. The elderly client is also more sensitive to central nervous system depressants used during the perioperative period; however, even elderly clients favorably tolerate extensive surgery when carefully assessed and managed.

LIFE SPAN CONSIDERATIONS

Surgery in the Elderly Client

Morbidity and mortality rates for surgical clients older than age 90 years are much higher than for those age 70 to 75 years (Hogstel, 2001). Elderly clients do not tolerate emergency or long, complicated surgery as well as do younger clients because of a lesser ability to adapt to physical and psychological stress.

Nutritional Status

Nutritional assessment includes evaluation of individual deficiencies or excesses that place the client at greater risk for complications during surgery. Surgery increases the body's need for nutrients necessary for tissue healing and resistance to infection.

Nutritional deficiencies place the client at greater risk for fluid and electrolyte imbalance, delayed wound healing, and wound infections. The malnourished individual has diminished stores of carbohydrates and fats; in such instances, proteins are used for energy instead of tissue building and restoration. In addition to carbohydrates and fats, vitamins B complex and C are also significant because these vitamins are essential to healing. Poor nutritional status also adversely affects liver and kidney function, leaving the client with a poor tolerance for anesthetic agents and a tendency for bleeding.

Nutritional excesses or obesity increase the risk for respiratory, cardiovascular, and gastrointestinal complications.

Obesity makes access to the surgical site more difficult, which prolongs surgical time and increases the amount of anesthetic agents required. Because inhalation anesthetics are absorbed by and stored in adipose tissue and released postoperatively, recovery time from anesthesia is slower in the overweight client. Adipose tissue is less vascular and more difficult to suture, which predisposes the client to wound infection, delayed wound healing, and increased incidence of wound complications, including postoperative incisional hernias. Failure to exercise and ambulate increases the chances of decreased respiratory function, accompanied by atelectasis and pneumonia, and also leads to decreased wound healing and an increased risk of thrombus formation. Often, obese clients also have other chronic conditions, such as hypertension or diabetes mellitus that increase the likelihood of surgical complications. In some surgical situations, such as joint replacement, surgery is delayed until nutritional status improves and the client loses weight.

Fluid and Electrolyte Status

Dehydration and hypovolemia, with correlating electrolyte disturbances, predispose a client to complications during and after surgery. Both are caused by diarrhea, excessive nasogastric suctioning, inadequate oral intake, vomiting, and/or bleeding. The complications of fluid and electrolyte imbalance are numerous and varied. Changes in fluid and electrolyte balance affect cellular metabolism, renal function, and oxygen concentration in the circulation. Nursing care focuses on administering parenteral fluids or blood products as prescribed, keeping a detailed intake and output record, and evaluating results of laboratory studies.

Respiratory Status

Respiratory assessment includes detection of acute and chronic problems. Because acute respiratory infections may lead to bronchospasms or laryngospasms, surgery for clients with these conditions is delayed or contraindicated. Chronic respiratory problems, such as asthma and chronic obstructive pulmonary disease, impair the client's gas exchange and increase the risk associated with inhalation anesthetic agents.

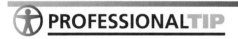

Client's Psychological Condition

The client "who fears dying while under anesthesia runs a greater risk of cardiac arrest on the operating table than [do] clients with known cardiac disease" (Phillips, 2007).

- The psychological condition of the client can have a stronger influence than does the physical condition.
- Encourage clients to express their feelings and fears about receiving anesthetic and having surgery.
- Observe the client for nonverbal clues indicating anxiety.
- To reduce client anxiety, explain what happens throughout the surgical experience.

Clients with chronic respiratory problems are more likely to develop atelectasis and pneumonia.

Respiratory assessment as performed by the nurse includes assessing breath sounds, color of the skin and mucous membranes, and for shortness of breath (dyspnea) and coughing. All clients, and especially those clients who smoke and have chronic lung disease, are taught deep breathing, use of incentive spirometry, coughing, and preoperative turning.

Cardiovascular Status

Cardiovascular assessment focuses on such diseases as angina, recent myocardial infarction or cardiac surgery, hemophilia, hypertension, and congestive heart failure. Clients with a history of cardiac disease are prone to developing complications such as dysrhythmias, hypotension, myocardial infarction, congestive heart failure, cardiac arrest, stroke, shock, deep vein thrombosis, thrombophlebitis, or pulmonary embolism.

Also assess for anxiety; elevated blood pressure; slow, rapid, or irregular pulse; chest pain; edema; coolness or cyanosis/discoloration of extremities; weakness; and shortness of breath (dyspnea). All clients are taught postoperative leg exercises to prevent thrombophlebitis. The goal of nursing care is to improve the client's cardiovascular condition to the highest degree possible by promoting rest alternated with activity; encouraging a low-sodium and low-cholesterol diet; administering heart medications; and judiciously administering parenteral fluids and recording intake and output.

Renal and Hepatic Status

Because many medications and anesthetic agents are detoxified by the liver and excreted by the kidneys, renal and hepatic sufficiency constitute a major concern. Renal disease affects fluid and electrolyte balance and protein equilibrium. Liver disease causes bleeding tendencies and carbohydrate, fat, and amino acid imbalances that impair wound healing and increase the risk of infection. Assess for symptoms of urinary frequency, dysuria, and anuria and record the color and amount of the urine. Also assess for a history of bleeding tendencies, easy bruising, nosebleeds, and use of anticoagulants. The most commonly ordered preoperative tests to assess renal function are urinalysis, blood urea nitrogen (BUN), and creatinine. The most common liver tests are prothrombin time (PT), partial thromboplastin time (PTT), bilirubin, and the liver enzymes alanine aminotransferase (ALT) and aspartate aminotransferase (AST). Nursing care focuses on administering fluids and adequate nutrition, monitoring fluid intake and output, and evaluating results of laboratory tests.

Neurological, Musculoskeletal, and Integumentary Status

Assess the client's overall mental status, including level of consciousness; orientation to person, place, and time; and the ability to understand and follow instructions. Note skin condition, including turgor and any rashes, bruises, lesions, or previous incisions. Assess client mobility and sensation through observation of both range of motion and ability to ambulate and through client statements. Note any abnormalities, injuries, or previous surgery and assess the risk for falls. The presence of internal or external prostheses or implants such as pacemakers, heart valves, or joint prosthesis is also

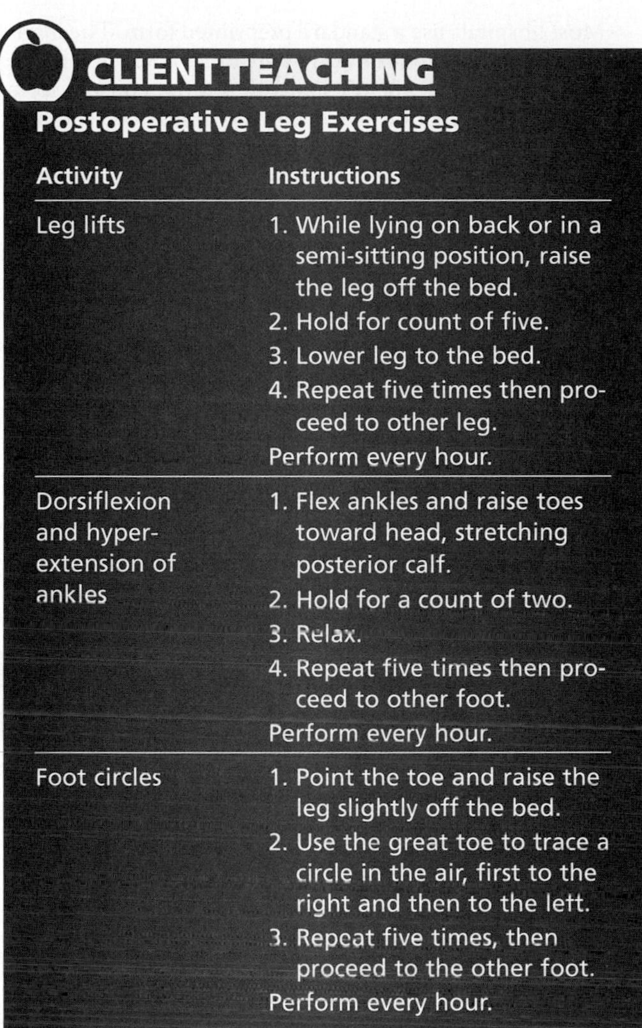

CLIENTTEACHING

Postoperative Leg Exercises

Activity	Instructions
Leg lifts	1. While lying on back or in a semi-sitting position, raise the leg off the bed. 2. Hold for count of five. 3. Lower leg to the bed. 4. Repeat five times then proceed to other leg. Perform every hour.
Dorsiflexion and hyper-extension of ankles	1. Flex ankles and raise toes toward head, stretching posterior calf. 2. Hold for a count of two. 3. Relax. 4. Repeat five times then proceed to other foot. Perform every hour.
Foot circles	1. Point the toe and raise the leg slightly off the bed. 2. Use the great toe to trace a circle in the air, first to the right and then to the left. 3. Repeat five times, then proceed to the other foot. Perform every hour.

noted, because the presence of these may necessitate preoperative antibiotics.

Thin clients, clients undergoing long surgical procedures or vascular procedures, and elderly clients are the most vulnerable to neurological, musculoskeletal, or integumentary injuries. Some underlying disease processes, such as edema, infection, cancer, osteoporosis, arthritic joints, or neck or back problems, also place a client at greater risk for injury. Clients who are malnourished, anemic, obese, hypovolemic, paralyzed, or diabetic are also prone to skin breakdown. Information gathered about the neurological, musculoskeletal, and integumentary systems is used to prepare the surgical site, for surgical positioning, and as a comparative basis for postoperative assessments and complication screening.

Endocrine and Immunological Status

Clients with diabetes are scheduled as early in the morning as possible, and a fasting glucose drawn immediately before surgery. Surgery is a stressor, and stress raises the serum glucose level in the client with diabetes. Thus the morning dose of insulin usually is adjusted.

When anesthetized during surgery, the diabetic client exhibits very few symptoms of glucose imbalance. Serum glucose must therefore be checked frequently during surgery, usually by the anesthesia provider. Stability is attained by the administration of insulin, glucose, or both. Besides hyperglycemia and hypoglycemia, a diabetic client is more prone to fluid and electrolyte imbalances, infection including respiratory and urinary tract infections, neurogenic bladder, impaired wound healing, ketoacidosis, deep vein thrombosis, thrombophlebitis, and pulmonary embolism.

Because the immunological system protects the client from infections, the immunocompromised surgical client is very prone to infection. Clients receiving steroids or chemotherapy, or who have systemic lupus erythematosus, Addison's disease, or acquired immunodeficiency syndrome (AIDS) are considered immunocompromised. The immune response in these clients is weakened or deficient, resulting in an increased incidence of infection. Because surgery breaks the integrity of the skin and the normal inflammatory response is suppressed, wound healing may be impaired. Strict adherence to aseptic technique (covered later in this chapter) is thus even more imperative. Prevention of infection is crucial in these clients. The role of the nurse is to communicate the presence of potential immunosuppression to other health care team members involved in the client's care and to prevent infection by practicing aseptic technique.

Medications

Knowledge of the client's use of drugs for recreational or therapeutic purposes is essential to preoperative assessment. The history of medication usage by the client should include type and frequency of use for over-the-counter, prescription, and street drugs. The use of certain drugs affects the client's reaction to anesthetic agents and surgery. Some drugs increase surgical risks; these medications usually are temporarily discontinued before surgery. Other medications, such as heart or hypoglycemic medications, may still be given even though the client is to undergo surgery; the surgeon or anesthesia provider writes specific orders in such instances. Dosages of medications may also be adjusted during the perioperative period.

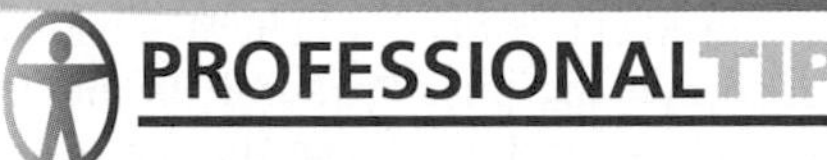

Questions to Assess Psychosocial Status

- Why are you having surgery?
- When did this problem start?
- What do you think caused this problem?
- Has this caused any problems in your relationships with others?
- Has your problem prevented you from working?
- Are you able to take care of your own needs?
- Are you experiencing any discomfort or pain?
- What are you expecting from this surgery?
- Is there anything that you do not understand regarding your surgery?
- Are you worried about anything?
- Will someone be available to assist you when you return home?

Chronic alcohol use increases surgical risk because it is often accompanied by impaired nutrition and liver disease. Postoperatively, the client may exhibit delirium tremens or acute withdrawal syndrome. Furthermore, pain medication may be less effective.

Psychosocial Health Assessment

The psychosocial health status of the client is also assessed. The nurse elicits the client's perceptions of surgery and the expected outcome. The nurse also ascertains the client's coping mechanisms and the client's knowledge level and ability to understand. The data collected are incorporated into nursing care throughout the perioperative experience.

Cultural beliefs can influence a client's perception of surgery. For example, some cultures believe that surgery is a "final effort" performed only when all other possible treatments have been of no avail. Furthermore, surgeries that cause changes in the appearance of the body can alter body image and self-esteem; the client may worry about being sexually attractive or active after surgery.

The nurse provides an opportunity for the client to express his spiritual values and beliefs. Many clients wish to see a member of the clergy before having surgery.

Surgical Consent

An **informed consent** is a legal form signed by the client and witnessed by another person that grants permission to the client's physician to perform the procedure described by the physician. An informed consent is needed whenever these situations occur:

- Anesthesia is used.
- The procedure is considered invasive.
- The procedure is nonsurgical but has more than a slight risk of complications (such as with an arteriogram).
- Radiation or cobalt therapy is used.

Informed consent protects both the client (against unauthorized procedures) and the physician and the health care facility and its employees (against claims that an unauthorized procedure was performed). Although the ultimate responsibility for obtaining the informed consent lies with the physician, the nurse often obtains and witnesses the client's signature and ensures that the client signs the consent form voluntarily and is alert and comprehending of the action.

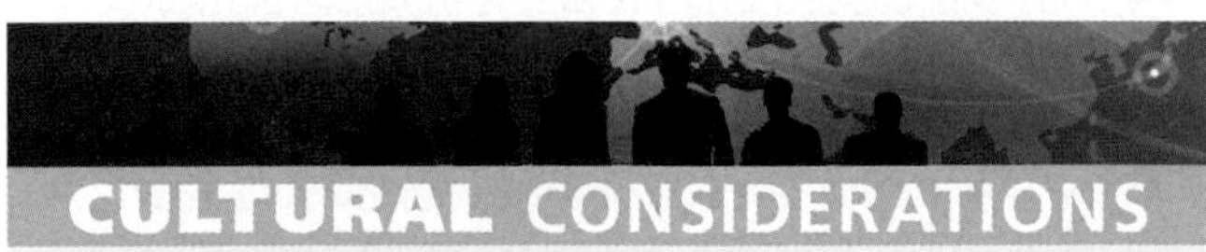

CULTURAL CONSIDERATIONS

Impending Surgery

- Some clients desire special religious rites before surgery.
- Some clients may not want to receive blood transfusions or other treatments.
- All client beliefs are respected.

Most hospitals use a standard preprinted form. The information written by the health care personnel is specific to the individual client. The client's signature on the consent form indicates the information has been read and is correct. The client has the right to refuse treatment even after signing the consent. When this occurs, the nurse informs the physician immediately of the client's decision.

Preoperative Teaching

The client about to have surgery is at risk for knowledge deficit related to preoperative procedures and protocols and postoperative expectations. The potential benefits of preoperative teaching include reduced anxiety and more rapid recovery with fewer complications and shorter hospitalization. Reduction in anxiety has a secondary benefit: The client usually requires less medication for pain. The purposes of preoperative teaching are to (1) answer questions and concerns about surgery, (2) ascertain the client's knowledge of the intended surgery, (3) ascertain the need or desire for additional information, and (4) provide information in a manner most conducive to learning.

One-on-one sessions constitute the most personal method of instruction, but try to include the family or significant other when possible. The level of learning increases when more than one teaching medium is used. For example, using materials such as videotapes, charts, tours, anatomic models, pictures, and brochures reinforces both visual and auditory learning. Demonstration followed by return demonstration is helpful. Written instructions serve as a reference for later use. Make instructions simple, using terms the client can understand. Any unfamiliar words or concepts are thoroughly explained.

Clients are often interested in any information that describes the sights, sounds, tastes, feelings, odors, and temperature of what they are about to experience. For example, the feeling of relaxation from preoperative medications; the sounds of instruments or equipment in the operating room (OR); the pressure from the automatic blood pressure cuff; the warmth or coolness of skin-preparation solutions; or the brightness of the OR lights are all sensations the client may experience. Analogies or stories of real or fictitious situations of sensory experiences help the client understand. The teaching methods used strongly influence the client's learning and retention of information.

Preoperative teaching begins as soon as surgery is agreed upon. Instructions given over the phone and/or mailed to the client during the time leading up to surgery are beneficial. Just before surgery, a brief review with additional information tailored to the needs of the client are given. Give the client an opportunity to ask questions.

Information always is targeted to the client's needs and according to the client's level of knowledge and anxiety. Mild-to-moderate anxiety actually heightens a person's alertness and motivates learning. Mildly anxious clients receive the most complete instructions. Moderately anxious clients receive less information but more attention to specific areas of concern. Severely anxious clients receive only basic information but are encouraged to verbalize their concerns. Clients in a state of panic are unable to learn; in such cases, no instruction is given, and the surgeon is notified.

Physical Preparation

Extremely close attention is given to identifying the proper client both verbally and by reading the identification name

CLIENT TEACHING

Preoperative Teaching

- Introduce self
  - Identify role in client's care
- Determine client's knowledge level and need or desire for addition information
- Explain the routine for the day of surgery
  - Restricted food or fluid intake
  - Intravenous fluids
  - Premedication
  - Time of surgery
  - Anticipated length of surgery
  - Transportation to the OR
  - Special skin preparations
  - Type of surgical incision (Figure 2-1)
- Familiarize client with the OR environment
  - Operating room lights and table
  - Accessory equipment
  - Monitoring equipment
  - Anesthesia induction
- Include significant others
  - Time to arrive at the hospital
  - Location of the surgical waiting area
  - What to expect when the client returns to the unit
- Explain postanesthesia care unit (PACU)
  - Location of recovery room
  - Purpose of recovery room
  - Routine of postanesthesia care
- Identify anticipated dressings, drains, catheters, casts, etc.
- Demonstrate and evaluate client's proficiency with:
  - Coughing and deep breathing exercises
  - Turning
  - Incentive spirometry
  - Extremity exercises
  - Any special transfer procedures or aids required after surgery
- Describe pain management strategies appropriate for the specific surgical procedure

band and to verifying the operative procedure. This is completed through client statements, surgeon verification, and the signed surgical consent form. *Particular attention is given to differentiating between right and left operative sites.*

Special care is given to the preparation of the operative site to lessen the chance of infection. The operative site is thoroughly cleansed with an antiseptic soap such as povidone-iodine to reduce the number of microorganisms on the skin.

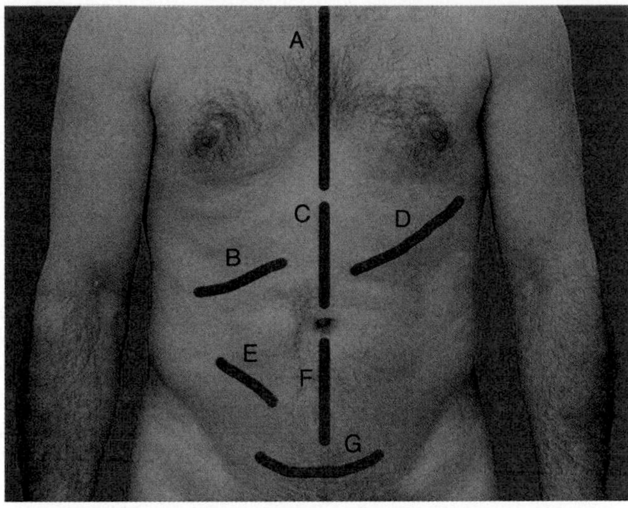

FIGURE 2-1 **Common Surgical Incisions; *A*, Sternal Split; *B*, Oblique Subcostal; *C*, Upper Vertical Midline; *D*, Thoracoabdominal; *E*, McBurney; *F*, Lower Vertical Midline; *G*, Pfannenstiel**

Typically, the operative site is not shaved, but if shaving is to be performed, it is done in the OR immediately before surgery. To reduce the number of bacteria in the gastrointestinal tract for gastrointestinal, peritoneal, perianal, or pelvic surgery, an enema is ordered. Enemas prevent contamination of the peritoneal area by fecal content passed during surgery. The reduction in colon size related to the loss of bulk also helps prevent colon injury and increases visualization of the operative site. Enemas are usually given the night before surgery. If the enema is done at home, give the client detailed instructions. Many types of surgery require special preparations. The specific protocol for each surgical procedure is available from the health care facility or the physician.

Check the client's vital signs, including blood pressure, temperature, pulse, and respirations. Some changes in vital signs are normal as a result of anxiety. If marked differences exist from the baseline data, however, the surgeon is notified.

Assist the client in putting on a hospital gown, hair cap and, if ordered, antiembolic hose sized according to client size. Institutional policy usually requires the removal of all jewelry, including body jewelry. Hairpins, wigs, and prostheses also are removed. The nurse is responsible for recording the disposition of any personal items removed for surgery. If policy requires, nail polish (from at least one nail, if dark polish) is removed to read oxygen saturation via pulse oximetry. Makeup is also removed so that skin color is observed.

SAFETY

Iodine Allergy, Latex Allergy

- Each client is asked about allergy to iodine and latex.
- If a client is allergic to either, document the allergy on the client's record and inform the surgeon and OR personnel so that an iodine-free solution and latex-free equipment is used.

Allergies to medication, food, and chemicals (including contrast agents) are verified, as are previous blood reactions. The nurse differentiates between a medication intolerance and a true allergic reaction. With an intolerance to certain medications, the client may experience side effects that are unpleasant. For example, many clients experience nausea when given morphine; although unpleasant, this is not a drug allergy. A true allergy produces a skin reaction or anaphylactic reaction, where the client experiences cardiorespiratory reactions that may be life threatening, such as hypotension and pulmonary edema. A client with multiple food allergies is also prone to hypersensitivities to medications. When allergies are identified, the client's chart is marked accordingly, and an allergy wrist band is put on the client. By being aware of and alerting other team members to the client's allergies, client safety and comfort are maintained.

Verify the NPO (nothing by mouth) status of the client for the time specified by the surgeon's order. Restricting oral intake reduces the possibility of aspiration. If surgery takes place in the afternoon, the client has a clear liquid breakfast if ordered by the surgeon. Careful client instruction is required because surgery may need to be postponed if the client eats or drinks.

In addition to the previously outlined preparations, remove dentures and bridgework to prevent loss, damage, and possible dislodgement and airway obstruction during the surgery. Ensure that the client has an empty bladder by allowing time for the client to void before transfer to surgery.

Identify any sensory deficits of the client and communicate this information to other health-care team members. Glasses, contact lenses, and hearing aids are usually removed to prevent loss or damage; if policy allows, however, it is best to leave these items in place so the client is better able to see and hear. Then the nurse is responsible for communicating the presence of these aids to the surgical team members.

The surgeon or anesthesiologist (a doctor trained in providing anesthesia) may order preoperative medication. The nurse gives the medication by the prescribed route (intramuscular, intravenous, or oral) at the specified time (typically 1 hour before surgery). Preoperative medications may be ordered "on call," which means that the nurse is notified by a member of the surgical team when the preoperative medication is to be given. Before administering the medication, ask the client to void. After administering the preoperative medication, raise the side rails of the gurney or bed, put the bed in the lowest position, and instruct the client not to get up without assistance.

PROFESSIONALTIP

Implementing NPO Status

- Explain reasons for NPO status to the client.
- Remove any food and water from the client's overbed table and nightstand.
- Mark the client's door and bed with an NPO sign.
- Mark the client's Kardex, electronic medical records, and other nursing information sources.
- Notify the dietary department.

LIFE SPAN CONSIDERATIONS

Preparation for Surgery

For pediatric clients:

- Provide physical and psychological preparation at the child's level of understanding.
- Listen carefully to the child to promote understanding.
- Ask the child to point to the operative site on self or doll.
- Be honest and truthful.

The elder client may have:

- Increased risk of complications including infection.
- Increased incidence of coexisting conditions.
- Unpredictable response to medications and anesthetics.
- Greater need for support from family and significant other.
- Increased skin and bone fragility.
- Nutritional and financial deficiencies.
- Impaired vision and hearing.
- Impaired or slowed thought processes and cognitive abilities.
- Fear of death, loss of independence, and change in lifestyle.

When the surgical team is ready, the client is transported on a gurney by a member of the OR team, typically an orderly. The client is always transported feet first and with the side rails up to ensure safety and minimize the likelihood of dizziness and nausea. The client may be taken to a preoperative holding area first (Figure 2-2). The nurse instructs the family or significant others where to wait.

The information collected as part of preoperative preparation is documented in the client record, usually on a preoperative checklist. Figure 2-3 (p. 23) illustrates a typical preoperative checklist. This checklist is completed before the

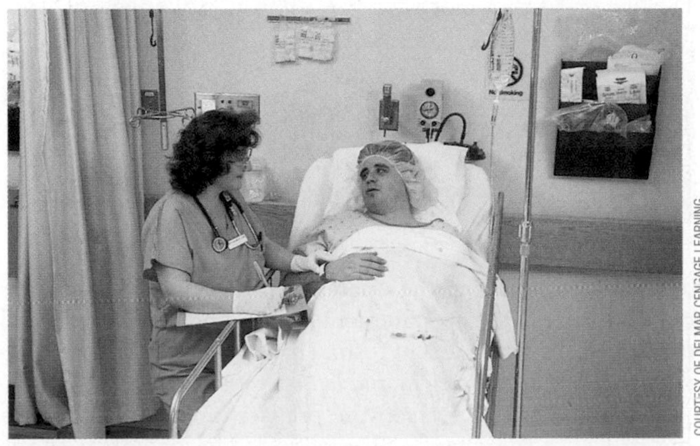

FIGURE 2-2 The holding area is used for clients who are waiting to have surgery.

	CK (✓)	COMMENTS	NURSE CK (✓)
COMPLETE NIGHT BEFORE SURGERY			
List allergies			
Procedure scheduled			
Surgical permit signed/witnessed			
History/physical on chart and/or dictated			
Preanesthetic evaluation done			
Able to state type and purpose			
Demonstrates ability to perform: Deep breathing, turning and coughing exercises			
Leg exercises			
P.M. care with shower or bath given			
Nail polish removed and makeup removed			
Old chart requested and obtained			
Type and crossmatch for ______ units of blood			
Blood consent signed and witnessed			
Labor work a. CBC ______ b. UA ______			
Tonsillectomy and adenoidectomy patients: a. ___PTT b. ___PT c. ___Platelets			
If ordered by MD: a. ECG ___ b. Chest X-ray ___			
Add other lab work ordered (specify)			
Notify surgeon of abnormal lab work			
New progress note and physician order sheet on chart			
Weight			
NPO after midnight (if applicable)			
Signature of Nurse ________________________		Date ____________	
COMPLETE DAY OF SURGERY			
Jewelry removed and secured with responsible party			
Dental prosthesis and contact lenses removed			
Voided on call to surgery			
Indwelling catheter ordered and inserted			
Tampon removed			
Identiband and/or bloodband on/checked for accuracy			
Time _______ Pulse _______ Resp _______ B/P _______ Temp. _______			
Pre-op medicine given medication ____________________ Time _______ AM PM			
Siderails up and bed to lowest level			
Patient instructed not to get out of bed without nursing assistance			
Addressograph plate/MARs on chart			
VS 30 minutes after pre-op (if remains on unit)			
BP _______ P _______ R _______ T _______			
Old chart sent to surgery per request			
Surgical prep done and checked			
To surgery Time _______ Via _______			
Signature of Nurse ________________________		Date ____________	
Holding Room Nurse Signature ________________________		Date ____________	

FIGURE 2-3 Sample Preoperative Checklist

client leaves the clinical unit or upon the client's admission to ambulatory surgery. The nurse also verbally communicates to other health-care members any necessary information collected.

INTRAOPERATIVE PHASE

The **intraoperative phase** is the time during the surgical experience that begins when the client is transferred to the OR table and ends when the client is admitted to the postanesthesia care unit (PACU).

Physical Description of the Operating Room Environment

For the purposes of preventing wound infections, the surgical suite is environmentally controlled. Personnel restriction and geographic isolation from other areas of the hospital or clinic are part of this control. Constant filtered airflow and positive air pressure in the OR also aid in environmental control. Clean areas and contaminated areas are separated within the suite. Equipment and supplies needed for each client are in the surgical suite so members of the surgical team do not have to leave the area.

ORs vary in size depending on the amount of equipment needed for each particular type of operation. Supplies and furniture are limited to prevent dust collection and are usually made of stainless steel to withstand corrosive disinfectants. Furniture and equipment are easily movable on wheels. In addition to general illumination from ceiling lights, the operative site is illuminated by overhead operating lights. Figure 2-4 shows a typical OR. The temperature of the room can be adjusted but usually is maintained at a cool 66°F to 68°F. This provides comfort for the surgical team (the members of which wear gowns, gloves, and masks under hot lights). This temperature also is an unfavorable environment for bacterial incubation and growth.

The client entering the OR is confronted with an environment that is most likely unfamiliar. The OR is cold. The surgical team members dress in surgical scrubs and have their hair covered by caps and their faces covered by surgical masks, making them appear impersonal and distant. The sounds of equipment being prepared can be unfamiliar and alarming. The terminology used in conversations among OR personnel may be foreign. These elements combined with the sight of ominous overhead lights and the feel of the hard OR table may increase the client's fear, anxiety, and feelings of powerlessness.

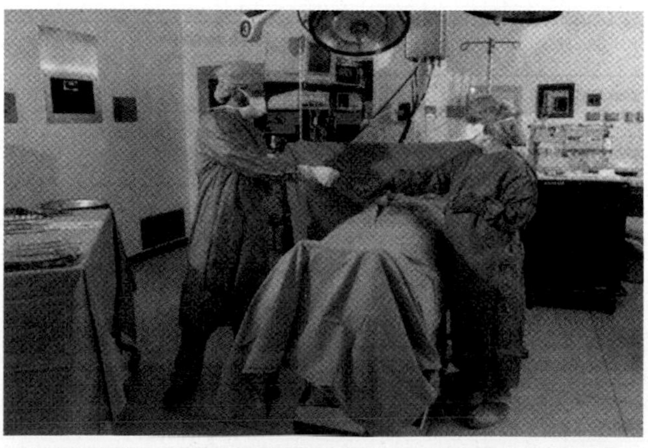

FIGURE 2-4 Typical Operating Room and Proper Surgical Attire (*Photo courtesy of the U.S. Army.*)

Members of the Surgical Team

The surgical team is a group of hospital personnel assigned to see a client successfully through an operative procedure. At no other time during hospitalization will the ratio of personnel to client be greater than when the client is undergoing surgery. The surgical team includes **sterile dressed** (without microorganisms) team members: the surgeon, the **first assistant** (a physician or RN who assists the surgeon in performing hemostasis, tissue retraction, and wound closure), and the **scrub nurse** (an LP/VN, RN, or surgical technologist who, under the direction of the circulating nurse, prepares and maintains the integrity, safety, and efficiency of the **sterile field** throughout the operation). These team members scrub their arms and hands, don sterile gowns and gloves, and then perform their duties in the sterile field. The sterile field is that area surrounding the client and the surgical site that is free from all microorganisms. It is created by using sterile drapes to drape the work area and the client. Other team members, dressed in nonsterile attire, include the anesthesia provider (an anesthesiologist or anesthetist) and **circulating nurse** (an RN responsible for management of personnel, equipment, supplies, environment, and communication throughout a surgical procedure). These team members perform their duties outside of the sterile field. Each team member has a clearly defined role and duties. Clear communication among team members and coordination of their activities improve the most favorable outcome for the client.

Asepsis

Prevention of infection is the responsibility of the entire surgical team. The environment of the surgical client contains both pathogenic (disease-producing) and nonpathogenic microorganisms. When the skin, a prime barrier to infection, is broken, as during surgery, susceptibility to a bacterial invasion increases. Bacteria carried by dust or nose and throat droplets are easily transported by air currents.

Asepsis is the absence of pathogenic microorganisms. **Aseptic technique** is a collection of principles used to control and/or prevent the transfer of pathogenic microorganisms from sources within (endogenous) and outside (exogenous) the client. For example, scrubbed persons wear sterile gowns and gloves; sterile drapes are used to create a sterile field; items used in a sterile field are sterilized; and those working within a sterile field maintain the integrity of the sterile field. Aseptic technique is applicable to other nursing functions such as changing dressings, inserting a Foley catheter, or preparing for an obstetrical delivery. Thus, the practice of aseptic technique is not confined to the OR, but applies to other clinical nursing units and other procedures as well.

The practice of aseptic technique requires the development of **sterile conscience**, an individual's personal sense of honesty and integrity with regard to adherence to the principles of aseptic technique. Aseptic technique must be strictly followed. Doing so requires constant assessment and monitoring of self and others. It is sometimes easier or less expensive to overlook an infraction of aseptic technique

CRITICAL THINKING

Sterile Conscience

How can you use a sterile conscience when providing nursing care?

rather than to correct that infraction. This must never be allowed. Compromising the principles of aseptic technique may increase the likelihood of infection and, thus, harm to the client.

Surgical Hand Scrub

An item is considered sterile when all microorganisms are removed. The skin, however, cannot be sterilized. For this reason, the sterile team members wear gloves as barriers between the sterile field and the skin. Because accidental tearing or puncturing of the surgical glove and resultant introduction of microorganisms into the surgical wound are possible, the sterile team members must take measures to lower the number of microorganisms on their hands and arms. The surgical hand scrub, performed before gowning and gloving, removes soil and transient (not always present and easily removed) microorganisms from the hands and forearms. The antimicrobial soap used lowers the count of resident (almost always present and not easily removed) microorganisms and continues to prevent sudden bacterial rebound or regrowth after the scrub is completed. The surgical scrub thus reduces the possibility of transmission of microorganisms from the surgical team to the client.

Watches, rings, and bracelets are removed before the surgical hand scrub. Fingernails must be short, clean, and healthy. Artificial nails cannot be worn (AORN, 2002a), although unchipped fingernail polish that has been applied within the last 4 days may be allowed (AORN, 2002b). The hands and forearms should be free of breaks in skin integrity.

Surgical Skin Preparation

Like the skin of the surgical team members, the skin surface at the client's incision site also cannot be sterilized. As with the surgical hand scrub, the goal of surgical skin preparation at the client's incision site is to lower the number of microorganisms on and near the incision site.

Typically, the client is asked to shower or to wash the operative site either before arriving at the surgical facility or immediately before surgery. The client is then transferred to the OR. After general anesthesia induction or regional block completion or before local infiltration of the operative site, the circulating nurse performs the surgical skin preparation. Using aseptic technique, the circulating nurse scrubs the area with an antimicrobial soap. Typically the soap used is povidone-iodine (containing iodine) or chlorhexidine, thus potential allergies to iodine must be verified. The circulating nurse scrubs a generous area surrounding the operative site to allow for extension of the surgical incision if the need arises. The scrub is completed in an ever-widening circular motion from the incision site, which is considered clean, to the periphery, which is considered dirty (Figure 2-5). Once the periphery is reached, the sponge is discarded, never brought back toward the center of the area. The concept of cleansing from the center (incision site) to the periphery also applies to skin preparation

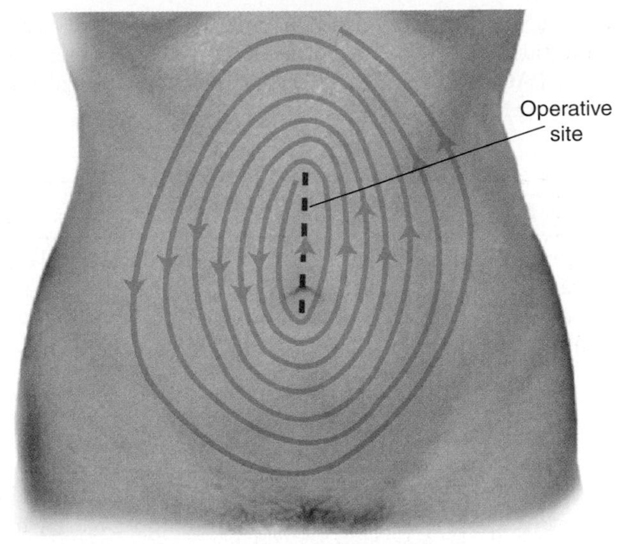

Figure 2-5 Skin Preparation at Operative Site

for other procedures such as intravenous (IV) insertion, chest tube insertion, thoracentesis, or subclavian catheter placement. Surgical skin preparation lasts 5 to 10 minutes. After the scrub is completed, the area is blotted dry with sterile towels. An antiseptic solution, often also iodine based, is then applied in the same manner.

Intraoperative Nursing Care

The success of nursing care in the OR is measured by client outcomes. The AORN has established client outcome standards for evaluating perioperative clients upon completion of surgery. These outcomes state that the client is to be free from infection and injury related to positioning, foreign objects, or chemical, physical, and electrical hazards. In addition, skin integrity and fluid and electrolyte balance are to be maintained. Consequently, nursing care in the OR strives to provide these standards to all clients undergoing surgery.

Although the responsibilities of the circulating nurse and scrub nurse may seem to be a series of tasks or duties, these same tasks and duties provide quality nursing care to the client. The nurse planning for surgery is involved in selection of equipment and supplies, room preparation, and formation of the sterile field before the delivery of actual nursing care.

After completion of surgery, the circulating nurse applies and secures the dressing. When the anesthesia provider is ready, the client is transferred to a stretcher or a gurney. The unconscious or semiconscious client is placed in a side-lying or semiprone position unless contraindicated by the surgical

SAFETY

Electrical Equipment

- Electrical equipment is plugged into grounded outlets.
- Electrical equipment is regularly checked by a bioelectronic technician.
- A grounding pad is placed under the client and in direct contact with the client's skin.

procedure. If the client is supine, the client's head is turned to the side in case the client vomits. The client is then taken to the PACU, accompanied by the anesthesia provider and another surgical team member.

POSTOPERATIVE PHASE

The **postoperative phase** is the time during the surgical experience that begins with the end of the surgical procedure and lasts until the client is discharged not just from the hospital or institution, but from medical care by the surgeon. Upon transfer from the OR, the client usually goes to the PACU (Figure 2-6). All clients who receive general anesthesia, spinal anesthesia, or regional anesthesia are admitted to the PACU. Occasionally, clients who have undergone surgery with local anesthesia or no anesthesia or who have received only IV sedation are placed in the PACU for a short period to be monitored closely until their conditions stabilize. The PACU is usually located next to the OR. Typically, it is one large room with individual units for clients along the perimeter of the room. Each of these units has an oxygen delivery system, suction, various other supplies, and cardiac, respiratory, and blood pressure monitoring devices. Curtains are pulled to provide privacy if needed, but an open view allows continual assessment of all clients.

Postoperative Nursing Care

The postanesthesia care nurse is an RN specially trained in caring for immediate postoperative clients. The goal of postanesthesia nursing care is to promote recovery from anesthesia and the immediate effects of surgery. The postanesthesia nurse has knowledge and skill in recognizing and treating anesthetic and surgical complications very quickly. The postanesthesia nurse is empathetic and is able to assess and manage pain for the client who is not able to express himself.

Upon the client's arrival in the PACU, the anesthesia provider verbally reviews the client's anesthesia and operative procedure with the postanesthesia nurse. The postanesthesia nurse begins the following nursing assessment and care in the immediate postoperative period:

- Time of arrival in recovery room
- Patency of airway
- Respirations
- Presence of artificial airway devices
  - Oral airway
  - Nasopharyngeal airway
  - Endotracheal airway
- Oxygen saturation
- Need for supplemental oxygen
  - Mode of administration
  - Flow rate
- Breath sounds
- Color of skin, nail beds, and lips
- Presence of cardiac dysrhythmias
- Other vital signs
  - Blood pressure, pulse
- Skin condition (moist or dry, warm or cool) and skin temperature
- Initiate Aldrete Score
- Intravenous infusion
  - Type of solution
  - Amount in bottle or bag
  - Flow rate
  - Appearance and location of IV site
- Dressings
  - Amount and character of drainage
- Drains and tubes
  - Intactness and function
  - Connection to drainage and/or suction
  - Amount and character of drainage
- Level of consciousness
- Activity level
- Other assessments according to surgical procedure
- Pain

The postanesthesia nurse notes the client's arrival time to the unit and immediately begins to assess the patency of the airway by placing a hand above the client's nose and mouth to feel exhalation. The quality and quantity of respirations are then immediately observed, as is the presence of an artificial airway. The client is attached to a pulse oximeter (Figure 2-7), and breath sounds are auscultated. The color and condition of the skin are noted as part of the respiratory assessment. The lips are checked for circumoral pallor.

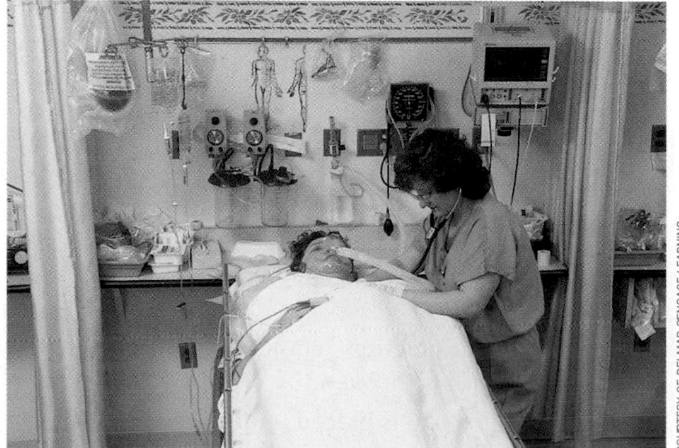
COURTESY OF DELMAR CENGAGE LEARNING

FIGURE 2-6 Postanesthesia Care Unit (PACU)

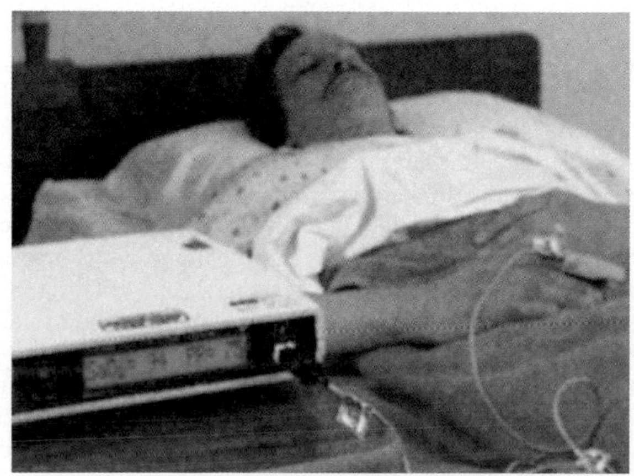
COURTESY OF DELMAR CENGAGE LEARNING

FIGURE 2-7 Client with Pulse Oximeter on Finger

Peripheral cyanosis may be an indication of hypothermia rather than respiratory distress. Thus, correlating with the "ABCs" of airway, breathing, and circulation, the respiratory system is assessed first.

Because most clients admitted are unconscious and have received muscle relaxants during surgery, respiratory exchange is often affected. Snoring, stridor, labored chest movement, sternal retractions, cyanosis, and apnea are all signs of respiratory distress. Respiratory distress is the gravest of all complications because respiratory crisis and subsequent death occurs in a matter of minutes if distress is not observed and treated quickly. In the event of any signs of respiratory distress, the postanesthesia nurse must be alert to the possibility of respiratory arrest and be ready to initiate cardiopulmonary resuscitation.

The **Aldrete Score**, also known as the Postanesthetic Recovery Score, is used in PACUs to objectively assess the physical status of clients recovering from anesthesia and serves as a basis for discharge from the PACU (Table 2-2). The Aldrete Score was adapted to also assess the readiness of clients for discharge from ambulatory surgery. The first five items are used for discharge from the PACU. Clients are assessed at the time of admission to the PACU and every 15 minutes until discharge. The first five items include assessing activity, respiration, consciousness, circulation, and color (oxygen saturation). Each of the five items is scored from 0 to 2, according to the degree of functional disturbance. The score is expressed as a total score, with 10 being the maximum. Typically, a minimum score of 8 is required for discharge from the PACU.

Fluid intake and output are assessed. The amounts and types of IV solutions hanging are identified, as are any added medications. The IV fluids are infused according to the surgeon's order and are run at a specified rate. The IV site is assessed for patency, redness, and swelling. The client is restrained as necessary to maintain patency of the IV site. All other infusions and irrigations are also assessed.

Dressings and/or peripads are checked for any evidence of bloody drainage and the amount noted so that any subsequent appearance of blood may be accurately evaluated. All drainage tubes are then connected, and the type of drain and the drainage amount are recorded according to physicians' orders. Table 2-3 outlines common types of drains placed in surgery. Urinary output is also monitored. Scanty urinary drainage (<50 mL/hour or as ordered) is reported to the surgeon.

Surgical drains are placed so the wound can drain freely of blood clots, body fluids, pus, and necrotic material that otherwise would collect in the wound and provide a rich medium for bacterial growth. Figure 2-8 illustrates common drainage devices. All drains are inserted at the operative site and exit through the incision or a separate stab wound adjacent to the incision. The type of drain is chosen according to the location of wound, size of wound, and type of drainage anticipated. The use of drains decreases pain and infection and aids wound healing; however, if the wound is draining, the skin is not closed, and a pathway exists for the entrance of microorganisms. Drain sites can thus also be a source of infection. Potential complications of drains include hemorrhage, sepsis, drain loss, and bowel herniation. Nursing care for drains includes assessing the color, character, and odor of drainage; ensuring the patency of the drain (making sure there are no kinks in the tubing); and ensuring that the drain does not accidentally become dislodged. Table 2-4 lists additional nursing care according to surgical procedure.

Part of the neurological assessment involves assessing the activity level or the ability to move extremities voluntarily. The ability to move extremities on command indicates voluntary movement. Hearing is the first sensation to return to the client after having been anesthetized. Clients in the

TABLE 2-2 Aldrete Score/Postanesthetic Recovery Score

Activity	Able to move 4 extremities voluntarily or on command	2
	Able to move 2 extremities voluntarily or on command	1
	Able to move 0 extremities voluntarily or on command	0
Respiration	Able to breathe deeply and cough freely	2
	Dyspnea or limited breathing	1
	Apneic	0
Consciousness	Fully awake	2
	Arousable on calling	1
	Not responding	0
Circulation	B/P ± 20% of preanesthetic level	2
	B/P ± 20% to 50% of preanesthetic level	1
	B/P ± 50% of preanesthetic level	0
Color	Normal	2
	Pale, dusky, blotchy, jaundiced, other	1
	Cyanotic	0
Additional Assessments: Aldrete Score/Postanesthetic Recovery Score for Clients Having Anesthesia on an Ambulatory Basis		
Dressing	Dry and clean	2
	Wet but stationary or marked	1
	Growing area of wetness	0
Pain	Pain free	2
	Mild pain handled by oral medication	1
	Severe pain requiring parenteral medication	0
Ambulation	Able to stand up and walk straight	2
	Vertigo when erect	1
	Dizziness when supine	0
Fasting/Feeding	Able to drink fluids	2
	Nauseated	1
	Nausea and vomiting	0
Urine Output	Has voided	2
	Unable to void but comfortable	1
	Unable to void and uncomfortable	0

Courtesy of J. Antonio Aldrete, M.D., M.S., Defuniak Springs, FL.

Table 2-3 Description, Uses, and Nursing Care of Common Drainage Devices Placed During Surgery

TYPE	EXAMPLE	DESCRIPTION	USES	NURSING CARE
Passive	Penrose	A single-lumen, soft latex tube that works with gravity directly from the surgical incision	To remove drainage when more than a minimal amount of drainage is expected	• Inspect dressing • Check underneath client to ensure drainage has not leaked from the side of the dressing • Always keep a dressing over drain • Check safety pin through end of drain
Active	Hemovac Jackson-Pratt J-Vac Relia Vac Surgivac	Closed wound drainage system with drain and reservoir having self-suction when reservoir is compressed	Used after multiple types of procedures; provides continuous gentle suction of the operative site to increase drainage of serosanguinous fluid and collapse tissue to facilitate healing	• Assess the drainage system as appropriate to client's condition for: 1. Continued drainage 2. Maintained decompression 3. Air-tight tubings 4. Need for emptying • To reactivate suction, wash hands and wear gloves and eye/face protection • Empty reservoirs every 8 hours, when drainage nears the full line, or as ordered by the physician
Passive or active	Davol Sump Axiom Sump	Large, multilumen tube with a larger main port for drainage and/or suction and with smaller side port(s) for irrigation and/or air venting to help prevent tissue from being suctioned against catheter and damaged	To drain intra-abdominal fluids from abscesses, cysts, or hematomas	• Use one of the smaller or sump ports for continuous irrigation • Calculate intake and output carefully with irrigations • Place impervious pads underneath client • Change dressings frequently when saturated • Attach to catheter drainage bag if not attached to suction; do not plug sump ports
	Chest tube ThoraKlex Pleure Vac	Large single-lumen drain attached to closed water-seal drainage system	To drain fluid or air from pleural cavity	• Assess breath sounds and respirations, including depth, rate, symmetry of chest expansion, color of mucous membranes, and presence of crepitus with suction off or tubing clamped • If present, assess amount and type of suction • Ensure that connections are tight and sealed with tape • Keep chest tube drainage reservoir lower than client's chest • Observe for air leaks in air leak indicator or drainage chamber of drainage reservoir • Place petroleum jelly gauze nearby for quick access should the tube become dislodged • Measure drainage at least every 8 hours (more frequently if in a critical care unit or client's condition warrants it) • Clamp or milk the chest tube only if ordered by surgeon • Notify surgeon if drainage is greater than 100 mL/hour • Change drainage system when 2/3 full

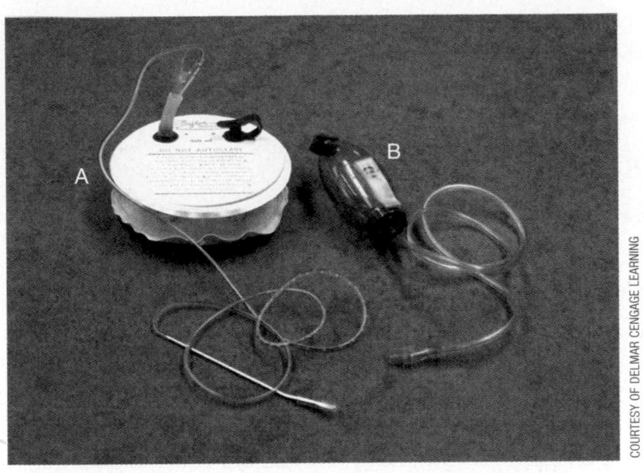

FIGURE 2-8 Common Drainage Devices; *A*, Hemovac; *B*, Jackson-Pratt

PACU are asked to squeeze the postanesthesia nurse's hands and to plantarflex and dorsiflex the feet.

CONTINUING NURSING CARE IN THE PACU

After the client has been admitted and assessed in PACU, the postanesthesia nurse checks the surgeon's and the anesthesia provider's orders and initiates any therapy designated for the PACU.

The postanesthesia nurse charts on a separate nursing record for the PACU. Anything unusual must be adequately documented. If vital signs are in the normal range, the postanesthesia nurse checks them every 15 minutes. If vital signs are unstable, they are checked every 5 minutes or as often as necessary until stable. If vital signs fail to stabilize, the surgeon and anesthesia provider are notified. The surgical site is checked at least every 30 minutes. If any initial bleeding has not subsided, the surgeon is notified. Routine checks are continued until the client is discharged from the PACU.

The postanesthesia nurse determines whether the client meets the criteria for discharge from the PACU. Typically, the client's vital signs are stable and within the client's normal limits. The Aldrete Score is 8 to 10. If the score is 7 or less, a surgeon's or anesthesia provider's order is required for discharge. Also before client discharge, the dressing is checked, changed, or reinforced according to orders. All other parameters are reassessed and charted. Institutional protocol dictates minimum stay in the PACU. Adults are typically kept in the PACU for a minimum of 1 hour, except outpatients, who go to the ambulatory surgery unit when they are awake and when postmedication time is fulfilled. Children are typically kept in the PACU until they are awake, stable, and have an Aldrete Score of 8 to 10. When criteria for discharge are met, the postanesthesia nurse calls the clinical unit or ambulatory surgery unit and reports the client's name, vitals, surgery, and any other pertinent information. The client is then transferred to the appropriate unit.

LATER POSTOPERATIVE NURSING CARE

Before the client's arrival in the clinical unit, the nurse prepares for the client. The linen is changed, the bed linen folded down, and the room cleared of clutter. Special required equipment, as directed by the postanesthesia nurse, is gathered. An emesis basin and tissue are available. The nurse is ready to assess the client in an organized manner, focusing on the body system affected by surgery.

Upon the client's arrival in the clinical unit, the nurse assists in transferring the client to the bed. Nursing assessment and care of the client upon admission to the clinical unit includes the following:

- Time of arrival in unit
- Transfer from cart to bed
  - Place bed in lowest, locked position, with side rails up
  - Place client in position of comfort, or as ordered
- Vital signs including airway assessment and breath sounds
- Color of skin, nail beds, and lips
- Skin condition (moist or dry, warm or cool)
- Level of consciousness
- Activity level
- Intravenous infusion
  - Type of solution
  - Amount in bottle or bag
  - Flow rate
  - Appearance and location of IV site
- Dressings
  - Amount and character of drainage
- Drains and tubes
  - Intactness and function
  - Connection to drainage and/or suction
  - Amount and character of drainage
- Urinary output
  - Need to void or time of voiding
  - Presence of patency and catheter; output/hour
- Pain
  - Last dose of analgesia
  - Current pain location, intensity, quality
- Compare assessment with PACU report
- Call light within reach
  - Reorient client to usage
- Location of family or significant others
- Postoperative orders

A brief assessment, including vital signs, is completed every 15 minutes for 1 hour; every 30 minutes for 2 hours; and every hour for 4 hours, or as prescribed by the physician. The possibilities of postanesthetic complications continue, but as time passes, different postsurgical complications may develop; the nurse is responsible for managing these.

1. The client is at risk for *Ineffective **Airway** Clearance* caused by atelectasis and hypostatic pneumonia. Respiratory complications can still occur with any anesthetized client. As in the PACU, the postoperative client is at risk for ineffective airway clearance, ineffective breathing patterns, and aspir.ation. Now, however, nursing measures are directed toward preventing ineffective airway clearance caused by atelectasis and hypostatic pneumonia, both of which usually occur within the first 48 hours postoperatively. In postoperative atelectasis, the

Table 2-4 Additional Nursing Care According to Classification or Type of Surgical Procedure

CLASSIFICATION OR TYPE OF SURGICAL PROCEDURE	NURSING CARE	
Orthopedic	• Expose wet casts to the air. • Check surgeon's orders for positioning of client; operated extremities typically are elevated. • Check for digital warmth, color, mobility, circulation (pulses), and sensation in affected extremity.	
Urologic	• Attach all catheters to drainage. • Closely monitor continuous irrigation to ensure that flow in and flow out are equal; if obstructed, the bladder could rupture. • Increase or decrease irrigation flow rate according to amount of bleeding. • Assess for chills or elevated pulse, possibly indicative of hemolysis or bacterial infection. • Assess abdomen for signs of distension and rigidity and report, especially if client complains.	
Oral	• Suction frequently and carefully around sutures. • Observe breathing; ensure that drainage or packing does not obstruct airway. • Apply ice bag, when ordered. • Remove dental packs as ordered and assess every 15 minutes for further bleeding.	
Eye, ears, nose, and throat (EENT)	*Eye surgery*	• Assess for facial paralysis. • Minimize head movement, coughing, vomiting, and restlessness.
	Ear surgery	• Assess edema and tracheal patency (listening for stridor and observing for restlessness).
	Nose surgery	• Maintain open airway; suction orally; and apply ice.
	Tonsillectomy	• Place on side to facilitate drainage: elevate head of bed; have suction available; and observe closely for bleeding, vomiting, and obstruction.
Neurologic	• Assess level of consciousness; be alert to drowsiness, slurred speech, disorientation, or irritability that differs from that exhibited in the preoperative state. • Observe for pupil changes: inequality, constriction, and nonreactivity to light. • Assess for respiratory changes such as snoring, retraction of cheeks and trachea, shallowness, and slowed rate. • Monitor blood pressure and pulse; an elevated blood pressure coupled with a lowered pulse leads to shock. • Observe extremity movement for weakness, paralysis, and rigidity; observe for unilateral drooping of facial features. • Use caution when medicating.	
	Laminectomy or discectomy	• Move only as ordered. • Assess sensation, circulation, and motion of extremities distal to incision.
	Craniotomy	• Position as ordered. • Complete a neurological check. • Use Trendelenburg position only with permission of the surgeon

Table 2-4 Additional Nursing Care According to Classification or Type of Surgical Procedure (Continued)

CLASSIFICATION OR TYPE OF SURGICAL PROCEDURE	NURSING CARE	
Vascular (all grafts, carotid endarterectomy, femoral-popliteal bypass)	• Assess color, sensation, warmth, and mobility of extremity. • Observe presence and strength of pedal and post-tibial pulses. • Complete a neurological check for carotid endarterectomy. • Frequently check all dressings and the area directly beneath the client. • Drainage can roll around a curved body part leaving the dressing appearing dry. However, check the area directly under curved body structures for bleeding.	
Thoracic	• Closely observe chest tube for patency, amount of bleeding, and air leaks. Tape all connections. Mark drainage container upon client's admission and discharge. Assess fluctuation of drainage in tubing. Attach suction as ordered. • Observe respirations closely with regard to color change, restlessness, apprehension, dyspnea, or mediastinal shift. • Elevate head of bed 30°, unless contraindicated. • Encourage coughing and deep breathing. • Use caution in administering narcotics, especially morphine sulfate, as client cannot afford respiratory depression.	
	Pneumonectomy	• Do not turn on nonoperative side. Alternately turn from back to operated side.
	Lobectomy and resection	• May turn client to either side.
Gynecologic	• Assess vaginal drainage.	

bronchioles of the lungs become plugged with mucus so that air cannot reach the alveoli. The alveoli then collapse. The client develops dyspnea, fever, tachypnea, tachycardia, and cyanosis. In postoperative hypostatic pneumonia, stagnant mucus promotes the growth of bacteria, and atelectasis then develops into a secondary infection. To prevent these complications, actively encourage the client to cough, deep breathe (with and without incentive spirometry), and turn as instructed preoperatively. Encourage the client to sit up and ambulate as soon and as often as ordered. Ensure adequate pain relief measures so that mobility is well tolerated.

2. The client is at risk for ***P****eripheral Neurovascular Dysfunction, Excess/Deficient* ***F****luid Volume, and* ***A****ctivity Intolerance*. The client continues to be at risk for decreased cardiac output and fluid volume deficit. Implement measures to prevent deep vein thrombosis, thrombophlebitis, pulmonary embolism, complications of fluid overload, fluid deficit, hypokalemia, and syncope.

The stress response to surgery, inactivity, pressure related to body position, obesity, and injury to pelvic veins during surgery contributes to the formation of deep vein thrombosis, thrombophlebitis, or pulmonary embolism. These complications may appear immediately after surgery or 1 to 2 weeks later. Routinely assess for a positive Homans' sign and for warm, tender, reddened, hardened areas in the calves. To assess for Homans' sign, ask the client to forcefully dorsiflex the foot. If pain is felt in the calf of the leg, it is considered a positive Homans' sign; if no pain is felt, it is considered a negative finding. A positive Homans' sign may indicate thrombophlebitis and is reported to the surgeon. Deep vein thrombosis and thrombophlebitis may lead to a pulmonary embolus, although there is no warning of pulmonary embolism. When pulmonary embolism occurs, the client experiences dyspnea, chest pain, cyanosis, cough, hemoptysis, tachycardia, and fever coupled with an elevated white blood cell count. If the embolism is large enough, shock develops rapidly. Pulmonary embolism may be fatal.

To prevent the formation of deep vein thrombosis, thrombophlebitis, and pulmonary embolism, encourage the client to ambulate to the extent the client is able. When in bed, encourage the client to perform postoperative leg exercises each hour. Antiembolism stockings are ordered, or a sequential compression device, which is a boot applied to the legs to simulate walking by alternate inflation. Remove the boots and antiembolism stockings every day to cleanse the skin. Antiembolism stockings and the sequential compression device are not substitutes for leg exercises. Encourage the client to perform leg exercises.

When ordered, low-molecular-weight heparin, enoxaparin (Lovenox), is administered to hemostatically stable clients who have undergone pelvic, abdominal, or thoracic surgery. It is given subcutaneously every 12 hours or daily as ordered until discharge. If preoperative INR levels were within normal range, no laboratory test is necessary to determine the drug's effect. The regimen is ordered at the surgeon's discretion.

Measure intake and output and monitor laboratory findings (e.g., electrolytes, hematocrit, hemoglobin, and serum osmolality) and signs and symptoms of hemorrhage by assessing vital signs, skin color and condition, dressings, drains, and tubes, as in the PACU.

Clients often experience syncope when changing from a lying position to a sitting or standing position. Assist the client to change positions slowly, proceed in steps, and allow time for the client's internal equilibrium to adjust. Check the radial pulse frequently and ask the client if he is dizzy or nauseated. If syncope occurs during ambulation, ask for assistance in obtaining a wheelchair for the client, use a nearby chair, or lower the client to the floor until the client recovers. Although frightening for the client, syncope is not physiologically threatening unless the client is injured in a fall.

3. The client may be at risk for *Imbalanced **N**utrition: Less than Body Requirements* related to nausea and vomiting, hiccups, abdominal distension, constipation, and NPO status. Gastrointestinal complications become more prevalent after immediate postoperative recovery. The client may also experience pain related to hiccups and slowed gastrointestinal function.

Anesthetic agents, narcotics, hypotension, and the manipulation of the bowel during surgery cause nausea and vomiting. Handling of the bowel during pelvic and abdominal surgery causes peristalsis to stop or severely slow. Bowel function normally returns 2 to 5 days after surgery. If bowel inactivity persists, a paralytic ileus develops. As bowel function resumes, continue to assess the client for bowel sounds and, if a nasogastric tube is present, a reduction in drainage. As peristalsis returns in a discontinuous fashion, the client experiences distention along with flatulence and gas pains. After bowel sounds resume in all quadrants, the client is removed from NPO status according to the surgeon's orders. Provide good oral hygiene when the client is NPO and administer antiemetics as needed for nausea and vomiting.

Hiccups are caused by irritation of the phrenic nerve. Impulses then cause the diaphragm to contract rhythmically and violently. Abdominal distention, gastric distention, and the presence of a nasogastric tube are common causes, but electrolyte and acid–base disturbances, intestinal obstruction, and intra-abdominal bleeding also initiate hiccups. Notify the surgeon when hiccups are prolonged.

Gas pains and signs and symptoms of abdominal distention are minimized by early and frequent ambulation and resumption of oral intake. Frequently repositioning the client encourages movement of air through the intestines, relieving gas pains. As air rises and peristalsis moves from right to left, the client is moved from lying on the left side (where air will rise on the right), to lying supine, to lying on the right side (where air will rise on the left). If the client can tolerate it and there are no contraindications, lying prone with the head turned to the side places pressure on the abdomen, forcing air to rise and move out through the rectum. Other nursing care measures to relieve abdominal distention might include irrigation of the nasogastric tube, if present. Irrigating the nasogastric tube may also relieve hiccups.

Constipation is a major source of discomfort for the client. Analgesics combined with decreased activity and NPO status are very constipating. Oral fluids and activity are encouraged. If ordered, the medical regimen of stool softeners and suppositories are indicated.

4. The client is at risk for developing ***U**rinary Retention* related to anesthesia, immobility, and pain. The client is also at *Risk for **I**nfection* related to Foley catheter placement. The quantity and quality of urine are more directly related to cardiac output and the perfusion of the kidneys than to anesthesia, immobility, and pain; although a stress response following surgery causes the body to retain fluids for 24 to 48 hours after surgery. Urine output should be at least 30 mL per hour if a catheter is in place. The catheter is assessed for patency. If not catheterized, the client should void at least 200 mL at the first postoperative voiding. Most clients void within 6 to 8 hours after surgery; however, urinary retention occurs frequently in the postoperative period, especially following abdominal or pelvic surgery. Anesthesia depresses the urge to void. Narcotics, vagolytic agents (anticholinergics), and spinal anesthesia also interfere with the ability to initiate voiding. Facilitate voiding by encouraging fluid intake and assisting the client to void in an anatomically correct position depending on the client's condition. Privacy, running water, indirect bladder pressure (placing a firm hand over the bladder), and warm water over the perineum may also encourage voiding.

If the client has not voided, use a noninvasive bladder ultrasound instrument to measure the bladder volume. If the facility does not have a bladder scanner, palpate, inspect, and percuss the bladder to check for distention. The surgeon orders a Foley catheter inserted if the client has a distended bladder or has not voided after 8-10 hours.

5. The client may become at risk for *Disturbed **S**ensory Perception* related to anesthesia, narcotics, change of environment, fluid and electrolyte imbalances, sleep deprivation, hypoxia, and sensory deprivation or overload. The client may also experience *Acute **P**ain* related to the surgical incision; ***H**ypothermia* related to anesthesia and surgical environment; and ***H**yperthermia* related to infection. Alterations in neurological function vary and manifest as pain, fever, or delirium. Assessing the level of consciousness is a priority. A change in level of consciousness may be the first indication of a stroke and/or increased intracranial pressure. Determining the level of consciousness is difficult, especially in the elderly client or at night, when clients are groggy from being awakened. Often, thoughts will clear if the client is given the opportunity to thoroughly awaken. Encouraging the presence of loved ones, offering explanations, and listening to the client decreases sensory perceptual alterations. Encouraging previous sleep patterns, providing uninterrupted sleep, and alternating rest and activity also is beneficial.

Assess and record subjective data regarding pain location, intensity on a scale of 0 to 10, quality, and duration as well as factors contributing to pain. Objective data such as grimacing and crying are also recorded. Analgesics are usually ordered for administration via patient-controlled analgesia (PCA) or epidural analgesia or intravenously, intramuscularly, or orally, all on a PRN (as needed) basis. Encourage the client to ask for medication before the pain becomes severe. Offer medication before activity or painful procedures such as wound irrigation. Attend to analgesic requests promptly. Ensuring comfort encourages the client's full participation in coughing, deep breathing, turning, and ambulation.

Hypothermia is common in the first few hours following surgery. Offer blankets as needed. Because of the normal inflammatory response, temperature may later elevate to a low-grade fever. If temperature rises higher than 101°F, notify the surgeon. Atelectasis and dehydration cause elevated temperature (higher than 101°F) in the first 24 to 48 hours after surgery. After 48 hours, temperature higher than 101°F indicates a wound, respiratory, or urinary tract infection; thrombophlebitis; or pulmonary embolism.

The nurse's primary role is to prevent infection by using aseptic technique. Once a fever has occurred, follow orders to ascertain the cause of the elevation by taking urine, wound, blood, or sputum cultures. Administer antipyretics as ordered. Providing light covers and clothing, performing frequent linen changes, offering cool washcloths, and ensuring a cool environment are measures that may increase comfort.

6. The surgical client is at *Risk for Impaired* ***S****kin Integrity and Risk for* ***I****nfection* related to surgical incision. The nurse generally does not remove the primary dressing without an order to do so. Bleeding is monitored by circling the drainage on the dressing and then reassessing later to ascertain whether the drainage area has increased in size. The dressing also is reinforced with additional absorbent dressings as needed. In some institutions, the dressing is changed as necessary after the first dressing change. Some surgeons prefer no dressing if there is no drainage or drains.

Drainage on dressings and in drains typically changes from sanguinous to serosanguinous to serous over several hours to several days, depending on the type of surgery. The amount also decreases over the same time period. Purulent, odorous drainage is a sign of infection. A sudden increase in drainage is a sign of impending wound separation. Always notify the surgeon of any excessive or abnormal drainage.

All wounds heal by primary, secondary, or tertiary intention. In primary intention, the wound layers are sutured together and have no gaping edges. The wound generally heals in 8 to 10 days but may take up to 3 months. There is minimal scar formation. Most surgical wounds are of this type.

In secondary intention, the wound heals by filling in with granulation tissue and by contracting where the skin edges are not approximated. This method is used for ulcers when there is not enough tissue to approximate the edges or for infected wounds when drainage is desirable. Wounds healing by secondary intention are assessed according to the presence of granulation tissue having a red, granular appearance. Wound healing is slow, possibly taking many months or years. Thus wound healing by primary intention is preferable.

In tertiary intention, the approximation of tissue edges is delayed. This allows an infection to drain or an area of extensive tissue removal to begin healing. The edges of the wound are closed 4 to 6 days later. Because areas of granulation tissue are brought together at this time, the scar is usually much wider (Figure 2-9).

Wound dehiscence and evisceration are serious complications of wound healing. **Dehiscence** occurs when the wound edges separate. **Evisceration** occurs when the wound separates completely and the viscera protrude from the wound (Figure 2-10). Both are more likely to occur 7 to 10 days after surgery and are preceded by a sudden spillage of serosanguinous drainage.

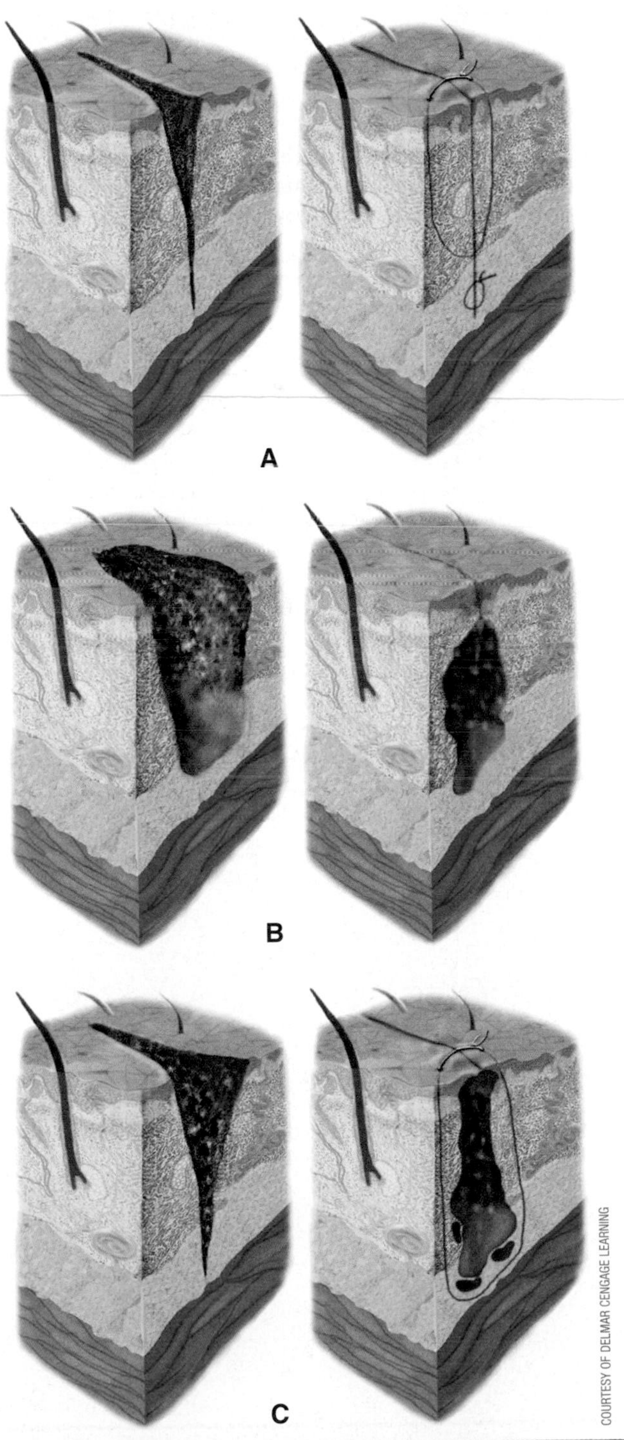

FIGURE 2-9 **Wound Healing; *A*, Primary Intention; *B*, Secondary Intention; and *C*, Tertiary Intention**

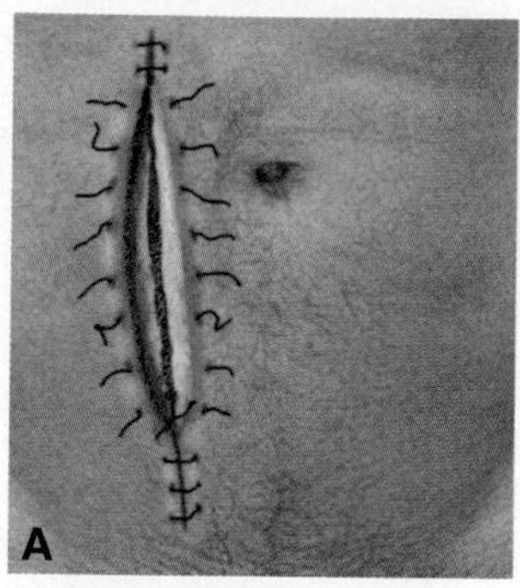

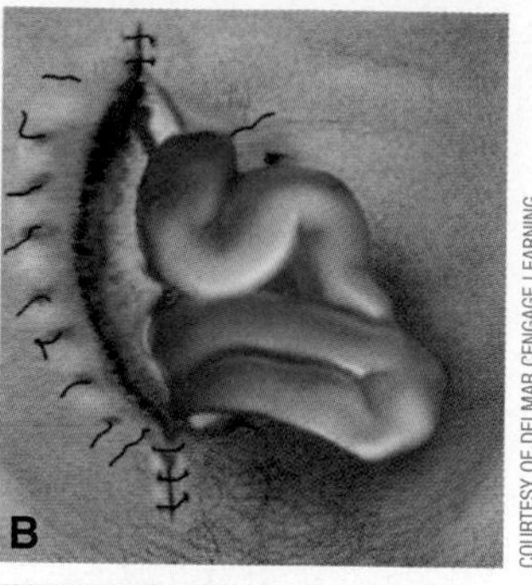

FIGURE 2-10 *A*, **Dehiscence;** *B*, **Evisceration**

Dehiscence and evisceration are more likely to occur in the very elderly client, the malnourished client, the client with an infection, or the client with abdominal distention who is straining severely. If evisceration occurs, the viscera is immediately covered with sterile saline dressings and the surgeon notified of the wound disruption.

When dressings are changed, the surgical incision is cleansed to remove debris and bacteria from the incision. The choice of cleansing agent depends on the physician's prescription as well as institutional protocol. It is recommended that isotonic solutions such as normal saline or lactated ringers be used.

The major principles to keep in mind when cleansing a surgical incision are:

- Use Standard Precautions at all times.
- Use a sterile swab or gauze and work from the clean area out toward the dirtier area. Begin over the incision line and swab downward from top to bottom. Change the swab and proceed again on either side of the incision, using a new swab each time (Figure 2-11).

The surface closures (staples or sutures) are removed as the incision heals. Continuous sutures are made with one thread and tied at the beginning and end of the suture line. Intermittent sutures are each tied individually. In blanket continuous sutures, the single thread is grounded again in the last suture exit (Figure 2-12). Some surgical wounds are closed with dissolvable sutures and special tape strips and others with special adhesive glue. The dissolvable sutures are not removed and the glue wears off. Sometimes no bandage is applied when the wound is closed with glue.

The incisional dressing keeps the incision clean and protects it from physical trauma and bacterial invasion. Generally, the same kind of dressing is put on as was taken off. As the incision heals and drainage lessens, a small, thinner dressing usually is applied. Bandages and binders are applied over the incision

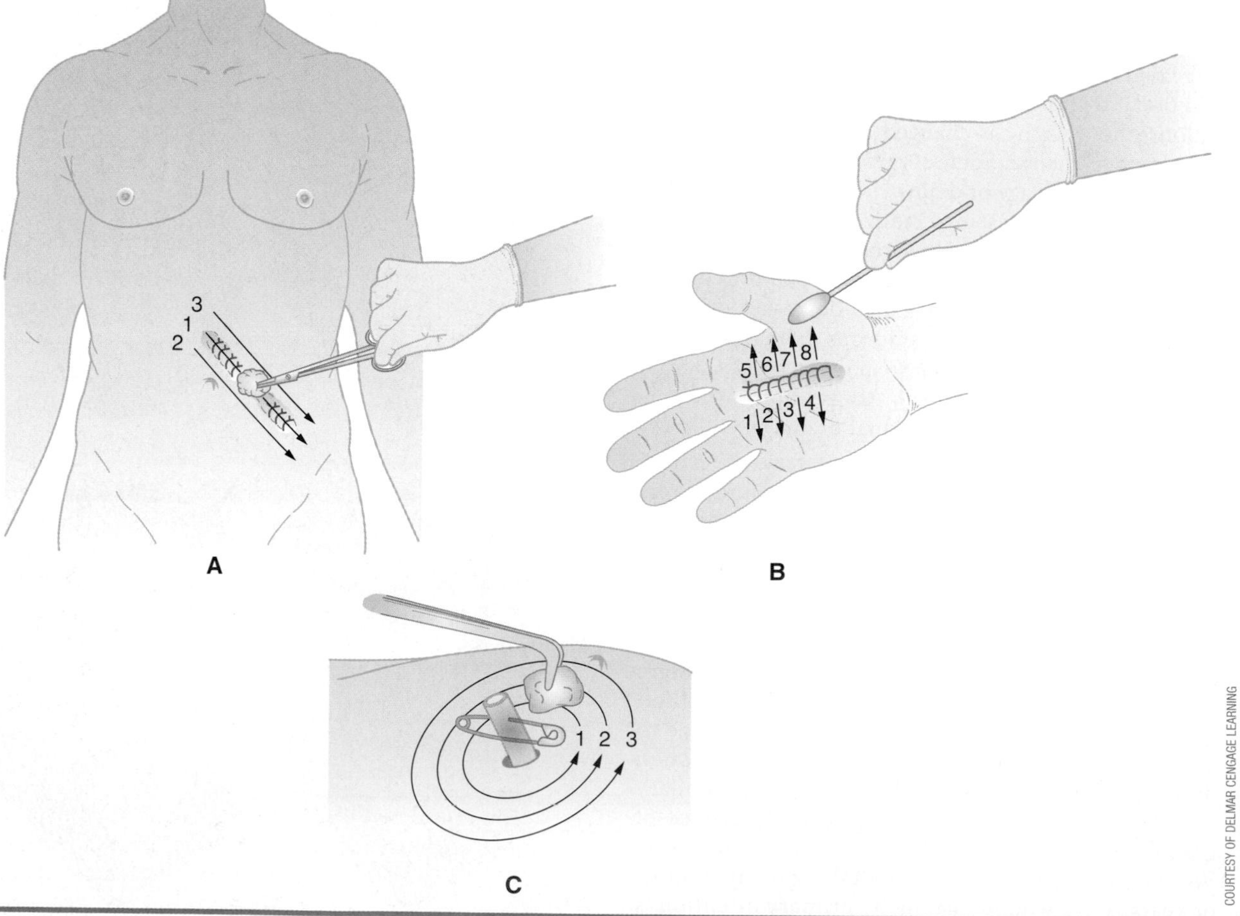

FIGURE 2-11 **Use a clean, sterile swab for each stroke when cleansing a surgical incision.** *A*, **Gently clean the incision, then each side alternately;** *B*, **Gently wipe swab outward, away from the incision;** *C*, **Clean around a drain site in a circular motion.**

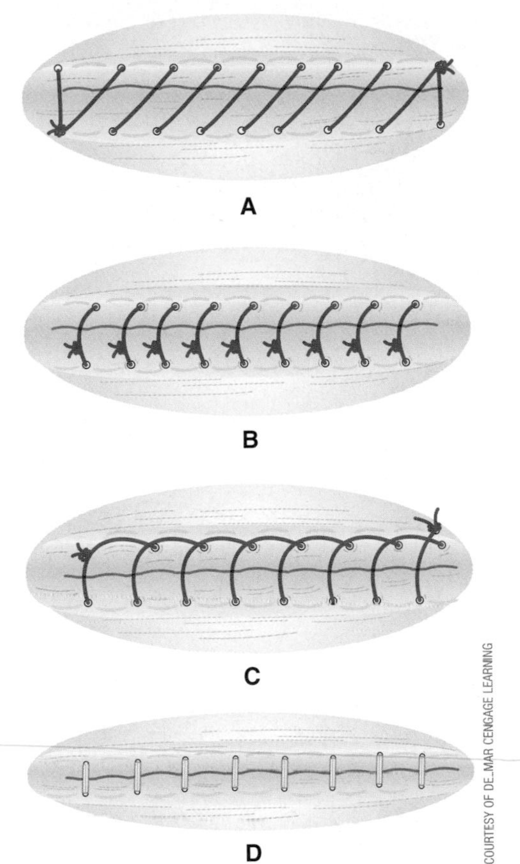

FIGURE 2-12 Skin Closure Methods; *A*, Continuous; *B*, Intermittent; *C*, Blanket Continuous; *D*, Staples

dressing to secure, immobilize, or support a body part; to hold the dressing in place; or to prevent or minimize swelling of a body part. Bandages are long rolls of material, such as gauze, webbing, or muslin, designed for wrapping around body parts. Figure 2-13 illustrates several different methods of bandaging.

COMMUNITY/HOME HEALTH CARE

Dressing Wounds

- Because of early discharge, clients are often sent home with incisions that need dressing changes.
- Ascertain the client's support system, including caregivers, the home environment, and available resources.
- Teach the client and/or home caregiver the correct method of changing the dressing.
- Have the client and/or home caregiver change the dressing before the client is discharged.
- Provide a list of signs and symptoms of complications of wound healing.
- At times, a referral for home care nursing is necessary.

COMMUNITY/HOME HEALTH CARE

Postoperative Care

For proper home care, the client and family must be given information about the following topics:

- Medication regimen
- Diet
- Activity restrictions
- Follow-up appointments
- Wound care
- Special instructions

The specifics for each topic will vary with each client and will depend on the surgical procedure and the client's age and physical condition.

Binders are bandages made for specific body parts, usually the abdomen or arm (sling) (Figure 2-14). Abdominal binders support the abdomen of an obese client following abdominal surgery. A sling is a cloth support with adjustable straps that wrap around the back to provide support for an injured arm; it maintains the arm in a set position.

During dressing changes and after the dressing has been removed, the surgical wound is assessed for skin edge approximation, edema, and bleeding. The skin edges may be slightly reddened and swollen from the normal inflammatory response. Possible signs of a wound infection include increased suture tension, warmth, erythema, drainage, odor, pain, and induration around the incision site. Wound healing is enhanced by promoting nutrition, discouraging smoking, and performing proper wound cleansing. The practice of aseptic technique cannot be emphasized enough in preventing nosocomial infections in a surgical incision.

7. Clients are at risk for ***Anxiety or Ineffective Coping*** related to disturbance in body image, change in lifestyle, financial strain, or a poor prognosis. Many clients undergo a psychological adjustment to surgery. Taking time to listen to the client as well as offering simple explanations and reassurances supports the client needs to combat anxiety.

As the client recovers and is ready for discharge from the hospital, the client is at risk for *Deficient Knowledge* related to home care. Ideally, the client receives home care instructions from the moment of admission. Adequate teaching about home care results in a quicker recovery, fewer complications, and greater independence.

Minimally invasive surgery (MIS) is replacing much of the traditional types of surgery. MIS is completed with three to five small incisions in which a videoscope and specialized instruments are inserted into the small incisions to complete the surgery (see Figure 2-15). The same traditional type of surgery would require a much longer incision through larger areas of tissue and muscle. The layout of the surgical

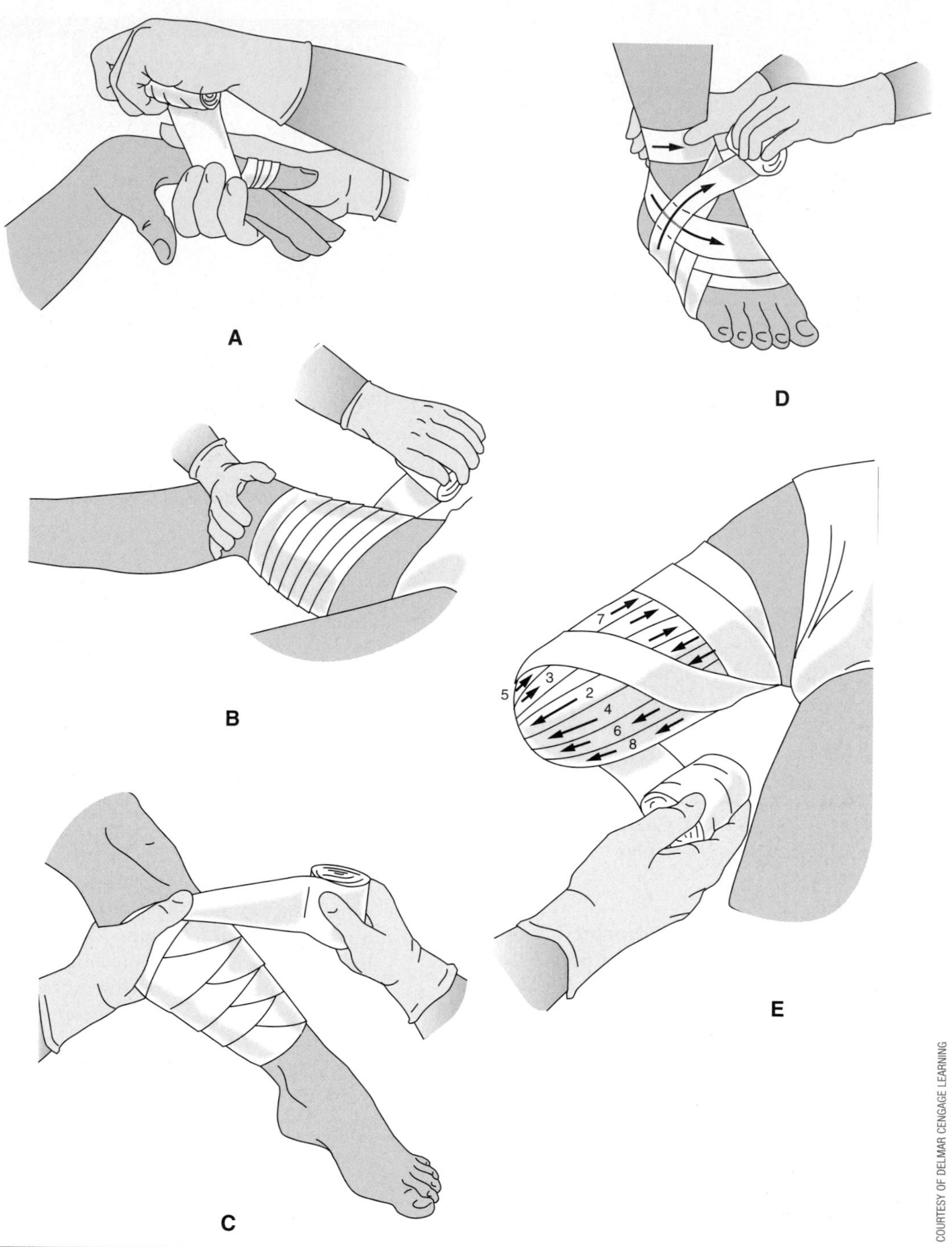

FIGURE 2-13 **Common Bandaging Methods; *A*, Circular turns are wrapped around a body part several times to anchor the bandage or supply support. *B*, Spiral turns begin with a circular turn and then proceed up the body part, with each turn covering two-thirds the width of the preceding turn. *C*, Spiral reverse turns begin with a circular turn. The bandage is then reversed or twisted, once each turn, to accommodate a limb that gets larger as the bandaging progresses. *D*, Figure-eight turns crisscross in the shape of a figure eight and are used on a joint that requires movement. *E*, Recurrent turns are anchored with circular turns, follow a back-and-forth motion, and are completed with circular turns; they are used to cover a fingertip, head, or residual limb.**

room is different than the usual surgery suite. See Figure 2-16 for a layout of the surgical room and surgical system of a console, patient cart, and vision cart. Abdominal, thoracic, pelvic, and spine surgeries are performed by MIS. The advantages of MIS are less postoperative pain, decreased hospital stay, less risk of infection, prompt return to normal activities and work, and less overall postoperative complications. Specific MIS surgery is discussed throughout the various system chapters (Ohio State University Medical Center, 2009; George Washington University Hospital, 2009).

AMBULATORY SURGERY

Ambulatory surgery is defined as surgical care performed under general, regional, or local anesthesia involving less than

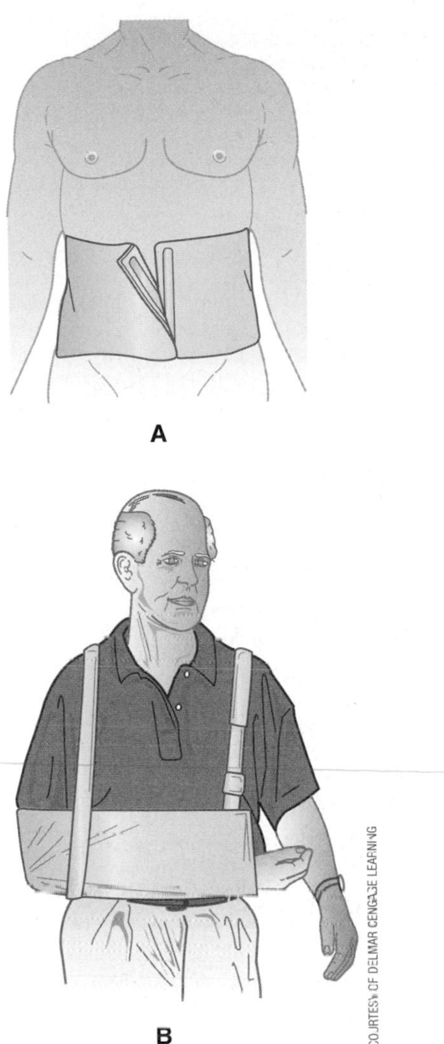

FIGURE 2-14 **Common Binders: *A*, Abdominal; *B*, Arm Sling**

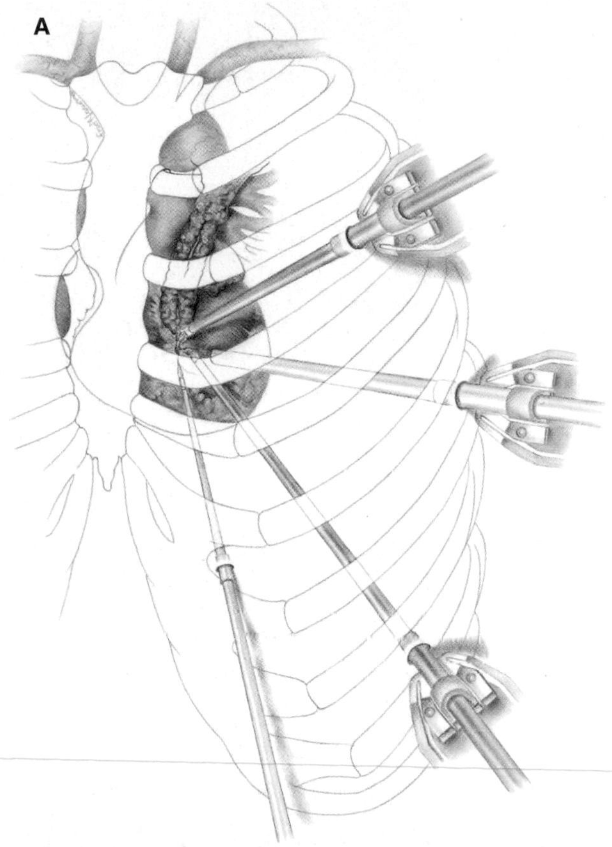

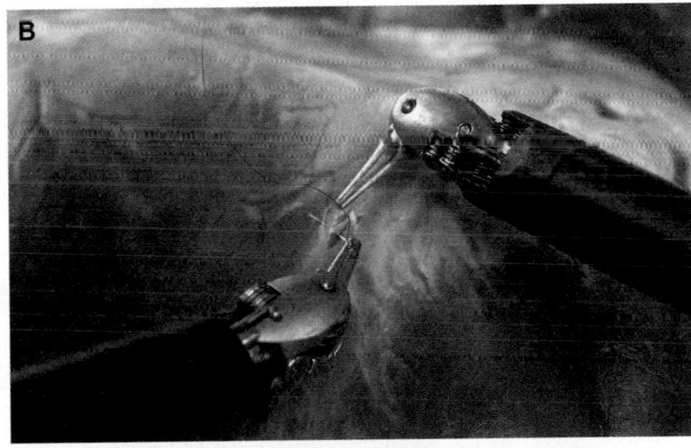

FIGURE 2-15 **Minimally invasive surgery (MIS); *A*, Surgeons, using small incisions, introduce specialized instruments into the body to perform surgery. *B*, Special instruments are manipulated by the surgeons to perform surgery. (© *2009 Intuitive Surgical, Inc.*)**

24 hours of hospitalization. Other names for ambulatory surgery include same-day, one-day, outpatient, in and out, or short-stay surgery.

The trend in health care is to promote wellness. Clients are encouraged to accept more personal responsibility for their state of health. In the past, the message sent to clients was that the client is sick, and the medical community will provide all care. Today, ambulatory surgery clients are sent an entirely different message: that the postoperative client is not sick and, except for a few minor limitations, can often resume normal daily activities soon after undergoing anesthesia and surgery.

Ambulatory surgery provides the longest period of time for the client to receive skilled postoperative care or monitoring without formal admission to the hospital. The practice of ambulatory surgery attempts to overcome the risk of premature dismissal while meeting fiscal requirements. The emphasis on cost containment coupled with government reductions in Medicare and Medicaid payments has further promoted the concept of ambulatory surgery.

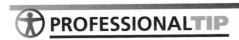

Ambulatory Surgery

- Precertification documents are approved before the preadmission visit.
- Preadmission diagnostic tests, preoperative nursing assessment, and initial teaching are usually performed the day before the scheduled surgery.
- On the day of surgery, care is focused on the immediate needs of the client.

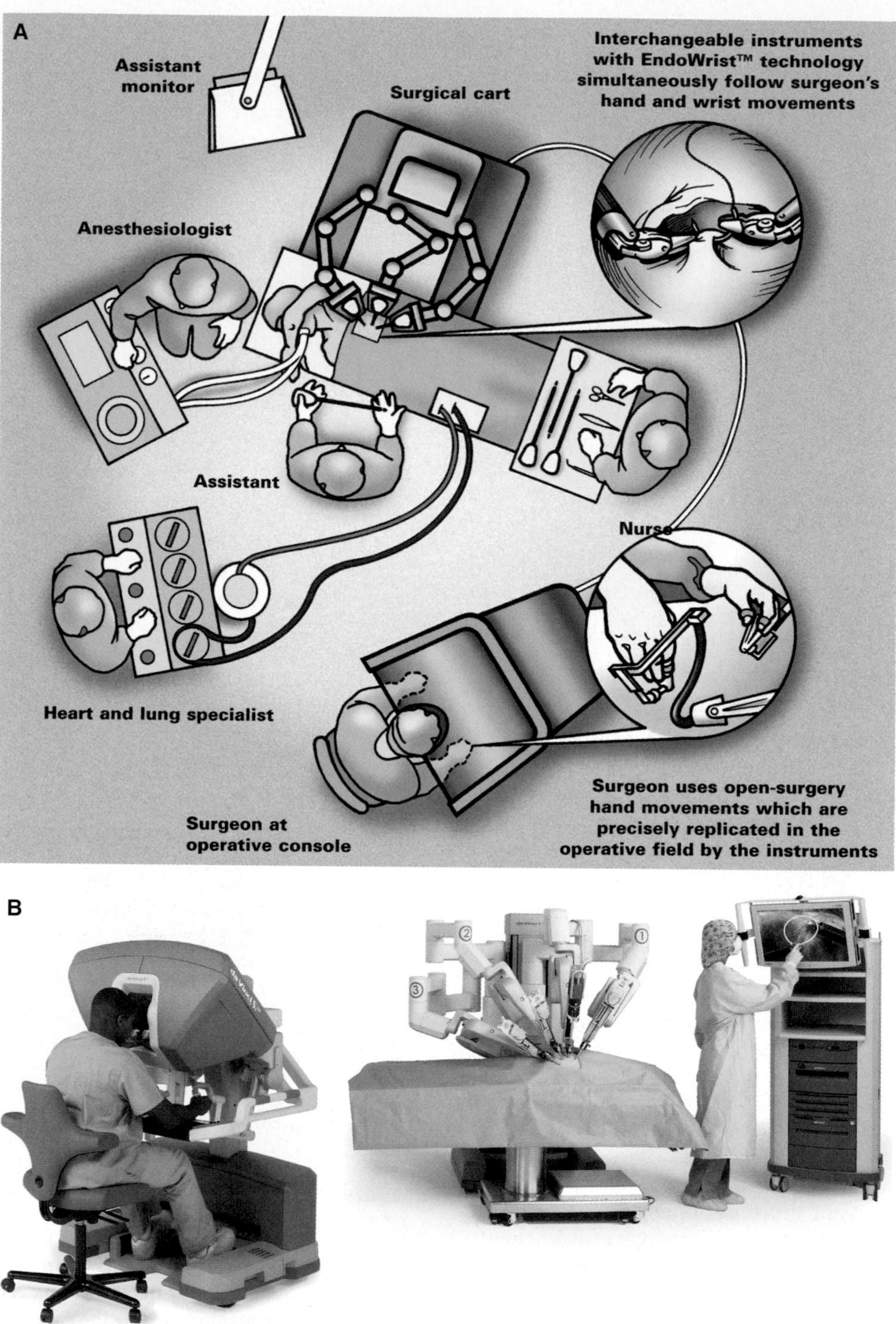

FIGURE 2-16 Minimally Invasive Surgical Suite; *A*, Typical Layout of a MIS Surgical Suite; *B*, Surgeon at the Da Vinci Si Console with Patient Cart and Surgical Nurse at the Vision Cart (© *2009 Intuitive Surgical, Inc.*)

To further reduce health care costs, few clients are admitted to the hospital before the day of surgery. Most surgical clients are processed through the ambulatory surgery unit. These clients are called "day of surgery" or "A.M. admit" clients. Necessary laboratory work, radiology tests, or other examinations are completed on an outpatient basis before the day of surgery. Even clients undergoing extensive surgeries such as open-heart surgery (a coronary artery bypass), craniotomy, or total joint replacement are admitted the day of surgery. Then, after discharge from the perioperative suite, the client either is admitted to the hospital as an inpatient or is sent home from the ambulatory surgery unit.

In addition to fiscal considerations, the growth of ambulatory surgery can also be traced to technological advances. Clients now require shorter recovery periods as a result of new procedural technology, such as laparoscopic cholecystectomy. The introduction of shorter-acting anesthetic agents also decreases the immediate postoperative recovery time, facilitating the client's ability to function independently upon discharge from the ambulatory surgery setting.

The benefits of ambulatory surgery are many. Ambulatory surgery decreases cost to the client, institution, insurance carriers, and governmental agencies. The risk of acquiring a nosocomial infection is also decreased. The client experiences less disruption to personal life and less psychological distress related to hospitalization. With ambulatory surgery, the client especially benefits from early postoperative ambulation.

Ambulatory surgery is performed in several different settings. Hospital-based integrated facilities are formal ambulatory surgery programs incorporated into existing inpatient surgery programs. Clients are cared for preoperatively and postoperatively in the ambulatory surgery unit but are mixed with inpatients on the OR schedule. This type of facility also allows preoperative processing of day-of-surgery clients. Hospital-affiliated facilities consist of a separate department with designated preoperative, intraoperative, and postoperative areas. Such a facility is located within the hospital, adjacent to the hospital, or at a satellite location. Freestanding facilities are independently owned and operated and are not affiliated with a hospital or medical center. In the past, physicians generally owned such facilities, but today the trend is for health care corporations to own these facilities. Some doctors' offices also have facilities for performing minor ambulatory surgery.

The Aldrete Score has been modified for use with clients having anesthesia on an ambulatory basis. Five assessments were added to the Aldrete Score for this purpose (Table 2-2). Attainment of these criteria indicates that clients can care for themselves at home and accomplish activities of daily living independently and safely. The points are totaled at regular intervals (usually every half hour), and clients are discharged home when their total score is 18 or higher.

ELDERLY CLIENTS HAVING SURGERY

Elderly clients (older than 65 years of age) are at risk for developing complications from surgery or anesthesia. Unfortunately, because an increased incidence of disease correlates with increasing age, more elderly clients require surgery than does any other age group. As the percentage of elderly persons in the whole population rises, the number of surgeries on elders is increasing. Because of the complex needs of the elderly client undergoing surgery, knowledge in promoting health and rehabilitation in the elderly client is necessary.

Surgery is a stressor. Because of depleted energy sources, the elderly client may not have sufficient resilience to react defensively to this stressor. The risk of complications from surgery further increases in elderly clients who have one or more chronic diseases. In these clients, surgery then can be the source of a downward spiraling effect toward debilitation or possibly death.

Elderly clients vary in their abilities to respond to the stress of surgery. Physiologic changes related to the aging process inhibit the elderly client from readily coping with surgery. The number of physiologic changes in the very elderly

Table 2-5 Physiologic Changes of Aging and Related Postoperative Nursing Interventions

BODY SYSTEM	CHANGES	NURSING INTERVENTIONS
Cardiovascular	• Decreased elasticity of the vascular system • Decreased cardiac output • Decreased peripheral circulation	• Closely monitor vital signs and peripheral pulses • Encourage early ambulation • Use antiembolism stockings • Monitor intake and output, including blood loss • Monitor preoperative response to activity and compare to postoperative response
Respiratory	• Decreased vital capacity • Decreased alveolar volume • Decreased movement of cilia	• Closely monitor respirations • Auscultate breath sounds frequently • Encourage coughing and deep breathing • Turn frequently • Monitor oxygen saturation

(Continues)

Table 2-5 Physiologic Changes of Aging and Related Postoperative Nursing Interventions (Continued)

BODY SYSTEM	CHANGES	NURSING INTERVENTIONS
Urinary	• Decreased glomerular filtration rate • Decreased bladder muscle tone • Weakened perineal muscles	• Monitor intake and output every 1 to 2 hours • Assist frequently with toileting • Monitor fluid and electrolyte status
Gastrointestinal	• Decreased gastric and intestinal motility • Altered digestion and absorption • Decreased food consumption	• Assess for obesity and malnutrition • Encourage fluids and activity • Encourage high-protein foods and supplements • Assist with meals as needed • Provide companionship during mealtime
Immunological	• Decreased level of gamma globulin • Decreased plasma proteins	• Follow strict aseptic technique • Monitor temperature • Assess incision site
Neurological	• Decreased conduction velocity • Decreased visual acuity • Loss of hearing • Decreased sensation	• Allow use of glasses and hearing aids • Orient to environment • Provide for safe environment • Repeat information as needed • Use medications sparingly • Provide written instructions • Allow for extra education time
Integumentary	• Lack of elasticity • Loss of collagen • Decreased subcutaneous fat	• To prevent shearing forces on skin when positioning client, lift rather than slide client • Pad bony prominences • Use tape that is easy to remove • Use warm prepping solutions, irrigating solutions, and IV solutions intraoperatively • Provide extra blankets • Ensure warm room temperature • Turn frequently • Encourage early ambulation

client (older than 80 years of age) is markedly greater than that in those in their sixties and seventies. Breathing capacity, renal blood flow, cardiac output, and conduction velocity of the nervous system all diminish. Table 2-5 lists the physiologic changes in the elderly client along with correlating nursing interventions for postoperative care. Aging affects all body systems, and the nurse's knowledge of these changes and the interventions geared toward each assist in preventing and detecting complications of surgery.

The elderly client has a lifetime of experiences that affects the response to surgery. A lifetime of watching family and friends experience surgery, illness, and death particularly influences personal reactions to impending surgery. Because of the variation in such experiences, each client reacts differently to similar situations. Simply talking with the client to provide information or listening to the client's fears helps prepare the client for upcoming surgery.

Third-party reimbursement policies often require elderly clients to undergo surgical procedures on an outpatient basis. Because many elderly clients have neurological deficits and other chronic disease processes, the elderly outpatient poses a particular challenge. Additional postoperative self-care deficits may result from the surgical procedure and the effects of anesthesia. Elderly clients often live alone and lack the support systems necessary for home care. In order to provide realistic discharge planning, the nurse assesses the ability of the client, family, and friends to provide care at home.

CASE STUDY

G.S., a 74-year-old retired school teacher who is married and the father of four and the grandfather of sixteen, weighs 275 lbs. He has undergone a right hemicolectomy, wherein the right side of his colon was removed because of cancer. He has a history of smoking but has no other health problems. The surgery was uncomplicated, and he is in the PACU. He has a midline incision with a Penrose drain and a stab wound with a Jackson-Pratt drain adjacent to the incision. He also has a nasogastric tube attached to low intermittent suction. He is alert and oriented and moves all four extremities freely. His blood pressure is normal for him in comparison to his preoperative levels. He is breathing regularly and easily at a rate of 16 breaths per minute, and his skin color is normal. His oxygen saturation, however, is 86% with additional oxygen given via mask.

The following questions will guide your development of a nursing care plan for the case study.

1. What risk factors for developing postoperative complications can you identify for G.S.?
2. What is his Aldrete Score at this point?
3. What nursing measures can you institute to promote oxygenation?
4. What type of drainage is expected from the incision and the drains during the first 1 to 2 days?
5. What nursing observations can be made and reported to indicate to the surgeon that the nasogastric tube can be removed?
6. What nursing measures can be implemented to prevent deep vein thrombosis, thrombophlebitis, and pulmonary embolism?
7. Write and prioritize three individualized nursing diagnoses and goals for G.S.
8. What information will G.S. need before discharge?

SUMMARY

- Surgery is a major stressor for all clients. Anxiety and fear are normal. Fear of the unknown is both the most prevalent fear before surgery and the fear easiest for the nurse to help the client overcome.
- The outcome of surgical treatment is tremendously enhanced by accurate preoperative nursing assessment and careful preoperative preparation. Information gathered through preoperative assessment and risk screening is later used to prepare the surgical site, for surgical positioning, and as a comparative basis for postoperative assessments and complication screening.
- The teaching methods that the nurse uses strongly influence the degree of learning and the retention of information.
- Aseptic technique is a collection of principles used to control and/or prevent the transfer of microorganisms from sources within (endogenous) and outside (exogenous) the client. All clinical nursing units practice these principles. The sterile conscience governs personal behavior with regard to adherence to aseptic technique.
- Nursing care in the OR focuses on the safety and protection of the client.
- Postoperative nursing assessments are completed in an organized manner, focusing first on the priorities of airway, breathing, and circulation, and then on the body system affected by surgery.
- The nurse prevents the formation of deep vein thrombosis, thrombophlebitis, and pulmonary embolism through encouraging early ambulation and postoperative leg exercises and by providing antiembolism stockings and/or sequential stockings, if ordered.
- Ambulatory surgery is defined as surgical care performed under general, regional, or local anesthesia and involving fewer than 24 hours of hospitalization. Cost containment, governmental changes, and technological advances promote the concept of ambulatory surgery.
- Because of the physiologic changes and complex needs of the elderly client undergoing surgery, the nurse's knowledge assists in promoting health and rehabilitation in the elderly surgical client.

REVIEW QUESTIONS

1. Client education is:
   1. completed when time allows.
   2. started when discharge is scheduled.
   3. always more beneficial when completed in a structured group setting.
   4. directed toward the client's family when the client is unable to learn.
2. A client is scheduled for surgery. The role of the nurse in obtaining consent includes:
   1. judging the quality of the explanation and ascertaining the client's understanding of the consent form.
   2. acting as a witness to the signature of the client.

3. administering the preoperative medication before the client signs the consent.
4. ensuring that coercion was used to obtain the client's signature on the consent.

3. Upon the client's admission to the PACU, the nurse knows to first:
   1. take the client's blood pressure.
   2. assess the airway.
   3. assess the client's level of consciousness.
   4. check the incision site.
4. The nurse is making a preoperative assessment on a client. Of the following findings, the most important item to know for a client who is having general anesthesia is:
   1. hearing impaired.
   2. a right-leg amputee.
   3. color blind.
   4. a smoker.
5. The nursing intervention that has the greatest impact on reducing overall surgical risk is:
   1. encouraging activity and early ambulation.
   2. assessing blood pressure.
   3. ensuring adequate nutrition.
   4. monitoring intake and output.
6. An elderly client is returning to the unit from surgery. The nursing interventions specifically geared toward elderly care are: (Select all that apply.)
   1. carefully monitoring vital signs and peripheral pulses.
   2. lifting the client rather than sliding client when repositioning.
   3. encouraging early ambulation.
   4. repeating information as needed.
   5. following strict aseptic technique.
   6. using tape that is easily removed.
7. The surgical client's most common fear is of the unknown. The nurse can ease the client's fears by:
   1. listening to the client's concerns about surgery.
   2. taking time from busy schedule and sitting beside the client for a few minutes.
   3. asking the client's family to stay with the client.
   4. teaching the client about the surgical process and answer questions.
8. A 73-year-old client is scheduled for prostate surgery. His vital signs are T 98.2, P 74, R 14, and BP160/92. He drinks heavily and smokes a pack of cigarettes a day. What is the client's risk factors pending his upcoming surgery? (Select all that apply.)
   1. Hepatic status.
   2. Fluid and electrolyte status.
   3. Age.
   4. Cardiovascular status.
   5. Respiratory status.
   6. Musculoskeletal system.
9. The PACU nurse asks a new surgical client if he has the ability to wiggle his toes and move his feet. She is assessing his: (Select all that apply.)
   1. hearing since that is the first sensation to return after anesthesia.
   2. ability to pull his drain from the wound.
   3. likeliness of becoming combative after surgery.
   4. ability to voluntarily move his extremity.
   5. Homans' sign in both lower extremities.
   6. circulation to the extremities.
10. A client returns to the PACU following a craniotomy. After assessing the airway, the first priority of the nurse is to:
    1. attach all tubes to drainage.
    2. place the client in Trendelenburg position.
    3. check abdomen for bowel sounds.
    4. assess level of consciousness and extremity movement.

REFERENCES/SUGGESTED READINGS

Aldrete, J. (1995). The post-anesthesia recovery score revisited. *Journal of Clinical Anesthesiology*, 7(1), 89–91.

Association of periOperative Registered Nurses (AORN). (2002a). Artificial nails. AORN Online Journal. [Online]. Available: www.aorn.org/journal/2002/juneci.htm

Association of periOperative Registered Nurses (2002b). Standards, recommended practices, and guidelines, Denver, CO: Author.

Brenner, Z. (1999). Preventing postoperative complications. *Nursing99*, 29(10), 34-39.

Bryant, R., & Nix, D. (2006). *Acute and chronic wounds: Current management concepts* (3rd ed.). St. Louis, MO: Mosby

Burden, N., Defazio-Quinn, D., & O'Brien, D. (2000). *Ambulatory surgical nursing*. Philadelphia: W. B. Saunders.

Cizzell, J. (1994). Back to basics: Test your wound assessment skills. *AJN*, 94(6), 34–35.

Crenshaw, J., & Winslow, E. (2002). Preoperative fasting: Old habits die hard. *AJN*, 102(5), 36–44.

Erwin-Toth, P., & Hocevar, B. (1995). Wound care: Selecting the right dressing. *AJN*, 95(2), 46–51.

Fort, C. (2002). Get pumped to prevent DVT. *Nursing2002*, 32(9), 50–52.

George Washington University Hospital. (2009). Thinking big about small incisions. *George Washington University Hospital Health News*. Retrieved on April 25, 2009 at http://gwashington.uhspublications.com/spring2009/story1.html

Gilchrist, B. (1990). Washing and dressings after surgery. *Journal of the Wound Care Society*, 86(50), 71.

Grogan, T. (1999). Bringing bloodless surgery into the mainstream. *Nursing99*, 29(11), 58–61.

Hogstel, M. (2001). *Gerontology: Nursing care of the older adult*. Clifton Park, NY: Delmar Cengage Learning.

Lewis, S., Collier, I., & Heitkemper, M. (2002). *Medical–surgical nursing: Assessment and management of clinical problems* (5th ed.). St. Louis, MO: Mosby.

Monahan, F., Sands, J., Neighbors, M., Marek, J., & Green-Nigro, C. (2006). *Phipps' medical-surgical nursing: Health and illness perspectives* (8th ed.). St. Louis, MO: Mosby.
Motta, G. (1993). How moisture retentive dressings promote healing. Nursing 93, 23(12), 26–33.
Ohio State Universtity Medical Center. (2009). What is minimally invasive surgery? Retrieved on April 25, 2009 at http://cmis.osu.edu/8880.cfm
Phillips, J. (1998). Wound dehiscence. *Nursing98*, 28(3), 33.
Phillips, N. (2007). *Berry and Kohn's operating room technique* (11th ed.). St. Louis, MO: C.V. Mosby Co.
Smeltzer, S., Bare, B. Hinkle, S., & Cheever, K. (2008). *Brunner and Suddarth's textbook of medical-surgical nursing* (11th ed.). Philadelphia: Lippincott Williams & Wilkins.
Surgical Associates at Virginia Hospital Center. (2009). Surgical wound care: Frequently asked questions. Retrieved on April 25, 2009 at http://www.SurgicalAssociatesVHC.com
Talabiska, D. (1995). *Malnutrition in the elderly. Newlines in Multi-Vitamin Infusion*, 4(2), 1, 2, 6.
Vernon, S., & Molnar-Pfeifer, G. (1997). Are you ready for bloodless surgery? *AJN*, 97(9), 40–47.
Winslow, E., & Jacobson, A. (2001). The case against artificial nails. *Nursing2001*, 31(10), 30.

RESOURCES

Association of periOperative Registered Nurses (AORN), http://www.aorn.org

Intuitive Surgical, Inc., http://www.intuitivesurgical.com

CHAPTER 3
Oncology

MAKING THE CONNECTION

Refer to the following chapters to increase your understanding of oncology nursing:

Adult Health Nursing

- *Surgery*
- *Hematologic and Lymphatic Systems*
- *Gastrointestinal System*
- *Neurological System*
- *Endocrine System*
- *Reproductive System*
- *Integumentary System*
- *Immune System*
- *The Older Adult*

LEARNING OBJECTIVES

Upon completion of this chapter, you should be able to:

- Define key terms.
- Explain how the behavior of cancer cells differs from that of normal cells.
- Describe the role of the nurse in cancer detection.
- Discuss three medical treatments for cancer.
- Describe four complications that can occur in advanced cancer.
- Discuss ways the licensed practical/vocational nurse can aid the client in coping with cancer.

KEY TERMS

alopecia
anorexia
antineoplastic
benign
biologic response modifier (BRM)
bone marrow transplantation (BMT)
cachexia
cancer
carcinogen
carcinoma
chemotherapy
curative surgery
differentiation
extravasation
leukemia
lymphoma
malignant
metastasis
neoplasm
oncology
palliative surgery
photodynamic therapy (PDT)
radiotherapy
reconstructive surgery
sarcoma
stomatitis
tumor marker
vesicant

INTRODUCTION

Cancer is a disease resulting from the uncontrolled growth of abnormal cells, which causes malignant cellular tumors. One in three Americans will develop some type of cancer during their lifetime. Cancer is the second-leading cause of death in the United States and can develop in individuals of any race, gender, age, socioeconomic status, or culture. It is not a single disease but, rather, a group of more than 200 different diseases that can attack any tissue or organ of the body.

According to the American Cancer Society (ACS), in the 1930s fewer than one in five cancer clients survived 5 years after diagnosis. In the 1940s, one in four survived 5 years. Today, 66% of people diagnosed with cancer will be alive in 5 years (ACS, 2003; ACS, 2008). Survival rates are influenced by the type of cancer, the progression of the disease at diagnosis, and the client's response to the treatment.

INCIDENCE

In the United States, men have a one in two lifetime risk of developing cancer, whereas women have a risk of one in three (ACS, 2008). Incidence and mortality rates are usually greater for African Americans than for Anglo Americans. The incidence of cancer is greater in the elderly population than in any other age group. In men, the most common cancers are prostate, lung, colorectal, and urinary bladder; in women, they are breast, lung, colorectal, and uterine cancer (Figure 3-1).

The ACS estimates that 1,437,180 new cancer cases were diagnosed in the United States in 2008. Not included in this estimate are basal- and squamous-cell skin cancers and noninvasive cancers except for urinary bladder cancer. More than 1 million cases of highly curable basal- and squamous-cell skin cancers were estimated to be diagnosed in 2008 (ACS, 2008).

In 2008, approximately 170,000 cancer deaths were estimated to be caused by tobacco. About one-third of the 565,650 cancer deaths estimated for 2008 are related to nutrition, physical inactivity, obesity, and other lifestyle factors and could be prevented (ACS, 2008).

PATHOPHYSIOLOGY

Cancer is a disease characterized by neoplasia, an uncontrolled growth of abnormal cells. Unlike normal cells, which reproduce in an orderly manner and grow for a purpose, cancer cells develop rapidly and undiscriminatingly, and they serve no useful function because they grow at the expense of healthy tissue. Neoplasms, any abnormal growth of new tissue, can be found in any body tissue. Neoplasms may be benign (not progressive and, thus, favorable for recovery) or malignant (becoming progressively worse and often resulting in death).

Benign neoplasms are not cancerous and are usually harmless. They grow slowly, are encapsulated and well-defined, and do not spread to neighboring tissues. Unless their location interferes with vital functions, benign neoplasms are associated with a favorable prognosis.

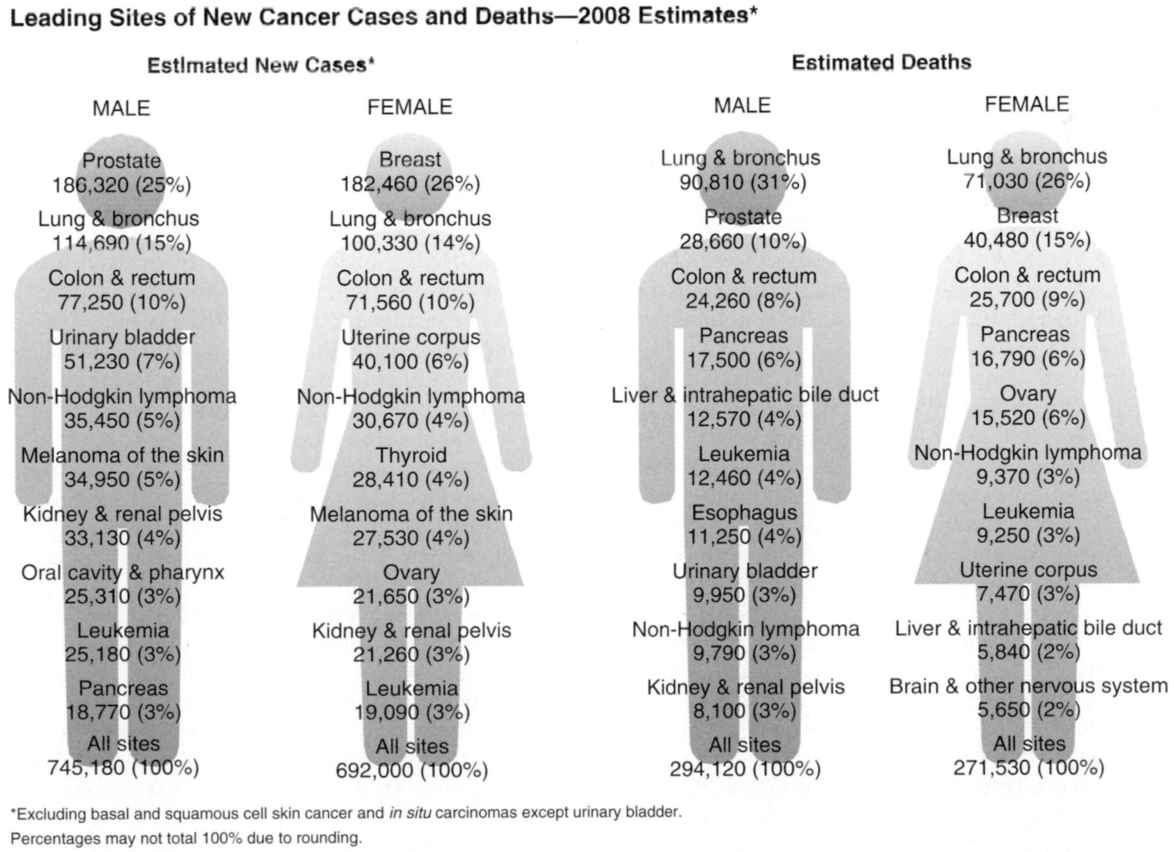

Leading Sites of New Cancer Cases and Deaths—2008 Estimates*

Estimated New Cases*		Estimated Deaths	
MALE	FEMALE	MALE	FEMALE
Prostate 186,320 (25%)	Breast 182,460 (26%)	Lung & bronchus 90,810 (31%)	Lung & bronchus 71,030 (26%)
Lung & bronchus 114,690 (15%)	Lung & bronchus 100,330 (14%)	Prostate 28,660 (10%)	Breast 40,480 (15%)
Colon & rectum 77,250 (10%)	Colon & rectum 71,560 (10%)	Colon & rectum 24,260 (8%)	Colon & rectum 25,700 (9%)
Urinary bladder 51,230 (7%)	Uterine corpus 40,100 (6%)	Pancreas 17,500 (6%)	Pancreas 16,790 (6%)
Non-Hodgkin lymphoma 35,450 (5%)	Non-Hodgkin lymphoma 30,670 (4%)	Liver & intrahepatic bile duct 12,570 (4%)	Ovary 15,520 (6%)
Melanoma of the skin 34,950 (5%)	Thyroid 28,410 (4%)	Leukemia 12,460 (4%)	Non-Hodgkin lymphoma 9,370 (3%)
Kidney & renal pelvis 33,130 (4%)	Melanoma of the skin 27,530 (4%)	Esophagus 11,250 (4%)	Leukemia 9,250 (3%)
Oral cavity & pharynx 25,310 (3%)	Ovary 21,650 (3%)	Urinary bladder 9,950 (3%)	Uterine corpus 7,470 (3%)
Leukemia 25,180 (3%)	Kidney & renal pelvis 21,260 (3%)	Non-Hodgkin lymphoma 9,790 (3%)	Liver & intrahepatic bile duct 5,840 (2%)
Pancreas 18,770 (3%)	Leukemia 19,090 (3%)	Kidney & renal pelvis 8,100 (3%)	Brain & other nervous system 5,650 (2%)
All sites 745,180 (100%)	All sites 692,000 (100%)	All sites 294,120 (100%)	All sites 271,530 (100%)

*Excluding basal and squamous cell skin cancer and *in situ* carcinomas except urinary bladder.
Percentages may not total 100% due to rounding.

FIGURE 3-1 Leading Sites of New Cancer Cases and Deaths—2008 Estimates (*American Cancer Society Cancer Facts and Figures, 2008. Reprinted with Permission.*)

Malignant neoplasms form irregularly shaped masses with fingerlike projections. They usually multiply quickly and spread to distant body parts through the bloodstream or the lymph system. This process is called metastasis. Patterns of metastasis will differ depending on the type of cancer.

Cancers are usually named according to the site of the primary tumor or to the type of tissue involved. There are four main classifications of cancer according to tissue type:

- **Lymphomas** (cancers occurring in infection-fighting organs, such as lymphatic tissue)
- **Leukemias** (cancers occurring in blood-forming organs, such as the spleen, and in bone marrow)
- **Sarcomas** (cancers occurring in connective tissue, such as bone)
- **Carcinomas** (cancers occurring in epithelial tissue, such as the skin)

The exact mechanism that causes cancer is unknown, but most authorities believe that cancer develops from a combination of factors rather than from a single factor. Environmental, genetic, and viral factors have been implicated in the development of cancer. Chemical substances that initiate or promote the development of cancer are known as carcinogens. These agents are thought to alter the DNA in the cell nucleus.

CLIENTTEACHING

Dietary Guidelines to Reduce the Risk of Cancer

- Choose most foods from plant sources.
  - Eat five or more servings of fruits and vegetables each day, especially green and dark-yellow vegetables and those in the cabbage family.
  - Consume other foods from plant sources including breads, cereals, pastas, beans (legumes), and soy products.
- Limit intake of high-fat foods, particularly from animal sources.
  - Choose foods low in fat.
  - Limit consumption of meats, especially red meats and high-fat meats.
- Be physically active and achieve and maintain a healthy weight.
  - Physical activity can help by balancing caloric intake with energy expenditures or by other mechanisms.
- Limit or eliminate consumption of alcoholic beverages.

(ACS, 2002; ACS, 2008)

RISK FACTORS

Many risk factors, such as environmental, lifestyle, genetic, and viral, may increase an individual's chances of developing cancer.

ENVIRONMENTAL FACTORS

The first environmental carcinogen was discovered in 1760, when Percival Pott noted that chimney sweeps had a very high rate of what is now known to be scrotal cancer because they were exposed to cancer-causing oils in the soot that was rubbed into their clothing. Since that time, hundreds of chemical carcinogens have been identified.

Many individuals come into contact with cancer-causing agents through occupational exposure. Industrial chemicals, such as asbestos or vinyl chlorides, have been found to be carcinogenic. For workers who handle these chemicals, the risk of developing cancers is greatly increased if occupational exposure is combined with cigarette smoking. Tobacco may act synergistically with other substances to promote cancer development. Occupational exposure to coal tar, creosote, arsenic compounds, or radium constitutes a risk factor for development of skin cancer. The effects of carcinogenic agents are usually dose dependent. The larger the dose or the longer the duration of exposure, the greater is the risk of cancer development. It is estimated that 80% of all cancers are associated with environmental exposures and might be prevented if exposure is avoided. Occupational Safety and Health Administration (OSHA) established safety standards and levels of exposure for those likely to be exposed to chemical carcinogens at work.

In 1993, the U.S. Environmental Protection Agency (EPA) declared secondhand smoke a human carcinogen. Approximately 3,000 nonsmoking adults die each year of lung cancer from breathing secondhand smoke (ACS, 2008).

LIFESTYLE FACTORS

Lifestyle factors include the use of tobacco, sun exposure, alcohol consumption, and diet. Tobacco accounts for nearly one in five deaths in the United States (ACS, 2008). Tobacco use includes cigarettes, cigars, pipes, and smokeless forms (e.g., snuff and chewing tobacco). The same carcinogens are found in all forms of tobacco, causing cancer of the oral cavity, esophagus, pharynx, and larynx. When tobacco is smoked, it can also cause cancer of the lung, pancreas, uterus, cervix, kidney, and bladder.

Overexposure to the sun's ultraviolet rays over long periods of time is the cause of many skin cancers. The most serious form of skin cancer is melanoma. The ACS (2008) estimates 62,480 newly diagnosed cases of melanoma in 2008. Other factors predisposing a person to skin cancer are family history, multiple nevi, and atypical nevi.

Heavy alcohol consumption has also been implicated in mouth, throat, esophageal, and liver cancers. Alcohol is hypothesized to cause 5% of cancer deaths. Alcohol and tobacco used together greatly increase the risk of oral and esophageal cancers. The combined effect of alcohol and tobacco is greater than the sum of their individual effects (ACS, 2008). Despite the epidemiological evidence linking alcohol to cancer, the exact carcinogen in alcohol is yet to be determined. Table 3-1 lists some risk factors for cancer.

Table 3-1 Risk Factors for Cancer

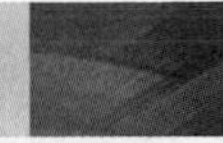

Breast Cancer

- Family history (immediate female relatives)
- High-fat diet
- Obesity after menopause
- Early menarche, late menopause
- Alcohol consumption
- Postmenopausal estrogen and progestin
- First child after age 30

Cervical Cancer

- Multiple sexual partners
- Having sex at early age
- Exposure to human papillomavirus
- Smoking

Colorectal Cancer

- Family history (immediate relatives)
- Low-fiber diet
- History of rectal polyps

Esophageal Cancer

- Heavy alcohol consumption
- Smoking

Lung Cancer

- Cigarette smoking
- Asbestos, arsenic, and radon exposure
- Secondhand smoke
- Tuberculosis

Skin Cancer

- Excessive exposure to ultraviolet radiation (sun)
- Fair complexion
- Work with coal, tar, pitch, or creosote
- Multiple or atypical nevi (males)

Stomach Cancer

- Family history
- Diet heavy in smoked, pickled, or salted foods

Testicular Cancer

- Undescended testicles
- Consumption of hormones by mother during pregnancy

Prostate Cancer

- Increasing age
- Family history
- Diet high in animal fat

Research suggests that an increase in dietary fiber may help prevent colon cancer. Some studies have suggested that obesity is a significant risk factor for breast, colon, endometrial, and prostate cancers. Studies have also shown that diets high in salt-cured, smoked, and nitrite-cured foods increase an individual's risk for cancer of the stomach and esophagus. Food substances that may reduce cancer risk include cruciferous vegetables (cabbage, broccoli, cauliflower, brussels sprouts, kohlrabi); possibly vitamins A, E, and C; and selenium. Some foods have been found to contain carcinogens in the forms of additives or as by-products of storage. On the basis of current knowledge, the ACS has offered dietary guidelines to reduce cancer risk.

Genetic Factors

Some families have a high incidence of certain types of cancer. Women whose mothers, grandmothers, or sisters have had breast cancer have twice the risk of developing cancer as those whose first-degree relatives have not had the disease (ACS, 2008). Leukemia and cancers of the colon, stomach, prostate, lung, and ovary may also run in families. Therefore, relatives of persons with these cancers should be carefully monitored.

Viral Factors

Although viruses have been linked to several cancers, their exact role is unclear. It has been theorized that they incorporate themselves into the genetic structure of the cell. Herpes simplex II virus and some of the human papillomaviruses that are transmitted sexually are known to predispose women to cervical cancer. Reducing the number of sexual partners can reduce the risk of contracting these viruses.

CLIENT TEACHING

Lifestyle Guidelines to Reduce the Risk of Cancer

- Do not smoke or use tobacco in any form.
- Avoid overexposure to the sun and indoor tanning.
- Eat a healthy diet.
- Get plenty of exercise.
- Have a physical examination on a routine basis, including a mammogram, Pap smear, testicular, and colon examinations.
- Get plenty of sleep (6 to 8 hours per night).
- Keep weight within normal limits.
- Practice regular self-examinations and see your physician if any changes are noted.
- Know and follow health and safety rules at the workplace.
- Avoid unprotected sexual behaviors.

DETECTION

When cancer develops, the earlier it is detected the more likely it is to be controlled. In some cases, a diagnosis is made before symptoms become apparent. Cancer is usually found by the affected individual, who notices a warning sign, or by a health-care provider during a checkup. A cancer checkup is recommended every 3 years for persons ages 20 to 39 years and annually for those ages 40 years and older. Risk assessment is the first step in cancer prevention. The cancer examination includes both a medical history of exposures to environmental agents and a comprehensive family history.

If cancer is suspected, various diagnostic studies are performed depending on the suspected primary or metastatic site of the cancer. They include laboratory studies or blood tests, radiologic studies, endoscopy, cytology, and biopsy. Nurses educate clients about such tests as well as assist in client preparation.

Although no one blood test can confirm a cancer diagnosis, some malignancies do alter the chemical composition of the blood. Specialized laboratory tests have been developed to detect **tumor markers**, substances such as specific proteins, antigens, genes, hormones, or enzymes that are found in the serum and indicate the possible presence of malignancy. Tumor markers are not 100% accurate because benign processes can also cause elevations; they are, however, useful in monitoring response to treatment or detecting a relapse. (See Table 3-2 for cancer-screening guidelines.)

CLIENT TEACHING

Warning Signs of Cancer

The professional nurse educates individuals about the warning signs of cancer. The seven warning signs can be easily remembered through an acronym, CAUTION.

C: Change in bladder or bowel habits, such as absence of urination or bowel movement or excessive urination or stool.

A: A sore that does not heal within a realistic period of time.

U: Unusual bleeding or discharge from any body orifice, such as the vagina, the nipple, or the penis. The unusual discharge can be bloody, purulent, clear, or viscous. The keywords are *unusual* and *any body orifice*.

T: Thickening or the presence of a lump of the breast, testicle, or any part of the body.

I: Indigestion or difficulty swallowing for a prolonged period of time.

O: Obvious change in a wart or mole, such as color, size, texture.

N: Nagging cough or hoarseness that is prolonged.

If any of these warning signs are observed, encourage client to see a health-care provider.

Courtesy of Daniels, R, Nosek, L., & Nicoll, L. (2010). Contemporary medical-surgical nursing. Clifton Park, NY: Delmar, Cengage Learning.

CRITICAL THINKING

Cancer Detection

Which diagnostic tests should a person have as part of a routine physical to detect cancer?

COMMON DIAGNOSTIC TESTS

Commonly used diagnostic tests for clients who present with symptoms of cancer are listed in Table 3-3. See Basic Nursing Diagnostic Tests, for explanation/normal values and nursing responsibilities related to each test.

STAGING OF TUMORS

Staging determines the extent of the spread of cancer. The TNM classification proposed by the American Joint Commission on Cancer is one of the most frequently used systems. The T refers to the anatomical size of the primary tumor; N, the extent of lymph node involvement; and M, the presence or absence of metastasis (Table 3-4). Use of this internationally recognized staging system for tumors ensures a reliable comparison of clients in many different hospitals. Staging is important because it influences decisions about treatment modalities and helps predict overall prognosis.

GRADING OF TUMORS

Normal body cells have individual characteristics that allow them to perform different body functions. This process is called **differentiation**. Tumor cells that retain many of the identifiable tissue characteristics of the original cell are termed *well differentiated*. Tumor cells having little similarity to the tissue of origin are termed *undifferentiated*. Tumor grading is based primarily on the degree of differentiation of malignant cells. Grading evaluates tumor cells in comparison with normal cells. Pathologists indicate tumor cell grades by using the Roman numerals I through IV; the higher the grade, the higher the number and the worse the prognosis. Thus, a grade I tumor is the most differentiated, and a grade IV tumor is the most undifferentiated (or least differentiated). Tumors containing poorly differentiated cells are more aggressive in growth and may display uncharacteristic behaviors, leading to a poorer prognosis. Grading criteria vary for different neoplasms.

Table 3-2 Screening Guidelines

SITE	AGE TO BEGIN	RECOMMENDATIONS	PREFERRED/ALTERNATIVE
Colorectal	50	One of the following initially: fecal occult blood or fecal immunochemical test annually; flexible sigmoidoscopy every 5 years; barium enema every 5 years; colonoscopy every 10 years.	Combination testing rather than a single diagnostic test.
Prostate	50	Protein-specific antigen (PSA) test and digital rectal exam (DRE) to men who have a life expectancy of at least 10 years	Begin at age 45 for African-American men and men with a strong family history.
Breast	20	Beginning at age 20, breast self-exams monthly and clinical breast exams every 3 years. Beginning at age 40, add annual mammograms and clinical breast exams.	Women at greater risk may begin mammograms at earlier age, or have additional tests performed (MRI, ultrasound, etc.).
Cervical	21, or 3 years after beginning vaginal intercourse	Pap test annually. After total hysterectomy with cervix removal screening is not necessary unless the surgery was performed as treatment for cervical cancer.	Pap test may be every 2 years, with a liquid-based test. A woman 30 or older with three normal test results in a row may be screened every 2–3 years. As an alternative HPV DNA testing and cytology could be done every 3 years. High-risk women may get screened more often. Women older than 70 years of age with three or more consecutive normal Pap tests in past 10 years may choose to stop screening.
Endometrium	35	Annual screening with biopsy for women with or at risk for HNPCC (hereditary nonpolyposis colon cancer).	All women at menopause should be educated about risks and symptoms and be encouraged to report any unexpected spotting or bleeding.

From *Cancer facts & figures*, by ACS Recommendations, 2006, Atlanta, GA: American Cancer Society; Understanding Neoplasms, *by R. Teasley, in press.*

TREATMENT MODALITIES

After cancer is diagnosed, staged, and graded, a medical treatment plan is developed. The most common treatment methods used are surgery, radiation therapy, and **chemotherapy** (use of drugs to treat illness); biotherapy/immunotherapy, hormone therapy, targeted therapy, photodynamic therapy, and bone marrow transplantation also are used. These methods may be used alone or in combination.

Surgery

Surgery is the oldest form of cancer treatment and remains the most common method of treatment today. Surgery is classified as curative, palliative, or reconstructive.

The goal of **curative surgery** is to heal or restore to health; this involves excising all of the tumor, the involved surrounding tissue, and the regional lymph nodes. Surgery most often has curative results when performed in the early stages of cervical, breast, or skin cancer.

CRITICAL THINKING

Teaching Risk Factors for Cancer

A neighbor, a 45-year-old female, asks you if there is anything she can do to "cancer-proof" her lifestyle. She tells you that there have been several incidences of cancer diagnosed in family members, although none have been in her immediate family. What is the best answer you can give her?

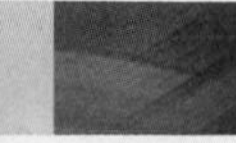

Table 3-3 Common Diagnostic Tests for Cancer Detection

Laboratory Tests
- Acid phosphatase (elevated)
- Alkaline phosphatase (elevated)
- Bence Jones protein
- CA-15-3
- CA-19-9
- CA-125
- CEA (carcinoembryonic antigen)
- Fecal occult blood test (FOBT) or fecal immunochemical test (FIT)
- PSA (prostate-specific antigen)
- Stool for occult blood (Guaiac)
- Serum calcitonin

Radiologic Studies
- X-ray studies
- Computerized axial tomography (CT scan or CAT scan)
- Magnetic resonance imaging (MRI)
- Scans (radioisotope test)
- Ultrasound
- Mammograms

Invasive Diagnostic Techniques
- Endoscopy
- Cytology
- Biopsy

Because 70% of clients show evidence of metastasis at diagnosis, cure is not always possible, and **palliative surgery** may be necessary. This surgery is effective in relieving symptoms in more advanced stages of cancer, although it does not alter the course of the disease. It is usually performed in an attempt to relieve complications such as obstructions or to surgically interrupt nerve pathways for intractable pain. It may also be used to insert special access devices or to place tubes for enteral nutrition.

Reconstructive surgery is performed to reestablish function or rebuild for a better cosmetic effect. Reconstructive surgery to areas such as the head, neck, breast, and extremities minimizes deformity. The surgery is completed all at once or done in stages.

RADIATION THERAPY

Radiation therapy is the second most common method of treating cancer. Radiation therapy, or **radiotherapy,** uses high-energy ionizing radiation to kill cancer. Ionizing radiation penetrates tissue cells and deposits energy within them. This intense energy causes breakage in chromosomes within the cell, thus preventing the ability of the cell to replicate. Cell death occurs hours, days, or even years after treatment, depending on the rate of mitosis.

The goal of radiation therapy is to eradicate malignant cells without causing harm to healthy tissues. Some cells are more sensitive to radiation than others. Better vascularized, better oxygenated cells and those that divide rapidly are the most sensitive.

It is used alone or as an adjunct to other therapies. As a single treatment modality, it is most often used when the disease is localized. Preoperative radiation is frequently used to reduce the tumor mass before surgery. Postoperative radiation therapy is frequently used to decrease the risk of local recurrence after surgery. Some chemotherapeutic drugs increase the sensitivity of cancer cells to radiation and thus are used together with radiation. Radiation therapy is classified as curative or palliative. It is frequently used to alleviate symptoms of metastasis, such as pain.

There are two types of radiation therapy: external radiation and internal radiation.

External Radiation

External radiation, or teletherapy, is performed with special equipment that can deliver high-energy radiation. Treatments are usually administered on an outpatient basis, divided over many days or weeks. Customized shielding blocks are created to protect healthy tissues, and immobilization devices are used to maintain the exact position for each treatment. Dyes or tattoos may be used to designate reference points on the skin.

Nursing care is directed toward client teaching, safety, and performing interventions that provide relief from side effects. Undesirable side effects that are most likely to occur include varying degrees of skin reactions and gastrointestinal discomfort, such as abdominal cramping, diarrhea, loss of appetite, and fatigue. Treatments have a cumulative effect and may thus produce symptoms after the therapy has been completed.

Internal Radiation

Internal radiation delivers radioactive isotopes directly within the body. Clients treated with internal sources of radiation are a source of radioactivity. Isotopes are introduced into the body by sealed or unsealed sources.

With sealed sources, radioactive elements are encapsulated in special containers such as tubes, wires, needles, seeds, or capsules. These containers are implanted close to the cancer cells to deliver a highly concentrated dose of radiation to the cancer cells. Radioactive implants are used in the treatment of

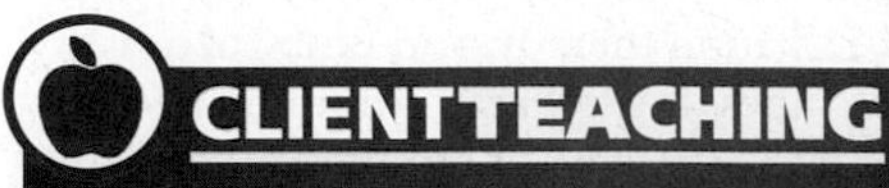

External Radiation

- Do not wash off the skin markings used to designate reference points for treatment.
- Client is alone in the room during treatment.
- Client must lie absolutely still.
- Treatment typically lasts 1 to 3 minutes.
- Treatment is usually painless.

Table 3-4 Staging of Tumors: TNM Classification

STAGE	TUMOR	LYMPH NODE	METASTASIS
I	<2 cm diameter Mobile Often superficial Confined to organ of origin	No involvement	No evidence
II	2 to 5 cm diameter No as mobile Extension into adjacent tissue	Palpable, mobile >2 to 3 cm diameter Firmer than normal	No evidence
III a	>5 cm diameter Not mobile Regional involvement	No involvement	No evidence
III b	<2 to >5 cm diameter Mobile or not mobile Localized or extended	>2 to 3 cm diameter Firmer than normal	No evidence
IV a	>10 cm diameter Extension into another organ; major arteries, veins, or nerves; or bone	No involvement or >2 to 3 cm diameter Firmer than normal	No evidence
IV b	No evidence to >10 cm diameter	3 to 5 cm diameter Partially mobile Firm to hard; or >5 cam diameter Extended and fixed to bone, large blood vessels, skin, or nerves	No evidence
IV c	No evidence to >10 cm diameter	No evidence to >10 cm diameter Fixed and destructive Extension to second or distant stations	Solitary or multiple

SAFETY

Internal Radiation

Client care is modified based on the three factors related to the degree of exposure to sealed-source radiation by:

- Preparing everything outside of the room so that as little time as possible is spent close to the client.
- Having several nurses assigned to care for the client so that the time of exposure for each nurse is lessened.
- Wearing a lead apron or other shielding device, as provided.

cancers of the tongue, lip, breast, vagina, cervix, endometrium, rectum, bladder, and brain.

Because sources are sealed, body fluids are not radioactive. Personnel caring for clients who have sealed sources must still be familiar with the hazards of radiation, however. Generally, the degree of exposure is dependent on three factors:

- The distance between the individual and the source (Figure 3-2)
- The amount of time an individual is exposed
- The type of shielding provided

Radioactive isotopes also are placed in suspensions or solutions as unsealed sources of radiation. They are given orally or parenterally or instilled into intrapleural or peritoneal spaces.

Some radioactive elements used in unsealed radiation sources are eliminated in body secretions, including urine and stool; thus health care workers must take special

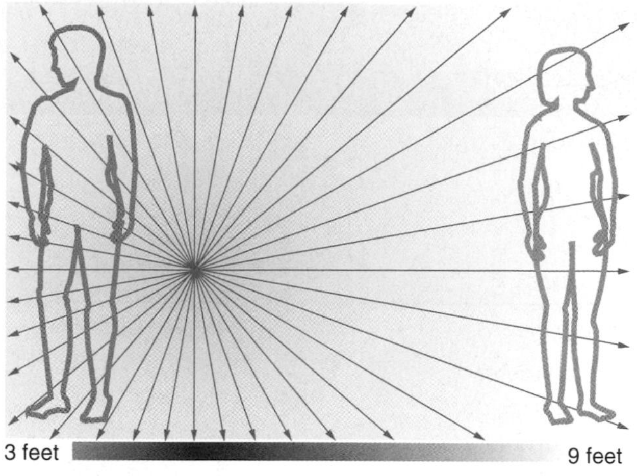

FIGURE 3-2 Radiation dose decreases with distance. (*Courtesy of the U.S. Nuclear Regulatory Commission.*)

precautions to avoid exposure. Agency policies and procedures as well as Standard Precautions are followed closely. Unsealed sources are not usually radioactive as long as the sealed sources.

CHEMOTHERAPY

Chemotherapy is used to cure, prevent, or relieve cancer symptoms. Drugs used in chemotherapy are called **antineoplastics** because they inhibit the growth and reproduction of malignant cells. To understand how anticancer drugs work, one must have a basic understanding of the cell cycle.

Almost all anticancer drugs kill cancer cells by affecting DNA synthesis or function, but they vary in how they exert their activity within the cell cycle. Most chemotherapeutic drugs are classified as cell-cycle specific (CCS) or cell-cycle nonspecific (CCNS).

CCS drugs attack cancer cells when the cells enter a certain phase of reproduction. These agents are most effective against rapidly growing tumors. Many of the drugs are "schedule dependent" because they produce a greater cell kill when given in multiple, repeated doses.

CCNS drugs can destroy cancer cells in any phase of the cell cycle and are used for large tumors that have fewer actively dividing cells. These drugs are not schedule dependent but, rather, dose dependent. This means that the number of cells destroyed is determined by the amount of drug given.

Anticancer agents are cytotoxic (toxic to cells) and destroy both normal and abnormal cells. They are most effective against cells that reproduce rapidly, such as those in bone marrow, gastrointestinal lining, hair follicles, and the ova and sperm. Because cells multiply at their most rapid rate at the beginning of the disease, the drugs work best against cancer in its earliest stages.

Many of these drugs are given in combination with or after radiation or surgery to achieve maximum effect. They are usually given intermittently over an extended period. Drug resistance can occur.

The most common routes of administration are oral and intravenous. A few drugs are given topically, subcutaneously, or intramuscularly. Recently, other methods have been introduced to increase the local concentration of the drug at the tumor site, including intrathecal injection and intracavity instillation. Table 3-5 lists some commonly used drugs.

Careful attention is given to intravenous administration. Leakage of fluid from the vein into the surrounding tissues during infusion is called **extravasation**. Because most chemotherapeutic drugs are irritating to the tissues, extravasation is a potentially serious problem, especially if the drugs administered are **vesicants**. These agents are so irritating that they can cause blistering and even necrosis. All sites must be monitored carefully. Pain, swelling, redness, and the presence of vesicles are all signs of extravasation. Additional signs include the following:

PROFESSIONAL TIP

Chemotherapy and Protective Equipment

- Because many chemotherapy drugs are carcinogenic, the nurse preparing and administering the chemotherapy wears protective equipment.
- All personnel involved in any aspect of handling chemotherapeutic agents receive instructions about the known risks of the drugs, the proper use of protective equipment, the applicable skill procedures, and the policies regarding pregnant personnel.

COMMUNITY/HOME HEALTH CARE

Home Care After Chemotherapy

Teach clients receiving chemotherapy to monitor the side effects of therapy at home.

- Inspect the skin daily for any signs of rash or dermatitis, which indicates hypersensitivity to a drug.
- Report taste loss and tingling in the face, fingers, or toes, which may signal peripheral neuropathy.
- Report signs of dizziness, headache, confusion, slurred speech, or convulsions, which are signs of central nervous system (CNS) toxicity.
- Report signs of unusual bleeding or bruising; fever; sore throat; or mouth sores, which may signal developing myelosuppression.
- Report signs of jaundice; yellowing of the eyes; clay-colored stools; or dark urine, which signals developing hepatic dysfunction.
- Report a continued cough or shortness of breath, which indicates developing pulmonary fibrosis.

Table 3-5 Drugs Commonly Used in Chemotherapy

Antimetabolites (CC5)	**Antibiotics (CCNS)**	**Antihormonal Agents (CCNS)**
cytarabine (Cytosar)	dactinomycin (Cosmegan)*	flutamide (Eulexin)
fluorouracil (Adrucil 5-FU)	daunorubicin (Cerubidine)*	goserelin acetate (Zoladex)
methotrexate (Mexate, Folex)	doxorubicin hydrochloride (Adriamycin)*	tamoxifen (Nolvadex)
6-mercaptopurine (Purinethol)	mitomycin (Mutamycin)*	
	mithramycin (Mithracin)	
	bleomycin (Blenoxane)	
Vinca Plant Alkaloids (CCS)	**Hormones (CCNS)**	**Nitrosureas (CCNS)**
vinblastine sulfate (Velban)*	diethylstilbestrol (DES)	carmustine (BiCNU)
vincristine sulfate (Oncovin)*	megestrol acetate (Megace)	lomustine (CeeNU)
	medroxyprogesterone acetate (Depo-Provera)	
	testosterone (Histerone, Testoderm)	
	tamoxifen citrate (Nolvadex)	
Alkylating Agents (CCNS)	**Corticosteroids**	**Miscellaneous Agents**
busulfan (Myleran)	dexamethasone (Decadron)	etoposide (VePesid)
chlorambucil (Leukeran)	hydrocortisone sodium succinate (Solu-Cortef)	L-asparaginase (Elspar)
cisplatin (Platinol)	prednisone (Deltasone)	procarbazine hydrochloride (Matulane)
cyclophosphamide (Cytoxan)		
mechlorethamine hydrochloride (Mustargen)*		
melphalan (Alkeran)		
thiotepa (Thiotepa)		

Frequently Used Combinations	
CAF	cyclophosphamide, doxorubicin, and fluorourcil (5-FU)
CHOP	cyclophosphamide, doxorubicin, vincristine (Oncovin), and prednisolone
C-VAMP	cyclophosphamide, vincristine, doxorubicin, and methyl-prednisolone
CVP	cyclophosphamide, vincristine, and prednisone
ECF	epirubicin, cisplatin, and fluorourcil
FEC	fluorourcil, epirubicin, and cyclophosphamide
MMM	mitomycin, methotrexate, and mitoxantrone
MOPP	mechlorethamine hydrochloride (Mustargen), vincristine, procarbazine, and prednisone
MVP	mitomycin, vinblastine, and cisplatin

*= vesicant drug

- Pain or burning at the site or along the vein
- Absent or sluggish blood return
- Redness 6 to 12 hours later
- Swelling
- Diffuse hardening

If extravasation occurs, the drug is stopped immediately and protocols for treatment initiated.

Improved infusion techniques, control of symptoms such as nausea and vomiting, and cost-containment restrictions have reduced the length of hospitalizations for clients undergoing chemotherapy. Teaching clients and family members to monitor side effects in the home setting is thus an essential function of the **oncology** (study of tumors) nurse.

Clients also are advised that their lifestyle may need adjustment to accommodate the side effects of chemotherapy. Clients are instructed to pace themselves according to their energy level and allow time for rest throughout the day. It is also important to inform clients that even between treatments they may not have the same amount of energy as before treatment initiation. Many clients do not experience any adverse effects, but some experience life-threatening toxicity. Nursing care of the client receiving chemotherapy requires not only a thorough understanding of the drugs used to destroy the cancer, but also skills in helping clients and families cope with the side effects of the therapy.

Biotherapy

Biotherapy/immunotherapy is performed with **biologic response modifiers (BRMs)**, agents that stimulate the body's natural immune system to control and destroy malignant cells. Some BRMs are being evaluated in trial studies. Biotherapy is used after surgery, radiation, and chemotherapy have removed the bulk of the tumor. Some agents currently used include interferons, monoclonal antibodies, interleukin-2, tumor necrosis factor, *bacillus Calmette-Guérin (BCG),* and colony-stimulating factors. Side effects are usually less severe than those seen in chemotherapy and include fever, malaise, myalgia, and headache. Because an anaphylactic reaction can occur, the client must be closely monitored.

Photodynamic Therapy

Photodynamic therapy (PDT) has a 90% effective rate when used for esophageal cancer and early-stage lung cancer (Cancer Treatment Centers of America, 2009b). PDT is also used as an investigation therapy for obstructive lung cancer, Barrett's esophagus, and head, neck and skin cancer. The client is injected with a light-activated drug (Photofrin) that targets cancerous cells. Twenty-four to 48 hours after injecting the drug, a low-power laser light is directed by a fiberoptic guide to the cancerous tissue area through an endoscope. The light stimulates the drug to destroy the cancerous cells, but the surrounding healthy tissue is not harmed. An advantage of PDT is the client has the procedure performed on an outpatient basis with slight sedation and is relatively pain free. There is less risk than with a surgical procedure, and there are fewer side effects. The side effects of PDT are discomfort from local swelling, nausea, fever, and constipation. The client experiences sunburn, redness, and swelling if the skin and eyes are exposed to a bright light or sunlight.

> **▼ SAFETY ▼**
>
> **Chemotherapy and Contamination**
>
> - Any personnel handling blood, vomitus, or excreta from clients who have received chemotherapy within the previous 48 hours wears disposable latex gloves and a disposable gown.
> - Place contaminated linen in specially marked laundry bags according to agency procedures.

Hormone Therapy

Some cancerous cells need estrogen, progesterone, or testosterone to grow. The goal of hormone therapy is to deprive the cancerous cells of these hormones. Clients may have the ovaries (**oophorectomy**) or testicles (**orchiectomy**) removed. Another method of depriving the cells of hormonal stimulation is to give women with early-stage breast cancer tamoxifen citrate (Nolvadex) and to give men luteinizing hormone-releasing hormone (LHRH). LHRH prevents the testes from producing testosterone. Tamoxifen is a systemic treatment and increases the chances for endometrial cancer. Hormone therapy is effective for a time in men, but eventually prostate cancer grows without hormone stimulation. The hormone therapy is no longer effective when this occurs (Cancer Treatment Centers of America, 2009c).

Targeted Cancer Therapy

Most targeted cancer therapies are in preclinical testing (animal research) and clinical trial (human research). Some drugs have been approved by the U.S. Food and Drug Administration (FDA). The goal of targeted cancer therapy is to stop the growth and spread of cancer cells by preventing normal cells from changing into cancerous cells at the molecular or cellular level. This therapy is more effective than present treatments and causes less harm to healthy cells. An example of targeted therapy is STI-571, or imatinib mesylate (Gleevac®), which is a small-molecule drug used to treat gastrointestinal stromal tumor and chronic myeloid leukemia (National Cancer Institute, 2006).

Bone Marrow Transplantation

Bone marrow transplantation (BMT) is used for cancers that respond to high doses of chemotherapy or radiation therapy. Treatment involves aspirating and storing a fraction of bone marrow, exposing the client to high-dose drug therapy or total-body irradiation, and then reinfusing the bone marrow after the treatment is complete.

The bone marrow used in transplantation can be the client's own marrow (autologous), marrow taken from an identical twin (syngeneic), or marrow taken from a histocompatibly matched donor, preferably a sibling (allogeneic).

Client expenses for BMT are high, ranging from $50,000 to $100,000 for an autologous transplant, and $100,000 to $200,000 for an allogeneic transplant unless covered or partially covered by insurance (NBMTLink, 2009). The average length of hospital stay is 35 to 40 days. Complications can be life-threatening and include infection, bleeding, gastrointestinal effects, renal insufficiency, veno-occlusive disease (deposits of fibrin obstruct venules of liver), and graft-versus-host disease (new bone marrow cells recognize environment as foreign and try to destroy the host). Clients who undergo autologous BMT do not experience graft-versus-host disease.

SYMPTOM MANAGEMENT

Cancer clients undergoing treatment experience a variety of secondary problems. One of the most important responsibilities of the oncology nurse is to formulate nursing interventions to manage these problems.

Bone Marrow Dysfunction

Cancer treatments kill both malignant cells and normal cells in bone marrow. Blood counts are monitored carefully during and after treatment.

A low white-cell count increases the risk of infection. A decreased neutrophil count ($<500\ mm^3$) is an indicator that special infection prevention measures should be initiated. Scrupulous hand hygiene is the most effective method of controlling bacterial infection. Personnel maintain strict asepsis when changing dressings or performing invasive procedures. Clients avoid contact with anyone who is ill. Antimicrobial soaps are used for bathing clients. The skin and mucous membranes are inspected daily for signs of infection. Vital signs are taken every 4 hours and the client observed for fever and chilling.

Clients with a platelet count of $<50{,}000\ mm^3$ are monitored for bleeding. Their skin is inspected daily for bruises or petechiae. Shaving is undertaken with an electric razor to minimize the chance of cutting the skin. Stool and urine are monitored for occult blood. Observe the client for bleeding from the vagina, rectum, nose, mouth, and venipuncture sites. If bleeding occurs, pressure is applied to the site for 5 minutes. Any bleeding that does not stop in 5 minutes is reported. A soft toothbrush is recommended for oral care. Aspirin or any medication containing acetylsalicylic acid is not given.

Nutritional Alterations

Cytokines are substances secreted by the tumor in an attempt to cannibalize the body and by the immune system to fight the tumor. Cytokines make the body digest muscle for energy instead of using stored fat for this purpose. This state of malnutrition and protein (muscle) wasting is called **cachexia**. It occurs in conjunction with lung, pancreatic, stomach, bowel, and prostate cancers but rarely with breast cancer.

In some cases, untreated cachexia, rather than the cancer itself, is the cause of death. Untreated cachexia also decreases the effectiveness of cancer treatments and increases the side effects of these treatments. Treating cachexia with drugs has met with little success.

A registered dietitian understands cancer cachexia and can identify appetizing foods that are nutrient and calorie dense. Foods that appeal to the client are eaten anytime. The use of liquid nutritional supplements and a multivitamin is often recommended (Wilkes, 2000).

Hallmarks of malnutrition are a weight loss of 10% or more or a serum albumin level <3.4 g/dL. Clients unable to maintain sufficient oral intake for long periods are given enteral or total parenteral nutrition (TPN). Nutritional problems associated with cachexia include anorexia, nausea and vomiting, altered taste sensation, mucosal inflammation, and dysphagia.

Anorexia

Anorexia, or the loss of appetite, is a common concern among individuals with cancer. It is generally best for these

CLIENTTEACHING

Increasing Nutritional Intake

- Drink 4 ounces of a nutritional supplement before breakfast.
- Eat breakfast (if desired), and then take a walk. Doing so will help build muscle and increase appetite.
- Drink another 4 ounces of nutritional supplement 1 hour before having a lunch consisting of whatever foods are appealing.
- Have another 4 ounces of nutritional supplement at midafternoon and at bedtime.
- If not hungry for dinner, take another walk.

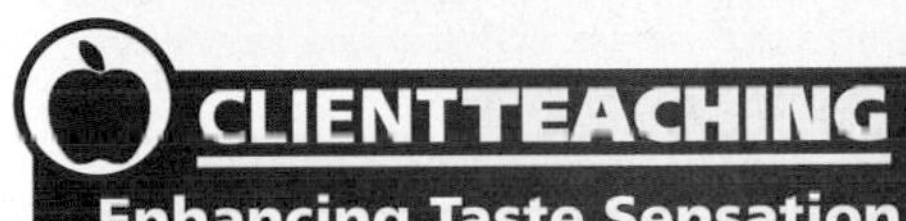

Enhancing Taste Sensation

- Tart food usually enhances taste sensation.
- Many foods taste better if they are cold or at room temperature.
- Using plastic utensils reduces metallic taste.

clients to eat small, frequent, high-calorie (carbohydrate and fat-rich) meals. Try to ascertain the client's likes and dislikes. Highly seasoned foods help increase taste. Clients are encouraged to eat when they are feeling best. Weight is monitored weekly.

Nausea and Vomiting

Nausea and vomiting usually occur within 3 to 4 hours after chemotherapy is administered and may last up to 72 hours. Antiemetics are given before chemotherapy and continued afterward as needed (Table 3-6). Small, frequent feedings of complex carbohydrates may be beneficial. Liquids are given 30 to 60 minutes before meals. Although highly seasoned foods may increase taste, they often also increase nausea and vomiting. Cool, bland foods are more easily tolerated. Avoid foods with strong odors. Frequent mouth care helps remove the taste of chemotherapy and increase the likelihood of the client's wanting to eat. The client should be monitored for dehydration and electrolyte imbalances.

Table 3-6 Commonly Used Antiemetics

Table 3-6 Commonly Used Antiemetics
prochlorperazine (Compazine)
metoclopramide (Reglan)
ondansetron hydrochloride (Zofron)
lorazepam (Ativan)
dolasetron (Anzemet)

PROFESSIONALTIP

Mucosal Inflammation

- The condition of the client's mouth provides a clue to the appearance and integrity of other areas of the gastrointestinal tract because mucosal inflammation caused by cancer treatments affects all mucosa.
- Mucositis (inflammation of the mucous membrane) in the esophagus, also called esophagitis, causes painful swallowing.
- In female clients, mucosal inflammation is found in the vagina, causing pain, itching, and discharge.

Altered Taste Sensation

Taste sensation is altered because cancer cells release substances that stimulate bitter taste buds, causing a bitter or metallic taste in the mouths of some clients. Some find they no longer enjoy the taste of red meat, and others say they have an aversion to sweets.

Mucosal Inflammation

Stomatitis, or inflammation of the mucous membrane of the oral cavity, occurs in one-half of cancer clients receiving treatment. It usually occurs 7 to 14 days after chemotherapy administration and lasts 2 to 3 weeks. To minimize stomatitis, assess for early signs and symptoms such as edema, ulceration, erythema, excessive saliva, and infection. If the client is receiving a chemotherapy drug that is known to cause stomatitis (e.g., methotrexate) oral care is administered at least four times a day.

Avoid rough, chewy foods and acidic foods. Straws are beneficial because food is taken in the back of the mouth and swallowed. Popsicles and frozen fruit bars sometimes help numb and lessen pain. Avoid commercial mouthwashes containing alcohol. A saline rinse may be helpful after meals. If the client has dentures, remove them at night. Viscous Xylocaine rinses are ordered for pain. Lemon and glycerine swabs are not used because lemon is irritating to mouth lesions.

Dysphagia

Dysphagia, difficulty in swallowing, often occurs in clients with esophageal cancers, or in those receiving radiotherapy.

Artificial saliva is ordered for severe dryness. A softer diet along with nutritional supplements is prescribed. Dry foods such as toast can scratch the delicate tissues of the throat. Food puréed in a blender is easier to tolerate. Encourage clients to take plenty of time to chew and swallow.

Pain

Approximately 60% to 90% of all individuals with progressive malignancy experience pain. The pain may be acute, but it is more likely to be chronic (>3 months in duration).

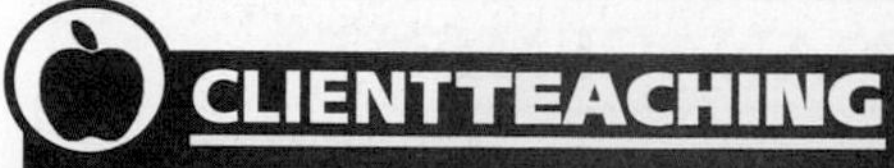

CLIENTTEACHING

Stomatitis

- Use soft bristle toothbrush.
- Avoid flossing if bleeding or discomfort occurs.
- Avoid tobacco products and alcohol because of their drying effects.

Pain usually does not occur until the advanced stages of the disease. The most common causes of pain are metastatic bone disease, venous or lymphatic obstruction, or nerve compression.

Pain causes anxiety, depression, and feelings of helplessness in addition to physical discomfort. It can affect the client's sleeping habits, eating patterns, work, family, and social relationships. Ultimately, pain can affect the client's quality of life.

Noninvasive pain-relief techniques are useful in pain management. They include cutaneous stimulation (heat, cold, massage); transcutaneous electrical nerve stimulation (TENS); relaxation techniques; imagery; and hypnosis. Most of these techniques are inexpensive and easy to perform. They have few side effects and can usually be done in any environment. They also give the client some control over the treatment of pain. Although not every client responds successfully to these measures, it is worthwhile to attempt them before using invasive techniques.

The Agency for Health Care Policy and Research (AHCPR, 1994) developed Cancer Pain Guidelines for clients, family members, and health care professionals. Some points emphasized by the guidelines include:

- Cancer pain can be managed effectively through relatively simple means in up to 90% of cancer clients in the United States. Skin patches, slow-release tablets, and client-controlled pumps are now available to complement standard drugs.
- The mainstay of pain assessment is the client self-report. Because there is no standard test for pain, the nurse must respect the client's report of pain and regard it as the single most reliable indicator.
- The simplest dosage schedules and least invasive pain management modalities are used first. Nonopioids are the first step in the analgesic ladder. They are tried first for mild to moderate pain.

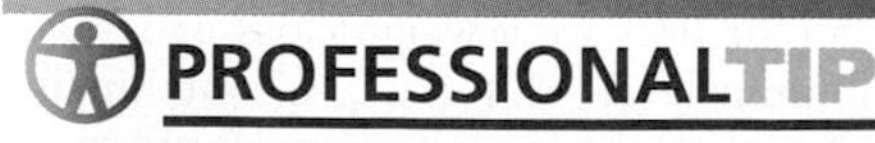

PROFESSIONALTIP

Inadequate Pain Control in the Cancer Client

A major reason given for inadequate pain control in the cancer client is the fear of inducing respiratory depression. This, however, is a rare occurrence in the cancer client.

- Morphine is the most commonly used opioid for moderate to severe pain because it is available in a wide variety of dosage forms, it has well-characterized pharmacokinetics and pharmacodynamics, and it is relatively low in cost. Morphine can be given orally, subcutaneously, intramuscularly, intravenously, rectally, and intraspinally. It can also be given in sustained-release preparations.
- Health-care providers work to prevent pain rather than try to treat pain after it has occurred. Analgesics work better when given regularly around the clock before pain becomes severe. A major nursing responsibility is to teach the client to request pain medication before the pain becomes severe. When medication is ordered around the clock, the nurse does not hesitate to wake the client to administer analgesics.

If pain control is not achieved with noninvasive techniques or medications, neurosurgical procedures such as nerve blocks are an option.

Fatigue

Fatigue occurs as a direct result of cancer treatment or because of anemia, chronic pain, stress, depression, insufficient rest, or inadequate nutritional intake. Although the etiology is not well understood, fatigue is often related to the effects of the tumor itself (Greifzu, 1998). Fatigue contributes to client noncompliance with the treatment regimen.

Frequent rest periods are provided for the client. Assess for the presence and pattern of fatigue. Proper planning allows the client to be active when energy level is higher, which in turn restore a greater sense of control. Evaluate factors that increase or decrease fatigue, such as nutritional intake. Blood count is monitored for anemia.

Alopecia

Alopecia, the thinning or loss of hair, is induced by chemotherapy or radiation treatments. The extent of hair loss depends on the dose and duration of the therapy. Scalp hair is most commonly affected, but pubic, axillary, and facial hair, even eyebrows and eyelashes, also are affected. The treatments cause hair loss by interfering with the growth processes in the hair follicle. This results in weakening of the hair shaft, thereby causing the hair to break off at the surface of the scalp. Hair loss usually begins 2 to 3 weeks after the initial treatment. Drug-induced alopecia is not permanent. Hair usually begins to grow back within 8 weeks after treatment is completed. The color and consistency of the hair may change.

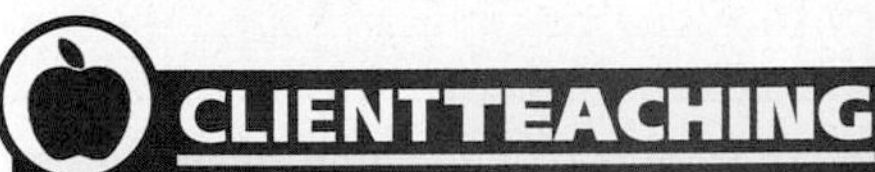

Alopecia, Threat to Body Image

Encourage client to:

- Buy a wig or hairpiece before treatment actually begins so that it will match the client's normal hair.
- Wear hats, scarves, or bandanas to cope with the change in body image caused by hair loss.
- Focus on other positive aspects rather than on just physical appearance.

Odors

Unpleasant odors emanating from the cancer client are a source of embarrassment. These odors are usually associated with drainage, exudates, or incontinence. Fortunately, meticulous nursing care can eliminate most offending odors. Change soiled linens, drainage pads, and dressings immediately. Wash the client's skin gently with soap and warm water. Protective creams are used if the areas are not receiving radiation. Room deodorizers are helpful but should be used cautiously because many clients experience nausea when exposed to the odors from room fresheners. Placing a drop of oil of wintergreen or oil of cloves on a cotton ball near the ventilation system can sometimes lend a light freshness to the environment.

Dyspnea

One-half of all clients with terminal cancer experience dyspnea, or difficulty in breathing. Possible causes include fluid accumulation in the chest, infection such as pneumonia, fibrosis caused by radiation, and anemia. Lungs are auscultated every 4 hours. Oxygen is ordered. Fluid is drained by an invasive procedure called a thoracentesis. High-Fowler positioning maximizes ventilation. Plan care to keep activity to a minimum to balance oxygen requirements and oxygen supply. Oxygen status is monitored with a pulse oximeter. Report a sustained reading of less than 90%. Avoid pulling the privacy curtain or shutting the client's door unless absolutely necessary because either of these actions reduces air flow and creates more anxiety.

Bowel Dysfunctions

Cancer clients frequently exhibit changes in bowel patterns. Constipation, diarrhea and subsequent perineal skin breakdown, and bowel obstructions are common elimination disorders.

Constipation results from decreased motility of the colon. It is frequently caused by chemotherapy, opioid analgesic, or inactivity. Monitor and record the frequency of the client's bowel movements. Constipation is an early sign of vincristine toxicity. Fluid consumption is encouraged and a stool softener is given daily. Clients at risk for constipation are started on a high-fiber diet, with increased intake of bran and prune juice.

Common causes of diarrhea include radiation therapy, chemotherapy, antibiotics, tube feedings, hyperosmolar dietary supplements, stress, and fecal impactions. Clients develop fluid and electrolyte imbalances from constant diarrhea. If the client is receiving a chemotherapy drug known to cause diarrhea (such as fluorouracil [Adrucil] or doxorubicin hydrochloride [Adriamycin]), a low-residue and lactose-free diet is encouraged. Instruct the client to avoid foods that stimulate the gastrointestinal tract, such as warm liquids and coffee.

Bananas (which are high in potassium) and sports drinks (which contain sodium and potassium) help replace lost fluids and electrolytes without irritating the gastrointestinal tract.

The perineum is kept clean and dry after each loose stool. Note signs of fluid and electrolyte imbalances, such as thirst, dry mucous membranes, and decreased skin turgor. The potassium level is monitored. Measure and record the amount, frequency, and characteristics of all client bowel movements.

Antidiarrheal medications such as Lomotil or Imodium are given for every loose stool. Sitz baths help soothe the sore or broken-down tissues.

Bowel obstructions occur more commonly in conjunction with advanced abdominal malignancies and are suspected if the client has received radiation or has adhesions from previous surgeries. Symptoms include nausea, vomiting, and abdominal pain. Surgery is required to relieve the obstruction.

Pathological Fractures

Pathological fractures are a major problem in cancers that metastasize to bone. These cancers weaken the bone to the point that normal activities cause painful breaks. Thus, limbs are supported and handled gently, and extreme care is taken when moving clients. Special devices such as splints are used for extra protection. Weight-bearing restrictions are ordered.

Ascites

Abdominal cancers cause ascites, or fluid accumulation in the abdomen. Clients experience abdominal swelling and difficult breathing. Symptoms are treated temporarily with an invasive procedure called a paracentesis, wherein a small, plastic tube is advanced through the abdominal wall and excess fluid is withdrawn. Chemotherapy drugs sometimes are instilled in an attempt to prevent the fluid from returning. Visually assess the abdomen. A protruding abdomen indicates ascites as well as intestinal distention and enlarged organs. Measure abdominal girth at the umbilicus daily with a tape measure to monitor changes, then auscultate the abdomen in all four quadrants. Gurgling bowel sounds heard every 5 to 15 seconds indicate normal peristalsis. Decreased or absent bowel sounds indicate peritonitis or paralytic ileus. Fluid accumulation is confirmed by percussing for shifting dullness. When a large amount of fluid is present, fluid waves are seen. Gentle palpation is used to detect pain and tenderness as well as abdominal masses. The nurse carefully documents any abnormal findings.

Weigh the client daily to monitor weight gain. Fluid consumption is restricted. Good skin care, especially to the abdomen, is essential. Fowler positioning maximizes ventilation. Clients are observed closely for electrolyte imbalance if large amounts of fluids are withdrawn via paracentesis.

Sexual Alterations

Many chemotherapy drugs interfere with sexual functioning and reproduction. Premenopausal women may become infertile. Those younger than 35 years of age may regain their fertility after therapy is completed. Men may experience impotence, decreased libido, interrupted sperm production, and ejaculation problems. Women experience vaginal dryness.

Encourage clients and their partners to express their feelings and concerns to each other and to explore other avenues of sexual expression, such as cuddling, kissing, and stroking. Birth control is practiced during therapy and for 1 or 2 years after therapy (depending on physician recommendation) to ensure that all chemotherapy drugs are eliminated and will have no ill effects on a pregnancy. Eggs and sperm may be saved before treatment.

MEDICAL EMERGENCIES

Medical emergencies occur in approximately 20% of clients with advanced-stage cancer. Early recognition and treatment can prevent irreversible complications and improve the quality of life. Four complications with which to be familiar are hypercalcemia, spinal cord compression, superior vena cava syndrome, and cardiac tamponade.

HYPERCALCEMIA

Hypercalcemia occurs commonly and can be a potentially fatal complication if not detected early. It is found most often in clients with malignant tumors that have metastasized to bone, such as breast cancer. The condition occurs when the serum calcium level rises >10.5 mg/dL.

Early symptoms of hypercalcemia, such as nausea, vomiting, constipation, and weakness, may be overlooked because these are common side effects of many cancer therapies. Later symptoms such as dehydration, renal failure, coma, and cardiac arrest develop swiftly.

Hypercalcemia is treated aggressively with intravenous normal saline and furosemide (Lasix), which increase calcium excretion. Clients also are given drugs to decrease bone reabsorption. Monitor the serum calcium level when Lasix is administered. Teach clients early symptoms of hypercalcemia so they recognize a recurrence. These clients are also at increased risk for pathological fractures because calcium has been released from the bones, leaving them very fragile.

SPINAL CORD COMPRESSION

Spinal cord compression can result in permanent paralysis if not treated promptly. Cancers of the lung, breast, and prostate carry the greatest risk of metastasizing to the spinal cord. The chief symptom of metastasis to the spinal cord is back pain. The discomfort is aggravated by lying down, coughing, or moving, and may be relieved by sitting upright.

Treatment is aimed at reducing tumor size to decrease pressure on the spinal cord. Radiation, surgery, and steroid therapy are used. Pain medications are given frequently, and clients are supported carefully during transfers.

SUPERIOR VENA CAVA SYNDROME

Superior vena cava syndrome is a collection of symptoms caused by an obstruction of the superior vena cava. It occurs more frequently in conjunction with lung cancer and lymphomas. Typically, clients experience dyspnea and swelling of the face and neck. Edema in the upper extremities, chest pain, and coughing may also occur. Central nervous system symptoms such as headache, visual disturbances, and alteration in consciousness rarely occur.

The goal of treatment is to reduce tumor size. Radiation along with diuretics is usually ordered. Administer oxygen as ordered and provide a calm, restful environment. Encourage the client to limit activities and lie in Fowler's position. Carefully monitor respirations. Lower extremities should not be elevated, as doing so will increase venous return to an already engorged area.

CARDIAC TAMPONADE

Cardiac tamponade is caused by the formation of pericardial fluid, which reduces cardiac output by compressing the heart. Tumor metastasis to the pericardium is associated with lung cancer, breast cancer, Hodgkin's disease, lymphoma, melanoma, gastrointestinal tumors, and sarcoma. Common symptoms of cardiac tamponade include a rapid, weak pulse; distended neck veins during inspiration; ankle or sacral edema; pleural effusion; ascites; enlarged spleen; lethargy; and altered consciousness.

Treatment is aimed at aspirating the fluid constricting the heart (pericardiocentesis). Reassure the client, explain the procedure, and administer medication for pain.

PSYCHOSOCIAL ALTERATIONS

Perhaps of all the problems that clients with cancer experience, none is more challenging than the associated psychosocial alterations. The mere diagnosis of cancer invokes fear and misunderstanding. A myriad of emotions may surface initially. These may range from deep depression to denial and total refusal of treatment. Anxiety, sadness, and withdrawal are common. Some clients feel that the disease is a punishment for some misguided deed. Each client responds differently to the diagnosis, depending on individual coping mechanisms and support systems.

Research has identified effective and ineffective coping mechanisms. Clients who seek information or share feelings tend to cope more effectively than do those who submit to treatment and procedures without asking questions or who use small talk to avoid discussing threatening issues.

Cancer affects not only the client, but the client's family as well. Responses of family members to the disease have a significant impact on the client's coping. The client and family face issues such as loss of control, changes in body image, and financial burdens, which can be a huge problem.

The nurse has several roles in this context. The client needs time and space to adjust to the diagnosis. Be available to offer support and reassurance. Answer questions, but do not bombard the client with information. Interpret information given by the physician and help the client formulate questions to ask the physician. Encourage the client to express feelings and fears about the illness.

The initial treatment is very frightening for most cancer clients. Allay anxiety by giving information about the treatment's purpose, adverse reactions, and signs and symptoms to report to the physician. Explaining procedures and answering questions in simple language help the client and family regain a feeling of some control. Treatment modalities cause many discomforts, but if the client knows what to expect, the distress can generally be handled. Symptom management is critical in preventing lifestyle disruptions.

Families and clients facing the terminal phase of cancer are confronted with a complex set of problems. The client and family face separation and impending death. Some families demand that extraordinary measures be taken to keep the client alive. Some search for meaning in life and experience a genuine closeness. Give the client and family privacy and time to share feelings. Sometimes, the only psychosocial support the client needs is to have someone sitting by the bedside. Touch, especially at times when words are hard to find, can often be the most comforting intervention.

As the client's condition deteriorates, physical needs become more pronounced. Focus on keeping the client comfortable and free of pain. Hospice care is designed to provide spiritual, emotional, and physical support during the final days of illness. The goal of hospice is to keep the client as comfortable as possible. Pain relief and symptom management are stressed. The focus is shifted from cure to care. Care is given in an institution, but most hospice care is given in the home. Hospice care is medically managed and nurse coordinated. Members of the hospice team typically include a chaplain, physician, nurse, social worker, physical therapist, and home health aide, as well as various volunteers. The team functions to ensure that the client's plan of care is carried out and that family members receive adequate support. The family is instructed in ways to provide care. Bereavement counseling is offered to help family members deal with their loss.

COMMUNITY/HOME HEALTH CARE

Psychosocial Aspects of Cancer

- Clients may see themselves as burdens to their families.
- Family caregivers may be angry that their own needs must go unmet.
- Family caregivers may feel inadequate with regard to caring for the client.
- Medical equipment such as a hospital bed, commode chair, or wheelchair may need to be brought into the home. These may have an impact on family member state of mind and disposition with regard to the family member with cancer.

NURSING PROCESS

ASSESSMENT

Subjective Data

The client interview serves as a forum for ascertaining the client's perception of the illness, treatment, and prognosis; health practices; and health concerns. The client's significant other also is interviewed to ascertain support systems.

Objective Data

Vital signs are measured, and a head-to-toe assessment is performed. Past hospital records are reviewed along with the current record. Laboratory reports, biopsy results, treatment modalities, and comments from other health care professionals are studied.

CRITICAL THINKING

Nursing Intervention Rationale

What is the rationale for each nursing intervention given for the possible nursing diagnoses identified in this chapter?

Nursing diagnoses for a client with cancer includes the following:

NURSING DIAGNOSES	PLANNING/OUTCOMES	NURSING INTERVENTIONS
Fear related to cancer diagnosis	The client will express anxieties and fears to family and/or health care providers.	Review the client's previous experience with cancer to ascertain any current misconceptions based on past beliefs. Encourage the client to share feelings regarding the diagnosis to facilitate identification of coping strategies. Explain hospital routines and focus on the recommended treatment, including its purpose and potential side effects. Accurate descriptions that convey what the client can expect eases fears associated with the unknown. A calm, reassuring environment also enhances coping abilities.
Anticipatory Grieving related to potential loss of body function	The client will express grief to family and/or health care providers.	Open, honest discussions help the client cope with the situation. Be aware that mood swings, hostility, and other negative behaviors often occur. Discuss the loss of body function with the client. Ask what the loss of body function means to the client. Encourage the client to seek help and support from close family members.
Imbalanced Nutrition: Less than Body Requirements related to side effects of chemotherapy	The client will maintain body weight.	Encourage the client to eat a high-calorie, nutrient-rich diet. Supplements are useful. Some clients benefit from frequent, small meals and snacks. Foods high in protein, such as cheese, fish, and poultry, are also recommended. Provide oral hygiene before and after meals. Administer antiemetics approximately 30 minutes before meals. Mints, hard candies, and saltine crackers may help if the client complains of metallic taste. Nondietary interventions include varying the surroundings, using small plates, eating at a table with friends, and minimizing food odors. Monitor intake and output along with daily weight.
Risk for Impaired Skin Integrity related to chemotherapy and radiation	The client will maintain skin integrity.	Assess skin frequently for side effects of cancer therapy. (A reddening or tanning effect develops with radiation. Skin reactions such as rashes, pruritus, and alopecia develop with chemotherapy.) Use lukewarm water and soap to gently wash the client's skin. Skin often becomes sensitive during radiation treatments.
Risk for Infection related to side effects of chemotherapy	The client will remain free of infection.	Monitor vital signs at least every shift. White blood count is monitored and protective isolation is instituted if the count falls $<500\ mm^3$. Educate the client, staff, and visitors in all aspects of infection prophylaxis. Thorough hand hygiene is the most important means of preventing and controlling the transmission of organisms. Fresh flowers and raw fruits and vegetables transmit microbes and therefore are eliminated. The client should not be exposed to anyone who has an infection or who has been recently vaccinated against or exposed to a communicable disease. Visitors are limited.

Nursing diagnoses for a client with cancer includes the following: (Continued)

NURSING DIAGNOSES	PLANNING/OUTCOMES	NURSING INTERVENTIONS
Risk for Injury related to altered clotting factors secondary to side effects of chemotherapy	The client will remain free of injury related to bleeding.	Every shift, assess the client for signs of bleeding (petechiae, ecchymoses, hematomas, bleeding gums, epistaxis, tarry stools, hematuria, frank or prolonged bleeding from puncture sites) because transfusions may be indicated. Monitor platelet count, which is an indicator of clotting ability. Institute special precautions if the count falls <50,000 mm^3. Apply pressure to all puncture sites for 3 to 5 minutes. Doing so prevents prolonged bleeding, which causes damage to underlying tissues such as nerves. Instruct the client to use a soft toothbrush or sponge for oral hygiene to prevent damage to oral mucosa, which is particularly susceptible to bleeding. Instruct the client to use an electric razor when shaving.
Fatigue related to analgesics, anemia, stress, increased metabolism, and chemotherapy	The client will experience less fatigue.	Plan frequent rest periods for the client to restore energy, and schedule activities when the client has the most energy. Monitor nutritional intake, as adequate nutrients are necessary to meet energy needs. Recognize that weakness places the client at increased risk for injury. Because fatigue may make activities of daily living difficult to complete, assistance may need to be provided.

Evaluation: Evaluate each outcome to determine how it has been met by the client.

SAMPLE NURSING CARE PLAN

The Client with Lung Cancer

H.S. is a 54-year-old carpenter. He is admitted with pain over his left scapula and radiating to his left arm. He describes having dyspnea and a productive cough. He denies any recent weight loss but does acknowledge experiencing extreme fatigue for the last 2 months. H.S. has been a chronic smoker for 20 years. A chest x-ray reveals an area of density in the left lung. A needle biopsy confirms small-cell lung cancer. A computed tomography (CT) scan confirms extrathoracic involvement. His physician referred H.S. to an oncologist for palliative chemotherapy. H.S. is to receive his first treatment of cisplatin (Platinol) and etoposide (VePesid). H.S. states that he is not sure about this treatment because it will not cure him and he does not know how he will keep breathing. He has never before been hospitalized.

NURSING DIAGNOSIS 1 *Death Anxiety* related to unfamiliar surroundings and uncertainty regarding change in health status as evidenced by H.S.'s statement that he does not know how he will keep breathing and the fact that he has never before been hospitalized

Nursing Outcomes Classification (NOC)
Anxiety Control
Acceptance: Health Status
Fear Control

Nursing Interventions Classification (NIC)
Anxiety Reduction
Coping Enhancement
Emotional Support

(Continues)

SAMPLE NURSING CARE PLAN (Continued)

PLANNING/OUTCOMES	NURSING INTERVENTIONS	RATIONALE
H.S. will share his feelings regarding his dyspnea.	Ascertain what the physician has told H.S. and what conclusions H.S. has reached. Encourage H.S. to share his feelings concerning cancer.	Helps decrease fear of the unknown. Identifies the source of any misconception that is increasing anxiety.
H.S. will express less anxiety about being in the hospital.	Maintain frequent contact with H.S. Explain the hospital routine and care H.S. will receive.	Reassures H.S. that he is not alone. An unfamiliar environment increases anxiety.

EVALUATION

H.S. shares his feelings about his diagnosis and treatment regimen. H.S. exhibits less anxiety about the change in his health status and hospitalization.

NURSING DIAGNOSIS 2 *Impaired **G**as Exchange* related to decreased lung capacity and increased secretions as evidenced by dyspnea, productive cough, and dense area in left lung

Nursing Outcomes Classification (NOC)
Respiratory Status: Gas Exchange
Respiratory Status: Ventilation
Tissue Perfusion: Pulmonary

Nursing Interventions Classification (NIC)
Airway Management
Respiratory Monitoring
Oxygen Therapy

PLANNING/OUTCOMES	NURSING INTERVENTIONS	RATIONALE
H.S. will report less dyspnea with oxygen saturation >90%.	Monitor pulmonary status by auscultating breath sounds; checking rate, depth, and pattern of respirations; evaluating skin color for cyanosis; and monitoring pulse oximetry.	Provides information regarding pulmonary status changes indicating either improvement or onset of complications.
	Position H.S. in Fowler's position.	Promotes expansion of lungs and respiratory muscles.
	Administer oxygen at prescribed level.	Corrects hypoxemia and provides oxygen for metabolic needs.
	Administer opioids with caution.	Opioids can depress the respiratory center.
	Monitor amount, color, and consistency of sputum.	Changes in sputum suggest infection or change in pulmonary status.
	Plan care and treatments within H.S.'s tolerance.	Oxygen demands increase with activity.

EVALUATION

Adequate ventilation with oxygen saturation >90% is maintained.

SAMPLE NURSING CARE PLAN (Continued)

NURSING DIAGNOSIS 3 *Acute **Pain*** related to tumor growth and tissue destruction as evidenced by verbal report of pain over left scapula radiating to left arm

Nursing Outcomes Classification (NOC)
Pain Control
Comfort Level

Nursing Interventions Classification (NIC)
Pain Management
Medication Management
Emotional Support

PLANNING/OUTCOMES	INTERVENTIONS	RATIONALE
H.S. will report less pain after pain-relief measures.	Provide routine comfort measures such as repositioning and backrub.	Noninvasive pain-relief techniques are helpful in pain management.
	Teach H.S. to request pain medication before onset of pain.	Keeps pain under control.
	Have H.S. rate pain on a scale of 0 to 10 (0 = no pain and 10 = worst pain).	Provides a method of evaluating the subjective experience of pain.
	Teach H.S. relaxation techniques.	Decreases the perception of pain.
	Document H.S.'s response to the pain-control regimen and adjust as needed.	Identifies effectiveness of pain-relief techniques.

EVALUATION

H.S. reports less pain; <2 on a scale of 0 to 10.

NURSING DIAGNOSIS 4 *Fatigue* related to chronic pain and dyspnea as evidenced by client's description of dyspnea and extreme fatigue for 2 months

Nursing Outcomes Classification (NOC)
Activity Tolerance
Energy Conservation

Nursing Interventions Classification (NIC)
Activity Therapy
Energy Management

PLANNING/OUTCOMES	INTERVENTIONS	RATIONALE
H.S. will report feeling less fatigued.	Plan care to allow for rest periods.	Helps conserve energy.
	Assess for related factors such as nutritional imbalances, lack of sleep, and causes of stress.	Reduces fatigue.
	Have H.S. rate fatigue on a scale of 0 to 10 (0 = not tired, 10 = total exhaustion) for a 24-hour period.	Identifies peak energy and exhaustion times.
	Teach energy-conservation strategies such as planning ahead, setting priorities, scheduling rest periods, and resting before a difficult task.	Decreases physical and psychological stress.

EVALUATION

H.S. exhibits less fatigue in light of having frequent rest periods daily.

NURSING DIAGNOSIS

*Anticipatory **Grieving*** related to loss of body function as evidenced by H.S.'s statement that he does not know how he will keep breathing

NOC: *Coping, Grief Resolution*
NIC: *Anticipatory Guidance, Coping Enhancement, Grief Work Facilitation*

NURSING GOAL

H.S. will verbalize his loss and develop coping skills as he acknowledges his illness as terminal.

NURSING INTERVENTIONS	SCIENTIFIC RATIONALES
1. Provide opportunities for H.S. to express his feelings.	1. Helps identify H.S.'s coping strategies.
2. Answer all of H.S.'s questions honestly.	2. Helps H.S. cope.
3. Encourage H.S.'s participation in his care.	3. Gives H.S. a greater sense of control.
4. Encourage family support and visits from friends.	4. Assures H.S. that he is not alone and provides time to discuss concerns openly.
5. Utilize appropriate referrals to professionals, such as clergy, as needed.	5. Facilitates the grief process and spiritual care.

EVALUATION

Has H.S. come to terms with the reality of his diagnosis and prognosis?

Concept Care Map 3-1

CASE STUDY

J.D. is a 70-year-old man with a history of prostate cancer, which was treated with palliative hormones and radiation. His admitting diagnosis is adenocarcinoma of the prostate with widespread bone metastasis. J.D. is married and has one grown daughter, who often helps with his care. His chief concern is severe back pain. The physician has ordered intrathecal morphine sulfate and aspirin 10 g for pain relief.

The following questions will guide your development of a nursing care plan for the case study.

1. List symptoms typically seen in clients diagnosed with prostate cancer.
2. Identify the population most at risk for developing prostate cancer.
3. List three possible risk factors for prostate cancer.
4. Discuss the rationale for the physician's orders including aspirin along with morphine sulfate.
5. Discuss the rationale for benzodiazepines not being used for pain relief.
6. List the subjective and objective data the nurse would want to obtain.
7. When you walk into J.D.'s room, he greets you with a smile and continues talking and joking with his daughter. While assessing him, you note that his vital signs are normal. You ask him to rate his pain on a scale of 0 to 10. He pauses to think about it, then rates the pain at 8. In the chart, you must record your nursing assessment by circling the appropriate number on the scale. Which number do you think you should circle?
8. Write three individualized nursing diagnoses and goals for J.D.
9. Discuss which oncological emergency J.D. is most likely to develop.

SUMMARY

- Cancer is the second most common cause of death in the United States.
- Most cancers are curable if treated early.
- Benign neoplasms are localized and encapsulated and do not spread.
- Malignant neoplasms spread to neighboring tissues via blood and lymph.
- Biopsy is the most accurate diagnostic test for cancer.
- The most common medical treatments for cancer are surgery, radiation, and chemotherapy. They may be used alone or in combination.
- Surgery is the treatment of choice for early cancers.
- Chemotherapy is the treatment of choice for metastatic cancers. It is also the treatment most responsible for increasing cancer cure rates in recent years.
- Lung cancer is the leading cause of cancer death among men and women. Eighty percent of all cases are related to smoking.
- Quality of life, not quantity of life, is the ultimate goal for clients living with cancer.

REVIEW QUESTIONS

1. The nurse carefully monitors the client's intravenous chemotherapy. An early indicator that extravasation may be occurring is when:
   1. the fluid stops infusing.
   2. edema is noted at the site.
   3. blood returns when the bottle is lowered.
   4. burning occurs at the site.
2. A breast cancer client states that the doctor says he is going to prescribe hormone therapy. Which of the following hormones would probably be ordered?
   1. Thyroxin.
   2. Parathormone.
   3. Progesterone.
   4. Testosterone.
3. A cancer client develops a low white-cell count. She is placed on neutropenic precautions. Which of the following menu selections would be best?
   1. Meat loaf, mashed potatoes, green beans, and fruit gelatin.
   2. Meat loaf, mashed potatoes, marinated carrots, and a garden salad.
   3. Meat loaf, mashed potatoes, chef salad, and tapioca.
   4. Meat loaf, mashed potatoes, green beans, fruit salad, and a cookie.
4. When stomatitis develops, it is best to encourage the client to:
   1. drink plenty of orange juice.
   2. use lemon and glycerine swabs frequently.
   3. brush teeth before and after eating.
   4. rinse with commercial mouthwash as needed.
5. Clients receiving radiation are encouraged to:
   1. wash and dry the skin carefully and apply lotion.
   2. not bathe.
   3. not apply deodorants or lotions.
   4. wash the skin with soap and apply baby powder.
6. The client asks the nurse to explain the implications of the TNM system. His physician told him "the news is not good; your tumor is classified as $T_2 N_2 M_1$." The nurse's response is based on the knowledge that:
   1. this is a local classification system used by the physicians at this particular hospital.
   2. this is an international system used by oncologists as a standardized method of defining a tumor and tumor activity.
   3. the numbers used are indicative of tumor growth and spread, with the smaller numbers meaning more aggressive growth.
   4. only the physician can interpret any findings to the client.
7. A difference between normal cells and cancer cells is that cancer cells:
   1. adhere to their area of origin.
   2. are well differentiated.
   3. multiply at will.
   4. cannot move freely around the body.
8. Choose risk factors for cancer: (Select all that apply.)
   1. use of oral birth control pills.
   2. consumption of a high fiber diet.
   3. heavy alcohol consumption.
   4. use of smokeless tobacco instead of smoking cigarettes.
   5. consumption of five servings of fruits and vegetables daily.
   6. multiple sexual partners with unprotected sex.
9. A nurse is caring for a client with advanced cancer. The first priority of nursing intervention is:
   1. support limbs and gently turn client to prevent a pathological fracture.
   2. monitor ascites by measuring abdominal girth at the umbilicus.
   3. listen to the client share her concerns about losing her hair.
   4. administer oral morphine sulfate for break through pain.

10. The nurse meets the psychosocial needs of the client with cancer and his family's needs by:
    1. conversing on a superficial level so she does not always have to think about her condition.
    2. allowing the client personal time to adjust to diagnosis but answer questions and provide support as needed.
    3. allaying anxiety by not giving any information about treatment options or adverse reactions.
    4. providing all the physical care for the client so the family is not involved with these needs.

REFERENCES/SUGGESTED READINGS

Agency for Health Care Policy and Research. (1994). *Clinical practice guidelines: Management of cancer pain* (AHCPR Publication No. 94-0592). Rockville, MD: U.S. Department of Health & Human Services.

American Cancer Society (ACS). (2000). Cancer Facts & Figures 2000. [Online]. Retrieved on May 2, 2009 from http://www.cancer.org/docroot/STT/stt_0_2000.asp?sitearea=STT&level=1

American Cancer Society (ACS). (2002). Cancer news roundup. *Nursing*2002, 32(10), 32hn6–32hn7.

American Cancer Society (ACS). (2003). Cancer Facts & Figures 2003. [Online]. Retrieved on May 2, 2009 from http://www.cancer.org/docroot/STT/stt_0_2003.asp?sitearea=STT&level=1

American Cancer Society (ACS). (2006). *Cancer facts & figures 2006.* Atlanta: American Cancer Society.

American Cancer Society (ACS). (2007). Global Cancer: Facts & Figures 2007. Retrieved on May 2, 2009 from http://www.cancer.org/downloads/STT/Global_Cancer_Facts_and_Figures_2007_rev.pdf

American Cancer Society (ACS). (2008). Cancer Facts & Figures 2008. Retrieved on May 2, 2009 from http://www.cancer.org/docroot/STT/stt_0_2008.asp?sitearea=STT&level=1

American Pain Society. (1992). *Principles of analgesic use in the treatment of acute and chronic cancer pain* (3rd ed.). Skokie, IL: Author.

Baird, S., Donehower, M., Stalsbroten, V., & Ades, T. (Eds.) (1997). *A cancer source book for nurses* (7th ed.). Atlanta, GA: American Cancer Society.

Belcher, A. (1992). *Cancer nursing*. St. Louis, MO: Mosby.

Blackburn, G. (1998). Wasting away: Cancer cachexia. *Health News*, 4(4), 4. Waltham, MA: Massachusetts Medical Society.

Bral, E. (1998). Caring for adults with chronic cancer pain. *AJN*, 4(98), 27–32.

Bulechek, G., Butcher, H., McCloskey, J., & Dochterman, J., eds. (2008). *Nursing Interventions Classification (NIC)* (5th ed.). St. Louis, MO: Mosby/Elsevier.

Cancerbackup. (2009). Combination chemotherapy regimen. Macmillan Cancer Support. Retrieved on May 5, 2009 from http://www.cancerbackup.org.uk/Treatments/Chemotherapy/Combinationregimen

Cancer Treatment Centers of America. (2009a). Biotherapy/Immunotherapy. Retrieved on May 1, 2009 from http://www.cancercneter.com/conventional-cancer-treatment/biotherapy-immunotherapy.cfm

Cancer Treatment Centers of America. (2009b). Photodynamic therapy. Retrieved on May 1, 2009 from http://www.cancercneter.com/conventional-cancer-treatment/photodynamic-therapy.cfm

Cancer Treatment Centers of America. (2009c). Hormone Therapy. Retrieved on May 1, 2009 from http://www.cancercneter.com/conventional-cancer-treatment/hormone-therapy.cfm

Chapman, D., & Goodman, M. (2000). *Cancer nursing principles* (5th ed.). Boston, MA: Jones & Bartlett.

Chiramannil, A. (1998). Lung cancer. *AJN*, 4(98), 46–47.

Dell, D. (2001). Regaining range of motion after breast surgery. *Nursing2001*, 31(10), 50–52.

Erickson, J. (1994, November). Update on Hodgkin's Disease. *Nurse Practitioner*, 63–67.

Estes, M. (2010). *Health assessment & physical examination* (4th ed.). Clifton Park, NY: Delmar Cengage Learning.

Fieler, B. (1997). Side effects and quality of life in patients receiving high-dose rate brachytherapy. *Oncology Nursing Forum*, 24(3), 545.

Galvan, T. (2001). Dysphagia: Going down and staying down. *AJN*, 101(1), 37–42.

Greifzu, S. (1998). Fighting cancer fatigue. *RN*, 61(8), 41–43.

Harris, L. (2002). Ovarian cancer: Screening for early detection. *AJN*, 102(10), 46–52.

Held-Warmkessel, J. (1998). Chemotherapy complications: Helping your patient cope with adverse reactions. *Nursing98* 4(28), 41–45.

Kediziera, P. (1998). The two faces of pain. *RN*, 61(2), 45–46.

Kohr, J. (1995). Measuring your patient's pain. *RN*, 58(4), 39–40.

Langhorne, M., Fulton, J., & Otto, S. (2007). *Oncology nursing* (5th ed.). St. Louis: Mosby.

Lewis, S., Heitkemper, M., & Dirksen, S. (2007). *Medical–surgical nursing: Assessment and management of clinical problems* (7th ed.). St. Louis, MO: Mosby.

Machia, J. (2001). Breast cancer: Risk, prevention & Tamoxifen. *AJN*, 101(4), 26–35.

McCaffery, M., & Ferrell, B. (1994, July). How to use the new AHCPR cancer pain guidelines. *AJN*, 42–47.

McCarron, E. (1995, June). Supporting the families of cancer patients. *Nursing95*, 48–51.

McConnell, E. (2001). Myth & Facts about dysphagia. *Nursing2001*, 31(7), 29.

Moorhead, S., Johnson, M., Maas, M., & Swanson, E. (2007). *Nursing Outcomes Classification (NOC)* (4th ed). St. Louis, MO: Elsevier—Health Sciences Division.

Monahan, F., Sands, J., Neighbors, M., & Marek, J. (2006). *Phipps' medical-surgical nursing: Health and illness perspectives* (8th ed.). St. Louis, MO: Mosby Elsevier.

Myers, J. (2000). Chemotherapy-induced hypersensitivity reaction. *AJN*, 100(4), 53–54.

National Bone Marrow Transplant Link (NBMTLink). (2009). Resource guide for bone marrow/stem cell transplant. Retrieved on April 30, 2009 from http://www.nbmtlink.org/resources_support/rg/rg_costs.htm

National Cancer Institute. (2006). Targeted cancer therapies: Questions and answers. National Cancer Institute Fact Sheet. Retrieved on May 4, 2009 from http://www.cancer.gov/cacncertopics/factsheet/Therapy/targeted/print?page=&keyword

Otto, S. (2001). *Oncology nursing* (4th ed.). St. Louis, MO: Mosby.

Porth, C., & Matfin, G. (2008). *Pathophysiology: Concepts of Altered Health States* (8th ed.). Philadelphia: Lippincott Williams & Wilkins.

Researchers say new drug may boost effects of cancer radiation. (1998, May 12). *Corpus Christi Caller Times.*

Resnick, B., & Belcher, A. (2002). Breast reconstruction. *AJN*, 102(4), 26–33.

Sargent, C., & Murphy, D. (2003). What you need to know about colorectal cancer. *Nursing2003*, 33(2), 36–41.

Schweid, L., & Werner-McCullough, M. (1994, September). Will you recognize these oncological crises? *RN*, 23–27.

Smeltzer, S., Bare, B., Hinkle, J., & Cheever, K. (2008). *Brunner & Suddarth's Textbook of Medical Surgical Nursing, North American Edition* (11th ed.) Philadelphia: Lippincott Williams & Wilkins

Tamoxifen for breast cancer prevention. (1998, December 15). *Healthnews*, 4(15).

Teasley, R. (in press). *Understanding Neoplasms.*

Thaler-DeMers, D. (2000). The cancer survival toolbox. *AJN*, 100(4), 52.

Timby, B., Smith, N., & Scherer, J. (2002) *Introductory Medical-Surgical Nursing* (8th ed.) Philadelphia: Lippincott Williams & Wilkins.

U.S. Preventive Services Task Force. (2002). Screening for colorectal cancer: Recommendations and rationale. *AJN*, 102(9), 107–114.

Watson, A., & Coyne, P. (2003). Recognizing the faces of cancer pain. *Nursing2003*, 33(4), 32hn1–32hn8.

Weber, M. (1995). Clinical snapshot: Chemotherapy-induced nausea and vomiting. *AJN*, 95(4).

White, L., & Spitz, M. (1994). Cancer risk and early detection assessment. *Capsules and Comments in Oncology Nursing*, 2(1), 2–3.

Wilkes, G. (2000). Nutrition: The forgotten ingredient in cancer care. *AJN*, 100(4), 46–51.

Woodward, W., & Thobaben, M. (1994). Special home health care nursing challenges: Patients with cancer. *Home Health Care Nurse*, 12(3), 33–37.

Zuckerman, D. (2002). The breast cancer information gap. *RN*, 65(2), 39–41.

RESOURCES

American Cancer Society (ACS), http://www.cancer.org

American Pain Society, http://www.ampainsoc.org/

Breast Cancer Network of Strength, http://www.networkofstrength.org/

National Cancer Institute, http://www.cancer.gov

National Coalition for Cancer Survivorship (NCCS), http://www.canceradvocacy.org

UNIT 2 Nursing Care of the Client: Oxygenation and Perfusion

CHAPTER 4
Respiratory System

MAKING THE CONNECTION

Refer to the following chapters to increase your understanding of the respiratory system:

Adult Health Nursing

- ***Oncology***
- ***Cardiovascular System***
- ***Hematologic and Lymphatic Systems***

Delmar's Heart & Lung Sounds on StudyWare CD™: Lung Sounds

LEARNING OBJECTIVES

Upon completion of this chapter, you should be able to:

- Define key terms.
- Describe components of a complete respiratory assessment.
- Identify normal parameters for common respiratory diagnostic studies.
- Discuss the etiology, medical–surgical management, and nursing care for clients with respiratory disorders.
- Prepare a nursing care plan for a client with a respiratory disorder.

KEY TERMS

adventitious breath sound
asthma
atelectasis
audible wheeze
bronchial sound
bronchiectasis
bronchitis
bronchovesicular sound
caseation
cavitation
chemoreceptor
coarse crackle
diffusion
emphysema
empyema
epistaxis
external respiration
fine crackle
hemopneumothorax
hemothorax
internal respiration
liquefaction necrosis
lung stretch receptor
perfusion
pleural effusion
pleural friction rub
pleurisy
pneumonia
pneumothorax
primary tubercle
respiration
sibilant wheeze
sonorous wheeze
status asthmaticus
stridor
surfactant
ventilation
vesicular sound

INTRODUCTION

Respiratory disorders account for millions of the dollars spent in the U.S. health care arena. From loss of time on the job because of the common cold to care for those with chronic respiratory disorders, the cost of respiratory disease is staggering. This chapter explores the various respiratory disorders, with a focus on the nursing process.

ANATOMY AND PHYSIOLOGY REVIEW

The primary function of the respiratory system is delivery of oxygen to the lungs and removal of carbon dioxide from the lungs.

THORACIC CAVITY

The chest cage is a closed compartment bounded on the top by the neck muscles and at the bottom by the diaphragm. The walls of the chest cage are formed by the ribs and intercostal muscles laterally, the thoracic vertebrae posteriorly, and the sternum anteriorly. The inside of the chest cage is called the *thoracic cavity*. Contained within the thoracic cavity are the lungs. The lungs are cone-shaped, porous organs separated from the other chest organs by the mediastinum. The lungs lie free, except for their attachment to the heart and trachea, and are encased in the pleura, a thin, transparent double-layered serous membrane lining the thoracic cavity. The layers of the pleura are the *parietal pleura*, which lie adjacent to the chest wall and produce pleural fluid, and the *visceral pleura*, which adhere to the surface of the lungs and absorb pleural fluid. The area between the two pleura is known as the *pleural space* or pleural cavity.

The pleural space contains 5 to 20 mL of fluid, which allows the layers of the pleura to slide on each other yet hold together. The pressure within the pleural space is less than that of outside air. This difference in pressure creates a suction that prevents the lungs from collapsing on exhalation.

The right lung is larger than the left and is divided into three sections, or lobes: upper, middle, and lower. The left lung is divided into two lobes: upper and lower (Figure 4-1). The upper portion of the lung is referred to as the apex (plural, apices). The lower portion is called the base. The lungs possess a dual blood supply: bronchial circulation and pulmonary circulation. Bronchial circulation begins with the bronchial artery, which provides the passageways of the lungs with blood to meet nutritional needs and ends when the venous blood enters the pulmonary veins. Pulmonary circulation is the route by which blood is delivered to the alveoli for gas exchange (Figure 4-2).

CONDUCTING AIRWAYS

The conducting airways are tube-like structures that provide a passageway for air as it travels to the lungs. These are the nasal passages, mouth, pharynx, larynx, trachea, bronchi, and bronchioles (Figure 4-1). The conducting airways are lined with

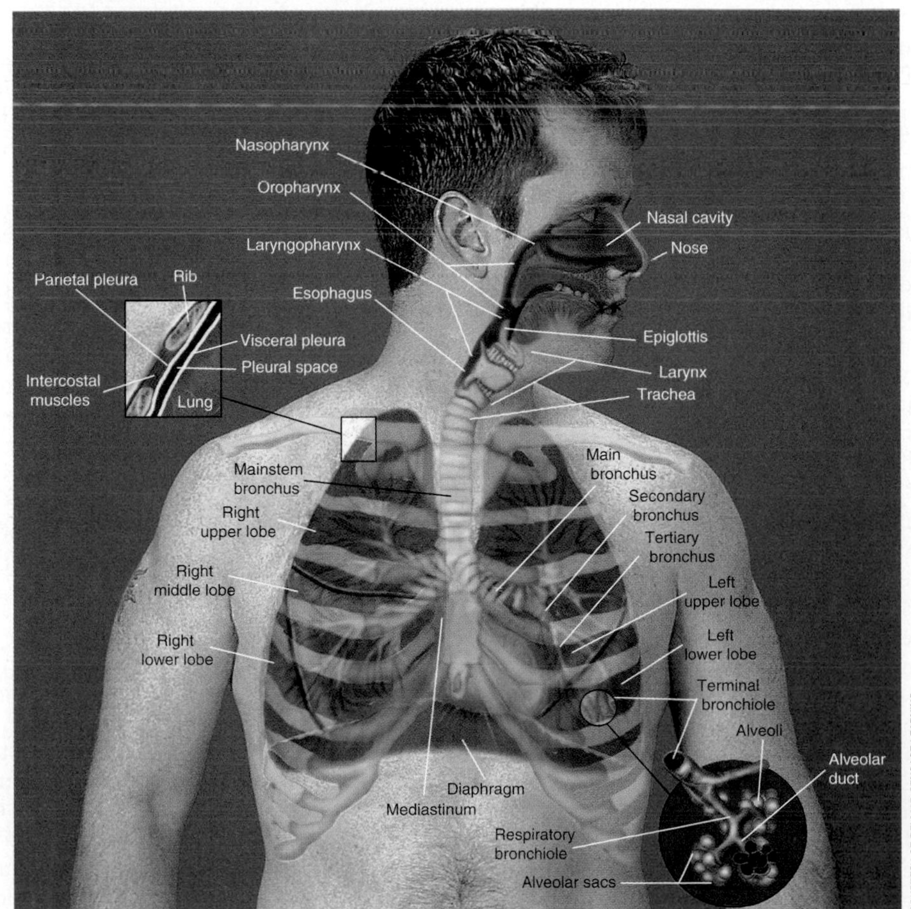

FIGURE 4-1 Structures of the Respiratory Tract

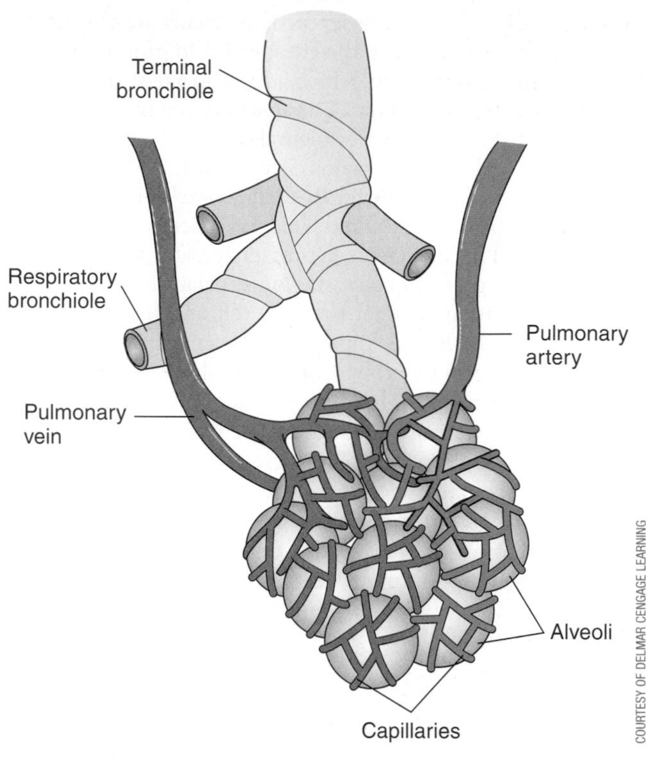

FIGURE 4-2 Gas exchange occurs at the alveolar capillary membrane.

epithelial tissue containing serous glands, mucus-secreting Goblet cells, and hair-like projections called *cilia*. The mucus of the Goblet cells together with the cilia form a mucociliary blanket that protects the respiratory system from foreign particles. The constant upward motion of the cilia propels the mucociliary blanket toward the pharynx, where foreign matter is expectorated or swallowed.

The nasal passages are the preferred route for air to enter the respiratory tract. In addition to the function of filtering inspired air, the nasal passages are richly supplied with blood vessels that warm and moisten the air. Because the mouth lacks cilia and abundant blood supply, breathing through the mouth reduces the ability to filter, warm, and moisten inspired air.

Connecting the nasal passages and mouth to the lower parts of the respiratory tract is the *pharynx*. Located behind the oral cavity, the pharynx serves as a passageway for both inspired air into the larynx and ingested food passing into the digestive system. At the distal portion of the pharynx is the larynx, also known as the voice box.

The *larynx* contains the vocal cords and is the passageway for air entering and leaving the trachea. The larynx is composed of four structures: the uppermost thyroid cartilage (Adam's apple), the cricoid cartilage (which lies at the lower edge of the larynx), the epiglottis (a leaf-shaped structure that covers the larynx during swallowing), and the glottis (the triangular space between relaxed vocal cords).

The *trachea*, commonly known as the windpipe, is a tube composed of connective tissue mucosa and smooth muscle supported by C-shaped rings of cartilage that extends into the bronchi. The trachea is 2.0 to 2.5 cm wide (approximately 1 inch) and 10 to 12 cm long (approximately 4 to 6 inches). The trachea terminates by branching into two tubes: the right and left primary bronchi. The *bronchi* are somewhat smaller in diameter than the trachea, and each passes into its respective lung.

The right bronchus is wider and more vertically positioned than the left. This difference in positioning allows foreign matter to enter the right bronchus more easily than the left. Within the lungs, the bronchi branch off into increasingly smaller diameter tubes until they become the terminal *bronchioles*. These branch further, forming alveolar ducts that end in numerous saclike, thin-walled structures called the *alveoli*. Collectively, the alveoli and the alveolar ducts resemble a cluster of grapes. The branching makes this portion of the respiratory tract resemble an inverted tree, giving rise to the term *bronchial tree* (Figure 4-1).

RESPIRATORY TISSUES

The respiratory tissues perform the function of gas exchange. The alveoli constitute the primary site of gas exchange. The alveolar ducts are smooth, muscular tubes containing abundant alveolar macrophages that remove foreign particles (e.g., bacteria). The alveoli, into which the alveolar ducts terminate, consist of interconnected spaces with thin walls, or septa, occupied by a network of capillaries called the *alveolar capillary membrane*.

The alveoli contain two specialized types of cells. Type I alveolar cells are flat, squamous, epithelial cells across which gas exchange occurs. Type II alveolar cells produce a phospholipid substance called **surfactant**. Surfactant coats the inner surfaces of the alveoli, reduces the surface tension of pulmonary fluids, allows gas exchange, and prevents the collapse of the airways. Each lung contains approximately 300 million alveoli.

RESPIRATION

Respiration is a process of gas exchange. This process is necessary to supply cells with oxygen for metabolism and to remove the waste by-product carbon dioxide. There are two types of respiration: external respiration and internal respiration. **External respiration** is the exchange of gases between the inhaled air, now in the alveoli, and the blood in the pulmonary capillaries. **Internal respiration** is the exchange of gases at the cellular level between tissue cells and blood in systemic capillaries (Figure 4-3). These functions depend on the adequacy of ventilation, perfusion, and diffusion. **Ventilation** is the movement of gases into and out of the lung. **Perfusion** is the flow of blood through the vessels of a specific organ or body part. Pertaining to the respiratory system, **diffusion** is the movement of gases across the alveolar capillary membrane from areas of high concentration to areas of lower concentration. Factors that affect ventilation, perfusion, and diffusion affect respiration (Table 4-1).

NEUROMUSCULAR CONTROL OF RESPIRATION

Unlike the heart muscle, the respiratory muscles must receive continuous neural stimuli to function. Regulation of respiration is integrated by neurons located in the pons and medulla of the brain. The control of respiration is influenced by involuntary (automatic) and voluntary components. Involuntary components include chemoreceptors, lung stretch receptors, and impulses from other sources. **Chemoreceptors** monitor the levels of carbon dioxide and

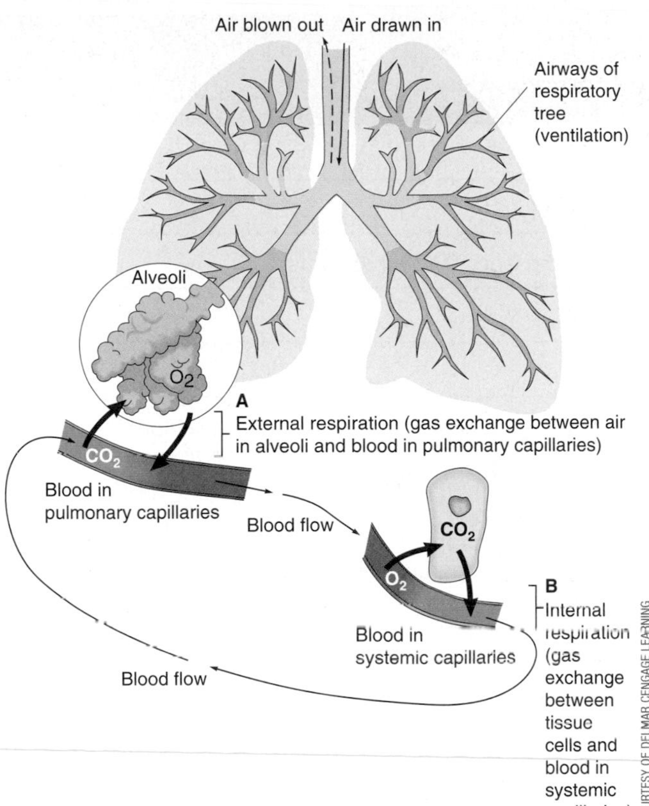

FIGURE 4-3 *A*, External Respiration; *B*, Internal Respiration

TABLE 4-1 Factors Affecting Ventilation, Perfusion, and Diffusion

Ventilation	Position: Dependent areas receive majority of air.
	Lung volume: Low volume results in shunting air to lung apices.
	Disease: Bronchial constriction and airway collapse decrease ventilation.
Perfusion	Position: Dependent areas receive majority of blood.
	Hypoxia: Results in vasoconstriction and decreased perfusion.
	Blockage: Results in decreased or absent perfusion to distal areas.
Diffusion	Alveolar capillary membrane: Alterations may occur in thickness and permeability of membrane.

COURTESY OF DELMAR CENGAGE LEARNING

oxygen and the acidity/alkalinity (pH) of the blood. Normally, chemoreceptors initiate respiration in response to an increase of carbon dioxide in the blood. With certain chronic pulmonary disorders, such as emphysema, chemoreceptors become more responsive to a low level of oxygen. This becomes significant when administering oxygen to persons whose drive to breathe depends on a low level of oxygen in the blood. **Lung stretch receptors** monitor the pattern of breathing and prevent overexpansion of the tissues. Many other sources involuntarily send impulses to the respiratory center. For example, if a person becomes frightened or angry, the respiratory rate increases in response to stimuli from the autonomic nervous system. Voluntary components of respiratory control integrate breathing with acts such as talking and speaking.

The diaphragm acts as the primary muscle of respiration. During inspiration, the diaphragm contracts and flattens out in response to stimuli from the respiratory center, increasing the length of the thoracic cavity. At the same time, the intercostal muscles contract, elevating the ribs and increasing the diameter of the thoracic cavity. The total thoracic space increases, reducing the pressure within the thoracic cavity. The pressure within the thoracic cavity then becomes negative in relation to that of atmospheric pressure, and air moves into the thoracic cavity. Upon expiration, the respiratory center signals the diaphragm and intercostal muscles to relax. The thoracic cavity returns to its original size. Aided by the elastic recoil of the lungs, the decrease in size of the thoracic cavity increases pressure, and air moves out of the lungs.

GAS EXCHANGE

Gas exchange occurs at the alveolar capillary membrane (Figure 4-2). Venous blood from the right ventricle is pumped into the pulmonary arteries and travels to the alveolar capillary network, where it is exposed to the inhaled air. Because of the higher concentration of oxygen in the alveoli, oxygen diffuses into the blood within the alveolar capillary network. The majority of oxygen binds to the iron atoms of the hemoglobin molecule in the red blood cells. Approximately 1% to 3% of oxygen dissolves into the blood plasma.

The exchange of carbon dioxide also occurs within the alveoli. Within the alveolar capillary network, the carbon dioxide detaches from hemoglobin and diffuses into the alveolar space. Carbon dioxide is removed from the alveolar space when exhalation occurs. The blood within the pulmonary capillary network is now oxygenated and travels to the heart via the pulmonary veins. Oxygenated blood is sent to the body via the aorta and the arterial network (Figure 4-3).

ASSESSMENT

To understand the assessment of the respiratory system, the student must be familiar with related terminology (Table 4-2).

HEALTH HISTORY

Nursing assessment begins with a complete history. The client is questioned regarding allergies, occupation, lifestyle, and health habits such as smoking or alcohol use (Box 4-1). Ask about other health problems that affect the respiratory system, such as pneumonia or cardiac problems. Symptoms such as dyspnea, decreased exercise tolerance, and cough are explored

TABLE 4-2 Respiratory Terms

TERM	DEFINITION
Eupnea	Normal breathing
Apnea	Cessation of breathing, possibly temporary in nature
Dyspnea	Labored or difficult breathing, possibly normal if associated with exercise
Bradypnea	Abnormally slow breathing
Tachypnea	Abnormally rapid breathing
Orthopnea	Discomfort or difficulty with breathing in any but an upright sitting or standing position
Kussmaul's respirations	Abnormal respiratory pattern characterized by irregular periods of increased rate and depth of respiration; most often seen with diabetic ketoacidosis
Biot's respirations	Abnormal respiratory pattern characterized by irregular periods of apnea alternating with short periods of respiration of equal depth; most commonly seen with increased intracranial pressure
Cheyne-Stokes respirations	Abnormal respiratory pattern characterized by initially slow, shallow respirations that increase in rapidity and depth and then gradually decrease until respiration stops for 10 to 60 seconds; pattern then repeats itself in the same manner
Anoxia	Without oxygen
Hypoxia	Lack of adequate oxygen in inspired air such as occurs at high altitude
Hypoxemia	Insufficient amount of oxygen in the blood possibly due to respiratory, cardiovascular, or anemia-related disorders
Cyanosis	Bluish, grayish, or purplish discoloration of the skin caused by abnormal amounts of reduced (oxygen-poor) hemoglobin in the blood; not always a reliable indicator of hypoxia
Acrocyanosis	Cyanosis of the fingertips and toes; often caused by vasomotor disturbances associated with vasoconstriction
Circumoral cyanosis	Bluish discoloration encircling the mouth
Oxygen saturation	Amount of oxygen combined with hemoglobin

in depth. Following a complete history, the nurse completes a physical assessment of the client.

Inspection

Physical assessment of the respiratory system starts with inspection. Note the client's color, level of consciousness, and emotional state. Respirations are observed for their rate, depth, quality, rhythm, and breathing pattern. Symmetry of chest wall movement is also noted. The nurse observes for use of accessory muscles to aid breathing. The position the client assumes provides information on respiratory status because individuals having trouble breathing often lean forward.

Palpation and Percussion

The next steps in the respiratory assessment are palpation and percussion. These are normally done by the registered nurse or physician. Through the use of palpation and percussion, areas of varying densities in the lung can be detected. The density of lung tissues changes with disease states such as pneumonia, pneumothorax, and pleural effusion.

Auscultation

The client should breathe slowly through the mouth while the listener assesses breath sounds at each location for the length of a complete inspiration and expiration. Breath sounds are assessed for duration, pitch, and intensity. Figure 4-4 illustrates the recommended stethoscope location for each auscultation.

Normal Breath Sounds

Under normal circumstances, **bronchial sounds** are heard over the sternum (Figure 4-5). These loud, high-pitched tubular, hollow-like sounds last longer during expiration than during inspiration. When heard in areas other than the sternum, bronchial sounds indicate fluid, exudate, or lung tissue

BOX 4-1 QUESTIONS TO ASK AND OBSERVATIONS TO MAKE WHEN COLLECTING DATA

Subjective Data

- Do you have seasonal or environmental allergies?
- Have you been coughing? If so, are you coughing up any mucous? What does it look like?
- Do you get frequent upper respiratory infections?
- Have you ever had pneumonia? If so, when and how often?
- Have you had the pneumonia vaccine?
- Do you get a flu shot annually?
- Do you have any chronic lung conditions such as asthma or emphysema?
- Are you experiencing any difficulty breathing?
- Have you experienced any shortness of breath with exertion or activity?
- Is your nose feeling stuffy and congested?
- Does your throat hurt or feel sore?
- Have you experienced changes in your voice?
- Do you currently or have you ever smoked?
- If you no longer smoke, when did you quit?
- If you smoke, how long have you smoked? What do you smoke? And, how much do you smoke each day?
- Does your chest feel tight when you breathe?
- Are you experiencing any chest pain or discomfort when breathing?

Objective Data

- Check vital signs.
- Check pulse oximetry levels.
- Observe respiratory effort.
- Observe use of accessory muscles.
- Assess color of mucous membranes and nail beds.
- Assess for sputum production.
- Record the quality, color, and odor of the sputum.
- Observe client's activity tolerance.
- Assess supplemental oxygen requirements.
- Auscultate lung sounds.
- Report chest x-ray results or other diagnostic test results.
- Record the quality, color, and odor of the sputum.

compression. **Bronchovesicular sounds** are heard over the anterior one-third of the chest near the sternum and also around the scapula posteriorly (Figure 4-5). Bronchovesicular sounds have a medium pitch and intensity with inspiration and expiration being equal in duration. They may be heard in the periphery of the lung when consolidation and fluid are present.

Vesicular sounds are heard over the majority of the lungs (Figure 4-5). These soft, low-pitched sounds are best heard during inspiration and may be inaudible during expiration.

Adventitious Breath Sounds

Abnormal breath sounds are called **adventitious breath sounds** and include **fine crackles** (rales), **coarse crackles** (rales), **sonorous wheezes** (rhonchi), **sibilant wheezes**, **pleural friction rub**, and **stridor**. Table 4-3 describes the general characteristics of these adventitious breath sounds.

COMMON DIAGNOSTIC TESTS

Commonly used diagnostic tests for clients with respiratory disorders are listed in Table 4-4. Table 4-5 lists normal values for arterial blood gases.

INFECTIOUS/INFLAMMATORY DISORDERS

Infectious/inflammatory disorders of the upper respiratory tract, pneumonia, tuberculosis, and pleurisy/pleural effusion are discussed in the following sections.

COURTESY OF DELMAR CENGAGE LEARNING

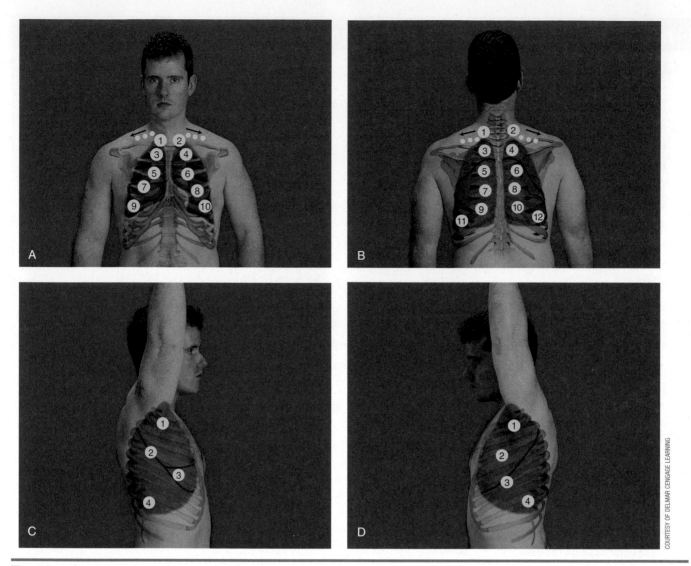

FIGURE 4-4 **Stethoscope Locations for Each Auscultation; *A*, Anterior Thorax; *B*, Posterior Thorax; *C*, Right Lateral Thorax; *D*, Left Lateral Thorax**

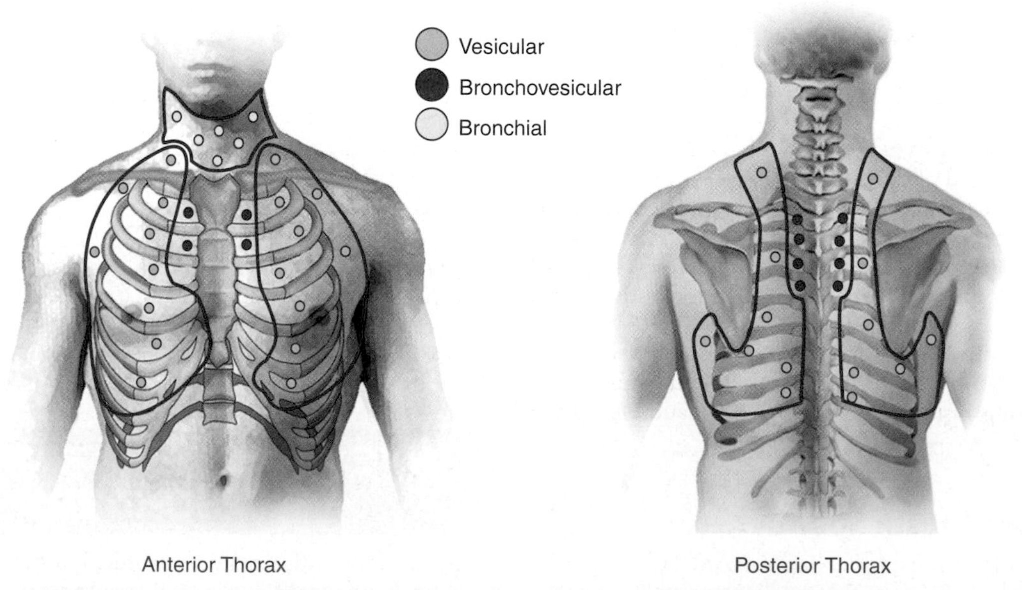

FIGURE 4-5 **Location of Breath Sounds**

TABLE 4-3 Characteristics of Adventitious Breath Sounds

BREATH SOUND	RESPIRATORY PHASE	TIMING	DESCRIPTION	CLEAR WITH COUGH	ETIOLOGY	CONDITIONS
Fine crackle (rale)	Predominantly inspiration	Discontinuous	Dry, high-pitched crackling, popping, short duration; roll hair near ears between your fingers to simulate this sound	No	Air passing through moisture in small airways that suddenly reinflate	COPD, congestive heart failure (CHF), pneumonia, pulmonary fibrosis, atelectasis
Coarse crackle (coarse rale)	Predominantly inspiration	Discontinuous	Moist, low-pitched crackling, gurgling; long duration	Possibly	Air passing through moisture in large airways that suddenly reinflate	Pneumonia, pulmonary edema, bronchitis, atelectasis
Sonorous wheeze (rhonchi)	Predominantly expiration	Continuous	Low pitched; snoring	Possibly	Narrowing of large airways or obstruction of bronchus	Asthma, bronchitis, airway edema, tumor, bronchiolar spasm, foreign body obstruction
Sibilant wheeze	Predominantly expiration	Continuous	High pitched; musical	Possibly	Narrowing of large airways or obstruction of bronchus	Asthma, chronic bronchitis, emphysema, tumor, foreign body obstruction
Pleural friction rub	Inspiration and expiration	Continuous	Creaking, grating	No	Inflamed parietal and visceral pleura; can occasionally be felt on thoracic wall as two pieces of dry leather rubbing against each other	Pleurisy, tuberculosis, pulmonary infarction, pneumonia, lung abscess
Stridor	Predominantly inspiration	Continuous	Crowing	No	Partial obstruction of the larynx, trachea	Croup, foreign body obstruction, large airway tumor

TABLE 4-4 Common Diagnostic Tests for Respiratory Disorders

Laboratory Tests

- Hemoglobin
- Arterial blood gases (ABGs)
- Pulmonary function tests (PFTs)
- Sputum analysis

Radiologic Studies

- Chest x-ray
- Ventilation-perfusion scan (V/Q scan)
- Computerized axial tomography (CAT scan)
- Pulmonary angiography

Other

- Pulse oximetry
- Bronchoscopy
- Thoracentesis
- Magnetic resonance imaging (MRI)

TABLE 4-5 Arterial Blood Gases: Normal Values

MEASUREMENT IN BLOOD	NORMAL VALUE
Acidity or alkalinity (pH)	7.35 to 7.45
Partial pressure of oxygen (PaO_2)	80 to 100 mm Hg
Partial pressure of carbon dioxide ($PaCO_2$)	35 to 45 mm Hg
Bicarbonate ion (HCO_3)	24 to 28 mm Hg
Arterial oxygen saturation (SaO_2)	95% to 100%

INFECTIOUS/INFLAMMATORY DISORDERS OF THE UPPER RESPIRATORY TRACT

Infectious and inflammatory disorders of the upper respiratory tract are common and usually self-limiting. Among the causal factors of infectious and inflammatory disorders are various viruses (rhino viruses, influenza viruses) and bacteria (*streptococci and pneumococci*). Group A *beta-hemolytic streptococci* infections of the upper respiratory system are associated with serious sequelae such as rheumatic fever. Allergic reactions frequently play a role in the development of sinusitis and pharyngitis. Laryngitis is associated with factors such as pollution, smoking, and excessive use of the voice. Breathing cold air decreases local immune responses of the respiratory tract. This fact coupled with closer and prolonged contact with others indoors during the colder months leads to an increased incidence of acute upper respiratory tract inflammatory disorders.

The signs and symptoms that occur with acute upper respiratory tract infection or inflammation are a result of the inflammatory process. Early signs and symptoms include general malaise, low-grade fever, localized redness, and edema of affected tissues. Joint pain is common with viral disorders. The client may complain of nasal or sinus congestion and headache. Drying of the mucous membranes coupled with edema cause local discomfort such as sore throat. Cough and nasal or sinus discharge may occur. Nasal secretions that are thick and purulent indicate bacterial infection.

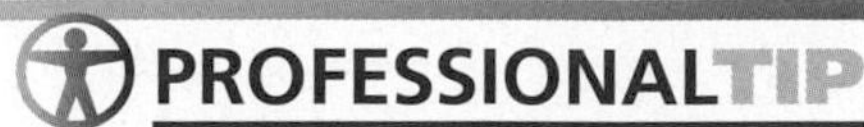

Influenza

Influenza (the flu) is a contagious respiratory illness caused by influenza viruses that lead to mild to severe illness and, at times, death. Influenza viruses are spread from person to person in respiratory droplets of coughs and sneezes. The Centers for Disease Control and Prevention (2009) estimates that 5% to 20% of Americans get the flu, more than 200,000 people are hospitalized from flu complications, and about 36,000 people die from influenza during each flu season, from November to March. The best way to prevent the flu is to get a flu vaccination each year. There are two types of influenza vaccines available: the "flu shot" and the nasal-spray flu vaccine. Currently there are four antiviral medications approved for treatment of influenza in the United States. Oseltamivir (Tamiflu) and zanamivir (Relenza) are recommended by the CDC due to the emerging influenza A resistance to the other two medications, amantadine (Symmetrel) and rimantadine (Flumadine) (National Institute of Allergy and Infectious Diseases, 2009). For more information on influenza, visit http://www.cdc.gov/flu/ or http://www3.niaid.nih.gov/topics/Flu/

MEDICAL–SURGICAL MANAGEMENT

Medical

Most clients with acute upper respiratory tract infections or inflammatory disorders are treated in a clinic or office setting. Unless the disorder becomes chronic or bacterial infection occurs, treatment is symptomatic. When infection is suspected, specimens for culture and sensitivity are obtained, and appropriate antibiotic therapy is initiated.

Surgical

Disorders that develop into chronic conditions (e.g., tonsillitis and sinusitis) may require surgical intervention to remove or drain affected tissues.

Pharmacological

Nonprescription antipyretic, analgesic, anti-inflammatory medications are used to reduce discomfort, fever, and inflammation. Antitussives are used to suppress cough and allow for rest. To aid in removal of secretions, expectorants are used. Bacterial infections are treated with various antibiotics according to culture and sensitivity studies. Comfort measures such as saline gargles may be useful.

time, the interior of the tubercle becomes soft and cheese-like as a result of decreased perfusion, a process known as **caseation**. Then the tubercle may become calcified and is called a Ghon's tubercle.

Liquefaction necrosis, where the tissue dies and changes to a liquid or semi-liquid state, may occur; this fluid may then be coughed up. A cavity is formed at the site where the primary tubercle liquefied and ruptured. This is called **cavitation**.

Following the advent of antitubercular medications in the 1950s, the incidence of TB decreased dramatically until 1985. From 1985 to 1992, TB cases increased 20%, but from 1992 have decreased 39%. In 2007, the total number of cases of TB (13,293 persons) in the United States was the lowest it has been since the study started in 1953 (ALA, 2009). New forms of TB, resistant to conventional drug therapy, have surfaced. Some of the factors that may be responsible for the increase in TB cases are increased numbers of persons with compromised immune systems (e.g., many AIDS clients also have TB); increased mobility of the world's population (persons from areas of high TB incidence moving to areas of low incidence); widespread IV drug abuse; increased numbers of those with poor access to health care; and increased numbers of those living in impoverished conditions. Direct health care costs for TB are $703.1 million each year (ALA, 2008a).

Symptoms of TB develop gradually following infection and include the following: low-grade fever that recurs in a specific pattern, persistent cough, hemoptysis, hoarseness, dyspnea on exertion, night sweats, fatigue, weight loss, and enlarged lymph nodes.

The Mantoux skin test is the preferred screening method for TB. Purified protein derivative (PPD) of killed tubercle bacilli 0.1 mL is injected intradermally in the inner forearm. The test is evaluated by measuring the area of induration (palpable swelling) that occurs 48 and 72 hours following injection. A reddened area with no induration is not considered positive. A positive skin test, however, indicates only that the client has been infected with and developed antibodies against the tubercle bacillus (Table 4-6). It is important for clients to know that the test will thereafter always be positive throughout the individual's lifetime. The Food and Drug Administration recently approved a new TB blood test called QuantoFERON-TB that is used for detecting TB and latent TB infection. The client receives the results from this test in less than 24 hours (ALA, 2008a).

The bacteria can remain alive but inactive in the body, often for a lifetime, so a client is given prophylactic treatment, usually isoniazid (INH), for 6 to 12 months. Other medications used against tuberculosis are outlined in Table 4-7. If INH has not been given and the person later in life is under physical or emotional stress, which weakens the immune system, the bacteria may become active and cause TB disease.

A negative reaction does not rule out the possibility of TB exposure. Individuals at high risk, such as those who are infected with HIV or who have compromised immune status, may have a negative reaction because they are unable to develop antibodies. Immediately following exposure to TB, a skin test may reveal a false-negative result because it can take up to 10 weeks for an infected individual to develop the antibodies. An additional skin test may be done in 10 to 12 weeks. If the second TB test is positive, the client's history is reviewed for the presence of symptoms suggesting TB, and further evaluation is indicated.

Chest x-ray and sputum specimens are utilized to confirm a diagnosis of TB. Inpatient clients are placed in airborne respiratory isolation until cultures are completed with results. Sputum is tested for the presence of acid-fast bacilli (AFB). The sputum specimen is collected when the client arises in the morning to prevent specimen contamination with ingested food and liquids. In most instances, three specimens collected on consecutive days and testing positive for AFB indicate a positive diagnosis of TB. The TB diagnosis is confirmed if

TABLE 4-6 Classification of the Tuberculin Reaction

CLASSIFIED AS POSITIVE	POPULATION
Induration of 5 mm or more	• HIV-positive persons • Recent contacts of TB case • Persons with chest x-rays consistent with old, healed TB • Clients with organ transplants or other immunosuppressed persons
Induration of 10 mm or more	• Injection drug users • Recent arrivals (<5 years) from high-prevalence countries • Residents and employees of high-risk congregate settings (prisons, nursing homes, mental institutions, residential facilities for AIDS patients, and homeless shelters) • Persons with medical conditions that have been shown to increase the risk of TB, such as silicosis; persons who are 10% or more below ideal body weight; and persons with some hematologic disorders (leukemias and lymphomas) and other malignancies • Mycobacteriology laboratory personnel • Children < 4 years of age, or children and adolescents exposed to adults in high-risk categories
Induration of 15 mm or more	*Persons with no risk factors for TB*

TABLE 4-7 Tuberculosis Medications

DRUG	MEDICATION PRECAUTIONS AND INFORMATION
First-Line Drugs	
ethambutol hydrochloride (Myambutol)	Monthly vision checks are important for acuity and distinction of red and green colors. Take medication with food.
isoniazid (INH) (Laniazid)	Alcohol ingestion interferes with metabolism and may cause hepatitis. Check baseline and monthly hepatic enzymes. Report signs of neuropathy and hepatitis. Have client take pyridoxine (vitamin B_6) to decrease side effects.
pyrazinamide (PMS Pyrazinamide)	Take medication with food and drink 2 liters of liquids daily. Check baseline and monthly uric acid and liver enzymes.
Rifamate	A combination of isoniazid and rifampin.
rifampin (Rifadin)	Body secretions (urine, sweat, tears) turn orange while taking the medication.
rifapentine (Priftin)	As effective as rifampin but taken less frequently. Body secretions (urine, sweat, tears) turn orange. Drug must be given with at least one other tuberculosis drug.
Rifater	A combination of isoniazid, rifampin, and pyrazinamide.
streptomycin sulfate	Have monthly audiograms to check auditory function. Check baseline and monthly renal function.
Second-Line Drugs	
cycloserine (Seromycin)	Observe for mental alertness. While taking the medication, monitor renal and liver function, drink 2 to 3 liters of fluid daily, and avoid alcohol.
ethionamide (Trecator-SC)	Given with other antitubercular drugs to prevent resistant organisms from developing.
kanamycin sulfate (Kantrex)	Drug may cause steatorrhea and electrolyte imbalance.
para-amino-salicylate (Sodium P.A.S.)	Must be taken with other antitubercular drugs; taken with meals.

the TB bacilli grow in a culture. Individuals who are unable to produce sputum, including children and older adults, may have stomach contents aspirated for AFB testing. Chest x-ray may reveal the presence of primary tubercles, calcified lesions, and cavitation in the lung.

MEDICAL–SURGICAL MANAGEMENT

Medical

Most clients are treated briefly in the hospital, with long-term treatment continuing at home. In the hospital, follow Airborne Precautions in addition to Standard Precautions. The precautions include placing the client in an isolation room with negative air pressure (air inflow is controlled through one vent and air outflow is exhausted through another vent directly to the outside and is not recirculated to other rooms.). The doors and windows of the client's room must be kept closed to maintain control of air flow. Caregivers should wear N95 particulate respirator masks because standard isolation masks do not prevent *Mycobacterium tuberculosis* from passing through (Figure 4-7). The Centers for Disease Control and Prevention recommend periodic TB skin testing for health care personnel.

Surgical

In the past, surgical intervention involving the removal of affected lung tissues was common. With the advent of effective chemotherapy (treatment with drugs), however, surgical intervention is now rarely utilized.

Pharmacological

Multidrug-resistant TB (MDR TB) can develop when a client does not complete the full therapy or is inadequately treated. A new strain of TB called extensively-drug resistant tuberculosis (XDR TB) is a strain with extensive resistance to second-line drugs. XDR TB is a public threat worldwide and is raising concerns of a future epidemic of TB that is virtually untreatable (ALA, 2008b). Active TB is treated with a combination of medications. Three medications—isoniazid (Laniazid, which is most effective), rifampin

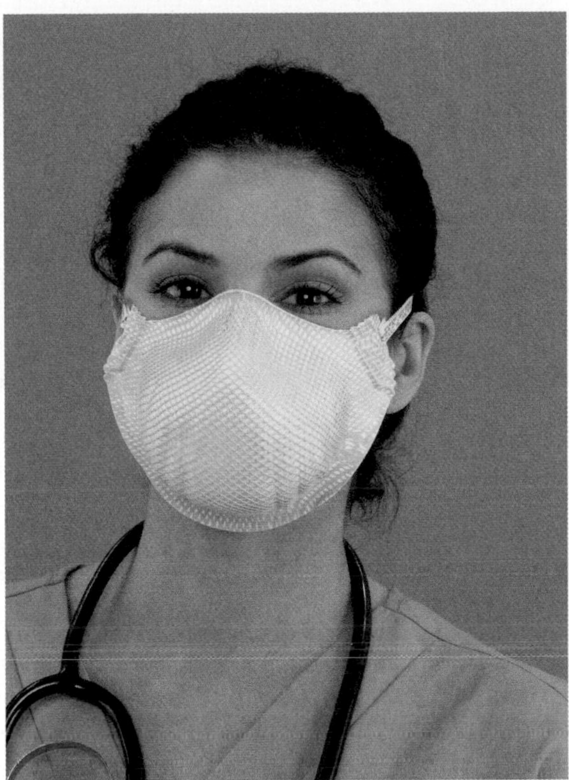

FIGURE 4-7 **A particulate respirator fits tightly around the nose and face.** (*Photo courtesy of Moldex Metric Inc; www.moldex.smugmug.com*)

(Rifadin), and pyrazinamide (PMS Pyrazinamide)—are given for several months. This is followed by a regimen of rifampin and isoniazid for an additional time. The combination of three drugs is given initially to rapidly decrease the number of active bacilli in the body and to prevent the development of MDR TB. Long-term therapy is required because TB bacilli have long periods of metabolic inactivity. Those clients with bone and joint infections, meningitis, or resistant forms of TB are treated for longer periods. Clients who are HIV positive require a longer regimen of isoniazid and pyrazinamide; prophylactic treatment with isoniazid is indicated from then on. Ethambutol hydrochloride (Myambutol) and streptomycin sulfate are added to the treatment regimen if the infecting organism is resistant to one of the three normally used medications. Infection with MDR TB requires the use of kanamycin sulfate (Kantrex), capreomycin sulfate (Capastat Sulfate), and cycloserine

SAFETY

Caregivers in Health Care Institutions

- Be aware of risks when caring for a client with TB.
- Follow Standard Precautions and Airborne Precautions.
- Use face and/or eye shield in addition to particulate mask when performing sputum-induction procedure.
- Plan care to limit prolonged exposure to client.
- Wash hands frequently and thoroughly.

MEMORY**TRICK**

MASK

A memory trick for the nurse to use to remember how to correctly wear and use an N95 particulate respirator mask when providing care for a TB client is the term **MASK**:

M = Make sure you are using the correct size mask.

A = Always wear an N95 particulate respirator mask (NOT a surgical mask).

S = Seal between face and respirator must be tightly fitted and intact.

K = Keep N95 particulate respirator mask on until after you leave the client's room.

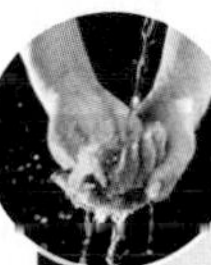

INFECTION CONTROL

Use of a Particulate Respirator

- Follow facility's procedure for fit-testing.
- Use the correct size mask.
- Put on respirator before entering client's room and remove after leaving client's room.
- Ensure that the respirator is free of holes.
- Check that the seal between face and respirator is intact.
- Discard soiled or damaged respirators.
- Have client wear N95 respirator when leaving the room.

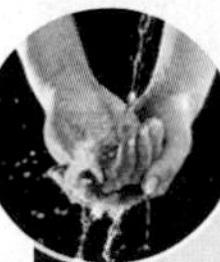

INFECTION CONTROL

Tuberculosis

- Instruct client to cover mouth and nose when coughing or sneezing.
- Double-bag secretions and dispose of them as infectious waste.
- Use disposable items for care when possible.
- Thoroughly clean and disinfect nondisposable items.

CLIENT TEACHING

Side Effects of Rifampin

- Urine, saliva, or tears may turn orange.
- May permanently discolor contact lenses.
- Birth control pills and implants become less effective. Use alternative methods of birth control.

CRITICAL THINKING

Tuberculosis Precautions

A nurse is working in a medical clinic when a client comes to the desk and informs her that one of his friends has TB, and that he was told to come to the clinic to get checked. The client is coughing continuously. The nurse knows that it will be 45 minutes before she can get him in to see the physician. What should the nurse do?

(Seromycin). The client is considered noninfectious following three negative AFB sputum specimens. At that point, the client may return to work and other normal activities. Prophylactic treatment of high-risk individuals is recommended to reduce their chances of developing the disease following their exposure.

Taking multiple drugs can be confusing and lead to noncompliance. The development of two new drugs has been valuable. These drugs are Rifater, a combination of isoniazid, rifampin, and pyrazinamide, and Rifamate, a combination of isoniazid and rifampin.

Diet

The client with TB often has nutritional deficits. Correcting these deficits assists the client in overcoming the disease process. Dietary management is based on the type of deficiency present. A well-balanced diet is encouraged for all clients with TB. Fluids are encouraged to aid in the liquefaction of respiratory secretions.

Activity

Activity is restricted based on the client's tolerance. The client who is severely compromised from a respiratory standpoint may be placed on bed rest. If the client's condition allows, activity is encouraged because it promotes lung expansion and aids in the removal of static secretions. The client in isolation whose condition permits it may ambulate in the hallways, as long as a particulate respirator mask is worn by the client while outside of the room.

COMMUNITY/HOME HEALTH CARE

The Client with Tuberculosis

Advise the client of the following:

- Keep all clinic appointments.
- Take all medications exactly as directed for duration of treatment.
- Until tested and noninfectious:
  - Put used tissues in a closed paper sack and throw away.
  - Avoid close contact with anyone; wear a mask.
  - Sleep alone in bedroom.
  - Air out bedroom often, using a fan in the window to blow air outside.
  - Thoroughly clean articles such as eating utensils.

Health Promotion

Prevention of TB is preferred to treatment. In areas where the disease remains endemic (seldom in the United States), a vaccine containing attenuated tubercle bacilli, *bacillus Calmette-Guérin* (BCG), may be given, but its effectiveness has not been proven. Individuals receiving it will test positive to the tuberculin skin test.

Any person who has had close contact with a client with TB without practicing appropriate protective measures should be tested. Other measures that decrease the likelihood of TB include adequate nutrition, housing, and health care access, and treatment of individuals who have or are at risk for developing TB.

Nursing Management

Assess client for low-grade fever, night sweats, and persistent cough. Teach client and family about the disease process and stress the importance of absolute compliance with the treatment plan.

NURSING PROCESS

Assessment

Subjective Data

The history includes questions about the presence of signs and symptoms of TB, such as night sweats, dyspnea on exertion or at rest in late disease, anorexia, loss of muscle strength, and fatigue. Pleuritic pain occurs when the pleura is involved.

Objective Data

Objective data include weight loss; persistent, low-grade fever; and persistent cough. The cough may be nonproductive early in the disease. Later, the cough is productive and yields thick, purulent sputum. Eventually, hemoptysis (blood spitting) occurs. Auscultation of breath sounds reveals coarse crackles. In the presence of cavitary disease, breath sounds are diminished or absent in the affected areas. Sputum is observed as to amount, color, odor, and consistency.

Nursing diagnoses for a client with TB include the following:

NURSING DIAGNOSES	PLANNING/OUTCOMES	NURSING INTERVENTIONS
*Ineffective **B**reathing Pattern* related to pulmonary infectious process	The client will have color and respiratory rate within normal limits and will not complain of dyspnea.	Assess client's color, respiratory rate, and respiratory effort and auscultate the breath sounds. Plan care activities to allow client uninterrupted periods of rest. Assist client in assuming the position that most aids respiratory effort. Administer medications as ordered. Encourage fluids if not otherwise contraindicated.
*Deficient **K**nowledge* related to disease process and its treatment	The client will verbalize an understanding of the disease process and its treatment.	Teach client and family about the basic pathophysiology of TB, how the infection is contracted, who is at risk of developing an infection, the signs and symptoms of TB infection, and complications that may arise. Present information regarding the actions, side effects, and untoward effects of the drugs being administered. Teach client signs and symptoms of adverse drug reactions to report to the physician. Emphasize the necessity of long-term therapy to cure TB. Inform client and family that symptoms decrease and are often gone long before the organism is eliminated from the body.
*Ineffective **T**herapeutic Regimen Management* related to client value system	The client will continue medication regimen for the prescribed length of time.	Include client and family in making decisions about care, when appropriate. Allow client to be an active participant in care decisions, to increase personal responsibility and accountability. Visits from public health or home care nurses may be necessary to monitor client for compliance. Explore reasons for noncompliance with client and family, and identify strategies to increase compliance. Refer client who is unable to afford the cost of medications to agencies such as the local health department for assistance. Begin directly observed therapy if the client continues to be noncompliant. Directly observed therapy involves sending the nurse or another health care worker to the client to administer the medications and verify that they are taken.

Evaluation: Evaluate each outcome to determine how it has been met by the client.

SAMPLE NURSING CARE PLAN

The Client with TB

R.D. is an 87-year-old man who is admitted to the hospital with a chief complaint of productive cough and fatigue. Four months ago, R.D. was placed in a long-term care facility because of his inability to care for himself at home after his wife's death 1 year previously. Since admission to the long-term care facility,

(Continues)

SAMPLE NURSING CARE PLAN (Continued)

R.D. has lost 15 pounds. The nurses at the facility report that R.D. has experienced progressive fatigue, dyspnea on exertion, cough, night sweats, and anorexia. Initially, his cough was nonproductive, but it is now productive of moderate amounts of thick, purulent sputum that is occasionally streaked with blood. Vital signs are temperature 99.8°F, pulse 108 beats/min, respirations 26 breaths/min, and blood pressure 138/86 mm Hg. A TB skin test done at the long-term care facility 1 week ago was evaluated as negative at 6 mm. Sputum specimens for AFB reveal the presence of active tubercle bacilli, and chest x-ray is positive for TB. Auscultation of breath sounds reveals crackles in the right lower half of the lung. R.D. says, "I don't understand why I can't breathe good and what all this fuss is about."

NURSING DIAGNOSIS 1 *Ineffective Breathing Pattern* related to infectious pulmonary process as evidenced by dyspnea on exertion and productive cough

Nursing Outcomes Classification (NOC)
Respiratory Status: Airway Patency
Respiratory Status: Ventilation
Energy Conservation

Nursing Interventions Classification (NIC)
Airway Management
Ventilation Assistance
Energy Management

PLANNING/OUTCOMES	NURSING INTERVENTIONS	RATIONALE
R.D. will have respiratory rate, oxygen saturation, and color within desired ranges and will not complain of dyspnea.	Initially and periodically assess R.D.'s respiratory status, including color, respiratory rate, respiratory effort, oxygen saturation, breath sounds, level of consciousness, cough, and sputum.	Provides a database from which the plan of care can be formulated and against which the effectiveness of treatment is evaluated. Subsequent assessments evaluate the effectiveness of interventions and may modify the care plan.
	Assist R.D. in assuming a position that most aids respiratory effort.	Allows for greater ease of respiration and lung expansion.
	Alternate care activities with periods of rest.	Allows R.D. to compensate for the increased oxygen demand required by activity.
	Encourage activity within R.D.'s tolerance.	Promotes expansion of the lungs.
	Encourage fluids.	Promotes liquefaction of respiratory secretions.
	Administer medications for fever as ordered.	Persistent fever leads to dehydration, which hinders the removal of respiratory secretions.
	Administer oxygen as ordered to maintain an SaO_2 of 95% or greater.	Necessary for optimal cellular function.
	Administer antitubercular drugs as ordered.	Decreases the number of viable tubercle bacilli.

EVALUATION

R.D. verbalizes a decrease in dyspnea and cough. R.D.'s color, respiratory rate, and oxygen saturation are within normal limits.

SAMPLE NURSING CARE PLAN (Continued)

NURSING DIAGNOSIS 2 *Risk for Infection* spread related to viable bacilli in secretions as evidenced by AFB in sputum

Nursing Outcomes Classification (NOC)
Knowledge: Infection Control

Nursing Interventions Classification (NIC)
Health Education

PLANNING/OUTCOMES	NURSING INTERVENTIONS	RATIONALE
R.D. will verbalize both those situations that allow for the transmission of the tubercle bacilli and the means to prevent their transmission.	Place R.D. in a negative air pressure, private room; keep door closed at all times. On the door, place Airborne Precaution signs indicating that R.D. has an infectious process and asking visitors to see nursing personnel before visiting. Instruct visitors to wear N95 respirators when in R.D.'s room, to limit the length of their visits, to avoid intimate contact, and to wash their hands when leaving the room.	Prevents transmission of the tubercle bacilli in air that has been circulated into and out of R.D.'s room. Prevents inadvertent contact and exposure. The nature of the infection is not revealed publicly to maintain client confidentiality. Visitors are informed of precautions to take to prevent exposure.
	Instruct R.D. to cover his mouth and nose when coughing and sneezing.	Aids in the containment of the tubercle bacilli.
	Instruct R.D. to cough up secretions in tissues and to place the tissues in a plastic bag. Dispose of contained secretions as infectious waste.	Aids in preventing the spread of the tubercle bacilli.
	Inform the long-term care facility and family/significant others of the positive results of the AFB studies. Instruct those persons who have been exposed to R.D. to have a TB skin test.	Known exposure to active tubercle bacilli necessitates testing to identify individuals who may have become infected.
	Observe Standard Precautions and Airborne Precautions.	Decreases the likelihood of transmitting the tubercle bacilli (and other infectious diseases) to staff and other clients.
	Wear a fitted N95 respirator when in R.D.'s room.	Prevents the inhalation of tubercle bacilli, which are able to pass through a simple surgical mask.

EVALUATION

Persons exposed to R.D. have been tested for TB. Those with TB are being treated.

(Continues)

SAMPLE NURSING CARE PLAN (Continued)

NURSING DIAGNOSIS 3 *Deficient Knowledge* related to disease process and its treatment as evidenced by client statement: "I don't understand why I can't breathe good and what all this fuss is about."

Nursing Outcomes Classification (NOC)
Knowledge: Disease Process
Knowledge: Treatment Regimen

Nursing Interventions Classification (NIC)
Teaching: Disease Process
Teaching: Individual

PLANNING/OUTCOMES	NURSING INTERVENTIONS	RATIONALE
R.D. will verbalize an understanding of the disease process and the required medication regimen.	Assess R.D.'s present level of knowledge regarding TB and its treatment.	Provides a database regarding R.D.'s present level of knowledge regarding TB and its treatment. Client education can then be individualized to build and expand on that knowledge base. Misinformation can also be corrected.
	Provide information in small amounts and use a variety of approaches (e.g., verbal, written, video).	Increases the likelihood of learning and stimulates the various senses.
	Encourage and allow time for R.D. to ask questions.	Provides a means to clarify information and for the nurse to evaluate learning and correct misconceptions.
	Have R.D. verbalize signs and symptoms of adverse medication effects to report to the staff.	Provides a means to clarify information and for the nurse to evaluate learning and correct misconceptions.

EVALUATION

R.D. verbalizes individual treatment regimen and its purpose. R.D. reports adverse effects of medication to health care personnel to allow for early intervention.

PLEURISY/PLEURAL EFFUSION

Pleurisy is a painful condition that arises from inflammation of the pleura, or sac that encases the lung. This pleuritic pain is sharp and stabbing in nature. Pain increases on inspiration as the irritated pleura rub over each other. Inflammation of the pleura occurs with many disorders, such as viral infections, cancer of the lung, trauma, tuberculosis, congestive heart failure, and pulmonary embolism. The inflamed pleura secrete increased amounts of pleural fluid into the pleural cavity, creating a **pleural effusion.** As fluid accumulates within the pleural space (cavity), it compresses the lung tissue (Figure 4-8). Collapse, or **atelectasis,** results if the effusion is left untreated. Those areas of collapsed lung tissue are unable to take part in gas exchange, thereby decreasing oxygenation. **Empyema** is the term to describe infected pleural exudate.

The primary manifestation of pleurisy is pain on inspiration. Signs and symptoms of pleural effusion depend on the amount of lung tissue compressed and the source of the effusion. With large pleural effusions, the mediastinum (heart, great vessels, and trachea) shifts toward the unaffected side; this can be detected by inspection, and heart sounds will move toward the unaffected side. Magnetic resonance imaging (MRI) or computerized tomography (CT) studies are useful in detecting pleural effusions, particularly small ones. A chest x-ray will show pleural effusions of 250 mL of fluid or more. If empyema is suspected, culture and sensitivity studies will identify the presence and type of infection. The client with empyema will also have an elevated temperature and white blood cell count.

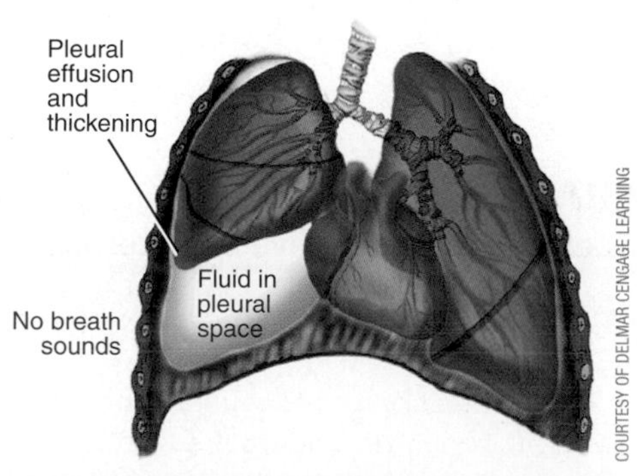

FIGURE 4-8 Pleural Effusion

PROFESSIONALTIP

Assessment of Client with a Chest Tube

- Obtain vital signs as ordered.
- Be alert for dyspnea.
- Record and describe amount of drainage.
- Look for loops of tubing containing drainage.
- Monitor water level in the water seal. Fluctuation (called tidaling) should occur with respirations and will stop when lung is reexpanded, tubing is kinked, connections are not tight, or chest tube becomes dislodged.
- Keep chest drainage system below the level of the client's chest.
- Every 2 hours, monitor client's response to coughing and deep breathing.
- If the chest tube is accidentally dislodged, cover opening with petrolatum gauze and tape only three sides of the dressing to create a one-way valve in which air can exit the pleural space on exhalation to prevent a tension pneumothorax from occurring (Daniels, Nosek, Nicoll, 2007).
- Assess for pain and discomfort.
- Ensure chest tube patency.
- Auscultate breath sounds in each lung lobe.
- Assess chest tube insertion site for signs of infection.
- Assess and palpate skin at chest tube insertion site for puffiness and crepitus (crackling).
- Observe for signs of subcutaneous emphysema.

MEDICAL–SURGICAL MANAGEMENT

Medical

Treatment is aimed at eliminating the underlying cause, maintaining adequate oxygenation to the tissues, and preventing complications such as atelectasis and pneumonia. Oxygenation is evaluated by ABGs and/or pulse oximetry. Supplemental oxygen is given to maintain an oxygen saturation of 95% or greater. Respiratory treatments to aid lung expansion such as incentive spirometry are used.

Surgical

Larger pleural effusions require that a thoracentesis be performed by the physician to remove accumulated fluid. After the overlying tissues are anesthetized, a large-bore needle is placed into the pleural space. Fluid is removed (no more than 1500 mL) and may be sent to the laboratory for diagnostic purposes (e.g., culture, cytology). If fluid accumulation continues, a thoracotomy tube is placed into the pleural space to drain fluid continuously. Following administration of local anesthetics, the physician places a large-bore catheter into the pleural space. This catheter is attached to an underwater seal chest tube drainage device (Figure 4-9). It prevents the negative pressure within the pleural space from pulling air into the pleural space, and

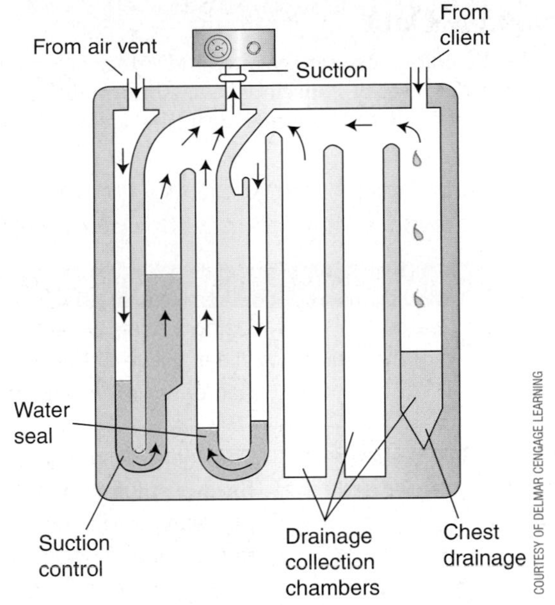

FIGURE 4-9 Underwater Seal Chest Drainage Device

allows for the drainage of accumulated fluid or air. Most chest tube devices have a chamber to which suction may be applied to assist in the removal of fluid or air from the pleural space. It can also be sealed with a Heimlich (one-way) valve. A chest x-ray is done to evaluate the chest tube's placement and effectiveness.

Pharmacological

If a pleural effusion is small and does not interfere greatly with respiratory function, diuretics are used to promote removal of fluid from the pleural space. Furosemide (Lasix) and bumetanide (Bumex) may be given for this purpose. If empyema is present, specific therapy is used once the causative agent is identified. Pain relief is a high priority. Analgesia that also decreases inflammation is preferred. Ketorolac tromethamine (Toradol) or other nonsteroidal anti-inflammatory drugs are often used. Severe pain may require narcotics. For extensive inflammation, corticosteroids may be utilized.

Activity

The client's activity is limited to prevent fatigue. High Fowler's position assists respirations.

NURSING MANAGEMENT

Assess the client's color, respiratory rate and effort, and level of consciousness. Monitor vital signs and breath sounds. If a chest tube is in place, watch that all tubes are in place and the drainage device is working properly. A variety of closed-drainage chest tube systems are available. Empty drainage per agency policy. Encourage the client to use the incentive spirometer.

NURSING PROCESS

ASSESSMENT

Subjective Data

A nursing history is obtained from the client regarding onset, duration, and severity of symptoms. The client usually describes both chest pain that increases with each inspiration and difficulty breathing.

Objective Data

The client's color, respiratory rate, and effort are evaluated along with the level of consciousness. Abnormalities in vital signs are noted. Breath sounds over the areas of involvement are diminished or absent. A pleural friction rub may be audible. Dyspnea, cyanosis, and hypoxia occur in proportion to the severity of the condition. If a chest tube is in place, the amount and color of drainage are assessed.

Nursing diagnoses for a client with a pleural effusion include the following:

NURSING DIAGNOSES	PLANNING/OUTCOMES	NURSING INTERVENTIONS
*Acute **P**ain* related to inflammation of the pleura	Using a scale of 0 to 10, the client will verbalize a decrease in the level of pain.	Administer pain medications as ordered. Assist the client in attaining the position that allows for greatest comfort. Elevate the head of the bed. Provide diversional activities.
*Impaired **G**as Exchange* related to compressed lung	The client will maintain an oxygen saturation of 95% or greater and a respiratory rate of 14 to 22 bpm and will have clear breath sounds.	Monitor vital signs and pulse oximetry. Provide supplemental oxygen as ordered. Encourage client to breathe deeply or use the incentive spirometer as ordered. Administer diuretics and anti-inflammatory medications as ordered. Assist physician with the thoracentesis or the placement of a thoracotomy tube. Collect specimen for culture and sensitivity and other studies as ordered.
*Risk for **A**ctivity Intolerance* related to hypoxia secondary to pleural effusion	The client will increase activity without complaining of fatigue.	Stagger periods of activity with periods of rest. To prevent fatigue, plan activities around therapies.
*Bathing/Hygiene **S**elf-care Deficit* related to mobility restriction	The client will increase self-care activities as mobility increases.	Assist client with hygiene and self-care needs, but encourage participation in self-care activities within the limits of the physician's orders.

Evaluation: Evaluate each outcome to determine how it has been met by the client.

SEVERE ACUTE RESPIRATORY SYNDROME

Severe acute respiratory syndrome (SARS) is a viral respiratory illness with flu-like symptoms that is caused by the SARS associated coronovirus (SARS-CoV). It was identified in China in late 2002, and first reported in Asia in February 2003 (CDC, 2008). A total of 8,098 people became sick with SARS, and 773 died worldwide during the outbreak (CDC, 2005a). SARS spread worldwide over several months before the outbreak ended (National Institutes of Health, 2009c).

It appears that SARS spreads by close personal contact or contact with infectious material (respiratory secretions). This happens when a client with SARS coughs or sneezes droplets onto themselves, others, or nearby surfaces.

The incubation period is generally 2 to 7 days. Then an elevated temperature of > 100.4°F (>38°C) occurs and may be associated with chills, headache, malaise, body aches, respiratory symptoms, pneumonia, and even respiratory failure. After 2 to 7 days, clients may develop a dry, nonproductive cough and dyspnea.

There is no specific treatment for SARS. Support treatment is provided based on the symptoms.

NURSING MANAGEMENT

Follow Standard Precautions (hand hygiene and eye protection), Contact Precautions (gown and gloves), and Airborne Precautions (isolation room with negative pressure and use of N-95 respirators). Monitor client's vital signs. Assess breath sounds. Provide routine care with uninterrupted rest periods.

ACUTE RESPIRATORY TRACT DISORDERS

Acute respiratory tract disorders include atelectasis, pulmonary embolism, pulmonary edema, acute respiratory distress syndrome, and acute respiratory failure.

ATELECTASIS

Atelectasis refers to the collapse of a lung or a portion of a lung. The most common cause of atelectasis is airway obstruction. A bronchiole becomes blocked with secretions, and the alveoli distal to it collapse (Figure 4-10). Airway obstruction of this nature is common after surgery and with immobility problems. Anesthesia, pain, narcotics, and immobility can cause hypoventilation and retention of secretions.

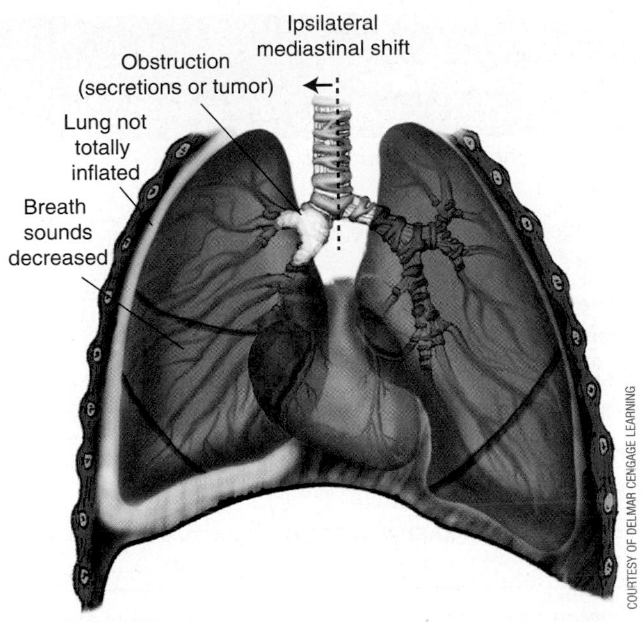

FIGURE 4-10 Atelectasis (Collapsed Lung)

Hypoventilation can cause atelectasis, which increases hypoventilation. Atelectasis can occur with compression of lung tissue, as in pleural effusion or pneumothorax. Insufficient surfactant results in increased recoil properties of the lungs, leading to atelectasis.

Signs of respiratory distress are proportional to the amount of lung tissue involved. When large areas of the lung are involved, orthopnea or cyanosis may develop. Breath sounds are diminished or absent over collapsed areas. Chest wall movement may decrease on the affected side. Oxygenation decreases as shown by ABGs or pulse oximetry. Pulse and respiratory rate increase as the heart and lungs work harder to meet the body's oxygen needs. Trapped secretions are a growth medium for microorganisms. An elevated temperature indicates secondary infection (pneumonia). Chest x-ray shows the areas of collapse. Bronchoscopy (insertion of a bronchoscope into the trachea) is used to directly visualize the area of obstruction and obtain a specimen for diagnostic purposes.

Medical–Surgical Management

Medical

The physician orders incentive spirometry and deep breathing and coughing exercises to promote expansion of the lungs. Postural drainage and percussion aids in the removal of any static secretions. If the client is unable to cough up secretions, suctioning of the respiratory tract is performed. Bronchoscopy may be done to remove secretions and obtain specimens. Arterial blood gases and pulse oximetry are utilized to evaluate the need for supplemental oxygen. Oxygen is administered to maintain an oxygen saturation of 95% or greater.

Surgical

Clients with pneumothorax or pleural effusion as the underlying cause of atelectasis require removal of trapped air or fluid via thoracentesis or placement of a thoracotomy tube (refer to the sections on pleural effusion and pneumothorax). Atelectasis resulting from the growth of a tumor requires removal of the tumor.

Pharmacological

Adequate pain control aids the client, particularly the surgical client, to breathe deeply and cough. Client-controlled analgesia or a routine schedule of pain medication may be used to provide effective pain management. Bronchodilators may be used to open the airways. Mucolytic agents are used to liquefy secretions. Bronchodilators, such as albuterol sulfate (Ventolin), and mucolytics, such as acetylcysteine (Mucomyst), may also be administered via updraft or nebulizer treatments. The client with an infection requires treatment with an appropriate antibiotic.

Diet

Unless otherwise contraindicated, fluids are encouraged to promote liquefaction of trapped respiratory secretions.

Activity

Activity promotes lung expansion. Immobile clients are turned a minimum of every 2 hours and assisted to do range-of-motion exercises. Surgical clients may do leg exercises as well as deep breathing and coughing. Ambulation is recommended if the client's condition allows. If the client is unable to walk, sitting up in a chair is encouraged. To prevent fatigue, rest periods are planned between activities.

Nursing Management

Monitor for pain, shortness of breath, fatigue, dyspnea, cyanosis, anxiety, and level of consciousness. Assess for Homans' sign. Teach client how to cough, deep breathe, and use the incentive spirometer. Encourage ambulation as client's condition allows. Turn immobile clients at least every 2 hours.

NURSING PROCESS

Assessment

Subjective Data

Clients who smoke, those who are immunocompromised, and those who have known chronic respiratory or cardiovascular diseases are at increased risk of developing atelectasis. The client is asked about the onset, duration, and severity of symptoms such as pain, cough, and dyspnea. The client may complain or show signs of air hunger, shortness of breath, fatigue, and anxiety.

Objective Data

Assess the client for changes in level of consciousness, an early sign of decreased oxygenation. Periodically evaluate for dyspnea, tachypnea, cyanosis, and restlessness. Measure vital signs frequently, with particular attention to respiratory rate and effort. Auscultation reveals diminished or absent breath sounds over the areas of atelectasis. Crackles (rales) or sonorous wheezes may be heard if pneumonia develops. Note objective indicators of pain such as facial grimacing, and validate by subjective questioning. Assess the effectiveness of the client's cough. A productive cough is evaluated for amount, color, consistency, and odor of secretions.

Nursing diagnoses for a client with atelectasis include the following:

NURSING DIAGNOSES	PLANNING/OUTCOMES	NURSING INTERVENTIONS
*Impaired **G**as Exchange* related to decreased alveolar–capillary surface	The client will have an oxygen saturation of 95% or greater, a respiratory rate of 14 to 22 bpm, and clear breath sounds.	Establish a schedule for coughing and deep breathing. Encourage client to ambulate and/or sit up in a chair three to four times daily. Turn the immobile client every 2 hours or more frequently. Assess client's vital signs and breath sounds every 4 hours or more frequently as situation warrants. Encourage fluids if client's condition allows. Administer respiratory treatments and medications as ordered. Assess secretions (sputum) for color, amount, consistency, and odor.
*Risk for **A**ctivity Intolerance* related to hypoxia secondary to atelectasis	The client will complete activity without complaints of shortness of breath, dyspnea, or fatigue.	Encourage some activity, such as walking, to promote lung expansion, and alternate with periods of rest to avoid client fatigue. Provide assistance with ADL as client's condition requires. Place client in a high or semi-Fowler's position to aid lung expansion. Position client on the unaffected side.
*Deficient **K**nowledge* related to the complications of surgery and/or immobility	The client will verbalize the purpose of deep breathing, coughing, and activity following surgery, and will demonstrate deep breathing and coughing.	Teach all preoperative and immobile clients to cough and breathe deeply at least every 2 hours and have the client demonstrate to ensure that learning has occurred. Teach the surgical client to splint the surgical incision to minimize discomfort that might occur with coughing and deep breathing. Instruct clients at risk for developing atelectasis in the use of incentive spirometry. Emphasize the importance of early ambulation and activity to promote lung expansion.

Evaluation: Evaluate each outcome to determine how it has been met by the client.

PULMONARY EMBOLISM

Pulmonary embolism (PE) develops when a bloodborne substance lodges in a branch of a pulmonary artery and obstructs flow. A common source of PE is deep vein thrombosis. Other sources are air from intravenous infusions; fat from long-bone fractures; and amniotic fluid. The size and location of the emboli determine the severity and outcome of the condition.

Pulmonary emboli rarely develop before adulthood. As age increases, the risk for pulmonary embolism becomes greater because of the development of arteriosclerosis and other vascular changes associated with aging. Other factors increasing the risk for PE are heredity, smoking, peripheral vascular disease, diabetes mellitus, and oral contraceptive use.

Emboli interfere with gas exchange to the pulmonary circulation distal to the emboli, resulting in hypoxemia. The client describes breathlessness and dyspnea. Pulse oximetry or ABGs will show the degree to which oxygenation has been affected. Obstruction of a main branch of a pulmonary artery can result in lung infarction, necrosis, and may even lead to death.

All clients at risk for PE are observed for signs and symptoms of deep vein thrombosis, such as localized calf tenderness or swelling. Measures to prevent thrombus formation are taken for these individuals. Any signs of thrombophlebitis are immediately reported to the physician.

Signs and symptoms of PE are abrupt in onset. The client becomes anxious and restless. Sudden, sharp chest pains or back pain of a pleuritic nature (worse on inspiration) develop. Dyspnea and cough, along with hemoptysis, occur. Venous return is diminished, resulting in jugular venous distention. The client becomes diaphoretic. A low-grade fever develops in response to inflammation. A high temperature indicates lung infarction. Diagnosis of PE is often done by a ventilation/perfusion lung scan, but the gold standard is pulmonary angiography. Arterial blood gases show hypoxia and respiratory alkalosis. A spiral CT scan of the lungs may be ordered, and can be performed within a few seconds.

Medical–Surgical Management

Medical

Preventive measures are instituted for the client at risk of developing deep vein thrombosis. Following surgery, antiembolism stockings, sequential compression devices (SCDs), intermittent pneumatic compression devices (e.g., PlexiPulse), and early ambulation are indicated. When hypoxia occurs, supplemental oxygen is given to increase oxygenation. The underlying cause of the PE is treated when identified.

Surgical

In severe cases, the physician may remove the clot via an embolectomy. This procedure is usually done at the time of angiography. Clients who experience successive episodes of PE may require a venacaval plication or filter. This surgical procedure involves placing a sieve-like device in the inferior vena cava to catch emboli before they enter pulmonary circulation (National Heart Lung and Blood Institute, 2009b).

Pharmacological

The client at risk of developing deep vein thrombosis and/or PE may be treated with enoxaparin (Lovenox). Lovenox is often used in the postoperative client to prevent clot formation. After PE has developed, anticoagulation is ordered to prevent the formation of further clots. Heparin sodium is initially used to establish anticoagulation and is administered parenterally by either the intravenous or subcutaneous route. After adequate anticoagulation is established, warfarin sodium (Coumadin) therapy is initiated and may be given concurrently with heparin while the client is hospitalized until Coumadin level is therapeutic. Coumadin alone is given orally when the client is discharged. If the clot is large or lies in a branch of a main pulmonary artery, fibrinolytic therapy may be used. Fibrinolytics lyse, or dissolve, the clot versus inhibiting the formation of new clots. Examples of fibrinolytic agents are alteplase recombinant (Activase) and streptokinase (Streptase). These agents may be administered intra-arterially at the site of the clot or intravenously to achieve a systemic effect. Narcotic analgesics such as morphine are used to control pain.

CLIENT TEACHING

Anticoagulant Therapy (Coumadin)

Stress the importance of:

- Follow-up laboratory testing
- Using a soft toothbrush to prevent trauma to the gums (bleeding)
- Inspecting the skin for bruises or petechiae
- Using an electric razor to avoid scratching skin
- Reporting nosebleeds, tarry stool, hematuria, or hematemesis to the physician
- Eating a consistent amount of green, leafy vegetables daily (differing amounts alter anticoagulant effects)
- Avoiding other medications including aspirin (it has an anticoagulant effect) without approval from physician
- In the female client, monitor menstrual flow for excessive amount

LIFE SPAN CONSIDERATIONS

Older Adults at Risk for Pulmonary Embolism

The risk of developing a pulmonary embolism increases with age. For each 10 years after age 60, the risk of developing a pulmonary embolism doubles (NHLBI, 2009c).

Diet

Fluids are encouraged to prevent hemoconcentration leading to clot formation. Unless contraindicated, fluids are encouraged for the client at risk of developing PE.

Activity

To prevent the formation of clots, activity is encouraged. After a clot has formed, however, the client's activity is restricted to prevent the clot from moving and becoming an embolus. Activities such as sitting, crossing the knees, or prolonged bending at the hips are to be avoided because they promote venous stasis.

Nursing Management

Assess the abrupt onset of pleuritic chest pain for location, duration, severity, and character. Assess lung sounds, monitor pulse oximetry, vital signs, jugular veins for distension, peripheral pulses, and capillary refill. Encourage deep breathing and provide supplemental oxygen as ordered. Monitor results of

APTT, INR, PT, hemoglobin, and hematocrit. Do not massage site if deep vein thrombosis (DVT) has occurred.

NURSING PROCESS

ASSESSMENT

Subjective Data

The client's history is obtained to identify potential risk factors for the development of PE. Ask the client about the onset, duration, and severity of symptoms. Shortness of breath, dyspnea, and severe pleuritic chest pain are abrupt in onset. Pain is evaluated as to onset, location, duration, severity, and character.

Objective Data

Pulse oximetry measurements are monitored. The client's respirations are rapid and shallow. Pallor progressing to cyanosis develops as oxygenation decreases. The client becomes diaphoretic. Increased anxiety or a change in level of consciousness may be the first indication of PE. The pulse increases in response to anxiety and in an attempt to supply oxygen to the body's cells. Blood pressure may increase or decrease in response to hypoxia, anxiety, and pain. Temperature may elevate in response to inflammation and tissue necrosis. On auscultation, breath sounds may or may not be decreased. The jugular veins may be distended.

Nursing diagnoses for a client with pulmonary embolism include the following:

NURSING DIAGNOSES	PLANNING/OUTCOMES	NURSING INTERVENTIONS
*Impaired **Gas** Exchange* related to alteration in pulmonary circulation	The client will maintain an oxygen saturation of 95% or greater, have a respiratory rate of 14 to 22 bpm, and have color within normal limits.	Assess client for indications of decreasing oxygenation. Auscultate breath sounds every 4 hours or more often. Assess peripheral pulses and capillary refill. Encourage deep breathing and coughing. Provide supplemental oxygen to maintain oxygen saturation at greater than 95% or as ordered. Administer anticoagulants (Heparin, Lovenox, Coumadin) as ordered. Encourage fluids, unless contraindicated, to prevent hemoconcentration.
*Acute **Pain*** related to decreased perfusion of lung tissue	Using a scale of 0 to 10, the client will indicate decreased pain.	Administer pain medication as ordered and monitor for relief. Assist client in assuming a position of comfort. If possible, place client in a high Fowler's position to aid respiratory effort.
*Risk for **Injury*** related to anticoagulation/fibrinolytic therapy	The client will be free of abnormal bleeding and maintain hemoglobin and hematocrit within normal limits.	Assess for evidence of bleeding. Monitor lab reports for activated partial thromboplastin time (APTT), international normalized ratio (INR), prothrombin time (PT), decrease in platelet count, and hemoglobin and hematocrit levels. Evaluate blood pressure and pulse for signs of bleeding (i.e., rapid pulse and low blood pressure). Check stool for occult blood. Assess gums for bleeding.

Evaluation: Evaluate each outcome to determine how it has been met by the client.

PULMONARY EDEMA

Acute pulmonary edema is a life-threatening condition characterized by a rapid shift of fluid from plasma into the pulmonary interstitial tissue and the alveoli (Figure 4-11). As a result, gas exchange is markedly impaired. Pulmonary edema generally has a cardiac cause such as left ventricular failure or myocardial infarction, or a noncardiac cause such as fluid overload, inhalation of noxious gases, opiate overdose, aspiration, sepsis, or radiation injury.

The hallmark of acute pulmonary edema is a cough producing a copious amount of frothy, blood-tinged sputum (hemoptysis), often appearing pinkish. The client rapidly becomes dyspneic, orthopneic, and cyanotic. Anxiety ranging from restlessness to panic occurs. Heart and respiratory rate increase. Progressive crackles (rales) are heard in the lung fields on auscultation. Initially, fine crackles (rales) are present in the posterior bases of the lung. As pulmonary edema progresses, the crackles (rales) become increasingly coarser, louder, and more diffuse. Wheezes are heard in the presence

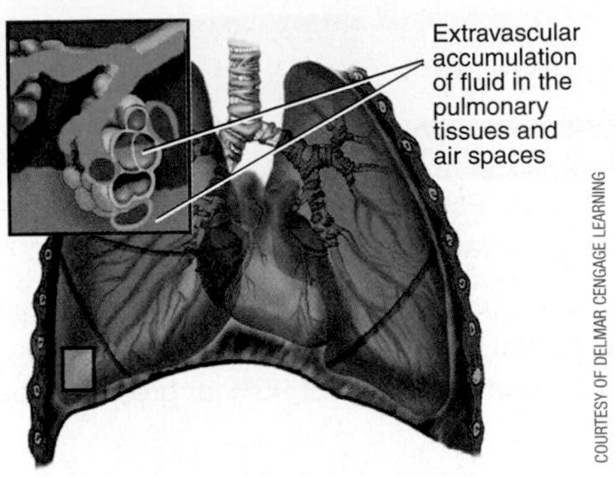

FIGURE 4-11 Pulmonary Edema

of significant airway obstruction by fluid. Left untreated, the client deteriorates rapidly as oxygenation decreases. The client's history is crucial to identify the cause. Noncardiogenic pulmonary edema can quickly become respiratory failure.

MEDICAL–SURGICAL MANAGEMENT

Medical

The goals of medical management are to remove fluid from the alveoli and pulmonary interstitial space, prevent further influx of fluid, improve oxygenation, and decrease workload of left ventricle. Arterial blood gases and pulse oximetry values are used to assess oxygenation. Oxygen is administered per physician's order when hypoxia is present. Noncardiogenic pulmonary edema often requires ventilation support and treatment of the cause.

Pharmacological

A diuretic such as furosemide (Lasix) is the primary treatment for cardiogenic pulmonary edema. When the pumping force of the left ventricle is impaired, a digitalis preparation is given to improve the contractile force of the myocardium. To prevent further influx of fluid into the lungs, venous pooling is enhanced. This also decreases the workload on the heart by limiting venous return. Morphine is used to promote vasodilation and, thus, venous pooling and to relieve anxiety. Bronchodilators are administered to dilate airways obstructed with fluid.

Diet

A sodium-restricted diet may be ordered to prevent fluid retention. Intake and output as well as daily weight are measured to monitor fluid balance.

Activity

Bed rest reduces the workload on the heart and lungs. High Fowler's position aids respiratory effort and enhances venous pooling. Activities are increased slowly according to the physician's orders and the client's ability to tolerate activity.

NURSING MANAGEMENT

Monitor ABGs and pulse oximetry and administer oxygen as ordered. Assess breath sounds, vital signs, and level of consciousness. Keep client in high Fowler's position. Keep an accurate intake and output record. Monitor client's weight daily.

NURSING PROCESS

ASSESSMENT

Subjective Data

The nurse must be aware of the conditions that predispose the client to pulmonary edema. The client may describe feeling anxious, breathless, and fatigued.

Objective Data

Breath sounds are auscultated for the presence of crackles (rales). Report increasingly coarse and diffuse crackles (rales) to the physician. Assess the client's level of consciousness, respiratory rate and effort, and color. Dyspnea, tachypnea, cyanosis and/or pallor may be present. Assess oxygenation via pulse oximetry or ABGs. A productive cough may be present, as may symptoms of CHF, such as rapid weight gain and peripheral edema. Pulse may be rapid and weak. Blood pressure may increase in response to anxiety and decreased oxygenation.

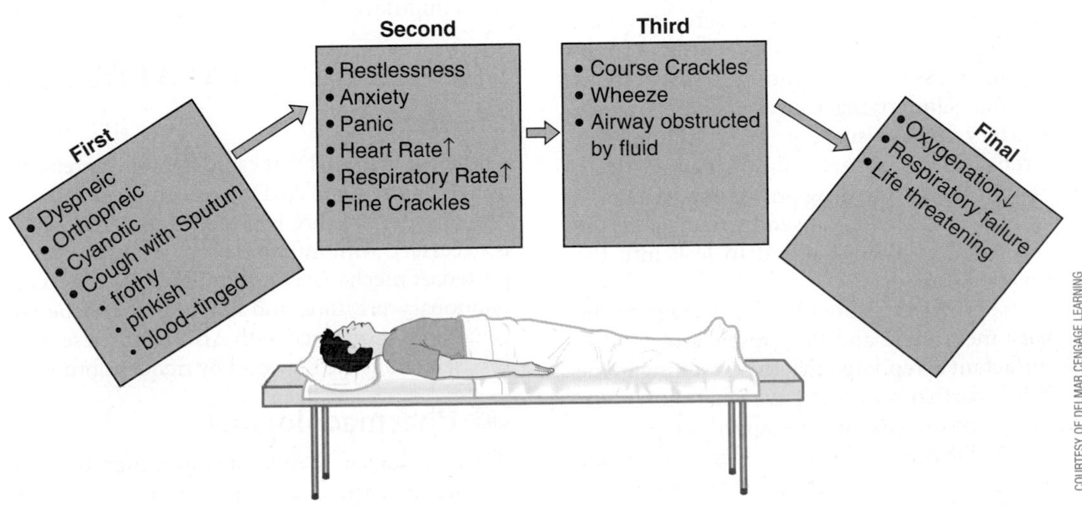

CONCEPT MAP 4-1 Progression of Pulmonary Edema

Nursing diagnoses for a client with pulmonary edema include the following:

NURSING DIAGNOSES	PLANNING/OUTCOMES	NURSING INTERVENTIONS
*Impaired **G**as Exchange* related to fluid in the lung tissue	The client will maintain an oxygen saturation of 95% or greater and will have respiratory rate, color, and blood gases within normal limits and clear breath sounds.	Place client in high Fowler's or orthopneic position (sitting upright leaning forward). Continually assess oxygenation with ABG or pulse oximetry measurements and provide supplemental oxygen to maintain an oxygen saturation of 95% or greater or per physician's order. Frequently assess respiratory rate, breath sounds, apical heart rate, and blood pressure. Administer respiratory treatments as ordered. Assist client with activities to reduce the workload on the heart and lungs, and alternate periods of activity with periods of rest to prevent client fatigue. Administer medications as ordered and evaluate the effectiveness of each. Monitor lab reports for electrolyte values.
*Excess **F**luid Volume* related to altered tissue permeability	The client's weight will return to normal.	Weigh client daily. Monitor I&O. Frequently assess the client for peripheral edema. Provide client with a low-sodium diet as ordered. Administer diuretics per order and evaluate their effectiveness. Monitor lab reports for electrolyte values. Monitor the rate at which intravenous fluids are given. Teach client and family symptoms of fluid excess, medication information, and dietary modifications.

Evaluation: Evaluate each outcome to determine how it has been met by the client.

ACUTE RESPIRATORY DISTRESS SYNDROME

Acute respiratory distress syndrome (ARDS; formerly called adult respiratory distress syndrome) is a life-threatening condition characterized by severe dyspnea, hypoxemia, and diffuse pulmonary edema. The condition usually follows a major assault on multiple body systems or severe lung trauma. Underlying causes include trauma, sepsis, coronary artery bypass surgery, major thoracic or vascular surgery, renal failure, severe pulmonary infections, inhalation lung injuries, and acute drug poisoning. ARDS is a noncardiogenic pulmonary edema, caused by damage to the alveolocapillary membranes allowing fluid to leak into the lungs under normal pressure.

Gas exchange is severely impaired by the damage to the pulmonary capillary membrane and the presence of fluid in the alveoli. The surfactant is rendered inactive, resulting in the collapse of the alveoli, further reducing gas exchange. Hypoxemia, resistant to conventional oxygen therapy, develops.

The client with ARDS is critically ill, as reflected by severe dyspnea, tachypnea, and cyanosis. Arterial blood gases will show $PaO_2 < 70$ mm Hg, $PaCO_2 > 35$ mm Hg, bicarbonate ion < 22 mEq/L, and initially elevated then steadily decreasing pH. The ABGs and pulse oximetry reveal severe hypoxemia and progressive respiratory and metabolic acidosis. On auscultation, the lung fields are filled with diffuse coarse crackles (rales) and sonorous wheezes. The client will have a productive cough yielding blood-tinged sputum. Chest x-ray shows widely scattered infiltrates, often referred to as a "white out."

MEDICAL–SURGICAL MANAGEMENT

Medical

The client with ARDS is cared for in the intensive care unit. The underlying cause of ARDS is ascertained and treated; until that time, supportive care is given. Mechanical ventilatory support is necessary, with multiple other systems often also being supported. A mechanical ventilator allows the oxygen percentage, pulmonary pressure, and lung volume to be controlled. Oxygenation is monitored with ABGs and pulse oximetry. Respiratory secretions are removed by frequent bronchial suctioning.

Pharmacological

Pharmacological therapy includes high doses of corticosteriods such as hydrocortisone sodium succinate (Solu-Cortef) or methylprednisolone sodium succinate (Solu-Medrol). Furosemide (Lasix) and other diuretics are given to remove fluids and increase urinary output. Aminophylline (Aminophyllin) is administered to open the bronchi. While the client is on the mechanical ventilator, pancuronium bromide (Pavulon) is given to suppress the client's own respiratory effort. Blood pressure can fall dangerously low, and vasopressors such as dopamine hydrochloride (Intropin) may be required to maintain the blood pressure within an acceptable range.

Diet

Total parenteral nutrition (TPN) may be given to the client, especially during the acute phase of the illness. When possible, enteral feedings are preferred.

Activity

The client with ARDS will be on bed rest. Special beds that provide movement and pressure adjustment prevent the complications associated with immobility. According to the ARDS Support Center (2009a), prone positioning improves oxygenation and may prevent further lung damage.

Nursing Management

Monitor client's level of consciousness, response to stimuli, vital signs, ABGs, pulse oximetry, and breath sounds. Suction excess secretions. Provide frequent oral care. Plan for uninterrupted rest periods. Assess for restlessness and anxiety.

NURSING PROCESS

Assessment

Subjective Data

The client history is typically gathered from family members or significant others because the client is usually too ill to communicate.

Objective Data

The client's level of consciousness and response to stimuli are assessed, and the client is observed for restlessness and anxiety. Vital signs are measured every 15 minutes or more often. Heart rate is increased, and arrhythmias may be present. Blood pressure is usually low. Respiratory rate, rhythm, and effort are assessed for signs of dyspnea, nasal flaring, cyanosis, tachypnea, and other indications of respiratory distress. Arterial blood gases and pulse oximetry values are assessed to evaluate oxygenation and acid–base balance. Diffuse, coarse crackles (rales) and wheezes are heard throughout the lung fields.

Nursing diagnoses for a client with ARDS include the following:

NURSING DIAGNOSES	PLANNING/OUTCOMES	NURSING INTERVENTIONS
*Impaired **G**as Exchange* related to pulmonary capillary membrane damage	The client will have an oxygen saturation of 95% or greater, ABGs within normal limits, and respiratory rate and effort within normal limits.	Provide adequate oxygenation and ventilation as ordered. Monitor ABGs and pulse oximetry to evaluate oxygenation and acid–base balance. Assess the client's respiratory rate and effort and auscultate the lungs frequently. Suction the respiratory tract as necessary to remove excess secretions, and provide oral care frequently.
***A**nxiety* related to difficulty breathing and mechanical ventilation	The client, if able, will verbalize a decrease in anxiety or will exhibit fewer objective signs of anxiety, such as restlessness and facial grimacing.	Describe care and purposes to the client. Allow rest periods between periods of activity to avoid overwhelming the client with stimuli. Plan care to allow for uninterrupted rest. Allow family and significant others to visit and participate in care, as appropriate. Assess client for signs of sensory overload/deprivation.

Evaluation: Evaluate each outcome to determine how it has been met by the client.

ACUTE RESPIRATORY FAILURE

Acute respiratory failure is not a disease entity in and of itself; rather, the term is used to refer to conditions wherein there is a failure of the respiratory system as a whole. This condition occurs as a result of the client literally becoming too tired to continue the "work" of breathing. Mechanical ventilatory support is required during the acute phase. Clients with preexisting pulmonary conditions coupled with acute respiratory tract infections are at risk for developing acute respiratory failure.

CHRONIC RESPIRATORY TRACT DISORDERS

Asthma, chronic obstructive pulmonary disease (COPD), chronic bronchitis, emphysema, and bronchiectasis are discussed following.

LIFE SPAN CONSIDERATIONS

Asthma and Age

In children:

- Asthma attacks often become less severe and less frequent as the child ages.
- Asthma attacks are usually associated with definite allergens.
- Oral bronchodilators should be taken 30 to 60 minutes before exercise, inhaled bronchodilators 15 to 20 minutes before exercise.

In adults:

- Asthma attacks usually become more severe and more frequent as the individual ages.
- Asthma attacks are usually not associated with definite allergens.

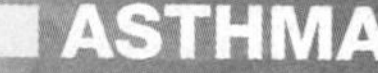

ASTHMA

Asthma is a condition characterized by intermittent airway obstruction in response to a variety of stimuli. The epithelial lining of the airways responds by becoming inflamed and edematous. Bronchospasm occurs in the smooth muscles of the bronchi and bronchioles. Secretions increase in viscosity. Elastic recoil decreases. All of these changes result in a reduction of the diameter of the airways, making breathing more difficult. Some clients who develop asthma in childhood experience spontaneous recovery.

Asthma is classified as extrinsic or intrinsic. Extrinsic asthma is caused by substances outside the body that precipitate the asthma response, such as pollen, house dust, or food additives. Intrinsic asthma is diagnosed when no extrinsic factor can be identified and the asthma is the result of internal factors such as emotional stress, exercise, or fatigue. An asthma attack that does not respond to treatment and persists is known as **status asthmaticus**.

The hallmark of an asthma attack is sudden onset of wheezing, increasing dyspnea, and chest tightness. Mild asthma usually is controlled by routine medication. Severe asthma attacks usually occur at night and require extra medication. With severe attacks, wheezing may be audible to the unaided ear. Expiratory wheezes are common as air attempts to escape through the narrowed airways. Both inspiratory and expiratory wheezes may be heard. *Absence of wheezing could indicate complete closure of the airway*. The respiratory rate rises initially, but as the client tires, the rate may decrease. Nasal flaring and costal and sternal retractions may be present, particularly in the young client. The client uses accessory muscles to assist respiratory effort. Cough occurs as the respiratory secretions become thick and block the airways. Cyanosis and a decrease in oxygen saturation occur. Heart rate elevates, as may blood pressure. The client becomes anxious and may complain of a sense of impending doom. These responses are thought to be caused by a release of catecholamines. Values of ABGs indicate hypoxia and respiratory acidosis. Chest x-ray shows hyperinflation of the lungs. Pulmonary function tests reveal an abnormal flow rate and lung volume. With a severe asthma attack, apnea and sudden death can occur in minutes.

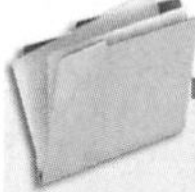

COLLABORATIVE CARE

Assessment and Teaching for Asthma

Respiratory therapists and nurses work together in assessing breath sounds and respiratory effort. Teaching the client how to use a nebulizer or inhalers and aerosol treatment is a collaborative effort of nurses and respiratory therapists.

MEDICAL–SURGICAL MANAGEMENT

Medical

The client with allergies should avoid specific antigens that might bring on an attack. Some clients with asthma are aided by controlling psychological stressors. Routine physical exercise is beneficial in treating exercise-induced asthma. The client with asthma should avoid other respiratory irritants such as cigarette smoke and air pollution. Clients who develop asthma later in life show more symptoms as they age.

Pharmacological

The primary treatment for an acute asthma attack is pharmacological. A combination of medications is used to open the narrowed airways. Medications used to dilate the bronchi include bronchodilators such as aminophylline (Aminophyllin) and terbutaline sulfate (Brethine, Bricanyl); beta agonists such as epinephrine (Primatene Mist) and albuterol sulfate (Ventolin); and anticholinergics such as atropine sulfate and ipratropium bromide (Atrovent). Corticosteroids such as prednisone (Delatsone) are utilized to decrease inflammation. Mucolytic agents such as acetylcysteine (Mucomyst) aid in liquefying secretions. Supplemental oxygen is given when indicated.

Diet

Adequate fluid intake is maintained to promote liquefaction of secretions. Foods, such as dairy products, which contribute to mucous production, should be avoided during or immediately following an asthma attack.

Activity

Incorporate several rest periods for the client. Use relaxation techniques to manage anxiety. The client should not overexert to the point of dyspnea, wheezing, or fatigue. If overexertion occurs, the client should sit down and sip warm water. This promotes slower, regular breathing; bronchodilation; and loosens secretions.

NURSING MANAGEMENT

Obtain history about previous asthma attacks. Evaluate wheezes for location, duration, and phase of respiration when they occur. Monitor pulse oximetry and ABGs for oxygenation and acid–base balance.

COMMUNITY/HOME HEALTH CARE

Asthma

- Prohibit smoking in the home, especially if a child has asthma.
- Use a humidifier, especially in the bedroom of the person with asthma.
- Use fans to circulate air.

NURSING PROCESS

ASSESSMENT

Subjective Data

A detailed history is taken regarding exposure to triggering stimuli before past asthma attacks. Also, the onset, duration, and severity of symptoms such as dyspnea are noted.

Objective Data

Note the effectiveness of ventilation. Wheezes are evaluated as to their duration, location, and the phase of respiration during which they occur (e.g., inspiration). Wheezes heard without the aid of a stethoscope are called **audible wheezes**. Respiratory rate, depth, rhythm and effort; position assumed; and client color are evaluated. Monitor pulse oximetry or lab reports of ABG values to determine oxygenation and acid–base balance. If sputum is produced, note its color, amount, viscosity, and odor.

Nursing diagnoses for a client with asthma include the following:

NURSING DIAGNOSES	PLANNING/OUTCOMES	NURSING INTERVENTIONS
*Inefficient **B**reathing Pattern* related to narrowed airways	The client will have respiratory rate and color within normal limits, clear breath sounds on auscultation, and ABG or pulse oximetry values within normal limits.	Assist client in assuming a position that facilitates ventilation. Administer medication as ordered. Assist client in the use of inhalers and aerosol treatments. Assess oxygenation by ABG or pulse oximetry values and administer supplemental oxygen, as ordered. Frequently assess respiratory rate and effort as well as color as client's condition dictates and auscultate the lung fields for presence of wheezes. If sputum is produced, note its color, amount, viscosity, and odor. Frequently assess vital signs as client's condition dictates. Unless otherwise contraindicated, encourage fluid intake to promote liquefaction of respiratory secretions.
*Deficient **K**nowledge* related to asthma, asthma treatment, and individual triggers for asthma attacks	The client will verbalize an understanding of both the pathophysiology and treatment of asthma, including the medications taken and their purposes and side effects. The client will also identify individual triggers and means of avoiding these triggers.	Teach client and family about the disease process; the purpose, effect, adverse effects, side effects, and use of all prescribed medications, especially inhalers and respiratory aerosol equipment. Assist client in establishing a medication schedule that will facilitate regular and timely taking of medications. Instruct client to use the inhaler prior to meals to aid in breathing while eating. If client is taking steroids, teach to rinse mouth after using the inhaler so as to prevent fungal infection. Encourage exercise because it increases respiratory reserve and improves overall physical condition. Assist client in identifying triggering stimuli and ways to avoid them. Teach client and family signs and symptoms of asthma attacks and respiratory tract infections. Teach client to avoid crowded areas and close contact with persons with infections.
Anxiety related to perceived threat of dying	The client will verbalize a decrease in anxiety.	Provide client with explanations for all care. Provide care in a calm, unhurried manner. Plan care to allow client uninterrupted periods of rest. Allow client to make decisions regarding care, if possible. Provide client with opportunities to discuss anxiety with staff, family, or significant others.

Evaluation: Evaluate each outcome to determine how it has been met by the client.

CHRONIC OBSTRUCTIVE PULMONARY DISEASE

Chronic obstructive pulmonary disease (COPD), also called chronic obstructive lung disease (COLD), is a term used for two closely related respiratory diseases: chronic bronchitis and emphysema. These two diseases often occur together. Most clients have a long history of heavy cigarette smoking (NHLBI, 2009a). First signs are chronic cough, sputum production, or shortness of breath. It gradually gets worse over time. There is no known cure. In the United States, about 12 million adults have COPD. It is the fourth leading cause of death. In 2007, the national cost for COPD was approximately $42.6 billion (ALA, 2007a).

CHRONIC BRONCHITIS

Bronchitis is an inflammation of the bronchial tree accompanied by hypersecretion of mucus. The condition becomes chronic if cough and sputum are present on most days for 3 months a year for 2 consecutive years or for 6 months in 1 year (NHLBI, 2001b). Constant irritation of the bronchi results in hypertrophy of the mucus-secreting glands. The bronchioles fill with exudate, and subsequent infections are common. There may be narrowing of large and small airways. Environmental factors, especially cigarette smoke, play an important role in the development of chronic bronchitis.

The client usually has a history of recurrent respiratory infections, dyspnea, cyanosis, and chronic or recurrent cough yielding copious amounts of sputum. Often, the sputum is purulent or green in color. Over the course of time, the chest wall configuration becomes slightly distended. Coarse crackles (rales) are present throughout the lung fields. Breath sounds may be diminished or absent over the periphery of the lung fields. Elevation of pulmonary artery pressure results in increased workload for the right ventricle and in signs and symptoms of right-sided congestive heart failure (CHF), such as peripheral edema and fatigue. Arterial blood gases reveal increased $PaCO_2$ and decreased PaO_2. The red blood cell count elevates, as do hemoglobin and hematocrit. The increases in the amounts of red blood cells and hemoglobin represent an attempt by the body to compensate for the lower oxygen level. Chest x-ray shows hyperexpansion of the lungs. When CHF occurs, the chest x-ray also shows an enlarged heart.

MEDICAL–SURGICAL MANAGEMENT

Medical

The goals of medical treatment are to decrease symptoms of airway irritation, decrease airway obstruction related to secretions and inflammation, prevent infection, maintain oxygenation, and increase the client's exercise tolerance. Respiratory therapy includes the use of updraft (nebulizer) and aerosol treatments, along with percussion and postural drainage. Humidification of inspired air helps liquefy secretions. Supplemental oxygen is administered based on ABG or pulse oximetry values. The neurological stimulus to breathe becomes altered in some clients with chronic bronchitis so that breathing is initiated when the blood level of oxygen falls instead of when the level of carbon dioxide rises. Consequently, when the level of oxygen in the blood is relatively high in relation to the level of carbon dioxide, the stimulus to breathe is reduced and further depresses the CNS. When supplemental oxygen is necessary, it is maintained at the lowest possible flow rate to maintain oxygenation and prevent depression of the client's respiratory drive. Evaluate the client with chronic bronchitis and CHF for signs of fluid overload. Daily weight, intake, and output are monitored.

Pharmacological

Current medications used include beta-adrenergic agonists, cholinergic antagonists, methylxanthines, corticosteroids, cromolyn sodium/nedocromil, and leukotriene modifiers. Bronchodilators such as theophylline (Theo-dur) given orally, and ipratropium bromide (Atrovent) given as an inhalation aerosol (metered dose inhaler [MDI]) or inhalation solution (nebulizer) are used to open airways. Tiotropium bromide (Spiriva) is a once-daily inhalation powder administered using a HandiHaler device. Salmeterol (Serevent), given by a dry powder inhaler (DPI) is a long-acting beta$_2$-selective agonist used for chronic maintenance therapy. Inhalation aerosol (MDI) or inhalation solution (nebulizer) treatments with bronchodilators such as albuterol (Proventil, Ventolin) or metaproterenol sulfate (Alupent) are often used in conjunction with oral medications. Prednisone (Meticorten), a corticosteroid, is given as short-term therapy for acute exacerbations. If steroids are required on a long-term basis, they may be given by inhalation to prevent some adverse systemic effects. Mucolytic medications such as acetylcysteine (Mucomyst) are given to reduce the viscosity of purulent and nonpurulent pulmonary secretions. Guaifenesin (Robitussin, Naldecon Senior EX, Mucinex) are expectorants given to loosen phlegm and thin bronchial secretions. If infection occurs, broad-spectrum antibiotics are given. Immunization against influenza viruses and *Streptococcus pneumoniae* is recommended.

The client with chronic bronchitis who also has CHF will receive medications to aid the function of the weakened heart. Digoxin (Lanoxin) strengthens the force of the contraction of the heart muscle. Diuretics such as furosemide (Lasix) are given to remove fluid by increasing urinary output. Supplemental potassium chloride (K-Dur, Kay-Ciel elixir) is given if the client's potassium level decreases from effect of the diuretic.

Diet

Encourage the client to eat a well-balanced diet. If the client also has CHF, sodium intake is restricted. Unless contraindicated, fluids are encouraged. Offer small, frequent meals to clients experiencing shortness of breath.

Activity

Activity is restricted to decrease the workload on the heart and lungs. With acute exacerbations, the client is placed on bed rest. The level of activity is then slowly increased based on the client's tolerance.

Programs of breathing exercises and graded (easy to difficult) exercise regimes assist the client to achieve the maximum level of activity tolerance. Breath-retaining exercises such as coughing techniques, pursed-lip breathing, and diaphragmatic or abdominal breathing are taught. The client is monitored from a respiratory standpoint while exercising. The goal is to increase the client's capacity for all ADLs.

NURSING MANAGEMENT

Obtain history of onset, duration, and severity of symptoms. Note changes in level of consciousness, mental status, respiratory rate and effort, color, and use of accessory muscles. Obtain sputum specimen for culture and sensitivity. Monitor vital signs. Assess for weight gain, peripheral edema, and neck vein distention.

NURSING PROCESS

ASSESSMENT

Subjective Data

A thorough past medical history is obtained, including information about the onset, duration, and severity of symptoms. The client may describe fatigue and difficult breathing.

Objective Data

Note changes in level of consciousness or mental status, color, respiratory rate and effort, the position the client assumes to aid respiratory effort, and the use of accessory muscles. Review ABGs or pulse oximetry values. Auscultate lung fields for crackles (rales) and diminished breath sounds. Note color, amount, viscosity, and odor of sputum. Obtain specimens for culture and sensitivity, if indicated. Frequently measure vital signs. The pulse may be elevated and irregular. Blood pressure may be elevated or low. An elevated temperature may indicate infection. Assess for peripheral edema, neck vein distention, and rapid weight gain.

Nursing diagnoses for a client with chronic bronchitis include the following:

NURSING DIAGNOSES	PLANNING/ OUTCOMES	NURSING INTERVENTIONS
*Ineffective **A**irway Clearance* related to thicker and increased amounts of respiratory secretions	The client's color, respiratory rate, and ABG values will be within normal limits.	Frequently assess level of consciousness, mental status, vital signs, respiratory effort, and color, and auscultate breath sounds at least every 4 hours.
		Obtain sputum specimens as ordered, and assess sputum for amount, viscosity, color, and odor.
		Assist client in assuming the position that most aids respiratory effort, usually an upright position.
		Administer oxygen and respiratory treatments as ordered and assess their effectiveness.
		Evaluate results of diagnostic and laboratory tests (ABGs) and notify the physician of abnormalities.
		Alternate care with periods of uninterrupted rest.
		Administer antibiotics and bronchodilators as ordered and evaluate their effectiveness.
		Provide client with a well-balanced diet and, unless otherwise contraindicated, encourage fluids.
		Assess client for signs and symptoms of CHF (i.e., fine crackles heard on auscultation, peripheral edema, weight gain, and fatigue).
		Report any signs and symptoms of CHF to the physician.
*Deficient **K**nowledge* related to chronic bronchitis and its treatment and prevention	The client will verbalize signs and symptoms to report to the physician, safety precautions to take with medication and equipment, medication and respiratory treatment regimen, and techniques for facilitating breathing.	Teach client to avoid respiratory infections, maintain adequate nutrition, increase fluid intake, and obtain adequate rest; the purpose, expected effects, and side effects of medications; and to administer respiratory treatments and medications prior to eating to aid in breathing.
		Instruct client to rinse mouth following use of inhaler.
		Teach client to self-administer oxygen.
		Provide information regarding both the use of equipment and safety measures for the equipment.
		Refer client to an established respiratory rehabilitation program. If such a program is not available, instruct client in breathing techniques.
		Encourage regular exercise within the client's limitations.
		Encourage client to obtain immunization against influenza viruses and *Streptococcus pneumoniae.*

Evaluation: Evaluate each outcome to determine how it has been met by the client.

EMPHYSEMA

Emphysema is a complex and destructive lung disease wherein air accumulates in the tissues of the lungs. The airways lose their elasticity and the walls thicken, resulting in narrower lumens. Airflow is impeded as it leaves the lungs (i.e., during expiration). The alveoli distal to these airways become overdistended with trapped air (Figure 4-12). Rupture of the alveolar wall may occur. The alveolar capillary membrane is destroyed, resulting in a loss of available area for gas exchange. Cigarette smoking is the most common cause of emphysema. Deficiency in alpha-1-antitrypsin is a familial disorder that leads to the development of emphysema. Alpha-1-antitrypsin is an enzyme that inhibits the activity of the enzyme elactase, which breaks down lung tissue.

Emphysema develops slowly over a period of years. The earliest symptom is a daily morning cough with clear sputum. Later, the client notes increasing dyspnea in response to activity. The degree of dyspnea corresponds to the degree of hypoxia, which is usually mild at rest but becomes increasingly severe in response to activity. In advanced stages of the disease, hypoxia is evident even at rest. With infection, a cough yielding purulent sputum occurs. The client's complexion appears ruddy, or reddish in color. The chest becomes barrel shaped (Figure 4-13) as the chest cage enlarges to accommodate distended lung tissues. The respiratory rate elevates. The expiratory phase of respiration becomes increasingly difficult. Accessory muscles are used to aid respiratory effort. Because of destruction of the alveoli, bronchial breath sounds are heard in the periphery of the lungs. As the disease progresses, breath sounds diminish and eventually disappear over the periphery of the lungs. Arterial blood gases reveal the degree of hypoxia depending on the severity of the disease. Hypercapnia, or retention of carbon dioxide, is not as likely as with chronic bronchitis. The extra effort required to breathe increases metabolic need, resulting in weight loss. Chest x-ray reveals hyperinflated lung tissue and a flattened diaphragm, which has been displaced by distended lung tissues. Pulmonary function studies reveal a decrease in expiratory volume. Polycythemia and elevation of hemoglobin and hematocrit occur in response to prolonged hypoxia.

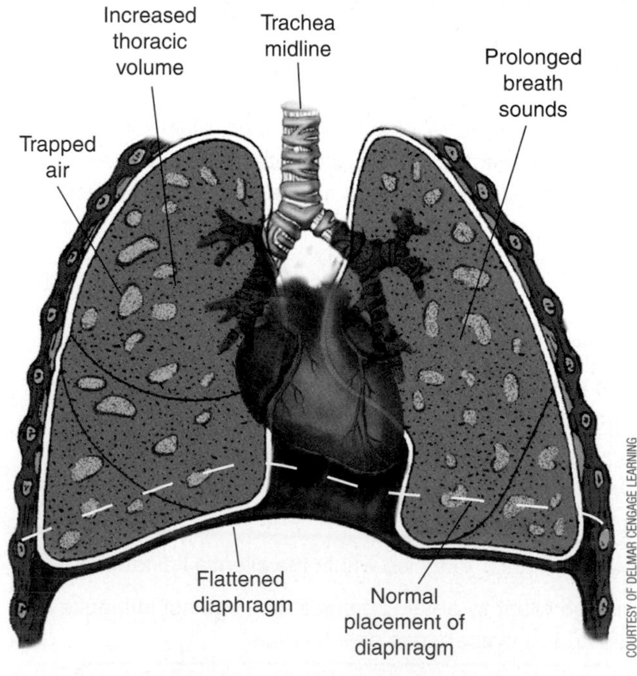

FIGURE 4-12 **Emphysema**

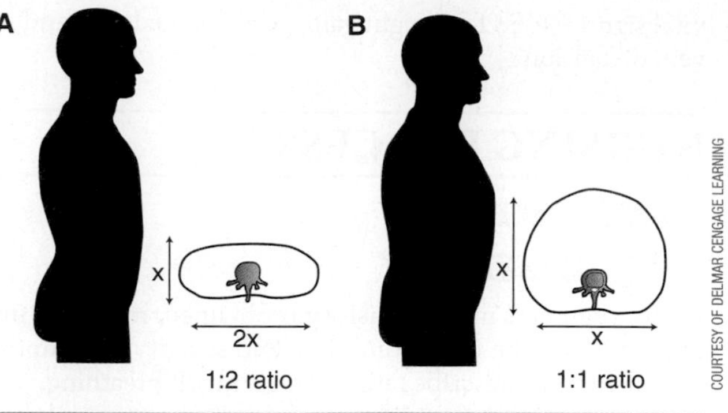

FIGURE 4-13 **Changes in Chest Configuration and Posture; *A*, The normal ratio of the anterior posterior diameter to the lateral diameter is 1:2; *B*, With a barrel chest, the ratio between the diameters is 1:1.**

MEDICAL–SURGICAL MANAGEMENT

Medical

The goals of treatment are to prevent further damage to the lung tissues, maintain adequate oxygenation, prevent infection, and improve the client's activity tolerance. The client who smokes should stop or, at least, decrease the number of cigarettes smoked daily. Supplemental oxygen is given to maintain oxygenation. The client with advanced emphysema and severe, chronic hypoxia may be maintained at PaO_2 of 55 to 59 mm Hg and/or oxygen saturation of 90% or greater. As with chronic bronchitis, the client with emphysema is given supplemental oxygen at the lowest possible flow rate, usually 2 to 3 L/min, to prevent respiratory and CNS depression.

Pharmacological

The client with emphysema receives many of the same medications used to treat chronic bronchitis. To open airways that have become fibrotic, theophylline and similar preparations are used. Steroids may be required for exacerbations. The client with emphysema usually does not need mucolytic agents, unless infection is present. Antibiotics are used to treat and prevent respiratory tract infections. The client should receive immunizations against influenza and *Streptococcus pneumoniae.* The client who smokes may use nicotine gum or transdermal patches to aid in smoking cessation.

Diet

The client with emphysema requires a diet high in carbohydrates to supply the energy necessary for breathing. If a negative nitrogen balance exists because of the client's using muscle tissue to provide energy, a diet high in protein is ordered. Dietary supplements such as Ensure may be needed to supply the necessary calories and nutrients. Unless contraindicated, fluids and small, frequent meals are encouraged.

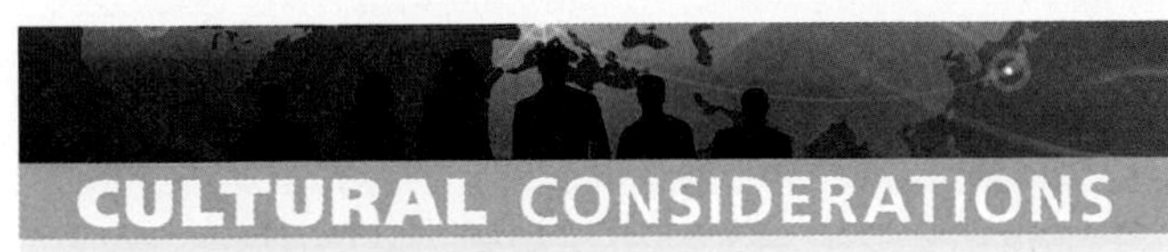

CULTURAL CONSIDERATIONS

Skin Color/Cyanosis

- For a client with highly pigmented skin, establish a baseline skin color.
- Observe skin surfaces that have the least amount of pigmentation, such as the palms, the soles of the feet, the abdomen, mucous membranes, or the inner aspect of forearms.

Activity

The client is placed on bed rest. Level of activity is increased based on the client's oxygenation. Oxygen saturation is evaluated periodically as the activity level is increased to determine the effect of activity on oxygenation.

Health Promotion

The client with emphysema benefits from a respiratory rehabilitation program. The client is taught breathing exercises similar to those taught to the client with chronic bronchitis. A graded exercise program is also used for the client with emphysema. Group programs that aid in smoking cessation are useful for the client who smokes.

Nursing Management

Review factors that increase client's dyspnea and those that relieve dyspnea. Evaluate client's nutritional status, vital signs, ABGs, pulse oximetry, color, and level of consciousness. Assist with ADL. Plan for uninterrupted periods of rest.

NURSING PROCESS

Assessment

Subjective Data

Included in the history is information regarding the timing of dyspnea, those factors that exacerbate dyspnea, and those factors that relieve dyspnea.

Objective Data

Assess sputum for color, amount, viscosity, odor, and vital signs. An elevated pulse may indicate hypoxia and/or infection. Auscultation of the lungs will reveal the presence of adventitious, diminished, or absent breath sounds. Note the client's position to aid respiratory effort, color, respiratory rate and effort, and use of accessory muscles to aid breathing. Evaluate the client's nutritional status by weighing the client and measuring nutrient and caloric intake. Review results of laboratory and diagnostic tests.

Nursing diagnoses for a client with emphysema include the following:

NURSING DIAGNOSES	PLANNING/OUTCOMES	NURSING INTERVENTIONS
*Impaired **G**as Exchange* related to destruction of the alveoli	The client's respiratory rate, color, and ABG values will be within normal limits.	Assess the client's level of consciousness and mental status. Frequently evaluate client's respiratory rate, respiratory effort, color, and oxygenation with ABG and/or pulse oximetry. Assess the effect of activity on oxygenation, particularly when activity is being increased and provide supplemental oxygen as ordered. Auscultate the lungs and report abnormalities to the physician. Assess client's vital signs: heart rate and temperature elevations may indicate infection, an elevated pulse may indicate hypoxia. Review results of diagnostic and laboratory tests and report abnormalities. Administer medications and respiratory treatments as ordered. Assist client in assuming the position that offers the most comfort and most aids respiratory effort. Instruct client in breathing techniques, such as pursed-lip breathing.
*Risk for **A**ctivity Intolerance* related to hypoxia	The client will complete activity without experiencing fatigue or dyspnea.	Assist client with ADL and hygiene needs. Plan care and treatments to allow client uninterrupted periods of rest. Allow rest before and after meals. As activity increases, assess the effects on oxygenation.

(Continues)

Nursing diagnoses for a client with emphysema include the following: (Continued)

NURSING DIAGNOSES	PLANNING/OUTCOMES	NURSING INTERVENTIONS
Imbalanced Nutrition: Less than Body Requirements related to increased energy requirements to maintain respiration	The client will achieve or maintain a weight within normal limits for height.	Assess client's weight and evaluate in relation to the client's height. Evaluate client's diet for nutritional adequacy and review client's food likes and dislikes. Provide a well-balanced diet based on client's likes and dislikes. Provide nutritional supplements as ordered. Avoid activities or procedures prior to meals that might reduce appetite (e.g., enemas). Administer medications and respiratory treatments prior to meals to aid in breathing.

Evaluation: Evaluate each outcome to determine how it has been met by the client.

BRONCHIECTASIS

Bronchiectasis is chronic dilation of the bronchi. The main causes of this disorder are pulmonary TB infection, chronic upper respiratory tract infections, and complications of other respiratory disorders of childhood, particularly cystic fibrosis. The bronchi become distended and eventually lose their elastic recoil property. The mucociliary blanket's function is impaired, and secretions thicken. Secretions accumulate in the bronchi, resulting in a medium for infection. Airflow is hindered, reducing gas exchange.

The client with bronchiectasis describes a frequent or chronic productive cough, dyspnea, weight loss, and fatigue. Sputum is thick and sometimes purulent when infection is present. Crackles, which clear on coughing, are heard scattered throughout the lungs and are more prominent early in the morning. Accessory muscles are used to aid respiration. Over a period of time, right-sided CHF and peripheral edema develop. Arterial blood gases reveal elevated $PaCO_2$, decreased PaO_2, and respiratory acidosis. Polycythemia and elevated hemoglobin and hematocrit levels are present. Chest x-ray shows slight hyperinflation of lung tissue and, in the presence of CHF, cardiomegaly. Respiratory flow rate decreases, and lung volume increases, as demonstrated by pulmonary function studies. Table 4-8 compares asthma, chronic bronchitis, emphysema, and bronchiectasis.

MEDICAL–SURGICAL MANAGEMENT

Medical

Medical treatment is aimed at removing respiratory secretions, preventing or eliminating infection, and maintaining adequate oxygenation. Percussion and postural drainage are used to aid in the removal of secretions. Aerosol and updraft respiratory treatments may be ordered before percussion and drainage. If the client is unable to expectorate secretions, bronchial suctioning is performed. The physician performs a bronchoscopy to remove especially tenacious and copious secretions. Arterial blood gases and/or pulse oximetry values are evaluated to assess the need for supplemental oxygen. Daily weight and I&O are performed to detect signs of CHF. Pulmonary function studies evaluate the severity of lung damage.

> **CRITICAL THINKING**
>
> **COPD Disorders**
>
> What are the differences and the similarities of the two disorders classified as COPD?

Pharmacological

Mucolytic agents are given to promote liquefaction of respiratory secretions. Antibiotics are ordered to treat and prevent infection. The client is immunized against influenza and against *Streptococcus pneumoniae* with the pneumococcal vaccine (Pneumovax 23). Bronchodilators are indicated to open the fibrotic airways. Inflammation is treated with oral steroids such as prednisone (Meticorten) and/or by inhalation with beclomethasone dipropionate (Beclovent). The client with cystic fibrosis is required to take pancreatic enzymes, pancrelipase (Pancrease capsules, Cotazym capsules), to replace those that are missing with this disorder. If CHF occurs, the client is treated with digoxin (Lanoxin), furosemide (Lasix), and potassium supplements, as indicated.

Diet

To provide energy for breathing, the diet should be high in carbohydrates and calories. Protein is supplemented if necessary. Dietary supplements such as Ensure may be needed. Fluids are encouraged, unless otherwise contraindicated. Sodium is restricted in the diet of the client with CHF to prevent fluid retention. The diet for the client with cystic fibrosis is restricted in fats because fats are not properly absorbed.

Activity

During acute exacerbations or in the presence of serious infection, activity is limited. The client is placed on bed rest. Activity is progressively increased depending on the client's

TABLE 4-8 Signs and Symptoms of Asthma, Chronic Bronchitis, Emphysema, and Bronchiectasis

	ASTHMA	CHRONIC BRONCHITIS	EMPHYSEMA	BRONCHIECTASIS
History	Intermittent attacks of dyspnea and wheezing	Recurrent respiratory infections, chronic cough	Insidious onset, dyspnea on exertion to dyspnea at rest	Cystic fibrosis, recurrent respiratory infections, TB
Cough	Present during attack	Chronic or recurrent productive cough	Present with infections	Frequent or chronic productive cough
Sputum	Thick	Copious, purulent, green	Scanty mucoid, unless infection present	Thick, tenacious, sometimes purulent secretions
Weight	No weight loss	Slight or no weight loss	Weight loss common	Commonly, weight loss or failure to gain
Appearance	Flushed then cyanotic	Commonly cyanosis ("blue bloater")	Ruddy complexion ("pink puffer")	Clubbing of fingernails
Chest Configuration	Slight overdistention	Slight overdistention	Overdistention prominent ("barrel chest")	Slight overdistention
Breath Sounds	Audible wheezing Prolonged expiration	Coarse crackles (rales)	Bronchial breath sounds in peripheral lung fields Diminished or absent in late disease	Crackles
Edema	Infrequent	Peripheral edema common, especially in ankles	Infrequent	Peripheral edema in late disease
Right-sided CHF (Cor Pulmonale)	Infrequent	Frequent	Infrequent	Frequent late in disease
CO Retention (Hypercapnia)	Sometimes	Common	Unlikely	Common in late disease
Hypoxemia	Depends on severity of attack	Possibly severe	Usually mild, especially at rest	Possibly severe in late disease and with infection
Dyspnea	Increases during attack	Progressive	Dyspnea on exertion to dyspnea at rest usually presenting symptom	With respiratory infection and late disease
Accessory Muscles Used for Respiration	Yes	Yes	Yes	Yes
Poly cythemia	Uncommon	Late in disease	Yes	In late disease
Respiratory Failure	Possible	Common	Possible	Common

tolerance. Respiratory rehabilitation and graded exercise programs are useful in the treatment of bronchiectasis. Regular exercise is encouraged, particularly for the pediatric client with cystic fibrosis.

NURSING MANAGEMENT

Review client's history for recent and past respiratory infections, TB, and cystic fibrosis. Monitor vital signs. An increased heart rate may indicate hypoxia and/or infection, and an

PROFESSIONALTIP

Cystic Fibrosis

Cystic fibrosis (CF) is an inherited life-threatening disorder that causes severe lung damage and nutritional deficiencies. Improvements in the treatment of CF have increased the life expectancy of a client with CF from 10 years of age in 1962 to 37 years of age in 2009 (National Institutes of Health, 2009a). Treatment for CF is aimed at relieving symptoms and complications. New antibiotics such as inhaled tobramycin sulfate (TOBI) are more effective in treating infections, and other drugs, such as dornase alfa recombinant (Pulmozyme) and azithromycin (Zithromax, Zmax) slow the progression of the lung disease. Mechanical chest physical therapy devices used daily, such as electric chest clappers and inflatable vibrating vests help loosen and remove thick mucus from the lungs. Lung transplantation may be an option for clients with severe lung damage. Respiratory failure is the most dangerous consequence of CF (Mayo Clinic, 2009). For more information about CF visit the Cystic Fibrosis Foundation at http://www.cff.org

elevated temperature may indicate infection. Note weight loss and muscle wasting. Monitor breath sounds and suction mucous as necessary.

CHEST TRAUMA

Pneumothorax/hemothorax is discussed following.

PNEUMOTHORAX/ HEMOTHORAX

Normally, the pleural space between the visceral and parietal pleura contains pleural fluid and is held together by surface tension. The pleural space is a closed compartment with a negative pressure compared to the lungs or the atmosphere. When the integrity of the pleura is interrupted, air from the atmosphere or from the lungs moves between the pleura, creating a space. This air in the pleural space is known as a **pneumothorax** (Figure 4-14). The lung tissue underlying the pneumothorax is compressed and unable to fully expand. If the pneumothorax is large enough, the entire lung may collapse from the compression.

A pneumothorax may be referred to as traumatic (closed or open), spontaneous, tension, or a hemopneumothorax. A closed pneumothorax occurs when there is no communication between the pleura and the external environment. An example of a closed pneumothorax is when blunt trauma to the chest causes a broken rib that pierces the pleura and lung, allowing air to enter between the pleura. An open pneumothorax exists when there is direct communication between the external environment and the pleural space as in a gunshot wound. A spontaneous pneumothorax occurs without an obvious underlying cause. A tension pneumothorax is a life-threatening condition wherein air enters the pleural space on inspiration but is unable to exit on expiration. The air thus continues to accumulate in the pleural space, compressing the underlying structures. If left untreated, a tension pneumothorax collapses the lung and encroaches on the structures on the opposite side. The structures of the mediastinum shift to the unaffected side as more and more air accumulates in the pleural space. Without intervention, tension pneumothorax will result in cardiopulmonary arrest. Tension pneumothorax is often associated with mechanical ventilation. The pressure exerted by the ventilator on compromised lung tissue interrupts the integrity of the pleura. Air continues to enter the pleural space but is unable to exit as mechanical ventilation continues. In the case of a pneumothorax associated with trauma or surgery, bleeding of adjacent vessels into the pleural cavity often occurs. Blood within the pleural space is referred to as a **hemothorax**. When accompanied by air, the condition is called a **hemopneumothorax**.

The severity of injury and the amount of lung tissue affected determine the signs and symptoms the client exhibits. The client with a small pneumothorax may be asymptomatic or may complain of minor dyspnea, whereas the client with a significant pneumothorax may exhibit signs of severe respiratory distress. Dyspnea, tachypnea, orthopnea, and cyanosis may be present. Oxygenation is impaired. Pleuritic pain is common. Breath sounds are absent in the area of the pneumothorax. The client with an accompanying hemothorax exhibits signs and symptoms of shock associated with blood loss.

MEDICAL–SURGICAL MANAGEMENT

Medical

For the affected lung to reexpand, the air and/or blood must be removed from the pleural space. When the blood loss

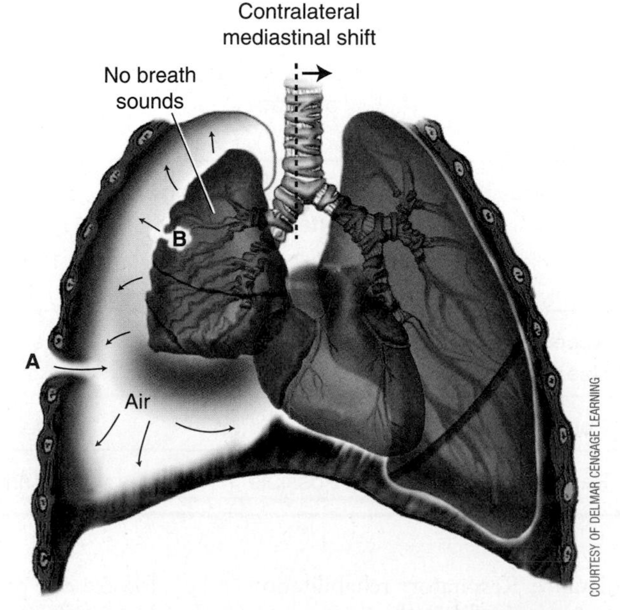

FIGURE 4-14 **Pneumothorax; *A*, Penetrating Wound; *B*, Ruptured Bleb on the Lung**

associated with a hemothorax is significant, fluid and blood replacement may be necessary.

Surgical

A thoracotomy tube, or chest tube, is inserted by the physician into the pleural space to drain fluid and air and allow the lung to reexpand. The tube is placed in the midaxillary line at approximately the fifth intercostal space. To drain air alone, the tube is placed in the anterior chest at the midclavicular line and the fourth intercostal space. The thoracotomy tube is connected to an underwater seal drainage device (refer back to Figure 4-9). The underlying cause of the hemopneumothorax then must be treated.

A recurrent spontaneous pneumothorax may require a pleural cortication to prevent further episodes. This involves roughing the adjacent surfaces of the visceral and parietal pleura so the resulting scar tissue will improve adhesion between the two surfaces. Emergency treatment for a tension pneumothorax that is severely compromising the function of the heart and lungs is placing a large-bore needle into the anterior chest at the fourth intercostal space. A thoracotomy tube is then inserted until the lung(s) are fully reexpanded and to prevent a recurrence.

Pharmacological

To control pleuritic pain, narcotic analgesics such as morphine sulfate or meperidine (Demerol) are prescribed. Analgesics may be given orally or parenterally depending on the severity of the pain. Before insertion of a thoracotomy tube, intravenous narcotics may be given prophylactically. Tissues adjacent to the area of the pneumothorax are injected with local anesthetics before insertion of a thoracotomy tube.

Diet

A well-balanced diet with sufficient amounts of protein is encouraged for healing. The client with other injuries and conditions may require TPN or enteral feedings.

Activity

If hypoxia is present, activity restrictions are necessary. The presence of other injuries or conditions may also necessitate activity restrictions. After the client is adequately oxygenated and stable, activity is encouraged to promote expansion of the lungs.

Nursing Management

Gather information about recent chest injuries or falls. Assess level of consciousness, mental status, color, respiratory effort, and chest wall movement. Monitor vital signs. Auscultate for breath sounds. When a chest tube is in place, assess function, patency, and amount and character of drainage.

NURSING PROCESS

Assessment

Subjective Data

Gather information about the source of the pneumothorax. Ask the client about previous pneumothoraces, recent chest injury, falls, and severe coughing. The client often describes being very anxious.

Objective Data

Assess the client's level of consciousness and mental status and the client's color, respiratory effort, and chest wall movement. Chest wall movement is decreased on the affected side. When a large pneumothorax is present, the trachea shifts toward the unaffected side. Dyspnea and cyanosis may occur. The cough is forceful and nonproductive. Respiratory rate and heart rate are elevated. Blood pressure may be elevated because of the presence of pain and anxiety or may be low because of blood loss. Breath sounds are diminished or absent over the affected areas. Note the location, duration, and severity of pain. When a chest tube is inflated, assess for function, patency, and amount and character of drainage.

Nursing diagnoses for a client with a pneumothorax include the following:

NURSING DIAGNOSES	PLANNING/OUTCOMES	NURSING INTERVENTIONS
*Ineffective **Breathing** Pattern* related to decreased lung expansion	The client's respiratory rate and color will be within normal limits, and the client will have clear breath sounds in affected area.	Monitor the amount and character of drainage from the chest tube and note chest tube drainage as output. Observe fluctuations (tidaling) in the water seal chamber, which indicates that the tube is in the pleural space. Investigate the absence of tidaling because this may indicate that the lung is fully reexpanded or that the tube is occluded or kinked. Observe for bubbling in the water seal chamber, which indicates an air leak. Assess the connections and chest tube to determine if leaks are present. If no air leaks are present, notify the physician because the air leak may be within the client's lungs. Encourage client to cough and deep breathe to prevent further respiratory complications.

(*Continues*)

Nursing diagnoses for a client with a pneumothorax include the following: (Continued)

NURSING DIAGNOSES	PLANNING/OUTCOMES	NURSING INTERVENTIONS
*Acute **Pain** related to pleural space irritation*	The client will verbalize a decrease in pain on a scale of 0 to 10.	Assist client in assuming the position that most aids respiration. Most clients find this to be the orthopneic position. Assess vital signs and respiratory status. Administer pain medications as ordered. Remember that respiratory depression is possible with narcotic medications. Provide diversional activities.

Evaluation: Evaluate each outcome to determine how it has been met by the client.

NEOPLASMS OF THE RESPIRATORY TRACT

Neoplasms discussed following include benign neoplasms, lung cancer, and laryngeal cancer.

BENIGN NEOPLASMS

A benign tumor or cyst in the lung has sharply defined edges, as revealed on an x-ray. Peripheral tumors usually have no symptoms. Bronchial tumors may cause obstruction, infection, or atelectasis.

LUNG CANCER

Malignant tumors (carcinomas) of the lung may originate within the lung or may result from metastasis from other tumor sites (e.g., breast, colon, or kidney). Men, especially those older than 40 years of age, are more likely to have lung cancer than are women. The number of deaths is still rising among women, but has reached a plateau for men (ALA, 2007c). Cigarette smoking is the most important risk factor for lung cancer. Air pollution and exposure to carcinogens such as asbestos are also risk factors, especially among smokers, for developing lung cancer. Exposure to radiation or radon is also known to cause lung cancer. Prognosis depends on the size of the tumor when diagnosed and the specific cell type (Figure 4-15).

Symptoms develop late in the course of lung cancers. Peripheral lesions generally have few symptoms. Initially, the client may complain of a chronic cough or wheezing. Central lesions cause obstruction and erosion of the bronchi. As the tumor grows and occludes the air passages, the client may experience shortness of breath, dyspnea, and blood-tinged sputum. Pain occurs relatively late in the course of the disease and indicates that the tumor has grown to a significant size to put pressure on adjacent nerves and other structures. Although some tumors can be seen on chest x-ray, many cannot. Low-dose helical CT scans and MRI scans are more reliable studies when assessing soft-tissue structures. To confirm a diagnosis, cytology studies are performed on specimens collected via bronchoscopy, needle biopsy, or mediastinoscopy. Lung scans are occasionally useful for diagnosis. Before initiating treatment, the client is evaluated for metastatic disease using bone and total body scans.

Family members and significant others often need assistance in coping with their feelings.

MEDICAL–SURGICAL MANAGEMENT

Medical

Treatment of lung cancer depends on the type and stage of the cancer.

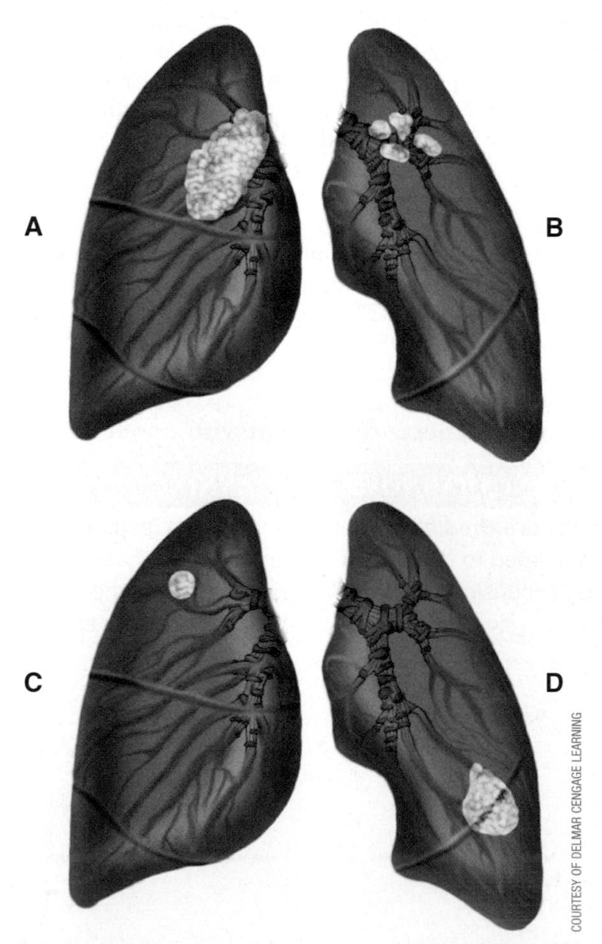

FIGURE 4-15 Lung Cancers; *A*, Small-Cell Carcinoma; *B*, Epidermoid (Squamous-Cell) Carcinoma; *C*, Adenocarcinoma; *D*, Large Cell (Undifferentiated) Carcinoma

COMMUNITY/HOME HEALTH CARE

Client with Laryngeal Stoma

- Humidify home, especially in winter.
- The client and family must know how to suction the respiratory tract and care for the respiratory equipment.
- Use warm water to clean around the stoma.
- Do not use tissues, linty cotton, or soap for cleansing.
- Wear a bib or dressing over the stoma to filter and warm incoming air.
- Do not swim or splash water in the stoma when showering or bathing.
- Notify the physician if any signs of respiratory infection develop, such as fever, cough, yellow or green mucus, or redness around the stoma.
- Keep follow-up appointments with physician.

Surgical

Surgical intervention involves the removal of the tumor and adjacent lung tissue. Pneumonectomy is the removal of an entire lung. Lobectomy is the removal of a lobe of a lung. Segmental resection is the removal of a segment of a lung. The client will have a thoracotomy tube on the operative side. Radiation and chemotherapy are often used in conjunction with surgery. The incidence of lung tumor recurrence following surgery is high. Surgery is often indicated for early non–small-cell carcinomas.

Pharmacological

The specific type of chemotherapy used depends on the cell type and the extent of tumor growth.

Health Promotion

The foremost method of preventing lung cancer is to avoid smoking or to cease smoking. Avoid the secondhand smoke of others.

NURSING MANAGEMENT

Review client's history for smoking, exposure to carcinogens, and other risk factors. Gather information about onset and severity of symptoms. Assess for pain. Monitor breath sounds, vital signs, and drainage from chest tube. Assist to semi-Fowler's position or lying on the affected side. Monitor ABGs and provide oxygen as indicated. When pain medication is given, monitor for respiratory depression. Aid client to express feelings of grief about diagnosis.

NURSING PROCESS

ASSESSMENT

Subjective Data

Review the client's history for smoking, exposure to carcinogens, and other risk factors. Gather information regarding the onset, duration, and severity of symptoms. The client may report hoarseness, chronic cough, pain, and shortness of breath. Assess pain for location, character, duration, and severity

Objective Data

Note the color, amount, consistency, and odor of sputum. Before surgery, wheezing or decreased breath sounds may be heard on the affected side. Following surgery, breath sounds are diminished or absent on the affected side. Monitor the amount and color of drainage from the thoracotomy tube. Assess the wound for hemorrhage and infection. Respiratory rate and effort may be increased. Pulse rate may be elevated as a result of a variety of factors including decreased oxygenation, hemorrhage, and infection. Hypotension occurs with significant blood loss. High blood pressure may indicate pain, anxiety, or other underlying pathology such as essential hypertension.

Nursing diagnoses for a client with lung cancer include the following:

NURSING DIAGNOSES	PLANNING/OUTCOMES	NURSING INTERVENTIONS
*Ineffective **Breathing** Pattern* related to disease process	The client's respiratory rate and color will be within normal limits.	Frequently monitor client's level of consciousness, vital signs, color, and respiratory effort. Auscultate breath sounds. Assess oxygenation and provide supplemental oxygen as indicated. Stagger activities with periods of rest to prevent overtaxing client's reserves. Assist client in assuming the position that maximizes respiratory effort by positioning client in semi-Fowler's position or lying on the affected side. Monitor lab reports for blood gas levels.

(*Continues*)

Nursing diagnoses for a client with lung cancer include the following: (Continued)

NURSING DIAGNOSES	PLANNING/OUTCOMES	NURSING INTERVENTIONS
*Chronic **Pain*** related to Lung cancer	The client will state pain is decreased on a scale of 0 to 10.	Administer pain medication and monitor for respiratory depression. Provide diversional activities. Assist client in assuming a position of comfort.
*Anticipatory **Grieving*** related to prognosis and perceived separation from significant others	The client will be able to express to significant others and/or staff feelings related to diagnosis and prognosis.	Aid the client in expressing feelings of grief related to the diagnosis. Hope should not be eliminated, but false hope should not be encouraged. Allow the client and family time to express their feelings.

Evaluation: Evaluate each outcome to determine how it has been met by the client.

LARYNGEAL CANCER

The American Cancer Society (2007) estimated that in 2008 approximately 12,250 Americans would be diagnosed with laryngeal cancer, and about 3,670 persons would die from it. Risk factors for cancer of the larynx include smoking, chronic alcohol abuse, chronic laryngitis, and overuse of the voice. Laryngeal cancer is relatively asymptomatic. The client may experience hoarseness or difficulty speaking above a whisper. If either persists for more than 2 weeks, medical care should be sought. Difficulty swallowing is sometimes present. Laryngeal pain radiating to the ear or a lump in the throat are often signs of metastasis.

MEDICAL–SURGICAL MANAGEMENT

Treatment is determined by the extent of tumor growth.

Surgical

Surgical removal of the larynx, a laryngectomy, is used to treat laryngeal cancer. A radical or modified radical neck dissection may be performed if the cancer has spread to surrounding tissues and lymph nodes. Radical neck dissection operations have been performed for almost 100 years and include the removal of lateral neck lymph nodes and tissues, the submandibular gland, the sternocleidomastoid muscle, the jugular vein and the spinal accessory nerve (Georgetown University Hospital, 2009). A modified radical neck dissection removes all the lymph nodes in one or both sides of the neck without removing neck muscles. The jugular vein and spinal accessory nerve may be removed (National Cancer Institute, 2009). Radiation may be used as an adjunct to surgery or as primary treatment if the tumor is detected in the early stages. Following surgery, a permanent tracheostomy is necessary to allow air to enter the respiratory tract. A small incision is made into the trachea and below the Adam's apple, and a plastic tracheostomy tube is inserted.

NURSING MANAGEMENT

Monitor respiratory status. Suction secretions and provide tracheostomy care. Teach client stoma protection. Keep head of bed elevated and provide extra humidity. Refer client to the American Cancer Society for support at www.cancer.org.

NURSING PROCESS

ASSESSMENT

Subjective Data

Obtain a history of the onset, duration, and severity of symptoms, such as hoarseness or laryngitis and alcohol and tobacco use. The client may describe ear pain and difficulty breathing and swallowing.

Objective Data

Evaluate the client's respiratory status for other respiratory problems that may accompany laryngeal cancer, such as COPD. Examine sputum for the presence of blood.

Nursing diagnoses for a client with laryngeal cancer include the following:

NURSING DIAGNOSES	PLANNING/OUTCOMES	NURSING INTERVENTIONS
*Ineffective **Airway** Clearance* related to tracheostomy tube	The client's respiratory rate and color will be within desired ranges, and the client will have clear breath sounds to auscultation.	Suction frequently following surgery to remove static secretions and provide routine tracheostomy care. Provide small, frequent feedings of liquid or pureed food to prevent choking. Assist client to turn, cough, and deep breathe two to four times an hour.

Nursing diagnoses for a client with laryngeal cancer include the following: (Continued)

NURSING DIAGNOSES	PLANNING/OUTCOMES	NURSING INTERVENTIONS
		Teach client stoma protection. Assess respirations two to four times an hour, if secretions are copious. Auscultate lung sounds. Keep head of bed elevated. Provide extra humidity.
Impaired Verbal Communication related to removal of the larynx	The client will be able to communicate needs.	Before surgery, establish a means of communication to be used afterward. If available, a manual or computer word/picture board works well. Keep call light by client's bed. Avoid mouthing communications, as this is frustrating to the client and is time consuming. As possible, ask questions that require only a "yes" or "no" answer. Refer client to the local support group (Lost Chord Club) or the American Cancer Society. Provide written information and materials.
Deficient Knowledge related to tracheostomy care	The client will verbalize precautions and safety measures for a tracheostomy, how to use equipment; how to suction the respiratory tract; how to change a tracheostomy tube; and actions to take in an emergency.	Teach client and family how to suction the respiratory tract, care for the tracheostomy, and use respiratory equipment. Instruct client and family in what to do in case of an emergency, such as secretions clogging the tracheostomy tube. Advise client not to swim and to avoid aspirating water when showering or bathing. Advise client to avoid extremely cold temperatures. Cover tracheostomy site for warming or cosmetic purposes with a porous material without frayed or loose threads.

Evaluation: Evaluate each outcome to determine how it has been met by the client.

DISORDERS OF THE NOSE

The most common disorder of the nose is epistaxis, or nose bleed.

EPISTAXIS

Epistaxis is hemorrhage of the nares or nostrils. It is either unilateral, which is most common, or bilateral. Epistaxis may be primary in nature, stemming from drying of the nasal mucosa, local irritation, or trauma, or may occur secondary to uncontrolled hypertension or coagulopathies (e.g., thrombocytopenia, anticoagulant therapy). The diffuse vascularity and proximity of blood vessels to the surface of the nasal mucosa make the nares a susceptible avenue for hemorrhage. Blood loss can be minimal to severe. With significant blood loss, hypovolemic shock occurs.

MEDICAL–SURGICAL MANAGEMENT

Medical

The client with epistaxis usually arrives at an urgent care facility or emergency room after unsuccessful attempts to stop the bleeding. Signs of airway obstruction or aspiration require immediate attention. The goals of treatment are to maintain airway, stop bleeding, identify the cause, and prevent recurrence. Nosebleeds are usually responsive to compression of the nares. Maintain firm pressure for 5 minutes. If bleeding persists, the client should blow the nose and clear the nasal passages. Resume pressure for a full 10 minutes. Epistaxis that continues following these measures requires more aggressive treatment. Bleeding sites that cannot be visualized require a sterile nasal packing inserted after application of a local anesthetic. In severe cases, a nasostat is inserted. This device resembles a Foley catheter and provides direct compression to the site of bleeding via

INFECTION CONTROL

Epistaxis

Wear gloves, goggles or a face mask, and a gown when caring for a client with epistaxis. A cough or sneeze can splatter blood.

a balloon. Clients with severe nosebleeds may require fluid and blood replacement to prevent hypovolemic shock. Persistent or recurrent epistaxis may require surgical ligation of the artery supplying the area.

Pharmacological

Sites of bleeding that can be visualized are cauterized by the physician using silver nitrate sticks. Hemostasis also is accomplished by packing the affected nostril with epinephrine 1:1000 on cotton packing.

Nursing Management

Evaluate overt blood flow and visually examine the posterior oropharynx for hidden bleeding. Monitor vital signs. Have client sit up with head bent slightly forward, breathe through the mouth, and allow blood to run freely from the nose into a container. Avoid tipping the head back as blood will flow down the esophagus causing nausea and vomiting. Then, wearing gloves, compress the nares for 5 minutes. Suction through the mouth to prevent aspiration. Monitor for nausea and vomiting caused by swallowed blood.

NURSING PROCESS

Assessment

Subjective Data

Ask about the onset, precipitating events, duration, and frequency of epistaxis, as well as associated symptoms such as nausea, vomiting, headache, and lightheadedness. The client with an occult bleeding in the back of the throat may complain of needing to swallow frequently.

Objective Data

Evaluate blood flow for amount, consistency, color, and rate (or severity). Overt bleeding from the nose may be present. This bleeding can vary in flow, from a continuous drip to a pulsating stream of blood. Visually examine the posterior oropharynx of the client with an occult epistaxis to assess blood flow. Vomiting may be present. Lowered blood pressure and rapid heart rate are signs of hypovolemic shock. Conversely, the client with uncontrolled hypertension has an abnormally high systolic blood pressure. Prothrombin time (PT), APTT, INR, and other clotting studies will be abnormal with underlying coagulopathies. Decreased red blood cell count, hemoglobin, and hematocrit are evidence of significant bleeding.

Nursing diagnoses for a client with epistaxis include the following:

NURSING DIAGNOSES	PLANNING/OUTCOMES	NURSING INTERVENTIONS
*Impaired **G**as Exchange* related to airway obstruction	The client's respiratory rate, color, and blood gases will be within normal limits.	Place client in a high Fowler's position, with the head bent slightly forward. Instruct client to breathe through the mouth and allow the blood to escape freely from the nose and into a container. This aids in preventing obstruction of the airway and swallowing of blood. Monitor client for signs and symptoms of airway obstruction. Assess client's color, respiratory rate and effort, and breath sounds. Monitor pulse oximetry and lab reports of ABGs and administer supplemental oxygen as indicated.
*Risk for **A**spiration* related to epistaxis	The client will develop no complications related to aspiration.	Place client in the position previously described to aid in preventing aspiration of blood. Assess client for signs of aspiration, such as choking, coarse crackles (rales) on auscultation, or elevated temperature. Suction the respiratory tract through the mouth to remove secretions and blood.
*Deficient Fluid **V**olume* related to blood loss	The client will maintain adequate fluid volume.	With a gloved hand, compress the nares for 5 minutes. If bleeding persists, have client blow nose to clear passages, then compress nares for 10 minutes. If bleeding continues following compression attempts, prepare to assist the physician with procedures such as cautery or insertion of nasal packing.

Nursing diagnoses for a client with epistaxis include the following: (Continued)

NURSING DIAGNOSES	PLANNING/OUTCOMES	NURSING INTERVENTIONS
		Administer medications to control blood pressure, as ordered. After hemostasis has been established, the clots formed should not be removed or dislodged, as this will lead to recurrence of bleeding. Every 30 minutes, evaluate the blood pressure and pulse of the client who shows signs of volume depletion. Assess for orthostatic hypotension as a means of measuring volume depletion. A decrease in systolic blood pressure of greater than 10 mm Hg when the position is changed from lying to sitting or standing indicates hypovolemia. Administer intravenous fluids, as ordered.

Evaluation: Evaluate each outcome to determine how it has been met by the client.

CASE STUDY

P.W. is a 77-year-old woman with a history of smoking two to three packs of cigarettes per day for the past 60 years. P.W. has been diagnosed with COPD for the past 4 years. She has required supplemental oxygen at 2 L/min for the last 18 months. Three days ago, P.W. was admitted with chief complaints of increasing dyspnea on exertion and a productive cough yielding thick, green-yellow sputum. She states that she does "not know why she is coughing up this awful stuff."

Physical examination of P.W. this morning revealed vital signs of T = 101.5°F, P = 124 beats/min, R = 38 breaths/min, BP = 168/74 mm Hg, and sonorous and sibilant wheezes on expiration and in the posterior lung fields, with superimposed coarse crackles heard in the right posterior lower lung field. She is unable to ambulate to the bathroom or complete other ADL because of the dyspnea. Chest x-ray showed a large area of consolidation in the right lower lobe. Sputum culture is still pending.

The following questions will guide your development of a nursing care plan for the case study.

1. List the clinical manifestations that indicate P.W. is experiencing an infection concomitant with her COPD.
2. Explain why COPD predisposes a client to respiratory infection.
3. Explain why the physician will increase P.W.'s oxygen flow to 3 to 4 L/min.
4. List the subjective and objective data the nurse should obtain during the nursing assessment.
5. Identify three nursing diagnoses and client goals that would be pertinent to P.W.'s care.
6. List the above diagnoses in order of priority, with number one being the highest.
7. Describe client outcomes indicating that P.W.'s treatment and nursing care regimen have been successful.

SUMMARY

- The primary function of the respiratory system is delivery of oxygen to the lungs and removal of carbon dioxide from the lungs.
- Pneumonia is a lung infection wherein infectious secretions accumulate in the air passages and interfere with gas exchange. Clients with chronic pulmonary disorders or problems of immobility are at increased risk of developing pneumonia.
- Pulmonary TB is an infection of the lung tissue caused by the *Mycobacterium tuberculosis*. Treatment of TB requires the long-term administration of pharmacological agents.

- A common respiratory tract disorder associated with immobility and the administration of anesthetic agents is atelectasis. Clients at risk are encouraged to cough and breathe deeply to aid in preventing atelectasis.
- Obstruction of a pulmonary artery by a bloodborne substance is known as pulmonary embolism. Deep vein thrombosis is a common cause of pulmonary emboli.
- Chronic obstructive pulmonary disease is a collective term used to refer to chronic bronchitis and emphysema, which often occur together.
- Traumatic disorders of the respiratory tract include pneumothorax and hemothorax, wherein the underlying lung tissue is compressed and eventually collapses.
- Cigarette smoking is indicated as a major causative factor in the development of respiratory disorders, such as lung cancer, cancer of the larynx, emphysema, and chronic bronchitis.

REVIEW QUESTIONS

1. The physician orders 2 to 3 L/min of oxygen to be delivered to the client with COPD because:
   1. no client ever requires more than 2 to 3 L/min of oxygen.
   2. the client requests it.
   3. a higher flow rate may suppress the client's drive to breathe.
   4. 2 to 3 L/min is the maximum flow that a nasal cannula can effectively deliver.
2. A particulate respirator mask is used by the nurse caring for a client with TB because:
   1. regular masks allow the tubercle bacilli to pass through.
   2. this mask is more comfortable for long-term use.
   3. this type of mask allows the nurse to be in close contact with the client for prolonged periods of time.
   4. there is no need for this type of mask when caring for clients with TB.
3. The nurse is teaching a client about lung cancer. Which statement best demonstrates the client correctly understands the risk factors for lung cancer?
   1. "I work with asbestos everyday and it is safe now."
   2. "Having asthma does not make me more at risk for getting lung cancer."
   3. "I should stop chewing tobacco and drinking alcohol."
   4. "My wife smokes and I do not, so I do not have to worry."
4. A client with severe epistaxis arrives at an urgent care clinic. When assessing this client, the nurse's initial action should be to:
   1. identify the cause of the bleeding.
   2. stop the bleeding.
   3. assess for a patent airway.
   4. teach the client how to prevent recurrence.
5. The nurse's assessment of a client with pulmonary edema indicates the following: thick frothy sputum, cough, and dyspnea. On the basis of these findings, the most appropriate nursing diagnosis is:
   1. ineffective airway clearance.
   2. activity Intolerance.
   3. altered tissue perfusion.
   4. acute pain.
6. A client needs to be tested for tuberculosis when the nurse takes a medical history that includes complaints of:
   1. cough, night sweats, hemoptysis.
   2. weight gain, diarrhea, vomiting.
   3. fever > 102°F, fatigue, dry mouth.
   4. weight loss, stridor, chills.
7. The health care provider has prescribed furosemide (Lasix) for a client with a pleural effusion as part of the treatment plan. Which of the following statements made by the client regarding furosemide (Lasix) indicates that further teaching is needed by the nurse?
   1. "I will probably need to urinate more frequently."
   2. "This medication will help remove fluid from my pleural space."
   3. "The nurse will monitor my intake and output each shift."
   4. "I should take this medication at bedtime."
8. Parents of a newly diagnosed 14-year-old asthmatic client ask the nurse what medications will be prescribed for their child. The nurse informs the parents that common medications for asthma include: (Select all that apply.)
   1. bronchodilators.
   2. antibiotics.
   3. corticosteroids.
   4. diuretics.
   5. mucolytic agents.
   6. beta agonists.
9. A client with a pneumothorax is brought to the emergency department. Which of the following assessments will the nurse be able to make?
   1. Decreased respirations, low blood pressure, constricted pupils.
   2. Cyanosis, dyspnea, tracheal shift, and tachycardia
   3. Clammy skin, dilated pupils, slow pulse, and low blood pressure.
   4. Dyspnea, agitation, visual hallucinations, and elevated blood pressure.

10. A client informs the nurse that she is not sure how to use her incentive spirometer. The most appropriate response from the nurse would be:
    1. "The incentive spirometer measures the amount of air inspired in one inhalation."
    2. "The incentive spirometer is a device that a client will use after surgery."
    3. "Would this be a good time for me to teach you and demonstrate?"
    4. "Did someone from the respiratory department teach you?"

REFERENCES/SUGGESTED READINGS

American Cancer Society (ACS). (2003). *Cancer facts and figures 2003.* Atlanta, GA: Author.

American Cancer Society (ACS). (2007). Overview: laryngeal and hypopharyngeal cancer. How many people get laryngeal and hypopharyngeal cancers? Retrieved April 1, 2009 from http://www.cancer.org/docroot/CRI/content/CRI_2_2_1X_How_many_people_get_these_cancers_23.asp?sitearea=

American Cancer Society (ACS). (2009). Lung cancer. Retrieved April 11, 2009 from http://www.cancer.org/docroot/PRO/content/PRO_1_1x_Lung_Cancer.pdf.asp?sitearea=PRO

American Lung Association (ALA). (2007a). Chronic obstructive pulmonary disease fact sheet. Retrieved April 11, 2009 from http://www.lungusa.org/site/apps/nlnet/content3.aspx?c=dvLUK9O0E&b=2058829&content_id={EE451F66-996B-4C23-874D-BF66586196FF}¬oc=1

American Lung Association (ALA). (2007b). HIV and tuberculosis fact sheet. Retrieved April 10, 2009 from http://www.lungusa.org/site/apps/nlnet/content3.aspx?c=dvLUK9O0E&b=2060731&content_id={A3132347-3F7C-4ED7-AB4C-34FBEE5B0D4C}¬oc=1

American Lung Association (ALA). (2007c). Lung cancer fact sheet. Retrieved April 11, 2009 from http://www.lungusa.org/site/apps/nlnet/content3.aspx?c=dvLUK9O0E&b=4294229&ct=3232839

American Lung Association (ALA). (2008a). Trends in tuberculosis morbidity and mortality. Retrieved April 10, 2009 from http://www.lungusa.org/atf/cf/{7a8d42c2-fcca-4604-8ade-7f5d5e762256}/TB_TRENDS_AUG_2008.PDF

American Lung Association (ALA). (2008b). Tuberculosis fact sheet. Retrieved April 10, 2009 from http://www.lungusa.org/site/apps/nlnet/content3.aspx?c=dvLUK9O0E&b=4294229&ct=3052619

American Lung Association (ALA). (2009). Influenza and pneumonia. Retrieved April 10, 2009 from http://www.lungusa.org/site/pp.asp?c=dvLUK9O0E&b=4074717

Andrews, C., & Kearney, K. (2002). Preventing air embolism. *AJN, 102*(1), 34–36.

ARDS Support Center. (2009a). Frequently asked questions about ARDS. Retrieved April 11, 2009 from http://www.ards.org/learnaboutards/whatisards/faq/

ARDS Support Center. (2009b). Learn about ARDS. Retrieved April 11, 2009 from http://ards.org/learnaboutards/

Avalos-Bock, S. (2001). The hard truth about the PPD skin test. *Nursing2001, 31*(6), 56–57.

Bulechek, G., Butcher, H., McCloskey, J., & Dochterman, J., eds. (2008). *Nursing Interventions Classification (NIC)* (5th ed.). St. Louis, MO: Mosby/Elsevier.

Carroll, P. (2001). How to intervene before asthma turns deadly. *RN, 64*(5), 52–58.

Centers for Disease Control and Prevention (CDC). (2005a). Basic information about SARS. Retrieved April 11, 2009 from http://www.cdc.gov/ncidod/sars/factsheet.htm

Centers for Disease Control and Prevention (CDC). (2005b). Current SARS situation. Retrieved April 11, 2009 from http://www.cdc.gov/ncidod/sars/situation.htm

Centers for Disease Control and Prevention (CDC). (2008). NIOSH topic area: Severe acute respiratory syndrome (SARS). Retrieved July 17, 2009 from http://www.cdc.gov/niosh/topics/SARS/

Centers for Disease Control and Prevention(CDC). (2009). Influenza: The disease. Retrieved July 20, 2009 from http://www.cdc.gov/flu/about/disease/index.htm

Chan, S., & Goldrick, B. (2003). Emerging infections. *AJN, 103*(6), 60–62.

Daniels, R., Nosek, L., & Nicoll, L. (2007). *Contemporary medical-surgical nursing*. Clifton Park, NY: Delmar Cengage Learning.

Davies, P. (2002). Guarding your patient against ARDS. *Nursing2002, 32*(3), 36–41.

Diehl-Oplinger, L., & Kaminski, M. F. (2002). Flash pulmonary edema. *Nursing2002*, 32(7), 96.

Dirkes, S., & Winklerprins, A. (2002). Help for ARDS patients. *RN, 65*(8), 52–58.

Dunn, N. (2001). Keeping COPD patients out of the ED. *RN, 64(2)*, 33–37.

Eckler, J. (2002). Keeping pulmonary tuberculosis at bay. *Nursing2002, 32*(12), 70.

Ellmers, K., & Criddle, L. (2002). Cystic fibrosis. *RN, 65*(9), 60–66.

Estes, M. E. Z. (2010). *Health assessment & physical examination* (4th ed.). Clifton Park, NY: Delmar Cengage Learning.

Finesilver, C. (2001). Perfecting your skills: Respiratory assessment. *Travel Nurse Today supplement to RN* (April) 16–26.

Georgetown University Hospital. (2009). Neck dissection patient information. Retrieved July 17, 2009 from http://www.georgetownuniversityhospital.org/body.cfm?id=1016#3

Goodfellow, L., & Jones, M. (2002). Bronchial hygiene therapy. *AJN, 102*(1), 37–43.

Hayes, D. (2001). Stemming the tide of pleural effusions. *Nursing2001, 31*(5), 49–52.

Lazzara, D. (2001). Respiratory distress. *Nursing2001, 31*(6), 58–63.

Lazzara, D. (2002). Eliminate the air of mystery from chest tubes. *Nursing2002, 32*(6), 36–43.

Lindell, K., & Jacobs, S. (2003). Idiopathic pulmonary fibrosis. *AJN, 103*(4), 32–41.

Little, C. (2002). Chronic bronchitis. *Nursing2001, 32*(9), 52–55.

Marion, B. (2001). A turn for the better: "Prone positioning" of patients with ARDS. *AJN, 101*(5), 26–33.

Marthaler, M., Keresztes, P., & Tazbir, J. (2003). SARS: What have we learned? *RN, 66*(8), 58–66.

Mayo Clinic. (2009). Cystic fibrosis. Retrieved July 20, 2009 from http://www.mayoclinic.com/health/cystic-fibrosis/DS00287

McConnell, E. (2002). Providing tracheostomy care. *Nursing2002, 32*(1), 17.

Miracle, V. (2002). Asthma attack. *Nursing2002, 32*(11), 104.

Moorhead, S., Johnson, M., Maas, M., & Swanson, E. (2007). *Nursing Outcomes Classification (NOC)* (4th ed.). St. Louis, MO: Mosby.

National Cancer Institute. (2009). Metastatic squamous neck cancer with occult primary treatment (PDQ). Retrieved July 17, 2009 from http://www.cancer.gov/cancertopics/pdq/treatment/metastatic-squamous-neck/Patient/page4

National Heart Lung and Blood Institute (NHLBI). (2009a). COPD: what causes COPD? Retrieved April 11, 2009 from http://www.nhlbi.nih.gov/health/dci/Diseases/Copd/Copd_Causes.html

National Heart Lung and Blood Institute (NHLBI). (2009b). How is pulmonary embolism treated? Retrieved April 11, 2009 from http://www.nhlbi.nih.gov/health/dci/Diseases/pe/pe_treatments.html

National Heart Lung and Blood Institute (NHLBI). (2009c). Who is at risk for pulmonary embolism? Retrieved April 11, 2009 from http://www.nhlbi.nih.gov/health/dci/Diseases/pe/pe_risk.html

National Institute of Allergy and Infectious Diseases. (2009). Flu (influenza). Retrieved July 20, 2009 from http://www3.niaid.nih.gov/topics/Flu/understandingFlu/DefinitionsOverview.htm

National Institutes of Health(NIH). (2009a). Fact sheet: Cystic fibrosis. Retrieved July 20, 2009 from http://www.nih.gov/about/researchresultsforthepublic/CysticFibrosis.pdf

National Institutes of Health (NIH). (2009b). Pleural disorders. Retrieved April 11, 2009 from http://www.nlm.nih.gov/medlineplus/pleuraldisorders.html

National Institutes of Health (NIH). (2009c). Severe acute respiratory syndrome. Retrieved April 11, 2009 from http://www.nlm.nih.gov/medlineplus/severeacuterespiratorysyndrome.html

Perkins, L., & Shortall, S. (2000). Ventilation without intubation. *RN, 63*(1), 34–38.

Phipps, W., Monahan, P., Sands, J., Marek, J., & Neighbors, M. (2003). *Medical–surgical nursing: Health and illness perspectives* (7th ed.). St. Louis, MO: Mosby.

Pope, B. (2002). Asthma. *Nursing2002, 32*(5), 44–45.

Pullen, R. (2003). Teaching bedside incentive spirometry. *Nursing2003, 33*(8), 24.

Schultz, T. (2002). Community-acquired pneumonia. *Nursing2002, 32*(1), 46–49.

Shortall, S., & Perkins, L. (1999). Interpreting the ins and outs of pulmonary function tests. *Nursing99, 29*(12), 41–47.

Spratto, G., & Woods, A. (2010). *2010 Delmar nurse's drug handbook.* Clifton Park, NY: Delmar Cengage Learning.

Tasota, F., & Davies, P. (2001). Diagnosing pulmonary embolism with spiral CT. *Nursing2001, 31*(5), 75.

Togger, D., & Brenner, P. (2001). Metered dose inhalers. *AJN, 101*(10), 26–32.

Wisniewski, A. (2003). Chronic bronchitis and emphysema: Clearing the air. *Nursing2003, 33*(5), 46–49.

Woods, A. (2002). Pneumonia. *Nursing2002, 32*(11), 56–57.

World Health Organization (WHO). (2009). Severe acute respiratory Syndrome. Retrieved April 11, 2009 from www.who.int/csr/sars/travel/en/index.html

Zorb, S. (2002). Transplantation offers hope. *RN, 65(9)*, 66–68.

RESOURCES

American Cancer Society (ACS), http://www.cancer.org

American Lung Association, http://www.lungusa.org

American Thoracic Society, http://www.thoracic.org

Centers for Disease Control and Prevention (CDC), http://www.cdc.gov

Cystic Fibrosis Foundation, http://www.cff.org

International Association of Laryngectomees, http://www.theial.com/ial/

CHAPTER 5
Cardiovascular System

MAKING THE CONNECTION

Refer to the following chapters to increase your understanding of the cardiovascular system:

Adult Health Nursing
- ***Respiratory System***
- ***Hematologic and Lymphatic Systems***
- ***Endocrine System***

Delmar's Heart & Lung Sounds on StudyWare™: Heart Sounds

LEARNING OBJECTIVES

Upon completion of this chapter, you should be able to:

- Define key terms.
- Describe the anatomy and physiology of the cardiovascular system.
- Relate laboratory results to each disorder.
- Describe basic heart dysrhythmias.
- Explain the pathophysiology of each disorder.
- Describe nursing interventions in caring for clients with cardiovascular conditions.

KEY TERMS

aneurysm
angina pectoris
annulus
arteriosclerosis
ascites
atherosclerosis
baseline level
bradycardia
cardiac cycle
cardiac output (CO)
cardiac tamponade
depolarization
dyspnea
dysrhythmia
embolus
heart sound
hemolysis
Homans' sign
hypertrophy
implantable cardioverter-defibrillator (ICD)
myocardial infarction
myocarditis
necrosis
orthopnea
palpitation

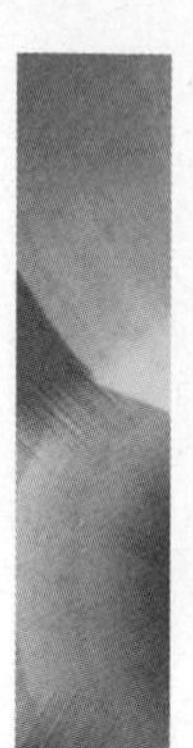

paroxysmal nocturnal dyspnea
pericardial friction rub
pericardiocentesis
pericarditis
peripheral resistance
phlebitis
phlebothrombosis
primary hypertension
repolarization
sclerotherapy
secondary hypertension
stasis dermatitis
stent
stroke volume (SV)
tachycardia
thrombectomy
thrombophlebitis
thrombosis
thrombus
transesophageal echocardiography (TEE)
varicosities
vasoconstrict
vasodilate
vein ligation
vein stripping
Virchow's triad

INTRODUCTION

Since 1900, heart disease has been the leading cause of death in the United States every year except in 1918 during the flu epidemic (AHA, 2007a). In 2003, 911,163 deaths were attributed to cardiovascular disease (CVD) compared to 869,724 deaths in 2007 (AHA, 2007a). The death rate for cardiovascular disease is declining because of public education in modifying and decreasing risk factors such as smoking, high-fat diets, and minimal exercise.

This chapter reviews the anatomy and physiology of the cardiovascular system. Pathophysiology, medical management, and nursing interventions related to cardiovascular conditions are discussed with an emphasis on decreasing risk factors and improving lifestyles.

ANATOMY AND PHYSIOLOGY REVIEW

The cardiovascular system consists of the heart and its vasculature and the peripheral vascular system. The heart is located in the lower anterior area of the mediastinum with the apex near the diaphragm. The heart apex tips forward and to the left of the client's chest cavity. In an average lifetime, the heart will pump 80 million gallons of blood.

The peripheral vascular system consists of arteries, arterioles, capillaries, venules, and veins. The arteries carry oxygenated blood away from the left side of the heart to the body tissues, and the veins carry deoxygenated blood back to the right side of the heart. The capillaries connect the arterioles to the venules. The venules and veins contain 60% to 70% of the body's total blood volume.

The cardiovascular system provides oxygen, nutrients, and hormones to the cells and removes carbon dioxide and waste products of cellular metabolism from body cells. Body temperature is maintained by the distribution of heat throughout the body produced by the metabolic activity of muscles and other body organs.

STRUCTURE OF THE HEART

The heart is encapsulated by a protective sac called the pericardium and consists of three layers: endocardium, myocardium, and epicardium. The endocardium is made of endothelium cells that line the inside of the heart, the four heart valves, and is continuous with the endothelial lining of the arteries, capillaries, and veins making the circulatory system a closed system. Therefore, if a person has a systemic blood infection the heart lining and valves are also affected. The myocardium consists of striated muscle and varies in thickness depending on the heart chamber. The left ventricle pumps blood to the body and is, therefore, the thickest chamber. The outside of the heart is surrounded by the epicardium. The pericardium consists of two layers: the parietal pericardium and visceral pericardium. The parietal layer (outer layer) is a fibrous loose sac that surrounds the heart and the visceral layer lines the great vessels and is also called the epicardium when it lines the heart. The pericardial space is between the two pericardium layers and is filled with fluid (see Figure 5-1).

The heart is a hollow muscular organ containing four chambers that fill and empty of blood with each contraction (**depolarization**) and recovery phase (**repolarization**) of the cardiac muscle. The upper chambers are the atria and the lower chambers are the ventricles (Figure 5-1). When the atria contract, blood is forced into the ventricles. Contraction of the right ventricle pumps blood into the pulmonary arteries and on to the lungs (pulmonary circulatory system). Contraction of the left ventricle pumps blood into the aorta and out to the entire body (systemic circulatory system). The myocardium of the left ventricle is thicker than the right ventricle because more force is needed to pump blood throughout the body.

There are four valves in the heart: tricuspid, bicuspid (mitral), pulmonic, and aortic. One end of fibrous cords called *chordae tendineae* is attached to the cusps of the tricuspid and mitral valves, and the other end is attached to papillary muscles on the ventricular walls. The chordae tendineae keep the valves from inverting when the ventricles contract, thus preventing blood from flowing back into the atrium. The pulmonic and aortic valves prevent blood from flowing back into the ventricles from the pulmonary artery and aorta during repolarization.

CIRCULATION OF BLOOD

Blood enters the heart through veins and leaves the heart through arteries. With the contraction of the right ventricle, blood is forced through the pulmonic valve into the pulmonary artery. Blood circulates through the pulmonary circulatory

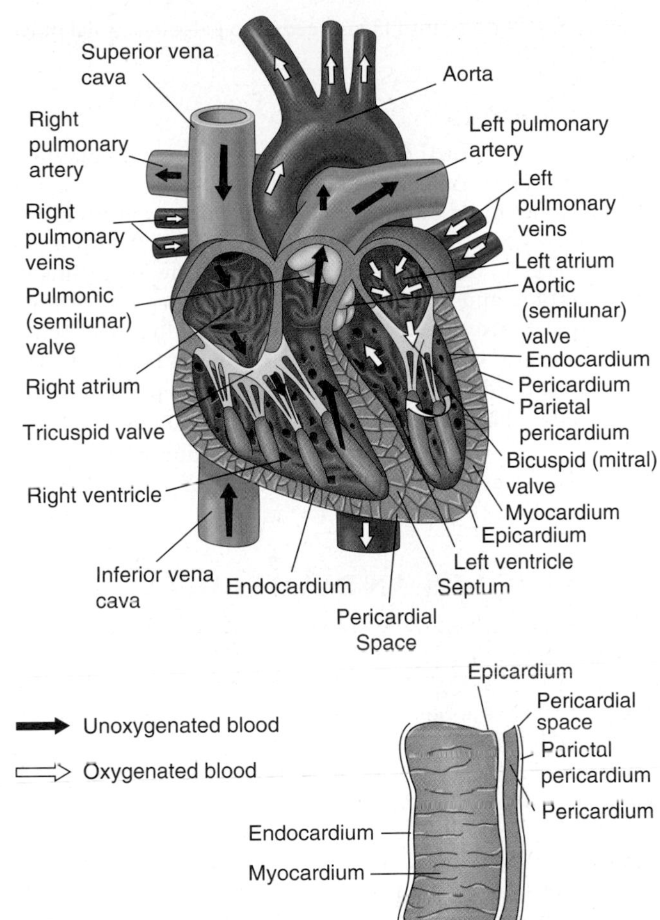

FIGURE 5-1 Internal View of the Heart with Aorta, Vena Cava, and Pulmonary Arteries and Veins

system, where carbon dioxide is exchanged for oxygen in the lungs. The blood then returns to the left atrium through the pulmonary veins, providing oxygenated blood for systemic circulation. When the left ventricle contracts, blood is forced through the aortic valve into the aorta, beginning systemic circulation. Blood is then distributed throughout the body and returns to the right atrium of the heart through the inferior and superior vena cava.

Stroke Volume and Cardiac Output

Heart rate (HR) is the number of ventricular contractions per minute as determined by auscultation of the heart or palpation of a pulse. Each time the heart beats, the ventricle pumps 60 to 80 mL of blood. The volume of blood ejected from the left ventricle with each contraction or systole is known as the **stroke volume (SV)**. Normal stroke volume is approximately 70 mL. The amount of blood ejected in 1 minute is known as the **cardiac output (CO)**. Therefore, CO is determined by multiplying HR for 1 minute by the stroke volume (CO = HR × SV) (Bender, 2008). If the heart has a strong ventricular contraction, more blood is pumped by the heart into the systemic circulatory system. Therefore, CO has a direct effect on the circulating volume of arterial blood.

Coronary Arteries

Coronary arteries supply nutrients and oxygen to the muscle tissue of the heart. The two coronary arteries, which branch off the aorta, are the right coronary artery and the left coronary artery (Figure 5-2). The right coronary artery divides into the posterior descending artery (interventricular artery) and the marginal artery and supplies blood to the anterior area of the right and left ventricles, the posterior area of the right ventricle, the AV node, and the posterior section of the interventricular septum. The left coronary artery divides into the anterior descending artery and the circumflex artery. The left anterior descending (LAD) artery supplies blood to the anterior section of the interventricular septum, anterior area of the left ventricle, and the lateral aspect of the left ventricle. The circumflex artery nourishes the left atrium and ventricle.

Conduction System

The specialized cardiac muscle cells are capable of conducting electrical impulses from one part of the heart to another. For the heart to beat regularly in a rhythmic sequence, electrical impulses follow a set pattern through the conduction system of the heart. The conduction system, consisting of the sinoatrial node (SA node), atrioventricular node (AV node), bundle of His, bundle branches, and Purkinje fibers, controls the heartbeat (Figure 5-3).

The SA node located in the superior aspect of the right atrium initiates electrical impulses that cause the heart to beat. It is called the pacemaker of the heart. Electrical impulses from the SA node pass through the muscle fibers of the right and left atria, causing the atria to contract almost simultaneously. Atrial impulses are transmitted to the AV node located in the lower part of the right atrium. There is a short delay in the impulse at the AV node that allows the atria

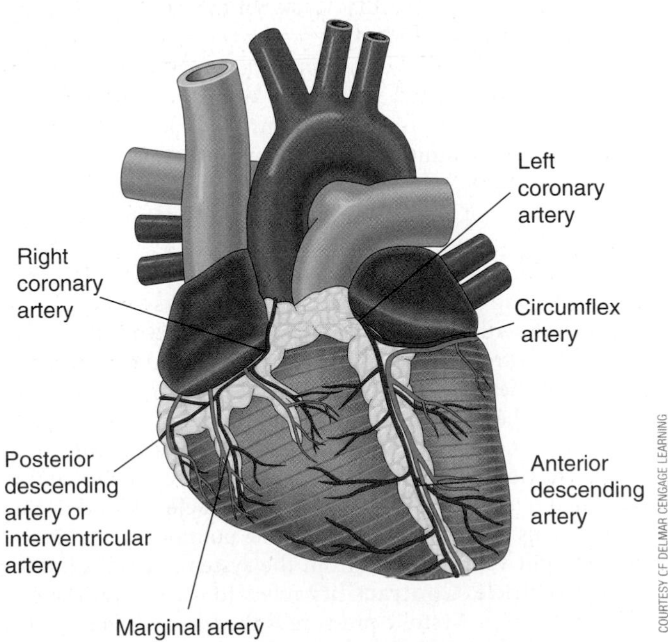

FIGURE 5-2 Coronary Arteries that Supply Blood to the Heart Tissue

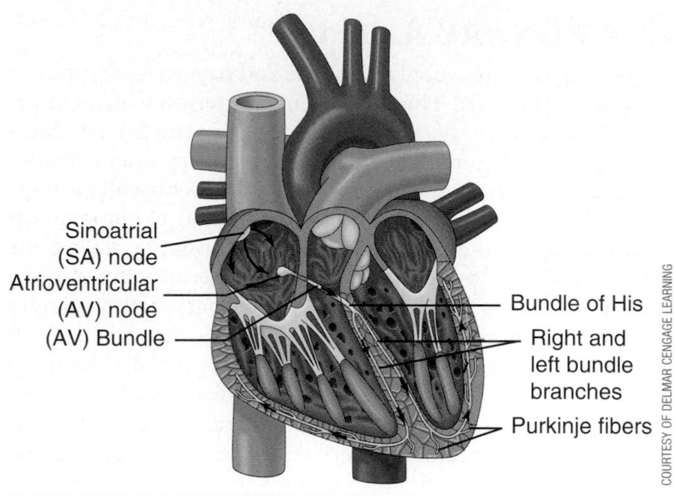

FIGURE 5-3 Conduction System of the Heart

to complete their contraction and empty the blood into the ventricles. The electrical impulse is transmitted from the AV node into a group of specialized conduction fibers called the AV bundle or the bundle of His. Once the impulse leaves the AV node, it travels down the fibers of the bundle of His into the interventricular septum. The fibers separate into right and left bundle branches dividing into smaller and smaller branches, called Purkinje fibers. These terminate in the ventricular muscle, causing the ventricles to contract. When an impulse has completely gone through the conduction system of the heart and the ventricles have contracted, a **cardiac cycle** is completed.

The end-diastolic volume (EDV) is the amount of blood in the ventricles after the ventricular rest and filling phase of the cardiac cycle. In the healthy heart, the EDV is usually around 120 mL. The end-systolic volume (ESV) is the amount of blood in the ventricles after the ventricular contraction and ejection phase of the cardiac cycle. In the healthy heart, the ESV is usually around 50 mL.

Ejection fraction (EF) is an indicator of ventricle functioning and is reduced in patients with myocardial infarction and diagnostic for heart failure (HF). To determine the EF, stroke volume is divided by end-diastolic volume (EF = SV/EDV). In healthy hearts, the EF is between 50% and 70% of the EDV. The EF is determined through echocardiography.

Four factors influence stroke volume and CO: preload, afterload, contractility, and HR. **Preload** refers to the amount of pressure within the ventricles. This is determined by the amount of stretch or tension derived from the ventricular filling and the pressure exerted by fluid volume on the myocardium at the end of diastole (ventricular end-diastolic pressure), or just before contraction. **Afterload** is the force that resists ejection of blood from the ventricles, or the force that is needed to open the semilunar valve and eject blood during systole. This resistance arises from the pulmonary circulation for the right ventricle, and from the systemic circulation for the left ventricle. **Contractility** refers to the strength of cardiac contraction. Systolic pressure is the force exerted against arterial walls during ventricular contraction. Diastolic pressure is the force exerted against arterial walls during ventricular relaxation. Blood pressure is expressed as systolic pressure/diastolic pressure (e.g., 120/80). A systolic blood pressure reading of at least 80 mm Hg is needed to palpate a radial pulse (Bender, 2008).

Heart Sounds

There are two normal **heart sounds** heard on auscultation; S_1 and S_2. They yield a sound like "lubb-dubb." S_1, or the "lubb," is the sound of the mitral and tricuspid valves closing simultaneously. The S_1 sound is heard on the left fifth intercostal space. S_2, or the "dubb," is the simultaneous closing of the pulmonic and aortic valves, heard on the right second intercostal space. There is a slight pause after the "lubb-dubb" is heard. Clients with congestive heart failure (CHF) may have a third sound known as S_3. The low-pitched sound occurs after the S_2 sound, or the "dubb," making the heart sound like the word "Kentucky" ("lubb-dubb-by"). The S_3 sound also is described as a gallop because of the similarity in sound to a horse's gallop.

ARTERIOLES AND ARTERIES

The arteries are thick-walled tubes consisting of three layers or tunics (Figure 5-4). The inner layer is called the *tunica intima* and consists of a single layer of smooth endothelial cells. The middle layer is the *tunica media* and is composed of smooth muscle cells. The smooth muscle layer of the artery receives nerve stimulation from the sympathetic nervous system. The suppleness of the smooth muscle allows the vessel to **vasoconstrict** (decrease in diameter) and **vasodilate** (increase in diameter). The outer layer, the *tunica adventitia* or *tunica externa*, consists of a connective tissue sheath with some of its collagen fibers fusing with those of the surrounding tissue to hold the vessels in place. The elastic connective tissue allows the artery to expand and recoil with each contraction of the ventricle as an increased volume of blood is pumped through the vessel. The arteries have thick walls, so they can withstand the increased pressure from the left ventricle pumping blood through the body.

The arteries divide and branch into smaller vessels called *arterioles*. The same three layers are present in the walls, but as the arterioles approach the capillaries their walls become thinner. The outer layer is reduced to a very thin layer of connective tissue.

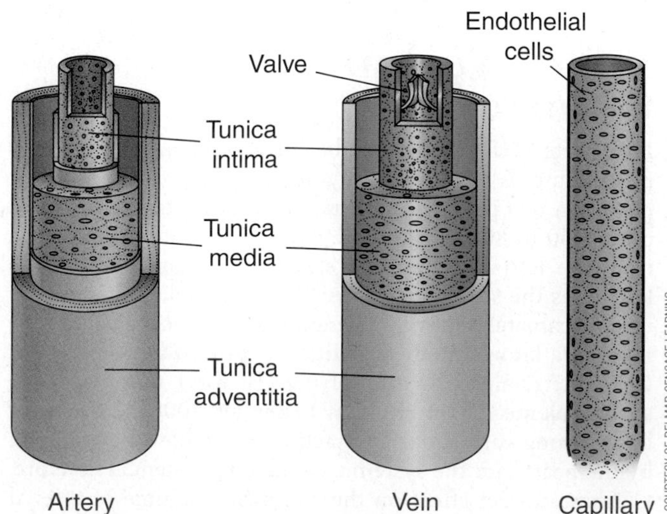

FIGURE 5-4 Tunic Layers of Each Type of Vessel

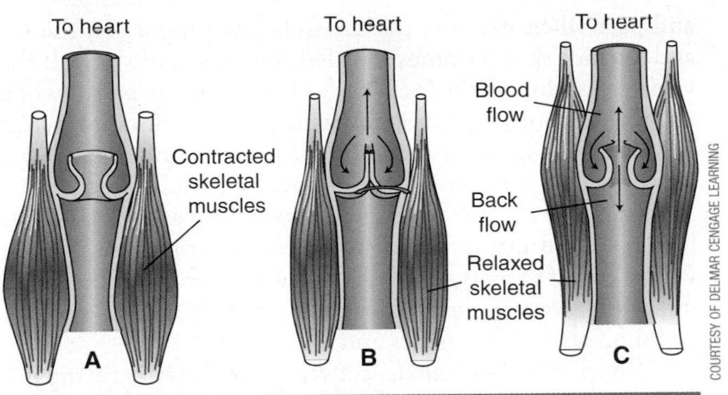

FIGURE 5-5 Valves in the veins hold the blood at a certain level in the vein. *A*, Contracted skeletal muscles apply pressure to veins and assist with the circulation of blood. *B*, Valves prevent the backflow of blood. *C*, Incompetent valves allow a backflow of blood.

CAPILLARIES

Capillaries are very tiny thin vessels that connect the smallest arterioles with the smallest venules. They have only one layer of endothelial cells whose cell membranes are the semipermeable membrane that allows the exchange of oxygen, nutrients, carbon dioxide, and waste products between the tissues of the body and the blood.

VENULES AND VEINS

Venules are small vessels that emerge from the capillaries and gradually increase in size to eventually form veins. Veins have three layers or tunics like the arteries, but the middle layer of a vein is thinner with less smooth muscle and elastic tissue. The elasticity of the smooth muscles allow the walls of the veins to dilate more easily. Endothelial flaps, called *valves*, are on the inside lining of veins. The valves open and close with each contraction of the surrounding skeletal muscles. The valves assist the blood in returning to the heart. Blood is held by the valves until skeletal muscle contractions move the blood toward the heart against gravity (Figure 5-5).

HEALTH HISTORY

There are three goals when obtaining a health history from a client: (1) identify present and potential health problems, (2) identify possible familial and lifestyle risk factors, and (3) involve the client in planning long-term health care.

Ascertain the onset of the symptoms, the predisposing factors that cause the symptoms, and the client's treatment of the symptoms. Ask about the client's activity level or limitations in activity. Determine if appetite has increased or decreased. Evaluate the client's ability to sleep, the need for the trunk of the body to be supported with pillows when sleeping, or the need to sleep in a chair.

Major risk factors associated with cardiovascular diseases are age, gender, heredity (including race), smoking, dyslipidemia (presence of increased total serum cholesterol and low-density lipoprotein [LDL]), high blood pressure, physical inactivity, overweight, obesity, and diabetes mellitus. An individual's response to stress may be a contributing factor. Additional contributing factors for women include menopause, use of birth control pills, and high triglyceride level.

Advancing age, male gender, diabetes, heredity, and family history of chest pain or myocardial infarctions are risk factors that cannot be altered. Alterable risk factors are physical inactivity, smoking, contraceptive method, dyslipidemia, overweight, obesity, and triglyceride level. A change in diet may alter the last four factors.

There are two objectives in assisting the client toward a healthier lifestyle: (1) to educate the client about the risk factors; and (2) to determine what risk factors the client would like to modify. Once this is determined, assist the client to establish goals and determine actions to achieve the goals.

ASSESSMENT

Assessment includes clients' self-report of symptoms as well as physical findings and confirming lab data.

SUBJECTIVE DATA

The typical concerns expressed by a client with a cardiac disorder are chest pain, **dyspnea** (difficulty breathing), edema, fainting, palpitations, diaphoresis, and fatigue. When a client talks about having chest pain, ascertain the time of onset, situation occurring at the onset of pain, location and radiation of pain, severity of chest pain, duration, past episodes of chest pain, and methods used to alleviate pain. Using the Memory Trick: Pain Assessment PQRST is an ideal way for a nurse to assess a client's pain. This method is described in the Memory Trick: Pain Assessment PQRST. Women are more likely to experience shortness of breath, fatigue, back or jaw pain, and atypical discomfort such as a feeling of indigestion or nausea and vomiting (Nagle & Nee, 2002; AHA, 2007b).

The client may be experiencing several types of dyspnea. Exertional dyspnea occurs when a person participates in moderate activity and becomes short of breath. This occurs in the early stages of HF and indicates that the heart is not able to meet the demands of the body during moderate activity. **Orthopnea** is when a client has difficulty breathing while lying down and must sit upright or stand to relieve the

MEMORY**TRICK**

Pain Assessment PQRST

P = Provoker of pain (aggravating factors) and palliative measures (alleviating factors)

Q = Quality of pain (gnawing, pounding, burning, stabbing, pinching, aching, throbbing, and crushing)

R = Region (location) and radiation to other body sites

S = Severity (quantity of pain on 0–10 scale, 0 = no pain and 10 = worst pain experienced) and setting (what causes the pain)

T = Timing (onset, duration, and frequency)

(Adapted from Estes, 2010)

dyspnea. This occurs in a more advanced stage of HF. **Paroxysmal nocturnal dyspnea** usually occurs 2 to 5 hours after an individual falls asleep. The person suddenly awakens, is sweating, and has difficulty breathing.

A client has fainting spells for various physical and psychological reasons. Cardiac clients faint because of decreased CO causing decreased blood flow to the brain.

A client may describe a "fluttering" or "pounding" sensation in the chest. This is known as **palpitations**. If these sensations occur during exercise, it is a sign that the heart has to work harder to meet the demands of the body. Palpitations may also be caused by anxiety, ingestion of a large meal, lack of adequate rest, or a large intake of caffeine.

A cardiac client will usually experience fatigue increasing throughout the day because the heart is not able to keep up with the demands of the body. Frequent rest periods will help alleviate some of the fatigue.

The typical concerns expressed by the client with a peripheral vascular disorder are pain, paresthesia (decreased sensation in an area), and/or paralysis in the hands, thigh, calf, ankles, foot, abdomen, or lower back. The quality of pain (aching, cramping, sharp, or throbbing) and any numbness or tingling is noted.

Objective Data

In a head-to-toe assessment on a cardiac client, the skin, neck veins, respirations, heart sounds, abdomen, and extremities are carefully assessed. Observe the skin for cyanosis in the earlobes, lips, mucous membranes, and finger-and toenails. Assessment of skin turgor may indicate fluid volume. If the skin is dry and has poor turgor, the client may be dehydrated from diuretics. If a client has distended internal and external jugular veins when the head of the bed is gradually elevated to a 45-degree angle or higher, there may be right-sided HF. Assess the quality of respirations for rate and ease of breathing, signs of dyspnea, and coughing. Heart sounds are assessed for the normal S_1 and S_2 sounds. If the typical lubb-dubb is heard, the valves are closing properly.

While listening to the heart, the radial pulse should be palpated to account for every heartbeat. If a heartbeat is heard through the stethoscope but not felt in the radial pulse, the heart has decreased CO to the extremities. If the abdomen is distended, the client may have **ascites**, which is excess fluid in the abdomen. After assessing the heart and lung sounds, check the peripheral pulses. Pulses on both sides of the body should be checked at the same time to determine adequate bilateral perfusion. It is important to check pedal pulses in both feet to determine blood flow to each foot. Pulse amplitude can be described as absent, diminished, normal, increased, and bounding (Gehring, 2002).

If the hands and feet are cold or have mottling, this indicates decreased CO. Capillary refill should be less than 3 seconds in the fingers and toes.

Note if the feet, ankles, or legs are edematous (Figure 5-6). A client may gain 10 pounds before edema is detected. Weigh cardiac clients with edema daily. The weight must be taken on the same scale, at the same time of day, with the client wearing the same amount of clothing.

Decreased circulation to an area results in coolness in the ischemic area, pallor, paresthesia, and paralysis. Paresthesia and paralysis result from a lack of oxygenated blood and nourishment to the nerves. Symptoms of paresthesia are numbness and tingling.

If an artery in the leg is occluded, the foot and/or leg become reddish in color when the leg is in a dependent position, and pale when elevated. As the ischemia progresses, the leg and/or foot skin becomes mottled, smooth, and shiny. If the veins are occluded, the foot and/or leg become cyanotic when in a dependent position, and has a normal coloration when elevated. The anterior area of the lower leg and ankle has a brown pigmentation with venous involvement.

Clients with decreased circulation to the extremities have hardened and brittle nails and less hair distribution. The leg will be cool if there is an arterial circulatory problem but warm if there is a venous circulatory problem. Skin ulcerations may be found around the ankles and toes.

Check the client's ankles for **stasis dermatitis**, an inflammation of the skin caused by decreased circulation. Waste products that normally are carried away by the circulatory system remain in the tissues, causing pruritus and irritation of the skin. At first, the ankle area is reddened and edematous, then vesicles form and start oozing. The skin becomes crusted, thickened, and brown.

A positive **Homans' sign** is present in some cases of deep vein thrombosis (DVT). To test for Homans' sign, dorsiflex the client's foot. If there is pain in the calf of the leg or behind the knee, the Homans' sign is positive and may indicate the presence of a venous clot. Do not do a Homans' sign if there is a diagnosis of a thrombus, because the clot may be dislodged with the procedure.

Refer to Box 5-1, "Questions to Ask and Observations to Make When Collecting Data" for guidance in completing client cardiac assessments.

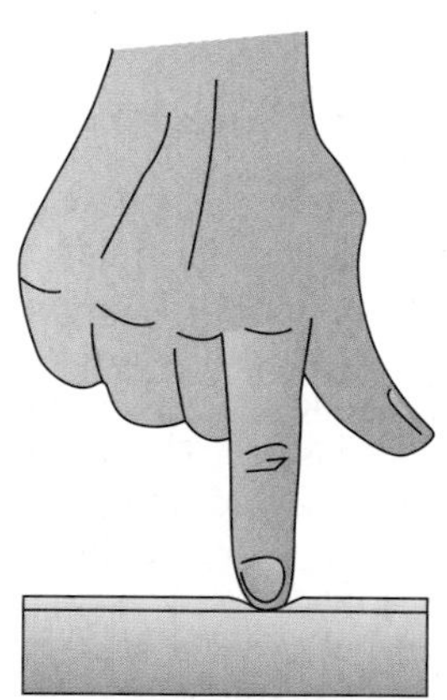

1+ = disappears rapidly

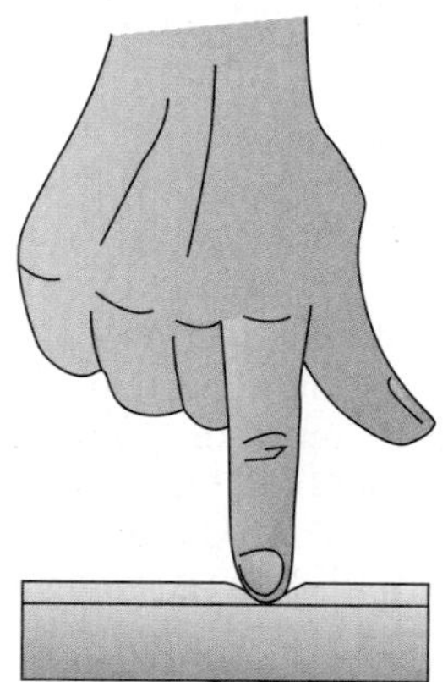

2+ = lasts 10 to 15 seconds

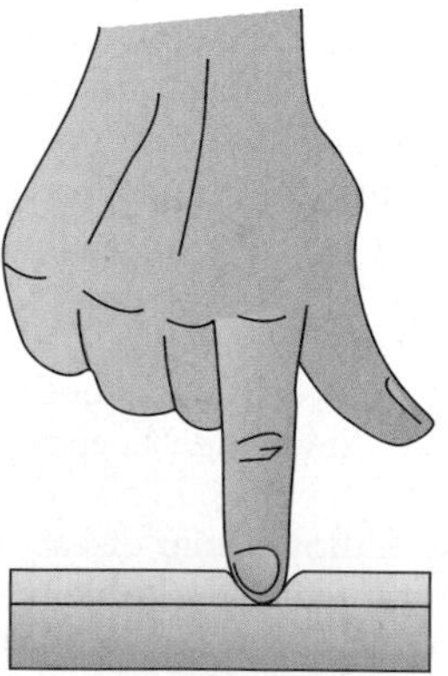

3+ = lasts more than 1 minute

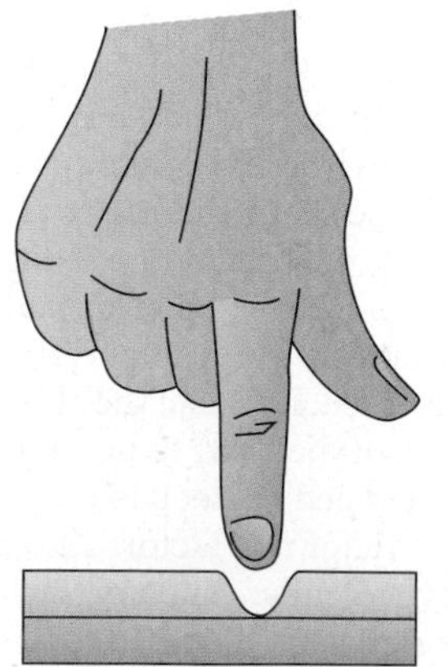

4+ = lasts 2 to 5 minutes

FIGURE 5-6 Edema Rating Scale: Press down for 5 seconds, then time how long indentation remains.

BOX 5-1 QUESTIONS TO ASK AND OBSERVATIONS TO MAKE WHEN COLLECTING DATA

SUBJECTIVE DATA

Have you experienced chest pain? Radiating pain? Nausea? Indigestion? Fatigue?

What activities cause chest pain?

Have you felt palpitations or your heart flutter?

Do you ever feel dizzy or lightheaded?

Tell me about your memory.

On how many pillows do you sleep?

Do you awaken short of breath?

List prescription and over the counter medications you are taking.

Do you use any herbal supplements?

Describe your daily exercise habits.

Are you on any specific type of diet?

Do you weigh yourself at regular intervals? Have you noticed a weight gain of 5 pounds or more from one day to the next?

How often do you urinate during the daytime? During the night?

Are you sexually active? Have there been any changes in the last year?

Do you experience swelling in your feet or ankles?

Can you climb a flight of stairs without becoming short of breath?

Can you walk a block without feeling cramps in your legs?

How do you cope with stress?

How do you relax?

OBJECTIVE DATA

Take vital signs; temperature, pulse, respirations, and pulse oximetry.

Check pupils.

Check capillary refill.

Check the skin, lips, fingers, and feet for cyanosis.

Listen to the apical pulse and palpate the radial pulse at the same time.

Listen to breath sounds on anterior and posterior aspects of chest

Listen to bowel sounds.

Palpate abdomen for edema or tautness.

Examine legs, ankles, and feet for swelling.

Examine legs for hair distribution.

Check for areas for decreased sensation.

Check peripheral pulses noting the quality, rhythm, and amplitude.

Check extremities for areas of brownish discoloration, ulcerations, and bruising.

Complete a Homans' sign.

COMMON DIAGNOSTIC TESTS

Commonly used diagnostic tests for clients with symptoms of cardiovascular system disorders are listed in Table 5-1. Cardiac biomarkers that diagnose, evaluate, and monitor clients with possible acute coronary syndrome (ACS) are troponin I, troponin T, CK, CK-MB, and myoglobin. AST and LDH are not specific for heart damage and are not recommended for clients suspected with ACS (American Association for Clinical Chemistry, 2008). Troponins are replacing CK and CK-MB in some settings because they are more specific for heart injury (versus skeletal muscle injury) and are elevated for a longer period of time. Troponins elevate within 3–4 hours after injury and may remain elevated for 10–14 days (see Table 5-2 for elevation times of biomarkers). The greater the tissue damage the greater the elevation. Muscular injection, strenuous exercise and drugs that affect muscles do not elevate troponin levels as they do with CK (Bender, 2008). Other general tests ordered with cardiac biomarkers are ABGs, comprehensive metabolic panel, basic metabolic panel, electrolytes, and CBC.

A newer cardiac biomarker test used with troponin and an ECG to identify clients at a greater risk of an MI is ischemia modified albumin (IMA). If IMA is not present in a client who has experienced chest pain for a few minutes to a few hours, it is not likely that the client has ischemia. IMA is not as valuable with a client who has experienced chest pain for several hours because the IMA level may have risen and returned to normal within that time frame.

CARDIAC RHYTHM/ DYSRHYTHMIA

As a basis for understanding cardiac dysrhythmias, the normal sinus rhythm must first be understood.

NORMAL SINUS RHYTHM

The electrical conduction of the heart begins with the SA (refer to Figure 5-7) node located in the superior section of the right atrium. From the SA node, the electrical impulse spreads in wave fashion through the atria similar to the ripples from a pebble dropped in water. The firing of the SA node and the electrical impulse spreading across both atria yields a P wave on the ECG. The P wave represents the electrical activity causing the contraction of both atria.

After the atria contract, the electrical impulse reaches the AV node, where it pauses for approximately one-tenth of a second, allowing blood to enter both ventricles. The electrical impulse then starts down the AV bundle that divides into right and left bundle branches in the interventricular septum. The electrical impulse continues from the right and the left bundle branches to the Purkinje fibers that transmit the electrical impulse to the myocardial cells resulting in depolarization or contraction of the ventricles. On an ECG the QRS complex represents the electrical impulse as it travels through the AV node, AV bundle, bundle branches, Purkinje fibers, and myocardial cells, ending with the

Table 5-1 Common Diagnostic Tests for Cardiovascular System Disorders

Laboratory Tests
Arterial blood gasses (ABGs)
Basic metabolic panel (BMP)
Cardiac biomarkers
- Creatine kinase (CK)
- CK-MB (CK_2)
- High-sensitivity C-reactive protein (hs-CRP)
- B-type natriuretic peptide (BNP)
- N-terminal pro BNP (NT-pro-BNP)
- Troponin
- Myoglobin
- Ischemia-Modified Albumin (IMA)

Complete blood count (CBC)
Comprehensive metabolic panel (CMP)
Cystatin C
Platelet count
Hemoglobin (Hgb)
Hematocrit (Hct)
Electrolytes
Erythrocyte sedimentation rate (ESR)
Glomerular filtration rate (GFR)
Glucose
Glycosylated hemoglobin (HbA_1c)
Liver function
Prothrombin time (PT)
Partial thromboplastin time (PTT)
International normalized ratio (INR)
Serum lipids (lipid profile)
- Cholesterol
- High-density lipoprotein (HDL)
- Low-density lipoprotein (LDL)
- Very low-density lipoprotein (VLDL)
- Triglycerides

Thyroid stimulating hormone (TSH)
Urinalysis (UA)

Radiologic Tests
Chest x-ray
Cardiac positron emission tomography scan
Radionuclide angiography (multiplegated radioisotope scan, multigated acquisition scanning, MUGA)
Technetium pyrophosphate scanning
Thalium scan

Other Diagnostic Tests
Cardiac biopsy
Cardiac catheterization
Echocardiogram
Electrocardiogram (ECG)
Holter monitor
Magnetic resonance imaging (MRI)
Pericardiocentesis
Pulse oximetry
Stress test
Arterial plethysmography (pulse volume recorder)
Venous plethysmography (cuff pressure test)

Table 5-2 Cardiac Biomarkers Elevation Times

CARDIAC BIOMARKER	ONSET OF ELEVATION	DURATION OF ELEVATION AFTER INJURY
Troponin I	4–6 hours	4–7 days
Troponin T	4–6 hours	10–14 days
Creatine kinase-MB (CK-MB)	4–6 hours	48–72 hours
Myoglobin	Less than 3 hours (Myoglobin is not specific to the heart. However, it is the first biomarker to elevate.)	
Ischemia modified albumin (IMA)	Few minutes to a few hours	IMA is not as valuable with a client who has experienced chest pain for several hours because the IMA level may have risen and returned to normal within that time frame.

ventricles contracting. The Q wave is not always present on the ECG strip.

The pause after the QRS complex is called the ST segment. This represents the period between the contraction and the beginning of the recovery or repolarization of the ventricular muscles. The T wave represents the repolarization of the ventricles.

After the repolarization of the ventricles, the entire cycle begins again at the SA node. In this way the P wave, QRS complex, and T waves are repeated with each

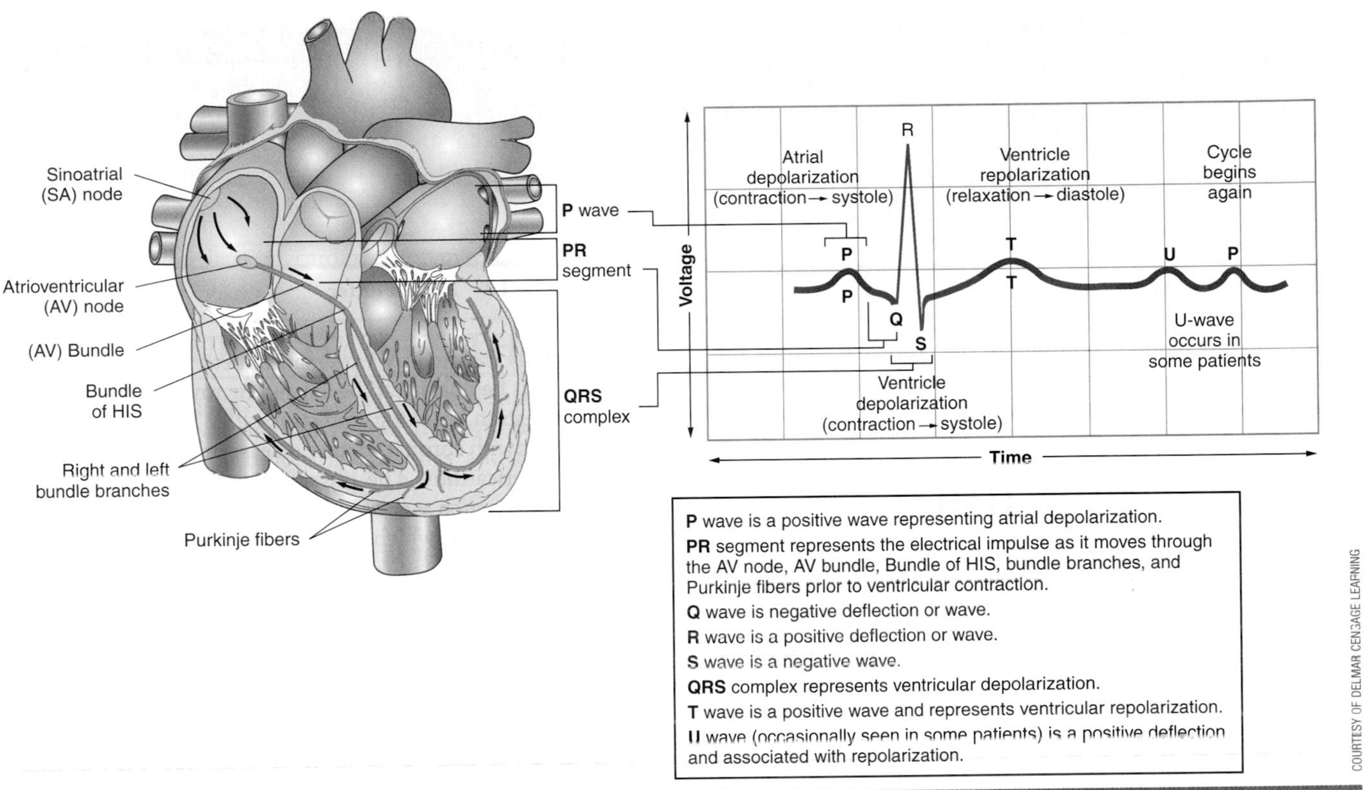
Sinoatrial (SA) node
Atrioventricular (AV) node
(AV) Bundle
Bundle of HIS
Right and left bundle branches
Purkinje fibers
P wave
PR segment
QRS complex
Voltage
Atrial depolarization (contraction → systole)
R
Ventricle repolarization (relaxation → diastole)
Cycle begins again
P
T
U
Q
S
U-wave occurs in some patients
Ventricle depolarization (contraction → systole)
Time
P wave is a positive wave representing atrial depolarization.
PR segment represents the electrical impulse as it moves through the AV node, AV bundle, Bundle of HIS, bundle branches, and Purkinje fibers prior to ventricular contraction.
Q wave is negative deflection or wave.
R wave is a positive deflection or wave.
S wave is a negative wave.
QRS complex represents ventricular depolarization.
T wave is a positive wave and represents ventricular repolarization.
U wave (occasionally seen in some patients) is a positive deflection and associated with repolarization.
COURTESY OF DELMAR CENGAGE LEARNING

FIGURE 5-7 Relationship of the Conduction System to an ECG Strip

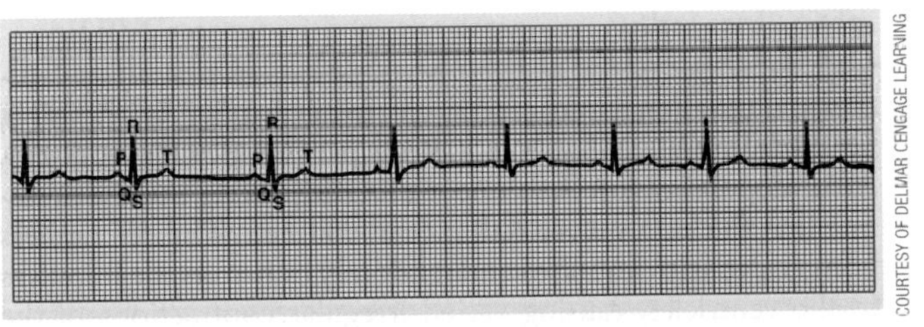
COURTESY OF DELMAR CENGAGE LEARNING

FIGURE 5-8 An ECG Strip Showing a Normal Sinus Rhythm with the P Wave, QRS Complex, and T Wave Identified

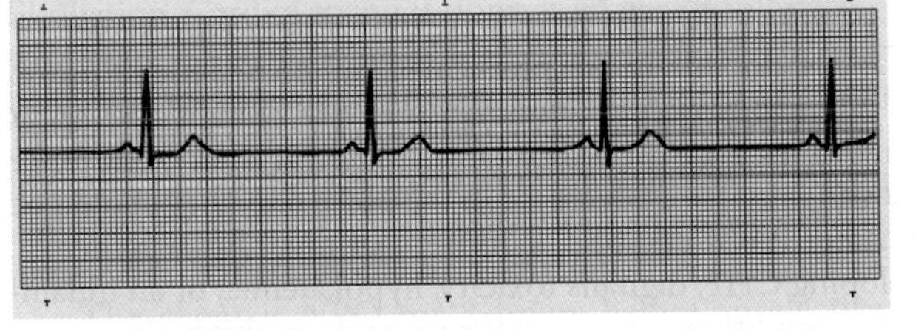
COURTESY OF DELMAR CENGAGE LEARNING

FIGURE 5-9 Sinus Bradycardia

heartbeat. Figure 5-8 shows an ECG strip of normal sinus rhythm.

DYSRHYTHMIAS

A **dysrhythmia** is an irregularity in the rate, rhythm, or conduction of the electrical system of the heart. Dysrhythmia can occur in the atria, ventricles, or any part of the conduction system. Specialized cells in the heart muscle have the ability to generate an electrical impulse. Under certain conditions these cells start sending impulses to other cells in the heart, causing irregular beats called *ectopic beats*. The most common causes of dysrhythmias are coronary artery disease (CAD), CHF, and myocardial infarction (MI). Other causes of dysrhythmias are electrolyte imbalances and drug toxicity.

Symptoms of a client experiencing a dysrhythmia vary from asymptomatic to cardiac arrest. The client experiences fainting, seizures, fatigue, decreased energy level, exertional dyspnea, chest pain, and palpitations.

BRADYCARDIA

Sinus bradycardia is a HR of 60 beats per minute or less (Figure 5-9). Causes of sinus bradycardia are myocardial ischemia, electrolyte imbalances, vagal stimulation, beta blockers, heart block, drug toxicity, intracranial tumors, sleep, and vomiting. The treatment for bradycardia is the administration of atropine. Some clients with bradycardia may require a permanent pacemaker. Asymptomatic bradycardia related to physical fitness is usually not treated.

TACHYCARDIA

Tachycardia is a sinus rhythm with a HR ranging from 100 to 150 beats per minute (Figure 5-10, following page). Causes of tachycardia are exercise, emotional stress, fever, medications, pain, anemia, thyrotoxicosis, pericarditis, HF, excessive caffeine intake, and tobacco use. When the heart is beating at this rate, there is limited time for the ventricles to fill with

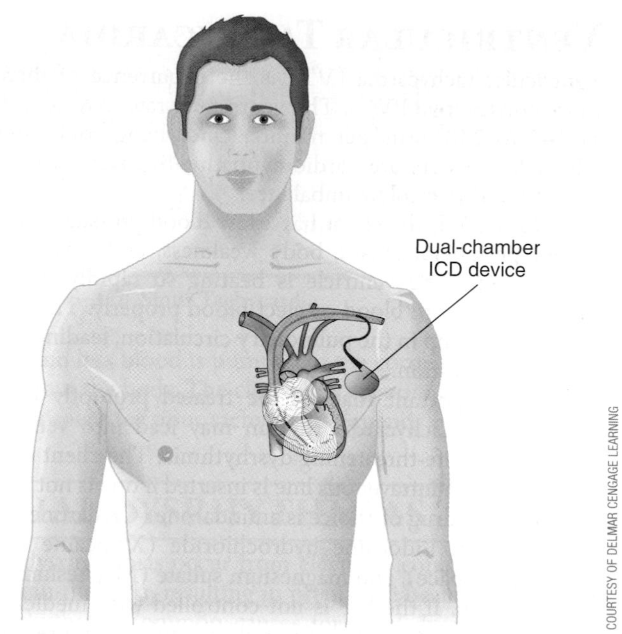

FIGURE 5-14 An Implantable Cardiovert-Defibrillator: A dual-chamber ICD device with a pulse generator is implanted below the collarbone and endocardial leads positioned in the heart through a vein.

electrical shock may be delivered in an attempt to convert the rhythm.

If conservative measures do not control the VT and the client has periodic episodes of VT, an **implantable cardioverter-defibrillator (ICD)** is implanted in the client (Figure 5-14). This device senses the dysrhythmia and automatically sends an electrical shock directly to the heart to defibrillate it.

Most ICDs have 1–3 endocardial leads that are guided through a vein into the right side of the heart where they become embedded into the heart tissue. The pulse generator is placed under the skin below the collarbone. The ICD detects VT and ventricular fibrillation (VF) through the leads attached to the heart muscle. Once VT or VF is detected, an electrical shock is sent from the pulse generator. The ICD is capable of delivering three more shocks to the heart muscle if the heart does not return to normal sinus rhythm (NSR). Usually, clients are converted to NSR with the first shock. Some ICDs also deliver cardiac resynchronization therapy (CRT) for clients with advanced HF. These devices have three leads; one lead is placed in the right atrium and one lead is placed in each of the ventricles. When this device functions as an ICD, it senses abnormal heart beats and delivers a shock to the heart to initiate a normal rhythm. When functioning as a CRT, it coordinates the beating of the ventricles so they effectively work together and pump blood throughout the body (FDA, 2002). Some ICDs also function as a pacemaker and an ICD; delivering shocks as needed to correct abnormal rhythms but also initiating heartbeats when the heartbeat is too slow. Another ICD, called antitachycardia pacing (ATP), sends a fast impulse to correct the rhythm after an ICD shock and detects and treats rapid atrial heartbeats (Stanford Hospital and Clinics, 2009; FDA, 2002). ICDs store the client's dysrhythmic activity and allow the health care practitioner to test the electrophysiologic activity noninvasively (AHA, 2007).

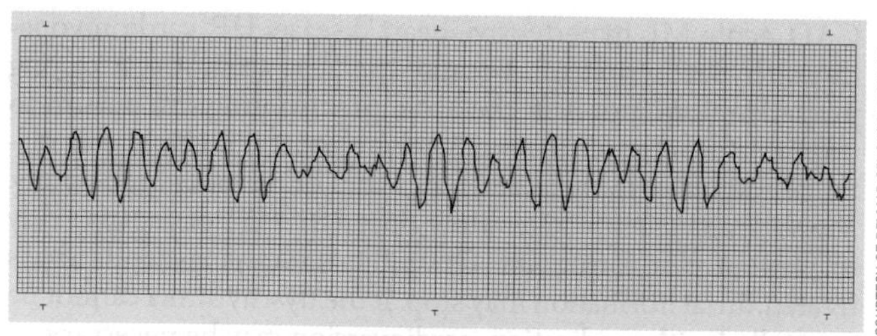

FIGURE 5-15 Ventricular Fibrillation (VF)

Complications after the insertion of an ICD are atelectasis, pneumonia, pneumothorax, thrombus, and a seroma at the generator site (a swelling from serum collecting around the device that initiates the shock). According to Shaffer (2002), anger and depression are common, expected side effects.

VENTRICULAR FIBRILLATION

The most common cause for VF is CAD. VF is a disorganized, chaotic quivering of the ventricles. The ventricles are unable to contract, and no blood is ejected into the circulatory system. The ECG reading is a series of jagged, unidentifiable waves (Figure 5-15). The client will not have a pulse, blood pressure, or respirations. This dysrhythmia is serious. Aggressive measures must be taken to initiate CPR and defibrillate the client immediately.

VENTRICULAR ASYSTOLE

Ventricular asystole is represented by a P wave or a straight line on the ECG (Figure 5-16). The ventricles are not contracting, and the client is in cardiac arrest. The client loses consciousness and has no pulse or respirations. Aggressive treatment should be initiated within 1 minute to prevent chemical changes within the body that jeopardize recovery. CPR is started, and the client is defibrillated. Atropine sulfate and epinephrine are given intravenously.

ATRIOVENTRICULAR BLOCKS

In atrioventricular blocks, the electrical conduction is interrupted to some degree between the atria and ventricles at the AV node. The extent of interruption is classified as first degree, second degree, or third degree.

FIRST-DEGREE AV BLOCK

In first-degree block, the impulse is delayed in traveling through the AV node. The impulse eventually reaches the

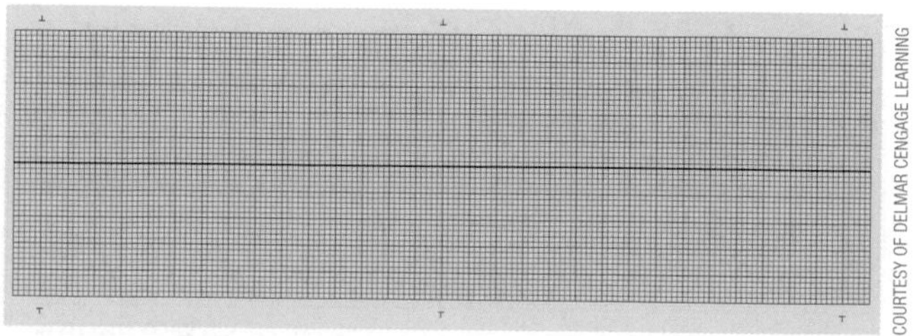

FIGURE 5-16 Asystole

ventricles but is delayed. There are no physical symptoms or treatment for first-degree block.

Second-Degree AV Block

In second-degree block, some of the impulses pass through the AV node to the ventricles and others are blocked. Symptoms include irregular pulse, vertigo, and weakness. A temporary pacemaker may be inserted until the conduction pattern is stabilized. If the dysrhythmia persists, a permanent pacemaker may be implanted. When the impulse is blocked, the ECG reveals an extended PR interval that is not followed by a QRS complex.

Third-Degree AV Block

Third-degree heart block is when no impulses are able to pass from the atria through the AV node to the ventricles. The atria and ventricles beat independently of each other. The causes of third-degree block are myocardial ischemia, drug toxicity, and electrolyte imbalances. Atropine sulfate may be given to improve conduction through the AV node. A permanent pacemaker is usually required to control the dysrhythmia.

A pacemaker is an electronic device that stimulates the heart to beat when the heartbeat is slow or drops below a set HR. It consists of one or two lead wires that are attached to the endocardium of the right atrium, right ventricle, or both, and a pulse generator that is "the 'brain' of the pacemaker" (Stanford Hospital and Clinics, 2009). The electrodes sense the heart's electrical activity and relay the information to the pulse generator. The purpose of the pacemaker is to regulate the HR and increase CO. When the heart beats slower than the programmed rate, an electrical impulse is sent to the lead that causes the heart to beat faster. Pacemakers are used for bradycardia, tachycardia, myocardial infarction, and heart block.

Some pacemakers have leads in the atrium, ventricle, or both to sense electrical activity and set the beating pace of one or both chambers. Sometimes in CHF the ventricles do not pump effectively together, decreasing the amount of blood pumped throughout the body. A biventricular pacemaker paces the ventricles together increasing the pumping effectiveness of the ventricles. The pacing of a biventricular pacemaker is called *cardiac resynchronization therapy* because it puts the ventricles back in synch.

A pacemaker is used either temporarily or permanently. A temporary pacemaker is used until a client's condition improves or until a permanent pacemaker is inserted. With a temporary pacemaker, the pulse generator remains outside of the body. The permanent pacemaker has a lead wire threaded through a vein to the heart and the pulse generator is implanted subcutaneously under the collarbone. An ECG of a client with a pacemaker shows the impulse from the pulse generator by a pacemaker spike, a vertical line before each QRS on the ECG strip.

Before discharge, teach clients to take accurate apical and radial pulses. Inform clients to report dizziness, fainting, or fever. Clients are taught to have regular pacemaker checks or transtelephonic monitoring in which an ECG strip is sent by phone to a designated hospital or physician's office.

SAFETY

Safety: Pacemaker and ICD

Encourage the client to carry an ID card and wear a medical identification tag indicating the presence of a pacemaker or ICD.

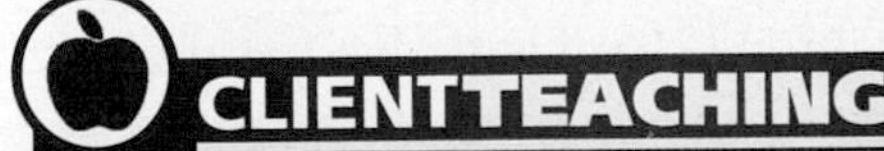

Pacemaker

- High-tension wires, high-voltage electrical generators, or MRIs may cause pacemaker malfunction.
- Avoid contact sports.
- Pacemakers may activate airport security alarms.

Medical–Surgical Management

Pharmacological

Dysrhythmias originating in the atria are treated with amiodarone (Cardarone), diltiazem hydrochloride (Cardizem, Dilacor, Tiazac), and digitalis (Digoxin). Dysrhythmias originating in the ventricles are treated with amiodarone (Cardarone), lidocaine hydrochloride (Xylocaine HCL), and magnesium sulfate.

Diet

The client is usually placed on a low-fat, low-cholesterol diet. Caffeine consumption is restricted.

Nursing Management

Monitor vital signs including apical pulse. Provide rest periods throughout the day. Explain all procedures and treatments. Encourage client to verbalize concerns about condition and potential complications. Teach relaxation methods.

NURSING PROCESS

Assessment

Subjective Data

Inquire if the client has experienced palpitations, lightheadedness, nausea, dyspnea, anxiety, fatigue, or chest discomfort.

Objective Data

If a client is experiencing dysrhythmias, check the HR, blood pressure, and respirations. While listening to the apical pulse and respirations, note abnormal heart sounds and monitor breath sounds for crackles. Crackles indicate the lungs are filling with fluid. Observe the skin for pallor and cyanosis, especially during and after activity/exercise. Urine output may decrease.

Nursing diagnoses for a client with dysrhythmias include the following:

NURSING DIAGNOSES	PLANNING/OUTCOMES	NURSING INTERVENTIONS
*Decreased **C**ardiac **O**utput* related to inadequate electrical conduction	The client will have increased CO.	Apply electrodes for telemetry monitoring. Balance activity with rest periods, and monitor vital signs during activity and at rest. Listen to the apical pulse, especially noting rate and rhythm. Elevate the extremities so they are not in a dependent position.
***A**nxiety* related to fear of potential diagnosis, treatment regimen, and death	The client will relate fears of potential cardiac problems.	Care for the client in a calm, confident, and efficient manner. Remain with the client and explain procedures and treatments. Encourage client input regarding the care. Encourage the client to verbalize concerns about the dysrhythmia and potential future complications. Teach the client relaxation activities.
*Deficient **K**nowledge* related to electrical conduction of the heart and treatment methods	The client will describe electrical disorder and treatment methods.	Explain medication administration times, action, side effects, and symptoms that need reporting. Provide written instructions to the client and family. Explain symptoms of dysrhythmias such as fatigue, edema, palpitations, lightheadedness, nausea, dyspnea, and anxiety. If a pacemaker is needed, explain to client and family the purpose, insertion procedures, and home care.

Evaluation: Evaluate each outcome to determine how it has been met by the client.

INFLAMMATORY DISORDERS

Inflammatory disorders include rheumatic heart disease, infective endocarditis, myocarditis, pericarditis, and valvular heart disease.

RHEUMATIC HEART DISEASE

Rheumatic heart disease is a complication of rheumatic fever and is also linked to group A streptococcus after an upper respiratory infection. Rheumatic fever is a systemic inflammatory disease that occurs 2 to 3 weeks after an inadequately treated pharyngitis caused by group *A beta-hemolytic streptococcus*. Symptoms of rheumatic fever are a mild fever, polyarthritis, carditis, chorea, and a rash. The endocardium, myocardium, and epicardium can become inflamed, with the most damage occurring to the mitral valve. The mitral valve becomes incompetent because of thickening and stenosis of the valve leaflets. Mitral prolapse (valve leaflets flip back into the left atrium during systole) may result.

A person who had rheumatic fever is more likely to have a recurrence. It is treated with intravenous antibiotics, anti-inflammatory agents, corticosteroids, and strict bed rest. The main goal is to treat the inflammation, prevent cardiac complications, and prevent the recurrence of the disease. These clients are placed on prophylactic antibiotic therapy before dental procedures or invasive surgery. Antibiotic therapy reduced the mortality from 15,000 in 1950 to 3,676 in 1999 (AHA, 2001c).

INFECTIVE ENDOCARDITIS

Infective endocarditis is an inflammation or infection of the inside lining of the heart, particularly the heart valves. The etiology of inflammatory endocarditis is a collagen-vascular disease or rheumatic fever. Infective endocarditis is caused by bacteria, fungi, or virus. As the microorganisms invade the valves, they form fibrinous substances called *vegetations*. The vegetations cause scar tissue on the valves resulting in hard, brittle valves that do not close properly and allow blood to flow back into the previous chamber. The valve is said to be insufficient. Sometimes the vegetations cause the valve flaps to grow together, resulting in a narrowing of the opening. This is called a *valvular stenosis*. The mitral valve is more frequently affected than any other. When the mitral valve is affected, it is termed *mitral insufficiency* or *mitral stenosis*.

Historically, rheumatic fever was the common cause of endocarditis. Clients at risk for endocarditis are individuals that use IV drugs, are immunosuppressed, have dental caries and abscesses, and a history of valvular heart disease. Goldrick (2003) reports that endocarditis is associated with body piercing.

There are two forms of endocarditis: acute and subacute. Symptoms of acute endocarditis are tachycardia, pallor, diaphoresis, and symptoms of a systemic infection, such as temperature of 103°F and shaking chills. Clients with subacute endocarditis have low-grade fever, malaise, weight loss, and anemia. Clients with both types may have murmurs and symptoms of CHF, such as dyspnea, peripheral edema, and pulmonary congestion.

Endocarditis is diagnosed by the client's history and symptoms. **Transesophageal echocardiography (TEE)** can confirm the diagnosis by ultrasonic imaging of the cardiac structures through the esophagus. The erythrocyte sedimentation rate (ESR) and WBC are elevated. A blood culture and sensitivity is done to determine the causative organism and the most effective antibiotic.

Medical–Surgical Management

Surgical

Surgical repair or replacement of a valve is done in severe cases.

Pharmacological

Clients are treated with antimicrobial drugs (endocarditis) and intravenous antibiotics. The antibiotics are usually continued for 2 to 6 weeks. The most commonly used antibiotics are penicillin V potassium (V-Cillin K), vancomycin hydrochloride (Vancocin), and gentamicin sulfate (Garamycin).

Diet

Provide the client with a well-balanced nutritious diet, with between-meal snacks.

Activity

The client is on bed rest to decrease the workload of the heart. Provide a calm, quiet environment.

Health Promotion

Clients who previously had endocarditis or have a mitral valve prolapse are more prone to develop endocarditis. They should take antibiotics prophylactically before having dental work and genitourinary or gastrointestinal invasive procedures. Amoxicillin trihydrate (Amoxil) 1 hour before the procedure and again after the procedure is the usual order.

Nursing Management

Administer oxygen as needed, and measure blood pressure and pulse before and after activity to monitor toleration. Note apical pulse rate and rhythm and assess breath sounds for adventitious sounds. Balance activity with rest periods. Monitor BUN and creatinine levels if a client is on vancomycin hydrochloride (Vancocin) or gentamicin sulfate (Garamycin) because both of these drugs are nephrotoxic.

MYOCARDITIS

Myocarditis is an inflammation of the myocardium of the heart. Lymphocytes and leukocytes invade the muscle fibers of the heart, causing the chambers to enlarge and the muscle to weaken. This can lead to CHF. Myocarditis is caused by bacteria, viruses, fungi, or parasites. It can also be an autoimmune reaction such as with rheumatic fever or lupus erythematosus. Usually the cause is a virus. Myocarditis is more prevalent in clients with AIDS.

Acute myocarditis presents with flulike symptoms of fever, pharyngitis, myalgias, and gastrointestinal complications. The client will also have chest pain and should be monitored for signs of CHF. A **pericardial friction rub** is often heard if the pericardium becomes involved. The friction rub is a "squeaky" sound heard through the stethoscope when the two inflamed pericardial surfaces rub together with the contraction of the heart.

Myocarditis diagnostic symptoms are nonspecific. They include elevated ESR and elevated LDH, CK, and SGOT levels. The diagnosis of myocarditis can be confirmed with an endomyocardial biopsy.

Medical–Surgical Management

Pharmacological

Digitalis preparations are given to try to prevent CHF. Broad-spectrum antibiotics are also given to treat the infection. Anti-inflammatory agents may be given to reduce the inflammation. Oxygen is administered as needed.

Activity

The client is placed on bed rest to decrease the workload of the heart.

Nursing Management

Monitor the client for symptoms of CHF or pericarditis. Place the client in a semi-Fowler's position to assist with breathing. Provide a quiet environment and frequent rest periods. Apply a pulse oximeter to monitor oxygen saturation.

PERICARDITIS

When the membranous sac surrounding the heart becomes inflamed, the condition is called **pericarditis**. Causative organisms are viral, bacterial, fungal, or parasitic. Inflammation can also occur from rheumatic or collagen-vascular conditions such as systemic lupus erythematosus. The most common cause of pericarditis is idiopathic, meaning no known cause. Symptoms of pericarditis are severe precordial pain (pain on the anterior surface of the chest over the heart) and a pericardial friction rub. The pain may radiate to the neck, back, or abdomen and become worse when the client coughs or lies on the left side. If the client sits erect and leans forward, the pain is relieved. Pericardial effusion (excess fluid in pericardial space) may develop. **Cardiac tamponade** will result if the fluid rapidly increases and hinders the functioning of the ventricle. The S_1 and S_2 sounds are often muffled and hard to hear because of fluid accumulation.

With inflammation, scar tissue develops in the pericardial sac. Heart movement is limited by the scar tissue and cardiac failure results.

Medical–Surgical Management

Medical

The physician performs a **pericardiocentesis** to aspirate the excess fluid from the pericardial sac. A needle is inserted through the chest wall into the pericardial space.

Surgical

If fibrotic scar tissue in the pericardium hinders heart performance, a pericardiectomy or pericardial window is done. Pericardiectomy is removal of the pericardium. When a pericardial window is done, a section of the parietal pericardium is cut and tacked back onto itself, allowing fluid to escape from the pericardial sac.

Pharmacological

Clients are given antipyretics, analgesics, and anti-inflammatory agents. The infection is combated with antibiotics. A digitalis preparation and diuretic are given to improve the pumping action of the heart and decrease fluid retention.

Nursing Management

Assess the client's apical pulse and blood pressure and monitor the ECG for dysrhythmias. Assess for signs of cardiac tamponade such as decreased pulse and blood pressure, muffled heart sounds, increased respirations, restlessness, and oliguria. Administer oxygen as needed, and assist the client to a position of comfort. Administer analgesics, antibiotics, and anti-inflammatory agents as ordered and monitor the client's responses. Encourage the client to verbalize concerns and fears.

VALVULAR HEART DISEASES

Valvular heart disease occurs when the valves do not open and close properly. When the valve does not close completely, blood leaks back into the chamber from which it was pumped. This is called regurgitation. The client with valvular heart disease often has a history of rheumatic fever.

STENOSIS AND INSUFFICIENCY

The definitions, symptoms, diagnostic findings, medical–surgical management, and nursing interventions for mitral and aortic valve conditions are covered in Table 5-3.

MITRAL VALVE PROLAPSE

Mitral insufficiency can lead to mitral valve prolapse in which the valve leaflets, chordae tendineae, and papillary muscle become damaged. The valve leaflets flip back into the left atrium when the left ventricle contracts. This condition affects more women than men. Often the client remains asymptomatic. The symptoms that a client may experience depend on how seriously the mitral valve is affected. Sometimes clients experience palpitations and fatigue caused by decreased CO. They also may experience angina, dizziness, and syncope. Some clients have panic attacks. Often a click or murmur is heard.

Medical–Surgical Management

Medical

Clients with valvular heart disease are to take antibiotics prophylactically before any dental procedures and genitourinary or gastrointestinal invasive procedures.

Table 5-3 Mitral and Aortic Valve Stenosis and Insufficiency

VALVE CONDITION	DEFINITION	SYMPTOMS	DIAGNOSTIC FINDINGS	MEDICAL-SURGICAL MANAGEMENT	NURSING INTERVENTIONS
Mitral stenosis	The diseased valve becomes narrowed and the leaflets thickened, preventing blood from freely flowing from the left atrium into the left ventricle.	Gradual onset of symptoms: exertional dyspnea, fatigue, orthopnea, paroxysmal nocturnal dyspnea, murmur. **Later symptoms:** peripheral edema, atrial fibrillation, jugular venous distention, hepatomegaly, abdominal distention, hypotension, thrombus from blood pooling in the left atrium.	**Chest x-ray:** hypertrophy and enlargement of left atrium and right ventricle. **ECG:** atrial fibrillation. **Echocardiogram:** fusion of valve leaflets, enlarged left atrium, decreased blood flow through valve.	**Medical management:** diuretics, digitalis, anticoagulants, antidysrhythmics, prophylactic antibiotics for invasive procedures, low-sodium diet, semi-Fowler's position, activity restrictions as needed. **Surgical management:** commissurotomy, percutaneous balloon mitral valvuloplasty, mitral valve replacement.	Encourage rest periods, administer oxygen, elevate head of bed, reposition frequently to decrease pressure points, elevate legs, low-sodium diet, monitor for signs of right and left-sided HF, teach stress reduction techniques, daily weight.

Table 5-3 Mitral and Aortic Valve Stenosis and Insufficiency (Continued)

VALVE CONDITION	DEFINITION	SYMPTOMS	DIAGNOSTIC FINDINGS	MEDICAL-SURGICAL MANAGEMENT	NURSING INTERVENTIONS
Mitral insufficiency	The valve leaflets become hard and do not close completely. Blood backs up in both the left atria and ventricle, causing both chambers to hypertrophy.	Gradual onset of symptoms: exertional dyspnea, palpitations, fatigue, atrial fibrillation, loud murmur and gallop.	**Chest x-ray:** hypertrophy and enlargement of left atrium and left ventricle. **ECG:** atrial fibrillation.	**Medical management:** same as mitral stenosis. **Surgical management:** valvuloplasty, mitral valve replacement.	Same as mitral stenosis, teach exercise modification.
Aortic stenosis	The valve cusps become hard and calcify due to rheumatic fever, syphilis, a congenital anomaly, or the aging process.	Syncope, exertional dyspnea, arrhythmias, angina, murmur, and gallop; sudden death may occur. **Later symptoms as the disease progresses:** paroxysmal atrial tachycardia, orthopnea.	**Chest x-ray:** enlargement of left ventricle, calcification of aortic valve. **ECG:** hypertrophy of left ventricle inverted T wave echocardiogram fusion of valve leaflets, regurgitation.	**Medical management:** same as mitral stenosis. **Surgical management:** percutaneous balloon aortic valvuloplasty, aortic valve replacement.	Same as mitral stenosis.
Aortic insufficiency	The valve cusps become so hardened they do not close completely. The blood no longer flows through the aorta but backs up into the left ventricle.	Palpitations, chest pain, exertional dyspnea, nocturnal angina, dizziness, fatigue, decreased activity, intolerance, paroxysmal nocturnal dyspnea, visible pulsation of the neck veins, murmur, lung congestion.	**Chest x-ray:** hypertrophy and enlargement of left ventricle.	**Medical management:** same as mitral stenosis. **Surgical management:** aortic valve replacement.	Same as mitral stenosis, teach exercise modification.

Surgical

When the activities of a client with valvular heart disease become curtailed because of decreased CO and the symptoms can no longer be controlled by medical means, surgery is performed. The type of surgery performed will depend on the client's overall condition and on the involved valve.

For the mitral valve, surgery alleviates the symptoms, but it does not cure the condition. Surgeries frequently have to be repeated. A commissurotomy is done for mitral stenosis, which surgically separates the valve leaflets. For mitral regurgitation or insufficiency, a valvuloplasty is becoming the treatment of choice. A percutaneous mitral valvuloplasty is a repair of perforated cusps or torn chordae tendineae. The risk of a thrombus is less with valvuloplasty than with grafts or prosthetic valves. An annuloplasty, a repair of an **annulus** or valvular ring, can also be done (see Figure 5-17A). The annulus is tightened with a purse-string suture or an annular ring. The mitral valve is replaced when other repair measures are not feasible.

The aortic valve is not repaired, only replaced, if the symptoms cannot be controlled by medical means. The preferred treatment for a client with an aortic stenosis is percutaneous aortic valvuloplasty. This treatment is often used in elderly or high risk surgical clients. A catheter is advanced to the affected valve and a balloon is inflated in the stenosed valve. The narrowed valvular space is expanded by the balloon, leaving a wider opening. Later, large balloons may be used to expand the opening as needed.

Mitral and tricuspid valves are now repaired or replaced with robotically-assisted closed-chest heart surgery. Cardiac surgeons perform these minimally invasive valve surgeries with a robot. Some valves are still repaired and replaced with the open chest method, but there are several advantages to robotically assisted surgery. They require smaller incisions with minimal scarring. The client experiences less trauma,

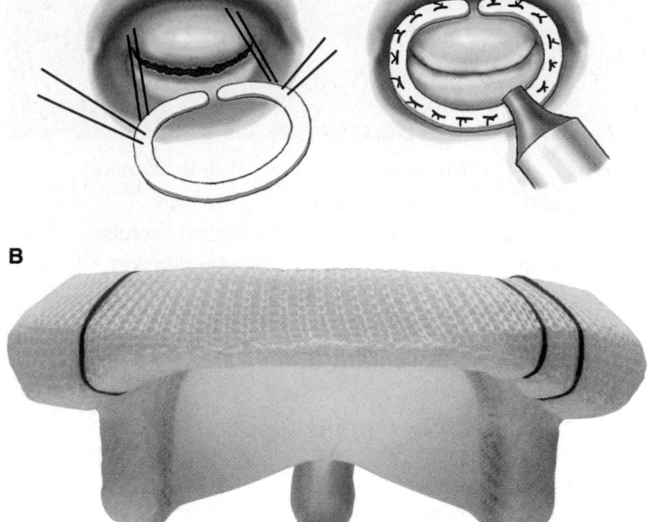

FIGURE 5-17 ***A,*** Annuloplasty ***B,*** Carpentier-Edwards Perimount Mitral Pericardial Bioprosthesis (*Image A courtesy of Delmar Cengage Learning; image B courtesy of Edwards LifeScience.*)

pain, and bleeding. Clients have a decreased need for pain medication and a decreased risk of infection. The hospital stay is shorter than open heart surgery and the recovery is quicker, with a prompt return to daily activities.

There are two types of replacement valves: mechanical and biological. The mechanical valve is the caged-ball valve (Figure 5-17B). There is a greater risk of a thromboembolism with a caged-ball valve. Clients remain on anticoagulant therapy with both types of valves. The biological valves come from calves, pigs, or humans. The disadvantage of the biological valves is tissue degeneration and calcification of the valve. Carpentier-Edwards produced the first biomechanical valve that consists of a mechanical device and natural tissue.

Nursing Management

Assess for dyspnea, fatigue, palpitations, lightheadedness, cough, and numbness and tingling in the extremities. Provide rest periods during the day. Encourage smokers to stop. Refer client and family to dietitian for information on low-sodium diets. Encourage client's input regarding care decisions.

NURSING PROCESS

Assessment

Subjective Data

Review past medical history for conditions such as rheumatic fever or streptococcal infections. Document if the client has experienced any dyspnea, palpitations, fatigue, cough, lightheadedness, or numbness and tingling in the extremities.

Objective Data

Take the vital signs and listen to the apical pulse for rate, rhythm, murmurs, and S_3 sound. Auscultate breath sounds for adventitious sounds. Note edema, jugular distention, cyanosis, and equality of peripheral pulses. Test for Homans' sign because dysrhythmias may produce clots.

Nursing diagnoses for a client with cardiac valvular disorders include the following:

NURSING DIAGNOSES	PLANNING/OUTCOMES	NURSING INTERVENTIONS
Decreased ***Cardiac*** *Output* related to structural changes in valves	The client will have increased CO.	Administer oxygen as needed. Help the client balance activities with rest periods. The pulse should return to the baseline within 10 minutes of activity; if not, activity has been excessive. Discourage smoking and refer clients to support groups to assist them to stop smoking.
Excess ***Fluid*** *Volume* related to decreased CO	The client will have a decrease in edema.	Administer diuretics as needed. Support extremities so they are not in a dependent position. Encourage the client to maintain a low-sodium diet.
Anxiety related to threat to or change in health status	The client will list ways to cope with stressors.	Calmly explain the procedures before doing them. Encourage the client's input to decisions regarding care. Assist the client and the client's family in identifying ways to cope with stressors. Teach relaxation techniques.

Nursing diagnoses for a client with cardiac valvular disorders include the following: (Continued)

NURSING DIAGNOSES	PLANNING/OUTCOMES	NURSING INTERVENTIONS
Deficient Knowledge related to disease process and treatment	The client will relate the disease process and needed self-care management.	Explain the valvular disease process, medication actions, dosage times, and medication side effects to report. Refer the client and family members to the dietitian for low-sodium diet instructions. Encourage the client to begin an appropriate exercise program.

Evaluation: Evaluate each outcome to determine how it has been met by the client.

OCCLUSIVE DISORDERS

Occlusive disorders include arteriosclerosis, angina pectoris, and myocardial infarction.

ARTERIOSCLEROSIS

Arteriosclerosis is a narrowing and hardening of arteries. A buildup of lipids, collagen, and smooth muscle cells narrows the lumen of the vessel. Decreased blood flow through the vessel causes decreased perfusion to cells beyond the narrowed or hardened area.

There are three types of arteriosclerosis: atherosclerosis, calcific sclerosis, and arteriolar sclerosis. **Atherosclerosis** is fatty deposits on the inner lining of vessel walls. The fat deposit is called *plaque*. In calcific sclerosis, calcium deposits are on the middle layer of the wall of the arteries. Hypertension causes a thickening of the arterioles and is called *arteriolar sclerosis*. With these conditions, vessels lose their elasticity, resulting in various conditions, such as arteriosclerotic heart disease, angina, myocardial infarction, stroke, and peripheral vascular disease.

ANGINA PECTORIS

When coronary arteries lose elasticity or become narrow as a result of plaque collection, the heart muscle receives less blood and oxygen. Physical exertion, emotional stress, smoking, exposure to extreme cold, heavy meals, or an arterial spasm may cause a temporary inadequate blood and oxygen supply to the heart. Myocardial ischemia and angina pectoris result. Myocardial ischemia is a temporary inadequate blood and oxygen supply to the myocardial tissues. When this temporary condition occurs, the person experiences chest pain or **angina pectoris.**

At first, the person may experience a squeezing pain under the sternum, which radiates to the left shoulder. For some, the pain may radiate to the right shoulder, jaw, or ear. The discomfort may vary from mild discomfort to immobilizing pain. Anginal attacks usually increase in frequency and severity over time. The severity of the condition depends on the development of collateral circulation.

Collateral circulation develops as larger vessels gradually narrow or harden. Blood that normally passes through the larger vessels is shunted into surrounding smaller vessels. These vessels enlarge in an attempt to supply blood to the affected area. Collateral circulation increases the blood supply to tissues with an inadequate blood supply.

Many people experiencing ischemic attacks do not experience angina. This is called silent myocardial infarct or ischemia. Symptoms are chest pressure or heaviness, restlessness, shortness of breath with increased respiratory rate, a sensation of epigastric fullness with noisy belching, numbness or tingling in both arms or shoulders, physical or mental fatigue, and dizziness. The person may also experience a change in sleep patterns and mental alertness. The person states that he or she "feels funny." Clients that are more likely to experience a silent myocardial infarction are women, older adults, and individuals with diabetes or a history of HF (Overbaugh, 2009).

Two other types of angina are unstable angina and Prinzmetal's angina. Unstable angina occurs at rest or with minimal exertion and is not relieved with nitroglycerin. The client is more susceptible to myocardial infarction and sudden death. Prinzmetal's angina is caused by a coronary artery spasm and occurs at rest.

There is a high incidence of angina pectoris in clients with hypertension and diabetes mellitus. The diagnosis of angina is made after reviewing the client's history, lifestyle, laboratory tests, and stress test. A lipid profile (cholesterol, HDL, LDL, and triglycerides), hs-CRP, and lipoprotein A [Lp(a)] are evaluated. Angina pectoris is diagnosed by a stress test, thallium scan, or a coronary arteriogram.

MEDICAL–SURGICAL MANAGEMENT

Medical

Treatment for angina includes measures to increase the blood supply to the affected area. Clients are administered 162 to 325 mg of chewed or crushed aspirin by mouth because it prevents platelet aggregation and vasoconstriction. Oxygen is given at 2 to 4 L/min per nasal cannula to maintain the SaO_2 >90%. Nitroglycerin tablets 0.3 to 0.4 mg are given sublingually every 5 minutes up to 3 doses because it is a vasodilator and increases the oxygen supply to the myocardium. If the pain is not relieved with the nitroglycerin, morphine sulfate 2 to 4 mg IV push is administered because it is a vasodilator and analgesic. The morphine dose can be repeated every 5 to 15 minutes until the pain is under control. The nurse should closely monitor the BP, respirations, and SaO_2 because the side effects

MEMORYTRICK

MONA for Anginal Pain

M = Morphine sulfate 2 to 4 mg IV push
O = Oxygen 2 to 4 L/min per nasal cannula to maintain SaO_2 above 90%
N = Nitroglycerin tablets 0.3 to 0.4 mg sublingually every 5 minutes up to 3 doses
A = Aspirin 162 to 325 mg by mouth (chewed or crushed)
(Overbaugh, 2009)

of morphine are hypotension and respiratory depression. A mnemonic to recall the treatment of angina is MONA (see Memory Trick: MONA). Even though the letters are not in the order of administration, it helps the nurse recall the treatment for angina (Overbaugh, 2009).

Silent ischemia is treated in the same way symptomatic ischemia is treated. The client needs to be educated about cardiac risk factors, the importance of following the prescribed medical regimen, and maintaining regular physical checkups.

Surgical

A percutaneous transluminal coronary angioplasty (PTCA) may be done if only one coronary artery is involved and if the atherosclerotic material is small and has not hardened. When a PTCA is done, atherosclerotic matter is pressed against the walls of the coronary vessels to improve circulation to myocardial tissue supplied by that coronary artery (Figure 5-18). A guidewire is inserted to the stenosed area, and a special balloon-tipped catheter is placed in the narrowed sclerotic area. When the balloon is inflated, the atherosclerotic material is pressed against the wall of the vessel. The vessel, now open, allows more blood to flow to the myocardial tissue. During this procedure, a piece of the atherosclerotic material may break off and occlude the vessel. If this occurs, the client would have to undergo immediate coronary artery bypass graft (CABG) surgery. Other complications of the procedure are occlusion of the vessel because of a vascular spasm.

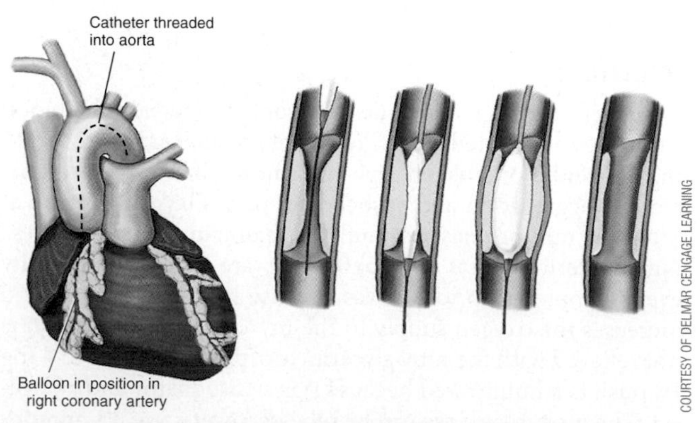

FIGURE 5-18 Demonstration of the Function of a Balloon-Tipped Catheter During a PTCA Procedure

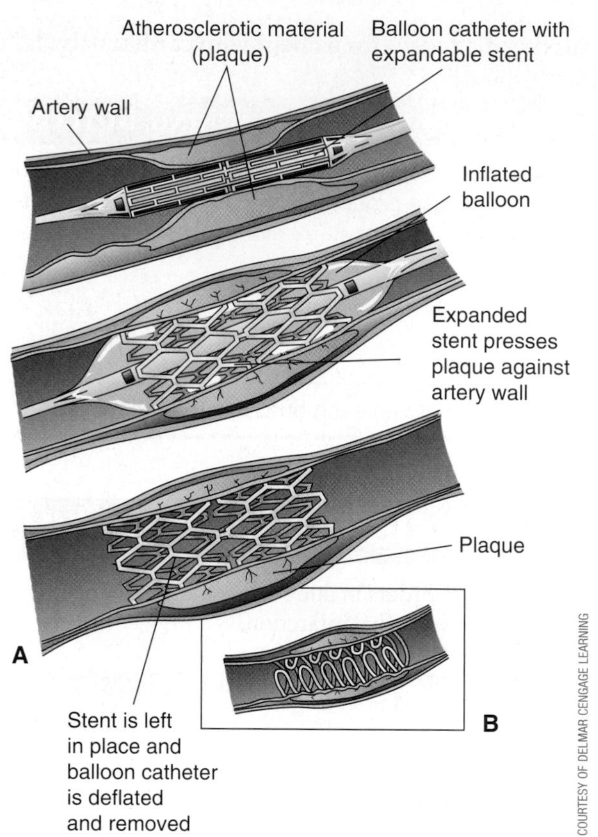

FIGURE 5-19 Placement of a Stent in a Coronary Artery; *A*, Palmaz-Schatz Stent; *B*, Gianturco-Roubin Ex-Stent

An intracoronary **stent** may be implanted into a stenosed vessel to prevent the vessel from collapsing and to keep the atherosclerotic plaque pressed against the vessel wall. A stent is a tiny metal tube with holes in it (Figure 5-19). The procedure is sometimes done when a vessel collapses after a PTCA or in place of a PTCA. The stent is tightly wrapped around a balloon catheter. When the balloon catheter has been threaded through a vessel to the stenosed area, the balloon is inflated and the stent expands and presses the plaque against the vessel wall. The stent remains in the vessel and the catheter is withdrawn.

If a CABG is performed, the internal mammary artery, the saphenous vein, or an accordion type of synthetic graft material is used. The vein or synthetic material is grafted to the aorta and passed beyond the obstruction in the coronary vessel (Figure 5-20). The graft provides an increased blood supply to the affected myocardium. The client then has less angina and an increased tolerance for activities.

A minimally invasive direct coronary artery bypass graft (MID CABG) surgery is now an option for clients whose surgeons use a left internal mammary artery to bypass an occlusion in the left anterior descending artery (see Figure 5-20B). With a MID CABG the client is not connected to a heart bypass machine and only small incisions (2–3 inches) are needed for the procedure. There is decreased risk of infection and the client experiences less bleeding and pain. The average recovery time is 2 to 4 weeks compared with 6 to 8 weeks with the traditional heart surgery.

Another recent advance in CABG surgery is Cardica's C-Port Flex-A System that completes the vessel anastomosis by arranging tiny, stainless steel staples attaching the bypass

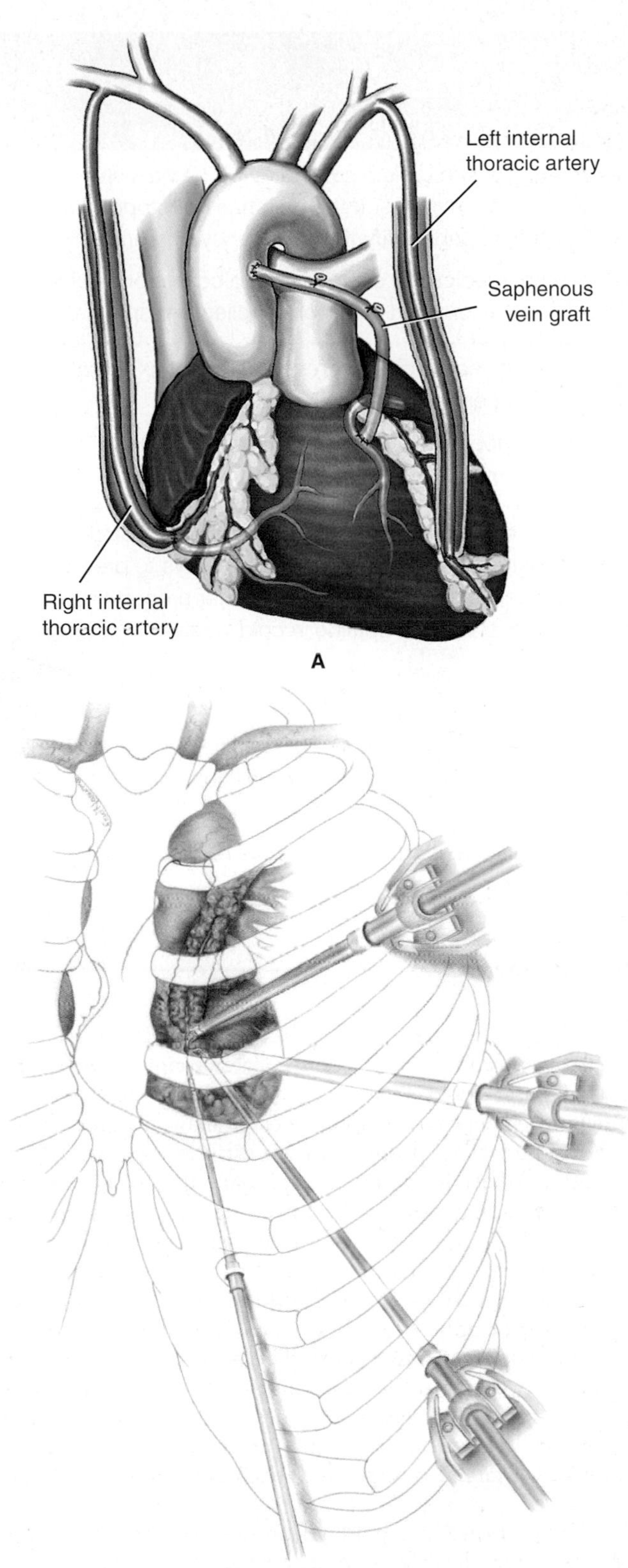

FIGURE 5-20 ***A*, Coronary Artery Bypass Graft (CABG) with the Saphenous Vein and Intern Mammary Vein; *B*, Robotic-assisted Surgery Completing a CABG (*Image A courtesy of Delmar Cengage Learning; image B courtesy of Intuitive Surgical, Inc. ©2005.*)**

vessel to the coronary artery. (To view the Cardica C-Port Flex-A System used in a robotic CABG or an animation of the C-Port Flex-A System, go to http://www.cardica.com.) The anastomosis is completed with robotic arms in a minimally invasive surgery while the heart is still beating. There is no need for a heart bypass machine or a sternotomy. This surgery has all the advantages of a minimally invasive surgery (Broadcast Newsroom, 2009).

Pharmacological

Vasodilators, such as nitroglycerin tablets, cause the blood vessels to dilate, providing an increased blood supply to tissues. The client may not need as much analgesic medication if beta blockers are given. Beta-adrenergic blockers and calcium channel blockers slow the HR and decrease the oxygen demand of the heart. Calcium channel blockers also dilate vessels and decrease spasms of the coronary vessels. All of these measures provide an increased blood supply to the myocardium.

Diet

The client is placed on a low-fat, low-cholesterol, sodium-restricted diet. Sodium restriction may vary from no salt to 4 grams daily depending on the ability of the client's kidneys to excrete excess sodium. An increase of fruits and vegetables is recommended in the diet.

Activity

Activity should be slower and for shorter periods of time with more rest periods.

Health Promotion

To prevent coronary artery disease from resulting in angina, it is recommended that a person limit fat intake to 30 grams or less per day and exercise 5 times per week for at least 30 minutes. Simple activities such as parking a car farther from an entrance to increase walking distance and taking stairs instead of an elevator improve circulation and help decrease cholesterol levels. Activities such as gardening or housework are also good.

NURSING MANAGEMENT

Assess pain and medicate client as ordered. Monitor vital signs. Emphasize taking rest periods. Encourage client to always carry nitroglycerin and to get regular exercise as recommended by the physician. Answer questions about the low-fat, low-cholesterol, sodium-restricted diet that is prescribed.

NURSING PROCESS

ASSESSMENT

Subjective Data

Ask the client to describe the pain regarding type, radiation, onset, duration, and precipitating factors.

Objective Data

Observe and document the client's actions during the anginal attack. Take vital signs and attach the client to an ECG monitor and observe for any dysrhythmias.

Nursing diagnoses for a client with angina include the following:

NURSING DIAGNOSES	PLANNING/OUTCOMES	NURSING INTERVENTIONS
*Acute **Pain*** related to decreased oxygen supply to the myocardium	The client will experience decreased episodes of angina.	Administer nitroglycerin tablets sublingually. The pain should be relieved within 1 to 2 minutes. If the pain has not stopped after 3 doses 5 minutes apart, notify the emergency personnel. Administer other medication such as beta blockers or calcium channel blockers as ordered and monitor client's response.
Anxiety related to perceived threat of death or change in lifestyle	The client will relate concerns and practice stress reduction techniques.	Assist the client in learning to decrease personal expectations and to live within personal activity limitations. Emphasize the importance of getting adequate rest and stopping before becoming too exhausted.
*Deficient **Knowledge*** related to disease process, medications, and treatment regimen	The client will explain the disease process, medication actions, dosage times and side effects, and self-care practices.	Explain the cause of angina. Teach the client to avoid stressful situations that may produce angina. Other ways to prevent angina are to sleep in a warm room, eat smaller proportions at mealtimes, and not exercise outside in cold weather. Inform the client to always carry nitroglycerin in a tightly closed container. Nitroglycerin may cause orthostatic hypotension, so inform the client to sit after taking it and to change position slowly after taking the medication. Encourage the client to start and maintain a regular exercise program as recommended by the physician.

Evaluation: Evaluate each outcome to determine how it has been met by the client.

MYOCARDIAL INFARCTION

In 2002, an estimated 1.1 million persons in the United States had an acute myocardial infarction (MI), and about 45% died. Half of those who died did so before arriving at a hospital (Nagle & Nee, 2002). The most common cause for myocardial infarction is atherosclerosis.

A **myocardial infarction** is caused by an obstruction in a coronary artery, resulting in necrosis (death) to the tissues supplied by the artery. The obstruction is usually caused by atherosclerotic plaque, a thrombus, or an embolism. The area most commonly affected is the left ventricle.

Obstruction of a large coronary artery damages the myocardial tissue and affects the pumping efficiency of the heart. A client's prognosis is better if a small coronary artery or arteriole is obstructed and there is good collateral circulation to the heart. If a large vessel is obstructed and the client does not have sufficient collateral circulation, the client may die immediately.

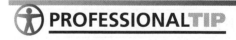

Risk Factors for Myocardial Infarction

- Overweight
- Cigarette smoking
- Hypertension
- Diabetes
- Family history of heart disease
- High cholesterol level
- High LDL

(Lab Tests Online, 2009)

The typical symptoms of men experiencing an MI are feelings of chest heaviness or tightness that progresses to a severe gripping pain in the lower sternal area. Pain also occurs in the arm, neck, back, or epigastric area and may or may not radiate to these areas. The pain is not relieved by rest or nitroglycerin, and the client becomes short of breath (dyspneic), diaphoretic, and anxious. The client frequently becomes nauseated and vomits. The pulse may be irregular, rapid, and weak, and the blood pressure is low. The skin is pale and then turns cyanotic. Even though a person may not experience the typical MI symptoms, the condition can still be serious or fatal. Complications such as HF and stroke may also occur.

Women experiencing an MI present with atypical symptoms that often delay an accurate diagnosis. Women are more likely to have upper abdominal pain, heartburn, nausea, dyspnea, fatigue, lethargy, dull pain, anxiety, as well as chest pain (Cheek & Cesan, 2003; Joy, 2006). Women have pain in the back or left side of the chest rather than substernally and report the symptoms as a numb, tingling, burning, or stabbing sensation (Overbaugh, 2009).

A myocardial infarction is diagnosed by client symptoms, ECG tracings, cardiac biomarker values, and a radioactive isotope scan; however, in women the ECG stress test has less diagnostic value than in men. An exercise echocardiography is more reliable for women (Cheek & Cesan, 2003). When an

MI is evolving in men, the ECG has an elevated ST segment, which eventually changes into an inverted T wave.

A CK-MB fraction that measures an isoenzyme specific to the cardiac muscle increases within 3 to 6 hours of the onset of a myocardial infarct, peaks in 18 to 24 hours, and returns to normal in 72 hours. CK studies are performed as soon as the client is admitted and then every 8 hours until four samples have been obtained. A CK-MB fraction >5% indicates myocardial damage.

Two other important lab values for diagnosing an MI are cardiac troponin I and myoglobin. Cardiac troponin I is a protein found in cardiac cells. When cardiac cells are damaged, the protein is released, resulting in an elevated level (normal level is <0.6 ng/mL) for 7 days. Within an hour of an MI, the myoglobin blood level increases, peaks in 4 to 12 hours, and returns to normal in 18 hours. If an MI is suspected, the lab value must be obtained quickly.

During the first 3 days after the infarction, the client may have a low-grade fever and an increased white cell count. The infarcted heart tissue is soft and necrotic and incapable of responding to electrical stimuli. Life-threatening dysrhythmias are most likely to occur at this time. Four to seven days after the infarction, the infarcted tissue is the softest and weakest. An aneurysm, or ballooning effect, can occur in the infarcted area with the potential of rupturing. There is a possibility of the ventricle rupturing from the time of the infarct to 2 weeks after the infarct. Collateral circulation begins forming around the edges of the infarct, but it will be 2 to 3 weeks before the collateral circulation functions effectively. Two to three months will pass before the heart muscle regains maximum strength.

Medical–Surgical Management

Medical

Medical–surgical management focuses on reducing oxygen demands, increasing oxygen supply to the myocardium, relieving pain, improving tissue perfusion, and preventing complications and further tissue damage. Immediately after an MI, a client is admitted into a coronary care unit. The client's heart is constantly monitored for dysrhythmias, and vital signs are monitored for any changes.

Three dysrhythmias that may occur after an MI are ventricular fibrillation, bradycardias, and tachycardias. Ventricular fibrillation is treated by defibrillation. Atropine and, if needed, a temporary pacer is inserted for bradycardias. Two tachycardias that may occur are atrial fibrillation and ventricular tachycardia. Atrial fibrillation is treated with digoxin (Lanoxin) diltiazem hydrochloride (Cardizem), or amiodarone hydrochloride (Cordarone). Ventricular tachycardia is treated with Cordarone, lidocaine hydrochloride (Xylocaine), or cardioversion. If dysrhythmias continue, magnesium may be given.

Medical complications that can occur following an MI are acute left ventricular failure, cardiogenic shock, pericarditis, embolism and/or thrombosis, and cardiac rupture. The health care team must closely monitor the client for signs of these complications. Women have a worse prognosis and die more often than men after a heart attack or bypass surgery (Cheek & Cesan, 2003).

Surgical

Primary treatment may be PTCA instead of thrombolytic therapy. Along with balloon compression, a stent(s) may be inserted. Clients with multiple vessels occluded, or for whom thrombolytic therapy and PTCA have not been effective, have the CABG procedure performed.

Pharmacological

Oxygen is given by a Venturi mask or nasal cannula. Morphine sulfate is given intravenously for pain. Medications include nitrates (IV or sublingually) to relieve pain and dilate coronary arteries, sedatives to calm and relax the client, and a stool softener to prevent rectal straining.

Thrombolytic therapy is sometimes used within 3 to 6 hours of the myocardial infarction to dissolve a clot blocking an artery and reperfuse the area. Medications such as streptokinase (Streptase), anistreplase (Eminase), and alteplase recombinant (Activase) are used. A possible complication from thrombolytic therapy is bleeding. Be alert for symptoms of hemorrhaging in the gastrointestinal tract (hematemesis and tarry stools), retroperitoneum (low back pain and numbness in lower extremities), or cerebrum (headache, vomiting, and confusion). Heparin therapy inhibits further clotting. Aspirin and/or clopidogrel (Plavix) is given to prevent vasoconstriction and platelet aggregation.

Diet

Until the client is stabilized, a diet is withheld in case a PTCA or CABG procedure is required. Fluids may be offered during the acute stage. A liquid diet is progressed to a regular low-fat, low-cholesterol, low-sodium diet. The client tolerates small frequent feedings better than three large meals. Avoid caffeine and extremely hot and cold foods.

Activity

It is vital that the client receive physical, mental, and emotional rest. Less stimuli places less demand on the heart. Explain procedures so the client understands the care provided.

The client is usually limited to bed rest during the first 24 hours and progressed to sitting in a chair by the second day. If pain returns or other complications occur, the client is back to bed rest. Early ambulation is encouraged to prevent thrombosis. During and after each activity, assess the client's tolerance by monitoring the HR for an increase of 20 beats per minute, checking for a decrease in systolic blood pressure, and observing for dyspnea and dysrhythmias. Document verbal and nonverbal statements of fatigue and chest pain.

Before discharge, low-intensity tests are performed to determine the types of activities in which the client may engage at home. When the client is able to climb two flights of stairs, sexual activity is resumed.

Health Promotion

A diet of less than 30 grams of fat per day reduces the progression of atherosclerosis, but there is no documented evidence that diet will prevent the disease in clients with hereditary hyperlipidemia. Regular exercise, 30 minutes at least 5 days per week, and smoking cessation help prevent an MI.

Participation in a cardiac rehabilitation program provides the client with monitored exercise sessions as well as education and counseling about reducing the risk of future heart problems and coping with a new lifestyle. Because women have a worse prognosis than men, it is critical for women to participate in a cardiac rehabilitation program.

NURSING MANAGEMENT

Assess for pain. Observe for verbal and nonverbal signs of pain. Have client describe symptoms. Monitor vital signs, breath sounds, pedal pulses, and ECG strips. Maintain client on bed rest with call light and other items within reach. Accurately record I&O. Provide a quiet, calm environment. Balance activity with rest periods.

NURSING PROCESS

ASSESSMENT

Subjective Data

Note the medications the client has taken, including over-the-counter medications, anticoagulants, and thrombolytic medications. Assess pain regarding onset, duration, intensity, location, radiation, and precipitating factors; ask the client to describe the symptoms. Not all persons having angina or an MI will experience or state having pain. Some may describe feelings of chest heaviness, indigestion, or "something not right." Explore these statements with the client so the client can explain them in more detail. Dizziness, weakness, and shortness of breath may be expressed. Ask how the client tried to relieve pain.

Objective Data

Assess vital signs, skin changes, breath sounds, and ECG rhythm strips. Monitor vital signs for an irregular or increased pulse, hypotension, or slight temperature elevation. The client may have pallor, cyanosis, diaphoresis, vomiting, cool clammy skin, or confusion. Assess breath sounds for lung congestion, and monitor the ECG for dysrhythmias. Note any client clenching of hands or clutching at the chest.

Nursing diagnoses for a client with myocardial infarction include the following:

NURSING DIAGNOSES	PLANNING/OUTCOMES	NURSING INTERVENTIONS
Decreased **Cardiac** *Output* related to damaged heart tissue	The client will have increased CO.	Maintain bed rest with head of bed elevated 30° until the condition is stabilized. Auscultate breath sounds and palpate pedal pulses every 4 hours. Administer oxygen per mask or nasal cannula at 2 to 4 L/min. Start an IV so medications such as morphine and antidysrhythmics can be administered. If beta blockers are administered, monitor closely for a drop in HR and blood pressure. Constantly monitor the client for dysrhythmias. Place a rhythm strip on the chart at least once per shift. Monitor I&O. Administer medications as prescribed by the physician.
Acute **Pain** related to decreased oxygenation of myocardial tissue	The client will verbalize decrease in frequency and intensity of chest pain.	Maintain client on bed rest and observe for verbal and nonverbal signs of pain such as grimacing, diaphoresis, or increased HR. Ask the client to rate the pain on a scale of 0 to 10, 0 being no pain and 10 extreme pain. Administer analgesic, usually morphine and oxygen, as ordered.
Risk for **Activity** *Intolerance* related to decreased circulation to body tissues	The client will increase activities with decreased symptoms of angina, dyspnea, cyanosis, and dysrhythmia.	Place objects within reach of the client. Balance activity with rest periods. Assist the client and partner to discuss their fears and feelings candidly about resuming sexual activity.
Death **Anxiety** related to change in health status and threat of death	The client will verbalize situations that are causing stress.	Encourage the family and client to verbalize their feelings. Provide a quiet, calm environment to relax the client and family. Administer sedatives to help the client relax and provide periods of uninterrupted rest. Since the myocardial client may be in denial, be aware of denial symptoms such as attempting to conduct business over the phone while hospitalized or statements that the pain is really nothing.

Evaluation: Evaluate each outcome to determine how it has been met by the client.

HEART FAILURE

HF is often the final stage of many other heart conditions. A weakened muscle wall from a myocardial infarction or a heart that has been stressed over a period of time to meet metabolic needs of the body can cause HF. HF develops when the heart is no longer capable of meeting the oxygen needs of the body. The muscles of the left ventricle **hypertrophy** (increases in muscle mass), and often the ventricular chamber enlarges in an attempt to meet the oxygen needs of the body.

Both the right and left ventricles act as pumps for the heart. Each of these pumps can fail separately, resulting in two types of HF: right-sided HF and left-sided HF. HF usually begins on the left side. Some of the causes of right-sided failure are untreated left ventricular failure, right ventricular myocardial infarction, chronic obstructive coronary disease, cor pulmonale, and pulmonic valve stenosis. Left-sided failure is caused by left ventricular myocardial infarction, aortic valve stenosis, prolapsed valve complications, and hypertension. Notice that right- and left-sided failure are caused by a defect of the ventricle or an increased resistance in the path of the blood pumped by the ventricles. This causes an increased workload for the involved ventricle.

When left-sided HF occurs, the left ventricle is not able to completely empty of blood or effectively pump blood out through the aorta to the body systems. Usually the right ventricle continues to pump adequate quantities of blood. This causes blood to back up in the left ventricle, left atrium, and pulmonary veins. The lungs become congested with fluid as fluid leaks through the capillaries and fills air spaces in the lungs. The client becomes cyanotic, dyspneic, restless, and coughs up blood-tinged sputum. The breath sounds have moist crackles. Often the client has tachycardia with low blood pressure because the heart is not able to pump sufficient blood to meet the body's demands. The client may have decreased urinary output because enough blood is not pumped through the kidneys. As the blood oxygen level decreases, the client becomes confused.

As the right side of the heart fails, blood becomes congested in the inferior vena cava, causing edema first in the extremities and then in the trunk of the body. As the condition progresses, the client experiences edema of the ankles, lower legs, thighs, and finally in the abdomen. The excess abdominal fluid causes the client to be anorectic. Hepatomegaly (enlargement of the liver) and splenomegaly (enlargement of the spleen) develop. The jugular veins in the neck become distended when the client is sitting or standing, and pitting edema occurs in the lower extremities. Refer to Figure 5-6. Oliguria occurs as decreased amounts of blood are pumped through the kidneys.

In the early stages of HF, the client experiences fatigue, dyspnea with slight exertion, pedal edema, and a slight cough with a small amount of expectoration. The client may also have paroxysmal nocturnal dyspnea.

CRITICAL THINKING

Lifestyle Changes for MI

What would you teach a client to assist him in decreasing risk factors for an MI?

What lifestyle changes could you take to decrease the risk factors for an MI?

MEDICAL–SURGICAL MANAGEMENT

Medical

Goals for treating HF are to improve circulation to the coronary arteries and decrease the workload of the left ventricle. To meet these goals, cardiac efficiency is increased with medication; oxygen requirements of the body are decreased by bed rest with the head elevated 45 degrees; edema and pulmonary congestion are treated with medications, diet, and restricted fluid intake; and fluid retention is monitored by weighing the client daily. A chest x-ray directly visualizes the ventricles and evidence of lung congestion. An ECG is done and arterial blood gases are evaluated. The client's oxygen saturation level is monitored by pulse oximetry. Depending on the seriousness of the client's condition, a pulmonary artery catheter (Swan-Ganz catheter) may be inserted to determine left ventricular function.

In right-sided failure, the symptoms of edema, hepatomegaly, and neck vein distention are significant diagnostic evidence.

Surgical

Two mechanical devices are available: an intra-aortic balloon pump and a ventricular assist device (VAD). An intra-aortic balloon is threaded through the femoral artery to the descending aorta (Figure 5-21). The pump is synchronized with the contractions of the left ventricle so the balloon inflates during diastole and deflates during systole. Inflation of the balloon increases the blood flow to the coronary arteries, thus increasing oxygenation of the myocardium. Deflation of the balloon allows the left ventricle to pump blood to the body tissues with less peripheral resistance.

The ventricular assist device (VAD) does not replace the heart, but it assists a weakened heart to pump sufficient blood throughout the body. It is referred to as "a bridge to transplant" because a client uses the VAD while waiting for a heart transplant. Some clients who are not transplant candidates may use the VAD until death. A left VAD takes blood from the left ventricle and delivers it to the aorta (see Figure 5-22); a right VAD takes blood from the right ventricle and delivers it to the pulmonary artery. Potential complications are bleeding, blood clots, respiratory failure, renal failure, infection, stroke, and device failure.

Pharmacological

Medications to reduce the heart's workload in moderate HF are angiotensin converting enzymes (ACE) inhibitors, angiotensin receptor blockers, vasodilators, nitrates, beta blockers, diuretics, digitalis, and aspirin (Table 5-4). The client with HF will receive diuretics such as furosemide (Lasix) to decrease fluid retention. ACE inhibitors, such as captopril (Capoten) or enalopril (Vasotec), are given to reduce blood pressure and peripheral arterial resistance and improve CO. Beta blockers carvedilol (Coreg) and metoprolol succinate (Toprol XL), the only beta-blockers approved for HF in the United States, are then added (Ammon, 2001). A digitalis preparation may be required to increase the strength and contractility of the heart muscle. Vasodilators such as nitroglycerin (Cardabid) are given to dilate the veins so the blood will stay in the peripheral vessels and decrease blood return to the right side of the heart, thereby decreasing the workload on the heart. Clients in severe HF who are already taking an ACE inhibitor may be given spironolactone (Aldactone) (Ahmed, 2008). Morphine sulfate is given in the acute phase to control pain and decrease anxiety.

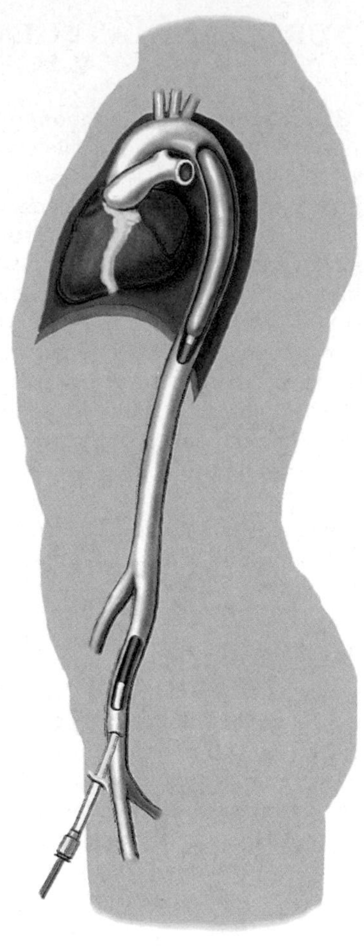

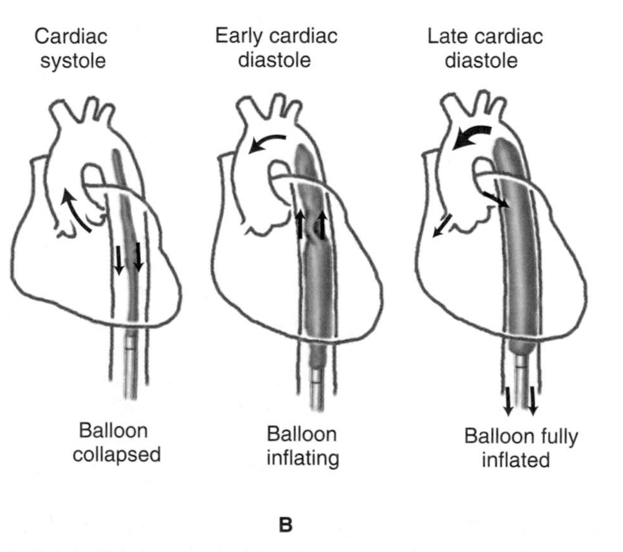

FIGURE 5-21 An intra-aortic balloon pump increases circulation to the coronary arteries and decreases the workload of the left ventricle.

Diet

A daily weight and strict intake and output are necessary to assess fluid retention. Sometimes fluid intake is limited. The client is generally on a low-sodium diet.

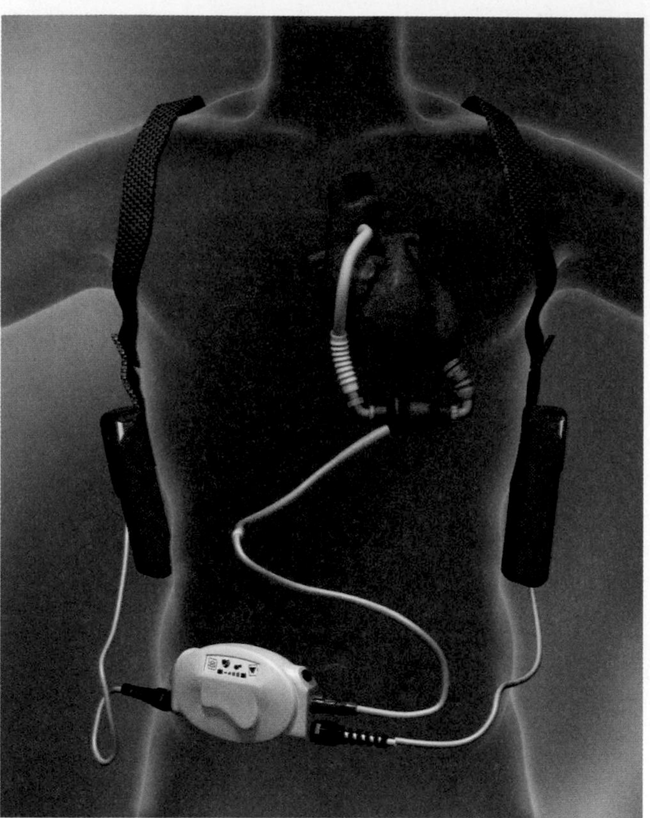

FIGURE 5-22 The cannula of the ventricular assist device (VAD) takes blood from the left atrium to the aorta, bypassing the ineffective left ventricle. (*Reprinted with permission from Thoratec Corporation.*)

PROFESSIONALTIP

Digoxin in Older Adults

HF is the leading cause of hospitalization in adults 65 years of age and older. New data indicates that a low dose (0.125 mg/day or lower) of digoxin decreases hospitalization due to HF and may also reduce mortality. Lower doses also decrease the risk of digoxin toxicity and the need for frequent serum digoxin levels. Digoxin in low doses is recommended for older adults with chronic HF (Ahmed, 2008).

Activity

Activity orders will depend on the client's activity tolerance. The client's activity may vary from strict bed rest to ambulation depending on the severity of the condition. When in bed, the head of the bed is elevated 45 degrees. Visitation privileges are monitored to provide rest periods.

Health Promotion

The most common cause of HF is left ventricular failure after a myocardial infarction. To prevent HF following coronary artery disease, a diet low in fat, high in fiber, and balanced in caloric intake to maintain optimum weight is recommended. Stress reduction and a regular exercise program will also decrease the risk of developing HF. Clients with congenital heart defects may not be able to prevent HF, but following the prescribed medical regimen may prevent the early development of HF.

TABLE 5-4 Recommended and Contraindicated Medications in Heart Failure

RECOMMENDED MEDICATIONS FOR HEART FAILURE THERAPY	CONTRAINDICATED MEDICATIONS FOR HEART FAILURE PATIENTS
• Loop diuretics for volume overload • ACE inhibitors (titrate upward to optimal dose) • Beta blockers (titrate upward to optimal dose with support and monitoring) • Digitalis • Spironolactone for advanced heart failure (with optimal doses of ACE inhibitors and beta blockers. Monitor for complications such as hyperkalemia) • ARBs if ACE inhibitors are not tolerated	• Alcohol • Cocaine • Antiarrhythmic agents except amiodarone • Calcium channel blockers except amlodipine • NSAIDs (associated with development of CHF and interact with ACE inhibitors) • Thiazolidinediones (may cause fluid retention) • Metformin

From State of the Science for Care of Older Adults with Heart Disease, by C. Deaton, J. Bennett, & B. Riegel, (2004). In *Nursing Clinics of North America, 39*(3), 495–528; Polypharmacy and Comorbidity in Heart Failure, by F. Masoudi & H. Krumholz, (2003), in *British Journal of Medicine, 327*(7414), 513–514.

NURSING MANAGEMENT

Monitor client's level of consciousness, skin color and turgor, and jugular veins for distension. Assess breath, heart, and bowel sounds. Check capillary refill and peripheral and abdominal edema. Weigh client daily at same time, on same scale, in same type of clothes. Monitor electrolytes and vital signs. Keep bed in semi-Fowler's position. Maintain accurate intake and output. Provide frequent rest periods and minimal interruptions at night. Teach about disease process, medications, and diet.

NURSING PROCESS

ASSESSMENT

Subjective Data

Ask the client about dyspnea, orthopnea, fatigue, anxiety, weight gain, edema, pain, or difficulty in performing activities of daily living.

Objective Data

Assess the client's level of consciousness to determine circulation of blood to the brain. Check skin color for pallor or cyanosis. Assess skin turgor to help determine the level of hydration. Jugular distention indicates right ventricle functioning. Assess breath sounds for adventitious sounds and heart sounds for gallop or murmurs. Bowel sounds may be hypoactive depending on the amount of fluid retention in the abdomen. Check peripheral pulses and capillary refill to assess the level of circulation to the extremities. Assess edema in the extremities and abdomen according to the edema rating scale. Monitor the client's weight daily for possible increase from fluid retention. The physician should be notified if there is a gain of more than 2 pounds in one day. Monitor I&O and assess for oliguria.

Nursing diagnoses for a client with HF include the following:

NURSING DIAGNOSES	PLANNING/OUTCOMES	NURSING INTERVENTIONS
Decreased **Cardiac** *Output* related to mechanical failure of heart muscle	The client's vital signs will remain stable. The client will have decreased adventitious breath sounds.	Take an apical pulse on all cardiac clients, especially checking the rate and rhythm. Monitor the client's HR and rhythm by telemetry. Auscultate breath sounds every 4 hours. Administer diuretics, digitalis, and vasodilators as prescribed. Closely monitor the electrolytes, especially the potassium level, as diuretics can deplete the potassium level. Administer potassium supplements as ordered. Take the apical pulse before giving a digitalis preparation. If the HR is below 60, withhold the medication and notify the physician. In some institutions the HR can drop to 50 before the physician is notified if the client is taking a calcium channel blocker or beta-blocker along with digitalis.

(*Continues*)

Nursing diagnoses for a client with HF include the following: (Continued)

NURSING DIAGNOSES	PLANNING/OUTCOMES	NURSING INTERVENTIONS
*Impaired **G**as Exchange* related to decreased CO and pulmonary edema	The client will have increased gas exchange.	Provide oxygen by mask or nasal cannula at 2 to 6 L/min. Apply a pulse oximeter and monitor the oxygenation status. If the pulse oximeter is ≤90%, notify the physician. Elevate the head of the bed to a semi-Fowler's or Fowler's position to relieve pressure on the diaphragm.
*Excess **F**luid Volume* related to decreased cardiac output and decreased renal output	The client will have less edema of the extremities.	Encourage elevation of the client's legs, not letting them hang in a dependent position. Maintain an accurate intake and output. Weigh daily at the same time each day, on the same scales, and with the client wearing the same type of clothing. If the client is on a fluid-restricted diet, offer hard candies to quench the thirst.
*Risk for **A**ctivity Intolerance* related to edema, dyspnea, and fatigue	The client will have an increased tolerance for activity.	Schedule nursing care so the client is given frequent rest periods with minimal interruptions at night. Teach the client to take frequent rest periods and to stop activities before becoming tired. Monitor the client's vital signs for an increase or decrease in HR or blood pressure, especially after periods of activity. Have an occupational therapist assist the client in energy saving methods. Instruct the client to call the physician if there is more dyspneic, fatigue, less activity tolerance, or weight gain or loss when at home.

Evaluation: Evaluate each outcome to determine how it has been met by the client.

COR PULMONALE

In this condition, the heart is affected because of a lung condition that interferes with the exchange of carbon dioxide and oxygen in the alveoli. The carbon dioxide level increases in the blood. For some unknown reason, the pulmonary arteries vasoconstrict, causing pulmonary hypertension. The right ventricle is forced to pump against increased pulmonary pressure. The right ventricle enlarges and finally weakens in the attempt to pump blood into the lungs. The symptoms the client experiences and medical and nursing care are the same as for right-sided HF.

CARDIAC TRANSPLANTATION

Cardiac transplantations are done for cardiomyopathy, end-stage coronary artery disease, and valvular disease. Recipients are evaluated for emotional stability, minimal disease involvement, and a good support system. The heart donor and the recipient's tissues are matched.

The transplant is performed by removing the recipient's heart except for posterior sections of the atria. The posterior sections of the atria are removed from the donor's heart, and then the heart is sutured to the recipient's posterior atria.

The recipient must remain on an immunosuppressant medication for the remainder of life so the donor heart is not rejected. Some immunosuppressant medications are azathioprine (Imuran), cyclosporine (Sandimmune), antithymocytic globulin, ATG (Atgam), antilymphocytic globulin (ALG), rapamycin, and FK 506 (Prograf).

PERIPHERAL VASCULAR DISORDERS

Disorders in this category include aneurysm, hypertension, venous thrombosis/thrombophlebitis, varicose veins, Buerger's disease, and Raynaud's disease.

ANEURYSM

An **aneurysm** is a localized dilation occurring in a weakened section of an artery's medial layer. The main cause for aneurysms is atherosclerosis (Mayo Clinic, 2002). Some aneurysms occur because of congenital conditions such as Marfan's syndrome or because of trauma to the vessel wall. Two other possible causes of an aneurysm are an increased turbulence in a section of the vessel and a slower production of smooth muscle cells. Clients have a higher tendency to develop an aneurysm if they smoke cigarettes and have hypertension.

Aneurysms can occur in any artery but occur most often in the abdominal aorta. Abdominal aneurysms occur more frequently in men over the age of 55 (Mayo Clinic, 2002). Other involved vessels are the ascending, transverse, and descending aorta, thoracic aorta, popliteal arteries, and femoral arteries.

Deposits of atherosclerotic plaque on the tunica intima cause a hardening of the vessel, and the media layer of the vessel loses elasticity. Atherosclerosis and a lack of elastin in the vessel wall predisposes the vessel to a weakened area, which develops into an aneurysm.

Symptoms of an aneurysm depend on its location. Aneurysms are often asymptomatic until they start leaking or pressing on other structures. A thoracic aneurysm may press on surrounding structures, causing dull upper back pain or deep, scattered chest pain. Pressure on the trachea and bronchus may cause dyspnea, coughing, wheezing,and hoarseness. Pressure on the esophagus causes dysphagia.

The most common location of an abdominal aortic aneurysm is between the renal and iliac arteries. There may be no symptoms, but as it enlarges and presses on other vessels, organs, and nerves, the client may experience abdominal, back, or flank pain. The client may feel a pulse in the abdomen when in a supine position. A tender pulsating mass may be palpated slightly left of the umbilicus. Popliteal and femoral aneurysms may cause decreased pedal pulses. Rupture of an aneurysm is an emergency situation. Signs of rupture may include hypotension, tachycardia, pallor, cool and clammy skin, and intense abdominal, back, or groin pain. An aneurysm is usually diagnosed when a client has an x-ray or ultrasound done for other conditions/symptoms.

MEDICAL–SURGICAL MANAGEMENT

Medical

If the client has hypertension, control of the hypertension is the focus of care. Aneurysms are monitored for enlargement. Thrombi formation and ischemia may also result.

Surgical

Before elective surgery, the status of the client's carotid arteries and peripheral vessels are checked with a Doppler ultrasound. Cardiac status is usually evaluated by a stress test or cardiac catheterization before surgery is scheduled. The surgeon often orders an angiogram, ultrasound, or CT scan of the affected vessel before surgery to assess the blood supply to the area surrounding the aneurysm. Before surgery, 4 to 8 units of blood are placed on hold because hemorrhage is a possibility. The surgeon clamps the aorta, removes the section of the vessel involving the aneurysm, and replaces it with a section of the client's saphenous vein or a synthetic graft (Figure 5-23). Complications that can occur from clamping the aorta are myocardial infarctions, strokes, and renal damage. Vessels below the repaired aneurysm may become occluded because of decreased blood flow during surgery or from plaque that has broken off from the wall of the vessel. A nasogastric tube may be inserted to decrease pressure on the aneurysm repair site and incision. After surgery, the client may be in the ICU with mechanical ventilator assistance in breathing.

Pharmacological

Clients with aortic aneurysms may be given propranolol hydrochloride (Inderal) to decrease the pressure of the blood coming from the heart. Clients with hypertension are given antihypertensive medications and diuretics. Analgesics are given to control pain.

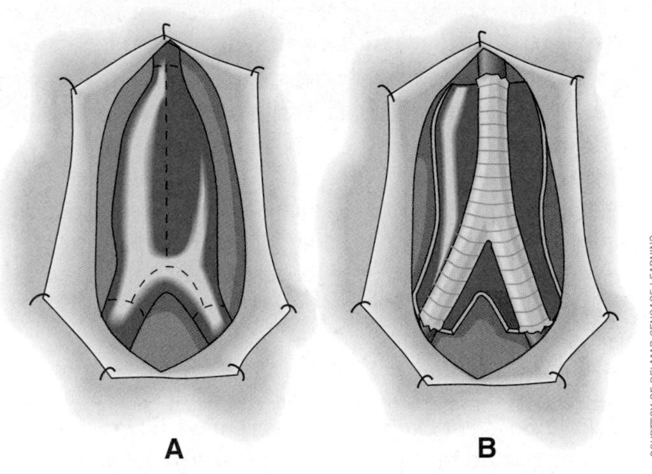

FIGURE 5-23 ***A*, Aortoiliac Aneurysm; *B*, Bifurcated Synthetic Graft**

Activity

Any activity that increases blood pressure, especially exercise and lifting, can increase pressure in the arteries and should be avoided.

Health Promotion

Clients are encouraged not to smoke. Education for the hypertensive client includes the importance of closely monitoring the blood pressure and taking antihypertensive medication as prescribed.

NURSING MANAGEMENT

Preoperatively, monitor vital signs and peripheral pulses. Assess capillary refill, feet for mottling, and for edema. Postoperatively, add checking operative site frequently. Check function and drainage of NG tube. Measure abdomen for increasing size indicating internal hemorrhage. Measure output hourly for at least 25 to 30 mL of urine.

NURSING PROCESS

ASSESSMENT

Subjective Data

Preoperatively, the client may be concerned about an abdominal pulsation when reclining. The client may have chest, back, abdominal, or flank pain depending on the aneurysm location. Postoperatively, listen for statements of pain and assess the level of pain according to a scale of 1 to 10 or the facility-approved scale.

Objective Data

Palpate the abdomen for a pulsating mass, and check vital signs. Immediate intervention is needed if symptoms of bleeding or a rupturing aneurysm occur. Check the peripheral pulses before surgery. Pulses can then be compared preoperatively and postoperatively. Postoperatively, assess the extremities for color, warmth, peripheral pulses, and sensation.

Nursing diagnoses for a client with an aneurysm include the following:

NURSING DIAGNOSES	PLANNING/OUTCOMES	NURSING INTERVENTIONS
*Ineffective **T**issue Perfusion (Peripheral)* related to decreased arterial blood flow	The client will have well-oxygenated tissues as manifested by strong pulses and the skin remaining baseline color and warm.	Monitor for symptoms of an occluded vessel (pain, paleness, cyanosis, and coldness). Monitor the temperature, color, and fullness of the peripheral pulses in both extremities and compare them to the preoperative pulses. Assess capillary refill and client's feet for mottling and darkened areas on the toes and soles of the feet. Notify physician immediately if any of these symptoms occur.
*Risk for Deficient **F**luid Volume* related to hemorrhage	The client will have adequate fluid volume.	Monitor vital signs closely for signs of hemorrhage. Check the operative site frequently to make sure the dressing is dry. Turn the client to make sure blood is not pooling under the client's body. Monitor for other signs of hemorrhaging. Measure the abdomen for increasing abdominal girth indicating internal bleeding. If the client has low back pain, there may be hemorrhaging in the retroperitoneal space. Other symptoms of hemorrhage are lightheadedness, dizziness, and tachycardia. Check for adequate functioning and drainage of the NG tube to decrease pressure on the aneurysm repair site and incision.
*Ineffective **T**issue Perfusion (Renal)* related to interruption of blood flow during surgery	The client will have a urine output above 25 mL/hour.	Measure hourly output to make sure the client has at least 25 to 30 mL of urine per hour. Assess for edema which could indicate fluid overload or a vessel occlusion. Provide fluids as ordered.

Evaluation: Evaluate each outcome to determine how it has been met by the client.

HYPERTENSION

Hypertension (HTN), also known as high blood pressure, is defined as an elevated arterial blood pressure. A systolic blood pressure at or above 140 or a diastolic blood pressure at or above 90 indicates hypertension. Fifty million adults in the United States have hypertension (NIH, 2002).

Before age 55, more men than women have hypertension, but after age 55, more women have hypertension (CDC, 2002). Unalterable risk factors include African-American race, male gender, aging, postmenopausal women, and family history of hypertension. Modifiable risk factors include smoking, lack of exercise, obesity, stress, low socioeconomic status, diet high in sodium and fat, alcohol intake, and oral contraceptives.

When the cause of hypertension is unknown, it is called **primary hypertension** or "essential hypertension." Eighty to ninety-five percent of clients with hypertension have primary hypertension (Klabunde, 2007). In 5% to 10% of the cases, the cause of hypertension is another condition within the body such as renal artery stenosis, chronic renal disease, primary hyperaldosteronism, sleep apnea, hyper- or hypothyroidism, pheochromocytoma, preeclampsia, or aortic coarctation (Klabunde, 2007); this is known as **secondary hypertension.** Arteriosclerosis, atherosclerosis, hypernatremia (increased sodium in the blood) or prolonged stress may also cause hypertension.

Malignant hypertension is a rapidly progressing, severe elevation of BP (diastolic 120 mm Hg). It damages small arterioles in the major organs. Arteriole inflammation in the eyes is the primary distinguishing finding. It is most common in black males younger than 40 years of age.

Renal diseases that interfere with blood flow to the kidneys cause them to release an enzyme called renin. The released renin interacts with plasma proteins, forming a vasopressor called *angiotensin*. Vasoconstriction caused by angiotensin increases blood pressure when more force is required to push the blood through the vessel. Vasodilation decreases vascular or **peripheral resistance** (pressure within a vessel that resists the flow of blood such as plaque buildup or vasoconstriction). Figure 5-24 depicts how renal disease causes hypertension.

Arteriosclerosis causes the vessel walls to have less elasticity, decreasing their ability to expand and recoil. Because the vessel is not able to expand, more pressure is needed to force the blood through the vessel. The plaque buildup causes resistance to blood flow through the vessel, and more pressure is needed to get the blood through the vessel. Hypernatremia (increased blood sodium) causes vasocongestion, and the heart must pump with more force, increasing the pressure in the arteries, thus causing HTN.

Stress stimulates the sympathetic nervous system, which supplies nerves to the smooth muscles of the arteries, arterioles, veins, and venules. Stimulation of these smooth muscles

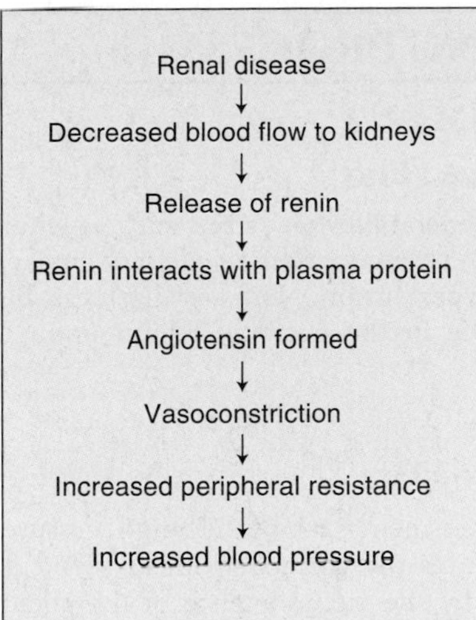

FIGURE 5-24 Pathophysiology of Renal Diseases and Hypertension

causes the vessels to constrict, leading to elevated blood pressure.

Some complications of HTN are cerebral vascular accident (stroke), myocardial infarction, HF, and renal failure. Table 5-5 lists the recognized classification of blood pressure.

MEDICAL–SURGICAL MANAGEMENT

Medical

The main goal for a client with HTN is keeping the blood pressure within normal limits. The regimen is referred to as a stepped-care approach. The first step is to encourage the client to try some diet and lifestyle changes, including losing weight if >15% over optimum weight; limiting sodium, saturated fat, cholesterol, and alcohol intake; exercising on a regular basis; stopping the use of nicotine; and maintaining an adequate intake of calcium, magnesium, and potassium. This step is tried for 3 to 6 months, and if the BP then is < 140/90 mm Hg, these steps are continued. If the BP still remains high, the second step is the addition of a diuretic or a beta-blocker to the client's care regimen. The client is again evaluated for a period of time, usually 2 months. If the BP is not <140/90 mm Hg, the third step of increasing the drug dosage, trying another drug, or adding a second antihypertensive drug from another class of drugs is implemented. If the BP is maintained at <140/90 mm Hg, the regimen is continued. If the BP is still high, the last step is implemented by adding a second or third antihypertensive drug.

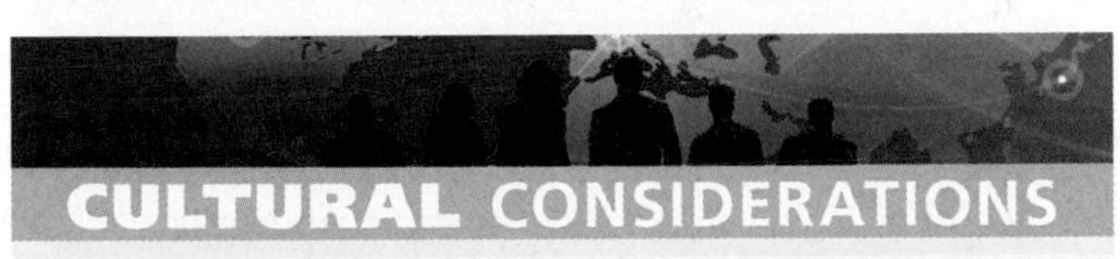

CULTURAL CONSIDERATIONS

Hypertension

African-American clients develop hypertension earlier in life, and it is more severe at any decade of life, than other ethnic groups.

Table 5-5 Classification Of Blood Pressure

CATEGORY	SYSTOLIC (MM HG)		DIASTOLIC (MM HG)
Normal	<120	and	<80
Prehypertension	120–139	or	80–89
Hypertension			
Stage 1	140–159	or	90–99
Stage 2	≥160	or	≥ 100

From *The Seventh Report of the Joint National Committee on Prevention, Detection, Evaluation, and Treatment of High Blood Pressure*, 2003, Bethesda, MD: National Institutes of Health.

Pharmacological

Diuretics are usually the first pharmacological step in treating HTN. Diuretics increase the renal excretion of sodium and water from the body, decreasing the total fluid volume. When less fluid is in the body, less pressure or force is needed to pump the blood through the body.

Beta-adrenergic blocking agents are given to block the epinephrine and norepinephrine receptor sites. With these receptor sites blocked, the vessels do not constrict and the blood has less resistance flowing through the vessel. Diuretics and antihypertensive medications may cause impotence.

Diet

A low-fat, low-cholesterol, and low-sodium diet is encouraged. Restricting sodium intake to 2.3 grams of sodium or 6 grams of sodium chloride per day assists in decreasing blood pressure. Avoiding processed foods, carbonated drinks, and most cereals helps decrease sodium intake. Encourage the client to have an adequate intake of potassium, magnesium, and calcium. These minerals are obtained by eating fresh oranges, bananas, broccoli, and collards. Fresh foods are better sources for minerals than frozen foods. Yogurt is a good calcium supplement. The National Committee on Prevention, Detection, Evaluation, and Treatment of High Blood Pressure recommends that clients with hypertension not consume more than 2 ounces of alcohol at a time and no more than twice a week.

Activity

A regular aerobic exercise regimen assists in lowering blood pressure. The client is to gradually increase the exercise period to

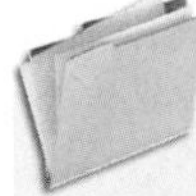

COLLABORATIVE CARE

Hypertension

Assisting a client to eliminate hypertension is a multidisciplinary task. Members of the care team most often include physician, nurses, dietitian, fitness center therapist, smoking cessation counselor, and stress management advisor.

CRITICAL THINKING

Lifestyle Changes for Hypertension

How can you best teach the hypertensive client ways to modify the present lifestyle?

30 to 45 minutes 3 to 5 times per week with a pulse rate at 75% of the target HR (target HR = 220 – age × 0.75). Walking, swimming, and jogging are excellent aerobic exercises.

Health Promotion

Measures to prevent hypertension are exercising regularly; reducing sodium in the diet; maintaining an optimum weight; reducing and managing stress; maintaining intake of potassium, calcium, and magnesium; decreasing alcohol consumption; and ceasing smoking.

Nursing Management

Monitor BP. Make referrals to assist in lifestyle changes. Explain pathophysiology, risk factors, suggested lifestyle changes, and complications.

NURSING PROCESS

Assessment

Subjective Data

Ask about general lifestyle habits such as smoking, alcohol consumption, exercise routine, dietary intake, and family history of hypertension. Note any dizziness, blurred vision, and headache in the occipital region upon rising in the morning.

Objective Data

The basic assessment is taking the blood pressure. An accurate reading requires the correct width of blood pressure cuff, determined by the circumference of the client's extremity. The cuff bladder should encircle 80% of the arm to obtain an accurate blood pressure (JNC 7 Express, 2003). The blood pressure is taken in both arms in supine and sitting positions. Before taking the blood pressure, the client should rest quietly in a chair, rather than on an exam table, for 5 minutes with both feet on the floor and the arm supported at heart level. If the client has an elevated BP, a repeat blood pressure is taken 15 minutes later and compared to previous readings. Measure client height and weight, heart sounds, and peripheral pulses.

Nursing diagnoses for a client with hypertension include the following:

NURSING DIAGNOSES	PLANNING/OUTCOMES	NURSING INTERVENTIONS
Ineffective Health Maintenance related to lack of knowledge about lifestyle habits contributing to hypertension	The client will relate needed changes in lifestyle habits to decrease blood pressure.	Make referrals to the appropriate personnel to teach the client lifestyle changes. These may include a dietitian, smoking cessation clinic, fitness center, or stress management seminars. Explain the pathophysiology, risk factors, lifestyle changes, medication actions and side effects, and complications of hypertension.
Noncompliance related to individual's value system (lack of physical symptoms and expense of medication)	The client will keep appointments for regular check-ups and take medications as prescribed.	Regularly inquire about the client's satisfaction in regard to the prescribed regimen of diet, exercise, and prescribed medication(s). If the client cannot afford needed medications, refer the client to financial assistance programs. Encourage the client to become an active participant in the treatment because this will give the client a sense of control over the condition. Encourage the client to record BP readings, weekly weight, exercise activities, and dietary intake as a way of giving a sense of control and encouraging compliance.
Imbalanced Nutrition: More than Body Requirements related to excess caloric intake and excess sodium intake	The client will maintain weight at no more than 15% over optimum weight and have no more than 2.3 grams of sodium per day.	Give basic dietary instructions as stated under medical management or make a referral to a dietitian. Weigh the client at scheduled appointments.

Nursing diagnoses for a client with hypertension include the following: (Continued)

NURSING DIAGNOSES	PLANNING/OUTCOMES	NURSING INTERVENTIONS
*Sexual **D**ysfunction* related to altered body structure or function and side effects of antihypertensive medications	The client will state satisfaction with sexual function while taking antihypertensive medications.	Because diuretics and antihypertensive medications may cause impotence, discuss this effect in an open and candid manner, so the client and spouse will be feel comfortable discussing sexual difficulties.

Evaluation: Evaluate each outcome to determine how it has been met by the client.

SAMPLE NURSING CARE PLAN

The Client with Hypertension

T.L., a 28-year-old African-American client, is in his last year of law school and is clerking for a prestigious law firm. He and his fiancé plan to marry as soon as he graduates. During the last week he has had four dizzy spells and a headache at the base of his skull upon awakening for the last 2 days. His father has a history of hypertension, so T.L. is aware that his symptoms may indicate high blood pressure. T.L. stops by the clinic on his way home from work and asks the nurse to check his blood pressure. The nursing assessment has the following data.

Subjective data: States he has had four dizzy spells and has awakened with a headache in the occipital lobe the last two mornings. T.L. has 1 glass of wine at lunch and 2–3 beers in the evening to relax from the tension of school and work. Most of his meals are at fast-food establishments and have a high fat content. T.L. does not smoke. He used to jog 4 mornings a week but quit when he started clerking. He has had nocturia for the last 3 weeks. He is not taking any medication. T.L. states he is concerned about having hypertension because he does not want to take medication.

Objective data: T 98.6°F, AP 78 beats/min, R 16 breaths/min, BP 142/92 mm Hg, Wt 190 lbs (optimum weight 160). No edema noted in hands, feet, or legs.

NURSING DIAGNOSIS 1 *Ineffective **H**ealth Maintenance* related to ineffective individual coping as evidenced by high-fat diet, lack of exercise, stressful job, and alcohol intake

Nursing Outcomes Classification (NOC)
Health-Promoting Behavior
Knowledge: Health Promotion

Nursing Interventions Classification (NIC)
Health Education
Self-Responsibility Facilitation
Risk Identification

PLANNING/OUTCOMES	NURSING INTERVENTIONS	RATIONALE
T.L. will change lifestyle habits by engaging in aerobic exercises at least 3 times a week for 30 to 45 minutes, stating three ways to reduce stress, and limiting alcohol consumption to 2 ounces twice a week.	Refer T.L. to a dietitian to learn ways to cut fat and sodium in his diet.	Knowledge encourages compliance.
	Discuss ways T.L. can exercise and still meet responsibilities of work, school, and personal and social life.	Encourages exercise if he sees ways that he can still meet responsibilities of life.
	Explain alcohol content in various beverages.	Encourages compliance.

EVALUATION

T.L. begins exercising with his fiancé 3 times a week. T.L. uses breathing techniques and a hot shower to reduce daily stress. T.L. limits alcohol consumption to 1 beer a day.

NURSING DIAGNOSIS 2 *Imbalanced **N**utrition:* More than Body Requirements, related to excessive caloric intake as evidenced by 30 pounds overweight and high-fat diet

(Continues)

SAMPLE NURSING CARE PLAN (Continued)

Nursing Outcomes Classification (NOC)
Nutritional Status
Teaching: Nutrition

Nursing Interventions Classification (NIC)
Nutrition Management
Nutrition Monitoring

PLANNING/OUTCOMES	NURSING INTERVENTIONS	RATIONALE
T.L. will lose 30 pounds and maintain a low-fat, low-sodium diet.	Refer T.L. to a weight support group.	It is easier to lose weight with support of others.
	Encourage T.L. to record a weekly weight and daily intake of fat.	Promotes self-care.

EVALUATION

T.L. is maintaining a diet low in sodium and no more than 30 grams of fat per day. T.L. keeps a weekly record of his weight.

NURSING DIAGNOSIS 3 *Anxiety* related to threat to or change in health status and stress as evidenced by alcohol consumption to relax and statement of not wanting to take medications

Nursing Outcomes Classification (NOC)
Anxiety Reduction
Coping

Nursing Interventions Classification (NIC)
Anxiety Reduction
Anticipatory Guidance

PLANNING/OUTCOMES	INTERVENTIONS	RATIONALE
T.L. states preventive measures to reduce blood pressure.	Have T.L. identify stress factors in life.	Action to cope with stressors can be taken only if stressors are identified.
	Discuss stress reduction techniques with T.L.	Knowledge promotes compliance.
	Discuss risk factors of hypertension and ways to reduce it.	Promotes identification of risk factors in personal life.
	Explain to T.L. and his fiancé that hypertension is a chronic condition, possibly without symptoms, but with some potentially serious complications.	Knowledge promotes compliance.

EVALUATION

T.L. states four ways to reduce blood pressure.

VENOUS THROMBOSIS/ THROMBOPHLEBITIS

The terms *phlebitis, thrombosis, phlebothrombosis,* and *thrombophlebitis* are often used interchangeably even though each word has a separate meaning and etiology. **Phlebitis** is an inflammation in the wall of a vein without clot formation. The formation of a clot in a vessel is a **thrombosis**, and a formed clot that remains at the site where it formed is a **thrombus**. If the thrombus moves, it becomes an **embolus**, a mass such as a blood clot or an air bubble that circulates in the bloodstream. **Phlebothrombosis** is the formation of a clot because of blood pooling in the vessel, trauma to the vessel's endothelial lining, or a coagulation problem with little or no inflammation in the vessel. **Thrombophlebitis** is the formation of a clot caused by an inflammation in the wall of the vessel.

In 1846, Virchow listed three factors leading to the formation of a clot: pooling of blood, vessel trauma, and a coagulation problem. These are known as **Virchow's triad**. Risk factors for thrombi formation are prolonged bed rest, leg trauma, oral contraceptives, obesity, varicose veins, hip fractures, and total hip and knee replacement.

There are two types of thrombi: a superficial thrombus and a deep vein thrombus (DVT). A superficial vein thrombus forms in a superficial vein such as the saphenous vein in the leg.

A DVT forms in the deep veins of the arms, pelvic area, or legs, but the legs are the most common site. Leg veins in which clots form are the femoral, popliteal, iliac, and deep veins of the calf.

Phlebitis can either form spontaneously or as a result of IV catheters or cannulas, IV medications such as potassium or antibiotics, or direct trauma to a vein. A clot may then form as red blood cells pass over the damaged area, rupture, and start the clotting process.

Phlebitis manifests as a reddened streak over a vein. If a clot is in a superficial vein, the site becomes reddened, warm, tender, and swollen. A hardening is palpated in a section of the vein. There are no symptoms with a deep vein thrombus, or there may be warmth and tenderness at the site, unilateral edema of the affected extremity, positive Homans' sign, dilation of superficial veins, and cyanosis of the foot. The client may say the leg feels "tight" or "heavy." If the clot is in the calf of the leg, the calf may feel tender. If the swelling restricts the arterial blood flow, the leg may be cool and pale. If there are obvious clinical signs of a thrombosis, Homans' sign should not be assessed because the clot may be dislodged and become an embolus.

A complication of a DVT is a pulmonary embolus that may result in death. Symptoms of a pulmonary embolus are sudden and severe chest pain, dyspnea, and tachypnea. Emboli may travel and block other vessels in the heart, brain, or peripheral vessels.

Medical–Surgical Management

Medical

A superficial phlebitis or thrombus may need no treatment, or warm soaks may be applied to the affected area. Acetaminophen or an NSAID is given for pain. Elevating the extremity decreases swelling and improves venous return. Some doctors recommend the application of elastic support hose. If a DVT is diagnosed, the client is placed on bed rest. Once the client improves and becomes ambulatory, below-the-knee compression stockings are recommended.

Surgical

If a clot has formed in a large vein and all conservative methods have failed, the clot may be removed surgically. This procedure is called a **thrombectomy** and is performed only if the tissue in the area becomes ischemic or gangrenous or if the client has a history of thromboemboli.

Another surgical procedure is a vena cava interruption surgery (venacaval plication) in which a Greenfield vena cava filter or umbrella filter is placed in the inferior vena cava to prevent thromboemboli from traveling from the lower extremities to the lungs, heart, or brain. Figure 5-25 shows these filters and their placement in the vena cava. The procedure is done on clients with a history of pulmonary emboli.

Pharmacological

If a client is at risk for a thrombus or phlebitis, anticoagulant therapy is initiated. A prophylactic heparin dose is given. Enoxaparin injection (Lovenox), a low-molecular-weight heparin, is used prophylactically after hip replacement surgery. It should be used cautiously with clients on oral anticoagulants.

If a clot forms, the client is immediately started on heparin as an IV bolus and then followed with a continuous IV drip of heparin. Before heparin is started, a partial thromboplastin time (PTT) or activated partial thromboplastin time (APTT) and a platelet count are drawn by the laboratory to establish a baseline level. The heparin dose is regulated by the PTT or the APTT. For effective heparin therapy, the client's PTT or APTT level should be 2.5 times the baseline. A **baseline level** is a value at a particular time that serves as a reference point for future value levels.

Clients are usually discharged on Coumadin. Because of rapid hospital discharges, clients are often started on Coumadin the next day after heparin has been initiated. Once the Coumadin dose is regulated, heparin is stopped.

CLIENT TEACHING

Thrombophlebitis

- Drink 2 to 3 quarts of water per day.
- Do not sit with legs crossed.
- Elevate both legs when sitting.
- Avoid sitting or standing for extended periods.
- Wear support hose.
- When standing, shift weight frequently and occasionally stand on tiptoes to stimulate the calf muscle to pump blood.
- Notify the physician immediately if leg pain, tenderness or swelling, difficulty breathing, or chest pain is experienced.

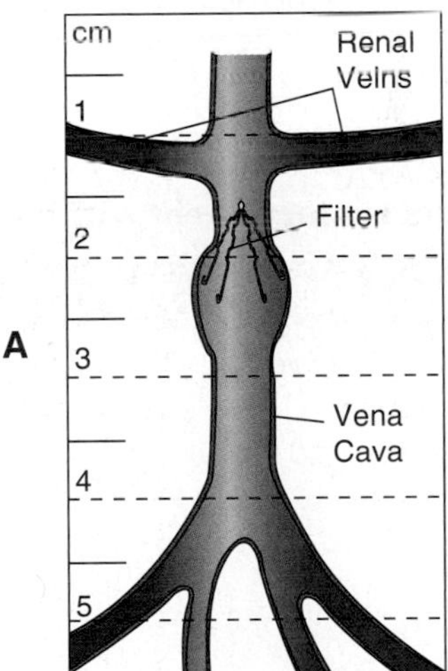

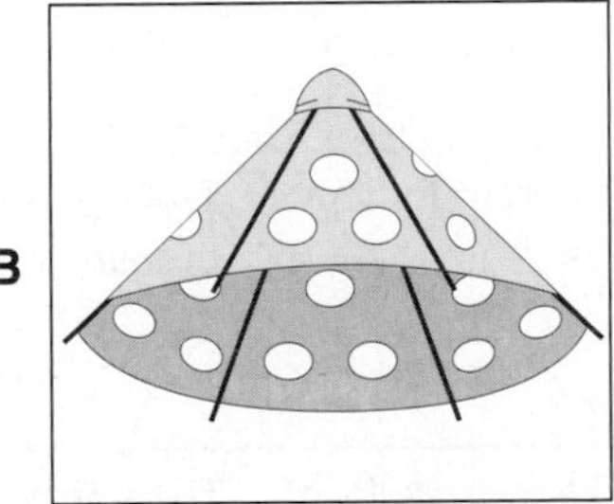

FIGURE 5-25 Filter in the Vena Cava Prevents an Embolus from Traveling to the Heart, Lungs, or Brain; *A*, Greenfield Filter in Place; *B*, Umbrella Filter

After the initial Coumadin dose, the daily Coumadin dose is regulated by the prothrombin time (PT) or the International Normalized Ratio (INR). The client generally remains on Coumadin for 3 to 6 months.

Thrombolytic drugs, urokinase (Abbokinase), streptokinase (Streptase), and tissue plasminogen activator, t-PA (Alteplase), are used locally and systemically if there is a massive DVT. Streptokinase should only be used on the same client once every 6 months. If the client has had a recent streptococcal infection, streptokinase may not be effective (Spratto & Woods, 2010). The main complication in a client receiving thrombolytic drugs is bleeding. Heparin and Coumadin are given after the thrombolytic drugs to prevent thrombi formation.

Diet

Adequate hydration is important for clients at risk for thrombi. This is accomplished orally or intravenously.

Activity

During the acute stage, the client is placed on bed rest to prevent the clot from dislodging and embolizing. Later, the leg is elevated periodically to improve venous return and decrease swelling. The client's leg should never be massaged because a clot could be dislodged and become an embolus.

Health Promotion

Prevention is the best way to treat a DVT. Early ambulation, adequate hydration, alternating pneumatic compression devices, prophylactic anticoagulants, elevation of legs, leg exercises, and deep breathing exercises all contribute to the prevention of thrombi.

Nursing Management

Monitor vital signs for changes and IV sites for redness and warmth. Do not do a Homans' sign if there is a diagnosis of a thrombus. Measure the circumference of the affected leg. Assess peripheral pulses and capillary refill. If on anticoagulant drugs, assess for signs of bleeding. When on bed rest, elevate the entire affected leg. Remove elastic support or pneumatic compression stockings daily for hygiene.

NURSING PROCESS

Assessment

Subjective Data

Ask the client if there was any recent injury to the extremity, if the affected area is tender to the touch, or if there have been clots previously. Note any chest pain, dyspnea, tachycardia, or hemoptysis.

Objective Data

Check IV sites at least once per shift to see if a phlebitis or reddened area is developing at the insertion site. If a positive Homans' sign is detected during an assessment, notify the physician and do not perform another Homans' sign until a clot has been ruled out. Assess the skin for redness, tenderness, hardness, or warmth, and measure both legs to determine baseline measurements. Measure the circumference of the affected leg every shift to determine an increase or decrease in swelling. Assess peripheral pulses every 4 hours and more frequently if the client experiences increased pain in the leg, cyanosis of the foot or extremity, or increased swelling. These are signs of an occlusion.

Nursing diagnoses for a client with a venous thrombosis include the following:

NURSING DIAGNOSES	PLANNING/OUTCOMES	NURSING INTERVENTIONS
*Ineffective **Tissue** Perfusion (Peripheral)* related to decreased venous blood flow and/or clot formation	The client will have adequate tissue perfusion.	Elevate the client's entire affected leg when on bed rest to improve venous return. When elevated, the leg should be slightly flexed at the knee with a pillow under the thigh and calf. Apply elastic support or intermittent pneumatic compression stockings on the client. Use intermittent pneumatic compression stockings only if a clot is not present. If the client has received thrombolytic or anticoagulant drugs, assess for signs of bleeding, which include hematuria, bruising, bleeding from the gums, and blood in the stool. Monitor pedal pulses and capillary refill and measure thigh or calf circumference daily.
*Acute **Pain*** related to inflammatory process	The client will state absence of pain.	If the client has phlebitis, apply warm moist soaks to the affected area as ordered. Administer acetaminophen or a nonsteroidal anti-inflammatory as ordered for discomfort.
Anxiety related to possibility of the clot becoming an embolus	The client will express anxiety about possible embolus.	Encourage client to discuss the possibility of embolus formation.

Evaluation: Evaluate each outcome to determine how it has been met by the client.

VARICOSE VEINS

Varicose veins, also called **varicosities**, are visibly prominent, dilated, and twisted veins, usually in the lower extremities, but the veins in the esophagus (esophageal varices) and anus (hemorrhoids) can also be affected. Usually, the saphenous vein is affected in the leg. Women are more prone to varicose veins than men. Risk factors for developing varicose veins are a familial tendency, congenital abnormalities, pregnancy, obesity, constrictive clothing, and occupations that require prolonged standing. Pregnancy and obesity cause more pressure in the veins of the legs.

The causes of varicose veins are incompetent valves and veins that have lost their elasticity. The wall of the vessel is weakened from a lack of elastin or collagen and is unable to support the normal pressure of the blood in the vessel. The vein dilates as the blood in it flows backward. As the walls of the vein dilate, the valves become incapable of holding the blood and allow blood to leak backward through the space between the valves. Refer to Figure 5-5C. The client has pain in the feet and ankles, swelling, and ulcers on the skin. Trendelenburg's test is used for diagnosis.

MEDICAL–SURGICAL MANAGEMENT

Medical

Varicose veins are usually treated conservatively with elastic support hose, elevation of the legs when sitting, not crossing legs, and ankle and leg exercises.

Sclerotherapy involves injecting a chemical into the vein, causing the vein to become sclerosed (hardened) so blood no longer flows through it. A compression bandage or elastic stocking is applied to the extremity for 4 to 5 days. The client wears support hose for 5 more weeks. Complications of the procedure are **necrosis** (tissue death) at the injection site, vasospasm, allergic responses, and **hemolysis** (destruction of red blood cells).

Surgical

In more severe cases, varicose veins can be ligated (tied off) or stripped. **Vein stripping** involves introducing a wire into a vein. The wire has collapsible claws on the end. As the wire is withdrawn, the claws expand and strip the walls of the vein. This measure is used when there is a threat of thrombus or leg ulcers. **Vein ligation** is tying off an involved section of a vein with suture. Endovenous laser ablation is another method of treating varicose veins.

Pharmacological

Analgesics are given for leg discomfort. Anticoagulants may be given to prevent clot formation.

Activity

The client is encouraged to exercise regularly. Walking is a very good exercise to improve circulation because the blood circulates faster in response to an increased heartbeat. Muscles in the legs apply pressure to the veins, forcing the blood toward the heart. Ankle exercises such as rotating the ankle in circular motions also improves circulation.

Health Promotion

Encourage clients with a familial tendency for varicose veins to elevate their legs 6 to 10 inches on a small stool when sitting in a chair. Frequent position changes and not standing in one spot for extended times also improve circulation.

NURSING MANAGEMENT

Assist the client in elevating the legs above the heart when in bed or elevating the feet 6 to 10 inches on a pillow or stool when sitting in a chair.

After sclerotherapy, the affected area may be tender and discolored. Most discoloration will disappear in a few weeks, but a darkened pigmentation may last for 6 to 8 months. Repeated sclerotherapy may be needed. Encourage the client to maintain a walking exercise program to improve circulation to the legs.

After a vein stripping, the client is on bed rest for the first 24 hours. Elastic hose are worn continuously for 5 days to compress the blood into the deeper veins and for 5 weeks after the surgery. Administer pain medication 30 minutes before the client ambulates until walking is tolerated without discomfort. Encourage walking and leg exercises.

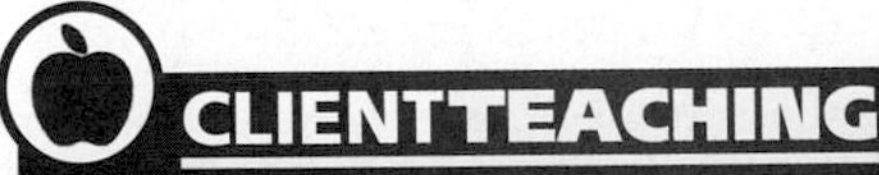

Varicose Veins

Apply support hose after the legs have been elevated for an extended time, 10 to 15 minutes, so the venous blood drains from the legs. Application before getting out of bed in the morning is ideal. Do not fold or roll hose down from the top because this would act like a tourniquet, causing pooling of blood. Smooth the hose on the legs because wrinkles or creases may cause extra pressure, leading to stasis or pooling of blood or pressure ulcers. Remove hose daily so the leg can be washed and dried before reapplication.

BUERGER'S DISEASE (THROMBOANGIITIS OBLITERANS)

Buerger's disease is an inflammatory disease of small and medium arteries and veins that leads to vascular obstruction. Inflammation occurs in the adventitia and media layers of the vessels and may affect only a portion of the vessel or the entire vessel. Hands and feet are mainly involved, but the wrists and lower extremities may also be affected. The distal tips of the hands and feet are pale, but as the disease progresses, the hands and feet become reddened when held in a dependent position. At first, pain in the palm of the hand and arch of the foot is the main symptom. Pain becomes more severe with disease progression, and as ischemia affects the nerves, the client may experience numbness, burning, pain when at rest, and decreased sensation in the hands and lower extremities. The dorsalis pedis, posterior tibia, and ulnar and radial pulses are weak or absent. Skin color changes, cold sensitivity, ulcers, and gangrene occur in the later stages.

Buerger's disease occurs primarily in men between the ages of 20 and 40 of Israeli, Indian, and Asian descent. There is a correlation between smoking and Buerger's disease. Tests for diagnosis include arteriography and Doppler ultrasound.

Medical–Surgical Management

Medical

The client is encouraged to stop smoking and is referred to a smoking clinic or seminar. Buerger-Allen exercises are recommended and explained. Buerger-Allen exercises consist of elevating the legs until they blanch and supporting them at that angle for 2 to 3 minutes. The legs are then lowered to a dependent position until they become red and supported at that level for 5 to 10 minutes. The legs are then placed flat on the bed with the client in a supine position for 10 minutes. The exercises are repeated as tolerated by the client.

Surgical

A sympathectomy (excision of a nerve, plexus, or ganglion of the sympathetic portion of the autonomic nervous system) is done to relieve pain and prevent vasospasm in the affected area. Digits and toes are amputated if gangrene occurs.

Pharmacological

Analgesics are given to control pain. Vasodilators are given to increase circulation to the affected area.

Nursing Management

Nursing diagnoses and interventions are the same as for other obstructive vascular conditions and are described under Raynaud's disease.

RAYNAUD'S DISEASE/ PHENOMENON

Raynaud's disease or primary Raynaud's is an intermittent spasm of the digital arteries and arterioles resulting in decreased circulation to the fingers and toes. Sometimes the tip of the nose and ears are also affected. The cause of the condition is unknown but seems to be related to vasospastic disorders, a disturbance with the innervation of the sympathetic nervous system, and angiography complications.

MEMORYTRICK

Peripheral Vascular Disorders Assessment

The nurse remembers 5 Ps when assessing clients with peripheral vascular disorders:

P = Pain
P = Pulse
P = Pallor
P = Paresthesia
P = Paralysis

During a spasm that lasts approximately 15 minutes, the fingers become pale and then cyanotic. As the circulation returns to the fingers, the fingertips become reddened and the person experiences a tingling or throbbing pain in the fingers. Some people experience only pallor and cyanosis. The episode may last 1 to 2 hours. Symptoms usually occur when the person is exposed to cold or experiences emotional stress. Gangrene is not common but can occur in the fingertips. Ulcerations can also occur and are difficult to heal because of decreased circulation in the fingers.

When associated with a connective tissue or collagen vascular disease, medications, or occupational trauma, the condition is called Raynaud's phenomenon or secondary Raynaud's. Raynaud symptoms may occur 10 years before the related disease is diagnosed. A 2-year history of signs and symptoms with no evidence of underlying disease, especially an autoimmune disease, is necessary for a diagnosis of Raynaud's disease.

Raynaud's is more prevalent in cold climates. Women are nine times more likely to be affected than men (Raynauds Association, 2008). Primary Raynaud's begins between the ages of 15 and 25 (NIAMS, 2006). Secondary Raynaud's begins later in life, between the ages of 35 to 40 (NIAMS, 2006). Persons who use vibrating hand tools such as air hammers or grinding wheels or who perform repetitive movements such as typing or playing the piano are at risk.

Diagnostic examinations include a complete blood count, digital blood pressure measurement, digital plethysmography waveforms, and a cold-challenge test. A digital blood pressure of 30 mm Hg below the brachial pressure indicates a digital artery obstruction. A sedimentation rate, antinuclear antibody, and rheumatoid factor determine the presence of autoimmune diseases. During a cold-challenge test, thermistors are placed on the fingers and a baseline temperature is taken. The hands are submerged into ice water for 20 seconds and then removed. The temperature of the hands is then taken every 5 minutes until it returns to the baseline level. Hand x-rays determine the presence of subcutaneous calcium deposits and narrowing of bone in the digits. The diagnostic tests distinguish between Raynaud's phenomenon and Raynaud's disease. If a client has unilateral or single-digit Raynaud's, an obstruction or emboli is suspected.

Medical–Surgical Management

Medical

Raynaud's phenomenon is treated conservatively. The client is assessed regularly for symptoms of autoimmune diseases. If the symptoms of Raynaud's are caused by a vasospastic disease, relief is best achieved with medications. Alternative therapies such as relaxation techniques and biofeedback may be beneficial.

Surgical

A sympathectomy is sometimes done to alleviate the client's symptoms; however, it usually provides temporary relief and is not a routine treatment.

Pharmacological

Calcium channel blockers, such as nifedipine (Adalat, Procardia), amlodipine (Norvasc), and diltiazem hydrochloride (Cardizem), improve symptoms in severe Raynaud's phenomenon by vasodilating small vessels in the hands and feet and decreasing the frequency and intensity of attacks (Mayo Clinic, 2008). Clients may be given nifedipine (Adalat, Procardia) at night for severe cases of Raynaud's phenomenon. Clients may also take the medication 1 to 2 hours before engaging in an outdoor activity during cold weather. They may not need to take the medication during warmer months. Alpha blockers, such as prazosin hydrochloride (Minipress) and doxazosin mesylate (Cardura), interfere with the effects of norepinephrine, a hormone causing vasoconstriction. Some clients benefit from topical nitroglycerin. Other drugs in Raynaud's research trials are losartan potassium (Cozaar), sildenafil citrate (Viagra), fluoxetine hydrochloride (Prozac), and prostaglandins (Mayo Clinic, 2008).

Beta blockers, birth control pills, cold medications, and diet pills cause some clients to have Raynaud's phenomenon. Chemotherapy drugs such as bleomycin sulfate (Blenoxane) and cisplatin, CDDP (Platinol), also cause secondary Raynaud's.

Health Promotion

Encourage the client to avoid decongestants, caffeine, exposure to cold, repetitive hand movements, and stressful situations. Also encourage the client to quit smoking and avoid secondary smoke because nicotine is a potent vasoconstrictor. Stress management techniques (e.g., biofeedback and tai chi) may assist in alleviating some distress from the condition. Wearing mittens in cold weather or when handling cold foods keeps fingers warmer than wearing gloves. Keeping the entire body warm is helpful.

Nursing Management

Assess digits for pallor, blanching, cyanosis, rubor, coldness, and texture. Encourage client to keep indoor temperature at a comfortable level. Teach relaxation exercises to enhance circulation. Encourage the use of mitts when pushing shopping carts and the wearing of wear mittens and socks to bed. Apply lotion regularly to prevent dry, chapped skin.

NURSING PROCESS

Assessment

Subjective Data

Ask the client how frequently the vasospastic episodes occur, what symptoms are experienced, what triggers the episodes, which digits are affected during an episode, and how long the incident lasts. Inquire about daily activities the client finds difficult, such as tying shoes, washing dishes, or handling frozen foods. Obtain a history of occupational activities.

Objective Data

Assess the digits for pallor, blanching, cyanosis, rubor, coldness, and texture. If the disease is longstanding, the digits may be tapered and the skin shiny in appearance. There may be ulcerated or gangrenous areas on the fingertips.

Nursing diagnoses for a client with Raynaud's disease include the following:

NURSING DIAGNOSES	PLANNING/OUTCOMES	NURSING INTERVENTIONS
*Ineffective **Tissue** Perfusion (Peripheral)* related to vasospasm of peripheral arteries	The client will have fewer vasospastic episodes and increased circulation in digits.	Encourage the client to use caution when engaging in activities that may cause a cut or scratch because healing may be impaired because of decreased circulation. If a client has ulcers, wash the areas with soap and water and administer prescribed medications such as ciprofloxacin (Cipro) and intravenous iloprost.
*Acute **Pain*** related to decreased circulation in digits	The client will experience decreased pain as vasospasms are controlled.	Teach client to keep the indoor temperature at a comfortable level to avoid ischemic attacks. Encourage client to avoid dramatic changes in environmental temperatures (e.g., entering a cold air-conditioned room during hot summer months). Encourage the client to wear woolen or wind-proof gloves or mittens and layered clothes when exposed to colder temperatures. Mittens may be better than gloves so the fingers can obtain warmth from each other. Chemical warming devices may be used inside gloves and shoes. Encourage the client to stop smoking and make a referral to a smoking cessation clinic. Teach the client relaxation exercises that may decrease the number of ischemic attacks.
*Situational Low **Self-esteem*** related to inability of hands to perform activities of daily living	The client will learn ways to handle activities of daily living.	Encourage client to use mitts or potholders when removing items from the freezer or handling cold food to decrease the risk of a Raynaud's episode. Clients can wear mittens or

(Continues)

Nursing diagnoses for a client with Raynaud's disease include the following: (Continued)

NURSING DIAGNOSES	PLANNING/OUTCOMES	NURSING INTERVENTIONS
		socks to bed. Use of insulated mugs, foam rubber holders, or stemware glasses may reduce ischemic attacks. Instruct client to wash vegetables under tepid water instead of cold, to bathe in lukewarm water, and to apply lotion regularly to prevent dry and chapped skin. Encourage client to use gloves when pushing shopping carts or operating some vibrating machines because this may decrease the cold sensation and soften the vibration.

Evaluation: Evaluate each outcome to determine how it has been met by the client.

CASE STUDY

L.J., a 55-year-old truck driver, is admitted to the emergency room with a feeling of heavy squeezing pressure in his sternal area. The pain is radiating to his left shoulder. He is diaphoretic, short of breath, and nauseated. He states the sternal pain came on suddenly while watching a football game. He had been mowing his yard and decided to rest. The emergency physician gives L.J. a nitroglycerin tablet and connects him to an ECG monitor. Cardiac biomarkers (CK-MB, troponin, and myoglobin) with an IMA and a chest x-ray are requested STAT. Morphine sulfate 2 mg is given intravenously. Oxygen is given by mask at 4 liters/minute. L.J.'s apical pulse is 102 beats/min and his blood pressure is 130/88 mm Hg. A cardiac catheterization with fluoroscopy is ordered to determine the patency of the coronary blood vessels and functioning of the heart muscle.

Three hours after admission, crackles are heard in the lungs.

The following questions will guide your development of a nursing care plan for the case study.

1. List symptoms/clinical manifestations, other than L.J.'s, that a client may experience when having a myocardial infarction.
2. List two reasons morphine sulfate was given to L.J.
3. List two other diagnostic tests that may have been ordered for L.J.
4. List subjective and objective data a nurse would want to obtain about L.J.
5. Write three individualized nursing diagnoses and goals for L.J.
6. L.J. is moved from the critical care unit. List pertinent nursing actions a nurse would do in caring for L.J. related to:

   oxygenation activity
   cardiac output medications
   comfort/rest teaching
7. List teaching that L.J. will need before his discharge.
8. List at least three successful client outcomes for L.J.
9. How might the MI symptoms for a woman differ from L.J.'s symptoms?

SUMMARY

- The function of the heart is to pump blood through the vascular system. Blood is the medium by which oxygen and nutrients are provided to the body cells and carbon dioxide and waste products are removed from the body cells.
- The coronary arteries supply blood to the heart. If the blood flow through these vessels becomes diminished or occluded, ischemia to the heart tissue occurs, resulting in angina or a myocardial infarction.
- Typical symptoms experienced by a person with cardiac problems include chest pain, dyspnea, edema, fainting, palpitations, diaphoresis, and fatigue.
- A lipid profile and cardiac biomarkers provide diagnostic information about the risk of heart disease and the occurrence of a myocardial infarction.
- A dysrhythmia is an irregularity in the rate, rhythm, or conduction of the electrical system of the heart.

- Inflammatory or infectious conditions of the heart include endocarditis, myocarditis, and pericarditis. Endocarditis may cause valvular heart disease with the possibility of the valve needing to be surgically repaired (valvuloplasty) or replaced with a mechanical (caged-ball valve or tilting-disk valve) or biological valve from a calf, pig, or human.
- Atherosclerosis causes a narrowing and occluding of vessels and is a primary cause of angina and myocardial infarction.
- Surgical treatment for angina includes a PTCA, intracoronary stent, transcatheter ablation, or a coronary artery bypass graft.
- Heart failure is often the final stage of many other heart conditions in which the heart is no longer able to fulfill the demands of the body.
- To assess the peripheral vascular system, the nurse assesses pain, pulse, pallor, paresthesia, and paralysis.
- Three factors leading to the formation of a clot—pooling of blood, vessel trauma, and a coagulation problem—are called Virchow's triad.
- A client with a DVT may be asymptomatic or may have warmth and tenderness at the site, edema of the extremity, a positive Homans' sign, cyanosis of the foot, and a sensation of heaviness or tightness in the extremity.
- It is important for the nurse to measure the leg circumference every shift and check peripheral pulses for the client with a thrombus.
- The cause of varicose veins is incompetent valves and veins that have lost their elasticity.
- Primary Raynaud's disease is an intermittent spasm of the digital arteries and arterioles, resulting in decreased circulation to the digits.
- Symptoms of an aneurysm depend on the location of the aneurysm in the body. Aneurysms are often asymptomatic until they start leaking or pressing on other structures.

REVIEW QUESTIONS

1. To assess a client with right-sided heart failure, the nurse would:
   1. listen for a pericardial friction rub.
   2. listen for a muffled S_1 and S_2 heart sound.
   3. check for distended neck veins with the bed at a 45-degree angle.
   4. assess for radiation of the squeezing sensation under the sternum.
2. It is important to teach a client with angina to:
   1. take antibiotics before having dental work.
   2. carry nitroglycerin tablets at all times.
   3. perform the Valsalva maneuver daily.
   4. massage the carotid sinuses in the neck.
3. A nursing intervention to improve cardiac output is:
   1. encouraging the client to verbalize fears.
   2. teaching the side effects of new medications.
   3. a referral to a dietitian for low-sodium diet instructions.
   4. administer oxygen per physician orders.
4. Instructions to a client on anticoagulant therapy include:
   1. taking Coumadin twice a day.
   2. watching for symptoms of bleeding.
   3. taking over-the-counter medications as needed.
   4. no dietary or activity limitations.
5. The first step of the stepped-care approach in treating hypertension is:
   1. lifestyle changes.
   2. diuretics.
   3. beta blockers.
   4. adding a second or third antihypertensive.
6. A client is admitted to the emergency room with chest pain. The first nursing intervention is:
   1. attach the client to an ECG monitor.
   2. administer oxygen.
   3. listen to the heart sounds.
   4. order cardio biomarkers.
7. A client is diagnosed with coronary artery disease and his physicians recommended a coronary bypass giving the client the option of a robotic CABG. The client and his wife ask the advantages of a robotic CABG as compared to a traditional CABG. The nurse states the advantages of robotic CABG as: (Select all that apply.)
   1. The client has less bleeding.
   2. The client's recovery is 6 to 8 weeks.
   3. The client will require less medication.
   4. The surgeon will do a complete sternotomy.
   5. The client has a risk of increased infection.
   6. The client's hospital stay is shorter.
8. What ECG wave represents ventricular repolarization?
   1. P wave.
   2. QRS complex.
   3. ST segment.
   4. T wave.
9. A client is admitted to the floor from an intensive care unit and has a pacemaker pulse generator lying beside his body. The client asks whether he will have to live the rest of his life with the pulse generator hanging from his body. The nurse's best response is:
   1. No, this is a temporary pacemaker. Your heart has maintained a regular rhythm for 2 days. As your heartbeat continues to stabilize, it will be removed.
   2. No, this is a temporary pacemaker. If you would need a permanent pacemaker, the energy source would be placed in a belt you will wear around your waist.

3. Yes. The pacemaker wires will be connected to an energy source and placed in a belt you will wear around your waist.
4. No, this pacemaker will be changed to an ICD that will regulate your heart with intermittent electrical shocks. It will also regulate the rhythm of your heart.

10. A client was admitted to the unit from the postoperative recovery room. He has a history of venous thrombus. Nursing measures to prevent the formation of a clot are to: (Select all that apply.)
    1. ambulate the client as soon as ordered.
    2. encourage the client to exercise his legs, such as making circular movements with his feet to increase circulation.
    3. encourage the client to rest in bed when he is dismissed.
    4. request an order for a pneumatic compression device if the client does not have one.
    5. check Homans' sign every shift.
    6. limit his fluid intake to 200 mL per shift.

REFERENCES/SUGGESTED READINGS

Ahmed, A. (2008). An update on the role of digoxin in older adults with chronic heart failure. *Geriatrics Aging, 11*(1), 37–41.

American Association for Clinical Chemistry. (2006). IMA. Retrieved on January 14, 2009 from http://labtestsonline.org/understanding/analytes/ima/multiprint.html

American Association for Clinical Chemistry. (2008). Cardiac biomarkers. Retrieved on January 14, 2009 from http://labtestsonline.org/understanding/analytes/a1c/glance.htmardiac_biomarkers/glance-2.html

American Association for Clinical Chemistry. (2009). Cardiac risk assessment. Retrieved on 1/19/09 from http://labtestsonline.org/understanding/analytes/cardiac_risk/glance.html

American Heart Association (AHA). (2001a). Rheumatic heart disease statistics. Retrieved from http://216. 185.112.5/presenter.jhtml?identifier=4712

American Heart Association (AHA). (2001b). Women, heart disease and stroke statistics. Retrieved from http://216. 185.112.5/presenter.jhtml?identifier=4787

American Heart Association (AHA). (2007). Implantable cardioverter defibrillator. Retrieved on January 16, 2009 at http://www.americanheart.org/presenter.jhtml?identifier=11227

American Heart Association (AHA). (2007a). Cardiovascular disease death rates decline, but risk factors still exact heavy toll. *AHA News.* Retrieved January 12, 2009 from http://www.americanheart.org/print_presenter.jhtml?identifier=3052670

American Heart Association (AHA). (2007b). Heart attack symptoms and warning signs. *AHA News.* Retrieved January 12, 2009 from http://www.americanheart.org/print_presneter.jhtml?identifier=4595

Ammon, S. (2001). Managing patients with heart failure. *AJN, 101*(12), 34–40.

Baker, S., & Graziano, J. (2003). A new device for heart failure. *RN, 66*(3), 32–35.

Beattie, S. (1999). Cut the risks for cardio cath patients. *RN, 62*(1), 50–54.

Beattie, S. (2002). New biomarkers may predict CAD. *RN, 65*(9), 47–54.

Bender, R. (in press). *Assessing the Cardiovascular System.*

Bither, C., & Apple, S. (2001). Home management of the failing heart. *AJN, 101*(12), 41–45.

Bond, E., Nelson, K., Germany, C., & Smart, A. (2003). The left ventricular assist device. *AJN, 103*(1), 32–39.

Breen, P. (2000). DVT: What every nurse should know. *RN, 63*(4), 58–62.

Broadcast Newsroom. (2009). Reminder: Cardica announces webcast of internationally renowned cardiothoracic surgeon, Dt. Sudhir Srivastava, performing robotic cardiac bypass surgery using revolutionary anastomosis device. Retrieved on January 19, 2009 from http://www.broadcastnewsroom.com/articles/viewarticle.jsp?id=622186

Bubien, R. (2000). A new beat on an old rhythm. *AJN, 100*(1), 42–50.

Bulechek, G., Butcher, H., McCloskey, J., & Dochterman, J., eds. (2008). *Nursing Interventions Classification (NIC)* (5th ed.). St. Louis, MO: Mosby/Elsevier.

Carelock, J., & Clark, A. (2001). Heart failure: Pathophysiologic mechanisms. *AJN, 101*(12), 26–33.

Centers for Disease Control and Prevention (CDC). (2002). Health, United States 2002. Retrieved from www.cdc. gov/nchs/data/hus/tables/2002/02hus068.pdf

Chase, S. (2000). Hypertensive crisis. *RN, 63*(6), 62–67.

Chavez, J., & Brewer, C. (2002). Stopping the shock slide. *RN, 65*(9), 30–34. Delmar Cengage Learning.

Cheek, D., & Cesan, A. (2003). What's different about heart disease in women? *Nursing2003, 33*(8), 36–42.

Cleveland Clinic. (2009a). Robotically assisted heart surgery. Retrieved on January 19, 2009 from http://my.clevelandclinic.org/heart/services/surgery/roboticallyassisted.aspx

Cleveland Clinic. (2009b). What is minimally invasive heart surgery. Retrieved on January 19, 2009 from http://my.clevelandclinic.org/heart/disorders/mini_invasivehs.aspx

Corona, G. (1999). Pacemakers: Keeping the beat today. *RN, 62*(12), 50–55.

Crumlish, C., Bracken, J., Hand, M., Keenan, K., Ruggiero, H., & Simmons, D. (2000). When time is muscle. *AJN, 100*(1), 26–35.

Dakin, C. (2008). New approaches to heart failure in the ED. *American Journal of Nursing, 108*(3), 68–71.

Daniels, R. (2010). Delmar's guide to laboratory and diagnostic tests, (2nd ed.). Clifton Park, NY: Delmar Cengage Learning.

Darty, S., Thomas, M., Neagle, C., Link, H., Wesley-Farrington, D., and Hundley, G. (2002). Cardiovascular magnetic resonance imaging. *AJN, 102*(12), 34–37.

Davis, S. (2002). How the heart failure picture has changed. *Nursing2002, 32*(11), 36–44.

Day, M. (2003). Recognizing and managing DVT. *Nursing 2003, 33*(5), 36–41.

deSouza, I. and Ward, C. (2008). *Ventricular tachycardia.* Retrieved January 16, 2009 from http://emedicine.medscape.com/article/760963-print

Fort, C. (2002). Get pumped to prevent DVT. *Nursing 2002, 32*(9), 50–52.

Freeman, J., & Hedges, C. (2003). Cardiac arrest: The effect on the brain. *AJN, 103*(6), 50–54.

Gehring, P. (April 2002). Perfecting your skills: Vascular assessment. *Travel Nursing Today (supplement to RN)* 16–24.

George, E., & Tasota, F. (2003). Predicting heart disease with C-reactive protein. *Nursing2003, 33*(5), 70–71.

Goldrick, B. (2003). Endocarditis associated with body piercing. *AJN, 103*(1), 26–27.

Goodreau, L. (2003). Coronary stenting—with a twist. *RN, 66*(1), 32–36.

Granger, B., & Miller, C. (2001). Acute coronary syndrome. *Nursing2001, 31*(11), 36–43.

Halm, M., & Penque, S. (1999). Heart disease in women. *AJN, 99*(4), 26–31.

Hays, D. (2003). Picturing reciprocal changes in an MI. *Nursing 2003, 33*(5), 53.

Hiller, G. (1999). Atrial fibrillation. *Nursing99, 29*(2), 27–31.

Hurley, M. (2003). The latest hypertension guidelines. *RN, 66*(8), 43–45.

Joint National Committee on Prevention, Detection, Evaluation, and Treatment of High Blood Pressure. (2003). The Seventh Report of the Joint National Committee on Prevention, Detection, Evaluation, and Treatment of High Blood Pressure. Retrieved from www.nhlbi.nih.gov/guidelines/ hypertension/index.htm

Joy, S. (2006). Women may delay treatment for acute myocardial infarction. *American Journal of Nursing, 107*(7), 16.

Klabunde, R. (2007). Cardiovascular physiology concepts. Retrieved on January 20, 2009 from http://www.cvphysiology.com/Blood%20Pressure/BP023.htm

Kowalczyk, T. (2002). A low-tech approach to venous congestion. *RN, 65*(10), 26–30.

Lab Tests Online. (2009). Cardiac Risk Assessment. Retrieved January 19, 2009 from http://labtestonline.org/understanding/analytes/cardiac_risk/glance.html

Lazzara, D. (1999). Shocking facts about semiautomatic defibrillation. *Nursing99, 29*(4), 55–57.

Lewis, A. (1999). Cardiovascular emergency. *Nursing99, 29*(6), 49–51.

Lewis, S., Heitkemper, M., & Dirksen, S. (2004). *Medical–surgical nursing: Assessment and management of clinical problems* (6th ed.). St. Louis, MO: Mosby.

Linton, A., Matteson, M., & Maebius, N. (2000). Introductory nursing care of adults (2nd ed.). Philadelphia: W. B. Saunders.

Lundberg, G. (2008). The Medscape medical minute: Recovery PVCs during treadmill testing tied to heart disease. *Medscape Journal of Medicine, 10*(4), 93. Retrieved on January 16, 2009 from http://www.medscape.com/viewarticle/571891_print

Macklin, D. (2003). Phlebitis. *AJN, 103*(2), 55–60.

Malacaria, B., & Feloney, C. (2003). Going with the flow of anticoagulant therapy. *Nursing2003, 33*(3), 36–42.

Mancini, M., & Kaye, W. (1999). AEDs: Changing the way you respond to cardiac arrest. *AJN, 99*(5), 26–30.

Marcolongo, E. (2003). Isolated systolic hypertension—not your usual silent killer. *Nursing2003, 33*(1), 32hn1–32hn3.

Martin, T. (2002). How heart failure complicates care. *Nursing2002, 32*(7), 32hn1–32hn5.

Mayo Clinic (2002). Aneurysms. Retrieved from www. mayoclinic.com/findinformation./invoke.cfm?objectid=FE3FE459-7DIE-405F-95E9339CD2E974B

Mayo Clinic. (2008). Raynaud's disease. Retrieved on January 21, 2009 from http://www.mayoclinic.com/health/raynauds-disease/DS00433/DSECTION=treatments-an

McAvoy, J. (2000). Cardiac pain: Discovering the unexpected. *Nursing2000, 30*(3), 34–39.

McConnell, E. (2002a). Applying antiembolism stockings. *Nursing2002, 32*(4), 17.

McConnell, E. (2002b). Using an automated external defibrillator. *Nursing2002, 32*(10), 18.

McCormick, J., & Deeg, M. (2000). Pharmacologic treatment of dyslipidemia. *AJN, 100*(2), 55–60.

McGrath, A. (1997). Clinical snapshot: Raynaud's syndrome. *AJN, 97*(1), 34–35.

McKinney, B. (1999). Solving the puzzle of heart failure. *Nursing99, 29*(5), 33–39.

Metules, T. (1999). Cardiac tamponade. *RN, 62*(12), 26–31.

Metules, T. (2003). IABP therapy: Getting patients treatment fast. *RN, 66*(5), 56–62.

Miracle, V. (2001a). Act fast during a hypertensive crisis. *Nursing 2001, 31*(9), 50–51.

Miracle, V. (2001b). Putting the brakes on pericarditis. *Nursing2001, 31*(4), 44–45.

Moorhead, S., Johnson, M., Maas, M., & Swanson, E. (2007). *Nursing Outcomes Classification (NOC)* (4th ed). St. Louis, MO: Elsevier–Health Sciences Division.

Mosley, M., Oenning, V., & Melinik, G. (1999). Methemoglobinemia. *AJN, 99*(5), 47.

Nagle, B., & Nee, C. (2002). Acute myocardial infarction. *Nursing2002, 32*(10), 50–54.

National Institute of Arthritis and Musculoskeletal and Skin Diseases (NIAMS). (2006). *Raynaud's Phenomenon* (NIH Publication No.06-4911). Retrieved on January 21, 2009 from http://www.niams.nih.gov/Health_Info/Raynauds_Phenomenon/default.asp

National Institutes of Health (NIH). (2002). New recommendations to prevent high blood pressure issues. Retrieved from http://www.nhlbi.nih.gov/news/press/02-10-15.htm

North American Nursing Diagnosis Association International. (2010). *NANDA-I nursing diagnoses: Definitions and classification 2009–2011*. Ames, IA: Wiley Blackwell.

Oliver-McNeil, S. (2001). Treating hypertrophic cardiomyopathy without surgery. *Nursing2001, 31*(2), 32cc1 32cc4.

Overbaugh, K. (2009). Acute coronary syndrome. *American Journal of Nursing, 109*(5), 42–60.

Palatnik, A. (2001). How cardiac drugs do what they do. *Nursing2001, 31*(5), 54–60.

Pope, B. (2002). Heart failure. *Nursing2002, 32*(8), 50–51.

Pope, W. (2002). Angioplasty & stenting in the carotid? *RN, 65*(6), 54–59.

Raynaud's Association, Inc. (2008). What is Raynaud's? Retrieved on January 21, 2009 from http://www.raynauds.org/raynauds/index.cfm

Reger, T., & Vargas, G. (1999). The return of the radial artery in CABG. *AJN, 99*(9), 26–30.

Ross, G., & DeJong, M. (1999). Pericardial tamponade. *AJN, 99*(2), 35.

Ryan, D. (2000). Is it an MI? A lab primer. *RN, 63*(1), 26–30.

Shaffer, R. (2002). ICD therapy: The patient's perspective. *AJN, 102*(2), 46–49.

Sims, J., & Miracle, V. (2001). Getting the lowdown on hypotension. *Nursing2001, 31*(10), 56–57.

Siomko, A. (2000). Demystifying cardiac markers. *AJN, 100*(1), 36–40.

Spratto, G., & Woods, A. (2010). 2010 Delmar's Nurses Drug Handbook. Clifton Park, NY: Delmar Cengage Learning.

Stanford Hospital and Clinics. (2009). Pacemaker/implantable cardioverter defibrillator (ICD) insertion. Stanford University Medical Center. Retrieved January 16, 2009 from http://www.stanfordhospital.com/healthLib/greystone/heartCenter/heartProcedures/cemakerImplantableCardioverterDefibrillatorICDInsertion

U.S. Food and Drug Administration (FDA). (2002). Medtronic In Sync ICD model 7272dual chamber implantable cardioverter defibrillator system with cardiac resynchronization therapy—P010031. Retrieved on January 16, 2009 from http://www.fda.gov/cdrh/mda/docs/p010031.html

U.S. Food and Drug Administration (FDA). (2004). Ventricular assist device (VAD). Retrieved on January, 19, 2009 from http://www.fda.gov/hearthealth/treatments/medialdevices/vad.html

Willis, K. (2001). Gaining perspective on peripheral vascular disease. *Nursing2001, 31*(2), 32hn1–32hn4.

Woods, A. (1999). Managing hypertension. *Nursing99, 29*(3), 41–46.

Woods, A. (2001). Improving the odds against hypertension. *Nursing2001, 31*(8), 36–41.

Woods, A. (2002). High blood pressure (hypertension). *Nursing2002, 32*(4), 54–55.

Zangerm, D., Solomon, A., & Gersh, B. (2000). Contemporary management of angina: Part II. Medical management of chronic stable angina. *American Family Physician, 61*(1), 129–138.

RESOURCES

American Heart Association, http://www.americanheart.org

National Heart, Lung, and Blood Institute, http://www.nhlbi.nih.gov

President's Council on Physical Fitness and Sports, http://www.fitness.gov

Raynaud's Association, Inc., http://www.raynauds.org

The Mended Hearts, Inc., http://www.mendedhearts.org

U.S. Food and Drug Administration, http://www.fda.gov

FDA heart health online illustration: Prosthetic heart valve, http://www.fda.gov/hearthealth/flash/fda_26.html

FDA heart health online illustration: Ventricular assist device, http://www.fda.gov/hearthealth/flash/fda_25.html

CHAPTER 6
Hematologic and Lymphatic Systems

MAKING THE CONNECTION

Refer to the following chapters to increase your understanding of the hematologic and lymphatic systems:

Adult Health Nursing

- ***Oncology***
- ***Respiratory System***
- ***Cardiovascular System***
- ***Endocrine System***
- ***Immune System***

LEARNING OBJECTIVES

Upon completion of this chapter, you should be able to:

- Define key terms.
- Relate anatomy and physiology of the blood and lymph systems to disease processes.
- Relate diagnostic test results to the blood and lymph disorders.
- Describe nursing interventions in caring for clients with blood and lymph disorders.
- Assist in developing a nursing care plan for clients with blood and lymph disorders.

KEY TERMS

agranulocytosis
apheresis
autologous
bands
blastic phase
erythrocytapheresis
fibrinolysis
hemarthrosis
hematocrit
hematopoiesis
hemolysis
hyperuricemia
idiopathic
leukocytosis
leukopenia
lymphoma
phlebotomy
purpura
reticulocyte
sickle
thrombocytopenia

INTRODUCTION

The hematologic system of the body consists of blood and blood-forming organs. Blood consists of formed elements (red blood cells, white blood cells, and platelets) and plasma. As blood is pumped through the body, it carries essential substances to the tissues and removes waste products from the tissues. Disorders of the hematologic system usually result from abnormal production or functioning of the cells. Some of these disorders are the result of genetics, environment, or pathogenic organisms.

The lymph system consists of lymph vessels, nodes, and organs. Lymph vessels collect and return lymph fluid to the blood vessels through the right and left lymphatic ducts at the right and left subclavian veins. The functions of the lymph system are assisting with immunity, controlling edema, and absorbing digested fats.

Medical management, nursing diagnoses, goals, and interventions are given for each blood and lymph disorder. A thorough understanding of the blood and lymph disorders equips the nurse to provide quality client care.

ANATOMY AND PHYSIOLOGY REVIEW

The anatomy and physiology of the blood and lymphatic systems are discussed in the following section.

BLOOD

The heart pumps 5 to 6 liters of blood per minute through the circulatory system of an adult. Blood is an aqueous mixture consisting of plasma and cells (Figure 6-1).

Plasma

Plasma is a straw-colored liquid consisting of approximately 90% water and 10% proteins. The water component assists in transporting body nutrients, hormones, antibodies, electrolytes, and waste; regulating blood volume; and controlling body temperature. The proteins are albumin, globulins, and fibrinogen. Albumin controls the volume of the blood and blood pressure by osmotic pressure that pulls tissue fluid into the capillary system. There are three types of globulins: alpha, beta, and gamma. Alpha and beta globulins are secreted by the liver and are carrier molecules for substances. Gamma globulins are antibodies important in the immune response of the body. Fibrinogen changes into fibrin, a solid that controls bleeding in the blood-clotting mechanism of the body. The formed elements in plasma are red blood cells (RBCs), white blood cells (WBCs), and platelets.

Red Blood Cells

Red blood cells, also called erythrocytes, are the most numerous blood cells in the body, generally 4.5 to 6.1 million/mm^3 in an adult. RBCs are biconcave disks that do not have a nucleus. They are about the size of the smallest capillary but are flexible and capable of changing shape so they can squeeze through the capillaries.

RBCs, in conjunction with the respiratory and circulatory systems, oxygenate body tissues. In the capillary bed of the

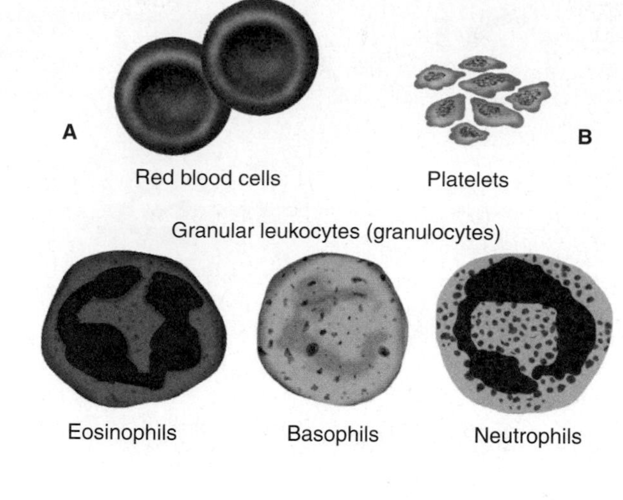

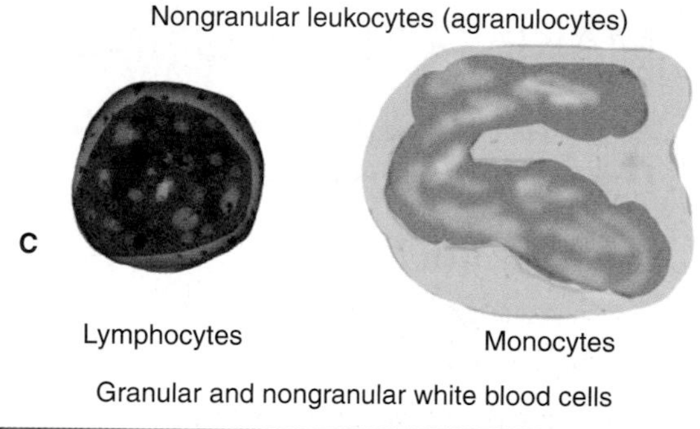

FIGURE 6-1 The Cells in Blood; *A,* Red Blood Cells (erythrocytes); *B,* Platelets (thrombocytes); *C,* White Blood Cells (leukocytes)

alveoli, blood receives oxygen (O_2), and carbon dioxide (CO_2) is eliminated. The O_2-enriched RBCs (oxyhemoglobin) carry O_2 to systemic capillaries, where O_2 is exchanged for carbon dioxide (CO_2). The CO_2-laden blood then returns the CO_2 to the alveoli in the lungs, where it is again exchanged for oxygen. The CO_2 is exhaled from the body with each breath. Hemoglobin is a protein in the RBC that carries O_2 and is responsible for the exchange of O_2 and CO_2.

The average life span for an RBC is 120 days. Blood cells originate from a single stem cell that proliferates and differentiates into lymphoid stem cells or blood stem cells (Figure 6-2). The lymphoid stem cells further divide and differentiate into T cells and B cells. The blood stem cells divide and differentiate

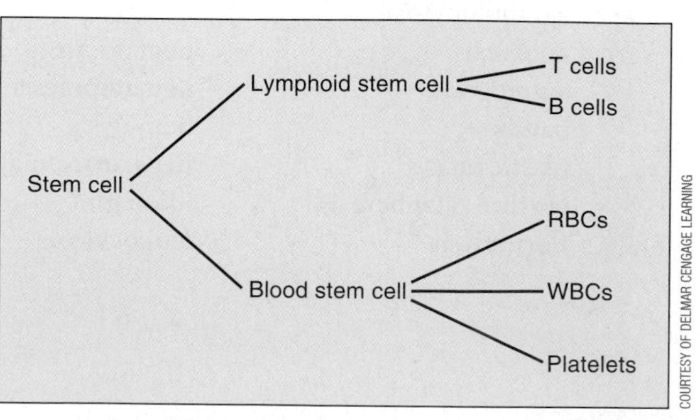

FIGURE 6-2 Origin of T Cells, B Cells, RBCs, WBCs, and Platelets

into RBCs, WBCs, and platelets. The process of blood cell production and development is called **hematopoiesis**. RBCs are produced daily by the bone marrow according to the demand of the body. When the partial pressure of O_2 decreases, a renal hormone, erythropoietin, stimulates the bone marrow to produce more immature RBCs (**reticulocytes**), which are released into the bloodstream. These reticulocytes develop into mature red blood cells. The number of circulating reticulocytes is used as a diagnostic tool for RBC disorders.

As RBCs age, their outer membrane deteriorates and they are destroyed by large macrophages in the liver and are filtered out of the body by the spleen. The iron from heme in the old RBCs is used in the production of new RBCs.

Hematocrit is the percentage of blood cells in a volume of blood. A normal hematocrit for a woman is 38% to 47% and, for a man, 40% to 54% (Daniels, 2009).

White Blood Cells

White blood cells (WBCs), also called leukocytes, fight infection and assist with immunity. The life span of a WBC varies, depending on the type of WBC. Neutrophils, basophils, and eosinophils live from a few hours to days, whereas lymphocytes and monocytes live from days to years. The normal WBC count is 4,100 to 10,800/mm^3 of blood (Daniels, 2009). An increased number of WBCs (**leukocytosis**) may signify the presence of an infection, inflammation, tissue necrosis, or leukemia. A decreased number of WBCs (**leukopenia**) may indicate bone marrow failure, a massive infection, dietary deficiencies, drug toxicity, or an autoimmune disease.

WBCs are classified as granulocytes or polymorphonuclear leukocytes (PMNs, or polys) and agranulocytes. The granulocytes have granules (grainy substances) in their cytoplasm, and the agranulocytes do not. Granulocytes are divided into three types: the neutrophils, eosinophils, and basophils. Agranulocytes are classified into two groups: monocytes and lymphocytes. Neutrophils are the most numerous, comprising approximately 60% of the total number of WBCs. The main function of neutrophils is to digest and kill microorganisms. If a client has an acute infection, the bone marrow is stimulated to produce more neutrophils, resulting in an increased circulation of immature neutrophils called **bands**. An increased production of neutrophils indicates the presence of an acute infection. An increased number of basophils and especially of eosinophils indicates an allergic response.

Monocytes become macrophages, cells that destroy dead and injured cells and bacteria. There are two types of lymphocytes, T cells and B cells, which are involved in the body's immune response.

Platelets

Platelets (thrombocytes) are not typical cells but nonnucleated, granular ovoid, or spindle-shaped cell fragments. The normal life span of a platelet is approximately 10 days. Platelets are active in the clotting mechanism of the body. When platelets flow over a rough or damaged area in a vessel, they adhere to the area and release thromboplastin and clotting factors that start the blood-clotting process. They also secrete prostaglandins and serotonin, which cause the vessel to constrict, thereby decreasing the blood flow through the area. Prothrombin, thromboplastin, and calcium ions form thrombin, which joins with fibrinogen to form fibrin. The fibrin strands seal the opening or area, and a clot is formed (Figure 6-3).

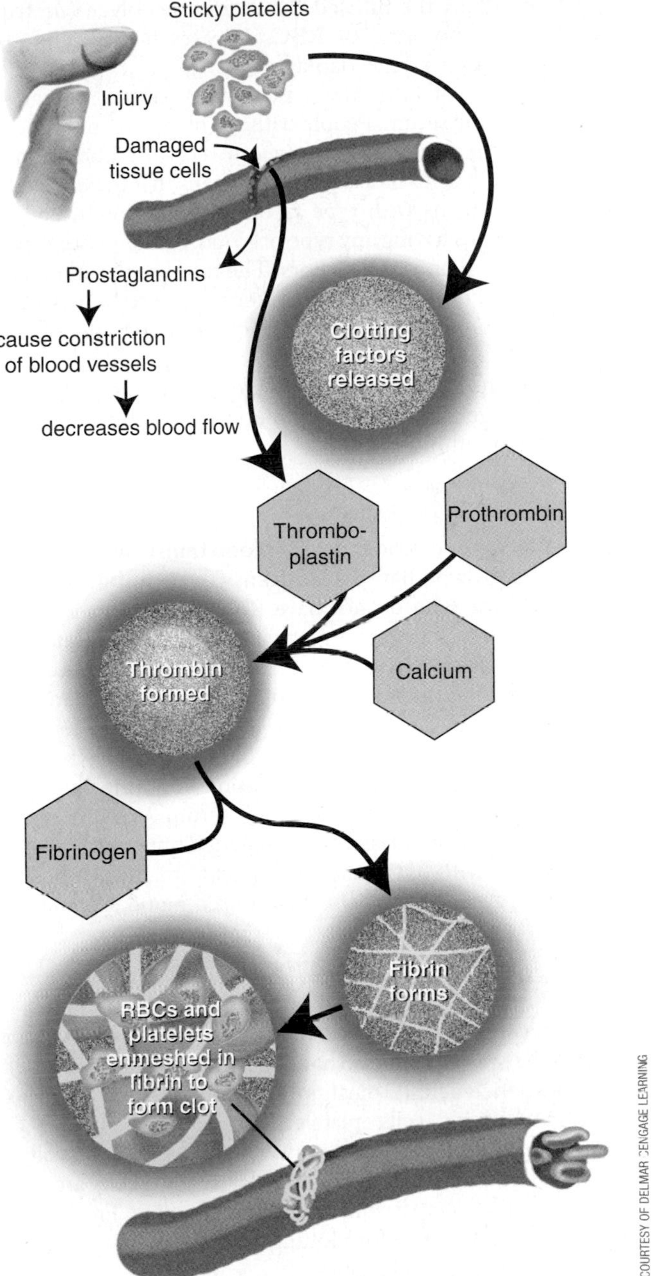

FIGURE 6-3 The Process of Clot Formation

Blood Types

Genetically determined antigens called agglutinogens are located on the surface of RBC membranes. The A and B antigens constitute the ABO blood group. If the A antigen is on the RBC membrane, the client has type A blood. If the B antigen is on the RBC membrane, the client has type B blood. If both an A and a B antigen are present, the client has type AB blood, and if no antigen is present, the client has type O blood.

Type A blood has anti-B antibodies in the serum, and type B blood has anti-A antibodies. If a person with type A blood receives type B blood during a transfusion, the anti-B antibodies attack the infused RBCs and hemolyze (destroy) them. The hemolyzing of RBCs releases hemoglobin that potentially causes kidney damage.

A person with AB blood has neither anti-A nor anti-B antibodies in the serum. People with AB blood are theoretically universal recipients because they can receive blood from all blood types. Type O blood has no antigens that the antibodies can attack. Persons with type O blood can theoretically give blood to persons having any type of blood. Persons with type O blood are called universal donors. The terms *universal recipient* and *universal donor* are only theoretical because during blood transfusions, blood incompatibilities can occur because of other types of antigens.

There are 14 different blood groups and more than 100 different antigens. The different blood groups vary in number with different ethnic groups.

Rh Factor

Another factor to consider during blood transfusions is the Rh factor. Persons who have Rh antigens (the D antigen) are Rh positive. Those who do not have Rh antigens on their RBC membranes are Rh negative. Approximately 85% of Caucasian people have Rh-positive blood and 15% have Rh-negative blood. The African-American population has 93% and 7%, respectively (Daniels, 2009).

If a person with Rh-negative blood is exposed to Rh-positive blood during a blood transfusion or during childbirth, anti-Rh antibodies form in the blood serum. When a person with Rh-negative blood is exposed a second time to Rh-positive blood, the anti-Rh antibodies will react with the Rh-positive blood and cause hemolysis of the infused blood and a severe blood reaction.

Blood Transfusions

Blood transfusions are given to replace needed blood components because of hemorrhage, anemia, clotting disorders, or blood deficiencies. Transfusable blood products are whole blood, packed red cells, platelets, fresh frozen plasma, and cryoprecipitate. Whole blood is given to increase blood volume and the various blood components. Packed red cells are given for anemia. Platelets assist in controlling bleeding. Fresh frozen plasma is administered for clotting disorders. Cryoprecipitate corrects fibrinogen deficiencies.

Before blood products are given, the lab does a type and crossmatch to check compatibility between the donor's blood type and Rh factor and the client's blood type and Rh factor. The lab also checks all blood products for HIV and hepatitis B and C viruses. When administering a blood transfusion, handle blood gently so the cells are not damaged. Administer blood within 30 minutes of obtaining it from the laboratory refrigerator. Take baseline vital signs—temperature, pulse, and blood pressure—before administering the blood product. Once the transfusion is started, temperature and pulse are measured after 15 minutes, 30 minutes, and then hourly; blood pressure is measured hourly during the transfusion. Blood is generally administered through a peripheral vein using an 18- or 19-gauge cannula. A large cannula is used so the blood cells do not break when passing through the cannula.

Before the transfusion, two nurses check the compatibility of the blood product with the client's blood. The first 50 mL is given within 5 to 10 minutes. The client is observed closely for a hemolytic blood reaction during this time. If a client experiences any symptoms of a reaction, the infusion is stopped immediately and the physician notified. Follow institutional protocol.

A blood transfusion should be completed within 4 hours of the start of administration. No medications are given at the blood administration site during infusion. Blood is administered with 0.9% sodium chloride solution since other solutions cause the blood to clot.

Autologous Transfusion If time and the client's condition permit, **autologous** ("from self") blood as opposed to homologous ("from a donor") blood is collected and saved for the client. This may be used for elective surgeries. An alternate procedure is to recover the blood lost during surgery and transfuse it back into the client. The use of autologous blood eliminates the possibility of a transfusion reaction and prevents the transmission of disease.

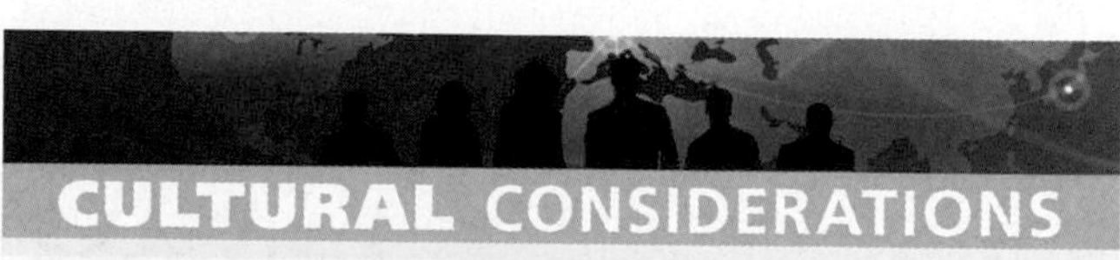

CULTURAL CONSIDERATIONS

Jehovah's Witnesses and Blood

- Many Jehovah's Witnesses agree to autologous blood transfusions.
- Some Jehovah's Witnesses allow the use of certain blood volume expanders and carry a card identifying the desired expanders.

Lymphatic System

The lymphatic, or lymph, system is a separate vessel system. The two main functions of the lymph system are to transport excess fluid from the interstitial spaces to the circulatory system and to protect the body against infectious organisms.

Lymph Fluid and Vessels

Lymph fluid is pale yellow. Fluid and substances move from the plasma through the capillary walls and become interstitial fluid (Figure 6-4). As fluid accumulates in the interstitial space, pressure within the interstitial space increases. The interstitial fluid then diffuses through the lymphatic vessel wall into the lymph vessel.

Semilunar valves in the lymphatic vessels assist the lymph system in returning the interstitial fluid, which is now called lymph, to the venous system. When the valves do not work properly or the vessels become obstructed, edema occurs. The pumping action or contractions of the skeletal muscles and the rhythmic action of the respiratory muscles assist in the movement of the lymph toward the subclavian veins. The right lymphatic duct drains lymph from the right side of the head, neck, thorax, and arm into the right subclavian vein. The lymph from the rest of the body drains into the left subclavian vein through the thoracic duct.

Lymph Nodes

Lymph nodes are scattered throughout the body along the lymph vessels (Figure 6-5) and contain dense patches of lymphocytes and macrophages. Lymphocytes act against such foreign particles as viruses and bacteria. Macrophages ingest and destroy foreign

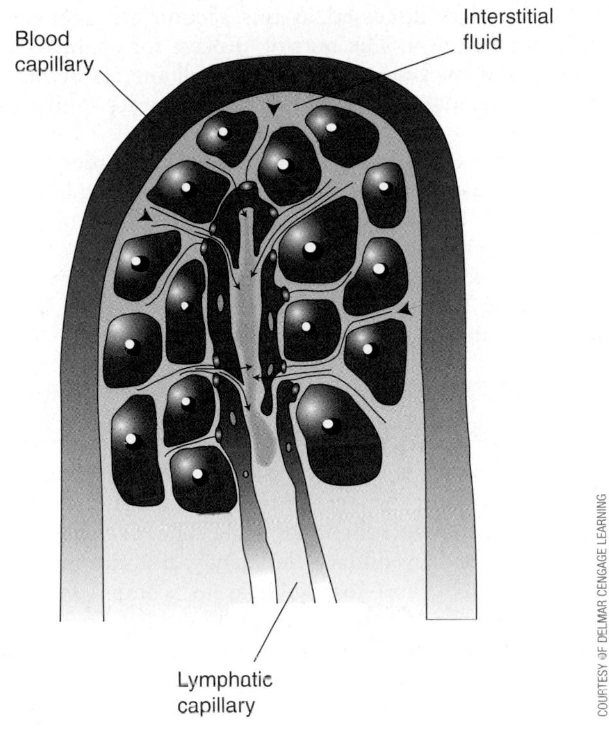

FIGURE 6-4 Flow of Fluid from the Blood into the Lymphatic System

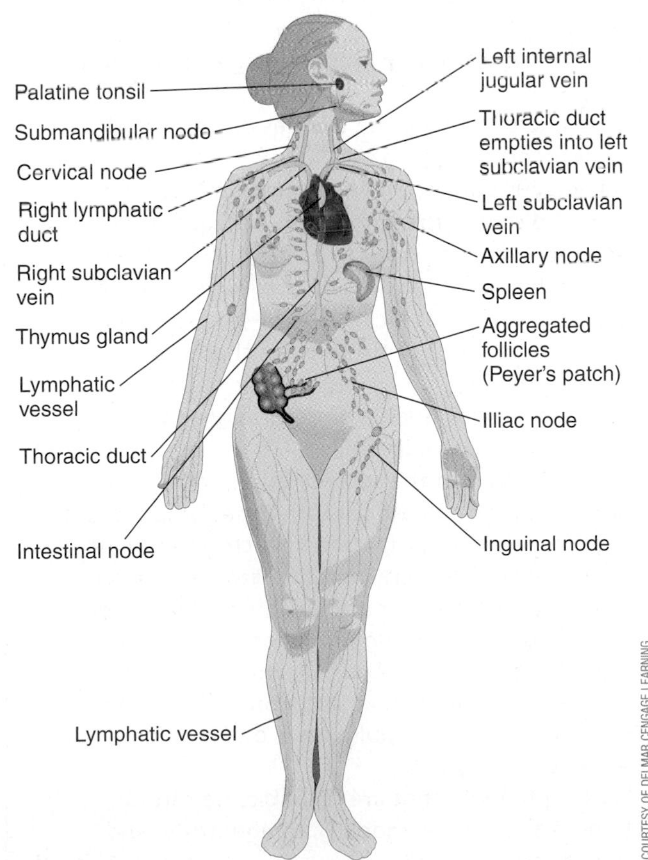

FIGURE 6-5 The Lymphatic System

substances, damaged cells, and cellular debris. The superficial lymph nodes in the neck, axilla, and groin can be palpated, especially when infected and swollen. The tonsils in the pharynx and Peyer's patch in the mucosal lining of the ileum are located deeper within the body and cannot be palpated.

As lymph is collected from body tissues, cancer cells enter the lymphatic system and escape into the circulation or to other body tissues, such as the lungs. Wherever the cancer cells collect, more cancer cells are produced. This is the way cancer spreads to other body parts. Lymph nodes are biopsied to check for the spread of cancer.

Lymph Organs

The spleen and thymus are lymph organs. The spleen removes old RBCs, platelets, and microorganisms from the blood. Approximately 350 mL of blood are stored in the spleen and approximately 200 mL can be pumped out within a minute into the body as needed (Thibodeau & Patton, 2009). During an infection, the spleen enlarges to produce and release monocytes and lymphocytes. Lymphocytes in the lymph tissue differentiate into T lymphocytes (T cells) and B lymphocytes (B cells).

In infancy and childhood, the thymus gland is large but decreases in size with age. In advanced age, it is replaced with fat and connective tissue. The thymus performs an important role in the special processing and proper functioning of the thymus-derived T lymphocytes (T cells). The T cells are actively involved in immunity.

ASSESSMENT

Information is based on client report, physical examination, and diagnostic tests.

Subjective Data

Biological and demographic data, including age, sex, ethnic background, and race, are important for many hematologic problems. Inquire about the client's occupation and hobbies because of possible exposure to radiation or chemicals. Past military experience is also important because some military personnel have been exposed to toxic chemicals. Obtain a medication history, including prescription and over-the-counter medications. Note recent or recurring infections, night sweats, palpitations, bleeding problems, previous blood transfusions, and any complications.

Assess neurological functioning by asking if the client has experienced any cognitive or mental difficulties or numbness and tingling of the extremities. A headache may indicate a low erythrocyte count or intracranial bleeding. Note hearing or vision difficulties.

Ask about past surgeries and any complications from surgeries; if the client has had a duodenal, gastric, or ileal resection, the absorption of iron and vitamin B12 may be affected. Alcohol use affects vitamin intake and is caustic to the gastrointestinal (GI) tract. Ask about the presence of blood in the stool or urine and any anorexia, nausea, vomiting, oral discomfort, or problems with taste perception. A diet history is helpful when reviewing the erythrocyte level. Inquire if the client has difficulty accomplishing ADLs because of decreased energy.

Objective Data

Begin by obtaining the client's height, weight, and vital signs. An elevated temperature is an indication of an infection. Note recent weight gains or losses.

Laboratory tests are very important when assessing the hematologic and lymphatic systems. The nurse compares past and present laboratory results.

Palpate the lymph nodes in the neck, axillae, and groin; normal findings include small (0.5–1.0 cm) nodes that are freely movable, firm, and nontender. Tender nodes indicate inflammation. Hard, fixed nodes may be malignant. See Table 6-2 for the general "Rules of Thumb" regarding abnormal lymph findings.

Next, inspect the skin and extremities for petechiae, bruises, lesions, and brittle nails. Check urine and stool for blood. Note dyspnea, an enlarged abdomen, or swollen joints. Refer to Box 6-1, Questions to Ask and Observations to Make When Collecting Data, for guidance in completing the client's hematology and lymphatic assessment.

COMMON DIAGNOSTIC TESTS

Commonly used diagnostic tests for clients with symptoms of blood and lymph system disorders are listed in Table 6-3.

RBC DISORDERS

Reduced production of RBCs results in anemia, of WBCs results in infections, and of platelets results in bleeding. RBC disorders discussed in this section are anemias and polycythemia vera. The nursing process for anemias is presented after the discussion of sickle cell anemia because the nursing diagnoses, goals, and interventions are similar for all anemias.

Anemia is a common hematopoietic disorder in which the client has a decreased number of RBCs and a low hemoglobin level. The causes for anemia are a decreased production of RBCs, an increased destruction of RBCs, or a loss of blood. Anemias discussed in this section are iron deficiency anemia, hypoplastic (aplastic) anemia, pernicious anemia, acquired hemolytic anemia, and sickle cell anemia.

IRON DEFICIENCY ANEMIA

Iron deficiency anemia is the most common type of anemia and occurs when the body does not have enough iron to synthesize functional Hgb. The decrease in iron may be caused by dietary deficiency, but the most common cause is blood loss such as in women with heavy menstrual periods or slow, chronic blood loss from a peptic ulcer, kidney or bladder tumor, colon polyp, or colorectal cancer (Mayo Clinic, 2009). Decreased iron absorption, menstruating women, or an increased need for iron such as

BOX 6-1 QUESTIONS TO ASK AND OBSERVATIONS TO MAKE WHEN COLLECTING DATA

Subjective Data

Do you smoke?
Have you gained or lost weight in the last six months?
Do you feel fatigued?
Have you noticed a decrease in your energy levels?
Do you get frequent colds or infections?
Do you ever have dizzy spells?
Do your teeth or gums bleed?
Have you experienced any changes in skin color or sensation? (See Table 6-1.)
Have you noticed any change in the sensation in your fingers and toes?
Do you experience numbness in your hands or feet?
Do you notice excessive bruising?
Do you have any swollen "glands"? If so, is the swelling always there or does it come and go? When is the swelling the worst? Is there any associated heat?
Do you have any sores that do not heal? Where are they?
Do you bruise easily?
Do you experience joint pain?
To your knowledge, have you been exposed to HIV?

Objective Data

Observe for apparent lymph nodes in the neck.
Inspect skin for lesions
Palpate the supraclavicular lymph bilaterally in the indentation just superior to the outer one third of the clavicle.
Inspect shoulder, elbow, wrist, and finger joints for edema, bruising, and deformity.
Examine the axillae bilaterally for redness and visible swelling.
Inspect and palpate lymph nodes.
Inspect for size and symmetry of extremities. If one extremity is asymmetrical and increased in size, it may be indicative of lymph drainage obstruction on that side.
Note and document any wounds or ulcerations, bruising or changes in vascular patterns.
While your patient is lying supine, palpate the liver and spleen for tenderness, nodules, or enlargement.
Inspect hip, knee, ankle, and toe joints for edema, bruising, and deformity.
Observe the backs of the legs for changes in vascular pattern.
Inspect joints for edema or deformity and symmetry in size and shape bilaterally.
Using the pads of the second, third, and fourth fingers, lightly palpate for superficial lymph nodes. Use a gentle circular motion in each lymph node area moving the overlying skin with your fingers. Note any enlargement or palpable nodes. Observe your client's face during palpation for any signs of discomfort with the exam. All lymph nodes should normally be nonpalpable and nontender. Lymph nodes do not have a pulse, so if one is palpated, it is definitely not lymph.
For lymph nodes that are palpable, be careful to note size, shape, mobility, temperature, and consistency.
Palpate the tissues around any enlarged nodes for changes adjacent to them.

TABLE 6-1 Common Skin Findings in the Presence of Blood Disorders

Pallor	Pale color of the skin. Lack of circulating oxygen to tissues. May indicate abnormal destruction of or lack of production of RBCs.
Purpura	Purplish discoloration greater than 0.5 cm in diameter resulting from bleeding under the skin. May be caused by intravascular defects, platelet disorders, or infection (Seidel, Ball, Dains, & Benedict, 2006).
Petechiae	Reddish discoloration less than 0.5 cm in diameter. Also caused by platelet disorders, infection, and vasculitis.
Ecchymosis	Red-purple bruising caused by tissue injury and bleeding underneath the skin.
Spider angioma	Small red center with red "spider leg" projections. May be caused by liver disease and vitamin B deficiency (Seidel, Ball, Dains, & Benedict, 2006).

COURTESY OF DELMAR CENGAGE LEARNING

during growth periods or pregnancy are also causes. Iron deficiency anemia is more frequently found in premature or low-birthweight infants, adolescent girls, alcoholic clients, and the elderly. The symptoms are fatigue, palpitations, tachycardia, exertional dyspnea, weakness, and pallor. Clients with chronic anemia have pica, stomatitis, glossitis, and brittle hair. Diagnostic tests reveal decreased RBCs, a low Hgb level, a low Hct, a low serum iron, and a high total iron-binding capacity (TIBC).

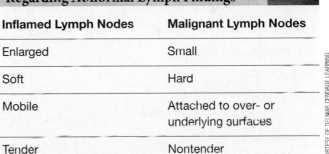

TABLE 6-2 General "Rules of Thumb" Regarding Abnormal Lymph Findings

Inflamed Lymph Nodes	Malignant Lymph Nodes
Enlarged	Small
Soft	Hard
Mobile	Attached to over- or underlying surfaces
Tender	Nontender

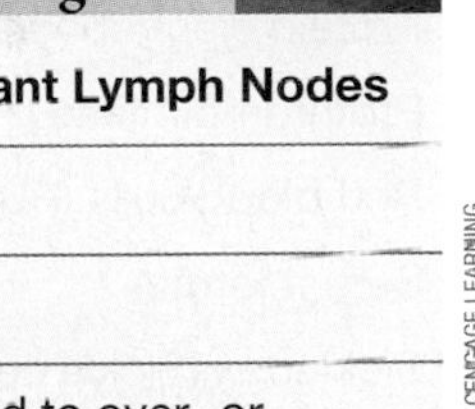

COURTESY OF DELMAR CENGAGE LEARNING

MEDICAL–SURGICAL MANAGEMENT

Pharmacological

An oral iron preparation, usually ferrous sulfate (Feosol) is ordered. These preparations are not given with food or milk because they interfere with iron absorption. The administration of iron with orange juice or vitamin C–rich drinks increases iron absorption. Iron dextran (InFeD), an intramuscular iron preparation, is given only in the upper, outer quadrant of the buttocks, deep IM with Z-track method.

Diet

A diet high in iron is encouraged. Foods rich in iron are red meats, fish, raisins, apricots, dried fruits, dark green vegetables, dried beans, eggs, and iron-enriched whole-grain breads. An increase of vitamin C in the diet assists in the absorption of iron. If the client has a loss of appetite, small frequent snacks are tolerated better than three large meals.

CRITICAL THINKING

Iron Deficiency Anemia

How are the symptoms of iron deficiency anemia related to a decreased red blood cell count and decreased hemoglobin?

Activity

Space daily activities to provide rest periods between times of exercise.

APLASTIC ANEMIA

The bone marrow decreases or stops functioning in a client with aplastic anemia. The client with aplastic anemia has pancytopenia, a decrease in the number of RBCs, WBCs, and platelets. In most cases the cause is unknown, but genetic factors are suspected. Secondary aplastic anemia is caused by exposure to viruses, chemicals (benzene or airplane glue), radiation, or medications. Some medications that cause aplastic anemia are chloramphenicol (Chloromycetin), mephenytoin (Mesantoin), trimethadione (Tridione), mechlorethamine or nitrogen mustard (Mustargen), methotrexate (Folex PFS), 6-mercaptopurine or 6-MP (Purinethol), and phenylbutazone (Butazolidin). Symptoms include fatigue, weakness, palpitvations, headaches, fever, mouth ulcers, petechiae, gingival bleeding, and epistaxis. These clients are extremely ill. Diagnosis is confirmed by a bone marrow aspiration.

TABLE 6-3 Common Diagnostic Tests for Blood and Lymphatic System Disorders
Partial thromboplastin time (PTT)
Activated partial thromboplastin time (APTT)
Bleeding time
Blood culture and sensitivity
Coombs' test (direct antiglobulin test)
D-dimer test (fragment D-dimer, fibrin degradation fragment)
Erythrocyte sedimentation rate (sed rate, ESR)
Folic acid (folate level)
Hematocrit (Hct)
Hemoglobin (Hgb)
Hemoglobin electrophoresis
International normalized ratio (INR)
Platelet count
Protein electrophoresis (immunofixation electrophoresis)
Prothrombin time (PT, protime)
Red blood cells (RBCs)
Serum ferritin
Sickledex (Sickle cell test)
Total iron binding capacity (TIBC)
White blood cells (WBCs)
Differential count
Granulocytes
Basophils
Eosinophils
Neutrophils
Bands
Agranulocytes
Lymphocytes
Monocytes
Bone marrow aspiration
Radiologic lymphangiogram

MEDICAL–SURGICAL MANAGEMENT

Medical

The cause of aplastic anemia is removed if possible. Immunosuppressive therapy with antithymocyte globulin or ATG (Atgam) and cyclosporine is given to suppress the reaction causing the aplastic anemia and to allow the client's bone marrow to recover. A client who has a good response will improve in 3 to 6 months. The response rate is 70% to 80% (Aplastic Anemia & MDS International Foundation, 2006). Transfusions of packed red cells and platelets are given as needed.

Surgical

A bone marrow transplant is performed if the client's bone marrow fails to respond to treatment. Cyclosporine (Sandimmune), an immunosuppressant, is given for a bone marrow transplant to decrease the graft rejection. The best response occurs in a young client who has not previously had a transfusion because transfusions increase bone marrow graft rejection. Bone marrow transplants from a human leukocyte antigen- (HLA-) matched sibling donor are the treatment of choice for clients younger than 30 years of age. The treatment of choice for an older adult or a client who does not have an HLA-matched sibling donor is immunosuppression with ATG and cyclosporine. (Bone marrow transplants are discussed in the section on acute myelocytic leukemia.)

Pharmacological

Infections are treated with antibiotics. Steroids and androgens are sometimes used to stimulate the bone marrow.

PERNICIOUS ANEMIA

The parietal cells of the gastric mucosa secrete a protein intrinsic factor that is essential for the proper absorption of vitamin B_{12}. Pernicious anemia is an autoimmune disease in which the parietal cells are destroyed and the gastric mucosa atrophies. Without the secretion of the intrinsic factor, vitamin B_{12} cannot be absorbed in the distal portion of the ileum.

The onset of the disease occurs around the age of 60. Pernicious anemia occurs most frequently in women of Northern European descent and some African Americans. Pernicious anemia occurs in clients who have had a gastrectomy with the section of the stomach removed that secretes the intrinsic factor. High levels of serum homocysteine and methylmalonic acid (MMA) are confirming diagnostic tests (NIH, 2009).

Pernicious anemia has an insidious onset because the body can store 3 to 5 years' worth of vitamin B_{12} in the liver. Neurologic changes, paresthesia, and numbness occur before lab tests identify vitamin B_{12} deficiency (Holcomb, 2001). Symptoms include extreme weakness, a sore tongue, edema of the legs, ataxia, dizziness, dyspnea, headache, fever, blurred vision, tinnitus, jaundice with pallor, poor memory, irritability, and loss of bladder and bowel control. The client has decreased sensitivity to heat and pain because of neurological involvement. Clients with pernicious anemia are highly susceptible to gastric carcinoma and are monitored closely for symptoms.

MEDICAL–SURGICAL MANAGEMENT

Pharmacological

Topical anesthetics are given to relieve oral discomfort during the acute phase of the disease. Vitamin B_{12}, cyanocobalamin crystalline (Rubesol-1000) is given IM until the Hct returns to normal. Then it is given monthly for the rest of the client's life. The frequency of administration depends on the client's

> **PROFESSIONAL TIP**
>
> **Vitamin B_{12} Deficiency**
>
> Strict vegetarians are at risk for vitamin B_{12} deficiency. A dietary supplement of vitamin B_{12} is the treatment.

symptoms and response to the medication. Oral administration of vitamin B_{12} is not effective because vitamin B_{12} cannot be absorbed without the intrinsic factor. Folic acid or folate (Folvite) is prescribed. Encourage the client to increase folic acid in the diet by eating green leafy vegetables, meat, fish, legumes, and whole grains. Iron is usually not prescribed because once the condition is corrected with regular administration of cyanocobalamin, erythrocytes are produced and the Hgb and Hct return to normal.

ACQUIRED HEMOLYTIC ANEMIA

In hemolytic anemias, **hemolysis**, or destruction of RBCs, occurs, and iron and hemoglobin are released. Several causes for acquired hemolytic anemia are an autoimmune reaction, radiation, blood transfusion, chemicals, arsenic, lead, or medications. Sulfisoxazole (Gantrisin), penicillin, and methyldopa (Aldomet) are medications that cause hemolysis. A substance produced by the bacterium *Clostridium perfringens* also causes hemolysis. Clients may not notice symptoms or experience a severe reaction. Symptoms are mild fatigue and pallor. More severe symptoms include jaundice, palpitations, hypotension, dyspnea, and back and joint pain. Diagnostic tests reveal a low Hgb and Hct and an increased level of lactate dehydrogenase (LDH). LDH is an enzyme in the heart, liver, kidneys, skeletal muscle, brain, RBCs, and lungs. As these tissues are damaged, LDH is released into the bloodstream, causing an elevated LDH.

MEDICAL–SURGICAL MANAGEMENT

Medical

Treatment is aimed at removing the cause, if possible. Clients are given blood transfusions or **erythrocytapheresis** (a procedure that removes abnormal RBCs and replaces them with healthy RBCs).

Surgical

The spleen destroys RBCs. In severe cases of hemolytic anemia, a splenectomy is performed in an attempt to stop the destruction of RBCs.

Pharmacological

Corticosteroids are administered to decrease the autoimmune response. Folic acid is given to increase the production of RBCs.

SICKLE CELL ANEMIA (INHERITED HEMOLYTIC ANEMIA)

Sickle cell anemia is also known as inherited hemolytic anemia or sickle cell disease. This genetic disorder has abnormal hemoglobin S rather than hemoglobin A in the RBCs. Sickle cell anemia is caused by a recessive gene or genes that are passed through the generations (Figure 6-6). The client with one s gene has sickle cell trait (Hb sA) and is asymptomatic but is a carrier of the disease. The client with sickle cell anemia has two s genes (Hb ss) and manifests symptoms.

The condition occurs most frequently in African-American clients, with an estimated 1,000 infants born with sickle cell disease each year in the United States (SCDAA, 2005). It also occurs in persons from Asia Minor, India, and the Mediterranean and Caribbean areas.

Sickle cell tests are done on infants to diagnose sickle cell trait or disease. A screening test to detect the presence of Hb S is Sickledex or sickle cell test. If Hb S is present, a hemoglobin electrophoresis is done to distinguish between sickle cell trait and sickle cell disease. If the hemoglobin electrophoresis test is negative, the client has the sickle cell trait and not sickle cell disease.

Situations that precipitate sickle cell crisis are dehydration, deoxygenation, acidosis, and temperature changes (Platt, Beasley, Miller, & Eckman, 2002). In these situations crystallization of hemoglobin is promoted, which forces the RBCs to **sickle**, i.e., become crescent-shaped and elongated

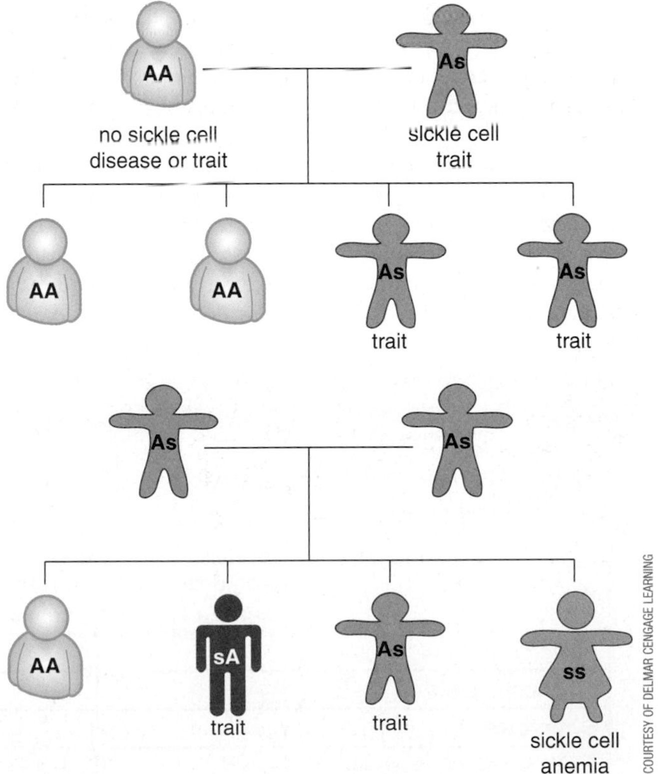

FIGURE 6-6 Inheritance of the Sickle Cell Trait and Sickle Cell Anemia

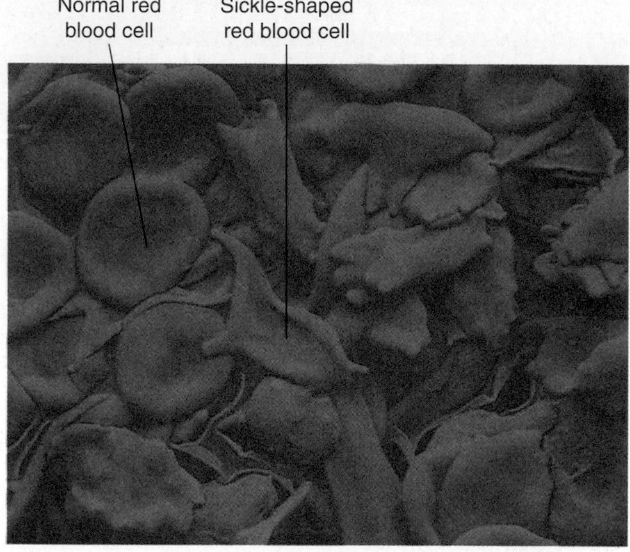

FIGURE 6-7 Blood Cells Magnified through a Scanning Electron Microscope Show Normal and Sickle-Shaped Red Blood Cells (*Courtesy of Phillips Electronic Instruments Company.*)

and obstruct vessels, especially capillaries (Figure 6-7) (Platt et al., 2002). The area normally supplied by these obstructed blood vessels becomes infarcted and ischemic. The destruction of sickled RBCs in 12 to 15 days causes chronic anemia; the heart enlarges in an attempt to circulate more blood for adequate oxygenation of body tissues. Other symptoms include fatigue, jaundice, chronic leg ulcers, tachypnea, dyspnea, and arrhythmias. When the client experiences a sickle cell crisis, there is fever, severe pain, and loss of blood supply to various organs because of obstructed vessels. Areas most frequently affected are the joints, bone, brain, lungs, liver, kidneys, and penis. Joints become painful, swollen, and immobile. Clients experience cerebrovascular accidents, renal failure, pulmonary infarction, shock, and priapism (a continuous, painful erection).

Assess extremity circulation frequently by doing capillary refill, peripheral pulses, and temperature. Application of warm compresses to painful areas relieves pain. Encourage the client to avoid restrictive clothing and anything that may restrict circulation. Teach clients to avoid high altitudes and have adequate fluid intake.

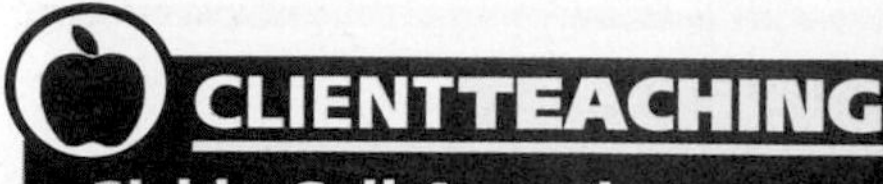

CLIENT TEACHING

Sickle Cell Anemia

- Encourage client to avoid high altitudes and nonpressurized airplanes.
- Encourage adequate fluid intake because dehydration causes a sickle cell crisis.
- Treat all infections promptly.
- Encourage client to tight-fitting, restrictive clothing, and strenuous exercise, smoking, and cold temperatures.
- Encourage client to receive yearly flu vaccine and pneumococcal vaccine.

MEDICAL–SURGICAL MANAGEMENT

Medical

Infections are treated promptly with antibiotics. Large amounts of oral and intravenous fluids (3–5 L/day) are given to remove the by-products of broken RBCs. Oxygen is administered based on pulse oximetry and ABGs to combat deoxygenation. Skin grafting is necessary for chronic leg ulcers.

Genetic counseling is recommended for clients with sickle cell trait and sickle cell anemia. There may be more openness to counseling if the counselor is from the same community as the client.

Pharmacological

Hydroxyurea (Droxia) reduces the frequency of painful crisis and the need for blood transfusions in adults (Spratto & Woods, 2004). Folic acid or folate (Folvite) is administered daily to assist in the production of RBCs. Pentoxifylline (Trental) reduces blood viscosity and increases RBC flexibility. Blood transfusions are given during a crisis.

Patient-controlled analgesia (PCA) with morphine is effective during a crisis. The client is progressed from narcotics to nonnarcotic analgesics as indicated.

CRITICAL THINKING

Anemias

Use the table and compare the etiologies, diagnostic tests, symptoms, treatments, and nursing interventions of the listed anemias.

	Iron deficiency anemia	Aplastic anemia	Pernicious anemia	Acquired hemolytic anemia	Sickle cell anemia
Etiology					
Diagnostic tests					
Symptoms					
Treatments					
Nursing interventions					

Nursing Management

Assess weight, vital signs, apical and peripheral pulses, breath sounds, color, abdominal tenderness, and signs of bruising or jaundice. Review client's history for possible familial illnesses. Encourage client to follow treatment regimen. Monitor laboratory test results. Administer blood products as ordered and monitor for a possible reaction.

NURSING PROCESS

Assessment

Subjective Data

Obtain a history of the client's medical problems, including a history of familial hematopoietic illnesses. Some anemias may be caused by drugs and environmental conditions, so information about medications taken and about environmental situations at work and in recreational settings is important. The client is asked about fatigue, dyspnea with exertion, palpitations, dizziness, pain, petechiae, tingling and numbness in the extremities, blurred vision, and oral discomfort.

Objective Data

The client's weight and vital signs; apical pulse and peripheral pulses; breath sounds; sensation and movement in the extremities; abdominal tenderness; and edema, pallor, and signs of bruising or jaundice are assessed. A thorough assessment of the cardiac system is completed because severe anemia causes cardiac enlargement and arrhythmias.

Nursing diagnoses for a client with decreased erythrocytes and hemoglobin may include the following:

NURSING DIAGNOSES	PLANNING/OUTCOMES	NURSING INTERVENTIONS
Deficient Knowledge related to prescribed treatment regimen	The client will relate the prescribed treatment regimen.	Teach the cause of the particular type of anemia and, if possible, ways to avoid the occurrence of that anemia in the future. For iron deficiency anemia, teach the importance of taking and increasing iron in the diet. Instruct clients with pernicious anemia to obtain a vitamin B_{12} injection at regularly scheduled times. Teach clients with hemolytic anemias the significance of following the prescribed regimens.
Activity intolerance related to imbalance between oxygen supply and demand	The client will increasingly tolerate activity.	Assist the client as needed with activities of daily living. Teach the client to alternate periods of rest with activity.
Ineffective Tissue Perfusion (Peripheral) related to a decreased hemoglobin concentration in the blood	The client will have increased tissue perfusion.	Administer oxygen as needed to relieve symptoms of dyspnea. Monitor Hgb, Hct, RBCs, pulse oximetry, electrolytes, vital signs, and mental alertness. Monitor for symptoms of obstructed vessels such as pain, leg ulcerations, abdominal tenderness, dyspnea, confusion, and blurred vision. Administer blood products as ordered and monitor the client closely after blood transfusions for possible reactions such as chills, fever, dyspnea, pruritus, wheezing, and pain in the lumbar region.

Evaluation: Evaluate each outcome to determine how it has been met by the client.

SAMPLE NURSING CARE PLAN

The Client with Sickle Cell Anemia

R.T., a 19-year-old African-American client, was diagnosed with sickle cell anemia 5 years ago. R.T. works for a computer company and has been working 12-hour days to get a system installed. He felt fatigued lately and decided to relax by playing golf on a warm Saturday morning. After the seventh hole, R.T. experienced dyspnea and tingling and numbness in his legs. After the next hole, he experienced severe pain in his ankles and knees. He was taken to the local medical center, where he was admitted. The physician ordered oxygen by nasal cannula, IV fluids, and a PCA pump with morphine sulfate.

NURSING DIAGNOSIS 1 *Acute Pain* related to occlusion of small vessels by sickled cells as evidenced by severe pain in the knees and ankles

Nursing Outcomes Classification (NOC)
Comfort Level
Pain Control

Nursing Interventions Classification (NIC)
Pain Management
Emotional Support
Heat/Cold Application

PLANNING/OUTCOMES	NURSING INTERVENTIONS	RATIONALE
R.T. will state pain has been relieved.	Assess pain type, location, and intensity.	Identifies where vessels may be occluded.
	Monitor analgesic administration by PCA pump.	Assesses relief from pain.
	Support joints and lower extremities with pillows.	Relieves joint pain.
	Keep bed linens off knees and ankles with a bed cradle.	Keeps linen from putting pressure on painful areas.

EVALUATION

The morphine in the PCA pump relieved R.T.'s pain, and oral analgesics were ordered.

NURSING DIAGNOSIS 2 *Ineffective Tissue Perfusion (Cardiopulmonary and Peripheral)* related to a decreased number of RBCs and decreased oxygenation as evidenced by dyspnea and tingling and numbness in his ankles and knees

Nursing Outcomes Classification (NOC)
Tissue Perfusion: Peripheral
Circulation Status

Nursing Interventions Classification (NIC)
Oxygen Therapy
Intravenous Therapy

PLANNING/OUTCOMES	NURSING INTERVENTIONS	RATIONALE
R.T. will experience improved circulation in his extremities.	Elevate the head of the bed.	Allows lungs to expand more fully.
	Administer oxygen as needed.	Oxygen increases blood oxygen level.
	Administer IV fluids as ordered.	Decreases the possibility of RBCs' sickling.
	Encourage R.T. to drink 8 to 10 glasses of water daily.	Prevents RBCs from sickling.
	Monitor for symptoms of obstructed vessels such as pain, leg ulcerations, abdominal tenderness, dyspnea, confusion, and blurred vision.	Vessels supplying blood to other vital organs can become obstructed.
	Administer blood products as ordered.	Improves the blood oxygen concentration.
	Closely monitor for possible blood transfusion reactions such as chills, fever, dyspnea, pruritus, wheezing, and pain in the lumbar region.	Administration of blood products may cause adverse reactions.

SAMPLE NURSING CARE PLAN (Continued)

EVALUATION

Circulation in lower extremities has improved as manifested by prompt capillary refill and strong pedal and popliteal pulses. Extremities are warm to touch.

NURSING DIAGNOSIS 3 *Deficient Knowledge* related to prescribed treatment regimen as evidenced by a lack of rest and working long hours

Nursing Outcomes Classification (NOC)	Nursing Interventions Classification (NIC)
Knowledge: Energy Conservation	*Self-Modification Assistance*
Knowledge: Treatment Regimen	*Teaching: Individual*

PLANNING/OUTCOMES	NURSING INTERVENTIONS	RATIONALE
R.T. will relate the prescribed treatment regimen before discharge.	Teach R.T. the pathophysiology related to sickle cell disease.	Improves compliance with the medical regimen.
	Encourage R.T. to take medications as ordered.	Improves circulation and postpones sickle cell crisis situations.
	Explain the importance of avoiding stressful situations and the symptoms of infection.	These situations increase oxygen demands.
	Explain the importance of adequate rest on a routine basis.	Allows adequate oxygenation and reduces stress.

EVALUATION

R.T. states his RBCs have Hgb S rather than Hgb A, and a lack of oxygen causes his RBCs to sickle. Sickling is caused by fatigue, lack of oral fluids, emotional and physical stress, infection, exposure to cold and anesthesia. He knows the purpose and side effects of each medication and the times he is to take them. R.T. states he is to avoid high altitudes. R.T. states that he will try to routinely have enough rest.

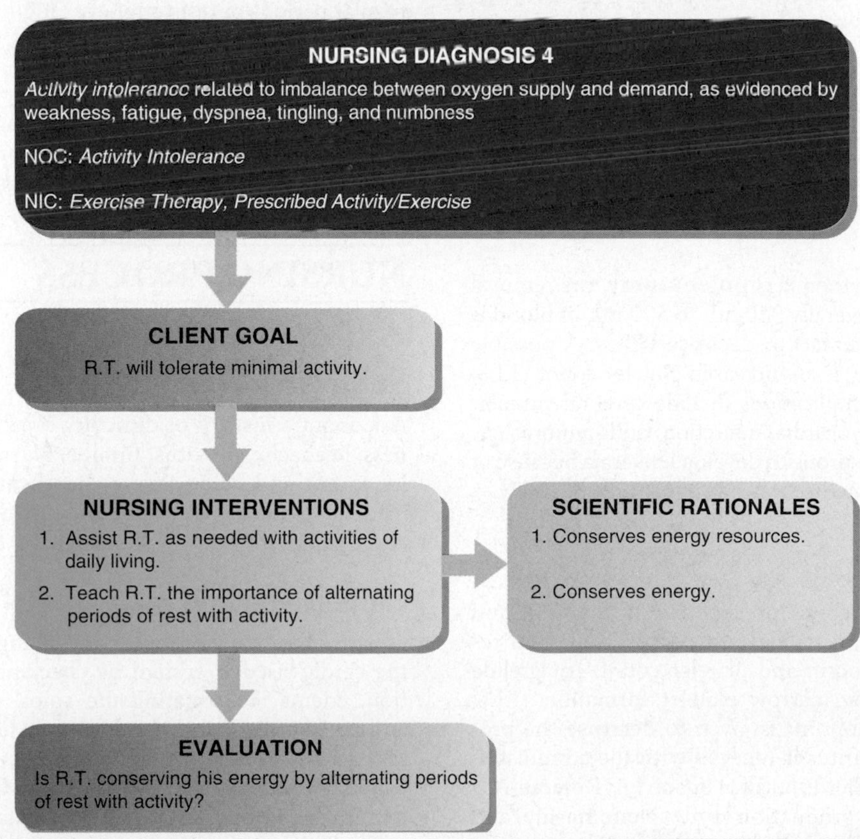
NURSING DIAGNOSIS 4
Activity intolerance related to imbalance between oxygen supply and demand, as evidenced by weakness, fatigue, dyspnea, tingling, and numbness
NOC: Activity Intolerance
NIC: Exercise Therapy, Prescribed Activity/Exercise
CLIENT GOAL
R.T. will tolerate minimal activity.
NURSING INTERVENTIONS
1. Assist R.T. as needed with activities of daily living.
2. Teach R.T. the importance of alternating periods of rest with activity.
SCIENTIFIC RATIONALES
1. Conserves energy resources.
2. Conserves energy.
EVALUATION
Is R.T. conserving his energy by alternating periods of rest with activity?

CONCEPT CARE MAP 6-1

POLYCYTHEMIA

Polycythemia is a disease in which there is an increased production of red blood cells. Usually the numbers of WBCs and platelets are also increased. The increase in RBCs increases the blood volume and viscosity and decreases the ability of the blood to circulate freely. There are two types of polycythemia: polycythemia vera (PV) (primary polycythemia) and secondary polycythemia. The average age for a diagnosis of polycythemia vera is between the ages of 60 and 65. It is more prevalent in Jewish men of Eastern European ancestry (The Leukemia and Lymphoma Society, 2007). Clients with PV have a mutation of the JAK2 (Janus kinase 2) gene, but the exact role of the mutated gene in the cause is not known. A DNA abnormality occurs in an early marrow cell that produces all of the blood cells in the individual. Secondary polycythemia is a compensatory mechanism as the body makes more red blood cells in response to low oxygenation caused by long-term hypoxia, as in chronic obstructive pulmonary disease, chronic heart failure, smoking, or living in a high altitude.

Symptoms of the two types are the same. As the blood viscosity and volume increase, the client experiences headaches, dizziness, tinnitus, blurred vision, fatigue, weakness, pruritus, exertional dyspnea, angina, and increased blood pressure and pulse. The client's complexion becomes ruddy (reddish), and the palms, earlobes, and cheeks are flushed. Some clients experience a burning sensation in the feet. The client is susceptible to thrombi formation because of the increased viscosity of the blood and increase in platelets. Even though there are more RBCs produced in polycythemia, the RBCs have a shorter life span than normal. When RBCs die, uric acid is released, causing **hyperuricemia** (increased uric acid blood level). The elevated uric acid levels cause or aggravate gout symptoms. The Hgb and Hct increase in the same proportion as the RBCs (Leukemia & Lymphoma Society, 2007).

MEDICAL–SURGICAL MANAGEMENT

Medical

The treatment for polycythemia is **phlebotomy**, the removal of blood from a vein. Generally 350 mL to 500 mL of blood is withdrawn at regular intervals to decrease RBCs. A possible side effect of phlebotomy is an increased platelet count (LLS, 2007). Polycythemia complications include cerebral vascular accident, thrombosis, myocardial infarction, and hemorrhage. Clients with PV are more prone to develop leukemia because of the disease process and medication side effects (LLS, 2007).

Pharmacological

Low-dose aspirin is given to prevent clot formation, and hydroxyurea (Hydrea®), a myelosuppressive agent, reduces the hemoglobin, hematocrit, and platelet count. Anagrelide (Agrylin®) reduces bone marrow platelet formation (LLS, 2007). Allopurinol (Zyloprim) is given to decrease the production of uric acid. Pruritus is relieved with the administration of antihistamines. Interferon alfa (Intron® A, Roferan-A®) reduces bone marrow production and splenomegaly and relieves pruritus. Interferon alfa is an option for younger clients with splenomegaly. However, interferon alfa is not used as often because of the expense and the side effects of the drugs (Stuart & Viera, 2004). Alkylating agents are not used as frequently because of the incidence of leukemia in clients using these drugs (Stuart & Viera, 2004). Radioactive phosphorus (32p) decreases the production of blood cells in the bone marrow and is used along with phlebotomy.

> **CLIENT TEACHING**
>
> **Polycythemia**
>
> - Drink at least 3 L of water daily.
> - Elevate feet when resting.
> - Avoid tight or restrictive clothing.
> - Wear support hose.
> - Take medications as ordered.
> - Report chest pain, joint pain, fever, or activity intolerance to physician.
> - Keep appointments for laboratory testing and physician checks.

Diet

The client is placed on a diet that has increased calories and protein. A diet low in sodium decreases fluid volume. Iron-containing foods are avoided.

Activity

Activities of daily living are adjusted so the client can have regular periods of rest to relieve fatigue.

NURSING MANAGEMENT

Monitor vital signs, nutritional status, and oxygenation. Keep accurate I&O. Initiate passive or active leg exercises or encourage ambulation. Encourage compliance with regimen.

NURSING PROCESS

ASSESSMENT

Subjective Data

Ask about a history of difficulty breathing, chest pain, dizziness, headache, pruritus, tinnitis, blurred vision, and sensitivity to hot and cold. Assess client's nutritional status for an inadequate dietary intake because of GI symptoms of fullness and dyspepsia.

Objective Data

Observe the skin for bruises and changes in skin color. Assess the cardiovascular system by checking for neck vein distention, edema, auscultating the apical pulse, palpating radial and pedal pulses, and checking for Homans' sign. Assess the respiratory system by observing for epistaxis and dyspnea and listening to the breath sounds. Check the central nervous system through pupil response, disorientation, and the presence of numbness or tingling.

Nursing diagnoses for a client with polycythemia include the following:

NURSING DIAGNOSES	PLANNING/OUTCOMES	NURSING INTERVENTIONS
*Deficient **Knowledge*** related to disease process and treatment	The client will relate disease process and treatment.	Explain the cause of the disease, possible symptoms, side effects of medications, and possible future complications to report. Teach client to report headache, chest pain, dyspnea, or redness, swelling, or tenderness in the arms or legs to the physician or nurse practitioner immediately.
*Ineffective **Tissue** Perfusion (Peripheral)* related to decreased blood circulation	The client will have 2+ peripheral pulses.	Administer oxygen as needed for dyspnea. Check vital signs frequently and assess Homans' sign and signs of thrombi formation. Explain phlebotomy process.
*Risk for **Injury*** related to dizziness	The client will relate measures to avoid injury.	Encourage the client to change positions slowly to prevent dizziness. Encourage activities of daily living when the client is feeling well. Teach client to avoid activities that cause bruising or trauma.

Evaluation: Evaluate each outcome to determine how it has been met by the client.

WBC DISORDERS

WBC disorders include leukemia and agranulocytosis.

LEUKEMIA

Leukemia is a malignancy of blood-forming tissues in which the bone marrow produces increased numbers of immature white blood cells that are incapable of protecting the body from infections. The increased number of WBCs crowds out the other cells in the bone marrow, causing a decreased production of RBCs and platelets. Anemia and bleeding result from the decreased number of RBCs and platelets.

Leukemia is divided into 4 categories: acute myelogenous leukemia (AML), acute lymphocytic leukemia (ALL), chronic myelogenous leukemia (CML), and chronic lymphocytic leukemia (CLL). An estimated 44,790 new cases of leukemia were diagnosed in 2009 (ACS, 2009a).

Because of the increased production of immature WBCs, clients with acute leukemia generally are fighting persistent infections and have fever and chills. The decreased number of RBCs causes symptoms of anemia such as fatigue, pallor, malaise, tachycardia, and tachypnea. The decreased platelet production causes bleeding tendencies, and the client experiences petechiae, bruising, epistaxis, melena, gingival bleeding, and increased menstrual bleeding. The client also experiences weight loss, night sweats, and swollen lymph nodes. As the malignant cells invade the central nervous system, the client experiences headaches, seizures, vomiting, blurred vision, and difficulty maintaining balance (ACS, 2007a). Some clients experience bone pain because the rapid production of WBCs crowds the cells in the bone marrow.

ACUTE LEUKEMIA

Acute leukemias have a rapid onset and must be treated quickly for a good prognosis. ALL has a more rapid onset than AML. ALL is the more common type of leukemia in childhood with most cases occurring between the ages of 2 and 4 years of age (LLS, ACS, 2009c). The 5-year survival rate for a child with ALL is more than 80%. (ACS, 2009c).

AML and CLL are more common in adults (LLS, 2009). AML in childhood occurs more frequently during the first 2 years of life and in teenage years. However, AML is more common in older people with the average age for a diagnosis at 67 years-of-age. The 5-year survival rate of a child with AML is more than 50%; more adults die from AML (ACS, 2009b).

Medical–Surgical Management

Medical

Diagnosis of acute leukemia is confirmed with a CBC and a bone marrow biopsy. A lumbar puncture determines the presence of malignant cells in the central nervous system. An x-ray, MRI, CT scan, or Gallium scan and bone scan of the chest and skeleton determine the presence of infection and bone marrow tissue involvement.

Bone marrow transplantation is used with relapsed ALL clients and AML clients. High doses of chemotherapy and radiation therapy are given to the client to destroy the bone marrow. Leukemic white blood cells and healthy bone marrow cells are both destroyed, placing the client at a high risk for infection and death. Identical human leukocyte antigen (HLA) bone marrow from a sibling, the client, or an antigen-matched donor is given intravenously in a manner similar to a blood transfusion. The transfused bone marrow finds its way to the client's bone marrow and starts producing WBCs, RBCs, and platelets. The bone marrow is matched in a process very similar to the process of crossmatching blood. If the client's own bone marrow is used, it is removed from the client, treated with chemotherapy, and then reinfused into the client.

Maningo (2002) describes a fast-emerging alternative to bone marrow transplantation, peripheral blood stem cell transplantation. The stem cell donor (client or HLA-matched donor) is given growth factors such as granulocyte colony-stimulating factor (filgrastim [Neupogen]) and granulocyte macrophage–colony-stimulating factor (sargramostim [Leukine]) to increase the number of circulating blood stem cells. The peripheral stem cells, collected with a large-bore central vascular access device, are separated out of the whole blood. The RBCs, platelets, WBCs, and plasma are returned to the donor. The stem cells are then infused. Engraftment occurs in 2 to 4 weeks.

Pharmacological

Initial doses of chemotherapy are called **induction doses**. Small doses of chemotherapy given every 3 to 4 weeks to maintain remission are called **maintenance therapy**.

Leukemic cells lie dormant in the brain and spinal area because the chemotherapeutic drugs are unable to pass through the blood–brain barrier. Intrathecal (within the spinal canal) administration of methotrexate has decreased recurrences of ALL. Methotrexate is given by a lumbar puncture into the cerebrospinal fluid or through a subcutaneous cerebrospinal reservoir. Sometimes radiation therapy is also used on the brain and spinal area.

AML is treated with chemotherapeutic agents, blood products, and antibiotics. Chemotherapeutic agents used in treating acute leukemia are listed in Table 6-4.

Diet

Avoid extremely hot or cold foods and drinks as well as alcohol. A bland, high-protein, high-carbohydrate diet is usually ordered.

Activity

Encourage clients to alternate periods of rest with activity and keep frequently used items nearby to conserve energy.

TABLE 6-4 Chemotherapeutic Agents to Treat Leukemia

LEUKEMIA	CHEMOTHERAPEUTIC AGENTS
Acute lymphocyctic leukemia (ALL)	vincristine (Oncovin) daunorubicin or daunomycin (Cerubidine) doxorubicin (Adriamycin) cytarabine (Cytosar) etoposide (VePesid) dexamethasone (Decadron) prednisone (Deltasone) 6-mercapotopurine or 6-MP (Purinethol) methotrexate (Methotrexate)
Acute myelogenous leukemia (AML)	daunorubicin HCl (Cerubidine) cytarabine or ara-C (Cytosar-U) 6-thioguanine or 6-TG (Thioguanine) vincristine (Oncovin) etoposide (VePesid)
Chronic myelogenous leukemia (CLL)	fludaravine (Fludara) pentostatine (Nipent) cladrivine (2-CdA, Leustatin) chlorambucil (Leukeran) COP (Cytoxan, Oncovin, and prednisone)
Chronic lymphocytic leukemia (CML)	Tyrosine kinase inhibitors are more effective than chemotherapy. hydroxyurea (Hydrea)

CHRONIC LEUKEMIA

Chronic leukemia generally occurs in adults with a gradual increase in the white cell count over months or years. The prognosis depends on the severity of the disease at the time of diagnosis.

CLL clients have increased abnormal B lymphocytes, with a WBC count between 20,000 and 100,000. CLL develops with advanced age and has a higher incident rate in men than in women (ACS, 2007e). There are two types of CLL. One type of CLL grows slowly, rarely needs treatment with a survival average of 15 years. The other type grows faster with a survival average of 8 years. The CLL cells have a protein called ZAP-70 and a substance called CD38. Clients with cells with lower levels of ZAP-70 and CD38 have a better survival rate (ACS, 2007f).

CML is characterized by the Philadelphia chromosome, indicating a possible genetic link. Treatment for CML has improved over the last few years and clients are surviving at least 5 years after diagnosis (ACS, 2008b). The WBC count ranges from 15,000 to 500,000. Most clients feel good and maintain a relatively normal life until later in the disease process, when the chronic recessed phase changes into an intensified stage that resembles an acute phase of leukemia. This acute phase is called a **blastic phase**, in which there is an increased production of WBCs. When this occurs, the general condition spirals downhill and the client soon dies. The most common cause of death in the leukemic client is viral and fungal pneumonia.

MEDICAL–SURGICAL MANAGEMENT

Medical

Diagnosis of chronic leukemia is confirmed with a CBC and a bone marrow biopsy.

In the CML chronic phase, the HLA-identical allogenic bone marrow is given, and the client's own treated bone marrow is given in the blastic phase. Autologous or allogenic peripheral blood stem cell transplantation is used.

Pharmacological

Refer to Table 6-4 for chemotherapeutic agents used in treating CLL and CML. Chemotherapy does not extend the length of life but seems to give a better quality of life by prolonging the chronic phase. Fludarabine (Fludara), a purine analog, is the most effective single drug used to treat CLL. Purine analogs have significant side effects and cause increase susceptibility to infections. Alkylating agents, such as chlorambucil (Leukeran), and cyclophosphamide (Cytoxan) are used in treating CLL clients who cannot tolerate aggressive treatment. Monoclonal antibodies are medications that boost the client's immune system to respond and kill cancer cells. These medications attach to specific targeted substances on the surface of the cancer cells. Alemtuxumab (Campath) attaches to the CD52 antigen on the B and T lymphocytes. Campath is used when the client is no longer responding to chemotherapy. It is given subcutaneously or intravenously. Since it increases the risk for infections, it is given with antibiotics and antiviral medications (ACS, 2007b). Rituximab (Rituxan), a monoclonal antibody, targets the CD20 antigen on the surface of B lymphocytes. It is used along with chemotherapy for CLL and is given intravenously once a week (ACS, 2007b).

Chemotherapy is no longer the main treatment for CML. Imatinib mesylate (Gleevec) is one of the main drugs to treat CML. Chemotherapy is used in treating CML after the tyrosine kinase inhibitors are no longer effective. Hydroxyurea (Hydrea) is an oral pill taken to decrease very high WBC counts and to decrease spleen enlargement.

Diet

The client is on a diet high in protein, carbohydrates, and vitamins. A bland, nonirritating diet prevents oral mucosal irritation. Alcohol is avoided.

Activity

It is important for the client to learn methods to conserve energy, such as placing frequently used items nearby.

Nursing Management

Assess for pain. Monitor for symptoms of infection and bleeding. Check platelet count results. Follow proper hand hygiene procedure and teach it to all visitors. Provide frequent oral care with soft toothbrush or cotton swabs. Assist with or provide daily personal hygiene with antimicrobial soap. Monitor vital signs and report any temperature over 100°F. Encourage client to use an electric razor. Administer antiemetics, stool softener, and vitamins as ordered. Encourage client to talk about concerns and fears.

NURSING PROCESS

Assessment

Subjective Data

Ask the client or family about chromosomal abnormalities, exposure to chemicals, viral infections, and previous chemotherapy or radiation therapy. Ask the client to describe the location, type, and duration of pain, especially in bones or joints. Note symptoms of infection such as the presence of a cough or pain or burning on urination. Document a history of bleeding such as epistaxis, gingival bleeding, melena, or hematuria. Fatigue, malaise, and irritability are often described.

Objective Data

Note signs of infection, bleeding, and chemotherapy complications. Common sites for infection include the mouth, pharynx, lungs, skin, bladder, and perianal area. During chemotherapy, the reduced white cell count may stop the formation of pus, so infection may manifest as redness, swelling, and pain.

Assess for bleeding by monitoring the platelet count because bleeding occurs easily if the platelet count falls below 50,000. Clients bleed from any orifice, so inspect all body discharge. Occult blood is present in the urine and stool.

Chemotherapy complications are nausea, vomiting, and stomatitis. Alopecia occurs 1 to 2 weeks after treatments are initiated.

Nursing diagnoses for a client with leukemia include the following:

NURSING DIAGNOSES	PLANNING/OUTCOMES	NURSING INTERVENTIONS
*Deficient **Knowledge*** related to disease process and treatment	The client will relate treatment methods and possible complications of chemotherapy.	Teach the client to observe for signs of infection and bleeding. Review side effects of chemotherapy and radiation with the client, family members, and significant others.
*Risk for **Infection*** related to increased production of immature white blood cells	The client will describe ways to prevent infection.	Follow good hand hygiene techniques. Teach proper hand hygiene to the family and friends who come into contact with the leukemic client. Use antimicrobial soaps for the client's daily bath. Provide frequent oral care with a soft toothbrush and nonirritating mouthwash to prevent open sores and stomatitis. Wash the perianal area after each bowel movement to decrease bacterial contamination and prevent rectal fissures.

(Continues)

Nursing diagnoses for a client with leukemia include the following: (Continued)

NURSING DIAGNOSES	PLANNING/OUTCOMES	NURSING INTERVENTIONS
		Avoid taking a rectal temperature and giving suppositories. Monitor the temperature every 4 hours for signs of infection. Report any temperature over 100°F to the physician. Administer antibiotics and antifungals as ordered. Closely monitor respiratory rate and breath sounds.
*Risk for **Injury*** related to decreased production of platelets	The client will identify ways to avoid injury and prevent bleeding.	Frequently observe the client for signs of bleeding such as epistaxis, gingival bleeding, petechiae, ecchymoses, hematemesis, enlarged abdomen, hematuria, melena, and confusion, which occur from intracranial hemorrhage. Administer stool softeners frequently to prevent anal irritation from hard stools. Use cotton swabs instead of a toothbrush for oral care. Encourage the client to use an electric razor. Avoid giving injections as much as possible. If a catheter is needed, lubricate it well to avoid trauma to the mucosal lining of the urethra.
*Imbalanced **Nutrition**: Less than Body Requirements* related to effects of disease process and chemotherapy on gastrointestinal tract	The client will choose nonirritating, high-protein, high-carbohydrate meals and snacks.	Administer antiemetics as ordered to relieve nausea and vomiting. Suggest that the client may tolerate small frequent feedings better than three large meals. Provide the client with a high-protein, high-carbohydrate diet to prevent infection and provide needed energy. Administer vitamin supplements as ordered. Teach the client to avoid raw fruits and vegetables as these foods contain more bacteria than cooked foods.
*Ineffective **Coping*** related to uncertainty about treatment of disease and prognosis	The client will identify ways to cope with concerns about disease process.	Inform the client of the possibility of alopecia from therapy treatments. Suggest client purchase a wig prior to initiation of chemotherapy treatments. Encourage the client to voice concerns and fears. Teach the client, family members, and significant others to monitor and report signs of infection and bleeding. Refer to support groups, social workers, and clergy as needed.

Evaluation: Evaluate each outcome to determine how it has been met by the client.

AGRANULOCYTOSIS

A severely reduced number of granulocytes (basophils, eosinophils, and neutrophils) is called **agranulocytosis** (see Memory Trick). The primary cause is an adverse reaction to medication or medication toxicity, especially with administration of phenylbutazone (Butazolidin), chloramphenical (Chloromycetin), penicillin derivatives, cephalosporins, phenytoin (Dilantin), antihistamines, vincristine (Oncovin), propythiouracil, diuretics, chlorpromazine hydrochloride (Thorazine), fluphenazene (Prolixin), promazene hydrochloride (Sparine), and sulfonamides and their derivatives. Other causes of agranulocytosis are neoplastic disease, chemotherapy, radiation therapy, and bacterial and viral infection. The causative agent suppresses the bone marrow, reducing the production of leukocytes.

The client exhibits the symptoms of infection: headache, fever, chills, and fatigue as well as mucous membrane ulcerations of the nose, mouth, pharynx, vagina, and rectum. The white blood count and neutrophils are low.

MEMORYTRICK

Granulocytes

There are three types of granulocytes: basophils, eosinophils, and neutrophils. A way to remember the granulocyte cells is to recall **G-BEN**:

G = Granulocytes
B = Basophils
E = Eosinophils
N = Neutrophils

MEDICAL–SURGICAL MANAGEMENT

Medical

The main goals of treatment are to remove the cause of the bone marrow suppression and either prevent or treat any infection. When the client's temperature is elevated, blood cultures are performed. Mucosal ulcerations are cultured. Blood transfusions are given to provide mature leukocytes. Filgrastim (Neupogen), a human granulocyte colony-stimulating factor, is given. Protective isolation is instituted.

Pharmacological

Antibiotics specific for cultured microorganisms are given.

Diet

A soft, bland diet high in calories, protein, and vitamins is ordered.

Activity

Periods of activity must be balanced with periods of rest to prevent weakness and fatigue.

INFECTION CONTROL

The Client with Agranulocytosis

- Perform hand hygiene frequently and follow aseptic technique when caring for the client.
- Keep client's environment very clean.
- The client should avoid crowds.
- Screen guests so no one with a cold or any type of infection visits the client.
- Teach client to avoid hot or cold environments.
- Ensure that the client reports any signs or symptoms of infection.

NURSING MANAGEMENT

Assess vital signs and monitor for temperature over 100.6°F. Auscultate lungs for crackles and wheezes. Balance periods of activity with periods of rest. Use strict asepsis for all procedures. Perform thorough hand hygiene before caring for client. Screen everyone coming into contact with the client for signs of infection. Encourage intake of adequate fluids. Monitor WBC count.

NURSING PROCESS

ASSESSMENT

Subjective Data

The client may describe having extreme fatigue, weakness, headache, chills, and fever. Inquire about all medications taken, including over-the-counter and prescription drugs.

Objective Data

Assess vital signs especially for a temperature over 100.6°F. Mucosal ulcerations may be reddened. Auscultate the lungs for crackles and wheezes.

A nursing diagnosis for a client with agranulocytosis includes the following:

NURSING DIAGNOSES	PLANNING/OUTCOME	NURSING INTERVENTIONS
Risk for Infection related to decreased leukocyte production	The client will not have signs and symptoms of infection.	Thoroughly cleanse hands before caring for the client. Screen all persons for signs of infection before allowing them near the client. Monitor vital signs for signs of infection. Use strict asepsis for all procedures. Encourage the client to drink an adequate amount of fluids. Monitor WBC count. Provide personal hygiene to prevent infection. Provide client with periods of rest between activities.

Evaluation: Evaluate each outcome to determine how it has been met by the client.

COAGULATION DISORDERS

Coagulation disorders include disseminated intravascular coagulation, hemophilia, and thrombocytopenia.

DISSEMINATED INTRAVASCULAR COAGULATION

Disseminated intravascular coagulation (DIC) is not a disease in itself but a syndrome that occurs because of a primary disease process or condition. A few of the conditions in which DIC may occur are burns, acute leukemia, metastatic cancer, polycythemia vera, pheochromocytoma, shock, acute infections, septic abortion, abruptio placenta, blood transfusion reactions, and trauma.

DIC is a condition of alternating clotting and hemorrhaging. The primary disease stimulates the clotting mechanism, causing many microthrombi (very small clots) to form and block the circulation in the arterioles and capillaries. With the formation of the numerous small clots, the body's fibrinolytic process responds in an attempt to stop the clot formation, thus causing hemorrhaging (Figure 6-8). This can be a very serious and potentially fatal condition.

The occlusion of blood vessels with the clots causes infarcts and necrosis of organs and tissues. The kidneys are the most commonly affected organ.

If a client with a predisposing condition develops **purpura** (reddish purple patches on the skin indicative of hemorrhage), bleeding tendencies, or renal impairment, the nurse assesses for DIC. Symptoms of DIC present as oozing from a venipuncture, mucus membrane, or surgical wound. The oozing progresses rapidly into a hemorrhage within a few hours to a day. The client has decreased urine output from decreased blood flow or renal infarction.

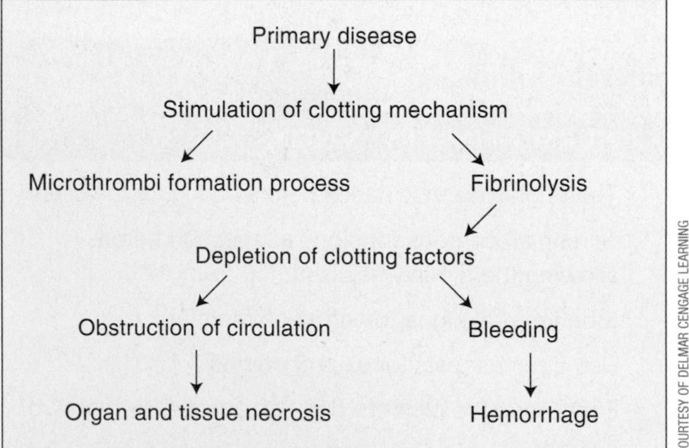

FIGURE 6-8 Pathophysiology of DIC

MEDICAL–SURGICAL MANAGEMENT

Medical

DIC is diagnosed by the client's symptoms and laboratory tests. With DIC there is an increased prothrombin time, partial thromboplastin time, thrombin time, and a decreased fibrinogen and platelet count. A laboratory test that confirms the diagnosis is the D dimer, which measures a fibrin split product that is released when a clot breaks.

The primary disease or condition must be treated. For example, if the primary disease is an infection, an antibiotic is given. If cancer is the primary disease, chemotherapy is given.

DIC is treated by administering whole blood or blood products to normalize the clotting factor level. Platelets and packed red cells are given to replace those lost during hemorrhage. Cryoprecipitate or fresh-frozen plasma is given to normalize clotting factor levels.

Pharmacological

Heparin has no effect on the thrombi that are already formed but is given to prevent the formation of more microthrombi. The administration of heparin is controversial because of the risk of hemorrhage. After thrombi formation is controlled with heparin, aminocaproic acid (Amicar) is given to stop the bleeding because it stops the fibrinolytic process. **Fibrinolysis** is the process of breaking fibrin apart.

NURSING MANAGEMENT

Be aware of precipitating conditions. Monitor I&O closely. Watch for purpura on the chest and abdomen, a common first sign. Monitor vital signs, peripheral pulses, and neurological checks. Avoid giving injections and venipunctures when possible.

NURSING PROCESS

ASSESSMENT

Subjective Data

Ask the client about previous conditions such as infectious processes, trauma, or cancer. Client statements of joint pain indicate bleeding into the joint. Document recent visual changes.

Objective Data

Observe and record the amount of bleeding from any wound or body orifice. Monitor I&O closely. Purpura on the chest and abdomen is a common first sign. Abdominal tenderness is often present. Note presence of pulmonary edema, hypotension, tachycardia, absence of peripheral pulses, confusion, restlessness, convulsions, and coma.

A nursing diagnosis for a client with DIC includes the following:

NURSING DIAGNOSES	PLANNING/OUTCOME	NURSING INTERVENTIONS
Risk for Injury related to altered clotting factors	The client will experience a minimal amount of injury.	Monitor vital signs, peripheral pulses, neurological checks, and urine output.
		Check urine and stool for the presence of blood.
		Assess for abdominal bleeding by checking for abdominal firmness or rigidity.
		If abdominal bleeding is suspected, measure the abdominal girth every 4 hours.
		Assess surgical wounds and all body orifices for bleeding and apply pressure to any oozing site.
		Assess color, warmth, sensation, and movement of extremities.
		Observe for changes in mental status.
		Avoid giving injections and venipunctures as much as possible.
		Observe for signs of orthostatic hypotension.

Evaluation: Evaluate each outcome to determine how it has been met by the client.

HEMOPHILIA

Hemophilia is an inherited bleeding disorder in which there is a lack of clotting factors. Approximately 18,000 persons in the United States have hemophilia (CDC, 2005). There are two types of hemophilia: hemophilia A is lacking clotting factor VIII, and hemophilia B (Christmas disease) is lacking clotting factor IX, along with an absence of a plasma protein, which results in nonformation of thromboplastin. The hemophilia trait is carried on the recessive X chromosome, so a mother is asymptomatic but can pass the trait to the son, who then manifests the symptoms of hemophilia (Figure 6-9). In the male population, hemophilia A occurs at the rate of 1:5,000 and hemophilia B occurs at the rate of 1:10,000 (NHF, 2006). Genetic counseling is often advantageous for clients who are carriers or who have hemophilia. There is no family history of hemophilia B in 33% of those with the disorder. These cases result from a new or spontaneous gene mutation (NHF, 2006). It is rare for a female to have hemophilia, but it can happen if the father has the disease and the mother is a carrier (NHF, 2002a).

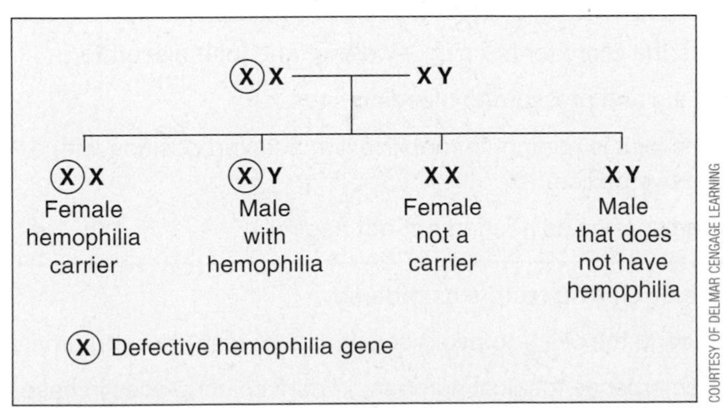

FIGURE 6-9 Hemophilia Inheritance Pattern between a Female Hemophilia Carrier and a Male without Hemophilia

There are three classifications of hemophilia: severe (factor level less than 1% of normal), moderate (factor level 1% to 5% of normal), and mild (factor level 40% of normal). The main symptom of hemophilia is bleeding. The client with severe hemophilia bleeds with minor trauma to an area but can also bleed spontaneously. **Hemarthrosis** (bleeding into the joints) occurs most frequently, causing pain, swelling, redness, and fever. Spontaneous ecchymoses and bleeding from the mouth and gastrointestinal and urinary tracts may occur. The most common cause of death is intracranial hemorrhage. Clients with mild hemophilia will not have spontaneous muscle and joint bleeding but will bleed after minor or major surgery. This condition could prove fatal if the diagnosis is not determined promptly.

MEDICAL–SURGICAL MANAGEMENT

Medical

Hemophilia is diagnosed by a deficient or absent blood level of factors VIII or IX. The prothrombin time (PT), thrombin time, platelet count, and bleeding time are normal, but the partial thromboplastin time (PTT) is usually prolonged.

The National Hemophilia Foundation's Medical and Scientific Advisory Council (MASAC) recommend that hemophilia A be treated with Recombinant (genetically engineered) factor VIII. Cryoprecipitate is not recommended because of the risk of hepatitis and HIV infections (NHF, 2002a). For hemophilia B, the MASAC recommends Recombinant factor IX concentrates. Plasma-derived factor VIII concentrates still has the possibility of transmitting HIV-1, HIV-2, or hepatitis B or C, even with the use of improved viral-depleting processes (NHF, 2009). About

COMMUNITY/HOME HEALTH CARE

Hemophilia

It is important for the client and family to understand the disease process, learn how to recognize signs and symptoms of bleeding, and be able to administer treatments at home. The client should:

- Obtain medical care for trauma, cuts, edema, or pain in muscles and joints.
- Wear a Medic-Alert tag.
- Not take aspirin.
- Use a soft-bristled toothbrush and carefully perform oral hygiene.
- Prevent injuries by wearing gloves and long-sleeved clothing when doing household chores and participating in noncontact sports and activities.

90% of hemophilia clients treated with plasma concentrates in the early 1980s were infected with HIV; more than 50% of these client have died (NHF, 2006).

Pharmacological

Desmopressin acetate is available in a parenteral form (DDAVP Injection) and a highly concentrated intranasal spray (Stimate Nasal Spray) in clients with mild hemophilia A. Desmopressin is not used in children under 2 years of age, pregnant women, or in hemophilia A clients who do not receive adequate Factor VIII levels with the medication (NHF, 2009).

NURSING MANAGEMENT

Assess for signs of bleeding: petechiae, ecchymoses, hematemesis, melena, epistaxis, hematuria, hemarthrosis, and abdominal rigidity. Note edematous or immobile joints. Encourage client to wear Medic-Alert bracelet and avoid activities that cause trauma. Advise not to take aspirin, and to use an electric razor and a soft toothbrush.

NURSING PROCESS

ASSESSMENT

Subjective Data

Assess the client for pain and ask what measures were used in the past to relieve pain and bleeding.

Objective Data

Assess the client for bleeding by checking for petechiae, ecchymoses, hematuria, hematemesis, melena, epistaxis, hemarthrosis, abdominal firmness and rigidity, and frank bleeding. Note edematous or immobile joints.

Nursing diagnoses for a client with hemophilia include the following:

NURSING DIAGNOSES	PLANNING/OUTCOMES	NURSING INTERVENTIONS
*Deficient **Knowledge*** related to disease process	The client will relate symptoms to report and treatment methods if bleeding occurs.	Discuss ways to improve the safety of the client's home environment. Advise client not to take aspirin and encourage the client to use an electric razor and soft-bristled toothbrush. Teach family members or significant others administration of clotting factors for prophylactic purposes and if injury occurs. Encourage client to wear Medic-Alert bracelet. Refer for genetic counseling. Refer client and family to a hemophilia treatment center.
*Acute **Pain*** related to bleeding into tissues and joints	The client will have minimal pain.	Assess the client for bruising, swelling, and joint discomfort. Apply ice and pressure to bleeding sites. When a joint is hurting, immobilize it in a flexed position with a supportive device. Give analgesics as needed but not aspirin.
*Risk for **Injury*** related to altered clotting factors	The client will take precautions to avoid injury.	Transfuse clotting factors as ordered. Encourage the client to avoid activities that may cause trauma. Post emergency medical numbers in convenient places in case of future need.

Evaluation: Evaluate each outcome to determine how it has been met by the client.

THROMBOCYTOPENIA

Thrombocytopenia is a decrease in the number of platelets in the blood. The decrease may be related to:

- Decreased platelet production as in aplastic anemia, tumors, leukemia, and chemotherapy
- Decreased platelet survival as in infection or viral illnesses
- Increased platelet destruction as in DIC or thrombocytopenic purpura that is either drug induced or **idiopathic** (occurring without a known cause)

Withdrawal of the causative drug usually allows the platelet count to return to normal in 1 to 2 weeks. The acute form of idiopathic thrombocytopenic purpura (ITP) is an autoimmune process caused by an autoantibody-destroying platelet antigen.

Petechiae, ecchymoses, and bleeding from mucous membranes are observed. Bleeding may occur in internal organs. The platelet count is very low; the bleeding time is prolonged; Hgb and Hct is low; and bone marrow aspiration shows mostly immature platelets.

MEDICAL–SURGICAL MANAGEMENT

Medical

Transfusions of platelet concentrates are given, or **apheresis** (removal of unwanted components) is performed on the client's blood to remove the autoantibodies.

Surgical

A splenectomy is performed because the spleen is the primary site of platelet destruction. This treatment is usually reserved until all other treatments have been unsuccessful.

Pharmacological

Corticosteroids are given to prolong platelet life and strengthen the capillaries. Immunosuppressive drugs, gamma globulin, and vitamin K are given.

Diet

A high-fiber diet is eaten to prevent constipation and the need to strain when having a bowel movement.

Activity

Activity is undertaken thoughtfully and carefully to prevent any trauma.

NURSING MANAGEMENT

Monitor for signs of bleeding (ecchymoses, petechiae, and rigid abdomen). Check laboratory reports for low platelet count, Hgb, and Hct, and prolonged bleeding time. Encourage a high-fiber diet to prevent constipation. Assess pain and administer analgesics as ordered. Monitor vital signs and mental status.

NURSING PROCESS

ASSESSMENT

Subjective Data

Ask the client about medications being taken and any recent infection.

Objective Data

Observe for petechiae, ecchymoses, and any signs of blood or internal bleeding.

Nursing diagnoses for a client with thrombocytopenia include the following:

NURSING DIAGNOSES	PLANNING/OUTCOMES	NURSING INTERVENTIONS
*Acute **Pain*** related to hemorrhage	The client will verbalize having less pain.	Assess client's pain on 0 (least) to 10 (most) pain scale and client's ability to cope with pain. Administer analgesic as ordered, and note client's response.
*Risk for **Injury*** related to thrombocytopenia	The client will have minimal injury.	Monitor client's vital signs and neurological and mental status. Assess client's skin and excretions for signs of bleeding. Handle client very carefully when turning, assisting out of bed, and in all other care situations.

Evaluation: Evaluate each outcome to determine how it has been met by the client.

LYMPH DISORDERS

A **lymphoma** is a tumor of the lymphatic system. Two malignant lymphomas discussed in this chapter are Hodgkin's disease and non-Hodgkin's lymphoma (NHL). The overview and medical management of each disease are presented separately. The nursing process for both diseases is presented together because the nursing diagnoses, goals, and interventions are the same.

HODGKIN'S DISEASE

Hodgkin's disease (Hodgkin's lymphoma) is a rare lymphoma that usually arises as a painless swelling in a lymph node. The diagnosis is confirmed when Reed-Sternberg cells (Hodgkin cells) are biopsied from the swollen lymph node. There are two types of Hodgkin's disease (HD), the classical Hodgkin's disease and the nodular lymphocyte predominance Hodgkin disease (NLPHD). HD has an abnormal B lymphocyte that is larger than normal lymphocytes. The abnormal B lymphocytes are known as Reed-Sternberg cells (Hodgkin cells) and confirm the diagnosis when biopsied from a swollen lymph node. NLPHD is confined to lymph nodes in the neck and under the arm (ACS, 2009d). HD affects children and adults, but occurs most frequently in early adulthood between the ages of 15–40 and in adults after 55 years of age (ACS, 2009d).

Risk factors are mostly unknown, but reduced immune function and certain infectious agents are involved. There is a slightly higher risk for HD in clients who had mono (infectious mononucleosis) caused by the Epstein-Barr virus (ACS, 2009d).

Clients with Hodgkin's disease most commonly have painless enlarged lymph nodes in the neck, in the area above the clavicles, and in the groin. Lymph nodes in the mediastinum may also be enlarged but are not usually diagnosed until the nodes enlarge and press on the mediastinal structures, causing dyspnea and a cough. A chest x-ray or a computed tomography (CT) scan confirms the involvement of the mediastinal lymph nodes. Other symptoms are weight loss, fatigue, pruritus, recurrent high fever, night sweats, anemia, thrombocytopenia, and lowered resistance to infections.

If a client has painless, enlarged lymph nodes and the symptoms of an elevated temperature of 100°F without any known cause other than HD, drenching night sweats, and weight loss of more than 10% of the body weight in a 6-month period, more intense treatment is recommended. Hodgkin's lymphoma spreads throughout the body in a predictable pattern. From the site of the original swollen gland, the disease spreads to nearby lymph nodes and then to other lymphatic tissue in the body such as the liver, spleen, and bone marrow. The invasion of other nodes and lymphatic tissue determines the prognosis of the disease. See Table 6-5 for the Ann Arbor Staging System for HD.

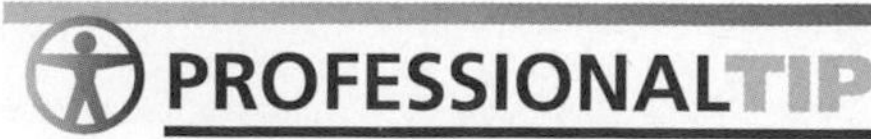

Serious HD Factors

If a client is male, older than 45 years of age, has tumors that are one-third as wide as the chest or tumors 4 inches across, a WBC >15,000, Hgb <10.5, lymphocyte count <600, and a low blood albumin level, the prognosis is worse, and more intense treatment is recommended.

MEDICAL–SURGICAL MANAGEMENT

Medical

Diagnostic tests include CBC, platelet count, bone marrow aspiration, chest x-ray, abdominal CT scan, lymphangiogram, and lymph node biopsy.

Localized Hodgkin's disease stages I and II are treated with radiation therapy. Clients with massive mediastinal involvement and those who have relapsed after radiation therapy alone are treated with radiation therapy and chemotherapy.

During radiation therapy, the client may experience weight loss, nausea and vomiting, skin reactions, esophagitis, fatigue, and bone marrow suppression. The client's blood count is monitored closely during therapy to check for infection and bleeding tendencies. If the WBC level drops too low, the client will be more susceptible to infections. A decrease in RBCs and platelets causes a bleeding tendency. Long-term complications from radiation therapy include hypothyroidism, radiation pneumonitis, immune system impairment, herpes zoster, and the development of a second cancer.

Generalized Hodgkin's disease stages III and IV are treated with combination chemotherapy, which is administering a series of combined drugs over a set period. Serious late complications of chemotherapy are infertility and a secondary malignancy or cancer.

Surgical

Sometimes a laparotomy is done to see if the liver and spleen are involved. The rationale of performing the procedure is being questioned since the overall treatment plan is not altered.

Pharmacological

During radiation therapy, antiemetics, such as ondansetron HCl (Zofran), are given for nausea and vomiting. Analgesics are given for esophagitis discomfort.

Chemotherapy drugs are often given in combinations. The main chemotherapy treatment for HD is ABVD, a combination of 4 drugs: adriamycin (Doxorubicin), bleomycin, vinblastine (Velban), and dacarbazine (DTIC). When the disease does not respond to other treatments, MOPP (nitrogen mustard (Mustargen), vincristine sulfate (Oncovin), procarbazine HCl (Matulane), and prednisone (Deltasone) is used. Sometimes MOPP alternating with ABVD or ABV (adriamycin, bleomycin, and vinblastine) are used. Zofran or Kytril are given for nausea and Zantac for an upset stomach with MOPP. These drugs are usually administered intravenously or through an implanted venous port. Allopurinol (Zyloprim) is given to prevent uric acid renal stones caused by the rapid destruction of cells during therapy.

If the disease process does not respond well to chemotherapy, an option for the client is a bone marrow or peripheral blood stem cell transplant with high-dose chemotherapy. Rituximab (Rituxan), a monoclonal antibody, is presently in trial for use with HD.

Diet

During therapy, the client is on a high-calorie, high-protein diet. Encourage an intake of 2,500 mL of fluid per day to prevent the formation of renal stones.

Activity

Extra rest periods may be necessary to cope with fatigue that occurs with Hodgkin's disease.

TABLE 6-5 Ann Arbor Staging System for Hodgkin's Disease with 5-Year Relative Survival Rate

STAGE	NODE AND ORGAN INVOLVEMENT	DESCRIPTION OF ANN ARBOR STAGING CLASSIFICATION	5-YEAR RELATIVE SURVIVAL RATE
I	Cervical nodes; Stage I	Enlargement of single lymph node region (I) or of a single extralymphatic organ (IE)	90% to 95%
II	Mediastinal nodes; Stage II	Involvement of two or more lymph node regions on the same side of the diaphragm (II) or involvement of extralymphatic organ and one or more lymph node region on the same side of the diaphragm (IIE)	90% to 95%
III	Splenic hilar nodes; Periaortic nodes; Iliac nodes; Mesenteric nodes; Inguinal nodes; Spleen; Splenic hilar nodes; Portahepatic nodes; Celiac nodes; Stage III	Involvement of lymph node region on both sides of the diaphragm (III) plus involvement of the spleen (IIIS) or with involvement of extralymphatic organ (IIIE) or both (IIISE)	80% to 85%
IV	Pulmonary infiltrates; Axillary nodes; Liver; Splenic hilar nodes; Small intestine; Bone; Stage IV	Scattered involvement of one or more extra-lymphatic organs with or without involving lymph nodes (IV)	Approximately 60% to 70%
If an organ outside of the lymph system but next to involved lymph nodes is affected, the letter "E" is added to the stage number, i.e., IE.			
If the spleen is involved, the letter "S" is added to the stage number, i.e., IIS.			
If the client has lost more than 10% of body weight in a 6-month time frame, has a temperature above 100°F without any known cause other than HD, and drenching night sweats, the letter "B" is added to the stage number, i.e., IIIB.			
If a client has tumors that are 1/3 as wide as the chest or 4 inches across, the letter "X" is added to the stage number, i.e., IIX.			

Adapted from Overview: Hodgkin's disease. By American Cancer Society (ACS), 2009d, retrieved May 13, 2009, from http://www.cancer.org/docroot/CRI/content/CRI_2_2_1X_What_is_Hodgkins_disease_20.asp?sitearea=CRI; Ann Arbor Staging Classification for Hodgkin Disease. By CureSearch, 2001, retrieved May 13, 2009, from http://www.curesearch.org/articleprint.aspx?ArticleId=3325

NON-HODGKIN'S LYMPHOMA

Non-Hodgkin's lymphoma (NHL) is more common than Hodgkin's disease and is the fifth most-common cancer in the United States. The incidence rate for NHL has almost doubled since the 1970s. Approximately 66,120 new cases are estimated for 2008. The 5-year relative survival rate is 63% and the 10-year rate is 51% (ACS, 2007g).

NHL originates from the B lymphocytes and the T lymphocytes. NHL arising from the B lymphocytes occurs in the older adult population; NHL arising from the T lymphocytes manifests in malignant skin diseases such as mycosis fungoides or Sezary syndrome. More men are affected than women. NHL does not have the Reed-Sternberg cell present.

Symptoms of NHL are enlarged painless lymph nodes in the neck, axillary, abdominal, and inguinal areas. Other symptoms include fever, night sweats, excessive tiredness, indigestion, abdominal pain, loss of appetite, and bone pain.

Medical–Surgical Management

Medical

The diagnosis of NHL is confirmed by a lymph node biopsy. Physicians use the same staging system as for Hodgkin's disease.

Pharmacological

There are two different chemotherapy regimens, CHOP and CVP: CHOP combines cyclophosphamide (Cytoxan), doxorubicin HCl (Adriamycin), vincristine sulfate (Oncovin), and prednisone (Deltasone); CVP combines cyclophosphamide (Cytoxan), vincristine sulfate (Oncovin), and prednisone (Deltasone). Other chemotherapy drugs used are chlorambucil (Leukeran), fludaravine (Fludara), and etoposide (VePesid). Bone marrow or peripheral blood stem cell transplantation is used for HD clients who have a relapse.

Nursing Management

Assess for enlarged, painless lymph nodes. Monitor vital signs, weight, and voice changes. Review blood test results. Encourage deep breathing and adequate fluid intake. Provide a high-calorie, high-protein diet in small, frequent meals.

NURSING PROCESS

Assessment

Subjective Data

Ask if the client is experiencing pruritus, night sweats, weight loss, decreased appetite, fever, fatigue, weakness, or chest pain.

Objective Data

Assess weight, vital signs, and for skin infections; dyspnea; cough; voice changes; enlarged lymph nodes in the neck, axilla, and groin; and edema in the extremities. Bone scan shows fractures and tumor infiltration. Review blood tests for hypercalcemia if bone lesions are present, and a CBC often indicates anemia. When the client is having radiation or chemotherapy treatments, the assessment includes observing for dysphagia, nausea and vomiting, skin rashes, and alopecia.

Nursing diagnoses for a client with Hodgkin's disease or non-Hodgkin's lymphoma include the following:

NURSING DIAGNOSES	PLANNING/OUTCOMES	NURSING INTERVENTIONS
*Ineffective **B**reathing Pattern* related to tracheobronchial obstruction from enlarged mediastinal nodes	The client will complete activities of daily living without dyspnea.	Elevate the head of the bed to assist the client's breathing. Encourage the client to take frequent deep breaths to expand the lungs and prevent infection; assess the client's breathing pattern every shift and as needed for dyspnea.
*Risk for **I**nfection* related to radiation/chemotherapy treatments, decreased WBCs and pruritus	The client will remain free of infection.	Monitor the lab results for lowered WBCs. Teach the client the importance of avoiding situations where there is exposure to infections. Provide cool sponge baths or oral medication to relieve pruritus. Assess the radiated skin areas for redness or breaks in the skin. Encourage the client to report symptoms of dyspnea, sore throat, and burning or frequency of urination.
*Imbalanced **N**utrition: Less than Body Requirements* related to decreased appetite	The client will consume an adequate amount of a nutritional diet.	Serve attractive high-calorie, high-protein meals in a pleasant environment. Offer six to eight smaller meals throughout the day to decrease a feeling of fullness. A soft, bland diet is more palatable during radiation or chemotherapy treatments. Avoid hot, spicy foods that are caustic to mucous membranes and lead to infection. Encourage an adequate intake of fluids to prevent constipation and renal stones. Weigh the client biweekly or more frequently if needed.

Nursing diagnoses for a client with Hodgkin's disease or non-Hodgkin's lymphoma include the following: (Continued)

NURSING DIAGNOSES	PLANNING/OUTCOMES	NURSING INTERVENTIONS
Anxiety related to disease and therapy treatments	The client will cope effectively with disease process and therapy treatments.	Listen to the concerns of the client regarding the effect of the disease on lifestyle, family, and finances. Encourage the family to express their concerns and discuss effective ways to deal with the diagnosis and treatment. Refer the client and family to clergy and social agencies when appropriate.

Evaluation: Evaluate each outcome to determine how it has been met by the client.

PLASMA CELL DISORDER

The main plasma cell disorder is myeloma.

MULTIPLE MYELOMA

There were an estimated 19,920 new cases of multiple myeloma diagnosed in 2008, and an estimated 10,690 persons died from it (ACS, 2009e). More cases occur in men older than age 65 (ACS, 2009e).

The plasma cells, mainly in bone marrow, become malignant, crowd out normal cell production, destroy normal bone tissue, and thereby cause pain. The normal production of antibodies is changed, making the client susceptible to infections. The first sign of myeloma is often bone pain, especially in the ribs, spine, and pelvis. The long bones ache; joints are swollen and tender; and a low-grade fever and general malaise are present. The client tires easily and has weakness from anemia. The weakened bones fracture easily. The cause of myeloma is not known.

Diagnosis is made with bone marrow biopsy showing large numbers of immature plasma cells and x-rays showing demineralization and osteoporosis. Bence Jones protein is found in the urine of many clients with myeloma. The client will also have hypercalcemia, hyperuricemia, anemia, and hypercalciuria.

MEDICAL–SURGICAL MANAGEMENT

Medical

Multiple myeloma is not curable, so treatment is symptomatic. Intensive chemotherapy followed by autologous peripheral blood stem cell transplantation may restore normal blood cell production.

Surgical

A laminectomy is required if any vertebrae collapse. If the client gets kidney stones from the large amount of calcium in the blood and urine, surgery may be required.

Pharmacological

Steroids such as prednisone and dexamethasone (Decadron) along with antineoplastic drugs such as cyclophosphamide (Cytoxan), meophalan (Alkeran), vincristine sulfate (Oncovin), and doxorubicin HCl (Adriamycin) are given. Some drugs are used in combination, such as VAD (vincristine, doxorubicin, and dexamethasone). Pamidronate (Aredia) and zoledronic acid (Zometa), bisphosphonates, are given intravenously for bone problems. Radiation therapy is used to treat bone pain or bone that is not responding to chemotherapy. Interferon is given when the client is in remission because it seems to extend the remission (ACS, 2009e).

If the serum calcium level increases above 10 mg/dL, the physician orders an IV of normal saline infused at a high rate followed by diuretics.

> **CLIENT TEACHING**
>
> **Myeloma**
>
> - Drink 3 to 4 L of fluids per day.
> - Exercise to decrease bone demineralization.
> - Monitor for symptoms of hypercalcemia and notify physician if symptoms occur.

Diet

Six small meals per day are often tolerated better than the usual three meals per day; nutritious meals based on the client's food preferences are recommended. A fluid intake of 3 to 4 L per day is essential to minimize the complications of excessive calcium in the blood and urine.

Activity

It is important to keep the client as mobile as possible. Walking stimulates calcium resorption and decreases demineralization. When the client is in bed, it is important to reposition the client frequently using a lift sheet to decrease the risk of pathological fractures.

NURSING MANAGEMENT

Assess for bone pain. Monitor laboratory test results for hypercalcemia. Provide six small meals each day of client's preferred foods. Encourage fluid intake to 3 to 4 L per day. Encourage ambulation. Monitor vital signs.

NURSING PROCESS

ASSESSMENT

Subjective Data

The client describes constant pain that increases with movement. The pain is usually in the back, ribs, or pelvis. Achiness in the long bones and joints and general malaise also is described.

Objective Data

Assess pain using a 0 (none) to 10 (most) pain scale. Temperature is elevated. The client's ability to perform activities of daily living is decreased. Monitor the level of blood calcium.

Nursing diagnoses for a client with multiple myeloma include the following:

NURSING DIAGNOSES	PLANNING/OUTCOMES	NURSING INTERVENTIONS
*Chronic **Pain*** related to disease process	The client will express a decrease in pain level.	Assess the client's pain level with pain scale. Administer analgesic as ordered and monitor the client's response.
*Risk for **Injury*** related to bone demineralization	The client will have minimal injuries.	Handle client gently and reposition the client using a lift sheet. Keep the client's personal items within easy reach.
*Risk for **Infection*** related to disease process and pharmaceutical agents	The client will have few infections.	Thoroughly cleanse hands before caring for the client. Teach the client and family proper hand hygiene. Assist the client with personal hygiene as needed. Screen visitors for signs of infections before allowing them to visit the client.

Evaluation: Evaluate each outcome to determine how it has been met by the client.

CASE STUDY

J.J., 46, owns a hobby shop. He has had a cold for 3 weeks that has recently settled in his chest. He has been tired lately and takes naps each evening before the evening meal. His wife noticed several bruises on his arms and legs, but J.J. could not recall any particular injury. J.J. has gradually lost 10 pounds during the last 3 months but has not been concerned about it. When J.J. went to the clinic for some antibiotics for his cold, the nurse practitioner completed a physical assessment and ordered a chest x-ray and CBC. The nurse practitioner noticed the WBCs were 250,000/mm^3; RBCs, 4.2 million/mm^3; and platelets, 100,000/mm^3. After several other tests were performed during the next few days, a diagnosis of chronic myelogenous leukemia (CML) was confirmed.

The following questions will guide your development of a nursing care plan for the case study.

1. List the symptoms occurring in J.J. that are typical of CML.
2. List five other typical symptoms of CML that were not stated in the case study.
3. List other diagnostic tests that could be done to confirm the diagnosis of CML.
4. List subjective and objective data the nurse would obtain about J.J.
5. Write three individualized nursing diagnoses and goals for J.J.
6. List nursing interventions for J.J.
7. List community resources specific to locale that could assist J.J. and his family during his illness with CML.
8. List discharge teaching the nurse would give to J.J. and his family.
9. List successful client outcomes for J.J.
10. List chemotherapeutic agents and side effects of the agents that may be prescribed for J.J.
11. List other medical treatments that may be ordered for J.J.
12. What measures could the nurse take to meet the emotional needs of J.J. and his family?

SUMMARY

- The main formed components of the blood are red blood cells, white blood cells, and platelets.
- The lymphatic system is composed of lymph vessels that drain lymph into the venous system; lymph nodes that filter microorganisms in the body; and lymph organs, the spleen and thymus.
- Sickledex and hemoglobin electrophoresis are diagnostic tests for sickle cell anemia.
- Some of the symptoms of anemia are fatigue, pallor, exertional dyspnea, and tachycardia.
- Symptoms of polycythemia vera are headache, epistaxis, dizziness, tinnitus, blurred vision, fatigue, weakness, pruritus, exertional dyspnea, angina, and increased blood pressure and pulse.
- Polycythemia vera is treated with chemotherapeutic agents.
- DIC is not a disease but a complication of a disease or condition that causes the client to alternate between forming many small clots and hemorrhaging.
- Hemophilia is a recessive X chromosome inherited bleeding disorder in which the client is lacking clotting

factors. The main symptom is spontaneous bleeding or bleeding caused by trauma.

- The two types of malignant lymphomas are Hodgkin's disease and non-Hodgkin's lymphoma. Clients with both types of lymphoma have enlarged lymph nodes.
- Hodgkin's disease is diagnosed by the presence of the Reed-Sternberg cell in the swollen lymph nodes. Non-Hodgkin's lymphoma arises from the B lymphocytes and T lymphocytes and does not have the Reed-Sternberg cell in the lymph system.

REVIEW QUESTIONS

1. A client has iron deficiency anemia. To improve iron absorption, the nurse serves Feosol with:
   1. milk.
   2. an orange.
   3. water.
   4. processed cheese.
2. A thorough assessment of the cardiac system on a client with sickle cell anemia is important because:
   1. the heart enlarges in an attempt to provide the oxygen needs to the body tissues.
   2. cells sickle more easily in the heart chambers.
   3. more cardiac force is needed to pump RBCs with Hbg S.
   4. people with sickle cell anemia are prone to bradycardia.
3. Clients with leukemia are prone to infections because:
   1. there are too many WBCs.
   2. the bone marrow is not producing WBCs.
   3. the bone marrow is producing too many cells.
   4. the WBCs are incapable of fighting infections.
4. Symptoms that alert a nurse that a client may have DIC are:
   1. tinnitus and numbness and tingling in the extremities.
   2. jaundice, palpitations, and dyspnea.
   3. purpura, bruising, and decreased urine output.
   4. ruddy complexion, epistaxis, and tinnitus.
5. A nurse teaches a client with non-Hodgkin's lymphoma about his disease condition. He knows that the teaching is successful when the client says:
   1. "I will use an electric razor."
   2. "I will take folic acid as prescribed."
   3. "I will apply ice and pressure to bleeding sites."
   4. "I will avoid exposure to infections."
6. A client had the axillary lymph nodes removed. Which one of the following activities is avoided in the affected arm?
   1. Using fingernail polish.
   2. Wearing rings.
   3. Blood pressure checks.
   4. Pulse checks.
7. A nurse examines a client's skin and notes multiple purplish areas randomly distributed over the abdomen. The areas measure more than 0.5 cm in diameter. The nurse records these areas as:
   1. purpura.
   2. petechiae.
   3. spider angioma.
   4. liver disease.
8. A Maine lobsterman was admitted to the unit with an infection in his right hand that he acquired while handling lobster bait. The nurse would most likely find palpable, tender lymph nodes in the:
   1. inguinal region.
   2. supraclavicular region.
   3. periaortic region.
   4. axillary region.
9. A client is at risk of developing a deep vein thrombosis. The nurse anticipates receiving an order for: (Select all that apply.)
   1. compression stockings.
   2. a sequential compression device.
   3. low molecular weight heparin.
   4. bed rest.
   5. a leg massage.
   6. a vitamin K injection.
10. What laboratory value confirms to the nurse that his client has DIC?
    1. Elevated white blood count.
    2. Elevated platelet count.
    3. Presence of fibrin degradation products.
    4. Elevated hematocrit.

REFERENCES/SUGGESTED READINGS

American Cancer Society (ACS). (2003). Cancer Facts & Figures 2003. [Online]. http://search.cancer.org/search?q=cancer+facts+and+figures+&start=30&num=10&access=p&entqr=0&restrict=cancer&output=xml_no_dtd&sort=date%3AD%3AL%3Ad1&ie=UTF-8&client=amcancer&ud=1&site=amcancer&oe=UTF-8&proxystylesheet=amcancer&ip=71.97.143.207

American Cancer Society (ACS). (2007a). How is acute lymphocytic leukemia diagnosed? Retrieved on May 12, 2009 at http://www.cancer.org/docroot/CRI/content/CRI_2_4_3X_How_Is_Acute_Lymphocytic_Leukemia_Diagnosed.asp?sitearea=

American Cancer Society (ACS). (2007b). Detailed Guide: Leukemia-Chronic lymphocytic (CLL) Monoclonal antibodies. Retrieved on

May 12, 2009 at http://www.cancer.org/docroot/CRI/content/CRI_2_4_4X_Monoclonal_Antibodies_62.asp?sitearea=

American Cancer Society (ACS). (2007c). Detailed Guide: Leukemia-Acute myeloid (AML) Chemotherapy (AML). Retrieved on May 12, 2009 at http://www.cancer.org/docroot/CRI/content/CRI_2_4_4x_Chemotherapy_AML.asp?sitearea=

American Cancer Society (ACS). (2007d). Detailed Guide: Leukemia-Acute lymphocytic (ALL) Chemotherapy (AML). Retrieved on May 12, 2009 at http://www.cancer.org/docroot/CRI/content/CRI_2_4_4X_Chemotherapy_57.asp?sitearea=

American Cancer Society (ACS). (2007e). Detailed Guide: Leukemia-Chronic lymphocytic (CLL). What are the key statistics about chronic lymphocytic leukemia? Retrieved on May 12, 2009 at http://www.cancer.org/docroot/CRI/content/CRI_2_4_1X_What_Are_the_Key_Statistics_About_Chronic_Lymphocytic_Leukemia.asp?sitearea=

American Cancer Society (ACS). (2007f). Detailed Guide: Leukemia-Chronic lymphocytic (CLL). What is chronic lymphocytic leukemia? Retrieved on May 12, 2009 at http://www.cancer.org/docroot/CRI/content/CRI_2_4_1X_What_Is_Chronic_Lymphocytic_Leukemia.asp?sitearea=

American Cancer Society (ACS). (2007g). Detailed Guide: Lymphoma, non-Hodgkin type. Retrieved on May 12, 2009 at http://www.cancer.org/docroot/CRI/content/CRI_2_4_1X_What_Is_Non_Hodgkins_Lymphoma_32.asp?sitearea=CRI

American Cancer Society (ACS). (2008a). Detailed Guide: Leukemia-Chronic myeloid (CML) Chemotherapy. Retrieved on May 12, 2009 at http://www.cancer.org/docroot/CRI/content/CRI_2_4_4x_Chemotherapy_CML.asp?sitearea=

American Cancer Society (ACS). (2008b). Detailed Guide: Leukemia-Chronic myeloid (CML). What are the key statistics about chronic myeloid leukemia (CML)? Retrieved on May 12, 2009 at http://www.cancer.org/docroot/CRI/content/CRI_2_4_1x_What_Are_the_Key_Statistics_About_Chronic_Myeloid_Leukemia_CML.asp?sitearea=

American Cancer Society (ACS). (2009a). Cancer Facts and Figures 2009. Retrieved on May 12, 2009 at http://www.cancer.org/downloads/STT/500809web.pdf

American Cancer Society (ACS). (2009b). Detailed Guide: Leukemia – Acute Myeloid (AML). What are the key statistics about acute myeloid leukemia (AML)? Retrieved on May 12, 2009 at http://www.cancer.org/docroot/CRI/content/CRI_2_4_1x_What_Are_the_Key_Statistics_About_Acute_Myeloid_Leukemia_AML.asp?sitearea=

American Cancer Society (ACS). (2009c). Detailed Guide: Leukemia-Acute myeloid (AML). What are the key statistics about childhood leukemia. Retrieved on May 12, 2009 at http://www.cancer.org/docroot/CRI/content/CRI_2_4_1X_What_are_the_key_statistics_about_childhood_leukemia_24.asp?rnav=cri

American Cancer Society (ACS). (2009d). Overview: Hodgkin's disease. Retrieved on May 13, 2009 at http://www.cancer.org/docroot/CRI/content/CRI_2_2_1X_What_is_Hodgkins_disease_20.asp?sitearea=CRI

American Cancer Society (ACS). (2009e). Detailed Guide: Multiple myeloma. Retrieved on May 12, 2009 at http://www.cancer.org/docroot/CRI/content/CRI_2_4_2X_What_are_the_risk_factors_for_multiple_myeloma_30.asp?rnav=cri

Aplastic Anemia & MDS International Foundation. (2006). Aplastic anemia. http://www.aamds.org/aplastic/disease_information/about_the_diseases/aplastic_anemia.php

Atassi, K., & Harris, M. (2001). Disseminated intravascular coagulation. *Nursing2001*, 31(3), 64.

Barry, D., & Schaefer, J. (2003). Hemophilia forces parents to make a tough decision: A nurse's child requires a venous access device implant. *AJN*, 103(1), 64A–64C.

Bulechek, G., Butcher, H., McCloskey, J., & Dochterman, J., eds. (2008). *Nursing Interventions Classification (NIC)* (5th ed.). St. Louis, MO: Mosby/Elsevier.

Centers for Disease Control and Prevention (CDC). (2005). Bleeding disorders. Retrieved on May 12, 2009 at http://www.cdc.gov/ncbddd/hbd/hemophilia.htm

Daniels, R. (2009). *Delmar's guide to laboratory and diagnostic tests* (2nd ed.). Clifton Park, NY: Delmar Cengage Learning.

Day, M. (2001). Sickle cell crisis. *Nursing2001*, 31(5), 88.

Gioia, K., Kleinert, D., & Hannon, M. (1999). What's wrong with this patient? *RN*, 62(2), 43–45.

Gorman, K. (1999). Sickle cell disease. *AJN*, 99(3), 38–43.

Hoffman, K. (2008). *Assessing the hematologic and lymphatic systems.* Manuscript submitted for publication.

Holcomb, S. (2001). Anemia: Pointing the way to a deeper problem. *Nursing2001*, 31(7), 36–42.

Leukemia & Lymphoma Society. (2007). Polycythemia Vera. Retrieved on May 14, 2009 at http://www.leukemia-lymphoma.org/attachments/National/br_1178803767.pdf

Leukemia & Lymphoma Society (LLS). (2009). Leukemia. Retrieved on May 11, 2009 at http://www.leukemia-lymphoma.org/all_page?item_id=7026&viewmode=print

LymphomaInfo. (2009). Hodgkin's chemotherapy – MOPP. 2009 Deep Dive Media, LLC. Retrieved on May 15, 2009 at http://www.lymphomainfo.net/therapy/chemotherapy/mopp.html

LymphomaInfo. (2009). Adult Hodgkin's lymphoma: Chemotherapy. 2009 Deep Dive Media, LLC. Retrieved on May 15, 2009 at http://www.lymphomainfo.net/hodgkins/chemo.html

Maningo, J. (2002). Peripheral blood stem cell transplant. *Nursing2002*, 32(12), 52–55.

Mayo Clinic. (2009). Iron deficiency anemia. Retrieved on May 9, 2009 at http://www.mayoclinic.com/health/iron-deficiency-anemia/DS00323/METHOD=print&DS

McBrien, N. (1997). Clinical snapshot: Thrombocytopenic purpura. *AJN*, 97(2), 28–29.

Mitchell, R. (1999). Sickle cell anemia. *AJN*, 99(5), 36–37.

Moorhead, S., Johnson, M., Maas, M., & Swanson, E. (2007). *Nursing outcomes classification (NOC)* (4th ed). St. Louis, MO: Elsevier – Health Sciences Division.

National Hemophilia Foundation (NHF). (2002a). Bleeding disorders information center/hemophilia A. Retrieved on May 14, 2009 at http://www.hemophilia.org/NHFWeb/MainPgs/MainNHF.aspx?menuid=180&contentid=45&rptname=bleeding

National Hemophilia Foundation (NHF). (2002b). Bleeding disorders information center/hemophilia B. Retrieved on May 14, 2009 at http://www.hemophilia.org/NHFWeb/MainPgs/MainNHF.aspx?menuid=181&contentid=46&rptname=bleeding

National Hemophilia Foundation (NHF). (2007). Fast facts. Retrieved on May 12, 2009 at http://www.hemophilia.org/NHFWeb/MainPgs/MainNHF.aspx?menuid=259&contentid=476

National Hemophilia Foundation (NHF). (2009). MASAC recommendations concerning products licensed for the treatment of hemophilia and other bleeding disorders (MASAC Document #190). Retrieved November 9, 2009 at www.hemophilia.org

National Institutes of Health (NIH). (2009). How is pernicious anemia diagnosed? Retrieved on May 10, 2009 at http://www.nhlbi.nih.gov/health/dci/Diseases/prnanmia/prnamia_diagnosis.html

North American Nursing Diagnosis Association International. (2010). *NANDA-I nursing diagnoses: Definitions and classification 2009-2011.* Ames, IA: Wiley-Blackwell.

Platt, A., Beasley, J., Miller, G., & Eckman, J. (2002). Managing sickle cell pain . . . and all that goes with it. *Nursing2002*, 32(12), 32hn1–32hn7.

Sickle Cell Disease Association of America, Inc. (SCDAA). (2005). Who is affected? Retrieved on May 10, 2009 at http://www.sicklecelldisease.org/about_scd/affected1.phtml

Sidel, H., Ball, J., Dains, J., & Benedict, G. (2006). *Mosby's guide to physical examination* (6th ed.). St. Louis, MO: Mosby Elsevier

Spratto, G., & Woods, A. (2008). *2009 edition Delmar's nurses drug handbook*. Clifton Park, NY: Delmar Cengage Learning.

Stuart, B., & Viera, A. (2004). Polycythemia vera. American Family Physician. Retrieved on May 11, 2009 at http://www.aafp.org/afp/AFPprinter/20040501/2139.html?print=yes

Thibodeau, G., & Patton, K. (2009). *Anatomy and physiology* (7th ed.) St. Louis, MO: Mosby.

Voshall, B. (2008). *Caring for clients with coagulation and lymphatic disorders*. Manuscript submitted for publication.

RESOURCES

American Cancer Society (ACS), http://www.cancer.org

Aplastic Anemia & MDS International Foundation, Inc., http://www.aamds.org

Blood and Marrow Transplant Information Network, http://www.bmtinfonet.org

Cancer Information Service (CIS), http://cis.nci.nih.gov/

Center for Sickle Cell Disease, http://www.sicklecell.howard.edu/

Cooley's Anemia Foundation, http://www.thalassemia.org/

Information for Sickle Cell and Thalassemic Disorders, http://sickle.bwh.harvard.edu/

National Cancer Institute, http://www.cancer.gov/

National Heart, Lung, and Blood Institute, http://www.nhlbi.nih.gov/

National Hemophilia Foundation, http://www.hemophilia.org

National Marrow Donor Program, http://www.marrow.org

Sickle Cell Disease Association of America, Inc., http://www.sicklecelldisease.org

The Leukemia & Lymphoma Society, http://www.leukemia_lymphoma.org

The Lymphoma Foundation, http://www.lymphomafoundation.org/

UNIT 3 Nursing Care of the Client: Digestion and Elimination

CHAPTER 7
Gastrointestinal System

MAKING THE CONNECTION

Refer to the following chapters to increase your understanding of the gastrointestinal system:

Adult Health Nursing

- ***Oncology***
- ***Endocrine System***
- ***Immune System***
- ***Mental Illness***
- ***The Older Adult***

LEARNING OBJECTIVES

Upon completion of this chapter, you should be able to:

- Define key terms.
- Discuss diagnostic tests associated with the digestive system.
- Discuss components necessary for a complete assessment of the digestive system.
- List medical and surgical management for clients with digestive disorders.
- Describe nursing interventions for clients with digestive disorders.
- Assist with the formulation of nursing care plans for clients with digestive disorders.

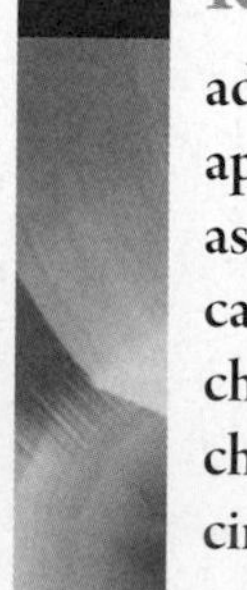

KEY TERMS

adhesion
appendicitis
ascites
calculi
cholecystitis
cholelithiasis
cirrhosis
colostomy
constipation
diverticula
diverticulitis
diverticulosis
effluent
gastric ulcer
gastritis
glycogenesis
glycogenolysis
hematemesis
hemorrhoid
hepatitis
ileostomy

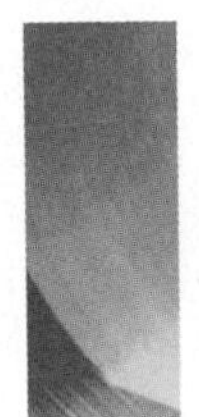

intussusception
jaundice
ligation
melena
occult blood test (guaiac)
pancreatitis
peptic ulcer
peristalsis
peritonitis
polyp
postprandial
steatorrhea
stoma
stomatitis
volvulus

INTRODUCTION

Disorders and diseases of the gastrointestinal system and accessory organs can affect not only the digestive process and nutrient absorption but the lifestyle of the individual as well.

ANATOMY AND PHYSIOLOGY REVIEW

The digestive system, also known as the *gastrointestinal (GI) tract or the alimentary system*, is responsible for breaking down complex food into simple nutrients the body can absorb and convert into energy (Figure 7-1). This process is known as digestion.

Mouth/Esophagus

Digestion begins in the mouth, where the teeth mechanically break food down into smaller pieces by chewing and mixing it with saliva. The chemical breakdown of cooked starches is begun in the mouth by the enzyme ptyalin, a salivary amylase. The food is then swallowed as a small ball or bolus and transported down the esophagus, a hollow, muscular tube approximately 10 inches long. **Peristalsis**, coordinated rhythmic contractions of the muscles, pushes the bolus through the esophagus. The cardiac sphincter, also called the *lower esophageal sphincter (LES)*, located at the distal end of the esophagus, relaxes and allows the food to pass into the stomach.

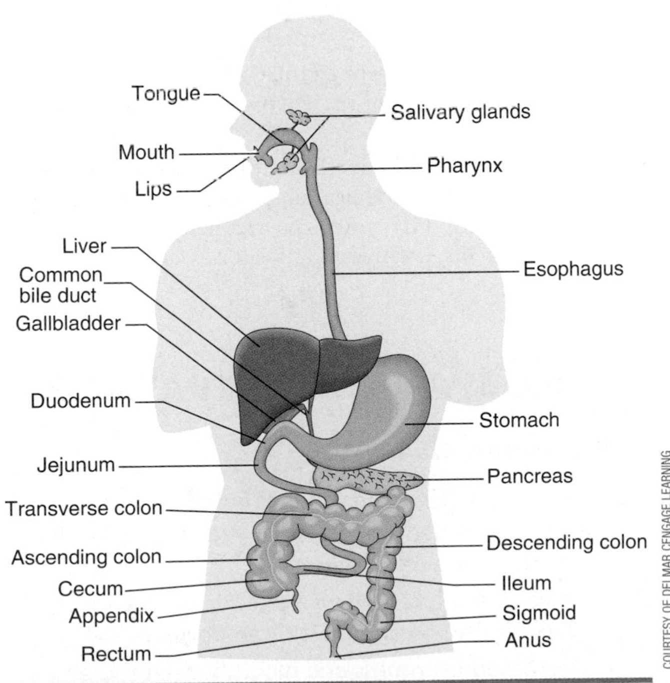

Figure 7-1 The Digestive System

Stomach

Further mechanical and chemical breakdown of the food occurs in the stomach, a J-shaped muscular organ located beneath the diaphragm. The stomach secretes gastric juices that contain hydrochloric acid (HCl) and pepsinogen, a nonactive form of the enzyme pepsin. HCl and pepsin are responsible for beginning the breakdown of protein and continuing the breakdown of starches. Starch digestion in the stomach gradually stops because of the acidic environment. Mucus is secreted to protect the lining of the stomach. The stomach also secretes an intrinsic factor necessary for vitamin B_{12} absorption and gastrin to stimulate HCl release.

The peristaltic movement of the stomach mixes the partially digested food and digestive enzymes into a semiliquid mass called **chyme**. The chyme will not pass into the small intestine until it is the proper consistency and particles are 1 millimeter or less. On average, the stomach empties in 3 to 4 hours. Carbohydrates are digested most readily, followed by proteins, with fats taking the longest to pass from the stomach. When the chyme has reached the proper consistency, the pyloric sphincter relaxes, releasing a portion at a time of the chyme into the small intestine.

Small Intestine

The small intestine is approximately 20 to 25 feet long and is responsible for absorbing nutrients from the chyme. The small intestine also secretes digestive enzymes, mucus to protect the mucosa, and hormones to aid in the absorption of nutrients.

The chyme enters the duodenum, the first 10 to 12 inches of the small intestine. The duodenum is responsible for absorbing calcium and iron as well as neutralizing the acids in the chyme. Enzymes from the pancreas and bile from the liver enter the duodenum from the common bile duct by way of the ampulla of vater; it is here that fats are digested.

The jejunum, the middle 8 to 10 feet of the small intestine, is responsible for absorption of fats, proteins, and carbohydrates. Vitamin B_{12} and bile salts are absorbed in the ileum, the distal 12 feet of the small bowel.

Large Intestine

The chyme enters the large intestine, also known as the *colon,* through the ileocecal valve into the cecum, a small pouch to which the appendix is attached. The colon is approximately 4 to 5 feet long and consists of the ascending or right colon, the transverse colon, the descending or left colon, and the sigmoid colon, an S-shaped segment before the rectum. The colon absorbs water, electrolytes, and bile salts.

The last 5 inches of the large intestine comprise the rectum. The distal end of the rectum forms the anal canal composed of muscles that control defecation. The opening to the anal canal is called the anus.

Accessory Organs

The digestive system also has accessory organs that aid in the digestion of food. The accessory organs include the pancreas, liver, and gallbladder (Figure 7-2).

Pancreas

The pancreas is a fish-shaped glandular organ 6 to 8 inches long extending from the duodenum across the abdomen behind the stomach. The pancreas has both endocrine and exocrine functions. The endocrine functions, which include the production of glucagon and insulin to regulate the blood sugar level, are presented in the endocrine system chapter.

The pancreas produces three main groups of enzymes in pancreatic juice for its exocrine function. The enzymes are:

amylase—converts carbohydrates into glucose
lipase—aids in fat digestion
protease—breaks down protein

Liver

The liver is the largest glandular organ of the body. It is located in the right upper quadrant of the abdomen. The liver is one of the most vascular organs, filtering 1,500 mL of blood per minute. Some of the many functions of the liver are to:

- Produce and secrete bile, which emulsifies fats
- Convert glucose into glycogen for storage (**glycogenesis**)
- Convert glycogen to glucose when blood sugar level drops (**glycogenolysis**)
- Metabolize hormones
- Break down nitrogenous wastes to urea
- Incorporate amino acids into proteins
- Filter blood and destroy bacteria
- Produce prothrombin and fibrinogen, which are necessary for blood clotting
- Manufacture cholesterol
- Produce heparin
- Store vitamin B_{12} and fat-soluble vitamins A, D, E, and K
- Detoxify poisonous substances

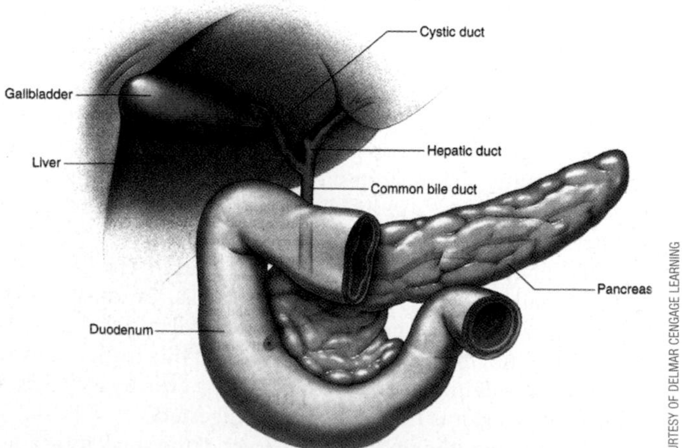

Figure 7-2 Accessory organs. Bile travels from the liver to the gallbladder via the hepatic and cystic ducts. The bile is released into the duodenum via the common bile duct. The pancreas releases its digestive juice into the duodenum.

Gallbladder

The gallbladder is a pear-shaped sac attached to the undersurface of the liver. The liver produces bile and transports the bile to the gallbladder through the hepatic and cystic ducts. The gallbladder stores and concentrates the bile until it is needed in the small intestine. When fats enter the small intestine, the gallbladder releases the bile through the cystic duct into the common bile duct and finally into the small intestine. The cystic duct, hepatic duct, and pancreatic duct combine to form the common bile duct.

Effects of Aging

As the body ages, several changes occur in the digestive system (Table 7-1). It is important to educate clients about these changes and ways they can adapt their lifestyles.

ASSESSMENT

A thorough assessment is necessary to collect data on which to make an accurate nursing diagnosis. For clients describing GI symptoms, the assessment should include the following:

1. History of the present complaint, including length and frequency of symptoms, when symptoms occur, as well as aggravating factors
2. Medication history, including prescribed and over-the-counter (OTC) medications, and their effectiveness. Clients with GI symptoms frequently self-medicate with antacids, laxatives, suppositories, and enemas.

LIFE SPAN CONSIDERATIONS

The Aging GI Tract

- Loss of elasticity and slowed motility of the GI tract, accompanied by lack of exercise, make the elderly prone to constipation.
- As the intestinal wall weakens, diverticuli, or scars on the intestinal wall, can develop.
- Decreased liver mass and blood flow alter the pharmacokinetics of various drugs.

TABLE 7-1 Changes in the Digestive System with Aging

COMMON CHANGES	RESULT	IMPLICATIONS FOR NURSES
Decrease in peristalsis	Food moves more slowly through digestive system. Bowel movements are more infrequent. Increase in constipation. Feeling full and bloated and may eat less.	Increase fiber and fluid intake. Encourage smaller, frequent meals. Offer fiber supplements.
Oral changes	Dentures are common. Chewing is more difficult. Eating and drinking time may be prolonged. Number of taste buds decreases.	Make sure dentures fit. Cut food into small bites. Teach that softer foods may be better tolerated. Some clients may start using more salt and seasonings to compensate for less flavor; monitor salt usage.
Decrease in enzyme secretion	Food is harder to digest. Increase in indigestion. Intolerance to some food and seasonings.	Encourage water between meals. Avoid foods that are not tolerated while ensuring adequate nutrient intake.
Decrease in saliva	Food is more difficult to chew. Swallowing becomes difficult.	Encourage fluid intake with meals. Have clients chew food well and do two swallows with each bite of food. Have clients sit up to eat.

3. A complete nutritional history; a note should be made of any foods that increase or decrease symptoms. Also, assess if meals aggravate symptoms or if symptoms occur within a specific time period after a meal. Note the fiber and fat content of the diet as well as the amount of fluids typically consumed.
4. Psychosocial factors, including compliance and noncompliance with health status. Meal patterns should be evaluated: note whether the client eats alone, eats large meals at regular intervals, or snacks all day.
5. Physical examination, including inspection, auscultation, percussion, and palpation of the abdomen. An evaluation of the client's ability to chew and swallow is also important.
6. Bowel elimination patterns, including frequency, consistency, and amounts of bowel movements.
7. Evaluation of diagnostic data, including laboratory analysis and radiologic and endoscopic examinations.

Refer to Box 7-1, Questions to Ask and Observations to Make When Collecting Data, for guidance in completing client gastrointestinal assessments.

COMMON DIAGNOSTIC TESTS

Commonly used diagnostic tests for clients with digestive disorders are listed in Table 7-2.

DISORDERS OF THE GASTROINTESTINAL TRACT

Disorders of the gastrointestinal tract include stomatitis, esophageal varices, gastroesophageal reflux disease, gastritis, ulcers, appendicitis, diverticulosis and diverticulitis, inflammatory bowel disease, irritable bowel syndrome, intestinal obstruction, hernias, peritonitis, hemorrhoids, and constipation.

STOMATITIS

Stomatitis is a painful condition characterized by inflammation and ulcerations in the mouth. Stomatitis can be caused by infections, damage to the mucous membranes by irritants, or chemotherapy.

MEDICAL–SURGICAL MANAGEMENT

Medical

Cultures may be done to determine whether an infectious process is present.

Pharmacological

Because the client's mouth can be sore, topical anesthetics such as xylocaine may be used. Analgesics may also be ordered. If an infection is present, the appropriate medication is ordered.

Diet

Dietary restrictions are based on what the client is able to tolerate. Bland, soft foods or liquids are usually tolerated best. As the sores heal, the diet may be advanced as tolerated. It is important to monitor dietary intake because caloric and fluid intake may be poor as a result of discomfort.

NURSING MANAGEMENT

Monitor caloric and fluid intake for adequacy. Encourage the client to eat soft, bland foods and liquids. Assess for mouth discomfort and check mouth for inflammation and ulcerations. Provide oral care and administer medications as ordered.

TABLE 7-2 Common Diagnostic Tests for Gastrointestinal Disorders

Laboratory Tests

- Complete blood count (CBC)
- Prothrombin time (PT)
- Partial thromboplastin time (PTT)
- Bilirubin
- Albumin
- Globulin
- Total protein
- Alkaline phosphatase
- Lactate hydrogenase (LDH-5)
- Gamma-glutamyl transpeptidase (GGT or GGTP)
- Aspartate aminotransferase (AST/SGOT)
- Alanine aminotransferase (ALT/SGPT)
- Cholesterol
- Triglycerides
- Amylase
- Carcinoembryonic antigen (CEA)
- HAA, now called hepatitis B surface antigen (HBsAG)
- Stool O & P
- Stool occult blood (guaiac)
- Fecal occult blood test (FOBT)
- Hemocult

Radiologic Studies

- Barium swallow
- Upper gastrointestinal tract (UGI) with small bowel follow-through
- Abdominal x-rays
- CT scans
- Ultrasound
- Barium enema
- Gallbladder series

Other

- Flexible sigmoidoscopy
- Esophagogastroduodenoscopy (EGD)
- Endoscopic retrograde cholangiopancreatogram (ERCP)
- Colonoscopy
- Esophageal motility studies (manometry)
- Gastric secretion analysis
- Liver biopsy
- Peritoneal aspiration

NURSING PROCESS

ASSESSMENT

Subjective Data

Clients usually describe pain in the mouth and difficulty swallowing.

Objective Data

Observations include inflamed mucosa of the mouth with ulcerations frequently present.

Nursing diagnoses for a client with stomatitis include the following:

NURSING DIAGNOSES	PLANNING/OUTCOMES	NURSING INTERVENTIONS
*Acute **Pain** related to* Stomatitis	The client will verbalize increase in comfort within 1 hour of initiation of treatment.	Assess the client frequently for discomfort. Administer medications such as topical xylocaine and analgesics as ordered. Allow for rest periods as indicated.
*Imbalanced **Nutrition**: Less than Body Requirements* related to inadequate caloric and fluid intake	The client will maintain caloric intake of 1,500 calories per day within 48 hours of treatment initiation. The client will maintain a fluid intake of 2,000 mL per day within 48 hours of treatment initiation.	Monitor daily caloric intake and consult with the dietitian to assist with food selection. Administer IV fluids as ordered and monitor I&O.
*Impaired **Oral** Mucous Membranes* related to stomatitis	The client will have less inflammation and a decrease in the size of the ulcers by 36 hours after treatment initiation.	Monitor the stomatitis every shift to assess status of condition. Provide oral care every 4 hours. Administer medications as ordered to combat the infection.

Evaluation: Evaluate each outcome to determine how it has been met by the client.

BOX 7-1 QUESTIONS TO ASK AND OBSERVATIONS TO MAKE WHEN COLLECTING DATA

Subjective Data

Do you wear dentures? If yes, do they fit properly?
Do you consume alcohol?
Obtain a history of alcohol use/abuse.
How much alcohol do you consume in a week?
Do you smoke cigarettes, cigars, or a pipe?
Do you chew tobacco?
Do you smoke, inhale, or ingest illicit drugs?
Do you have pain or discomfort in your mouth?
Do you have difficulty swallowing?
What kind of foods and liquids do you consume?
Do you consume acidic foods?
What is your ideal weight? Do you have unexplained weight loss? Weight gain?
Have you ever vomited bloody stomach contents?
Have you vomited stomach contents that look like coffee grounds?
Are you easily fatigued?
Describe your energy level now compared to 6 months ago.
Do you have a history of liver disease?
Do your bowel movements appear black and tarry?
Are your bowel movements constipated, watery?
Do you have diarrhea? Persistent or occasional?
Have you passed blood clots in your stool?
Have you ever experienced bloody diarrhea alternating with normal bowel movements?
Do you experience heartburn? How often do you have heartburn?
Do you take any OTC medications to treat the heartburn? Do you get relief from these medications?
Do you have heartburn, acid regurgitation into the throat or mouth, or increased salivation after bending over to tie your shoes or retrieve something from the floor?
Do you have increased difficulty swallowing when lying down, bending over, or straining?
Have you experienced a burning sensation in the chest, throat, or behind the sternum?
Do you belch frequently?
Do you have a burning or squeezing pain when swallowing?
Have you experienced the sensation of food being caught in your throat or like you are choking?
Have others mentioned that you frequently have bad breath?
Do you have frequent chest pain? Describe the chest pain. How long does it last?
Is the chest pain related to any particular activity? Does it seem to occur after a heavy meal?
Are you hoarse in the morning?
Do you have difficulty breathing in the morning?
Do you cough in the morning? During the night?
Do any foods irritate your stomach, cause indigestion, belching, or bloating? Do you take any medications to relieve stomach discomfort, pain, or indigestion?
Do you take NSAIDs?
What do you think causes the discomfort, pain, or indigestion?
What relieves the discomfort, pain, or indigestion?
Do you notice more discomfort or pain at one time more than another?
Have you missed work because of stomach discomfort, pain, or indigestion?

Objective Data

Inspect the oral mucosa for ulcers or lesions.
Assess the mucous membranes for dryness, cracked lips, erythema, bleeding, and presence and appearance of saliva.
Assess the surface of the tongue.
Inspect the gingiva for redness and swelling.
Assess the teeth for caries and firmness within the gums.
Assess vital signs.
Guaiac all stools for occult blood.
Observe for hematemesis and melena.
Assess and measure amount of blood vomited.
Assess lab data for H & H, liver profiles, albumin, pre-albumin, bilirubin, WBCs, and neutrophils.
Assess the skin and sclera for presence of jaundice.
Weigh the client every day and evaluate BMI.
Assess for recent weight loss and/or weight gain.
Assess eating habits for types of food/beverages consumed, and time and frequency of meals.
Assess breath odor for halitosis.
Assess voice for hoarseness.
Assess for frequent belching.
Assess breath sounds for cough and wheezing.
Inspect the abdomen for distention.
Assess for presence of bowel sounds.
Assess for presence and location of abdominal pain.
Assess for rebound abdominal tenderness.
Keep client NPO as ordered.
Monitor I&O.
Maintain IV fluids for hydration.

ESOPHAGEAL VARICES

A varix is an enlarged, tortuous vein or, occasionally, an artery. Although varices can occur in any part of the digestive system, they occur most frequently in the distal veins of the esophagus. The varices are often associated with cirrhosis of the liver or any other condition that causes chronic obstruction of drainage from the esophageal veins into the portal veins. Swelling of the veins causes the walls to weaken, making them prone to ulceration and bleeding. Anything that causes increased abdominal venous pressure, such as sneezing, coughing, vomiting, the Valsalva maneuver, swallowing large, poorly chewed pieces of food, and the erosion of vessel walls by gastric acid, can cause the varices to rupture.

Varices have no symptoms, so clients may not be aware of them until they start bleeding. Death may ensue rapidly if the hemorrhaging varix is not treated immediately.

Medical–Surgical Management

Medical

The varices may be treated with sclerotherapy, ligation, or balloon tamponade. Sclerotherapy is a procedure in which a caustic substance is injected into the varix. An esophagogastroduodenoscopy (EGD) is performed and a sclerosing agent is injected through a special needle. Several treatments are necessary to cause formation of scar tissue and to stop the bleeding. After the bleeding has stopped and the client has stabilized, the remaining treatments may be done on an outpatient basis.

Complications to sclerotherapy include mediastinal inflammation secondary to extra esophageal injection, perforation, ulceration, stricture secondary to scar formation, and rebleeding.

Esophageal **ligation**, also called banding, involves placing a rubber band, tie, or O-ring on the varix (Figure 7-3). An EGD is performed to guide the placement of the bands. The complications include rebleeding and stricture formation.

In a case where varices are actively bleeding, a three- or four-lumen balloon tamponade, known as a Minnesota or Sengstaken-Blakemore tube, is passed into the esophagus. The balloon is then inflated in the esophagus to put direct pressure onto the bleeding varices. The balloon is periodically deflated to prevent necrosis of the esophageal tissue. Isotonic saline lavages also are administered through the tube. During the procedure, the client must be kept NPO with the head of the bed elevated 30 to 45 degrees. Complications include perforation of the esophagus from the balloon pressure and necrosis of the surrounding tissue.

Surgical

A portosystemic shunt is performed to relieve the pressure on the esophageal veins by redirecting blood from the portal vein to the inferior mesenteric vein. Some of the blood bypasses the liver and reenters the circulatory system (Figure 7-4).

A nonsurgical but invasive procedure, transjugular intrahepatic portosystemic shunt (TIPS), may also be performed. With this procedure, the right internal jugular vein is used to place a cannula into the hepatic and portal veins. A connection is made through the liver tissue between the hepatic and portal veins. A stent is placed in the connection. This allows some of the blood to bypass the liver and relieve pressure in the portal vein. This procedure is done in x-ray and is used with clients who are too unstable for surgery (also refer to Figure 7-9.)

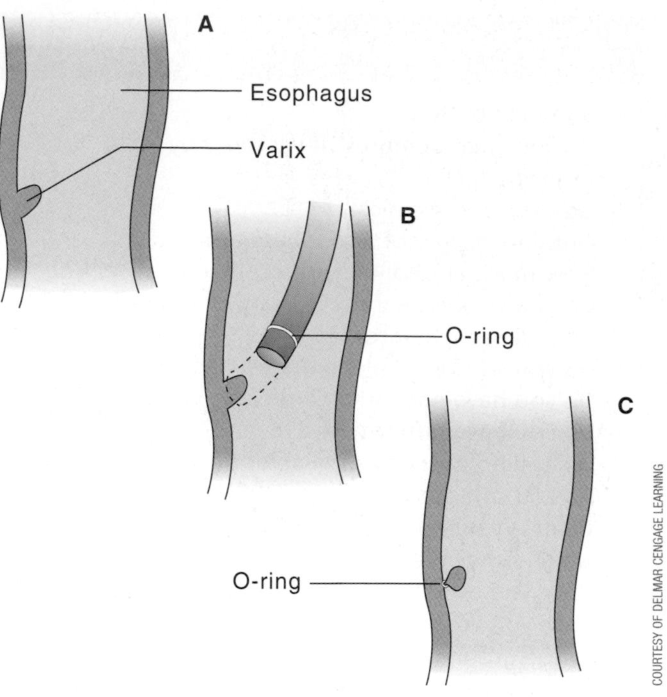

FIGURE 7-3 **Banding of an Esophageal Varix; *A*, Varix; *B*, Insertion of Tube with O-Ring; *C*, O-Ring is Placed around the Varix**

Pharmacological

Octreotide (Sandostatin) is given by IV to help control the bleeding by decreasing blood flow to the gut, thus lowering pressure in the portal system. Analgesics may be necessary following sclerotherapy if clients have chest discomfort. Clients should avoid NSAIDs, aspirin, and all anticoagulants. Sucralfate (Carafate) liquid may be given to coat the esophagus, protecting it from erosion by gastric acid. IV rehydration as well as blood transfusions may be necessary for clients with active bleeding.

Activity

If varices are bleeding or have recently bled, the client should remain on bed rest. If no active bleeding is present, the client may be ambulatory but should avoid strenuous exercise.

Nursing Management

Monitor vital signs. Explain tests and procedures. Allow time for client to express fears and concerns about the varices. Check laboratory test results for changes. Explain reasons to avoid strenuous activity. Assess for nausea and dizziness.

NURSING PROCESS

Assessment

Subjective Data

Assessment includes history of liver disease or alcohol abuse and nausea. With esophageal varices there is no abdominal pain. The symptom of abdominal pain helps distinguish esophageal

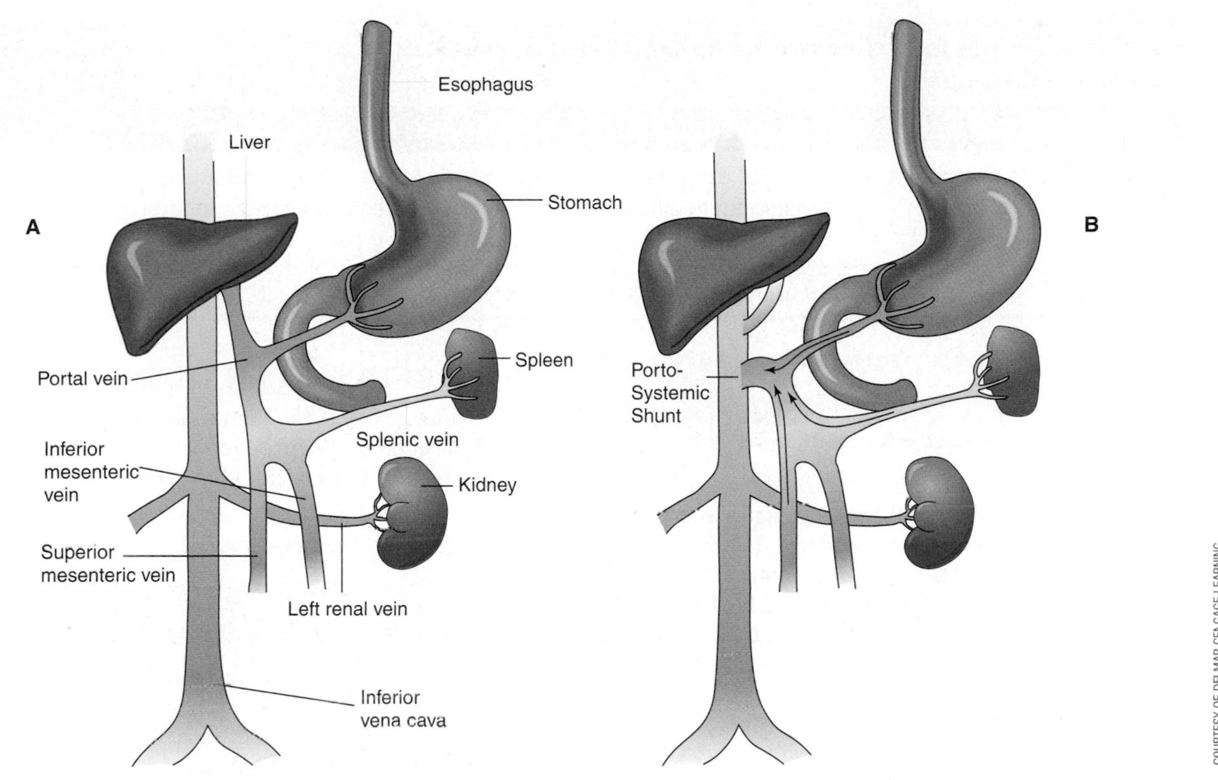

FIGURE 7-4 *A,* **Normal Circulation of Abdominal Organs;** *B,* **An Example of a Portosystemic Shunt (May be Performed in Clients with Elevated Portal Vein Pressure That Is Resistant to Medical Management)**

varices from bleeding gastric ulcers, which generally do cause pain that worsens after eating (Movius, 2006).

Objective Data

Assessment includes testing stools for **occult blood (guaiac)** and **melena** (black, sticky, tar-like stools containing partially broken-down blood), and assessing for **hematemesis**, or vomiting blood. Review hemoglobin and hematocrit (H & H) to evaluate anemia and liver profile for elevated bilirubin and globulin levels and a decrease in albumin.

If cirrhosis of the liver is present, **jaundice**, a yellowing of the skin, mucous membranes, and sclerae of the eyes, is present. Jaundice results when the liver is unable to fully remove bilirubin from the blood. Nutritional status may be poor if the client abuses alcohol.

Nursing diagnoses for a client with esophageal varices include the following:

NURSING DIAGNOSES	PLANNING/OUTCOMES	NURSING INTERVENTIONS
*Risk for Deficient **Fluid** Volume* related to bleeding esophageal varices (if the varices are not actively bleeding)	The client will maintain adequate fluid volume.	Monitor vital signs every 4 hours including orthostatic blood pressures. Orthostatic blood pressure is obtained by taking the blood pressure when the client is lying down and then when standing. A 20 mm Hg difference in blood pressures from lying to standing would indicate a change in fluid volume, possibly indicating varix bleeding. Monitor for nausea and dizziness. Monitor H & H every 4 to 8 hours as ordered. A decrease in H & H values would indicate bleeding.
*Deficient **Fluid** Volume* related to bleeding esophageal varices and gastric loss from vomiting	The client will maintain an H & H within normal limits. The client's blood pressure will be within 20 mm Hg of baseline with no orthostatic changes.	Monitor H & H. Frequently monitor vital signs. Administer IV fluids, electrolyte replacement, and blood transfusions as ordered.

(*Continues*)

Nursing diagnoses for a client with esophageal varices include the following: (Continued)

NURSING DIAGNOSES	PLANNING/OUTCOMES	NURSING INTERVENTIONS
Anxiety related to change in health status, threat of death	The client will discuss concerns about health status.	Explain all tests and procedures to decrease anxiety. Allow client to express fears and concerns regarding condition.

Evaluation: Evaluate each outcome to determine how it has been met by the client.

GASTROESOPHAGEAL REFLUX DISEASE

In gastroesophageal reflux disease (GERD), gastric secretions flow upward into the esophagus, damaging the tissues. An inability of the lower esophageal sphincter (LES) to fully close contributes to this condition. Environmental and physical factors contribute to decreased pressure in the LES. Fatty foods, caffeine, nicotine, calcium channel blockers, and NSAIDs decrease the tightness of the sphincter. Symptoms include belching, dysphagia, esophagitis, epigastric pain, heartburn, flatulence, melena, and bleeding. Diagnosis is made by symptoms, a 24-hour pH monitoring, and an esophageal motility test. An endoscopy determines the extent of esophagitis and rules out a malignancy.

MEDICAL–SURGICAL MANAGEMENT

Medical

GERD is generally treated conservatively with diet and medications. Clients are encouraged to lose weight if they are overweight.

Surgical

A fundoplication is done to alleviate symptoms. A fundoplication is a laparoscopic procedure in which the LES is tightened by wrapping and suturing the fundus of the stomach around the esophagus.

Pharmacological

GERD is treated conservatively with antacids, H_2 receptor antagonists, proton pump inhibitors, cytoprotective agents, and gastrointestinal motility agents.

Diet

A low-fat, high-protein diet is recommended. The client is encouraged to avoid caffeine, milk products, alcohol, peppermint, licorice, and spicy foods.

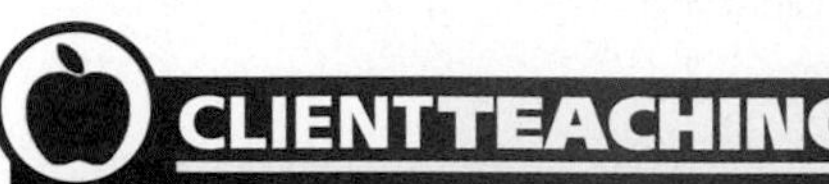

CLIENT TEACHING

GERD

- Lose weight as needed.
- Avoid fatty foods, alcohol, nicotine, caffeine, and spicy foods.
- Take medications as instructed.
- Elevate head of the bed 2 to 4 inches on blocks.
- Avoid wearing constrictive clothing.

NURSING MANAGEMENT

Encourage client to avoid foods that increase the symptoms (e.g., caffeine, milk products, alcohol, and fatty foods). Obtain diet history from client. Observe for melena and signs of discomfort or pain.

GASTRITIS

Gastritis is an inflammation of the stomach mucosa occurring when the stomach has been exposed to irritating substances such as medications, smoke, food allergens, or toxic chemicals. Another contributing factor to gastritis is impaired mucosal defenses, which occur when the epithelial cells of the stomach are not able to secrete an adequate quantity or quality of mucus to protect the stomach. The presence of the bacteria *Helicobactor pylori* (*H. pylori*) has also been associated with gastritis.

MEDICAL–SURGICAL MANAGEMENT

Medical

Diagnosis of gastritis is based on history and symptoms. An UGI or EGD is done to help diagnose the condition. If *H. pylori* is suspected, a biopsy is obtained during an EGD and a culture is performed.

Pharmacological

Treatment for gastritis is primarily pharmacological involving antacids and histamine (H_2) receptor antagonists (also call H_2 blockers). A proton pump inhibitor such as omeprazole (Prilosec) or prostaglandins is used. If *H. pylori* is present, bismuth preparations are used to inhibit *H. pylori* growth and antibiotics to eliminate the bacteria (Table 7-3).

NSAIDs such as ibuprofen (Motrin) and indomethacin (Indocin) have been shown to compromise mucosal defenses and increase acid secretion. Clients who are on NSAIDs chronically, such as clients with arthritis, need to be evaluated to determine whether other analgesics would be effective or if a prostaglandin should be taken with the NSAIDs.

Diet

Although studies have shown that dietary modifications have little impact on the rate of gastritis healing, some modifications are indicated. Any foods that aggravate symptoms are eliminated. Also, foods that increase acid secretions, such as milk, coffee, decaffeinated coffee, tea, colas, and chocolate, should be consumed only in small amounts or eliminated if possible. Eating before bedtime is avoided because it increases nocturnal acid secretions.

TABLE 7-3 Medications Used for Ulcers and Gastritis

MEDICATION	PURPOSE	NURSING IMPLICATIONS
Antacids • aluminum hydroxide (Amphogel) • aluminum hydroxide and magnesium hydroxide (Maalox) • dihydroxyaluminum sodium carbonate (Rolaids)	Seal impaired mucosa. Neutralize acids.	Antacids containing aluminum hydroxide may cause constipation. Antacids containing magnesium hydroxide may cause diarrhea; monitor serum electrolytes; do not give with other meds.
H_2 Receptor Antagonists • ranitadine HCl (Zantac) • cimetidine (Tagamet)	Decrease gastric acid secretion.	Do not give within 1 hour of antacids.
Proton Pump Inhibitor • omeprazole (Prilosec)	Stop gastric acid secretion.	Give with food. Suspend granules in an acid liquid. Takes 4 days to achieve blood level.
Prostaglandins • misoprostol (Cytotec)	Decrease gastric acid secretion. Enhance mucosal defenses.	Give when NSAIDs need to be continued.
Bismuth Compounds • bismuth subsalicylate (Pepto-Bismol)	Enhance mucosal barriers. Inhibit *H. pylori* growth.	Do not give within 1 hour of H_2 blockers.
Antibiotics • ampicillin (Omnipen) • metronidazole (Flagyl)	Eliminate *H. pylori*.	Some antibiotics will cause N/V if taken with alcohol. Do not give with antacids or meals with the exception of Flagyl, which must be taken with food. Clients are usually placed on two different antibiotics simultaneously.

Health Promotion

Smoking and alcohol aggravate the mucosal lining of the stomach and significantly impair gastritis healing. Smoking and alcohol consumption are minimized or eliminated if possible.

NURSING MANAGEMENT

Encourage client to minimize or eliminate smoking and alcohol consumption (if applicable) and any foods that aggravate symptoms. Teach client about medications.

NURSING PROCESS

ASSESSMENT

Subjective Data

Clients with gastritis may have no symptoms or may describe epigastric pain or burning, or nausea. They may also state that certain foods aggravate symptoms.

Objective Data

Stools may test positive for blood.

Nursing diagnoses for a client with gastritis include the following:

NURSING DIAGNOSES	PLANNING/OUTCOMES	NURSING INTERVENTIONS
*Acute **Pain*** related to gastric acid on inflammation	The client will experience less pain within 24 hours of onset of treatment as identified by pain scale.	Administer medications and provide diet as ordered. Assess client for improvement of symptoms. Implement education about lifestyle changes.
*Deficient **Knowledge*** related to condition, therapy, and symptoms of potential complications	The client will verbalize understanding of condition and symptoms of complications and will comply with treatment regimen.	Educate regarding medication regimen and lifestyle changes. If the client smokes or drinks alcohol, provide information on smoking and drinking cessation. Discuss dietary modifications.

Evaluation: Evaluate each outcome to determine how it has been met by the client.

ULCERS

Peptic ulcers are erosions that form in the esophagus, stomach, or duodenum resulting from an acid/pepsin imbalance. **Gastric ulcers** refer to erosions in the stomach and are correlated to exposure to irritants such as NSAIDs, smoking, alcohol, food allergens, toxic chemicals, *H. pylori* infections, and impaired mucosal defenses. Impaired mucosal defenses occur when the epithelial cells of the stomach are not able to secrete an adequate quantity or quality of mucus to protect the stomach.

Clients with gastric ulcers frequently complain of pain 1 to 2 hours after eating. Eating may not relieve pain or may even increase pain. Weight loss is common. Risk factors include alcohol use, stress, and NSAID use.

Stress ulcers are a type of gastric ulcer that form when gastritis becomes erosive and starts bleeding. As the name implies, stress ulcers occur in clients whose bodies are experiencing stress, such as clients who have experienced major surgery, trauma, burns, chemotherapy, or radiation therapy. Clients with chronic respiratory disorders also experience stress ulcers because hypoxia can lead to impaired mucosa. Bleeding may be massive resulting in significant blood loss or can be slow and insidious. Because of the multiple sites of bleeding, stress ulcers are difficult to manage.

Duodenal ulcers refer to ulcers in the duodenum. Incidents of duodenal ulcers have been correlated to a high secretion of HCl. Clients with duodenal ulcers frequently complain of pain 2 to 4 hours after eating. Nocturnal pain may be present, occurring between midnight and 3:00 a.m. Eating frequently relieves symptoms. Weight gain is common. Risk factors include a history of pulmonary disease, cirrhosis, chronic pancreatitis, and/or chronic renal failure.

If an ulcer erodes through a blood vessel, the client may experience a life-threatening hemorrhage. A perforation occurs if the ulcer erodes through the wall of the stomach or small intestine resulting in gastric or intestinal contents entering the abdominal cavity and causing peritonitis.

Diagnosis of ulcers is based on symptoms, history, and an UGI or EGD performed to visualize the ulcer. If an *H. pylori* infection is suspected, a biopsy is obtained during an EGD and a culture is performed.

MEDICAL–SURGICAL MANAGEMENT

Medical

If an ulcer bleeds, an EGD may be performed, and the ulcer is either injected with epinephrine to cause vasoconstriction or a special electrical probe is used to cauterize or burn the tissue that is bleeding. A nasogastric (NG) tube is inserted to remove gastric contents and blood, and iced isotonic saline is instilled to help cause vasoconstriction and stop the bleeding.

Surgical

The most commonly performed surgery for peptic ulcers is a vagotomy, in which a section of the vagus nerve is cut removing vagal innervation to the fundus of the stomach. This eliminates the production of hydrochloric acid, decreases function of the gastrin hormone, and slows motility of the stomach. A vagotomy eliminates the complications of the more aggressive surgeries, such as gastrectomies.

If the ulcer continues to bleed or if the ulcer has perforated, the client is taken to surgery and a gastrectomy is performed. The portion of the stomach or duodenum that is perforated is removed and the bowel is reconnected with an anastomosis.

Complications from gastrectomies include gastric dumping in which the stomach experiences **postprandial** (after eating) rapid gastric emptying. Clients experience abdominal pain, nausea, vomiting, explosive diarrhea, weakness, and dizziness. Clients with gastric dumping have malabsorption of nutrients because the food passes too quickly to permit absorption, thus leading to malnutrition. In addition, many clients with significant symptoms limit dietary intake to avoid symptoms, compounding the malnutrition and weight loss issues.

Management of gastric dumping includes small, frequent meals of high fiber and high protein and avoidance of simple carbohydrates.

Pharmacological

Treatment of ulcers is primarily pharmacological involving antacids, histamine (H_2) receptor antagonists (also called H_2 blockers), proton pump inhibitors, or prostaglandins. If *H. pylori* is present, bismuth preparations are generally used to inhibit its growth and antibiotics to eliminate the bacteria (refer to Table 7-3).

NSAIDs such as ibuprofen (Motrin) and indomethacin (Indocin) have been shown to compromise mucosal defenses and increase acid secretion. For clients who are on NSAIDs chronically, such as clients with arthritis, one needs to evaluate whether other analgesics would be effective or whether a prostaglandin should be taken with the NSAIDs.

Diet

Although studies have shown that dietary modifications have little impact on the rate of ulcer healing, some modifications are indicated. Foods that aggravate symptoms are eliminated. Also, foods that increase acid secretions, such as milk, coffee, decaffeinated coffee, tea, colas, and chocolate, should be consumed only in small amounts or eliminated if possible. Eating close to bedtime is avoided because it increases nocturnal acid secretions.

Health Promotion

Smoking and alcohol aggravate the mucosal lining of the stomach and duodenum and significantly impair ulcer healing. Smokers also experience a higher ulcer recurrence rate. Stress has been shown to increase the rate of peptic ulcers. Although the type or severity of stress may not be significant, the client's interpretation of the events as stressful is. Clients need to develop mechanisms for reducing stress such as exercise, biofeedback, and relaxation.

NURSING MANAGEMENT

Encourage lifestyle changes when necessary regarding smoking, alcohol, and stress. Teach relaxation techniques. Monitor weight and laboratory test results. Discourage having a bedtime snack to prevent acid secretions at night. Assess pain including relationship to eating a meal.

NURSING PROCESS

Assessment

Subjective Data

Clients with gastric ulcers are often asymptomatic or may describe epigastric pain or burning 1 to 2 hours after eating, and nausea or bloating. Clients may experience an increase of symptoms when they eat and therefore may decrease dietary intake. When questioned about lifestyle, NSAID usage, stress, smoking, and alcohol use may be discovered.

Clients with duodenal ulcers may exhibit no symptoms or may complain of pain 2 to 4 hours after eating. Eating will frequently decrease symptoms, so clients will often eat more frequently. When questioned about lifestyle, stress, smoking, and alcohol consumption may be discovered. The client may also have a history of pulmonary disease, cirrhosis, chronic pancreatitis, and/or chronic renal failure.

A client who is actively bleeding from an ulcer will experience an acute onset of epigastric pain, shortness of breath, and nausea.

Objective Data

Clients with gastric ulcers may show a weight loss and stools may test positive for blood. An H & H may show anemia.

Clients with duodenal ulcers may show a weight gain and stools may test positive for blood. An H & H may show anemia.

The client who is actively bleeding from an ulcer will show signs of shock: pale clammy skin, an elevated pulse rate, and a drop in blood pressure. The client may also have hematemesis. Laboratory tests show a low H & H and stools test positive for blood.

Nursing diagnoses for a client with ulcers include the following:

NURSING DIAGNOSES	PLANNING/OUTCOMES	NURSING INTERVENTIONS
*Acute **Pain*** related to gastric acid on ulcerated mucosa	The client will experience less pain within 24 hours of onset of treatment as identified on pain scale.	Assess clients for decrease of pain. Administer medications as ordered. Assess for elevated BP.
*Deficient **Knowledge*** related to condition, therapy, and symptoms of complications	The client will verbalize understanding of factors related to condition and symptoms of complications. Client will comply with treatment regimen.	Identify client's learning style and provide information in a manner compatible with the learning style. Educate regarding medication regimen, lifestyle changes, and signs and symptoms of possible complications. If indicated, provide client with smoking cessation information and stress reduction techniques such as exercise and biofeedback.
*Deficient Fluid **Volume*** related to bleeding ulcer	The client will exhibit normal fluid volume as evidenced by stable H & H and blood pressure within 20 mm Hg of baseline.	Check vital signs every 4 hours and PRN including orthostatic blood pressure. Monitor for dizziness and nausea. Check stool for blood. Administer IV fluids, electrolyte replacement, and blood transfusions as ordered.

Evaluation: Evaluate each outcome to determine how it has been met by the client.

APPENDICITIS

Appendicitis is the inflammation of the vermiform appendix, a 10-cm small, slender tube attached to the cecum. The appendix may be inflamed, gangrenous, or ruptured. If the opening to the appendix becomes blocked with feces, the *E. coli* multiply in the appendix and infection develops with pus formation. If it ruptures, fecal content spills into the abdominal cavity causing peritonitis, which may be fatal. It is most common in young adults, but can occur at any age (Atassi, 2002a). A barium enema or an ultrasound is ordered to confirm inflammation in the appendiceal area.

Medical–Surgical Management

Early diagnosis and treatment are necessary for the best client outcome. A white blood count and differential will usually show a WBC >10,000/mm^3 and neutrophils >75%. An elevated temperature indicates infection. Rebound tenderness in the right lower quadrant (RLQ) of the abdomen (at McBurney's point) is a positive diagnostic finding. An appendectomy is performed along with other abdominal surgeries as a preventive measure.

Surgical

A surgical procedure called an appendectomy is necessary before the appendix ruptures. Appendectomies are the most common emergency surgery and require a hospital stay of a few days if the appendix has ruptured. If no rupture has occurred, a laparoscopic appendectomy, in which the appendix is removed through a scope, may be done. This requires only a small incision and allows the client to be discharged 24 hours after the surgery.

Pharmacological

Preoperatively, no analgesics are administered so that symptoms will not be masked by the medication. Fluids and electrolytes may need to be replaced before surgery. Antibiotics are usually given preoperatively. Postoperatively, analgesics are administered for relief of incisional discomfort. Antibiotics are usually given postoperatively, especially if a perforation is present.

Diet

Preoperatively and initially postoperatively, the client is NPO. If a perforation with peritonitis occurred, the client is kept NPO longer, and an NG tube is inserted until bowel sounds return. Clear liquids and then full liquids and finally a regular diet is given as normal bowel function returns.

Activity

Initially postoperatively, the client is encouraged to turn, cough, and deep breathe every 2 hours. Next, the client is encouraged to increase ambulation gradually. Activity restrictions depend on the severity of the appendicitis. Driving, exercise, and lifting will be limited for a few weeks to allow for incisional healing.

NURSING MANAGEMENT

Assess pain. Keep client NPO. Monitor vital signs, especially temperature. Assess bowel sounds. Monitor the results of the CBC, especially WBC and neutrophils. Postoperatively, encourage client to turn, cough, and deep breathe every 2 hours. Encourage ambulation. Advance diet from liquid to regular as bowel function returns.

NURSING PROCESS

ASSESSMENT

Subjective Data

Clients with appendicitis describe abdominal pain, typically located in the RLQ around McBurney's point (halfway between the umbilicus and the right iliac crest). Clients also complain of anorexia (a loss of appetite) and nausea.

Objective Data

Clients may have vomiting and fever. Bowel sounds may be diminished or absent. Rebound tenderness, pain that occurs when fingers are pressed into the RLQ and then released suddenly, may be present. A CBC will show WBCs elevated $> 10{,}000/mm^3$ with neutrophils $> 75\%$.

Nursing diagnoses for a client with appendicitis include the following:

NURSING DIAGNOSES	PLANNING/OUTCOMES	NURSING INTERVENTIONS
*Acute **Pain** related to appendicitis/ appendectomy*	The client will experience a decrease in pain as evidenced by improved mobility and as identified on pain scale.	Preoperatively, monitor client's pain and check abdomen for rigidity. Provide an ice pack to help relieve pain as ordered; never use heat. Postoperatively, give analgesics as ordered and medicate prior to activities such as ambulation. Teach client to use a pillow to splint the incision when coughing. If client is having difficulty passing flatus, administer enemas or a rectal tube as ordered, and encourage ambulation.
*Impaired **Skin** Integrity* related to the abdominal incision	The client will verbalize signs and symptoms of infection and factors that enhance wound healing, by discharge.	Administer antibiotics as ordered. Educate the client that incision may be left open to the air after 24 hours; that showers may be taken, per physician instruction; and signs and symptoms of infection and activity restrictions. If adhesive strips are present, leave in place until they no longer cover the incision (approximately 10 days to 2 weeks).

Evaluation: Evaluate each outcome to determine how it has been met by the client.

DIVERTICULOSIS AND DIVERTICULITIS

Diverticula are saclike protrusions of the intestinal wall. **Diverticulosis** refers to a condition of the colon in which multiple diverticula are present (Figure 7-5). The exact cause of diverticulosis is not known; however, a diet low in fiber is believed to contribute to the formation of the pouches. Diverticulosis affects >50% of the elderly population (Marrs, 2006). It is asymptomatic unless perforation or hemorrhage occur.

Diverticulitis refers to the inflammation of one or more diverticula generally in the sigmoid colon. It is a complication of diverticulosis and is thought to be caused by stool impacted in the diverticula.

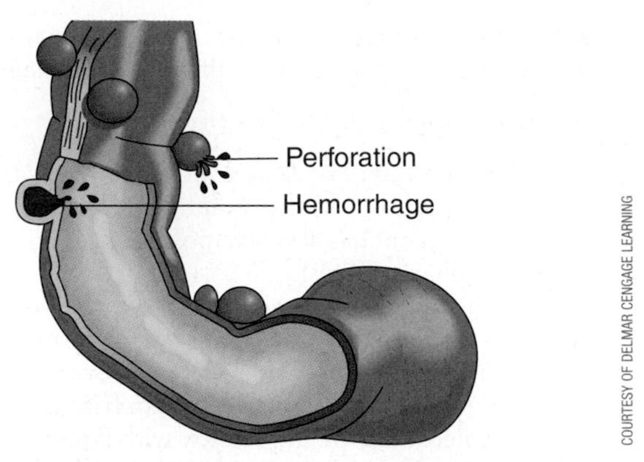

FIGURE 7-5 Diverticula in the sigmoid colon. Diverticulosis is almost always located in the descending or sigmoid colon.

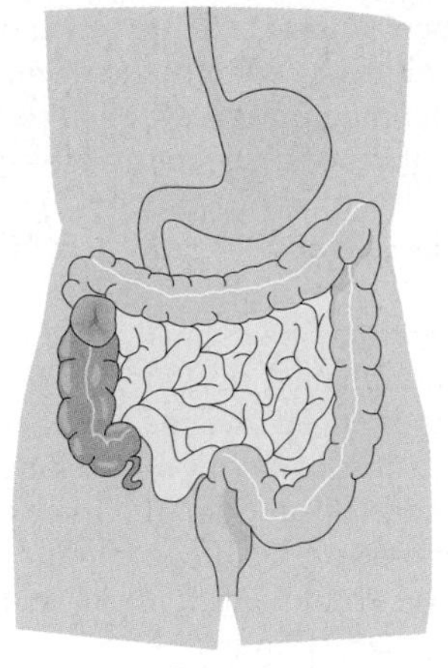

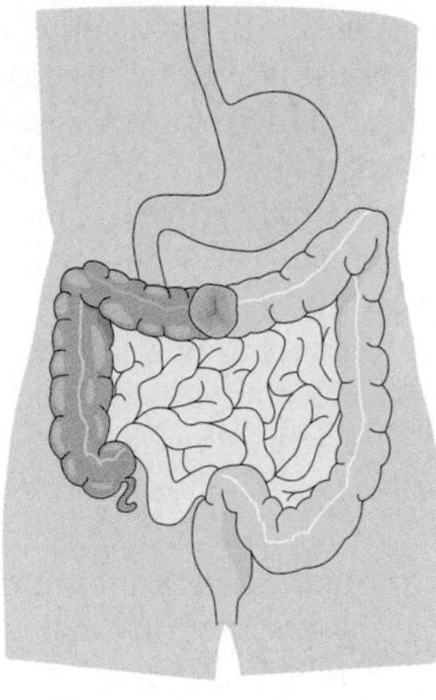

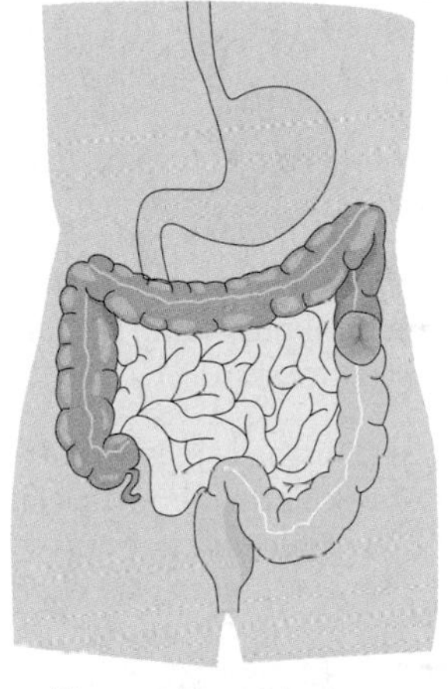

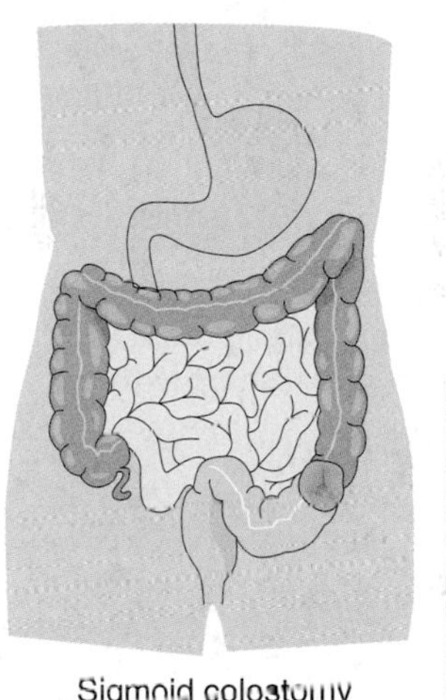

FIGURE 7-6 Colostomy Sites (Blue Area Is Colon Removed)

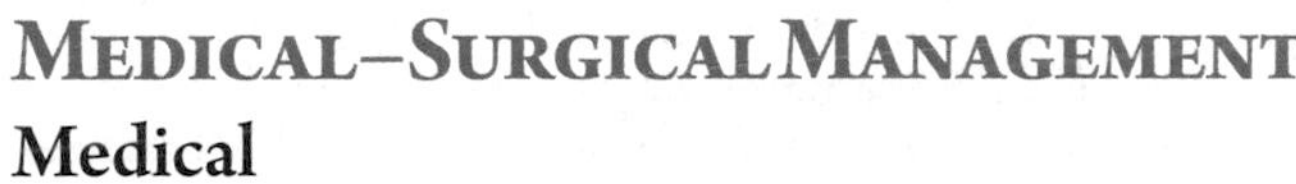

MEDICAL–SURGICAL MANAGEMENT

Medical

Diverticulosis is typically asymptomatic and needs no intervention. Most cases of diverticulitis are treated with analgesics, antibiotics, bed rest, NPO to rest the bowel, and IV fluid hydration.

A barium enema or abdominal ultrasound is usually ordered when diverticulitis is suspected. A flexible sigmoidoscopy is also performed.

Surgical

If bleeding or perforation of the diverticula occurs, or if an abscess forms, surgery is required to remove the affected portion of the bowel. A colon resection is performed. A **colostomy** may be required. A colostomy is a surgically created opening from the colon through the abdominal wall to relieve either a disease or functional problem in the large intestine.

Stool consistency depends on the placement of the **stoma** (surgical opening between a cavity and the surface of the body) in the colon. A colostomy is named for the part of the colon where it is located. An ascending colostomy takes its name from the ascending colon and would be on the right side of the abdomen. It has a liquid output. A transverse colostomy would be more toward the midline of the abdomen and has a pasty liquid output. A descending colostomy or sigmoid colostomy has a more solid output. Figure 7-6 shows the different colostomy sites.

If a large amount of inflammation is present, a temporary colostomy is performed to allow the colon to heal. The colon is reconnected at a later time. Sometimes a permanent colostomy needs to be performed.

Pharmacological

Clients who have been identified as having diverticulosis are usually placed on fiber supplements or stool softeners. Clients with diverticulitis are treated with sulfa antibiotics and other antimicrobial agents. Analgesics also are ordered for discomfort.

Diet

A high-fiber diet is believed to help reduce the occurrence of diverticulosis and diverticulitis. Clients experiencing diverticulitis will be NPO to rest the bowel. Once the diverticulitis begins healing, the client is placed on clear liquids and then advanced to a bland, low-residue diet while the diverticulitis heals.

If surgery is performed, the client is NPO until bowel sounds return. The client is then started on clear liquids, advanced to full liquids as more bowel function returns, and then finally advanced to a regular diet. A high-fiber diet is encouraged for clients once the diverticulitis episode has resolved.

Activity

For clients experiencing diverticulitis, bed rest and decreased mobility are encouraged to allow the bowel to rest. In clients who have had a bowel resection, activity will gradually be progressed postoperatively.

STOMA/OSTOMY MANAGEMENT

Assessment

Provide the client with an opportunity to ask questions and begin coping with a possible altered body image. Before ostomy surgery, the surgeon and the enterostomal (ET) nurse talk with the client and explain the reason for the surgery and the possibilities of ostomy surgery. Choosing the site or placement of the stoma depends on the type of ostomy being created, the lifestyle of the client, and the contours of the client's abdomen.

On return from surgery, the new stoma is edematous and ranges from deep red to dusky in color. The color of the stoma is checked with a penlight and documented at least once per shift. Color is important because it reveals the status of the blood supply to the stoma. If blood supply to the stoma is inadequate, the stoma will turn black. Notify the physician if the stoma becomes black.

Immediately after surgery there may be a small amount of serosanguineous drainage in the appliance, the stool-collection device. When the appliance is changed and the stoma is cleaned or touched when swollen, a small amount of bleeding may occur. Reassure the client that a small amount of bleeding is normal. Bowel function is checked every shift to monitor for any obstruction or ileus. Bowel sounds, distention, and abdominal tenderness are checked every 4 hours.

Complications

Hemorrhage Bleeding or hemorrhage may occur at the incision site or stoma site. It is important to check the incision and stoma site for bleeding and to check the blood pressure and pulse frequently after surgery.

Infection The risk of infection around the stoma is great because of the presence of stool around the new suture line.

Hernia A hernia is the most frequent complication of an ostomy and is caused when a loop of bowel pushes up through the muscle next to the stoma and under the skin.

Obstruction Obstruction of the bowel ostomy may occur as a complication after surgery. Ileostomy clients are instructed to chew their food well before swallowing because large pieces of food such as an olive or large piece of meat may get caught at the opening of the ostomy.

Prolapse The bowel may sometimes telescope out through the stoma, resembling an elephant's trunk. If the bowel continues to work, this is not an emergency. The physician or ET nurse may be able to replace the bowel back into the abdomen; if not, the mucosa of the bowel may become injured, so the prolapse is corrected surgically. Prolapse can be frightening for the client, and its possibility is discussed in postoperative teaching.

Electrolyte Imbalance An ileostomy with a high output of effluent can cause electrolyte imbalances by loss of large amounts of potassium and protein. The client may have difficulty learning to cope with an appliance that is always filling and the need to take in enough fluid, protein, and potassium to replace the lost nutrients.

Skin Excoriation The skin around a high-output ostomy may become excoriated if an appliance that protects the skin cannot be found. Ileostomy effluent contains digestive juices that, if left on the skin, will start to digest the skin, resulting in red, open areas. To prevent this problem, correct appliance fitting that will stay in place is important for these clients.

Discharge Teaching for the Ostomy Client

Assessment

As the client prepares to go home, it is important to assess the client's or the family's ability to handle ostomy care at home. The client may still be dealing with an altered body image and not want to look at or touch the stoma. The family may have to help with care and be supportive until the client can assume the care.

Appliances

If the client has only one bowel movement per day, a closed appliance that is taken off and emptied once a day is all that is needed. If the client has several stools per day, an open-ended drainable appliance is best.

For ileostomies, the one- or two-piece open-end appliance offers ease in emptying. Effluent usually varies from liquid to pasty, so an appliance that can be drained several times per day without taking it off is important. A skin barrier is also necessary for the ileostomy or any ostomy with liquid output.

Irrigation

Irrigation is a means of regulating some colostomies. Descending or sigmoid colostomies are irrigated daily or every other day for control of evacuation. After irrigation, the client may wear a small security appliance or a gauze pad over the stoma the rest of the day. The disadvantage of irrigation is that it takes about an hour or more to perform. The decision to irrigate is made by the client, with the consent of the surgeon, after healing has taken place. To irrigate a colostomy, a cone tip is needed on the end of the irrigation catheter. Using the cone on the tip of the tubing prevents the end of the tube from poking into the side of the bowel and injuring the bowel and helps hold the fluid in the bowel. The cone needs to be lubricated liberally with water-soluble lubricating jelly.

Support Person

Upon discharge, the client and family receive the telephone number of the hospital and unit where treatment was received so they may call if questions arise. Seeing the ET nurse again in 4 to 6 weeks is sometimes recommended to check how the client is doing with ostomy care. If there is a local stoma support group, a person from the group may call or visit the client at home and invite the client and family to come to the group sessions.

Having ostomy surgery is no reason to stop any life activity. People with ostomies live full, active, productive lives.

Nursing Management

Assess bowel sounds frequently. Monitor severity of symptoms such as pain, diarrhea, constipation, abdominal distention, anorexia, nausea, vomiting, and fever. Check CBC reports for increased WBC and low H & H. Explain all tests and treatments and answer questions.

NURSING PROCESS

Assessment

Diverticulosis often has no symptoms, and therefore, clients may not be aware they have it.

Subjective Data

Clients with diverticulitis frequently describe left lower abdominal pain, constipation or diarrhea, bloating, anorexia, and nausea.

Objective Data

Assessment shows abdominal distention with tenderness on palpation, decreased bowel sounds, fever, vomiting, and stools that test positive for blood. A CBC will show an increased WBC and, if bleeding is present, a low H & H.

Nursing diagnoses for a client with diverticulosis or diverticulitis include the following:

NURSING DIAGNOSES	PLANNING/OUTCOMES	NURSING INTERVENTIONS
*Acute **Pain*** related to diverticulitis	The client will verbalize a decrease in pain within 24 hours after intervention as measured by the pain scale.	Encourage bed rest to allow healing. Maintain client as NPO. Administer analgesics and antibiotics as ordered.
*Risk for **Infection*** related to abscess formation or perforation	The client will verbalize understanding of signs and symptoms of possible complications.	Monitor vital signs and pain level every 4 hours and assess abdomen every 4 hours for increased tenderness and distention. Educate the client to notify staff of chills, shortness of breath, or increasing pain.
Anxiety related to possible surgery	The client will verbalize fears related to surgery and exhibit decreased anxiety regarding the procedure and follow-up treatment.	Explain all tests and treatments to decrease the client's anxiety level. Answer all concerns and questions. Allow the client to verbalize fears and concerns. If a colostomy is planned, arrange a consult with an enterostomal therapist to help answer concerns.
Evaluation: Evaluate each outcome to determine how it has been met by the client.		

SAMPLE NURSING CARE PLAN

The Client with Diverticulitis

W.D. is a 67-year-old man admitted to the hospital with abdominal pain that started 2 days ago. The pain has been increasing in intensity and is now accompanied by nausea and anorexia. Physical assessment reveals temperature 101.7°F, pulse 96, respirations 24, and blood pressure of 162/90. W.D.'s abdomen is tender on palpation. He is in obvious discomfort and is unable to lie on his back. W.D. states he has not been eating any food or drinking adequate fluids for 24 hours. Skin turgor is poor. An abdominal ultrasound is ordered and identifies diverticulitis. An IV of D5 1/2 NS with 20 mEq KCl, droperidol (Inapsine) IV for nausea, meperidine (Demerol) IM for pain, and IV antibiotics are ordered. W.D. is placed on I&O, bed rest with bathroom privileges, and is made NPO. W.D. states that he does not understand why all this is being done. His first two voidings are 50 mL each and very concentrated (dark-gold colored).

NURSING DIAGNOSIS 1 *Deficient **K**nowledge* related to diagnosis and treatment regimen, as evidenced by W.D.'s statement that he does not understand why all this is being done

Nursing Outcomes Classification (NOC)
Knowledge: Disease Process
Knowledge: Treatment Regimen

Nursing Interventions Classification (NIC)
Teaching: Disease Process
Teaching: Individual

PLANNING/OUTCOMES	NURSING INTERVENTIONS	RATIONALE
W.D. will verbalize understanding of treatment plan.	Assess W.D.'s knowledge level of diverticulosis/diverticulitis.	Helps client relate new information and integrate it into his behavior.
	Assess W.D.'s learning style and present information in a compatible manner.	Increases understanding and retention.
	Monitor for signs of pain and fatigue.	They impair learning.
	Answer questions and reinforce information.	Reinforces the new information learned.

(Continues)

SAMPLE NURSING CARE PLAN (Continued)

EVALUATION

W.D. verbalizes understanding of the disease process and treatment regimen.

NURSING DIAGNOSIS 2 *Acute* ***Pain*** related to diverticulitis as evidenced by tender abdomen

Nursing Outcomes Classification (NOC)
Comfort Control
Pain Control

Nursing Interventions Classification (NIC)
Pain Management
Medication Management

PLANNING/OUTCOMES	NURSING INTERVENTIONS	RATIONALE
W.D. will verbalize a decrease in pain within 24 hours of pain intervention.	Assess pain by the use of a scale of 1 (no pain) to 10 (extreme pain).	Provides objective measure of the client's perceived discomfort and effectiveness of analgesics.
	Medicate with analgesics as ordered.	Provides pain relief.
	Encourage W.D. to request analgesics before pain becomes intense.	Provides better control of pain.
	Monitor effectiveness of the pain medication by reassessing the pain 45 minutes after the analgesic is given.	Provides a measure of analgesic effectiveness.

EVALUATION

W.D. demonstrates adequate pain relief as demonstrated by a decrease in pain scale.

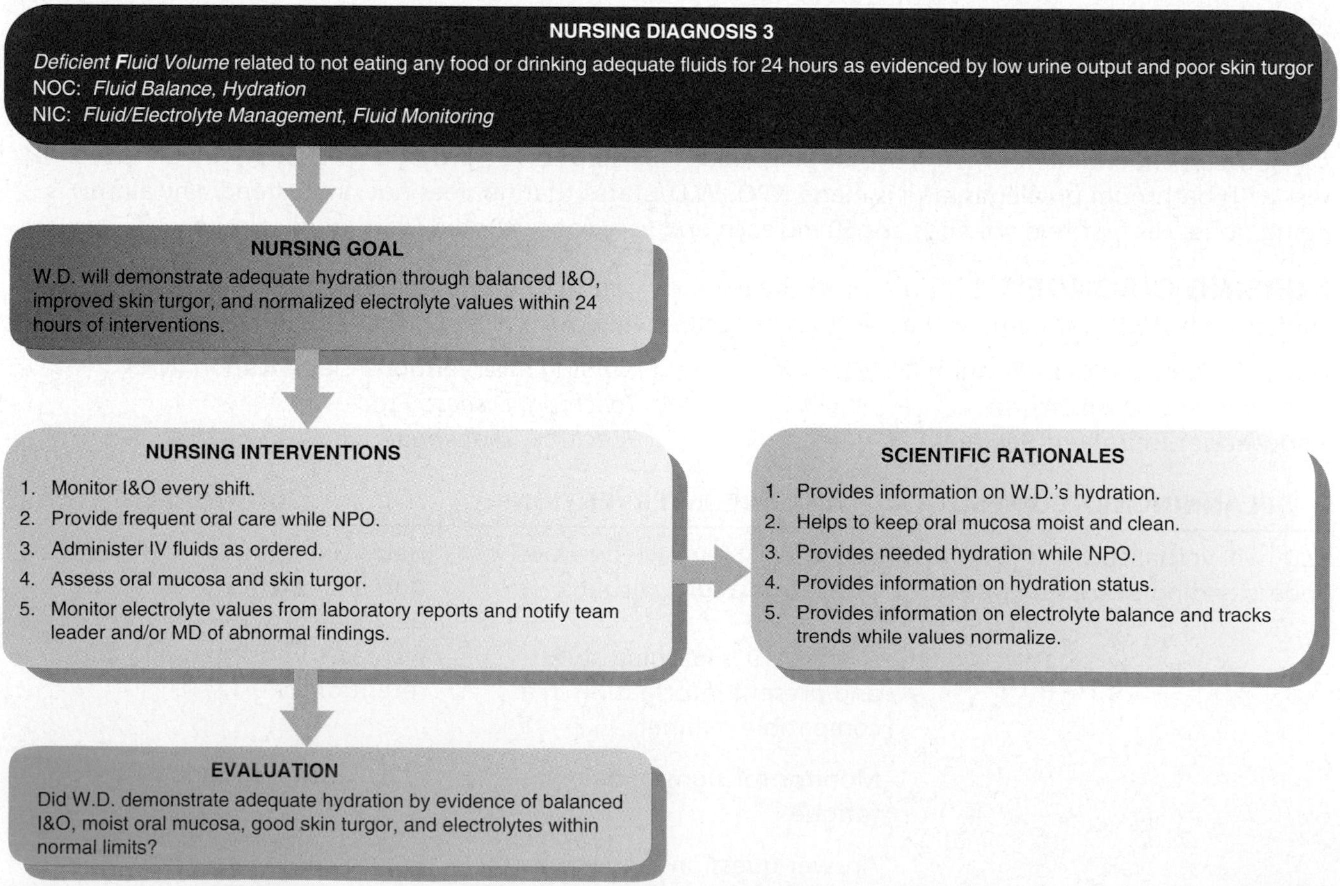

NURSING DIAGNOSIS 3

Deficient ***Fluid*** *Volume* related to not eating any food or drinking adequate fluids for 24 hours as evidenced by low urine output and poor skin turgor
NOC: *Fluid Balance, Hydration*
NIC: *Fluid/Electrolyte Management, Fluid Monitoring*

NURSING GOAL

W.D. will demonstrate adequate hydration through balanced I&O, improved skin turgor, and normalized electrolyte values within 24 hours of interventions.

NURSING INTERVENTIONS

1. Monitor I&O every shift.
2. Provide frequent oral care while NPO.
3. Administer IV fluids as ordered.
4. Assess oral mucosa and skin turgor.
5. Monitor electrolyte values from laboratory reports and notify team leader and/or MD of abnormal findings.

SCIENTIFIC RATIONALES

1. Provides information on W.D.'s hydration.
2. Helps to keep oral mucosa moist and clean.
3. Provides needed hydration while NPO.
4. Provides information on hydration status.
5. Provides information on electrolyte balance and tracks trends while values normalize.

EVALUATION

Did W.D. demonstrate adequate hydration by evidence of balanced I&O, moist oral mucosa, good skin turgor, and electrolytes within normal limits?

CONCEPT CARE MAP 7-1

INFLAMMATORY BOWEL DISEASE

Inflammatory bowel disease (IBD) is the term used to describe Crohn's disease and ulcerative colitis (UC), which are diseases characterized by inflammation and ulcerations of the bowel (Table 7-4). The symptoms of IBD are not confined to the bowel but can affect many of the body's systems, such as uveitis and inflammatory process in the eye (Cox, Evans, Withers, and Titmuss, 2008). Potential extraintestinal manifestations may be found in other internal organs, eyes, blood, skin, and musculoskeletal system. Thirty percent of IBD clients have at least one extraintestinal manifestation (Rayhorn & Rayhorn, 2002).

Crohn's disease is characterized by lesions that affect the entire thickness of the bowel and can occur anywhere throughout the colon and small intestine. Symptoms include abdominal pain, diarrhea that usually does not contain blood, fever, anorexia, weight loss, and **steatorrhea** (fatty stools). Electrolyte imbalance, iron-deficiency anemia, and amino acid malabsorption occur when the disease involves the jejunum and the ileum. Long-term complications of Crohn's disease include bowel obstructions, fistulas, abscesses, and perforation. The risk for colorectal cancer, although not as high as in UC, is still increased. There is malabsorption of fat and fat-soluble vitamins.

UC is characterized by mucosal lesions occurring typically in the rectal area and sigmoid colon and progressing throughout the colon. Symptoms include fever, anorexia, weight loss, cramping, spasms, abdominal pain, and bloody diarrhea. Long-term complications include fissures, abscesses, and an increased risk for colorectal cancer.

The gold standard for diagnosing IBD is an endoscopic examination with a biopsy.

MEDICAL–SURGICAL MANAGEMENT

Medical

Treatment for Crohn's disease and UC is similar. Crohn's disease, however, is more debilitating because it involves more of the GI tract. UC is more limited but can still produce significant symptoms.

An endoscopy done on a UC client reveals continuous mucosal inflammation and ulceration, loss of mucosal vascularity, diffuse erythema, and often purulent exudate. Any granuloma found in the biopsy confirms Crohn's disease (Rayhorn & Rayhorn, 2002). The goals of treatment are to control inflammation, relieve symptoms, maintain fluid and electrolyte balance, provide adequate nutrition, and prevent complications.

Surgical

In severe cases of UC resistant to medical management, the colon is removed and an ileostomy is performed, curing the disease. An **ileostomy** is an opening created in the small intestine (ileum). The output from an ileostomy is a thin liquid, usually of a yellowish-green color. This thin output is called **effluent**. It generally has no odor, and it may get thicker in time as the body adapts to the need to retain moisture. Many ileostomies have almost constant effluent output. The Kock continent ileostomy has a pouch made inside the abdomen to hold the effluent until the client is ready to empty the pouch. Figure 7-7 illustrates a Kock continent ileostomy.

Most clients with Crohn's disease need surgery at some point to repair the structural damage caused by scarring. Intestinal obstructions and perforations may also occur in Crohn's disease, necessitating further surgery. Surgical intervention, however, does not cure the disease.

TABLE 7-4 Comparison of Crohn's disease and ulcerative colitis

PARAMETER	CROHN'S DISEASE	ULCERATIVE COLITIS (UC)
Involvement	Patchy areas. Can involve small and large intestine.	Starts in lower colon and spreads progressively throughout colon. Affects only the colon.
Tissue affected	Affects entire thickness of bowel.	Affects mucosal lining of bowel.
Long-term complications	Intestinal obstruction, fistulas, abscesses, perforations; cancer risk increases with age.	Fissures, abscesses, increased risk for colorectal cancer.
Surgical intervention	Usually needed at some point to repair structural damage. Does not cure or limit the progress of the disease.	Ileostomy performed in approximately 20% of cases to remove the colon. Cures the disease.
Cause	Unknown: possibly altered immune state.	Unknown: possibly enteric bacterium *E. coli*.
Stools	3 to 4 semisoft/day; rarely bloody; steatorrhea and mucus present.	15 to 20 liquid/day; blood present; no steatorrhea.

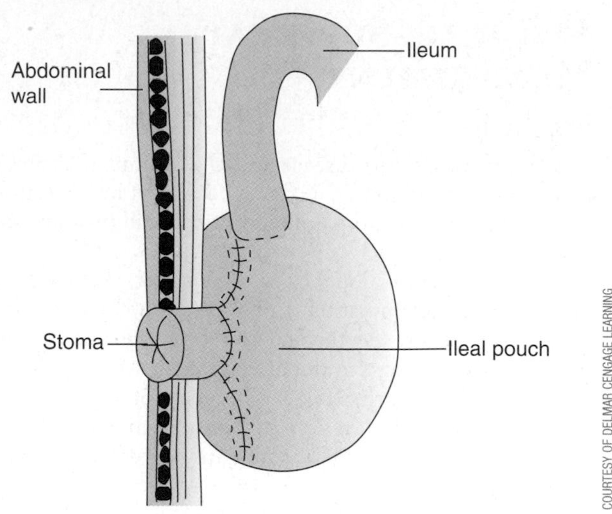

FIGURE 7-7 Kock Continent Ileostomy

Pharmacological

Treatment for both UC and Crohn's disease includes 5-ASA compounds such as sulfasalazine (Azulfidine) or salicylates such as mesalamine (Rowasa) or olsalazine sodium (Dipentum). If inflammation is severe, corticosteroids also are administered. In cases resistant to the 5-ASA compounds and corticosteroids, immunosuppressors are used. If an infection is present, antibiotics are administered. According to Rayhorn and Rayhorn (2002), clients are seldom given antidiarrheal medications because they may predispose the client to toxic megacolon.

Clients need IV fluid and electrolyte replacement during severe flare-ups. In the most severe cases, clients are placed on total parenteral nutrition (TPN) to allow for complete bowel rest and to improve nutritional status.

Diet

Protein and calorie malnutrition is a concern in clients with IBD. Because of the severe cramping, pain, and diarrhea brought on by foods, these clients typically put themselves on a very restrictive diet that is not nutritionally balanced. Clients with Crohn's disease may also have malabsorption of iron and vitamin B_{12}.

Nutritional support includes modifying the diet to eliminate foods that exacerbate symptoms while maintaining a balanced diet. A high-calorie, low-residue, high-protein, low-fat diet is recommended (Rayhorn & Rayhorn, 2002).

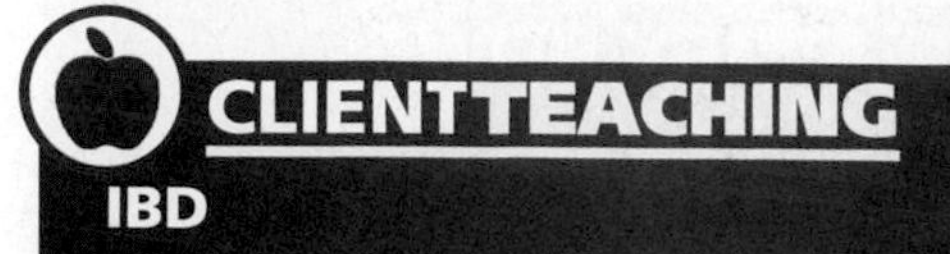

CLIENT TEACHING

IBD

- Schedule a colon cancer screening regularly.
- When taking oral corticosteroids, strictly adhere to the prescribed schedule.

Health Promotion

Although stress has not been shown to exacerbate the symptoms of Crohn's disease or UC, the impact on the client's lifestyle can be significant, especially with Crohn's disease. Support groups can be beneficial. Encourage clients to develop mechanisms to help them cope with the disease process. Exercise, meditation, and biofeedback may be helpful.

NURSING MANAGEMENT

Assess the abdomen for tenderness, distention, and bowel sounds. Monitor weight, vital signs, and stools. Maintain an accurate I&O and calorie count. Provide high-calorie, high-protein small, frequent meals and snacks. Encourage verbalization of feelings.

NURSING PROCESS

ASSESSMENT

Subjective Data

Clients describe mild abdominal spasms and cramping, which may increase to severe abdominal pain, nausea, and anorexia. Clients with UC have an urge to defecate with the cramping.

Objective Data

Clients have abdominal tenderness on palpation, guarding, distention, weight loss, diarrhea, an elevated WBC count, and fever. In clients with Crohn's disease, steatorrhea and iron-deficiency anemia may be present. In clients with UC, stools may be positive for blood and the H & H may be low. The serum potassium, magnesium, and albumin levels are usually low. Because Crohn's disease is so debilitating, clients may become depressed.

Nursing diagnoses for a client with Crohn's disease or UC include the following:

NURSING DIAGNOSES	PLANNING/OUTCOMES	NURSING INTERVENTIONS
*Imbalanced **N**utrition: Less than Body Requirements* related to postprandial pain, bowel hypermobility, and decreased absorption	The client will demonstrate adequate nutritional status as exhibited by maintaining weight within range for height and body type.	Monitor I&O every shift; caloric count and weight daily. Administer IV fluid and electrolyte replacement as ordered. Provide high-calorie, high-protein supplements as ordered along with small, frequent meals. Administer TPN, a high-calorie and nutrient-dense IV solution, as ordered. Closely monitor lab reports for electrolytes and glucose level.

Nursing diagnoses for a client with Crohn's disease or UC include the following: (Continued)

NURSING DIAGNOSES	PLANNING/OUTCOMES	NURSING INTERVENTIONS
*Risk for Deficient **Fluid** Volume* related to diarrhea and altered intake	The client will exhibit adequate hydration as evidenced by electrolytes within normal range, moist mucous membranes, and I&O nearly equal within 48 hours of intervention. The frequency and amount of diarrhea will decrease within 48 hours of intervention.	Administer 5-ASA compounds, corticosteroids, and immunosuppressors as ordered. Monitor I&O every shift. Administer IV fluid and electrolyte rehydration as ordered.
***P**owerlessness* related to impairment in lifestyle secondary to disease process	The client will verbalize a plan to seek support, by discharge.	Provide client with information on national organizations and local support groups. Arrange social work consult if needed. Allow client to verbalize feelings.

Evaluation: Evaluate each outcome to determine how it has been met by the client.

IRRITABLE BOWEL SYNDROME

Irritable bowel syndrome (IBS) refers to a group of symptoms—cramping, abdominal pain, bloating, constipation, or diarrhea. Some clients have both constipation and diarrhea which alternate in appearance. There is no organic cause, but the movement of feces and gas through the colon and the absorption of fluids are affected. When feces stay in the colon too long and too much water is absorbed, constipation results. When feces is pushed through the colon too fast by spasms, little water is absorbed and diarrhea results. Spasms also temporarily trap gas or feces, preventing them from moving forward, and therefore causing pain.

The colon seems to be more sensitive and reactive especially to certain foods and stress. Since the colon is partly controlled by the autonomic nervous system, it responds to stress. It may contract too much or too little, and too much water or too little water may be absorbed.

In the United States, one in five persons has IBS, making it one of the most common gastrointestinal disorders. Only a small proportion of people seek medical treatment, while most will treat the symptoms themselves. IBS occurs more frequently in women than in men, and usually begins around age 20 (NIDDK, 2009b).

There is no diagnostic test for IBS, but clients presenting with the aforementioned symptoms often undergo testing to rule out other disorders. Criteria for a diagnosis of IBS include:

1. Abdominal pain or discomfort for at least 12 weeks (not necessarily consecutive) out of the previous 12 months.
2. At least two of the following three features must be present:
   - Abdominal pain or discomfort is relieved by having a bowel movement.
   - When abdominal pain or discomfort begins, there is a change in how often the client has a bowel movement.
   - When abdominal pain or discomfort begins, there is a change in the form of the stool or the way it looks.

MEDICAL-SURGICAL MANAGEMENT

Medical

The goal of treatment is to relieve the symptoms. Foods that make the symptoms worse are eliminated from the diet. Increasing dietary fiber is often helpful. Anxiety-reducing measures often relieve symptoms. If the client has severe anxiety or depression, counseling may be required.

Pharmacological

Anticholinergic medications are administered before meals. Clients with constipation may be given tegaserod maleate (Zelnorm), usually for 4 weeks. Bulk-forming psyllium hydrophilic muciloid (Metamucil) may also be used.

Clients who primarily have diarrhea and have not responded to other therapies may be given alosetron hydrochloride (Lotronex). It should be used with caution because it can have serious side effects, such as severe constipation or decreased blood flow to the colon.

Diet

The client is instructed to eliminate from the diet those foods that aggravate the symptoms and discomfort. Foods often associated with making IBS symptoms worse include wheat, rye, barley, chocolate, milk products, alcohol, and caffeinated drinks. Foods high in fiber such as bran, cereal, beans, fruits, and vegetables may reduce symptoms. Large meals cause cramping and diarrhea.

Activity

Regular exercise may help relieve symptoms. Seldom is weight loss a problem.

Nursing Management

Encourage the client to write down what is eaten, what symptoms are present and when they occur, and which foods always make the client feel bad. Then eliminate those foods causing symptoms or making the client feel bad. Suggest that the client eat five or six small meals instead of three large meals each day. Encourage the client to exercise regularly and practice stress-relieving measures such as progressive relaxation or guided imagery.

NURSING PROCESS

Assessment

Subjective Data

Some clients describe cramping, abdominal pain, and diarrhea during or soon after a meal, others complain of constipation, and still others report alternating diarrhea and constipation. Abdominal fullness, gas, and bloating also often occur.

Objective Data

The client's stools will be either very loose (diarrhea) or very hard and difficult to pass (constipation). Mucus may be passed with the bowel movement. ***No** weight loss, bleeding, or fever is associated with IBS.*

Nursing diagnoses for a client with irritable bowel syndrome include the following:

NURSING DIAGNOSES	PLANNING/OUTCOMES	NURSING INTERVENTIONS
***D**iarrhea* related to rapid movement of feces through the colon with too little fluid being absorbed	The client will have normally formed stools.	Encourage frequent meals. Add high-fiber foods gradually to meals. Teach client to eliminate gas-forming foods and other foods causing symptoms from the diet. Teach stress-reducing measures.
***C**onstipation* related to delayed movement of feces through the colon with too much fluid being absorbed	The client will have regularly passed, soft, formed stools.	Encourage increased fluid intake unless contraindicated, and increase consumption of high-fiber foods. Encourage regular exercise such as walking. Administer medications as prescribed. Teach stress-reducing measures.

Evaluation: Evaluate each outcome to determine how it has been met by the client.

INTESTINAL OBSTRUCTION

An intestinal obstruction occurs when the contents cannot pass through the intestine. Obstructions occur in the large or the small intestine, with most occurring in the ileum. Obstructions may be mechanical, neurogenic, or vascular in origin.

A mechanical obstruction may be a partial or complete obstruction caused by a tumor; fecal impaction; hernia; **volvulus**, a twisting of the bowel on itself; **intussusception**, a telescoping of the bowel where the bowel slides inside itself (Figure 7-8); or **adhesions**, scar tissue in the abdomen from previous surgeries or disease process such as Crohn's disease.

A neurogenic obstruction, known as a *paralytic ileus*, occurs when nerve transmission to the bowel is interrupted by trauma, infection, or medications, resulting in a portion of the bowel being paralyzed.

A vascular obstruction occurs when blood flow to a portion of the bowel is interrupted, as in atherosclerosis, and that portion of the bowel becomes necrotic.

When the small intestine becomes obstructed, large amounts of fluid, bacteria, and swallowed air build up in the bowel proximal to the obstruction. The normal process of

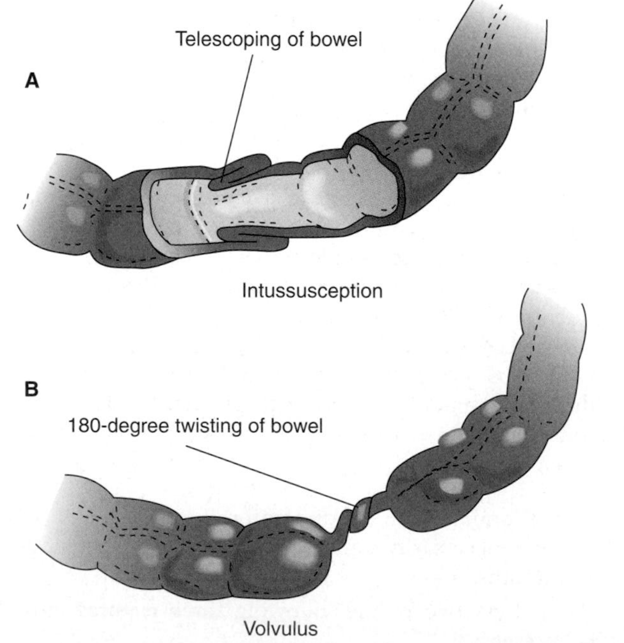

FIGURE 7-8 Bowel obstructions can be caused by *A*, an intussusception; or *B*, a volvulus.

secretion and absorption of the electrolyte-rich fluid is interrupted. Distention and poor absorption occur when water and salts move from the circulatory system to the lumen of the intestine.

An abdominal x-ray and a barium enema or UGI with small bowel follow-through are ordered when a bowel obstruction is suspected.

Medical–Surgical Management

Medical

Treatment of the obstruction depends on the cause and location. Some can be treated medically by inserting an NG tube for decompression, providing IV fluids for rehydration, and treating the cause, such as the use of enemas for fecal impaction.

Surgical

Most bowel obstructions require surgery. A bowel resection is performed to remove the portion of the bowel affected by the obstruction.

Pharmacological

Nonnarcotic analgesics are used to avoid the intestinal motility decrease caused by opioids. Antibiotics also are ordered.

Diet

Clients are kept NPO until the obstruction is cleared and then slowly progressed from a clear liquid diet to a regular diet as more bowel function returns.

Activity

In cases of paralytic ileus, ambulation is encouraged to help bowel function return. Encourage clients who have had a bowel resection to turn, cough, and deep breathe every 2 hours initially postoperatively. Activity is progressed the next day.

Nursing Management

Assess abdomen for tenderness, distention, and bowel sounds. Monitor vomiting for fecal material. Assess weight daily. Accurately record I&O and limit ice chips when NPO. Check laboratory reports for low sodium and potassium and elevated BUN, amylase, and H & H.

NURSING PROCESS

Assessment

Subjective Data

Clients report symptoms of colicky abdominal pain, nausea, constipation, and bloating.

Objective Data

Objective assessment includes abdominal distention and tenderness on palpation. Vomiting temporarily relieves the abdominal pain. Vomitus may include fecal material, which is a poor prognostic sign (Lynch and Sarazine, 2006).

Laboratory analysis demonstrates decreased levels of sodium and potassium, elevated BUN, elevated amylase, and elevated H & H caused by hemoconcentration.

Nursing diagnoses for a client with intestinal obstruction include the following:

NURSING DIAGNOSES	PLANNING/OUTCOMES	NURSING INTERVENTIONS
*Deficient **Fluid Volume*** related to vomiting, shift in fluids, and NPO status	The client will exhibit adequate hydration within 48 hours of initiation of treatment as evidenced by moist mucous membranes, electrolytes within normal limits, and I&O approximately equal.	Monitor I&O every shift. Administer IV fluid and electrolyte replacements as ordered. Allow limited ice chips to prevent further electrolyte imbalance in clients with NG tubes. Assess weight daily.
*Acute **Pain*** related to distention, edema, or ischemia	The client will verbalize increased comfort within 1 hour of analgesic administration as measured on pain scale.	Administer nonnarcotic analgesics as ordered. In clients with a paralytic ileus, encourage ambulation to encourage return of bowel function. Maintain and monitor NG tube as ordered for abdominal decompression. Check bowel sounds every 4 hours or PRN.
*Deficient **Knowledge*** related to disease process, treatment regimen, and possible surgery	The client will verbalize treatment course, possible complications, and possible need for surgery.	Identify client's learning style and present information in a manner compatible with learning style. Include intestinal decompression, need for ambulation, need for good oral care due to fecal drainage, and surgery.

Evaluation: Evaluate each outcome to determine how it has been met by the client.

HERNIAS

A hernia occurs when the wall of a muscle weakens and the intestine protrudes through the muscle wall. Hernias that do not return to the abdominal cavity with rest or manipulation and cause complete bowel obstruction are said to be *incarcerated*. If the blood supply to the hernia is cut off, the hernia is said to be *strangulated*. Immediate surgery is required to restore blood flow. If not done, gangrene develops, which may be fatal.

Several types of hernias exist. In an umbilical hernia, a portion of the bowel protrudes through the umbilicus. In children, these generally resolve on their own once the child begins to walk. Umbilical hernias most commonly occur in multiparous women or in adults with cirrhosis and **ascites** (abnormal accumulation of fluid in the peritoneal cavity). Because of a high risk for strangulation in adults with umbilical hernias, surgery is usually performed.

Abdominal hernias occur in the midline of the abdomen between the umbilicus and the xyphoid process. Most are asymptomatic, with a few causing pain on exertion that resolves with reclining and rest. Inguinal hernias, the most common hernia, occur in the groin area. Inguinal hernias frequently occur after activities, such as lifting, that increase intraabdominal pressure; they subside with relaxation. Pain is located lower than in the abdominal hernia. Femoral hernias occur when the intestine pushes into the passageway carrying blood vessels and nerves to the legs and are more common in women than in men. A hiatal hernia occurs when a portion of the stomach protrudes into the mediastinal cavity through the diaphragm. Symptoms of hiatal hernias include indigestion and heartburn, especially after eating a large meal.

Upon evaluation and recommendation of a physician, some hernias can be reduced or pushed back into place. This can be accomplished by having the client recline, applying direct pressure to the hernia, and, in some cases, having the client exhale to decrease intraabdominal pressure. The nurse should never try to reduce a hernia.

MEDICAL–SURGICAL MANAGEMENT

Medical

Some hernias have no symptoms or minimal symptoms, so clients may not be aware they have one or may learn to live with it by reducing it when needed. Clients who are a poor surgical risk may use a truss, a device that applies pressure to the hernia, thus keeping the intestine in the abdominal cavity.

Surgical

Hernias are repaired with surgery called herniorrhaphy. The surgery is typically performed on an outpatient basis, with clients going home the same day. If the surgery is more complicated because the hernia is incarcerated, the client may stay overnight. If the hernia is strangulated, a bowel resection may be required.

Surgical repair of a hiatal hernia involves reinforcing the esophagus with a portion of the stomach. The surgery is performed laparoscopically, with the client remaining in the hospital 3 to 5 days postoperatively. Initially, the client will have an NG tube. The NG tube is removed 24 to 48 hours later and the diet gradually progressed to a soft diet.

Diet

Clients with hiatal hernias modify their dietary patterns by eating small frequent meals. Clients are encouraged not to eat after the evening meal, lie down for 2 hours after eating, or consume aggravating foods.

NURSING MANAGEMENT

Assess abdomen for bowel sounds and bulge in abdominal wall. Encourage client with hernia to eat small, frequent meals and avoid lying down for 2 hours after eating.

NURSING PROCESS

ASSESSMENT

Subjective Data

Clients may describe pain at the site of the hernia.

Objective Data

Assessment may show a bulge through the abdominal wall. If the hernia is strangulated, the client will have the symptoms of a bowel obstruction.

Nursing diagnoses for a client with a hernia include the following:

NURSING DIAGNOSES	PLANNING/OUTCOMES	NURSING INTERVENTIONS
Acute ***Pain*** related to tissue edema	The client will experience less pain within 1 hour of intervention as measured on the pain scale.	Administer analgesics as ordered. Evaluate aggravating activities (e.g., straining to have a bowel movement) and provide information on modification if indicated. Educate regarding signs of complications and when to notify staff of symptoms.
Ineffective ***Tissue Perfusion*** *(Gastrointestinal)* related to strangulation	The client will have minimal tissue necrosis.	Assess abdomen for bowel sounds every 4 hours. Insert NG tube to decrease abdominal distention as ordered. Administer IV hydration as ordered. Prepare client for surgery as ordered. Keep client NPO.

Evaluation: Evaluate each outcome to determine how it has been met by the client.

PERITONITIS

Peritonitis is the inflammation of the peritoneum, the membranous covering of the abdomen. Peritonitis is caused by irritating substances such as feces, gastric acids, bacteria, or blood in the abdominal cavity. A ruptured portion of the digestive system (such as the appendix), a ruptured tubal pregnancy, or invasion of tumors through the gastric wall can lead to peritonitis. Peritonitis is a serious, life-threatening condition. Complications of peritonitis include adhesions (scar tissue), paralytic ileus, and pneumonia.

MEDICAL–SURGICAL MANAGEMENT

Surgical

Treatment is primarily surgical with repair of the cause and irrigation of the abdominal cavity with saline and antibiotic solutions. Drains are left in the abdomen for several days postoperatively to allow any remaining fluid to drain. Because bowel function usually stops as a result of the irritating substances, an NG tube is placed to decompress the abdomen and relieve nausea.

Pharmacological

Analgesics are ordered postoperatively for discomfort. If an ileus develops, nonnarcotic analgesics are ordered. Antibiotics are ordered preoperatively and postoperatively.

Diet

Clients are NPO preoperatively and postoperatively until bowel sounds return. Clients are then placed on a clear liquid diet and slowly progressed to a regular diet as more bowel function returns.

Activity

Preoperatively, clients are placed on bed rest and encouraged to turn, cough, and deep breathe. Because clients tend to breathe shallowly with peritoneal inflammation, pulmonary hygiene is important. Activity is increased postoperatively, as soon as tolerated, to increase lung expansion and to encourage bowel function return. Exercise, lifting, and driving are restricted until the incision heals.

NURSING MANAGEMENT

Assess vital signs and administer antipyretics as ordered. Monitor I&O, signs of dehydration, and fluid and electrolyte replacement. Provide comfort measures (cool cloth, oral hygiene, back rub). Maintain patency of NG tube. Encourage coughing and deep breathing and teach incision splinting. Keep client in semi-Fowler's position to help localize purulent exudate. Follow surgical asepsis for wound care. Empty drainage devices as required. If drainage does not flow into a device, change dressings frequently to keep drainage off the skin. If the wound is still draining when the client is discharged, teach client/family aseptic technique for changing dressings.

NURSING PROCESS

ASSESSMENT

Subjective Data

Clients describe abdominal pain, nausea, and constipation.

Objective Data

Assessment reveals vomiting, absent bowel sounds, a tense or distended abdomen with tenderness on palpation, shallow and rapid respirations, weak and rapid pulse, dry mucous membranes, low urine output, fever, and limited mobility because of pain. Laboratory analysis will show an increased WBC. If the client is bleeding, the H & H will be low. Sodium, potassium, and chloride may be low.

Nursing diagnoses for a client with peritonitis include the following:

NURSING DIAGNOSES	PLANNING/OUTCOMES	NURSING INTERVENTIONS
*Deficient **Fluid** Volume* related to gastric losses and restricted intake	The client will maintain hydration as indicated by an I&O that is nearly equal and electrolytes within normal limits.	Monitor I&O every shift. Monitor for signs of dehydration: dry mucous membranes, poor skin turgor, and low urine output. Monitor electrolytes as ordered. Administer IV rehydration and electrolyte replacement as ordered.
Hyperthermia related to inflammatory process and dehydration	The client will maintain temperature within normal limits.	Assess VS including temperature every 4 hours. Administer antipyretics as ordered; probably rectal suppositories due to NPO status. Monitor for dehydration: decrease in urine output, dry mucous membranes, and poor skin turgor. Provide comfort measures: cool cloth to the head or neck, assistance to turn, and a back rub with cooling lotion.

(*Continues*)

Nursing diagnoses for a client with peritonitis include the following: (Continued)

NURSING DIAGNOSES	PLANNING/OUTCOMES	NURSING INTERVENTIONS
*Acute **Pain** related to abdominal distention*	The client will have less pain and improved mobility within 1 hour of receiving analgesics as measured on the pain scale.	Administer analgesics as ordered. Encourage activity such as coughing and deep breathing after analgesics. Teach splinting of incision for cough and deep breathing. Monitor NG tube to decompress abdomen. Maintain patency of NG tube.

Evaluation: Evaluate each outcome to determine how it has been met by the client.

HEMORRHOIDS

Hemorrhoids are swollen vascular tissues in the rectal area. They may be internal or external. Hemorrhoids may be caused by straining with constipation or sitting on the toilet (reading) for an extended time. Hemorrhoids frequently occur with pregnancy. Hemorrhoids can cause burning, pruritis, and pain with defecation. At times, they can bleed, leading to anemia.

MEDICAL–SURGICAL MANAGEMENT

Medical

Sitz baths or warm compresses on the rectal area for 20 minutes, 4 times a day, often helps decrease swelling.

Surgical

If bleeding continues despite medical intervention, or if discomfort is significant, hemorrhoids can be surgically removed by a hemorrhoidectomy. For external hemorrhoids, surgery is performed on an outpatient basis by placing a band around the hemorrhoid as for esophageal varices, allowing it to necrose and fall off. For internal hemorrhoids, sclerotherapy, cryotherapy, or laser is performed. This usually requires that the patient stay overnight in the hospital. Hemorrhoids can recur after surgical removal if the cause is not eliminated.

Pharmacological

Treatment includes the administration of creams and suppositories to decrease inflammation, some with cortisone to decrease swelling. Fiber supplements and stool softeners are ordered to keep bowel movements soft.

Diet

Bowel movements are kept soft with a high-fiber diet of 20 to 30 grams of fiber per day and at least 2,500 mL of fluid intake daily.

NURSING MANAGEMENT

Teach client to modify bowel habits (sit on toilet only for short periods), increase fiber in diet to 20 or 30 grams per day, and increase fluid intake to 2,500 mL per day. Provide sitz baths several times a day or teach client how to do it.

NURSING PROCESS

ASSESSMENT

Subjective Data

Clients describe rectal burning, pain, and pruritis with bowel movements; constipation; and, occasionally, bright red bleeding. A dietary history is obtained to determine fiber and fluid intake.

Objective Data

If hemorrhoids are external, they can be visualized during a physical examination. If chronic bleeding is present, laboratory analysis may show a low H & H.

Nursing diagnoses for a client with hemorrhoids include the following:

NURSING DIAGNOSES	PLANNING/OUTCOMES	NURSING INTERVENTIONS
*Acute **Pain*** related to edema and inflammation of swollen vascular tissues	The client will verbalize a decrease in discomfort within 48 hours of initiation of treatment.	Provide sitz baths or warm compresses for 20 minutes, 4 times a day. Administer creams and suppositories as ordered. Increase fiber and fluids in diet to keep stools soft to avoid straining.
*Deficient **Knowledge*** related to diet, causes of condition, treatment, and potential complications	The client will be able to verbalize treatment regimen and long-term management of hemorrhoids.	Determine client's learning style and present information in a manner compatible with learning style. Educate client about increasing fiber in diet to 20 to 30 grams per day, increasing fluid intake to 2,500 mL per day, causes of hemorrhoids, possible complications such as anemia, and modification of bowel habits (such as not sitting on the toilet for long periods).

Evaluation: Evaluate each outcome to determine how it has been met by the client.

CONSTIPATION

Constipation is characterized by hard, infrequent stools that are difficult and/or painful to pass. Constipation can be caused by tumors, low-fiber diet, inactivity, some diseases that interfere with the mechanical functioning of the bowel (such as multiple sclerosis), or some medications (such as narcotics, antidepressants, or anti-Parkinson drugs).

MEDICAL–SURGICAL MANAGEMENT

Pharmacological

Fiber supplements and stool softeners are ordered. Laxatives and enemas may be ordered, but long-term use is avoided because they interrupt normal bowel function. If constipation is caused by medications the client is taking, the client should discuss other options with the physician, such as modifying the dosage or changing medications.

Diet

Fiber is increased to 20 to 30 grams per day. Fluid intake is increased to 2,500 mL per day.

Activity

Increase activity level if possible because exercise, such as walking, increases motility in the colon.

LIFE SPAN CONSIDERATIONS

Constipation in the Older Client

The slowing of peristalsis, which is part of the aging process, leads to constipation in the older client. An increase in dietary fiber and fluid intake (water) helps to prevent constipation. A regular schedule for bowel evacuation also helps.

NURSING MANAGEMENT

Assess dietary intake of fiber and fluids and activity/exercise level. Review medications client is taking for any causing constipation. Encourage regular schedule for bowel evacuation.

NURSING PROCESS

ASSESSMENT

Subjective Data

Clients describe infrequent, difficult to pass stools. Dietary assessment of fiber and fluids usually reveals inadequate intake. Ask client to describe activity/exercise level.

Objective Data

Bowel movements are hard-formed.

Nursing diagnoses for a client with constipation include the following:

NURSING DIAGNOSES	PLANNING/OUTCOMES	NURSING INTERVENTIONS
Constipation related to inadequate intake of fiber and fluids	The client will have soft stools every other day by one week from intervention.	Encourage client to increase fiber in the diet to 20 to 30 grams a day and fluid intake to 2,500 mL a day. Administer fiber supplements and stool softeners as ordered. Determine fluid preferences of client and always have fluids at client's bedside within reach. Help the client establish a regular schedule for bowel movements, usually 30 minutes after a meal.
Deficient Knowledge related to dietary sources of fiber and the importance of adequate fluid intake and exercise	The client will be able to select a menu high in fiber and fluids utilizing nutrients from the food pyramid within 48 hours and verbalize the need for adequate exercise.	Assess client's learning style and present information in a manner compatible with learning style. Teach client about foods that are high in fiber (fruits, vegetables, whole grains) as well as importance of fluid intake. Discuss with client the importance of exercise in maintaining bowel function.

Evaluation: Evaluate each outcome to determine how it has been met by the client.

DISORDERS OF THE ACCESSORY ORGANS

Disorders of the accessory organs include cirrhosis, hepatitis, pancreatitis, and cholecystitis/cholelithiasis.

CIRRHOSIS

Cirrhosis refers to the chronic, degenerative changes in the liver cells and thickening of surrounding tissue that result from the liver repairing itself after chronic inflammation.

Causes of cirrhosis include chronic hepatitis, repeated exposure to toxic substances, disease processes (such as sclerosing cholangitis and hemochromatosis), cancer, and chronic alcohol abuse. Alcohol abuse accounts for most cases of cirrhosis.

Because the liver is responsible for so many functions, complications of cirrhosis can be significant and include malnutrition, hypoglycemia, clotting disorders, jaundice, portal hypertension, ascites, hepatic encephalopathy, and hepatorenal syndrome.

Liver dysfunction causes several organ-related complications. Malnutrition results from the liver's inability to absorb fat and fat-soluble vitamins and leads to muscle wasting, weight loss, and fatigue. Hypoglycemia occurs when the liver is unable to perform glycogenolysis efficiently. When the liver is not able to produce sufficient amounts of prothrombin and fibrinogen, clotting disorders arise.

Portal hypertension results when blood flow through the cirrhotic liver is inhibited, resulting in blood backflowing in the portal vein. Portal hypertension leads to distention of the esophageal veins, resulting in esophageal varices; distention of rectal veins, resulting in hemorrhoids; and distention of the splenic vein, resulting in splenomegaly.

Because the liver is responsible for metabolizing medications, clients frequently become intolerant to some medications. Jaundice, a yellow discoloration of the skin, is usually present. Jaundice occurs when the liver is unable to convert bilirubin, an end product of red blood cell breakdown, into a water-soluble form that can be excreted in the bile. The extra bilirubin collects in areas that contain elastin, such as the sclera of the eyes, the skin, and the nail beds.

Fluid accumulates in the pleural cavity in the form of pleural effusions. Fluid may also accumulate in the peritoneal cavity. This condition is called ascites. The cause of ascites is the congestion of blood in the portal system.

Hepatic encephalopathy is a condition in which ammonia accumulates in the brain. Fluid is pulled into the extracellular compartment, accelerating brain stem herniation. Confusion, lethargy, and/or coma may occur. Symptoms of impending hepatic encephalopathy are disorientation and *asterixis* (liver flap), a flapping tremor of the hands. When the client extends the arms and hands in front of the body, the hands rapidly flex and extend.

Hepatorenal syndrome is a complication of cirrhosis in which the client goes into renal failure. Symptoms include oliguria (diminished production of urine), azotemia (excess nitrogen in the blood), anorexia, fatigue, and weakness.

Cirrhosis is a form of end-stage liver disease for which there is no cure. The process of cirrhosis can be slowed by removing the cause (i.e., abstaining from alcohol), but the damage cannot be reversed. Clients in end-stage liver disease are evaluated to determine whether they qualify for a liver transplant.

Medical–Surgical Management

Medical

The physician performs a paracentesis to remove the fluid from the abdomen and relieve pressure on the diaphragm and lungs. A small incision is made and a trochar inserted into the abdomen to drain the fluid. Albumin may be infused at the same time to pull excess fluid back into the vascular system.

Surgical

If the client continues to develop ascites after medical treatment, a LeVeen or Denver peritoneal venous shunt is used. The pressure-regulated shunt is implanted in the peritoneal cavity and threaded through the subcutaneous tissue into the superior vena cava, returning the fluid back to the vascular system. As fluid pressure builds in the peritoneal cavity, a valve opens and drains the fluid into the superior vena cava.

If esophageal varices are present, an EGD with sclerotherapy or banding is done to prevent hemorrhage (refer to Figure 7-3).

If portal hypertension cannot be controlled with medications, a portosystemic shunt or a transjugular intrahepatic portosystemic shunt (TIPS) may be performed. The shunt redirects the blood flow, thereby relieving the portal hypertension, and decreases the risk of rupturing distended veins in the esophagus (Figure 7-9).

Pharmacological

A potassium-sparing diuretic, such as spironolactone (Aldactone), decreases ascites and pleural effusion. Lactulose (Cholac) moves ammonia from the blood into the bowel. The lactulose acts as a laxative and causes the body to excrete the stool containing ammonia. Tap water enemas may also be ordered to help the body eliminate the ammonia.

Propranolol hydrochloride (Inderal), an antihypertensive medication, is ordered to lower portal hypertension. All unnecessary medications are avoided because the liver cannot metabolize them.

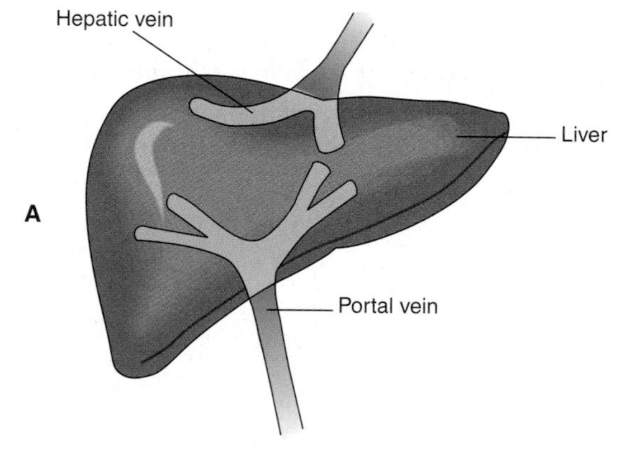

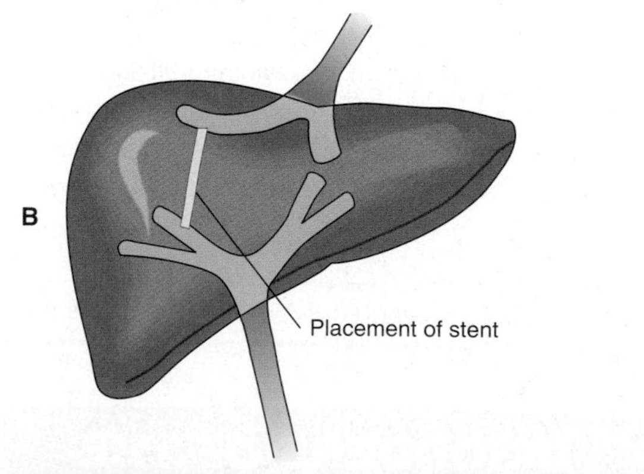

FIGURE 7-9 ***A,*** **Blood Flow before TIPS;** ***B,*** **TIPS is performed in radiology on clients deemed too unstable for the surgery necessary for a portosystemic shunt. A stent is placed to redirect the blood flow.**

Diet

Clients with cirrhosis are placed on a low-protein diet, usually 40 grams per day. If ascites is present, sodium will also be restricted to 2 grams or less per day to decrease the amount of fluid retained by the body. Fluids also are restricted to 1,000 mL to 2,000 mL per day depending on the severity of fluid accumulation.

Activity

Because fatigue is such a common symptom of cirrhosis, the client's tolerance for activity will be diminished. Plan rest periods during the day, and schedule activities between rests.

SAFETY

Cirrhosis

If hepatic encephalopathy is present, precautions are taken to ensure the client's safety, such as elevating bedrails and allowing the client to ambulate only with assistance, especially if the client's gait is unsteady.

Nursing Management

Monitor vital signs and mental status. Restrict fluid intake as ordered. Accurately record I&O. Weigh client daily and measure abdominal girth. Provide low-sodium, low-protein diet. Turn client every 2 hours and monitor for redness and skin breakdown. Assist with or provide frequent oral hygiene.

NURSING PROCESS

Assessment

Subjective Data

Clients describe fatigue, nausea, anorexia, weakness, and indigestion.

Objective Data

Assessment shows ascites, jaundice, enlarged liver and spleen, petechiae (small bruises on the skin), vomiting, weight loss, fever, epistaxis, and decreased breath sounds. Lethargy, confusion, or coma is present if encephalopathy has occurred.

Laboratory analysis includes a CBC, which will demonstrate low WBCs, RBCs, Hgb, and platelets. A liver panel will show an elevated bilirubin, alkaline phosphatase, GGT, ALT, and AST. Albumin will be low. PT, PTT, and clotting times will be delayed.

Nursing diagnoses for a client with cirrhosis include the following:

NURSING DIAGNOSES	PLANNING/OUTCOMES	NURSING INTERVENTIONS
Disturbed Thought Processes related to elevated serum ammonia level and hepatic coma	The client will experience an improved level of orientation within 48 hours of initiation of treatment.	Administer tap water enemas and lactulose as ordered to eliminate ammonia-rich stools. An NG tube may be placed to give lactulose if the client is comatose. Monitor ammonia level. Elevate bedrails to prevent injury. As coma lessens, reorient client frequently.
Excess Fluid Volume related to ascites	The client will have less ascites by discharge.	Weigh daily. Educate client to notify physician of weight gain of 1½ lbs or more in 1 week. Measure abdominal girth daily. Restrict fluid to 1,000 to 2,000 mL per day depending on the severity of the ascites. Provide low-sodium diet of 500 to 2,000 mg a day depending on severity of the ascites. Teach client how to measure fluids and calculate sodium in diet. If a paracentesis is done, check vital signs every 15 minutes during the procedure and after the procedure until the vitals are stable. The amount of fluid removed from the abdomen is measured and sent to the laboratory.
Risk for Impaired Skin Integrity related to accumulation of bile salts in skin, poor skin turgor, ascites, and edema	The client will not experience skin breakdown while hospitalized.	Provide egg crate mattress. Turn client every 2 hours. Monitor skin closely for redness and skin breakdown. Apply lotion to skin frequently, especially to pressure areas. Assist with ADLs to promote good hygiene and conserve client's energy.

(Continues)

Nursing diagnoses for a client with cirrhosis include the following: (Continued)

NURSING DIAGNOSES	PLANNING/OUTCOMES	NURSING INTERVENTIONS
*Imbalanced **N**utrition: Less than Body Requirements* related to inadequate diet, anorexia, or vomiting	The client will eat a balanced diet of 1,500 calories a day.	Offer small, high-calorie meals frequently. Offer high-nutrient supplements if client is unable to maintain adequate caloric intake. Assist and encourage client to eat. Provide frequent oral hygiene. Observe for changes in mental status that would interfere with caloric intake (e.g., increased lethargy).

Evaluation: Evaluate each outcome to determine how it has been met by the client.

HEPATITIS

Hepatitis is a chronic or acute inflammation of the liver caused by a virus, bacteria, drugs, alcohol abuse, or other toxic substances. There is a diffuse inflammatory reaction with liver cells degenerating and dying. The functions of the liver slow down. Because viral infections are the most common cause of hepatitis, emphasis will be placed on viral hepatitis within the chapter.

Researchers are still learning about the viruses that cause hepatitis. Seven viruses are known to cause hepatitis: A, B, C, D, E, F, and G.

Dustia (2005) describes hepatitis F as similar to hepatitis A and E and hepatitis G usually as a coinfection with hepatitis C. Hepatitis F has no serologic test and is diagnosed by seeing the virus with an electron microscope. Hepatitis G is transmitted by blood. Most clients have no symptoms, and 90% to 100% develop chronic infection. The viruses are similar and have almost identical signs and symptoms. Incubation period, mode of transmission, treatment and prognosis vary. See Table 7-5 for a summary of hepatitis viruses A–E.

Medical–Surgical Management

Treatment is focused on resting the liver and early detection of complications. The liver is rested by modifying the diet so that less bile is needed to digest the food. Treatment is related to the signs and symptoms present and the prevention of transmission.

Pharmacological

Antiemetics such as hydroxyzine hydrochloride (Atarax, also Vistaril) or trimethobenzamide hydrochloride (Tigan) are given before meals for nausea. IV hydration with vitamin C for healing may be ordered. A vitamin B complex also is ordered to help clients absorb fat-soluble vitamins. Vitamin K may be ordered if clotting time is prolonged. All unnecessary medications, especially sedatives, are avoided.

Those exposed to hepatitis B by needle puncture or sexual contact should have hepatitis B immunoglobin (HBIG). Vaccines for hepatitis A (HAV) and hepatitis B (HBV) are available. HAV vaccine is recommended for persons 2 years of age and older at risk for exposure to hepatitis A such as homosexuals, IV drug users, travelers to countries with poor sanitation conditions, and laboratory workers who handle live hepatitis A virus (CDC, 2009). HBV vaccine is recommended as a routine vaccination for all 0 to 18 years olds and for those in high-risk groups (CDC, 2009). The Food and Drug Administration approved a combined hepatitis A and B vaccine in September 2001. It is recommended for persons younger than age 18 years and those in a high-risk group.

Diet

Diet modifications include decreasing fat intake to decrease the amount of bile needed in the digestive tract. A low-protein diet is needed if the client's liver is no longer able to metabolize the protein. Anorexia is a common symptom that can be treated with small, frequent, high-calorie meals. Fluids are restricted if the client retains fluids. No alcoholic beverages are recommended for at least 1 year or longer.

Activity

Bed rest is usually recommended for the first several weeks, generally at home unless the serum bilirubin is greater than 10 mg/dL or the PT is prolonged. If either occurs, hospitalization is usually recommended. Once bed rest is no longer necessary, activity is increased gradually because fatigue will be present for up to several months. Rest periods are included throughout the day.

Nursing Management

Follow Standard Precautions with all clients and Enteric Precautions for hepatitis A and E. Teach clients to always follow proper hand hygiene. For hepatitis A and E, be careful about consuming contaminated food and/or water. Hepatitis B spreads through blood and body fluids. Health care workers are at risk for hepatitis B and C. Most clients with hepatitis have flu-like symptoms, weight loss, hepatomegaly, jaundice, dark yellow urine, and light stools. Monitor laboratory test results for increased levels of bilirubin, GGT, AST, ALT, LDH, and alkaline phosphatase. Clotting time and PT are prolonged. Encourage low-fat, low-protein, high-calorie frequent small meals and fluid intake of 2,500 to 3,000 mL daily. Bed rest is important for the first several weeks and then a gradual increase in activity with rest periods several times a day.

TABLE 7-5 Comparison of Different Types of Viral Hepatitis

	A	B	C	D	E
Etiologic Agent	Hepatitis A virus (HAV)	Hepatitis B virus (HBV)	Hepatitis C virus (HCV)	Hepatitis D virus (HDV)	Hepatitis E virus (HEV)
Transmission	Fecal-oral; contaminated water or food; person to person	Blood or body fluids from infected person	Blood	Only persons with hepatitis B can get hepatitis D; blood and blood products; needlesticks; seldom sexual; rarely perinatal	Oral-fecal route; contaminated water; person to person uncommon
Risk Groups	Household/sexual contact with infected person; international travelers	Intravenous drug users; sexual/household contact with infected person; infants born to infected mothers; health care workers; multiple sex partners	Blood transfusions or organ transplants prior to 1992; sharing needles; exposure to blood and blood products	Needle sharing; needlesticks	Mainly travel to countries where endemic
Incubation Period	15–50 days	45–160 days	14–180 days	15–60 days	15–60 days
Infectious Period	Usually less than 2 months	Before symptoms appear; lifetime if chronic	Before symptoms appear; lifetime if chronic	Not determined	Not determined
Diagnostic Tests	IgM anti-HAV	HBsAg	EIA-3; RIBA serum ALT increased 10x; HCVRNA-PCR	IgG anti HDV and/or Igm anti-HDV	None available
Symptoms	Flu-like; jaundice; dark yellow urine; light colored stools	Flu-like; may have jaundice; dark yellow urine; light colored stools	80% have no symptoms; flu-like	Flu-like; may have jaundice; dark yellow urine; light colored stools	Abdominal pain; anorexia; dark yellow urine; jaundice; fever
Prevention	Standard Precautions; Enteric Precautions; hepatitis A vaccine (entire series); immune globulin (for short term)	Standard Precautions; reduce risk behaviors; hepatitis B vaccine (entire series); immune globulin (for short term)	Standard Precautions; reduce risk behaviors; no vaccine	Standard Precautions; reduce risk behaviors; hepatitis B vaccine; if client already has hepatitis B, no prevention for hepatitis D	Standard Precautions; be sure water safe when traveling; no vaccine
Treatment	Immune globulin within 2 weeks of exposure	Immune globulin (HBIg); alpha interferon; lamivudine (Epivir-HBV); adefovirdipivoxil (Hepsera)	Peginterferon alfa-2a (Pegasys); ribavirin (Virazole)	Alpha interferon	None given

(Continues)

TABLE 7-5 Comparison of Different Types of Viral Hepatitis (Continued)

	A	B	C	D	E
Prognosis	Rarely fatal; no chronicity; resolves on its own in several weeks	No cure; may become chronic	75% to 85% have chronic infection; 70% develop chronic liver disease	Low risk of chronicity	No evidence of chronicity

Data from Viral Hepatitis A. By Centers for Disease Control and Prevention (CDC), 2009a, retrieved from www.cdc.gov/ncidod/diseases/hepatitis/a/fact.htm; Viral Hepatitis B. By CDC, 2009b, retrieved from www.cdc.gov/ncidod/diseases/hepatitis/b/fact.htm; Viral Hepatitis C. By CDC, 2009c, retrieved from www.cdc.gov/ncidod/diseases/hepatitis/c/fact.htm; Viral Hepatitis D. By CDC, 2009d, retrieved from www.cdc.gov/ncidod/diseases/hepatitis/slideset/hep-d.htm; Viral Hepatitis E. By CDC, 2009e, retreived from www.cdc.gov/ncidod/diseases/hepatitis/slideset/hep-e.htm; Peginterferon alfa-2a plus ribavirin for chronic hepatitis C virus infection, by M. W. Fried, M. L. Shiffman, et al., 2002e, *New England Journal of Medicine, 347*(13), 975; Resolution of chronic delta hepatitis after 12 years of interferon alpha therapy. By D. T. Lau, D. E. Kleiner, Y. Park, A. M. DiBisceglie, & J. H. Hoofnagle, 1999, *Gastroenterology, 117*(5), 1229-33; What I need to know about hepatitis C. By NIDDK, 2006, retrieved from www.niddk.nih.gov/health/digest/pubs/hep/hepc/hepc.htm; Viral hepatitis A to E and Beyond. By National Institute of Diabetes and Digestive and Kidney Diseases (NIDDK) 2008a, retrieved from www.niddk.nih.gov/health/digest/pubs/hep/hepa-e/hepa-e.htm; What I need to know about hepatitis A. By NIDDK, 2008b, retrieved from www.niddk.nih.gov/health/digest/pubs/hep/hepa/hepa.htm; What I need to know about hepatitis B. By NIDDK, 2008c, retrieved from www.niddk.nih.gov/health/digest/ pubs/hep/hepb/hepb.htm; Speaking out about the silent epidemic, by S. Parini, 2001, *Nursing 2001,* 31(3), 36–42; FDA approves new treatment for chronic hepatitis B. By U.S. Food and Drug Administration, 2002, retrieved from www.fda.gov/bbs/topics/ANSWERS/2002/ANS01163.html.

NURSING PROCESS

ASSESSMENT

Subjective Data

Symptoms include fatigue, anorexia, photophobia, nausea, headaches, abdominal pain, generalized muscle aches, chills, pruritis, and bloating.

Objective Data

The client may have weight loss, hepatomegaly, fever, jaundice, dark amber urine, and clay-colored stools.

Laboratory analysis shows an increased level of bilirubin, GGT, AST, ALT, LDH, and alkaline phosphatase. Clotting time and PT are prolonged. Specific hepatitis test is elevated (refer to Table 7-5).

CRITICAL THINKING

Hepatitis and Lifestyle

What lifestyle changes are necessary with a diagnosis of hepatitis A, B, C, or D?

Nursing diagnoses for a client with hepatitis include the following:

NURSING DIAGNOSES	PLANNING/OUTCOMES	NURSING INTERVENTIONS
Deficient Knowledge related to disease process, treatment regimen, and mode of transmission	The client will be able to explain disease process, incubation period, and mode of transmission, by discharge. The client will practice precautions to prevent spread of disease. The client will be able to select a menu using foods from the food guide pyramid and maintain a low-fat, low-protein diet.	Assess client's learning style and present information in a manner compatible with learning style. Educate about disease process and incubation period. Teach proper hand hygiene technique and emphasize importance of washing hands after using the bathroom. Emphasize that client cannot donate blood. Emphasize importance of follow-up laboratory analysis. Instruct in selection of low-fat, low-protein diet. For clients with hepatitis A, teach client to disinfect articles contaminated with feces (such as the toilet), not to prepare food for others, and not to share articles such as eating utensils or toothbrushes. For clients with hepatitis B, teach to avoid sexual contact until they test negative for HBsAg or their partners are immunized with the HBV vaccine.

Nursing diagnoses for a client with hepatitis include the following: (Continued)

NURSING DIAGNOSES	PLANNING/OUTCOMES	NURSING INTERVENTIONS
		For clients with hepatitis C, teach that it is unknown whether it can be transmitted through sexual contact, so precautions are recommended until more is known.
*Imbalanced **Nutrition**: Less than Body Requirements* related to inadequate caloric intake, fat intolerance, nausea, and vomiting	The client will maintain a caloric intake of 2,000 calories/day.	Monitor I&O every shift. Weigh daily. Offer small, frequent, high-calorie, low-fat meals. Encourage low-protein diet of 40 gm of protein. Monitor daily calorie count. Offer largest meal in morning, as food tends to be tolerated better in the morning. Encourage fluid intake of 2,500 to 3,000 mL daily. Note color and consistency of stools and color of urine. Administer antiemetic 30 minutes before meals as ordered.
Fatigue related to decreased energy production and altered body chemistry	The client will verbalize plan to modify activity, by discharge.	Educate client regarding reasons for fatigue and that fatigue may be present for several months. Encourage client to maintain bed rest for several weeks. Advise client that when resuming normal activity, rest periods should be included until stamina returns.

Evaluation: Evaluate each outcome to determine how it has been met by the client.

PANCREATITIS

Pancreatitis is an acute or chronic inflammation of the pancreas caused when pancreatic enzymes digest the lining of the pancreas. Pancreatitis occurs when obstruction of the pancreatic duct occurs as a result of gallstones, tumors, exposure to chemicals or alcohol, or injury to the pancreas. In severe cases, the pancreas can hemorrhage, resulting in a life-threatening condition.

MEDICAL–SURGICAL MANAGEMENT

Medical

Treatment depends on the cause of the pancreatitis. If the pancreatitis results from exposure to chemical or alcohol abuse, treatment is primarily medical. An NG tube is inserted to rest the bowel and relieve abdominal distention.

Surgical

If the pancreatitis is caused by structural changes such as gallstones, an endoscopic retrograde cholangiopancreatogram (ERCP) with stone removal is performed. Surgery to relieve the pancreatic duct obstruction is necessary in cases where tumors or injury are the causes of the pancreatitis.

Pharmacological

Insulin is administered if the client's pancreas is unable to secrete enough to maintain normal blood sugar level. If nausea and vomiting are present, antiemetics are ordered. Meperidine (Demerol) is ordered for analgesia because morphine sulfate may cause spasms of the sphincter of Oddi. Atropine sulfate or propantheline bromide (Pro-Banthine) is ordered to decrease pancreatic activity. Antacids or an H_2 receptor antagonist is ordered to prevent stress ulcers.

Diet

Clients are kept NPO while the serum amylase level is elevated to decrease the demand for digestive enzymes in the bowel. An NG tube is inserted to decrease pancreatic activity and to prevent nausea, vomiting, and abdominal distention. As the serum amylase level begins to decrease, clients are started on clear liquids and slowly advanced to a bland, low-fat, high-protein, high-carbohydrate diet. No coffee or alcohol is allowed.

IV rehydration is necessary while the client is NPO. If the pancreatitis is severe and the client must be NPO for a prolonged period, TPN, a high-calorie, high-nutrient IV solution, is administered.

Activity

Clients are generally placed on bed rest to decrease metabolic rate. Activity is increased as the serum amylase decreases.

NURSING MANAGEMENT

Monitor and maintain NG tube. Weigh client daily and maintain client on bed rest. Assess pain and administer an analgesic. Monitor vital signs. Provide personal hygiene. Assess and maintain IV hydration and TPN if ordered. Accurately record

I&O. Monitor laboratory results, especially serum amylase, bilirubin, electrolytes, and H & H.

NURSING PROCESS

ASSESSMENT

Subjective Data

Clients describe excruciating epigastric pain that radiates to the back. Pain may decrease by leaning forward or lying in a fetal position. Nausea and anorexia are also present.

Objective Data

Assessment includes steatorrhea, vomiting, low-grade fever, tachycardia, and jaundice. Laboratory analysis shows an elevated serum amylase followed by an elevated urine amylase and serum lipase, leukocytosis, and an increased Hct. Glucose, alkaline phosphatase, and bilirubin may also be elevated.

Nursing diagnoses for a client with pancreatitis include the following:

NURSING DIAGNOSES	PLANNING/OUTCOMES	NURSING INTERVENTIONS
*Acute **Pain*** related to inflammation and edema of the pancreas	The client will verbalize a decrease in pain as evidenced by pain scale by 1 hour after initiation of interventions.	Monitor NG tube to decompress the abdomen. Position client in most comfortable position. Assess pain for increasing severity that would indicate worsening pancreatitis. Administer analgesics as ordered and monitor for relief. Monitor serum amylase, WBCs, and H & H for signs of increasing severity of pancreatitis or hemorrhage.
*Imbalanced **Nutrition**: Less than Body Requirements* related to NPO status, nausea, vomiting, and altered ability to digest nutrients	The client will experience no further weight loss during hospitalization.	Monitor I&O every shift. Administer IV rehydration or TPN as ordered. Weigh client daily. Maintain bed rest to decrease the metabolic rate. Insert NG tube to decompress the abdomen as ordered.
*Risk for Deficient **Fluid** Volume* related to vomiting, NG tube, or hemorrhage	The client will maintain adequate hydration as evidenced by I&O that is nearly equal, electrolytes within normal limits, and moist mucous membranes.	Monitor I&O every shift. Administer IV hydration or TPN as ordered. Monitor electrolyte levels and H & H as ordered.

Evaluation: Evaluate each outcome to determine how it has been met by the client.

CHOLECYSTITIS AND CHOLELITHIASIS

Cholecystitis is an inflammation of the gallbladder. In >90% of the cases, gallstones are present. **Cholelithiasis** is the presence of gallstones or **calculi** (concentration of mineral salts) in the gallbladder. Not all gallstones cause cholecystitis. Some gallstones pass out of the gallbladder and into the duodenum with the client unaware of the stones. Sometimes gallstones migrate into the cystic or common bile duct causing an obstruction that, in turn, leads to cholecystitis. The exact cause of the formation of these stones is not known.

These two diseases are more common in multiparous women, age 45 and older; obese people; those who use birth control pills or control cholesterol with gemfibrozil (Lopid); and people with a history of a disease of the small intestine such as Crohn's disease. Also, clients on sudden weight reduction diets that are low in fat will cause the bile to pool in the gallbladder, increasing the risk for gallstone formation.

Ultrasound of the gallbladder is ordered if gallstones are suspected.

MEDICAL–SURGICAL MANAGEMENT

In asymptomatic clients, no intervention is necessary.

Medical

If stones are lodged in the common bile duct, an ERCP is performed.

Surgical

A sphincterotomy, an incision in the ampulla of vater, is performed to enlarge the opening of the common bile duct. Stones are then removed or crushed. If the stones are too large or in the case of clients with repeated episodes of cholelithiasis, a cholecystectomy, the surgical removal of the gallbladder, is performed. The cholecystectomy is performed laparoscopically or by making a large abdominal incision.

Laparoscopic cholecystectomies have become the surgery of choice for cholelithiasis and cholecystitis. The gallbladder is removed by making four small incisions and extracting the gallbladder through an endoscope. If the cholecystectomy is performed laparoscopically, it is more difficult to perform an exploration of the common bile duct, especially in clients with cholecystitis. An ERCP may need to be performed if stones remain in the common bile duct (CBD). Clients are ready for discharge 24 hours after the surgery.

The cholecystectomy can also be performed by making a large abdominal incision. A cholangiogram can be performed easily, and therefore this type of procedure is more common in clients with much inflammation of the gallbladder. If damage has occurred to the CBD from severe inflammation or a stone, a T-tube will be left in place to allow the bile to drain into a collection bag. This allows the CBD to heal. Clients are typically ready for discharge 3 to 7 days after surgery.

Pharmacological

In acute cholecystitis, analgesics are ordered to relieve discomfort. Meperidine (Demerol) is preferred because morphine sulfate is believed to increase sphincter spasms. IV hydration is ordered if the client is unable to maintain hydration. Antiemetics are ordered for nausea and vomiting. In clients who have surgery, analgesics are ordered after surgery to control discomfort.

Diet

In clients with mild or moderate symptoms, a clear liquid diet to rest the bowel, followed by small frequent meals low in fat, may resolve the symptoms.

If clients are to have surgery, they will be NPO before surgery and initially after surgery until bowel sounds return. They are started on clear liquids first and then advanced, as tolerated, to a regular diet.

Activity

In acute cases of cholecystitis, bed rest is recommended to decrease metabolic rate. If surgery is performed, the client is encouraged to turn, cough, and deep breathe every 2 hours initially after surgery. On the day after surgery, the client is assisted out of bed and encouraged to gradually increase activity. Clients who have a laparoscopic cholecystectomy are ambulated within hours of returning from the recovery room. Clients usually leave the hospital later on the day of surgery, but may stay overnight depending on their overall condition (University of Michigan Health System, 2009). Clients return to normal activities within 4-5 days and typically return to previous activity level 2 weeks after surgery. Clients who have an incision restrict lifting, driving, and exercise until incisional healing is complete, usually 4 to 6 weeks.

Nursing Management

Monitor vital signs and bowel sounds. Assess pain, nausea, and vomiting and administer analgesic and/or antiemetic. Prepare for surgery by teaching deep breathing, coughing, splinting incision, incentive spirometry use, and leg exercises. Monitor and maintain NG tube if used. Accurately record I&O.

NURSING PROCESS

Assessment

Subjective Data

Clients describe pain in the right upper quadrant radiating to the right scapular area that occurs 2 to 4 hours after a meal containing significant amounts of fat, nausea, flatulence, and indigestion.

Objective Data

Assessment shows vomiting, occasionally a fever, jaundice, steatorrhea, clay-colored stools, and dark amber urine. Laboratory analysis shows increased alkaline phosphatase, GGT, WBCs, and bilirubin.

Nursing diagnoses for a client with cholecystitis and cholelithiasis include the following:

NURSING DIAGNOSES	PLANNING/OUTCOMES	NURSING INTERVENTIONS
*Acute **Pain*** related to inflammation or blocked bile duct	The client will experience less pain as evidenced by pain scale within 1 hour of initiation of treatment.	Keep client NPO or on a clear liquid diet as ordered. Administer analgesics as ordered. Monitor NG tube to decompress the abdomen as ordered. Observe for jaundice and bile flow obstruction.
*Ineffective **Breathing** Pattern* related to decreased lung expansion because of pain	The client will demonstrate appropriate breathing pattern and will not have respiratory complications while hospitalized.	Assist client to cough and breathe deeply every 2 hours. Teach use of incentive spirometer. Teach splinting techniques for comfort and to facilitate breathing. Turn client every 2 hours and ambulate as soon as indicated.
*Risk for Deficient **Fluid** Volume* related to nausea, NG tube, NPO, or bile drainage	The client will maintain adequate hydration as evidenced by I&O that is nearly equal and moist mucous membranes.	Monitor I&O every shift including NG drainage and T-tube drainage if present. Administer IV hydration as ordered. Maintain patency of NG tube.

Evaluation: Evaluate each outcome to determine how it has been met by the client.

NEOPLASMS OF THE GASTROINTESTINAL SYSTEM

Neoplasms of the gastrointestinal system may occur anyplace in the GI system. Signs, symptoms, and treatment vary according to where the cancer occurs. Oral cancer, colorectal cancer, and liver cancer are discussed following.

ORAL CANCER

Oral cancer refers to cancers of the lips, tongue, oral cavity, and pharynx. According to the American Cancer Society (ACS, 2009), 35,720 new cases are expected that year. Risk factors are tobacco use and excessive consumption of alcohol. Symptoms include a mouth sore that bleeds easily and does not heal, a lump, or difficulty chewing, swallowing, or moving tongue or jaw. On the lips, the cancer may be a growth.

MEDICAL–SURGICAL MANAGEMENT

Surgical

Treatment is primarily surgical and involves removal of the cancer with excision of tissue and lymph nodes surrounding the cancer. In cases of cancer involving the pharynx, a radical neck dissection is performed, which requires reconstruction of the pharynx. Clients undergoing radical neck dissection frequently have a tracheostomy.

Pharmacological

Chemotherapy is not effective against most oral cancers and is, therefore, used only in the most severe cases with metastases. Medications ordered are based on the client's symptoms. If the client is experiencing side effects from the radiation such as nausea, antiemetics are ordered.

If a client has surgery, analgesics are ordered postoperatively. Analgesics are also ordered if the cancer has progressed and is causing discomfort.

Diet

Because the surgery is in the oral area, it may be difficult to maintain adequate nutrition. Depending on the extent of the surgery, clients require a soft diet or, in some cases, nutritional supplements to allow the surgical area to heal. Tube feedings, either by a feeding tube or by a gastrostomy tube (a special tube inserted through the abdomen into the stomach), are frequently needed in clients who have undergone a radical neck dissection.

Activity

If the surgery is minor, no activity restrictions are necessary. If surgery is extensive, postoperatively, the client will need to turn, cough, and deep breathe. Activity is increased postoperatively. Clients receiving radiation treatments frequently experience fatigue and need scheduled rest periods.

Other Therapies

In cases where the lesion cannot be surgically removed, radiation and/or radium implants is/are used. High-energy radiation is used to destroy cancer cells. Clients may experience irritated skin, swallowing difficulties, dry mouth, nausea, diarrhea, hair loss, or fatigue. Radiation is usually administered daily for a specified period. If radium implants are used, a radioactive capsule is implanted into the area.

NURSING MANAGEMENT

Encourage all clients to refrain from tobacco use and excessive alcohol consumption. Maintain feeding tube and administer tube feedings as ordered. Preoperatively, teach client to turn, cough, and deep breathe, and encourage client to practice postoperatively. Weigh client daily and accurately record I&O.

NURSING PROCESS

ASSESSMENT

Subjective Data

Clients describe a sore throat, difficulty swallowing, or a painful area in the mouth.

Objective Data

Assessment reveals a sore or lesion of the lips or in the oral cavity, and hoarseness.

Nursing diagnoses for a client with oral cancer include the following:

NURSING DIAGNOSES	PLANNING/OUTCOMES	NURSING INTERVENTIONS
Fear related to diagnosis and long-term prognosis	The client will verbalize fear and express plan to cope with diagnosis.	Allow client time alone and with significant others and client and family to express fears and concerns.
		Answer questions.
		Encourage contact with support system (e.g., clergy).
		Discuss past experiences with stress and individual responses to those situations.

Nursing diagnoses for a client with oral cancer include the following: (Continued)

NURSING DIAGNOSES	PLANNING/OUTCOMES	NURSING INTERVENTIONS
*Imbalanced **Nutrition**: Less than Body Requirements* related to oral surgery or radical neck dissection	The client will maintain weight while hospitalized.	Monitor I&O every shift. Weigh client daily. Administer tube feedings and IV rehydration as ordered and introduce fluids, when indicated. Monitor for aspiration.
*Disturbed **Body** Image* related to disfiguring surgery	The client will verbalize feelings regarding surgery and altered body image.	Allow client time to verbalize feelings. Answer questions. Discuss options (e.g., plastic surgery or makeup). Provide information on support groups.

Evaluation: Evaluate each outcome to determine how it has been met by the client.

COLORECTAL CANCER

Colorectal cancer is the third most common site of new cancers and deaths in the United States (ACS, 2009). Almost all colorectal cancers arise from **polyps**, an abnormal growth of tissue that protrudes into the colon. Risk factors for colorectal cancer include age 50 or older, history of polyps, family history of polyps and/or colorectal cancer, a history of ulcerative colitis, and a diet high in fat and low in fiber.

Prognosis is very good if the cancer is caught in the early stages. Recommended routine screenings for early detection include fecal occult blood testing and colonoscopy depending on personal and family history.

A colonoscopy or barium enema may demonstrate the disease. A CBC may show anemia if the cancer is bleeding. A CEA may be effective in detecting recurrent cancer but is not a valid screening test. Signs and symptoms include a change in bowel habits, guaiac-positive stools, and abdominal pain.

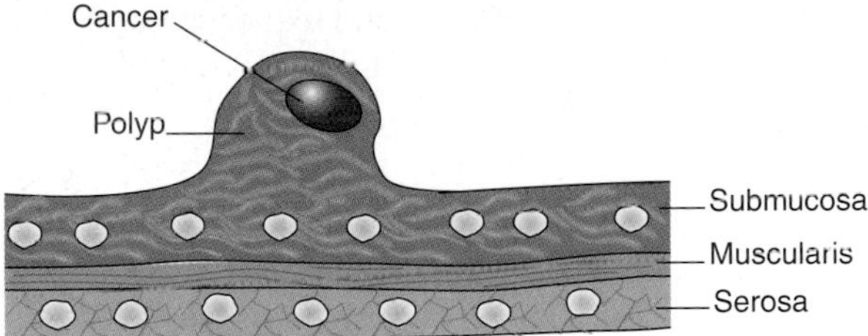

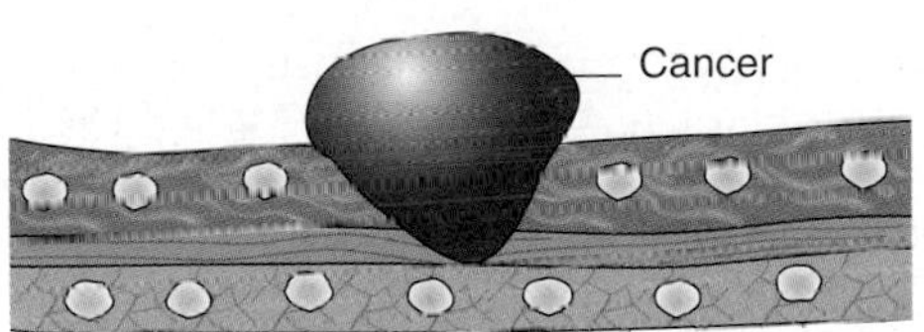

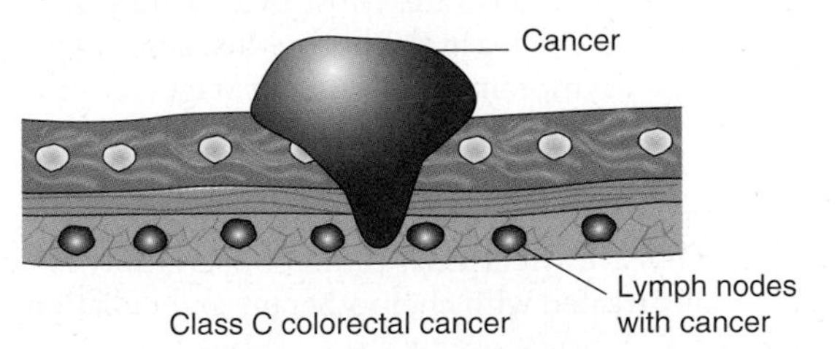

FIGURE 7-10 Classes of Colorectal Cancer

MEDICAL–SURGICAL MANAGEMENT

Surgical

Treatment is surgical to remove the cancer. In class A tumors, a colonoscopy is performed with a polypectomy, the removal of the polyp. In class B or C tumors, a colon resection is done (Figure 7-10). In some cases, a colostomy, either temporary or permanent, is performed. In class D tumors, surgery is done only to relieve symptoms (e.g., bowel obstruction). Follow-up colonoscopies must be performed throughout the client's life to monitor for recurrence of the disease.

Pharmacological

In cases of class B, C, and D tumors, chemotherapy is given after the surgery. Side effects of chemotherapy include nausea, vomiting, weight loss, hair loss, fatigue, and dry skin. Medications to combat some side effects of the chemotherapy are ordered. Immunotherapy as an adjunct therapy for class C and D tumors is ordered to boost the immune system.

Diet

Preoperatively, the client is NPO. Postoperatively, the client is NPO and an NG tube is in place until bowel sounds return. The client is then started on a clear liquid diet and progressed to a high-fiber, low-fat diet.

Activity

Postoperatively, the client is encouraged to turn, cough, and deep breathe every 2 hours. The client is ambulated the next day and activity is progressed.

Other Therapies

No significant benefits have been found with the use of radiation on colorectal cancer; however, radiation may be used on metastatic sites in class D tumors.

Nursing Management

Encourage all clients to have recommended routine screenings, fecal occult blood test, and colonoscopy, based on their personal and family history. Prepare client for side effects (hair loss, fatigue, nausea, and dry skin) when chemotherapy is used. Postoperatively, maintain the NG tube. Assess bowel sounds. Encourage turning, coughing, deep breathing, use of incentive spirometer, leg exercises, and ambulation.

NURSING PROCESS

Assessment

Subjective Data

Clients describe a change in bowel habits and possibly abdominal pain.

Objective Data

Stools may be guaiac positive for blood. An H & H may show anemia.

Nursing diagnoses for a client with colorectal cancer include the following:

NURSING DIAGNOSES	PLANNING/OUTCOMES	NURSING INTERVENTIONS
Fear related to diagnosis and long-term prognosis	The client will verbalize fear and express plan to cope with diagnosis.	Allow client time alone and with significant others and allow client and family to express fears and concerns. Answer questions and encourage contact with support system (e.g., clergy). Discuss past experiences with stress and identify individual responses to those situations.
Deficient Knowledge related to disease process, treatment options, and follow-up	The client will be able to explain disease process, treatment, and follow-up care.	Determine client's learning style and present information in a manner compatible with the learning style. Educate client regarding disease process and discuss treatment options. Recognize that information may need to be presented more than once.

Evaluation: Evaluate each outcome to determine how it has been met by the client.

LIVER CANCER

Primary liver cancer is rare. Most liver tumors are metastatic from other sites in the body. Most cases of primary liver cancer are asymptomatic until later stages. Risk factors for primary liver cancer include a history of cirrhosis, hepatitis B, and exposure to toxic chemicals.

A primary liver tumor can be removed surgically if the disease is not extensive. Metastases cannot be surgically removed and are usually treated with chemotherapy and radiation.

Obesity

According to the National Heart Lung and Blood Institute (NHLBI), the body mass index (BMI) measures body fat in relation to an individual's height and weight. The BMI determines an individual's weight according to categories of underweight, normal weight, overweight, or obese. According to the World Health Organization, an individual is overweight with a BMI of 30 or greater and morbidly obese with a BMI of 40 or greater. The NHLBI website provides a formula to automatically calculate an individual's BMI: http://www.nhlbisupport.com/bmi/

The National Center for Health Statistics (2007) reported that more than one third of adult Americans (>72 million people) were obese in 2005 to 2006 (Ogden, Carrol, McDowell, & Flegal, 2007). Between 2000 and 2005, the number of obese cases rose 24% and morbidly obese cases with a BMI of >40 and 50 increased 50% and 75%, respectively.

A 1990 study by Blumberg and Mellis reported that 78% of preoperative bariatric clients felt health care professionals "always" or "usually" treated them with disrespect. Another study 12 years later in 2002 by Kaminsky and Gadaleta revealed very similar results. Kaminsky and Gadaleta concluded their results were because health care providers do not understand the disease of obesity, its causes, or the medical consequences if not treated. Little data suggest that health care providers' attitudes affected their delivery of care. In other words, the medical/nursing care was provided but the "caring" attitude was not perceived. Clients having bariatric surgery deserve respect for privacy and deserve kind, compassionate care. To provide clients with compassionate, quality care, health care providers may desire to analyze personal attitudes toward obesity and take appropriate steps to care for each individual as a valued person of worth.

The obese client presents challenges to the health care provider. The extra soft tissue makes it difficult to assess heart and lung sounds, and significant abnormalities can be missed. A nurse needs the appropriate equipment to assess and care for the obese client, such as an extra large blood pressure cuff to obtain an accurate reading. A blood pressure cuff that is too small gives an elevated reading. An echocardiograph may be more accurate than an EKG. Fatigue and

▼ SAFETY ▼

Weight Limitations with Equipment

When caring for an obese client, consider the weight limits on equipment such as stretchers, toilets, and bedside commodes. If these weight limitations are not considered, staff and clients are at risk for injury (Wolf, 2008).

lethargy along with nausea and vomiting are possible symptoms of a cardiac or glycemic emergency (Wolf, 2008). Obese clients have more difficulty breathing and present issues with intubation. A guided ultrasonography assists with IV insertion, and an extra long needle is used for central venous catheter placement. Obese clients are at risk for rapid skin breakdown, hypercoagulopathy leading to venous thromboembolism, and pulmonary emboli after surgery. Pneumonia is a risk because of immobility, difficulty taking deep breaths, and extra soft tissue on the chest (Wolf, 2008). Signs of hypoxia are lethargy, mental status changes, and restlessness. Regular-size stretchers are not safe because the client makes the stretcher top-heavy and causes it to tip over. Skin pressure sores also may occur from the side rails. Therefore, bariatric stretchers and beds provide stability and client safety.

Medical-Surgical Management

Health care professionals are reluctant to discuss weight loss with clients. In a national study of adults with a BMI of ≥30 only 42% reported that a health care provider discussed the need for weight loss (Calonge, 2004). The health care provider could suggest a monitored weight-loss program with nutritional counseling and exercise to assist the overweight client. If these interventions do not work and the client desires to lose weight, the health care provider makes a referral to a bariatrician (a specialist in the treatment of obesity and obese diseases).

Bariatric surgery may be a client option and includes a restrictive or malabsorptive surgery. The laparoscopic adjustable gastric band is a restrictive surgery. A band is placed laproscopically around the proximal stomach distal to the gastroesophagel junction as shown in Figure 7-11A. A tube is connected to the band and threaded through the abdomen to the abdominal wall, where it is connected to an access port. The access port is anchored to the fascia. Throughout the next year, the physician injects saline into the access port to restrict the stomach size so the client loses weight.

The Roux-en-Y gastric bypass is a malabsorptive surgery. A section of the stomach close to the gastroesophageal junction is divided from the remaining stomach by stapling along the dividing line as shown in Figure 7-11B. A section of the jejunum is anastomosed to the stomach pouch. The remaining stomach, duodenum, and proximal jejunum are anastomosed distally on the jejunum. Weight loss occurs for 2 reasons: the restricted stomach area cannot hold as much food and the bypassed bowel section cannot absorb as many calories and nutrients from ingested food. Thus, it is called a malabsorptive surgery. This surgery bypasses the part of the small intestine that absorbs calcium, iron, and other nutrients placing the client at risk for chronic nutritional deficits and vitamin B_{12} anemias. After the surgery, the client is placed on multivitamin and mineral supplements.

Nursing Management

Postoperatively the nurse maintains the client's oxygen saturation at 92% by administering 2 to 4 L of oxygen by nasal cannula or, if client tolerates it, room air. Encourage the client to use the incentive spirometer every 2 hours. The head of the bed is elevated to 45° to enhance breathing. If the client uses a continuous positive airway pressure device (CPAP),

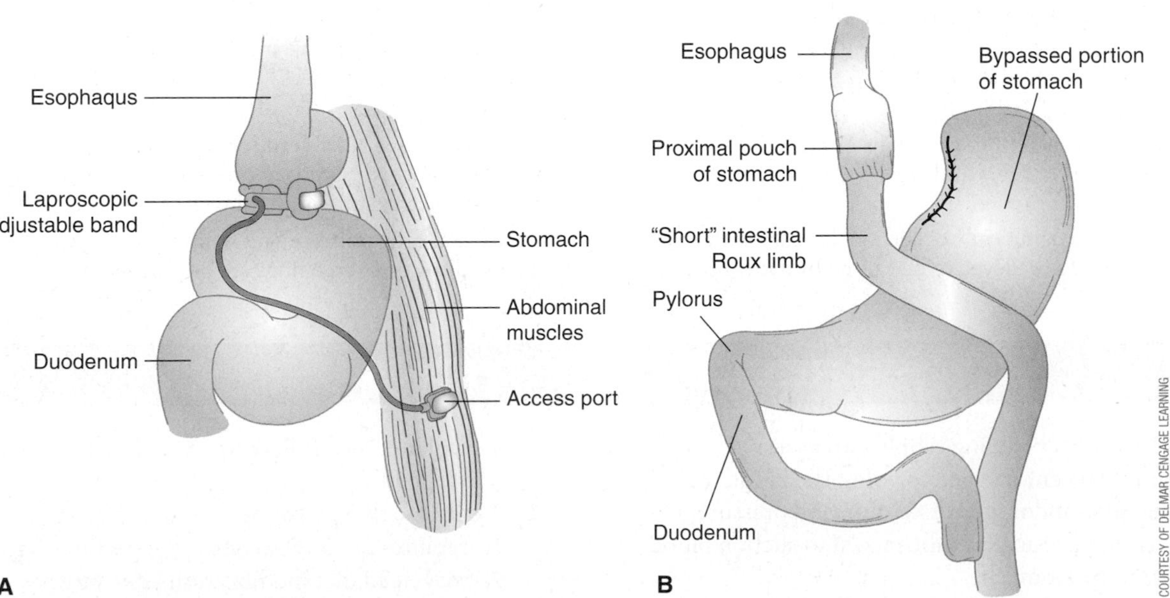

Figure 7-11 Types of Bariatric Surgery; *A*, Laparoscopic Adjustable Gastric Banding; *B*, Roux-en-Y Gastric Bypass

continue using it in the hospital. The nurse assesses pain regularly, monitors PCA use, and obtains appropriate orders to manage pain (Sammons, 2002). If an NG tube is in place, the nurse does not reposition the NG tube as the movement may damage the suture line. The client takes sips of water and, if tolerated, slowly progresses to eating very small portions of pureed food or juices. The nurse teaches diet modifications and exercise to assist the client in controlling weight. Weight loss is a lifetime challenge.

Postoperative complications are nausea and dumping syndrome. The nurse assesses for abdominal distension, diarrhea, cramping, hypotension, flushing, and tachycardia indicating symptoms of dumping syndrome that last 20 to 30 minutes. Dumping syndrome is a common side effect caused by eating simple sugars. It is a benign problem that possibly can be modified by decreasing the ingestion of simple sugar.

CASE STUDY

R.J. is a 52-year-old woman admitted to the hospital with acute abdominal pain. R.J. complains of right upper quadrant pain radiating to the back. She has had previous episodes, usually occurring about 2 hours after eating. This episode, however, is not resolving. R.J. also complains of nausea. Her vital signs are BP 152/88 mm Hg, pulse 92 beats/min, and respirations 24 breaths/min and shallow. R.J. is a slightly obese female who states she has recently been dieting to lose weight. Laboratory analysis includes a CBC with slightly elevated WBCs, elevated bilirubin, and elevated alkaline phosphatase. An IV is started, and R.J. is given meperidine (Demerol) IM for pain. R.J. has been made NPO. An ultrasound of the gallbladder is ordered.

The following questions will guide your development of a nursing care plan for this case study.

1. List subjective and objective data a nurse would want to obtain about R.J.
2. List risk factors other than those R.J. has that would put a client at risk for developing cholecystitis.
3. List two nursing diagnoses and goals for R.J.
4. The ERCP is successful in removing the CBD stone. The decision is made to perform a laparoscopic cholecystectomy. What teaching will R.J. need?
5. Why is meperidine (Demerol) the medication of choice for pain control?
6. List at least three successful outcomes for R.J.

SUMMARY

- The gastrointestinal system is a complex system composed of the digestive tract as well as accessory organs.
- Disorders of the GI tract affect the breakdown and absorption of nutrients, breakdown of wastes and by-products, and the lifestyle of the individual.
- Because the liver is responsible for so many functions in the body, disorders of the liver can affect other systems significantly.
- Peptic ulcers may be either gastric or duodenal. *H. pylori* is a common cause of ulcers and can be treated with antibiotics.
- Diverticulosis is a commonly occurring disorder in the United States and is believed to be caused by a low-fiber diet.
- Inflammatory bowel disease includes both Crohn's disease and ulcerative colitis. IBD can lead to nutritional imbalances, bowel obstructions, alterations in the structure of the intestine, and affected lifestyle.
- Bowel obstructions have multiple causes and can lead to electrolyte imbalances, dehydration, and possibly sepsis.
- Viral hepatitis is a concern for health care professionals at risk for exposure. Standard precautions must be used to prevent the transmission of the virus.
- Colorectal cancer is one of the most preventable forms of cancer if routine screenings are performed.

REVIEW QUESTIONS

1. A client with a bleeding esophageal varix:
   1. should be encouraged to vomit the blood to decrease abdominal distention and pressure.
   2. should have an NG tube placed to suction blood from the stomach.
   3. should have the Minnesota tube deflated every 4 hours.
   4. will not need follow-up once the bleeding has stopped.

2. A client with a perforated duodenal ulcer:
   1. requires an EGD to repair the perforation.
   2. may need diet modification after surgery.
   3. will have a vagotomy performed.
   4. may experience an increased risk for cholecystitis.

3. Clients with hepatitis C:
   1. should be instructed that all the mechanisms of transmission are not known.
   2. will have a negative HCV if they are a carrier.
   3. should be instructed that recombinant interferon alpha-2b will cure the hepatitis C.
   4. are not contagious until symptoms develop.
4. Crohn's disease:
   1. can be cured by removing the colon.
   2. usually causes clients to gain weight from the slower metabolism of nutrients.
   3. can be a debilitating disease leading to depression.
   4. is cured as long as the clients remain on 5-ASA compounds.
5. Hernias are a protrusion through the muscle wall and:
   1. can be easily reduced by the nurse applying gentle pressure.
   2. are benign occurrences that do not need any intervention.
   3. can lead to bowel obstructions.
   4. are caused by a lack of exercise.
6. Postoperative care of clients who have undergone gastric bypass surgery includes:
   1. immobilization of abdominal wound to stabilize the incision areas.
   2. keeping the head of the bed flat to avoid stressing the incision.
   3. allowing only sips of fluids and small amounts of food in soft consistency.
   4. bed rest to prevent complications from surgery in obese patients.
7. An excessively overweight client expressing a desire to lose weight must be advised initially to:
   1. decrease caloric intake.
   2. follow a weight loss diet and increase activity level.
   3. consider a referral for surgical intervention.
   4. participate in vigorous exercise.
8. A nurse gave dietary instructions to a client recently diagnosed with ulcerative colitis. What dietary choice indicates the client understands the appropriate foods to eat? (Select all that apply.)
   1. Apple.
   2. Lettuce salad.
   3. Refined pasta.
   4. Chunky peanut butter.
   5. Cream of asparagus soup.
   6. Cottage cheese.
9. A client is returning to the unit with a bowel resection from an intestinal obstruction. What is the nurse's first action when the client returns to the room?
   1. Encourage ambulation to stimulate the return of bowel function.
   2. Connect NG tube to suction to decompress the abdomen.
   3. Identify client's learning style and teach information in a manner compatible with learning style.
   4. Assess for pain and administer an analgesic as ordered.
10. A client is admitted to the unit with the diagnosis of a peptic ulcer. When assessing the client, the nurse would most likely find:
    1. epigastric pain that increases when the stomach is empty.
    2. stools that are fatty and foul smelling.
    3. alternating episodes of diarrhea and constipation.
    4. pain in the upper quadrant radiating to the right scapular area that occurs 2–4 hours after eating fatty foods.

REFERENCES/SUGGESTED READINGS

Ables, A., Simon, I., & Melton, E. (2007). Update on Helicobacter pylori treatment. *American Family Physician, 75*(3), 351–358.

American Cancer Society. (2007). What are the risk factors for stomach cancer? Retrieved March 28, 2008 from http://www.cancer.org/docroot/cri/content/cri

American Cancer Society. (2009a). Cancer facts & figures 2009. Retrieved from http://www.cancer.org/docroot/home/index.asp

American Cancer Society. (2009b). Colorectal cancer: Statistics and incidences. Retrieved from http://www.cancer.org/docroot/CRI/CRI_2_3x.asp?dt=10

Atassi, K. (2002a). Appendicitis. *Nursing2002, 32*(8), 96.

Atassi, K. (2002b). Bleeding esophageal varices. *Nursing2002, 32*(4), 96.

Barba, K., Fitzgerald, P., & Wood, S. (2007). Managing peptic ulcer disease: Learn how it develops and how to help your patient heal. *Nursing2007*, July, 1–4.

Bazensky, I., Shoobridge-Moran, C., & Yoder, L. (2007). Colorectal cancer: An overview of the epidemiology, risk factors, symptoms, and screening guidelines. *MedSurg Nursing, The Journal of Adult Health, 16*(1), 46–51.

Beattie, S. (2007). Bedside emergency: Hemorrhage. *RN, 70*(8), 30–35.

Blumberg, P., & Mellis, L. (1985). Medical students' attitudes toward the obese and the morbidly obese. *International Journal of Eating Disorders, 4*(2), 169–175.

Boekhold, K. (2000). Who's afraid of hepatitis C? *AJN, 100*(5), 26–31.

Bulechek, G., Butcher, H., McCloskey, J., & Dochterman, J., eds. (2008). *Nursing Interventions Classification (NIC)* (5th ed.). St. Louis, MO: Mosby/Elsevier.

Bunting, T. (2001). Putting the lid on gastroesophageal reflux. *Nursing2001, 31*(6), 46–49.

Calonge, N. (2004). Screening for obesity in adults: Recommendations and rationale. *American Journal of Nursing, 104*(5), 94–105.

Cameron, C., & Sawatzky, J. (2008). Postoperative pain management: The challenges of the patient with Crohn's disease. *MedSurg Nursing, The Journal of Adult Health, 17*(2), 85–91.

Cameron, J. (1998). *Current surgical therapy* (6th ed.). St. Louis, MO: Mosby.

Centers for Disease Control and Prevention (CDC). (2001). FDA approval for a combined hepatitis A and B vaccine. *MMWR, 50*(37), 806–807. Retrieved May 28, 2009 from www.cdc.gov/mmwr/preview/mmwrhtml/mm5037a4.htm

Centers for Disease Control and Prevention (CDC). (2009a). Viral hepatitis A. Retrieved May 28, 2009 from www.cdc.gov/ncidod/diseases/hepatitis/a/fact.htm

Centers for Disease Control and Prevention (CDC). (2009b). Viral hepatitis B. Retrieved May 28, 2009 from www.cdc.gov/ncidod/diseases/hepatitis/b/fact.htm

Centers for Disease Control and Prevention (CDC). (2009c). Viral hepatitis C. Retrieved May 28, 2009 from www.cdc.gov/ncidod/diseases/hepatitis/c/fact.htm

Centers for Disease Control and Prevention (CDC). (2009d). Viral hepatitis D. Retrieved May 28, 2009 from www.cdc.gov/ncidod/diseases/hepatitis/slideset/hep-d.htm

Centers for Disease Control and Prevention (CDC). (2009e). Viral hepatitis E. Retrieved May 28, 2009 from www.cdc.gov/ncidod/diseases/hepatitis/slideset/hep-e/htm

Chene, B., & Decker, A. (2001). Battling hepatitis C. *RN, 64*(4), 54–58.

Clinical Rounds. (2003). Acetaminophen linked to most liver failure cases. *Nursing2003, 33*(3), 34.

Cole, L. (2001). Unraveling the mystery of acute pancreatitis. *Nursing2001, 31*(12), 58–63.

Cox, C., Evans, P., Withers, T., & Titmuss, K. (2008). The importance of gastrointestinal nurses being HLA-B27 aware. *Gastrointestinal Nursing, 6*(9), 32–40.

Daniels, R. (2009). *Delmar's guide to laboratory and diagnostic tests* (2nd ed.). Clifton Park, NY: Delmar Cengage Learning.

Day, M. (2008). Fight back against inflammatory bowel disease. *Nursing2008, 38*(11), 34–42.

Durston, S. (2005). What you need to know about viral hepatitis. *Nursing2005, 35*(8), 36–42.

Edmondson, D. (2008). Esophageal cancer—A tough pill to swallow. *Nursing2008*, April, 44–51. http://www.nursingcenter.com/ce/nursing

Erwin-Toth, P. (2001). Caring for a stoma. *Nursing2001, 31*(5), 36–40.

Estes, M. (2010). *Health assessment & physical examination* (4th ed.). Clifton Park, NY: Delmar Cengage Learning.

Farrar, J. (2001). Acute cholycystitis. *AJN, 101*(1), 35–36.

Framp, A. (2006). Diffuse gastric cancer. Retrieved from http://gateway.ut.ovid.com/gw1/ovidweb.cgi

Frazzoni, M., DeMicheli, E., Zentilin, P., & Savarino, V. (2004). Pathophysiological characteristics of patients with non-erosive reflux disease differ from those of patients with functional heartburn. *Alimentary Pharmacological Therapy, 20*, 81–88.

Fried, M., Shiffman, M., et al. (2002). Peginterferon alfa-2a plus ribavirin for chronic hepatitis C virus infection. *New England Journal of Medicine, 347*(13), 975.

Galvan, T. (2001). Dysphagia: Going down and staying down. *AJN, 101*(1), 37–42.

Hairon, N. (2008). New IBS guidance focuses on improving diagnosis and care. *Nursing Times, 104*(9), 23–24.

Harris, T. (2009). Does cigarette smoking increase the risk of developing ulcerative colitis or Crohn's disease? *Internet Journal of Academic Physician Assistants, 6*(2).

Heitkemper, M., & Jarrett, M. (2001). It's not all in your head: Irritable bowel syndrome. *AJN, 101*(1), 26–33.

Kaminsky, J., & Gadaleta, D. (2002). A study of discrimination within the medical community as viewed by obese patients. *Obese Surgery Journal, 12*(1), 14–18.

Klonowski, E., & Masoodi, J. (1999). The patient with Crohn's disease. *RN, 62*(3), 32–37.

Krumberger, J. (2002). When the liver fails. *RN, 65*(2), 26–29.

Krupp, K., & Heximer, B. (1998). Going with the flow: How to prevent feeding tubes from clogging. *Nursing98, 28*(4), 54–55.

Lau, D., Kleiner, D., Park, Y., DiBisceglie, A., & Hoofnagle, J. (1999). Resolution of chronic delta hepatitis after 12 years of interferon alpha therapy. *Gastroenterology, 117*(5), 1229–33.

Lee, C., Kelly, J., & Wassef, W. (2007). Complications of bariatric surgery. *Current Opinion in Gastroenterology, 23*(6), 636–643. Retrieved July 15, 2009 from http://www.medscape.com/viewarticle/565072_print

Lee, L., & Grap, M. (2008). Care and management of the patient with ascites. *MedSurg Nursing, The Journal of Adult Health, 17*(6), 376–381.

Lord, L. (2001). How to insert a large-bore nasogastric tube. *Nursing2001, 31*(9), 46–48.

Lynch, B., & Sarazine, J. (2006). A guide to understanding malignant bowel obstruction. *International Journal of Palliative Nursing, 12*(4), 164–171.

McConnell, E. (2001a). Administering total parenteral nutrition. *Nursing2001, 31*(11), 17.

McConnell, E. (2001b). Myths & facts . . . about dysphagia. *Nursing2001, 31*(7), 29.

McConnell, E. (2001c). What's behind intestinal obstruction? *Nursing2001, 31*(10), 58–63.

Marrs, J. (2006). Abdominal complaints: Diverticular disease. *Clinical Journal of Oncology Nursing, 10*(2), 155–157.

Mehta, M. (2003). Assessing the abdomen. *Nursing2003, 33*(5), 54–55.

Metheny, N., & Titler, M. (2001). Assessing placement of feeding tubes. *AJN, 101*(5), 36–45.

Moorhead, S., Johnson, M., Maas, M., & Swanson, E. (2007). *Nursing Outcomes Classification (NOC)* (4th ed). St. Louis, MO: Elsevier – Health Sciences Division.

Movius, M. (2006). What's causing that gut pain? Appendicitis? Diverticulitis? Constipation? MI? *RN, 69*(7), 25–29.

National Cancer Institute. (2008a). *U.S. National Institutes of Health: Esophageal cancer*. Retrieved July 14, 2008 from http://www.cancer.gov/cancertopics/types/esophageal/

National Cancer Institute. (2008b). *U.S. National Institutes of Health: Stomach (gastric) cancer screening*. Retrieved July 26, 2008 from http://www.cancer.gov/cancertopics/types/stomach

National Heart Lung and Blood Institute (NHLBI). (2009). *Calculate your body mass index*. Retrieved July 15, 2009 from http://www.nhlbisupport.com/bmi/

National Institute of Diabetes and Digestive and Kidney Diseases. (2006). Chronic hepatitis C: Current disease management. Retrieved July 14, 2008 from www.niddk.nih.gov/health/digest/pubs/chrnhepc/chrnhepc.htm

National Institute of Diabetes and Digestive and Kidney Diseases. (2008a). Viral hepatitis A to E and beyond. Retrieved May 29, 2009 from www.niddk.nih.gov/health/digest/pubs/hep/ hepa-e/hepa-e.htm

National Institute of Diabetes and Digestive and Kidney Diseases. (2008b). What I need to know about hepatitis A. Retrieved May 29, 2009 from http://digestive.niddk.nih.gov/ddiseases/pubs/viralhepatitis/index.htm

National Institute of Diabetes and Digestive and Kidney Diseases. (2008c). What I need to know about hepatitis B. Retrieved May 29, 2009 from http://digestive.niddk.nih.gov/ddiseases/pubs/viralhepatitis/index.htm

National Institute of Diabetes and Digestive and Kidney Diseases. (2009a). What I need to know about hepatitis C. Retrieved July 14, 2008 from www.niddk.nih.gov/health/digest/pubs/hep/hepc/hepc.htm

National Institute of Diabetes and Digestive and Kidney Diseases. (2009b). NIDDK recent advances and emerging opportunities: Digestive diseases and nutrition. Retrieved July 14, 2009 from www2.niddk.nih.gov/NR/rdonlyres/B36A7E82-C94A-4599-A749-7D2609F8A09E/0/DDN_508compliant.pdf

North American Nursing Diagnosis Association International. (2010). *NANDA-I nursing diagnoses: Definitions and classification 2009–2011*. Ames, IA: Wiley-Blackwell.

Ogden, C., Carrol, M., McDowell, M., & Flegal, K. (2007). Obesity among adults in the United States–No statistically significant change since 2003–2004. Centers for Disease Control and Prevention National Center for Health Statistics. Retrieved July 15, 2005 from http://www.cdc.gov/nchs/data/databriefs/db01.pdf

Parini, S. (2001). Hepatitis C: Speaking out about the silent epidemic. *Nursing2001, 31*(3), 36–42.

Parini, S. (2003). Hepatitis C: Update your knowledge of this silent stalker. *Nursing2003, 33*(4), 57–63.

Perry, J., Jagger, J., & Parker, G. (2003). Statistically, your risk of HCV infection has dropped. *Nursing2003, 33*(6), 82.

Rayhorn, N., & Rayhorn, D. (2002). An in-depth look at inflammatory bowel disease. *Nursing2002, 32*(7), 36–42.

Sammons, D. (2002). Roux-en-Y gastric bypass. *American Journal of Nursing, 102*(10), 24A–24D.

Sargent, C., & Murphy, D. (2003). What you need to know about colorectal cancer. *Nursing2003, 33*(2), 36–41.

Schlapman, N. (2001). Spotting acute pancreatitis. *RN, 64*(11), 54–58.

Snyder, D. (2005). Evidence-based recommendations for older adults with Helicobacter pylori or those using nonsteroidal anti-inflammatory drugs. *Gastroenterology Nursing, 28*(4), 309–314.

Spratto, G., & Woods, A. (2009). *2009 PDR nurse's drug handbook*. Clifton Park, NY: Thomson Learning Center.

University of Michigan Health System. (2009). Laproscopic cholecystectomy. Retrieved November 30, 2009 from http://www.med.umich.edu/1libr/aha/aha_llapch_crs.htm

U.S. Food and Drug Administration. (2002). FDA approves new treatment for chronic hepatitis B. Retrieved from www. fda.gov/bbs/topics/ANSWERS/2002/ANS01163.html

Wolf, L. (2008). The obese patient in the ED. *American Journal of Nursing, 108*(12), 77–80.

RESOURCES

American Liver Foundation, http://go.liverfoundation.org/

Crohn and Colitis Foundation of America, Inc., www.ccfa.org

Hepatitis Foundation International (HFI), www.hepfi.org

National Digestive Diseases Information Clearinghouse (NDDIC), http://digestive.niddk.nih.gov/

National Institute of Diabetes and Digestive and Kidney Diseases, http://www2.niddk.nih.gov/

United Ostomy Associations of America — Ostomy, Colostomy, http://www.uoaa.org/

CHAPTER 8
Urinary System

MAKING THE CONNECTION

Refer to the following chapters to increase your understanding of the urinary system:

Adult Health Nursing
- ***Cardiovascular System***
- ***Reproductive System***
- ***The Older Adult***

LEARNING OBJECTIVES

Upon completion of this chapter, you should be able to:

- Define key terms.
- Describe the anatomy and physiology of the urinary system.
- Relate diagnostic test results to urinary disorders.
- Discuss the pros and cons of peritoneal dialysis/hemodialysis and kidney transplantation, including lifestyle changes for the client receiving dialysis.
- List four drug classifications and two examples of each used in the treatment of urinary disorders.
- State two changes in the urinary system related to the normal aging process.
- Compare and contrast acute and chronic renal failure, including nursing care.
- Assist in formulating a nursing care plan for clients with urinary disorders.

KEY TERMS

anasarca
azotemia
cachectic
calculus
cystitis
dialysate
dialysis
dysuria
erythropoiesis
fulguration
glomerular filtration rate (GFR)
hematuria
ileal conduit
intravesical
litholapaxy
lithotripsy
micturition
nephrotoxic
nocturia
nocturnal enuresis
oliguria
overflow incontinence
polyuria
pyelonephritis
pyuria
renal colic
residual urine
retroperitoneal
stress incontinence
urge incontinence
urgency
urinary incontinence (UI)
urinary retention
urolithiasis

INTRODUCTION

Urology is the study of disorders of the urinary system. The National Kidney Foundation estimates that more than 26 million Americans have chronic kidney disease and more than 26 million more are at increased risk (National Kidney Foundation [NKF], 2008). Disorders of the urinary system may seriously affect an individual's health and, thereby, affect the lives of family members. Clients are treated by a urologist, specialist in urinary tract disorders, or a nephrologist, specialist in structure, function, and diseases of the kidney.

According to the National Kidney Foundation (2009b), the warning signs of kidney disease are:

- Burning or difficulty during urination
- Increase in the frequency of urination, especially at night (**nocturia**)
- Passage of bloody appearing urine
- Puffiness around the eyes, or swelling of the hands and feet, especially in children
- Pain in the small of the back just below the ribs (not aggravated by movement)
- High blood pressure

ANATOMY AND PHYSIOLOGY REVIEW

The urinary system consists of two kidneys, two ureters (upper urinary tract), a urinary bladder, and a urethra (lower urinary tract) (Figure 8-1). The kidneys manufacture urine (Figure 8-2). Urine normally consists of 95% water; the nitrogenous waste products of protein, which are urea, uric acid, and creatinine; the excessive electrolytes sodium, calcium, potassium, and phosphates; bile pigments; hormones; and metabolized drugs and toxins. Urine moves steadily by peristalsis through the ureters into the urinary bladder (Figure 8-3). The urine remains in the urinary bladder until capacity has been reached (about 500 mL) or until the body feels the **urgency** or desire to urinate (about 250 mL). The urine is then expelled from the bladder through the urethra, which is shorter in females than in males. **Micturition**, the process of expelling urine from the urinary bladder, is also called urination or voiding.

The kidneys are located beneath the false ribs, in the **retroperitoneal** space (behind the peritoneum outside the peritoneal cavity) of the abdominal cavity. The kidneys also assist in acid–base balance, raise blood pressure by secreting the enzyme renin, and produce the hormone erythropoietin, which is responsible for **erythropoiesis** (the production of red blood cells and their release by the red bone marrow).

Within the kidneys are microscopic units called nephrons, which are responsible for urine formation (Figure 8-4). The nephron winds into the cortex and medulla of the kidney. Each nephron includes a renal corpuscle, which consists of a glomerulus, a ball-like network of capillaries formed from an arteriole and held within a cuplike Bowman's capsule. The Bowman's capsule is attached to a long, intricate, ultrathin looped and coiled tubular structure called the renal tubule. Continuing on from the glomerulus is an arteriole that forms a capillary network around the tubule. Blood flowing through this system is collected by venioles.

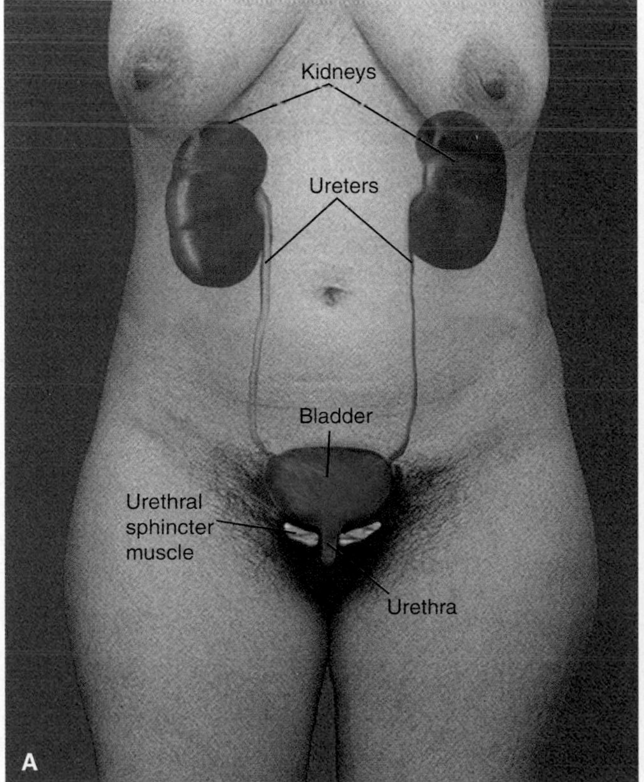

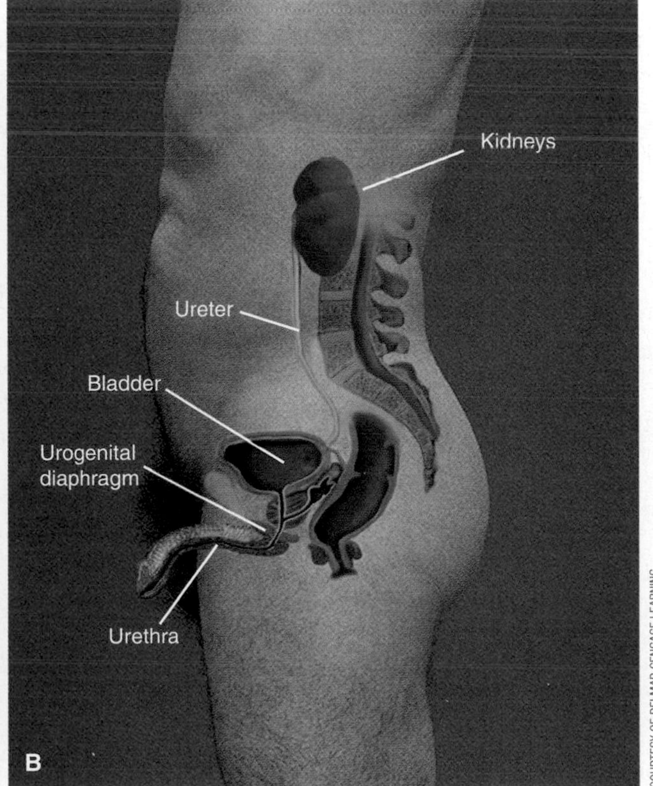

FIGURE 8-1 Urinary Tract; *A*, Female; *B*, Male

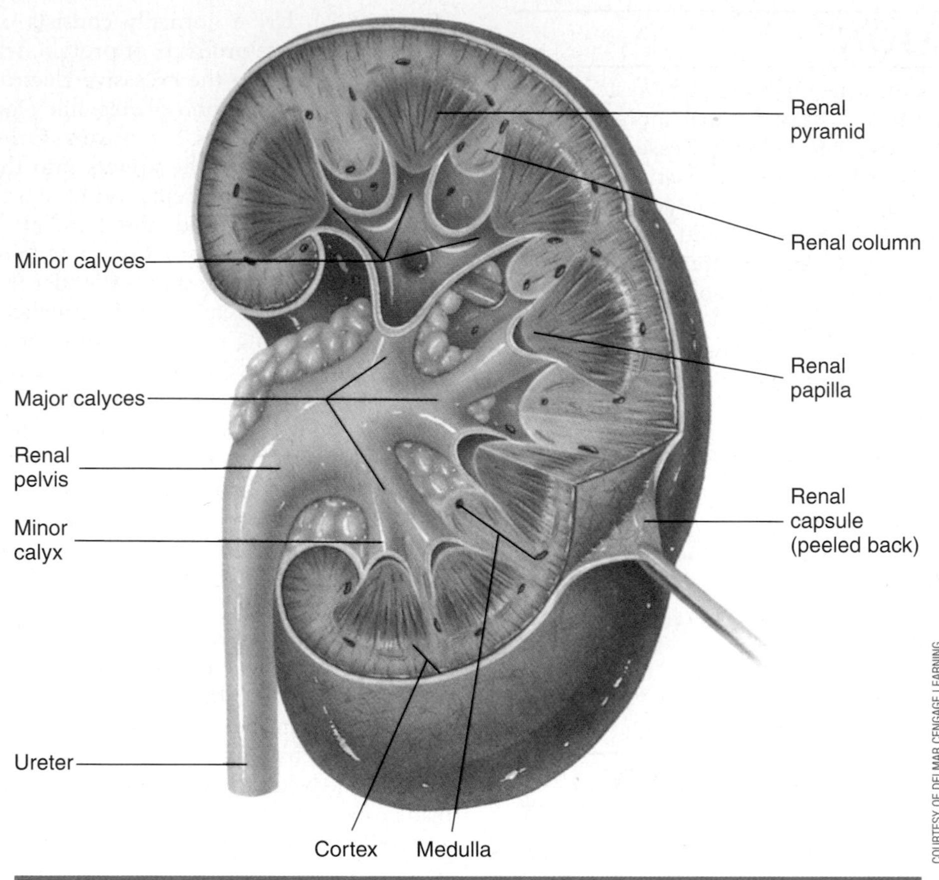

FIGURE 8-2 The Internal Anatomy of the Kidney

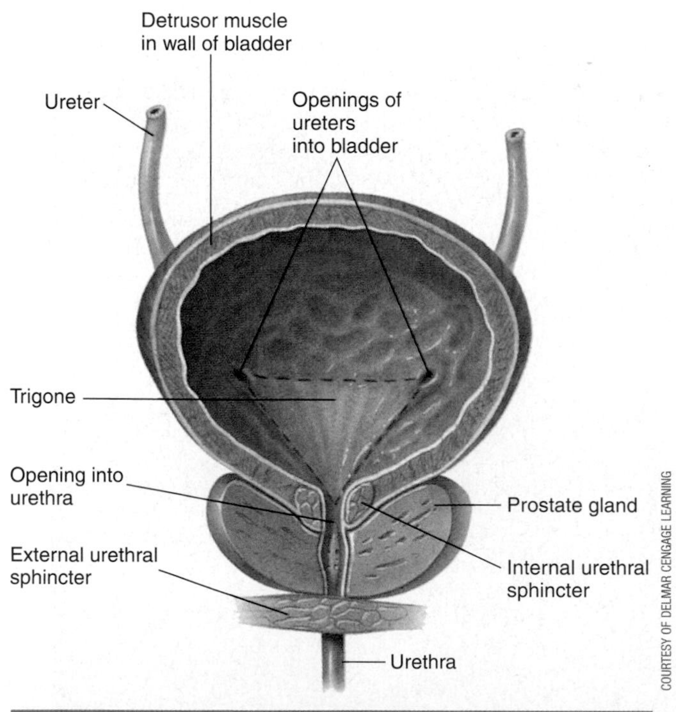

FIGURE 8-3 The Anatomy of the Urinary Bladder

Most of the contents of the blood, except for large molecules and blood cells, are forced out of the blood from the capillaries of the glomerulus and into the Bowman's capsule (glomerulofiltration). This occurs because of the high capillary blood pressure within the glomerulus. The glomerular basement membrane assists with the process of filtration. The **glomerular filtration rate (GFR)** is the amount of fluid filtered from the blood into the capsule per minute and an accurate measure of the functioning status of the kidneys. The material filtered from the blood is called glomerular filtrate, which contains water, electrolytes, glucose, various toxic substances, waste products (urea and creatinine), and just about everything else in the blood except large protein molecules and blood cells. As the filtrate passes through the first parts of the tubular structure, various substances such as necessary amounts of electrolytes, glucose, and water are reabsorbed (tubular reabsorption) back into the circulatory system through the capillaries or into the interstitial fluid. Tubular secretion then removes certain ions, nitrogen waste products, and drugs from the blood in the capillaries and adds it to the filtrate. The remaining filtrate—water, urea, excess electrolytes, toxic substances, and wastes, all of which constitute urine—continues through the tubules into the collecting duct, which collects urine from many nephrons. The urine passes from the collecting duct into the pelvis of the kidney, then through the ureter into the bladder and out of the body through the urethra. The kidneys process about 200 quarts of blood a day to eliminate 2 quarts of waste products and extra water as urine (NIDDK, 2006).

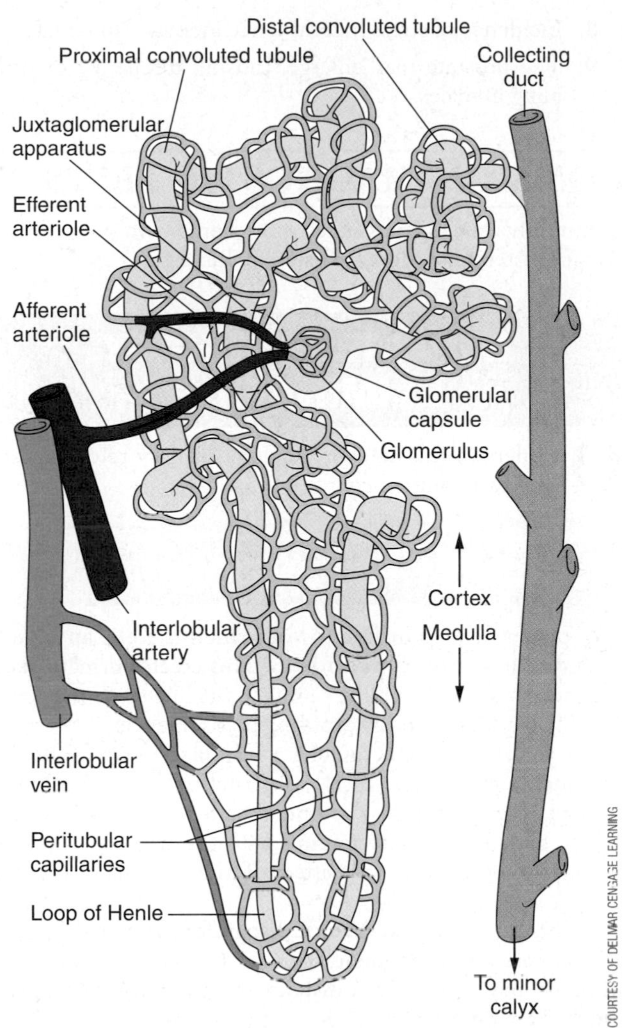

FIGURE 8-4 The Anatomy of a Nephron

ASSESSMENT

Assessment of the urinary system is included in the baseline data for all clients. The client may be reluctant to discuss urinary problems. Assist the individual to relax by asking open-ended questions, using familiar terms, and making sure the client understands the medical terms (Table 8-1).

A more in-depth assessment is performed when clients are at high risk for renal disease because of exposure to nephrotoxins; an altered health state such as diabetes mellitus, pregnancy, or hypertension; trauma, dehydration, or fluid retention, which can compromise renal function; and those with suspected or active renal disease.

SUBJECTIVE DATA

Ask the client to describe how the symptoms developed and progressed. Is there pain? Is it sharp or a dull ache? Constant or intermittent? Does it radiate to the groin, genital area, or leg? Is the pain associated with urination? Have headaches been experienced?

TABLE 8-1 Urinary Terms

TERMS	DEFINITION
Anuria	Cessation of urine production or urine output <100 mL/day
Dysuria	Painful or difficult urination
Hematuria	Blood in the urine
Nocturia	Excessive urination at night
Oliguria	Diminished capacity to form and excrete urine (<500 mL/day)
Polyuria	Excreting an abnormally large quantity of urine
Urgency	Feeling the need to urinate immediately

COURTESY OF DELMAR CENGAGE LEARNING

CRITICAL THINKING

Clinical Setting Activity: Urinalysis Results

Research and evaluate the urinalysis results of a client in the clinical setting. Were abnormal results detected? If so, what course of treatment was ordered for the client? What nursing interventions should be implemented?

Next, the client can describe the urine and urination pattern. Is there difficulty starting the stream? Is there urgency, frequency, incontinence, or hematuria? Does the bladder feel empty after voiding? Does the client have pruritis or dry skin?

OBJECTIVE DATA

If edema is present, ask the client if it is always present or if it disappears during the night. Monitor I&O and vital signs, and palpate the client's bladder for retention. Weigh the client. Assess mucous membranes for moisture and the skin for dryness and uremic frost. Evaluate urine for color, clarity, and odor. Review diagnostic tests.

CHANGES WITH AGING

The following changes are found in the urinary system as a result of aging:

1. Nephrons decrease, resulting in decreased filtration and gradual decrease in excretory and reabsorptive functions of renal tubules.
2. Glomerular filtration rate decreases, resulting in decreased renal clearance of drugs.

Box 8-1 QUESTIONS TO ASK AND OBSERVATIONS TO MAKE WHEN COLLECTING DATA

Subjective Data

Do you have any urinary health problems?

Do you have any family members with any urinary health problems?

How do you view your overall urinary health?

What was different today than any other day that brought you here?

How often do you urinate in the day and at night?

Are you urinating as much as you are drinking?

How many glasses of water do you drink a day?

Does it ever hurt or burn when you urinate?

Do you leak urine when you cough or exercise?

Do you have trouble starting your urine stream?

Does your urine have a strong odor or appear dark yellow?

Do you ever see blood in your urine?

Are you experiencing sleep disturbances?

Do you experience shortness of breath on exertion?

Objective Data

Check vital signs

Inspect color, odor, and consistency of the urine

Observe client for signs of anorexia

Observe client's activity tolerance and for signs of fatigue

Assess client for nausea and/or metallic taste in the mouth

Assess skin condition for pruritus

Measure and record intake and output

Weigh client daily

Monitor client for impaired cognition

Report diagnostic test results

3. Blood urea nitrogen (BUN) increases 20% by age 70. The creatinine clearance test is a better index than the BUN of renal function in the elderly.
4. Sodium-conserving ability is diminished.
5. Bladder capacity decreases, causing increased frequency of urination and nocturia.
6. Renal function increases when the client is lying down, sometimes causing a need to void shortly after going to bed.
7. Bladder and perineal muscles weaken, resulting in inability to empty the bladder. This results in residual urine and predisposes the elderly to cystitis.
8. Incidence of stress incontinence increases in females.
9. The prostate may enlarge, causing frequency or dribbling in males.

COMMON DIAGNOSTIC TESTS

Commonly used diagnostic tests for clients with symptoms of urinary system disorders are listed in Table 8-2.

IMPAIRED URINARY ELIMINATION

Disorders in this category include urinary retention and urinary incontinence.

URINARY RETENTION

A person who is unable to void when there is an urge to void has **urinary retention**. This creates urinary stasis and increases the possibility of infection. The urine may overflow the bladder's capacity, causing incontinence.

A variety of causes include a response to stress; benign prostatic hypertrophy (BPH), obstruction of the urethra by **calculi** (concentration of mineral salts, known as stones), tumor, or infection; interference with the sphincter muscles during surgery; or as a side effect of medications or perineal trauma.

The client may experience discomfort and anxiety from urinary retention. Frequency of urination and voiding small amounts may also occur. A distended bladder can be palpated above the symphysis.

Treatment may include urinary analgesics and antispasmodics to help the client relax. Cholinergic medications such as bethanechol chloride (Urecholine) may be ordered to promote detrusor muscle contraction and bladder emptying. A urinary catheter may be used to empty the bladder, or surgery may be performed to remove any obstruction.

When a client is unable to void, check for residual urine. Immediately after the client voids, use a bladder scan or insert an intermittent straight catheter, if ordered, and measure the urine output. The bladder scan is preferred because it reduces the risk of urinary tract infection (UTI). The urine left in the bladder, **residual urine**, should be less than 50 mL.

URINARY INCONTINENCE

Urinary incontinence (UI) is the involuntary loss of urine from the bladder. UI may be a complication of urinary tract problems or neurologic disorders and may be permanent or temporary. Medications such as sedatives, hypnotics, diuretics, anticholinergics, antipsychotics, and alpha antagonists may be associated with UI.

More than 25 million men and women in the United States experience UI, with women twice as often as men (National Association for Continence, 2008). This is not just a physiological problem but also affects the client's emotional, psychological, and social well-being. UI can occur in clients of any age but is more common in older adults. All

TABLE 8-2 Common Diagnostic Tests for Urinary System Disorders

URINALYSIS	
Urinalysis	
Color	Bilirubin
Odor	Glucose
Albumin (protein)	Specific gravity
Acetone (ketone)	Bacteria
RBCs	Casts
WBCs	pH
Culture and sensitivity (C & S)	
Creatinine clearance	
Residual urine (postvoiding residual urine)	
BLOOD TESTS	
Blood urea nitrogen (BUN)	
Serum creatinine	
Antistreptolysin O titer (ASO titer)	
Serum electrolytes	
Sodium	Calcium
Potassium	Phosphorus
Chloride	Uric acid
URINE TESTS	
Voiding cystourethrography	
Kidney-ureter-bladder (KUB) x-ray	
Computed tomography (CT; spiral CT)	
Magnetic resonance imaging (MRI)	
Intravenous pyelogram (IVP)	
Renal angiography	
Renal scan	
Ultrasound	
Portable ultrasonic bladder scan	
Retrograde pyelogram	
URODYNAMIC TESTS	
Uroflowmetry	
Cystometrogram (CMG)	
Urethra pressure profile (UPP)	
ENDOSCOPIC EXAMS	
Cystoscopy	
Biopsy	
Renal biopsy	

types of incontinence can be treated at any age. Keeping the perineal area dry and intact is a goal for all clients. UI is classified as stress, urge, overflow, total, or nocturnal enuresis.

STRESS INCONTINENCE

Stress incontinence is the most common type of incontinence. It is not a disease or a natural, inevitable effect of aging. Anyone can be affected; however, women are more likely to have this condition than men. In stress incontinence there is leakage of urine when a person does anything that strains the pelvic floor, such as coughing, laughing, jogging, dancing, sneezing, lifting, making a quick movement, or even walking. Medical management depends on the underlying cause. Treatment may include bladder retraining, medicines such as conjugated estrogens (Premarin Vaginal Cream), or surgery. Surgery may be necessary to restore the support of the pelvic floor muscles or to reconstruct the sphincter but is used after other treatments are unsuccessful. Another possible treatment is having collagen injected into the tissues surrounding the urethra thus causing the urethra to close enough to prevent urine from leaking out. The procedure is done in a nonsurgical outpatient setting. Surgical procedures include internal mesh support of the urethra, formation of a urethral sling to elevate and compress the urethra, and implantation of an artificial sphincter. Several support prostheses and external barriers are available.

The client can be taught pelvic floor exercises (Kegel exercises) to strengthen the muscles, thereby preventing or minimizing stress incontinence. Kegel exercises involve having the client tighten the pelvic floor muscles to stop the flow of urine when urinating, and then releasing the muscles to start the flow of urine again. Once the client can do this, the exercise may be done anytime, anyplace. Practicing the exercise 10 times, 7 or 8 times a day strengthens the pelvic floor muscles.

CLIENT TEACHING

Performing Pelvic Muscle Exercises (Kegel Exercises)

The nurse instructs the client to do the following when learning Kegel exercises:

- To learn how to control the pelvic floor muscles, tighten the pelvic floor muscles to stop the flow of urine when urinating.
- Then, release the pelvic floor muscles to start the flow of urine again.
- Now, practice (without urinating) tightening and holding the pelvic floor muscles for a count of 3 to 5 seconds and then release the muscles.
- Perform each contraction 10 times, three times daily.
- This exercise can be done anytime, anyplace.
- Develop a schedule or routine to remember to do daily Kegel exercises (e.g., when drinking morning coffee, working at the kitchen sink, waiting at a stoplight).

LIFE SPAN CONSIDERATIONS

Elderly Clients and UTIs

- Elderly clients are more prone to UTIs because of incomplete emptying of the bladder, fecal incontinence with perineal soiling, and a decrease in urine acidity.
- Incomplete emptying of the bladder in women is caused by bladder or uterine prolapse or loss of pelvic muscle tone; in men it is caused by an enlarged prostate gland.
- In elderly clients, sometimes the only sign of a UTI or urosepsis is new onset of mental changes or confusion (National Institutes of Health, 2006).

Bladder retraining begins with assessing the client's voiding pattern and encouraging the client to void 30 minutes before the projected time of incontinence. The schedule is extended until the client can stay dry for 2 hours, gradually increasing the time between voidings until a 3- to 4-hour schedule is achieved.

URGE INCONTINENCE

Urge incontinence occurs when a person is unable to suppress the sudden urge or need to urinate. Sometimes urine may leak without any warning. An irritated bladder is often the cause. Infection or very concentrated urine may irritate the bladder.

Treatment includes clearing up an infection, if present, and encouraging the client to have a fluid intake of 3,000 mL per day. This prevents the urine from becoming concentrated. Less fluid does not prevent incontinence but may promote infection.

OVERFLOW INCONTINENCE

When the bladder becomes so full and distended that urine leaks out, it is called **overflow incontinence**. This occurs when a blocked urethra or bladder weakness prevents normal emptying. The blockage may be an enlarged prostate. The distended bladder cannot contract with enough force to expel a stream of urine. Bladder weakness occurs most often in persons who have diabetes, drink a large quantity of alcohol, and have decreased nerve function. Bladder retraining may alleviate the situation.

TOTAL INCONTINENCE

When no urine can be retained in the bladder, it is termed total incontinence. The client may be able to manage with an indwelling catheter. A neurologic problem is usually the cause. Surgery to make a temporary or permanent urinary diversion may be required. Kobayashi, Nomura, Yamada, Fujimoto, and Matsumoto (2005) surgically performed the Mitrofanoff procedure, which creates a catheterizable channel between an abdominal stoma and the bladder. Clients can then empty their bladder with a catheter.

MEMORY TRICK

DRIP

There are several causes of incontinence that can be reversed or corrected. A memory trick to easily identify the reversible causes of incontinence is **DRIP**:

D = Delirium (a new onset of delirium)
R = Restriction (restricted mobility)
I = Infection (a new infection)
P = Polyuria (increase in urination as seen in diabetes)

NOCTURNAL ENURESIS

Incontinence that occurs during sleep is called **nocturnal enuresis**. Limiting fluid intake after 6 p.m. helps the client remain continent during the night. The total fluid intake for 24 hours, however, should remain the same. The bladder should be emptied immediately before going to bed.

NURSING MANAGEMENT

Identify impaired urinary elimination based on subjective and objective data. Assess vital signs. Encourage adequate fluid intake. Teach Kegel exercises. Initiate bladder retraining.

INFECTIOUS DISORDERS

Infectious disorders of the urinary system are called urinary tract infections (UTIs). There are two types: lower UTIs affect the bladder (cystitis) and urethra, and upper UTIs affect the kidneys (pyelonephritis, and acute and chronic glomerulonephritis) and ureters.

CYSTITIS

Cystitis is an inflammation of the urinary bladder. It is more common in females because their short urethra allows bacteria to ascend through the urethra from the vagina or rectum to the urinary bladder. Also, bacteria from an infected kidney can descend through the ureter into the urinary bladder. Most urinary tract infections are caused by *Escherichia coli*, but some are caused by *Candida albicans*. Other common causes of cystitis are coitus, prostatitis, and diabetes mellitus.

As women age, pelvic floor muscles relax, leading to a decreased ability to empty the bladder completely. This contributes to stasis of urine and promotion of bacterial growth, as in pregnancy or benign prostatic hypertrophy. In men, cystitis usually occurs secondary to another infection such as epididymitis or prostatitis.

Once bacteria enter the bladder, they multiply, causing redness and swelling of the wall of the bladder. These changes result in urinary frequency, dysuria, pyuria, hematuria, and sometimes burning and urgency with urination. These symptoms increase as the bladder distends with even a small volume of urine.

A clean-catch midstream urinalysis showing a bacteria count greater than 100,000 organisms/mL confirms the diagnosis. Microscopic examination of the urine also shows **hematuria** (blood in the urine) and pus.

Medical–Surgical Management

Medical

Treatment of cystitis includes medication and fluids. Recurrence of a UTI usually occurs when it is not effectively treated. Obtaining and sending a urine specimen for C & S before the administration of any urinary antimicrobial is necessary to determine the most effective medication. A repeat urinalysis after 2 or 3 days on medication confirms its effectiveness. Chronic lower urinary tract infections are often a factor in the development of pyelonephritis.

Diet

Encourage fluid intake. Clients are usually asked to drink between 3 and 4 liters of noncaffeinated fluid per day. The intake of meats and whole grains makes the urine more acidic and may discourage the growth of bacteria in the urinary bladder. Drinking cranberry juice has been advised for years, but how it worked was not understood. Research suggests that condensed tannins in the juice prevent E. coli from sticking to the urinary tract (Lynch, 2004).

Pharmacological

Cystitis treatment entails the use of antimicrobial medication in conjunction with urinary tract analgesics. Cystitis is generally treated with trimethoprim-sulfamethoxazole (TMP-SMZ, Bactrim), ciprofloxacin (Cipro), cephalexin (Keflex), nitrofurantoin (Macrobid, Macrodantin), Amoxicillin (Amoxil), doxycycline calcium (Vibramycin), and Augmentin. Determine whether the client is allergic to sulfonamides or penicillins before administering the medication. The antimicrobial ordered is determined by the results of the urine culture and sensitivity. The length of treatment is related to the type of cystitis, acute or chronic. Some physicians may order a single dose or short course (3 or 4 days) of antimicrobial therapy rather than the traditional 7- to 10-day course. **Dysuria** (difficult or painful urination) related to a burning sensation when voiding can be alleviated with the use of the urinary tract analgesic phenazopyridine hydrochloride (Pyridium), which causes red-orange urine and stains clothing and toilets.

Activity

Because cystitis causes frequency of urination, call lights must be answered promptly for clients on bed rest or those in need of assistance to the bathroom. Clients on bed rest are generally not able to empty their bladder completely when using a bedpan. Encourage orders for bathroom privileges or using a commode chair. Help allay the client's fears of being incontinent with properly timed bladder management.

Nursing Management

Monitor vital signs. Accurately record intake and output. Encourage fluid intake, especially water and cranberry juice. Encourage the client to void more frequently and women to void after intercourse. Teach clients that when taking Pyridium the urine will be red-orange and will stain clothing. Encourage cotton-crotch undergarments. Teach those who wear an incontinence control product to change it frequently.

NURSING PROCESS

Assessment

Subjective Data

The client will usually describe having frequency or urgency of urination or nocturia. This is annoying and embarrassing, regardless of age or sex. Burning and pain when voiding are common reasons clients seek medical care. Even clients with an indwelling catheter may complain of dysuria, burning, and frequency. Clients often feel body discomfort and malaise.

Objective Data

Perineal irritation may be noticed when the client with a catheter pulls on it in hopes of alleviating the bladder pain. The urine will smell foul and appear cloudy. Hematuria may be present (Figure 8-5). The elderly population in particular may become anorexic and develop a low-grade fever. The urinalysis will indicate the presence of bacteria, and the C & S will identify the specific microorganism causing the UTI and the medication to which the pathogen is most sensitive.

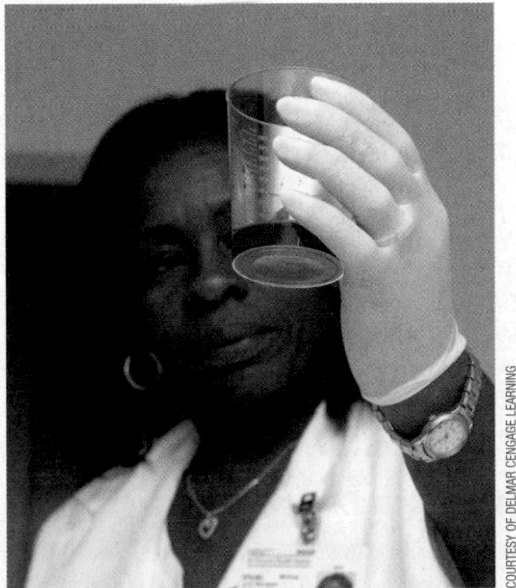

FIGURE 8-5 Nurse Examining and Measuring Hematuria Sample from Client with a UTI

Nursing diagnoses for a client with cystitis include the following:

NURSING DIAGNOSES	PLANNING/OUTCOMES	NURSING INTERVENTIONS
*Impaired **U**rinary Elimination* related to UTI	The client will return to usual pattern of urinary elimination.	Encourage a large amount of fluid intake, at least 3,000 mL each day, especially water and cranberry juice twice a day. Administer urinary tract analgesics and antimicrobial medications as ordered. Alert the client, if Pyridium is being taken, that the urine will be red-orange and will stain clothing.
*Deficient **K**nowledge* related to treatment regimen and prevention of recurrence	The client will comply with treatment regimen and practice preventive habits.	Discuss the importance of taking all medication ordered even after the symptoms are relieved. Teach or reinforce the following preventive measures. Clean the perineum from front to back. If nylon undergarments are worn, they should have a cotton crotch. Wearing tight-fitting jeans and thongs, and taking long bike rides may be irritating to the perineum. Perfumed perineal products such as menstrual products, douches, powder, or bubble bath may also be contributing factors to bladder infections. Spermicidal contraceptive products can be irritating, thus contributing to a lower UTI. Advise the client to void more frequently and not retain urine in the bladder. Advise women to void after sexual intercourse. Teach the elderly client who uses incontinence control products, to change the product frequently to prevent cystitis. When this client is hospitalized, plan time for frequent ambulation to the bathroom or commode chair.

Evaluation: Evaluate each outcome to determine how it has been met by the client.

CRITICAL THINKING

Assessment Scenario

A 24-year-old female client comes into the emergency department complaining of frequency and dysuria on urination.

1. What assessment should the nurse perform?
2. What tests might be ordered?
3. What instructions should the nurse teach the client?

PYELONEPHRITIS

Pyelonephritis, also known as pyelitis or nephropyelitis, is a bacterial infection of the renal pelvis, tubules, and interstitial tissue of one or both kidneys. Bacteria generally ascend from the urinary bladder through the ureter and enter the kidney in the renal pelvis. Bacteria can also enter from the blood and lymph. Pyelonephritis can be secondary to ureterovesicular reflux (backflow of urine from the bladder into the ureters) or when urine cannot drain from the pelvis of the kidney because of an obstruction blocking the kidney or ureter. Pyelonephritis may occur during pregnancy, with prostatitis, when bacteria are introduced during a cystoscopy or catheterization, or from trauma to the urinary tract. Pyelonephritis can be an acute illness or a chronic condition leading to the development of high blood pressure and/or chronic renal failure.

Escherichia coli is the microorganism most often cultured. The inflamed kidney becomes edematous and the renal blood vessels become congested. Sometimes abscesses form in the kidney. The urine is usually cloudy, containing mucus, blood, and pus.

MEDICAL–SURGICAL MANAGEMENT

Medical

Diagnostic tests that may be ordered include a CT scan, an ultrasound (when CT scan is contraindicated), a urinalysis with a C&S, complete blood count [CBC], BUN, and serum creatinine.

Collect urine specimens before the administration of any antimicrobial medication. Medical treatment and care are focused on preventing pyelonephritis from becoming chronic. Follow-up care and treatment may be necessary for up to 6 months.

Pharmacological

Pyelonephritis is generally treated with sulfonamides, such as trimethoprim-sulfamethoxazole (TMP-SMZ, Bactrim) or the antimicrobial ciprofloxacin hydrochloride (Cipro). Cipro may not be indicated if the client has renal damage. Antipyretics are used to reduce fever and analgesics to manage pain.

Diet

As with infections in general, the individual's diet should be light during the febrile stage. Fluids must be increased to 3,000 mL per day by mouth and supplemented intravenously when indicated.

Activity

Because the disease process causes fatigue, bed rest is maintained during the acute phase of pyelonephritis. Diversionary activities are important while on bed rest. When the client is allowed to ambulate, dizziness related to the analgesic medication taken for pain may be a problem.

NURSING MANAGEMENT

Encourage client to verbalize concerns and fears. Answer questions honestly. Monitor I&O and observe output. Encourage fluid intake to 3,000 mL per day and cranberry juice twice a day. Cleanse perineum from front to back. Encourage client to empty bladder frequently. Promote rest periods during the day. Weigh client daily. Monitor adequate pain management. Monitor and record diagnostic test results.

NURSING PROCESS

ASSESSMENT

Subjective Data

In acute pyelonephritis the client is acutely ill with malaise, urgency in urination, and pain during voiding and in the flank area. **Renal colic**, severe pain in the kidney that radiates to the groin, may occur, impairing urination. The client may describe being hot, with or without chills. In chronic pyelonephritis, only a general symptom of nausea may be present. The client may be very anxious that this kidney infection will cause permanent kidney damage.

Objective Data

Assessment may find the client tender on one or both sides of the lower back. Temperature, pulse, and respiratory rate may all be elevated. The urine is foul smelling, cloudy, and often hematuria is noted. The urinalysis results show bacteria and **pyuria** (pus in the urine), and the CBC indicates leukocytosis. The client with chronic disease will have the systemic signs of vomiting, diarrhea, and elevated blood pressure. Some clients with pyelonephritis may be asymptomatic.

Nursing diagnoses for a client with pyelonephritis include the following:

NURSING DIAGNOSES	PLANNING/OUTCOMES	NURSING INTERVENTIONS
Anxiety related to unknown prognosis	The client will verbalize fears and concerns to family and health care team.	Encourage the client to verbalize fears and concerns. Use active listening and observe for behavioral signs of anxiety. Answer questions honestly.
*Impaired **U**rinary Elimination* related to UTI	The client will regain normal urinary pattern.	Encourage drinking cranberry juice in the morning and evening. Encourage fluid intake to 3,000 mL per day, especially water. Monitor intake and output. Evaluate kidney function by measuring and observing urine output and monitoring the results of blood and urine tests.
*Deficient **K**nowledge* related to disease process, treatment regimen, and prevention	The client will verbalize understanding of disease process, treatment regimen, and preventive measures.	Teach or reinforce the hygiene measure of cleansing the perineum from front to back and practice this when doing perineal care on any client. Instruct the client on the importance of taking all the antimicrobial medication as prescribed in order to eliminate the bacteria. Teach the client to refrain from using perfumed perineal products such as menstrual pads, tampons, or douches, and avoid bubble baths and hot tubs because they can be irritating to the tissues of the genital area.

(Continues)

Nursing diagnoses for a client with pyelonephritis include the following: (Continued)

NURSING DIAGNOSES	PLANNING/OUTCOMES	NURSING INTERVENTIONS
		Encourage the client to empty the bladder frequently to avoid distention.
		Promote rest periods, which aid the healing process.
		Inform the client to call the physician immediately if there is a decrease in urine output or signs of infection (elevated temperature, chills, flank pain, urgency, fatigue, nausea, and vomiting).
		Teach client to weigh daily and report sudden weight gain (2 pounds/week) to the physician.
		Emphasize the importance of keeping all appointments with the physician for follow-up care and when signs of infection appear.
		Teach the client the importance of long-term treatment and monitoring for chronic pyelonephritis.

Evaluation: Evaluate each outcome to determine how it has been met by the client.

ACUTE GLOMERULONEPHRITIS

Glomerulonephritis is a condition that can affect one or both kidneys. In both acute and chronic disease, the glomerulus within the nephron unit becomes inflamed. It is predominantly a disease of children and young adults when the cause is bacterial. The viral form can affect all ages. The prognosis for most clients is a full recovery; however, some may develop chronic glomerulonephritis. Acute glomerulonephritis during childhood is known as Bright's disease.

Clients may develop symptoms 1 to 3 weeks after an upper respiratory infection (tonsillitis or pharyngitis with fever) or skin infection caused most commonly by group A *β-hemolytic streptococcus*. The infection triggers an autoimmune response and the glomeruli are attacked by antibodies at the site of the glomerular basement membrane, resulting in inflammation. Some clients are asymptomatic. A nephrotoxic drug or systemic disease such as diabetes or lupus may also be a cause (NIDDK, 2006).

Immunologic effects on the body are not completely understood. Direct effects on the glomeruli result in the reduced ability of the glomeruli to function. The glomeruli become more permeable, resulting in the loss of red blood cells and protein from the blood. These substances escape from the body in the urine. The inflammatory process causes thickening of the membrane of the glomeruli and potential scarring.

Diagnostic tests on blood and urine as well as KUB x-rays will be performed. BUN, serum creatinine, potassium, erythrocyte sedimentation rate (ESR), and antistreptolysin O titer (ASO titer) will be elevated. Urinalysis will show proteinuria and red blood cells. A CBC and electrolytes are ordered. Cultures of the throat and skin may be ordered to rule out *Streptococcus*.

MEDICAL–SURGICAL MANAGEMENT

Medical

Prevention of renal complications and complications to cardiac and cerebral functioning is the focus of care. Medical treatment must start as soon as the client is diagnosed to restore kidney function. Management includes drug therapy, diet, and rest. Treatment is correlated with the blood pressure and the results of urine testing for red blood cells and protein. The client is not considered to be free from the disease until the urine tests negative for protein and red blood cells for 6 months.

Plasmapheresis may be indicated if there is no response from other treatments and if the client also has Goodpasture's syndrome. Between 150 and 400 mL of blood is removed from the client and put in a cell separator. Here the blood is divided into plasma and formed elements which are mixed with a plasma replacement and returned to the client through a vein. Another technique filters the client's own plasma to remove a specific disease mediator (antibody) and then returns the plasma to the client.

Pharmacological

Prophylactic antimicrobial therapy may be administered. The drug of choice is penicillin. If the client is allergic to penicillin, erythromycin is ordered. Diuretic and antihypertensive medication furosemide (Lasix) may be ordered. Corticosteroids, chemotherapeutic drugs such as cyclophosphamide (Cytoxan), and/or immunosuppressive agents such as azathioprine (Imuran) may be ordered to control the inflammatory response. Corticosteroids and immunosuppressive drugs may be prescribed to treat the underlying causes of glomerulonephritis, such as lupus or vasculitis (Mayo Clinic, 2009).

Diet

Fluid retention often requires fluid restriction. The restriction is adjusted according to the client's I&O record and daily weight. Protein in the client's diet will be regulated according to the BUN and the creatinine blood levels. The kidneys need to rest; however, particularly in children, it may not be necessary to restrict protein. Potassium will need to be replaced if the diuretic promotes its excretion. Sodium may be restricted to prevent fluid retention. Strict intake and output are necessary to monitor kidney function.

COMMUNITY/HOME HEALTH CARE

Sodium Restriction

When water at home is naturally high in sodium or if water is chemically softened, teach the client to use low-sodium bottled water in cooking and for the drinking allowance.

Activity

Physical and emotional rest are essential. Compliance with bed rest may be difficult, especially for a child or the client who feels well. Bed rest is indicated until the inflammation subsides, urinary flow increases, and as long as the client has hematuria or proteinuria. During this time a strict turning schedule needs to be followed because skin breakdown is more likely in the presence of edema. When ambulation is allowed, the client may feel weak from the effects of anemia and inactivity.

NURSING MANAGEMENT

Monitor vital signs and I&O. Blood pressure should be monitored closely. Assess for headache, flank pain, and edema. Weigh client daily. Assess heart and lung sounds. Monitor results of diagnostic tests. If fluids are restricted, work with client on fluid intake schedule. Encourage client to follow schedule. Assist with or provide oral hygiene several times a day. Refer for dietary consultation if protein and sodium are restricted.

NURSING PROCESS

ASSESSMENT

Subjective Data

The health history will likely reveal a recent sore throat, skin infection, flulike symptoms, and a headache. The client describes flank pain as the kidneys become congested. Other symptoms the client may describe are headache, malaise, anorexia, cola-colored "smokey" urine, and a marked decrease in the amount of urine (**oliguria**). Facial edema may be the first sign noticed, may impair vision, and may cause the client to have negative feelings about body image.

Objective Data

Vital signs will generally show an increase in body temperature and blood pressure. Facial (periorbital) edema is present. The edema will progress to dependent areas such as the sacral area and the legs. Monitor daily the location and degree of edema. Ascites may also develop. Assess the general condition of the skin and skin integrity. Weigh the client to establish a baseline weight. Assess heart and lung sounds for signs of heart failure and pulmonary edema (unusual heart sounds and crackles in the lungs). Neck veins may be distended. Dyspnea on exertion or when recumbent, and shortness of breath, may both be noted. Urine output is decreased and cola colored to red colored urine is present.

Monitor results of diagnostic tests: urine for red blood cells and protein (albumin) and blood for BUN, serum creatinine, potassium, ESR, ASO titer, and specific gravity, all of which will be elevated.

Nursing diagnoses for a client with acute glomerulonephritis include the following:

NURSING DIAGNOSES	PLANNING/OUTCOMES	NURSING INTERVENTIONS
Fear related to potential permanent damage to the kidneys	The client will communicate fears of kidney damage to the family and the health care personnel.	Provide client and family with support and understanding. Encourage client to discuss fears. Explain the importance of protecting the client from other infections. Allow no one with an upper respiratory infection to visit the client. Discuss the importance of compliance with medications, bed rest, and diet to prevent permanent damage to kidneys. Emphasize the importance of keeping the follow-up visits to the laboratory for tests and to the physician's office. Arrange consultation with social services to assist the client in arranging time off from work and to help the client and family with their financial needs.
Excess Fluid Volume related to compromised regulatory mechanism secondary to renal dysfunction	The client will have decreased edema and adequate urinary output.	Fluids will be restricted with specific amounts designated throughout the day. For example, 900 mL of fluids for a day might be divided in the following manner: 7 a.m. to 3 p.m. 600 mL; 3 p.m. to 11 p.m. 200 mL; 11 p.m. to 7 a.m. 100 mL. Encourage compliance to the fluid amounts. Maintain accurate intake and output records hourly.

(*Continues*)

Nursing diagnoses for a client with acute glomerulonephritis include the following: (Continued)

NURSING DIAGNOSES	PLANNING/OUTCOMES	NURSING INTERVENTIONS
		Provide oral hygiene several times a day. Advise that thirst may be relieved by sucking on hard candy or, if allowed, a few ice chips. Provide eye care with normal saline to promote comfort from the periorbital edema.
Impaired Social Interaction related to changes in body image	The client will resume social interaction.	Encourage client to keep in contact with friends and relatives by telephone. Encourage keeping appointments with the physician and laboratory.
Imbalanced Nutrition: More than Body Requirements related to the disease process	The client will comply with nutritional restrictions.	Once the client's condition warrants solid foods, arrange a dietary consultation to incorporate food preferences and religious and/or cultural needs. Finances may be an issue if the family has to incorporate foods that are not usually part of its budget. Teach client to plan menus and to read food labels in order to comply with the dietary restrictions. Before discharge, teach client and family about diet, fluids, and activity restrictions and measuring fluid intake and urine output. Provide client with guidelines listing reasons to call the physician.

Evaluation: Evaluate each outcome to determine how it has been met by the client.

CHRONIC GLOMERULONEPHRITIS

The prognosis for acute glomerulonephritis is often good when treatment is begun early; however, chronic glomerulonephritis generally leads to permanent kidney damage. Those who develop chronic glomerulonephritis may have neither symptoms nor a recent history of an infection. Chronic diseases, such as diabetes mellitus or systemic lupus erythematosus, often mask renal symptoms and the client does not seek medical care until kidney function is impaired. It may take up to 30 years for the signs of renal insufficiency to develop.

Chronic glomerulonephritis is a slowly progressive, destructive process affecting the glomeruli, causing loss of kidney function. The kidney decreases in size as glomeruli are destroyed. If end-stage renal disease (ESRD) develops, the client may die quickly.

Nephrons lose their ability to filter nitrogenous wastes from the blood. Protein (albumin) and red blood cells escape into the urine and are present on a urinalysis. Nitrogenous waste remains in the blood, and the BUN level increases. As glomeruli are destroyed, the serum level of creatinine also increases. BUN and serum creatinine are checked on a regular basis to monitor renal function. Serum electrolyte levels are also monitored. Anemia is evaluated with a CBC.

MEDICAL–SURGICAL MANAGEMENT

Medical

Prevention of further renal damage as well as heart or cerebral complications is the focus of care. Management includes drug therapy, diet, and bed rest. Exposure of the client to infection of any kind must be avoided. Blood transfusion may be required for severe anemia. The client may be transferred to a facility where dialysis and/or kidney transplantation can be performed.

Pharmacological

Diuretic and antihypertensive medications are ordered. Antimicrobial therapy is generally given prophylactically. Monitor for side effects from all medications and report to the physician immediately.

Diet

Fluid intake is adjusted according to urinary output. Protein allowed in the diet will be regulated according to the BUN and the creatinine blood levels. As these levels increase, protein will be restricted to decrease the nitrogenous wastes. Sodium and potassium restrictions will be determined by the serum electrolyte levels. Carbohydrates are usually increased in the diet to provide adequate energy.

Activity

Bed rest is indicated when the client has hematuria or albuminuria.

Nursing Management

Assist client with ADLs and encourage bed rest with diversional activities. Monitor vital signs and I&O. Measure urine hourly or as ordered. Assess color and consistency of urine. Assess lung sounds, edema, speech, and mental functioning. Assist client to reposition frequently and assess skin. Weigh client daily. Monitor laboratory reports.

NURSING PROCESS

Assessment

Subjective Data

Clients may describe a morning headache, pruritis, a decreased ability to concentrate, fatigue, and dyspnea making it difficult to perform ADLs. Facial edema and/or blurring of vision caused by retinal edema may also be reported by clients.

Objective Data

As chronic glomerulonephritis develops, fluid retention becomes evident, leading to shortness of breath, especially at night. Monitor vital signs; hypertension is usually present. Assess lung sounds every shift for crackles, a sign of fluid retention. Monitor weight daily, and note the degree of edema, its location, and if it is pitting or nonpitting. **Anasarca** is generalized edema that appears as the client's condition deteriorates. Assess skin for color, presence of ecchymosis or rash, dryness, and evidence of scratching. Note mental functioning, irritability, tremors, ataxia, or slurred speech.

As nephrons lose their ability to concentrate urine, the urine becomes pale and dilute. Closely monitor I&O because initially, polyuria develops, giving the client a false sense that recovery will be soon. Monitor results of blood and urine tests.

Nursing diagnoses for a client with chronic glomerulonephritis include the following:

NURSING DIAGNOSES	PLANNING/OUTCOMES	NURSING INTERVENTIONS
*Impaired **Urinary** Elimination* related to the failing kidney function	The client will have adequate urine output.	Measure urine output hourly, or every 4 or 8 hours as ordered. Parameters will be set by the physician for immediate notification. Assess and document the color and consistency of the urine. Measure intake to determine compliance with the amount of fluids permitted. Weigh client daily at the same time each day, on the same scale and with the same clothes.
*Excess **Fluid** Volume* related to compromised regulatory mechanism	The client will have decreased edema.	Assess and describe the location of the edema. Administer medications as ordered for treatment of the edema. Monitor electrolyte values. Maintain fluid intake at restricted amount. Document I&O.
Anxiety related to threat to or change in health status (potential dialysis treatment)	The client will communicate less anxiety about possible treatment with dialysis.	Assist client to express concerns about possible treatment with dialysis. Arrange for a dialysis nurse to visit client. Provide written information about dialysis.
*Risk for Impaired **Skin** Integrity* related to immobility and edema	The client will maintain skin integrity.	Assess skin every time the client is repositioned. Cleanse the skin frequently, especially when crystals of urea form on the skin, causing itching and dryness.

Evaluation: Evaluate each outcome to determine how it has been met by the client.

OBSTRUCTIVE DISORDERS

Disorders of this type include urolithiasis, urinary bladder tumors, renal tumors, and polycystic kidney.

URINARY CALCULI

Approximately 1 million Americans each year have kidneystones (NKF, 2009c). **Urolithiasis** is a calculus, or

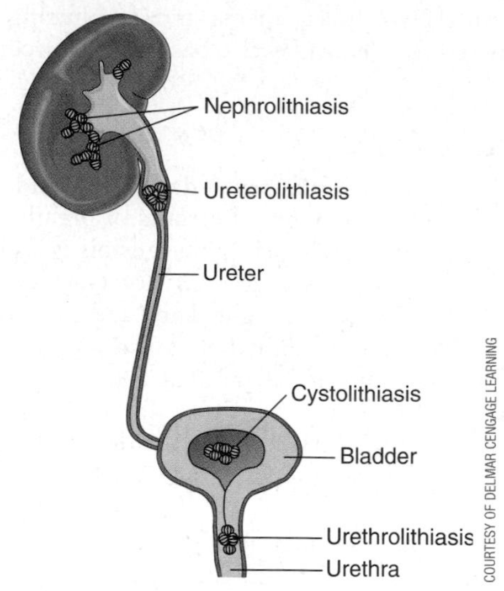

FIGURE 8-6 Common Locations of Urinary Calculi Formation

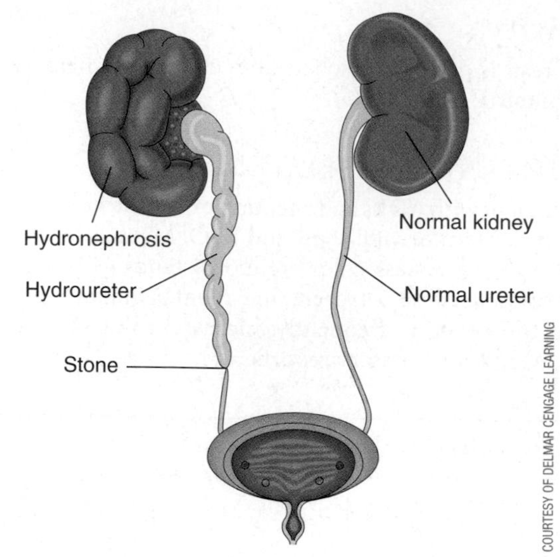

FIGURE 8-7 Hydronephrosis and Hydroureter Resulting from a Stone in the Ureter

stone, formed in the urinary tract. A **calculus** (plural—calculi) is a solid mass of mineral salts occurring within a hollow organ such as the renal pelvis, ureters, bladder, or urethra (Figure 8-6). A urinary calculus can range in size from microscopic to 10 to 20 mm in diameter.

Calculi are formed when minerals precipitate out of solution and collect within hollow areas. The reason stones form has not yet been identified, but individuals who are immobile, hyperparathyroid, or have recurrent UTIs are predisposed. When a person is immobile for long periods, calcium is pulled from the bones into the blood. The nephrons filter the excess calcium out of the blood into the urine. Calculi can also lodge in and obstruct an indwelling catheter. The size and location of the stone within the urinary system greatly affects the degree of pain and other symptoms present. When the stone is in the kidney, the pain is dull and constant mainly in the back just below the ribs near the spine. Stones in the ureter often cause ureteral colic, an excruciating, intermittent pain that begins in the flank and radiates into the groin, inner thigh, or genitalia. It is caused by spasm of the ureter as the calculus moves down the ureter. The client often has nausea and vomiting.

If a calculus becomes lodged anyplace along the ureter and urine cannot pass, a condition called hydronephrosis and/or hydroureter occurs. The kidney and/or ureter become enlarged with the accumulated urine (Figure 8-7).

Tests to confirm the diagnosis and determine the size and location of the stone include spiral CT scan, KUB, IVP, cystoscopy, and ultrasound. A BUN and serum creatinine indicate whether the calculus has damaged kidney function. A urinalysis with a culture and a CBC may be ordered to determine whether an infection is present. A 24-hour urine may be sent to the laboratory to determine whether there is abnormal excretion of calcium oxalate, phosphorus, and uric acid.

MEDICAL–SURGICAL MANAGEMENT

Medical

All urine is strained whether voided or from an indwelling catheter drainage bag. Urine from a catheter drainage bag is drained and strained every 2 to 4 hours. All strained particles are saved for the physician or sent to the laboratory.

A very small calculus may be flushed out by peristalsis and fluids. The client is encouraged to drink at least 4,000 mL of fluid per day, unless contraindicated by other health problems. The urologist may insert a small, pliable catheter stent into the ureter or urethra to allow temporary drainage of urine around the calculus.

PROFESSIONALTIP

Risk Factors for Kidney Stone Development

The following factors may increase a client's risk of developing kidney stones:

- Diet: high protein, high sodium, foods containing oxalate
- Lack of fluids: causes a higher concentration of substances that can form stones
- Family/personal history
- Age/sex: common between 20 to 70 years of age, men more likely to develop
- Limited activity: on bed rest or sedentary for long periods of time
- Hypertension: doubles the risk of forming stones
- Obesity: higher body mass index (particularly in women)
- Gastric bypass surgery, inflammatory bowel disease, or chronic diarrhea: changes in digestive process that affect absorption of calcium increase the level of substances in urine that form stones

Adapted from Mayo Clinic, 2009, Kidney Stones Risk Factors, from http://www.mayoclinic.com/health/kidney-stones/DS00282/DSECTION=risk-factors

Extracorporeal shock wave **lithotripsy** (ESWL) is a noninvasive method of crushing a calculus in the urinary system with ultrasonic waves to shatter or pulverize the stones into tiny pieces that are small enough to be passed in the urine. Sedation or light anesthesia is used to maintain comfort during the procedure due to the pain caused by the shock waves. The procedure requires 30 minutes to 2 hours to complete. The client is placed in a warm-water bath, and ultrasonic waves aimed at the stone break the stone into small pieces. An alternate method is to appropriately place a fluid-filled bag on the client's body and aim the ultrasonic waves at the stone through the bag, or the client is placed on a soft cushion. There is some discomfort and the client may be bruised where the ultrasonic waves hit the body. The urine will be slightly bloody for 24 to 48 hours and must be strained. The client should drink large amounts of fluids (3,000 mL to 4,000 mL per day) unless contraindicated. Clients should avoid taking aspirin and other drugs that affect blood clotting for several weeks before the procedure (NIDDK, 2007a).

Ureteroscopy is used for mid- and lower-ureter stones. The small fiber-optic ureteroscope is passed through the urethra and bladder into the ureter. The stone is either removed in a cage-like device or shattered with a shock wave and the pieces removed (NIDDK, 2007b).

Surgical

The surgeon may choose from several surgical procedures, depending on the location and size of the calculus. These include nephroscopic removal, pyelolithotomy, or nephrolithotomy (Figure 8-8).

Percutaneous nephrolithotomy is an endoscopic procedure in which a small incision is made in the fleshy area on the client's side between the ribs and the hip. A catheter is inserted and an ultrasonic probe is inserted through the catheter. Ultrasound waves directed at the stone break it into small pieces that can be withdrawn through the catheter. The catheter is left in place until the edema subsides, usually 1 or 2 days.

A bladder calculus may be crushed with special surgical instruments and the fragments washed out through a catheter. This is called a **litholapaxy**.

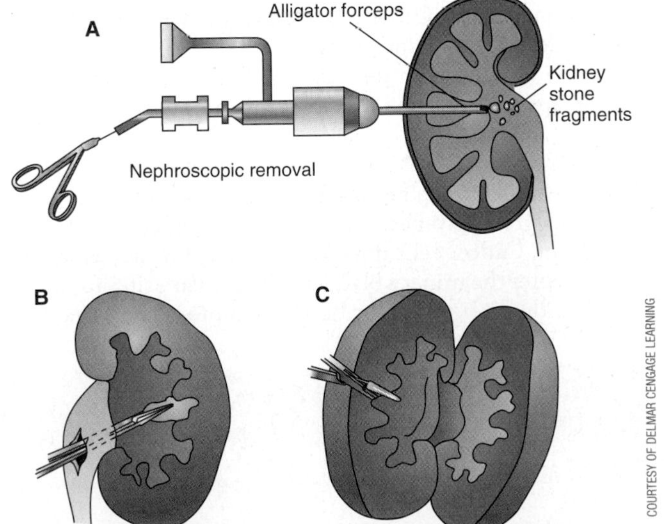

FIGURE 8-8 Methods of Removing Urinary Stones; *A*, Nephroscopic Removal (percutaneous nephrolithotomy); *B*, Pyelolithotomy, Removal Through the Renal Pelvis; *C*, Nephrolithotomy, Removal Through Incision into the Kidney

Pharmacological

Narcotic analgesics are generally prescribed for the severe pain often called renal colic. Antispasmodics such as propantheline bromide (Pro-Banthine) or belladonna preparations may be ordered to relieve ureteral spasms. Antibiotics may be ordered prophylactically.

Drug therapy is specific to stone composition. Allopurinol (Zyloprim) reduces the serum urate level, preventing calcium oxalate stones. Diuretics, such as hydrochlorothiazide (Esidrex, Ezide, Hydro-Par), are prescribed to decrease the amount of calcium released by the kidneys in the urine. Tiopronin (Thiola) and penicillamine (Cuprimine) are given to prevent the formation of cystine stones by reducing the amount of cystine in the urine. Aluminum hydroxide gel (Amphojel) binds with excess phosphates in the gastrointestinal tract. The phosphates are then excreted. Rarely, clients with hypercalciuria are given sodium cellulose phosphate (Calcibind) to bind with calcium in the intestines and facilitate excretion of calcium and prevent it from leaking into the urine.

Diet

In the past, clients who formed calcium stones were told to avoid foods high in calcium. It was believed that foods high in calcium, including dairy products, may contribute to the formation of calcium stones. Recent studies have shown that eating foods high in calcium may help prevent calcium stones, but taking calcium in pill form may increase the risk of developing stones (NIDDK, 2007a). When the stones contain uric acid, purine-rich foods (meat, fish, and poultry) are restricted, and organ meats, anchovies, and sardines avoided. Foods rich in oxalic acid (broccoli, asparagus, chocolate, tea, rhubarb, and spinach) are restricted when oxalate stones form. A deficiency of pyridoxine, thiamin, and magnesium may also contribute to the formation of oxalate stones.

Sometimes an effort is made to change the pH of the urine and thus prevent the formation of calculi. Acid-ash or alkaline-ash diets are used. Acid-ash foods are meats, fish, poultry, eggs, cereals, cranberries, and plums. Alkaline-ash foods are vegetables and all other fruits. These diets are often difficult for the client to maintain.

Drinking large amounts of fluid, at least half of it water, dilutes the urine and helps move any microscopic calculi through the system. Up to 4,000 mL per day of fluid is indicated for a client with renal calculi, unless contraindicated by another health problem such as heart failure.

Activity

Exercising regularly helps reduce the formation of calculi and keeps calculi moving through the urinary tract. Clients on bed rest should perform active range-of-motion (ROM) exercises daily in addition to frequent turning and positioning.

Nursing Management

Strain all urine. Monitor I&O. Encourage 4,000 mL per day of fluid intake unless contraindicated. Refer to dietitian for special acid-ash or alkaline-ash diet. Encourage active ROM exercises for clients on bed rest. Assess for pain and administer analgesic as ordered.

NURSING PROCESS

ASSESSMENT

Subjective Data

Many individuals are asymptomatic until the calculus begins to move or becomes too large. When the stone moves, the client usually describes intractable pain (pain not relieved by ordinary measures). The pain is often described as beginning in the flank and radiating down to the groin and inner thigh. Nonverbal client behaviors may indicate pain by tossing and turning when in bed or the inability to sit still when out of bed. If the calculus is not moving, the client may describe symptoms of infection such as lethargy, frequency of urination, persistent urge to urinate, dysuria, burning on urination, or feeling very warm. Nausea and vomiting are often reported. The client may express feelings of frustration related to the inability to complete daily tasks.

Objective Data

Assess hematuria, vomiting, intake and output, and vital signs. Elevated pulse and blood pressure may indicate pain. Check urine for stones when it is strained. Assess for cloudy, foul smelling urine and fever and chills if infection is present.

Nursing diagnoses for a client with urolithiasis include the following:

NURSING DIAGNOSES	PLANNING/OUTCOMES	NURSING INTERVENTIONS
Acute **Pain** related to irritation of the urinary tract and the mobility of calculi	The client will verbalize a reduction in pain.	Develop a pain management plan. Inquire about intensity, location, duration, and alleviating factors of pain. Observe for nonverbal signs of pain. Provide comfort measures and diversionary activities and administer analgesics and antispasmodics as ordered.
Impaired ***U**rinary Elimination* related to blockage of urine flow by the calculi	The client will return to normal urine elimination.	Encourage fluids to dilute the urine and flush out the calculi. Monitor urine for color and amount. Assist client to ambulate, if able. Accurately monitor intake and output. If a ureteral catheter is in place, measure and record the urine output from it separately from the urine output from the bladder.

Evaluation: Evaluate each outcome to determine how it has been met by the client.

URINARY BLADDER TUMORS

The American Cancer Society estimates approximately 70,980 new cases of urinary bladder cancer in 2009 (ACS, 2009b). Men are affected four times more often than women. Bladder cancer occurs most frequently after the age of 50. The only early warning signs are increased urinary frequency and painless, intermittent hematuria. As the disease progresses, the client may present with a UTI, painful urination, back pain, and abdominal pain. The main risk factor is cigarette smoking. Those individuals who smoke nicotine products have twice the risk of developing bladder cancer as do nonsmokers. Other risk factors are working with dyes, rubber, leather, or paint products; arsenic in drinking water; genetics; bladder birth defects; low fluid consumption; chemotherapy and radiation therapy; and chronic bladder inflammation (ACS, 2009d).

Benign papillomas are the most common urinary bladder tumor. Although papillomas are quite small, they should be treated aggressively because they are considered to be premalignant. Cancer cells develop mainly in the area where the ureters enter the urinary bladder. The primary sites for metastasis are the liver, lungs, or bones. Symptoms resulting from

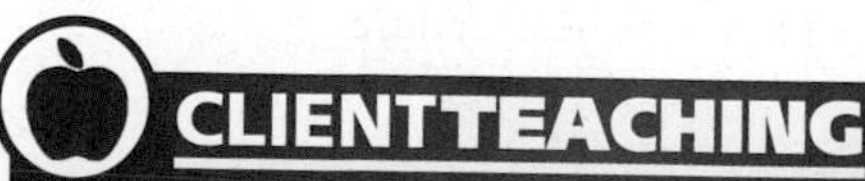

Urinary System Calculi

A person with a family history of stones or who has had more than one stone is at risk to develop another stone. Instruct these clients to:

- Drink plenty of fluids—water is best—to prevent stone formation.
- Avoid immobility.
- Take medications and modify diet as prescribed.
- Keep a record of intake and output.
- Learn how to strain urine.

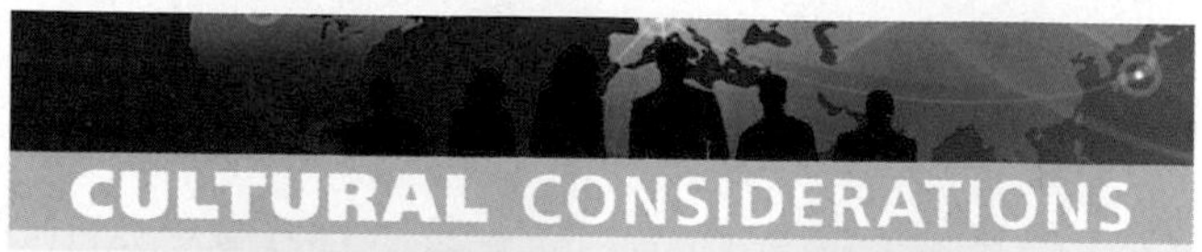

CULTURAL CONSIDERATIONS

Bladder Cancer

Caucasians are almost 2 times as likely to have bladder cancer as African Americans (ACS, 2009).

POLYCYSTIC KIDNEY

Approximately 600,000 Americans have polycystic kidney disease (PKD), which is the fourth leading cause of kidney failure (NIDDK, 2007c). Two major inherited forms of PKD include autosomal-dominant PKD, about 90 % of all cases, and autosomal recessive PKD, a rare form. Acquired cystic kidney disease (ACKD) is associated with kidney failure and dialysis. Approximately 90% of clients on dialysis for 5 years develop ACKD (NKF, 2009d). In PKD, multiple grape-like clusters of fluid-filled cysts develop in and greatly enlarge both kidneys. They compress and eventually replace functioning kidney tissue. PKD has an insidious onset that becomes obvious between 30 and 50 years of age.

Early symptoms include hypertension, polyuria, and urinary tract infections. Flank pain and headache are common. Recurrent hematuria and proteinuria develop. Diagnosis is made by x-ray or sonogram showing the cysts. BUN and creatinine are used to monitor kidney function.

The goal of medical management is to preserve kidney function, prevent infections, and relieve pain. Hypertension is carefully managed with antihypertensive medications, diuretics, and fluid and dietary modifications. Eventually, dialysis or renal transplantation may be needed.

RENAL FAILURE

According to the NIDDK (2006), any acute or chronic loss of kidney function is called renal failure and is the term used when some kidney function remains. Total, or nearly total, and permanent kidney failure is called ESRD. It may take only a few days or weeks to lose renal function or it may deteriorate slowly over decades. Disorders of renal failure are either acute or chronic.

ACUTE RENAL FAILURE

The rapid deterioration of renal function with rising blood levels of urea and other nitrogenous wastes (**azotemia**) is termed acute renal failure (ARF). The nephrons are unable to regulate the fluid and electrolyte or the acid–base balance of the blood. Predisposing factors include acute glomerular disease; severe, acute kidney infection; decreased cardiac output; trauma; or hemorrhage.

There are three major forms depending on the location of the cause: postrenal ARF (disrupted urine flow), prerenal ARF (disrupted blood flow to the kidney), and intrarenal ARF (renal tissue damage). Both postrenal ARF and prerenal ARF are reversible situations if they are identified early and treatment is begun. Undiagnosed postrenal ARF and prerenal ARF lead to intrarenal ARF. Diagnostic testing to identify the cause of ARF includes an ultrasound, CT scan, MRI, and, on occasion, a kidney tissue biopsy.

POSTRENAL ARF

Postrenal ARF is caused by an obstruction. It should be checked out first when a client has an unexplained decrease in urine output or has anuria. Kidney function can be easily restored by removing the obstruction. Urine volume will vary depending on the location and degree of obstruction. Catheterization, ultrasound, and retrograde pyelogram are used to diagnose an obstruction. An obstruction may be caused by renal calculi, blood clots, edema, tumors, urethral strictures, benign prostatic hypertrophy (BPH), pregnancy, or a nerve disorder. Postrenal failure can be ruled out if there is no obstruction. If an obstruction is confirmed, relief of the obstruction is imperative to minimize renal damage and resolve azotemia. When postrenal failure is prolonged, both blood creatinine and BUN will rise.

PRERENAL ARF

Any abnormal decline in kidney perfusion that reduces glomerular perfusion can cause prerenal failure. Common causes include extremely low blood pressure from severe bleeding, infection, shock, congestive heart failure, myocardial infarction, or severe dehydration. Fluid volume status does not indicate perfusion. Effective arterial blood volume (EABV) is the amount of fluid in the vascular space that effectively perfuses the kidneys. Even in fluid volume excess situations, such as low cardiac output caused by heart failure, the EABV falls, causing prerenal failure. The kidney interprets a fall in EABV as fluid volume deficit.

The glomeruli are then unable to filter waste from the blood. The renal tubules are structurally intact, and the kidneys can resume normal functioning if perfusion is restored fairly quickly. Ischemia results from prolonged inadequate perfusion, which can cause acute tubular necrosis (ATN).

The client generally has pale, cool skin; orthostatic hypotension; and oliguria. The BUN-to-creatinine ratio increases from 10:1 to more than 20:1. This increase occurs because of greater reabsorption of urea when fluids flow slowly through the tubules. A urinalysis shows a low sodium level (<20 mEq/L), high osmolality (>500 mOsm/L), and high specific gravity (>1.020). This results because the kidneys are retaining sodium and water in an attempt to correct the perceived fluid volume deficit.

When the client truly has a fluid volume deficit, treatment consists of intravenous fluids and albumin, plasma, or blood to restore the EABV. When the cause is inadequate cardiac output, inotropic agents such as dobutamine hydrochloride (Dobutrex) or amrinone lactate (Inocor) are used.

INTRARENAL ARF

Tissue damage of the glomeruli and/or tubules causes a loss of renal function known as intrarenal ARF. Glomerulonephritis and ATN are the main reasons for renal tissue damage. The antigen/antibody complexes formed in glomerulonephritis become trapped in the basement membrane, where they cause inflammation. The glomeruli then become more permeable, so red blood cells and protein are allowed to enter the filtrate and ultimately the urine.

Most intrarenal failure cases are caused by ATN and are the most common cause of nosocomial acute renal failure. ATN is the result of ischemia or toxic insult to the renal tubules. Ischemia may result from untreated prerenal failure or severe hypoxemia. Radiographic contrast dye, pigments (myoglobin and hemoglobin), aminoglycoside and cephalosporin antibiotics, and NSAIDs are all **nephrotoxic** (substances that causes kidney tissue damage) and can cause acute tubular necrosis.

The BUN-to-creatinine ratio in acute tubular necrosis is usually normal between 10:1 and 15:1; however, both the BUN and creatinine are greatly elevated. For example, the BUN may be 70 mg/dL and the creatinine 7 mg/dL. Urine sodium is more than 40 mEq/L, urine osmolality less than

CLIENTTEACHING

Acute Renal Failure

Teach clients at risk for ARF (older clients; diabetic clients; and clients with renal, heart, or liver disease) to:

- Immediately report to health care provider signs of fluid retention, pain on urination, and changes in urine output (amount or appearance).
- Avoid chronic use of and high doses of NSAIDs.
- Follow sodium and fluid restrictions as prescribed.
- Advise all health care providers of condition.

300 mOsm/L, and specific gravity less than 1.010. There are three phases to the clinical course of ATN: oliguric/nonoliguric, diuretic, and recovery. The first phase is either oliguric or nonoliguric depending on the causative factor.

Oliguric/Nonoliguric Phase

A nonoliguric phase is usually seen when nephrotoxic agents are the causative factor. When adequate urine output is maintained, dialysis is needed less often, and the morbidity and mortality rates are lower.

An oliguric phase, which may last 1 to 2 weeks, is seen more often when ischemia is the causative factor. Oliguria, voiding less than 400 mL/24 hours, can cause fluid volume overload; electrolyte imbalance, specifically high potassium and phosphorus, and low sodium and calcium; metabolic acidosis; and uremia.

Diuretic Phase

The diuretic phase is seldom seen because early dialysis keeps extracellular fluid volume at a fairly normal level. If it were seen, there would be a tremendous increase in urine output.

Recovery Phase

As renal function begins to improve, the client's urine output returns to normal and serum and urine laboratory test values move closer to normal. There is usually a short period of rapid improvement and then a period (may be several months) of slower improvement. Some clients will have residual renal insufficiency and a few will require long-term dialysis.

Medical–Surgical Management

Medical

Acute renal failure is often reversible, and complications can be prevented with early diagnosis and treatment. The goal is to have kidney function stabilized and returned to normal. Problems to be alert for are fluid volume overload, electrolyte imbalances, metabolic acidosis, high rate of catabolism, uremia, hemotologic abnormalities, and infection.

Dialysis is now an early treatment in ATN. Homeostasis is maintained while the cause of ATN is determined and treated. Permanent kidney damage may thus be averted. See the section on dialysis later in this chapter.

Surgical

The obstructions causing postrenal failure are often removed surgically. The exact procedure will depend on what type of obstruction is present and its location.

Pharmacological

Drugs used to treat acute renal failure include antihypertensives, diuretics, cardiotonics (inotropics), phosphate-binding antacids, potassium-lowering agents, and electrolyte replacement. It is important to ensure that drugs used are not nephrotoxic. See Table 8-3 for drugs used in acute renal failure.

Table 8-3 Drugs Used in Acute Renal Failure

DRUGS	NURSING RESPONSIBILITIES
Antihypertensives methyldopa (Aldomet) minoxidil (Loniten) clonidine HCl (Catapres) hydralazine HCl (Apresoline)	Monitor BP and pulse, weigh daily, monitor for postural hypotension and K, Na, Cl, and CO_2 levels, I&O.
Diuretics furosemide (Lasix) hydrochlorothiazide (HydroDiuril)	Monitor output, maintain fluid restrictions, weigh client daily.
Cardiotonics/inotropics digoxin (Lanoxin) amrinone lactate (Inocor)	Assess apical pulse before giving, report blood level of digoxin, monitor BP and P, monitor blood level of potassium.
Phosphate-binding antacids aluminum hydroxide gel (Amphojel)	Monitor serum potassium, assess BP and P, and for constipation.
Potassium exchange sodium polystyrene sulfonate (Kayexalate)	Monitor serum potassium, assess BP and P, and for constipation.
Electrolyte replacement calcitrol (Rocaltrol) calcifediol (Calderol)	Monitor blood calcium and phosphate levels, report metallic taste.

Diet

Restrictions generally include sodium, potassium, phosphorus, protein, and fluids. The amounts allowed are based on the laboratory tests results. Carbohydrates and fats are increased to be sure energy needs are met and protein will be spared as a source of energy. Clients with a high rate of catabolism often require total parenteral nutrition (TPN) to provide adequate nutrition.

Activity

Because the client is often weak and may also be confused, activity is restricted during the initial phase of acute renal failure. As recovery becomes evident, ambulation is begun.

Nursing Management

Accurately record I&O (often hourly). Monitor vital signs, BUN, creatinine, and serum electrolytes and protein. Weigh client daily. Assess skin turgor, lung sounds, and jugular vein distention. Provide fluids within prescribed limits. Ask dietitian to discuss dietary restrictions with client. Provide or assist with oral hygiene before meals. Listen to client's concerns.

NURSING PROCESS

Assessment

Subjective Data

The client may describe diarrhea; nausea, possibly with vomiting; swelling; loss of appetite; headache; increasing fatigue; and/or a change in mental alertness. Anxiety and fear related to not knowing what is happening is often expressed.

CRITICAL THINKING

Assessment Scenario

A 52-year-old male client has been admitted to the hospital for chest pain. After a couple of days in the hospital, the nurse notices the client has a total urinary output of 325 mL in 24 hours and has edema in both ankles. The lab results for this client are: sodium 130 mEq/L, BUN 28, and serum creatinine 2.5.

1. What might be going on with the client at this time?
2. What is significant about the client's lab results?
3. What type of diet may this client need to be on? Why?

Objective Data

Physical findings will depend on how far the disease process has progressed. Assess for hypertension, GI bleeding and/or bruising, reduction in urine output, anasarca, poor skin turgor, and dry mucous membranes because vomiting or diarrhea can cause dehydration. In a severe stage, the client may be drowsy and have muscle twitching and convulsions.

The BUN and serum creatinine will be elevated, as are the serum electrolytes potassium and phosphorus. The serum electrolyte calcium will be low. Blood level of red blood cells will decrease as the production of erythropoietin decreases. Leukocyte level will increase in the presence of an infection.

Nursing diagnoses for a client with acute renal failure include the following:

NURSING DIAGNOSES	PLANNING/OUTCOMES	NURSING INTERVENTIONS
*Excess **Fluid** Volume* related to sodium and water retention	The client will maintain a stable fluid volume.	Monitor BUN, creatinine, and serum electrolyte and protein levels. Accurately measure urine output, often on an hourly basis. Parameters are often set for notification of the physician. Weigh daily to identify weight gain related to fluid retention. One pound of weight gain is equivalent to 500 mL of retained fluid. Assess skin turgor, edema, BP, lung sounds, jugular vein distention, pulse and respiratory rate and quality. Provide fluids within the prescribed limits. Teach client about importance of fluid restrictions.
*Impaired **Nutrition**: Less than Body Requirements* related to anorexia, dietary restrictions, and increased catabolism	The client will have stabilized weight within normal limits.	Arrange for a dietary consultation to provide food in keeping with the prescribed restrictions and client preferences, including cultural and religious factors. Suggest 6 small meals throughout the day. Offer antinausea medications before meals. Provide or assist with oral hygiene prior to meals. Monitor weight and serum albumin level weekly

(Continues)

Nursing diagnoses for a client with acute renal failure include the following: (Continued)

NURSING DIAGNOSES	PLANNING/OUTCOMES	NURSING INTERVENTIONS
***A**nxiety* related to the disease process	The client will verbalize anxieties with the family and health care workers.	Establish rapport with the client. Listen to the client's concerns. Maintain open communications to foster expression of anxieties.

Evaluation: Evaluate each outcome to determine how it has been met by the client.

SAMPLE NURSING CARE PLAN

The Client with Acute Renal Failure

R.H., age 65, has had a history of heart trouble for several years. He is admitted because he has urinated very little for 2 days, he gets dizzy when he gets up from lying down, and he cannot get his shoes on because his feet are "fat." He states that he does not know what is happening to him. Results of laboratory tests are BUN 90 mg/dL, creatinine 4 mg/dL, urine sodium 15 mEq/L, and urine specific gravity 1.030.

NURSING DIAGNOSIS 1 *Excess Fluid Volume* related to sodium and water retention as evidenced by "fat feet," urine sodium 15 mEq/L, and urine specific gravity 1.030

Nursing Outcomes Classification (NOC)
Fluid Balance
Electrolyte & Acid–Base Balance

Nursing Interventions Classification (NIC)
Electrolyte Management
Fluid Management

PLANNING/OUTCOMES	INTERVENTION	RATIONALE
R.H. will have reduced fluid volume excess.	Accurately measure and record intake and output.	Provides information about retention of intake.
	Weigh R.H. daily—same time, scale, clothes.	Allows weight comparisons.
	Assess skin turgor, edema, BP, lung sounds for crackles.	Provides information about fluid in tissue, lungs, or vascular system.
	Monitor BUN, creatinine, and serum electrolyte and protein levels.	Gives insight to kidney functioning.
	Administer inotropics or cardiotonic medications as ordered.	Strengthens heartbeat, which will give better perfusion to kidneys.
	Provide fluids within prescribed limits.	Prevents fluid excess.

EVALUATION

R.H.'s feet are no longer "fat." His urine sodium is 18 mEq/L and urine specific gravity is 1.027

NURSING DIAGNOSIS 2 *Impaired urinary Elimination* related to decreased perfusion as evidenced by his urinating very little for 2 days and BUN–creatinine ratio of 22.5:1

Nursing Outcomes Classification (NOC)
Urinary Elimination
Knowledge: Disease Process

Nursing Interventions Classification (NIC)
Urinary Elimination Management
Teaching: Disease Process

SAMPLE NURSING CARE PLAN (Continued)

PLANNING/OUTCOMES	NURSING INTERVENTIONS	RATIONALE
R.H. will increase amount of urination to 1,200 mL/day.	Administer diuretics as ordered.	Increases water elimination by enhancing sodium excretion by the kidneys.
	Accurately measure and record intake and output.	Provides information about fluid movement through the body.

EVALUATION

R.H. is urinating 1,000 mL/day. His BUN is 50 mg/dL and creatinine is 3 mg/dL.

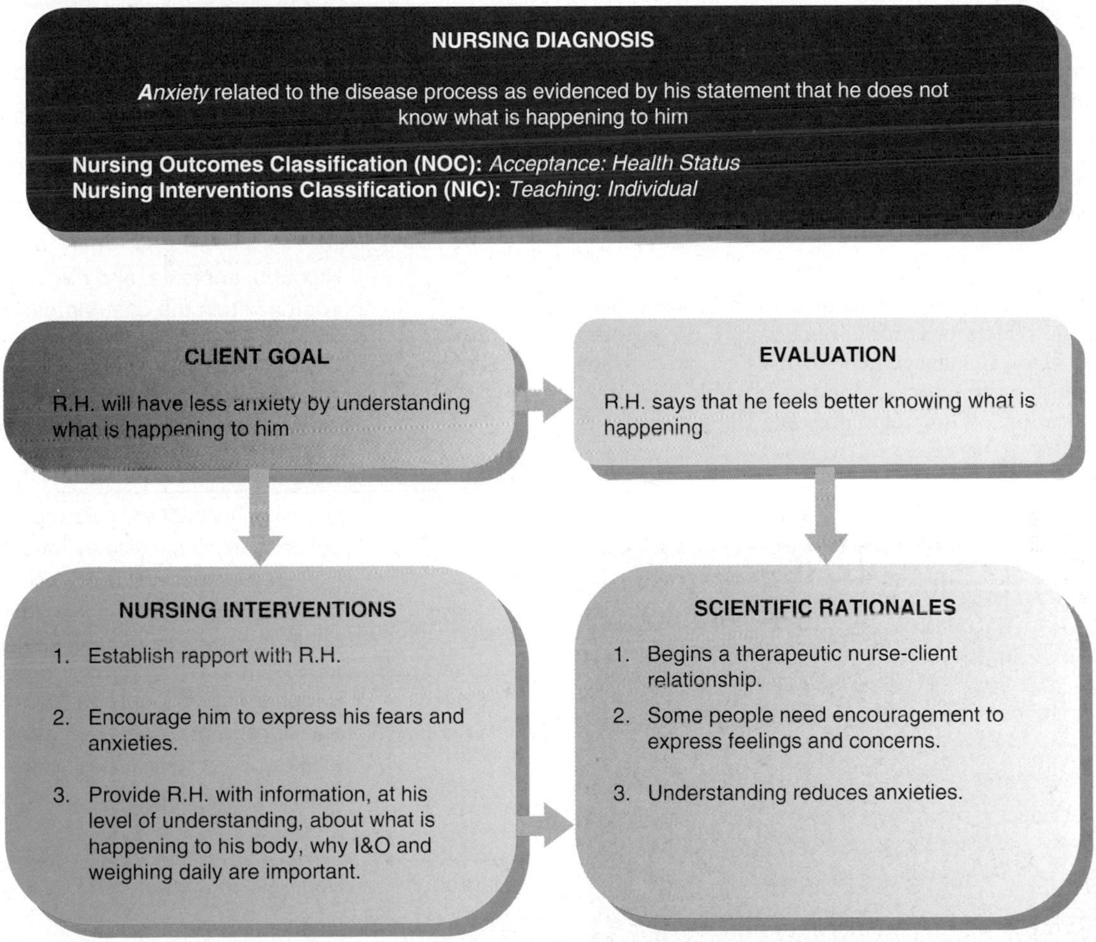

NURSING DIAGNOSIS

Anxiety related to the disease process as evidenced by his statement that he does not know what is happening to him

Nursing Outcomes Classification (NOC): *Acceptance: Health Status*
Nursing Interventions Classification (NIC): *Teaching: Individual*

CLIENT GOAL

R.H. will have less anxiety by understanding what is happening to him

EVALUATION

R.H. says that he feels better knowing what is happening

NURSING INTERVENTIONS

1. Establish rapport with R.H.
2. Encourage him to express his fears and anxieties.
3. Provide R.H. with information, at his level of understanding, about what is happening to his body, why I&O and weighing daily are important.

SCIENTIFIC RATIONALES

1. Begins a therapeutic nurse-client relationship.
2. Some people need encouragement to express feelings and concerns.
3. Understanding reduces anxieties.

Concept Care Map 8-1

CHRONIC RENAL FAILURE/ END-STAGE RENAL DISEASE

Chronic renal failure is a slow, progressive condition in which the kidney's ability to function ultimately deteriorates. This condition is not reversible. The kidneys have an amazing capability to perform effectively, even though most of the nephrons are destroyed.

Renal erythropoietin decreases, causing anemia. Hypertension, acidosis, and glucose intolerance usually are also present. Urea in the blood is extremely elevated. As the disease progresses, uremia develops.

There are three stages of chronic renal failure: reduced renal reserve, renal insufficiency, and end-stage renal disease (ESRD). Symptoms of reduced renal reserve are not apparent until more than 40% of the nephrons fail. A prolonged urine concentration test or a decline in GFR may be the only evidence of reduced renal reserve. When 75% of the nephrons stop functioning, renal insufficiency occurs. BUN and creatinine are above normal, and the client may have nocturia and polyuria. The onset of ESRD occurs when at least 90% of the nephrons fail: BUN and creatinine levels rise, polyuria changes to oliguria, and severe fluid and electrolyte imbalances are evident.

When the kidneys become unable to filter blood, an alternate method for filtration is necessary. Lifetime dialysis becomes inevitable unless kidney transplantation is performed and is successful. Life expectancy varies with the initial cause of chronic renal failure and the person's overall health at the time of diagnosis.

According to the National Kidney Foundation (2008), 485,000 Americans have ESRD. There are numerous causes of chronic renal failure. The four leading causes are diabetes mellitus 45%, hypertension 27%, glomerulonephritis 8.2%, and polycystic kidney 2.2% (NKF, 2008). Nephrotoxic drugs, including some over-the-counter drugs, aggravate the situation.

The diagnosis is confirmed when the BUN is at least 50 mg/dL and the serum creatinine level is greater than 5 mg/dL.

MEDICAL–SURGICAL MANAGEMENT

Medical

Chronic renal failure is a multisystem disease process. See Table 8-4 for the effects of chronic renal failure on various body systems. Medical management focuses on preserving the remaining kidney function as long as possible and preventing complications. This helps preserve the integrity of

CLIENT TEACHING

Herbal Facts for Renal Clients

Use of herbal supplements may be unsafe for renal clients because their bodies are unable to clear waste products effectively. Listed below are facts about herbs that every renal client should know (NKF, 2009e):

- The government does not regulate herbal supplements, so the exact contents and affects are unknown.
- Many herbs can interact with prescription drugs.
- Check with the physician, dietitian, or pharmacist regarding safety, dosage, duration of use, interaction with prescription drugs, etc. for all herbal products.
- Any interaction between herbs and medications could potentially put a transplant client at risk for rejection or losing the kidney.
- Herbs that may be toxic to the kidneys are artemisia absinthium (wormwood plant), periwinkle, autumn crocus, tung shueh, chuifong tuokuwan (Black Pearl), vandelia cordifolia, and horse chestnut.

TABLE 8-4 Effects of Chronic Renal Failure by Body System

SYSTEM	EFFECT
Urinary	Oliguria from renal insufficiency Azotemia
Blood	Anemia from decreased red blood cell production Decreased platelet activity, causing bleeding tendency
Cardiovascular	Hypervolemia and tachycardia Hypertension and dysrhythmias from hyperkalemia
Respiratory	Dyspnea, pulmonary edema Hyperventilation from metabolic acidosis Eventually Kussmaul respirations
Gastrointestinal	Urea in the blood is converted to ammonia by the mouth, causing uremic halitosis Hiccups, anorexia, and nausea from edema within the gastrointestinal tract
Skin	Dry skin with pruritis from uremic frost (excretion of urea through the skin with an odor of urine); pallor with anemia, yellowish-brown skin color
Nervous	Lethargy, headaches, confusion, impaired concentration with disorientation, depression, decreased level of consciousness, sleep disturbances, and uremic encephalopathy resulting in seizures and coma
Sensory	Peripheral neuropathy with numbness and tingling of extremities with complaints of a prickly, crawling feeling in the feet and legs, especially at night, sleep problems
Reproductive	Decrease in libido Decreased sperm count Amenorrhea Impotence Delayed puberty
Musculoskeletal	Joint pain and muscle cramping/twitching Bone demineralization from Hypocalcemia
Immune	Greater chance of infections from immunosuppression Decrease in antibody production

the person's life. Fluid retention increases the risk of complications such as edema (ascites), hypertension, and heart failure. Electrolytes are monitored and regulated.

Pharmacological

Antihypertensives such as methyldopa (Aldomet) and propranolol hydrochloride (Inderal) are used to control hypertension. Diuretics such as furosemide (Lasix) are used to treat fluid retention; anticonvulsants, phenytoin (Dilantin) to control seizures; antiemetics, prochlorperazine (Compazine) to control vomiting; and antipruritics, cyproheptadine hydrochloride (Periactin) to control itching. Calcium acetate (Phos-Lo) is used to lower the phosphate level in the blood; however, it can be constipating. A low renal erythropoietin level causing anemia is often treated with epoetin alpha (Epogen). An iron supplement is used to decrease the anemia-related symptoms. Multivitamins with folic acid are used because dialysis promotes the loss of water-soluble vitamins.

Diet

Diet restrictions are similar to those in acute renal failure. Sodium, potassium, phosphorus, and protein are restricted. Fluids are also limited. Modifications are made as kidney function deteriorates. With consistent compliance, symptoms decrease, resulting in fewer complications. Resources are available for clients to obtain assistance with dietary restrictions. Meal ideas are published in newsletters such as *NephroNotes*. Long-term dietary compliance is a challenge, and daily activities as well as special events during the year are a continual reminder of the client's dietary restrictions. As with other chronic diseases, those with renal failure need to have all family members and friends encouraging them to adapt to their restrictions. Dietitians can assist the family to incorporate religious and cultural dietary practices. The person with chronic renal failure may also have to incorporate dietary guidelines for additional diagnoses such as diabetes mellitus and/or coronary artery disease.

With the progression of chronic renal disease, dialysis becomes necessary. Fluid restrictions must be followed, and the amount allowed divided throughout the day. The greatest amount of fluid should be allowed during the day, incorporating enough fluids with oral medications. Some fluids should be planned for the evening meal, with a small amount to be allowed during the night; for example, days—500 mL, evenings—200 mL, and nights—100 mL. Protein restriction is closely monitored and regulated with the blood albumin level. The development of hyperkalemia will lead to a diet restricted in potassium. Foods high in potassium include dried fruits or dried beans and peas, peanuts, bananas, sweet potatoes, spinach, products with tomatoes, oranges, chocolate, artichokes, avocados, pumpkins, and mushrooms.

Activity

The client is encouraged to participate in activities of daily living. Safety becomes a significant factor during periods when the client has weakness, fatigue, or mental confusion. Confusion is seen in clients who have uremic encephalopathy. When bed rest is required, turning, ROM exercises, and skin care are important. As symptoms continue to become more severe, the client will need total assistance for all ADLs.

NURSING MANAGEMENT

Monitor daily weight, skin turgor, vital signs, and lung sounds. Provide prescribed amount of fluids and accurately record intake and output (sometimes hourly). Assist with or provide oral hygiene before meals and as needed. Administer an antiemetic 30 minutes before meals. Arrange for a dietitian to plan meals with the client. Assist with or provide bathing frequently, followed by applying lotion on the skin. Encourage repositioning at least every 2 hours, ROM exercises, and use of an egg-crate mattress or Clinitron bed. Monitor for mental confusion. Refer client and family to the National Kidney Foundation website at www.kidney.org for more information.

NURSING PROCESS

ASSESSMENT

Subjective Data

Inquire about the client's past medical history including treatments for maintenance of renal disease. Take a complete medication history, including the use of over-the-counter drugs. Description of fatigue, joint pain, severe headaches, nausea, anorexia, some chest pain, intractable singultus (hiccups), decreased libido, menstrual irregularities, and impaired concentration is given by the client. The client may feel uncomfortable talking directly to the nurse if uremic halitosis is a problem.

Objective Data

Note changes in the client's neurological status such as reduced alertness and awareness. Kussmaul respirations appear as coma develops. Halitosis with a urine odor and "uremic frost," a white powder on the skin, result from the accumulation of urates. Observe for dark-colored urine and bloody or tarry stools, which could indicate bleeding in the intestinal tract.

Nursing diagnoses for a client with ESRD include the following:

NURSING DIAGNOSES	PLANNING/OUTCOMES	NURSING INTERVENTIONS
Excess Fluid Volume related to compromised renal mechanism	The client will understand the importance of prescribed (restricted) fluid amounts.	Monitor daily weight, intake and output (maybe hourly), skin turgor, edema, blood pressure, respirations, and lung sounds. Provide prescribed amounts of fluids. Teach client to plan nutritional and fluid intake within the prescribed amounts. Monitor laboratory reports for serum albumin level and serum electrolyte levels.

(*Continues*)

Nursing diagnoses for a client with ESRD include the following: (Continued)

NURSING DIAGNOSES	PLANNING/OUTCOMES	NURSING INTERVENTIONS
*Imbalanced **N**utrition: Less than Body Requirements* related to dietary restrictions, GI distress, anorexia	The client will stabilize weight within normal limits and participate in dietary plan.	Provide or assist with complete mouth care before meals because uremic halitosis leaves a metallic taste in the client's mouth. Provide a clean, quiet, odor-free environment for meals. Suggest 6 small meals throughout the day. Encourage self-feeding. Arrange a consultation with the dietitian to plan alternate ways to prepare foods allowed on the diet. Ask the family to bring favorite foods, within the dietary restrictions, from home. Administer antiemetics 30 minutes before meals to control nausea.
*Risk for Impaired **S**kin Integrity* related to altered metabolic state leading to pruritis from "uremic frost"	The client will maintain skin integrity.	Bathe skin frequently to remove "uremic frost." Encourage the use of emollients and lotions on the skin. Administer antihistamines, as ordered, for the temporary relief of itching. Assist the client to change position every 2 hours. Provide an egg-crate mattress or Clinitron bed.
*Ineffective **C**oping* related to uncertainty of long-term compliance of the treatment regimen	The client will verbalize feelings and intention to comply with treatment.	Encourage the client to discuss feelings about long-term lifestyle changes. Refer client to the National Kidney Foundation website at www.kidney.org for information about client services and treatments for diseases of the kidney. Include the client and family in rehabilitation and discharge planning to ensure compliance. Topics for these sessions include diet, rest, medications, fluid restrictions, intake and output, activities, dialysis, required lab tests, and frequent visits to the physician. Incorporate into the discharge planning and teaching the client's socioeconomic needs, cultural background, role in the family unit, accessibility to medical care, and anticipated follow-up care. Complete referrals before discharge to lessen client anxiety.
		Consider future needs of a newly diagnosed client with end-stage renal disease and include the availability of dialysis, vocational rehabilitation, home health care, financial assistance with medical needs, and psychological therapy for the client and family.

Evaluation: Evaluate each outcome to determine how it has been met by the client.

DIALYSIS

As the kidneys continue to deteriorate, nitrogenous waste products accumulate in the circulatory system. These waste products need to be removed artificially with **dialysis**, a mechanical means of removing nitrogenous waste from the blood by imitating the function of the nephrons. It involves filtration and diffusion of wastes, drugs, and excess electrolytes and/or osmosis of water across a semipermeable membrane into a dialysate solution. The **dialysate** is a solution designed to approximate the normal electrolyte structure of plasma and extracellular fluid.

There are two types of dialysis: hemodialysis and peritoneal dialysis. These treatments can be obtained throughout the country at dialysis centers or at hospital dialysis units.

HEMODIALYSIS

Hemodialysis is performed by a machine with an artificial semipermeable membrane used to filter the blood. This machine is often referred to as an artificial kidney. A graft or fistula is surgically prepared to access the client's circulatory system. Figure 8-11 illustrates several ways this can be done. With each hemodialysis treatment, a catheter is inserted into the graft or fistula. The client's blood is circulated through the semipermeable membrane (Figures 8-12 and 8-13). Excess fluids are removed by osmosis, and by-products of protein metabolism, especially urea and uric acid, as well as creatinine, drugs, and excess electrolytes, are removed from the blood by diffusion or filtration. In return, the client receives fluids, electrolytes, and blood products, as necessary. The solution (dialysate) is especially prescribed to meet the client's metabolic needs.

For the entire process, Standard Precautions must be followed and strict asepsis maintained. The client is weighed before and after each dialysis session to determine if fluid is being retained. It is important to keep the client comfortable and provide diversionary activities during the treatment. Hemodialysis is usually performed 3 times a week and takes 3 to 4 hours each time.

The graft or fistula site requires strict aseptic care and must be assessed daily for signs of infection: redness, swelling, or drainage. Assess circulation through the site by palpation or feeling the area and/or listening with a (Doppler) stethoscope. A thrill should be felt and/or a bruit should be heard. Lack of these signs may indicate a blood clot, which requires immediate surgical attention. Patency must be documented. Assess pulses peripheral to the graft site.

Blood pressure and blood draws are never done on the extremity where the graft or fistula is placed. Also, restraints or intravenous solutions are never applied to or inserted into that extremity. All health care personnel should know the location of the hemodialysis access site. These sites should not be used for any other purpose than dialysis.

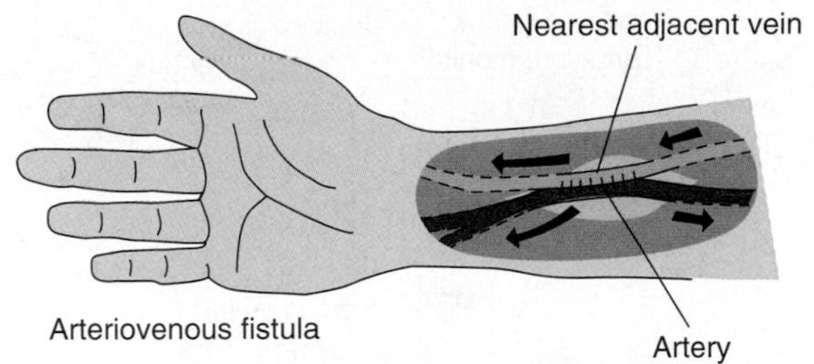

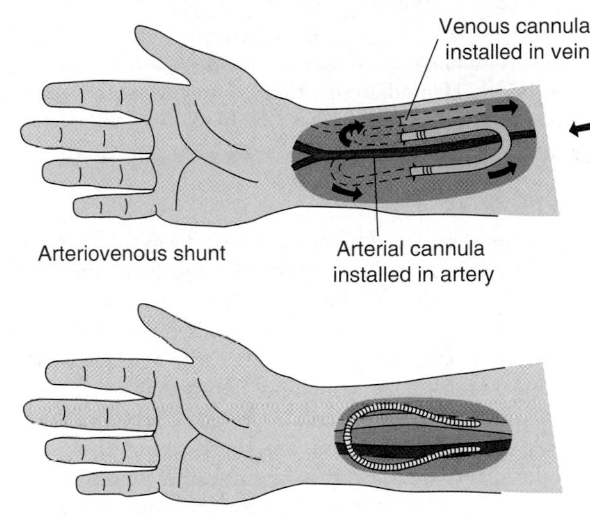

FIGURE 8-11 Types of Hemodialysis Access Sites

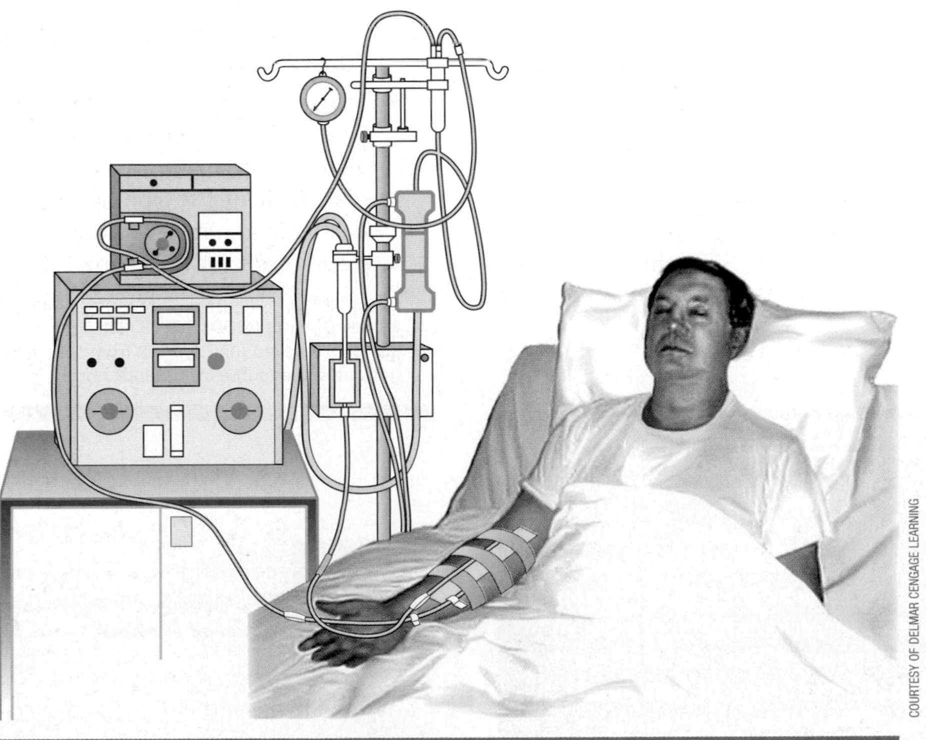

FIGURE 8-12 Client Receiving Hemodialysis

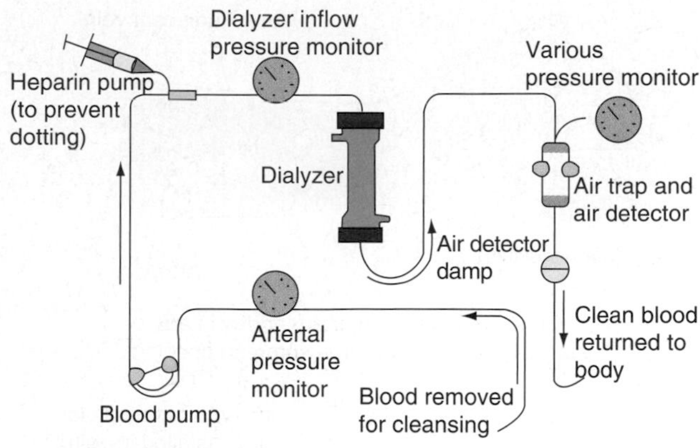

FIGURE 8-13 Hemodialysis (*Adapted from National Institute of Diabetes and Digestive and Kidney Diseases 2006, Treatment Methods for Kidney Failure: Hemodialysis.*)

Because most medications are removed during dialysis, they are generally not administered until after the dialysis session. Vancomycin hydrochloride (Vancocin) is not removed during dialysis and so is often used. If the client is hypertensive before dialysis, nifedipine (Procardia) is given because of its fast action.

Possible complications include hemorrhage, infection, and emboli formation. Some factors for the client and family to consider about hemodialysis are the distance they must travel to the dialysis center, the expense, the time involved, and the presence of a permanent arteriovenous (AV) line. Clients can be taught to do their own hemodialysis at a center. Portable units are being developed to make hemodialysis more usable in the client's home. This is a growing trend with home health care.

Continuous renal replacement therapy (CRRT), a slow, gentle form of dialysis, is available.

PERITONEAL DIALYSIS

Peritoneal dialysis uses the peritoneal lining of the abdominal cavity as the membrane through which diffusion and osmosis occur instead of the artificial kidney machine. It is usually performed 4 times a day or overnight 7 days a week. A Tenckhoff or a flanged-collar catheter is placed by the physician, under aseptic conditions, into the client's peritoneal space. The client must void just before catheter insertion to prevent accidental puncture of the bladder. As with hemodialysis, weigh the client before and after each dialysis session. Also auscultate bowel sounds.

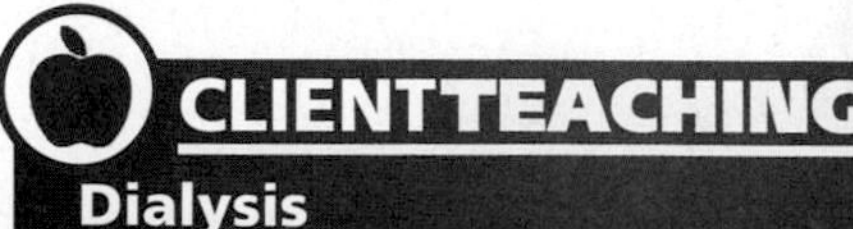

Dialysis

Clients who are receiving dialysis need a significant amount of teaching. All clients should have the process thoroughly explained. Other teaching topics are the importance of physician and laboratory visits, and observations for which the physician needs to be notified. Clients undergoing dialysis should wear Medic Alert tags stating their condition.

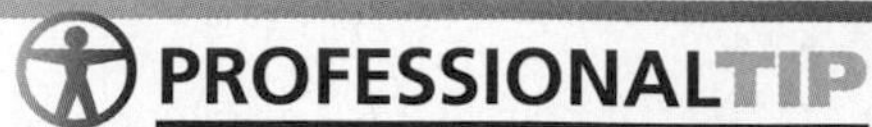

Nutrition for Dialysis Clients

Dialysis clients need to follow strict dietary and fluid guidelines. Listed below is information and discussion of several of these guidelines.

- Refer the client to a dietitian. A dietitian with special training in care for kidney health is called a renal dietitian.
- Monitor and record how much fluid the client drinks and ensure that fluid restrictions are followed as ordered by the physician.
- Teach client to limit or avoid sodium and to eat fresh foods that are naturally low in sodium.
- Potassium levels can rise between dialysis sessions and affect the client's heartbeat. Evaluate serum potassium levels and assess client for cardiac arrhythmias.
- Educate client that foods high in potassium must be avoided or limited as ordered (refer to Chapter 24 for a listing of foods high in potassium). Potassium can be reduced from potatoes and other vegetables by peeling and soaking them in a large container of water for several hours, then dicing or shredding, and cooking in fresh water (Figure 8-14).
- Teach client that foods high in phosphorus should be avoided. The client will probably need to take a phosphate binder such as Renagel, PhosLo, Tums, or calcium carbonate with food to control the serum phosphorus level between dialysis sessions.
- Clients on dialysis are encouraged to eat high-quality protein.
- Instruct client to not take over-the-counter vitamin supplements as they may contain vitamins and minerals that are harmful to dialysis clients. The physician may prescribe a vitamin and mineral supplement such as Nephrocaps for the client.

Adapted from National Institute of Diabetes and Digestive and Kidney Diseases (NIDDK), 2008, Eat right to feel right on hemodialysis, retrieved July 26, 2009 from http://kidney.niddk.nih.gov/kudiseases/pubs/eatright/index.htm

CRITICAL THINKING

Peritoneal Dialysis, Hemodialysis, and Kidney Transplantation

What are the pros and cons for peritoneal dialysis, hemodialysis, and kidney transplantation?

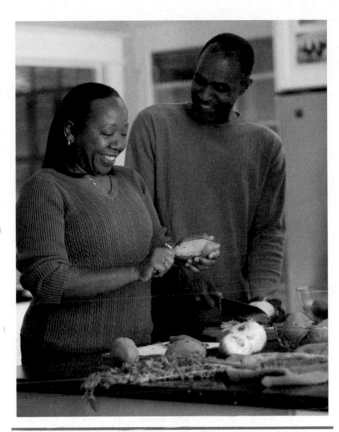

FIGURE 8-14 **Hemodialysis clients need to follow strict dietary guidelines.** (*Courtesy of Centers for Disease Control and Prevention/photo by Cade Martin.*)

The dialysate, held within a sterile soft container similar to an IV bag, is instilled aseptically through the catheter into the abdominal cavity. *To decrease client discomfort, the dialysate should be at body temperature and not instilled too rapidly.* Severe pain should not be experienced. The container, still connected to the catheter, is then rolled up and the dialysate remains in the abdominal cavity for a specified length of time. The client is free to ambulate during this time. The container is then unrolled and lowered below the abdominal cavity to allow the dialysate to drain, by gravity, back into the container. The dialysate now contains excess fluids, nitrogenous waste, and other impurities. The outflow of dialysate is inspected for color, sediments, and amount. The fluid should be light yellow and clear enough to read the printing on the bag when placed on a white towel. Usually 2 liters of dialysate are exchanged each time. If the outflow does not at least equal the inflow, the client is asked to turn from side to side to increase the outflow.

Peritoneal dialysis may be performed manually by the nurse, client, or family member as just described; by a cycler machine; or by continuous ambulatory peritoneal dialysis (CAPD). The cycler machine automatically completes dialysis after sterile setup and connection; CAPD is performed by the client. After the dialysate is aseptically installed, the empty bag is rolled up under the clothing, and the client can go about normal activities. Every 6 to 8 hours, the solution is drained into the bag, which is then discarded following standard precaution guidelines. A new bag of dialysate is attached and instilled. This provides continuous dialysis 24 hours per day, 7 days per week. The client's lifestyle is only minimally disrupted. Peritoneal dialysis is less expensive, easier to perform, less stressful for the client, and almost as effective as hemodialysis.

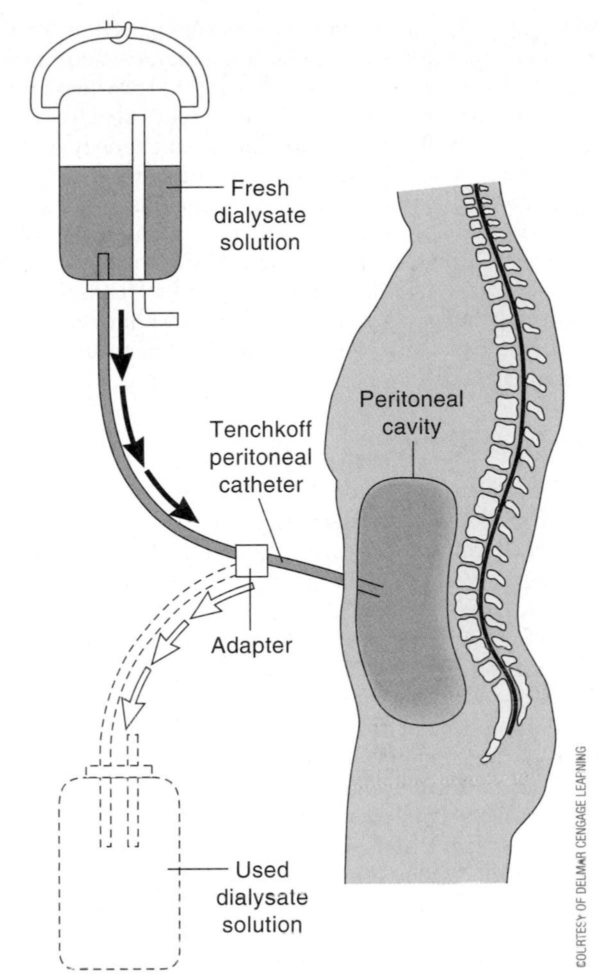

FIGURE 8-15 **Peritoneal Dialysis Setup**

The main complication of peritoneal dialysis is infection. Strict aseptic care of the catheter site is necessary. Standard Precautions are essential in caring for the dialysis client. Figure 8-15 shows a peritoneal dialysis setup.

KIDNEY TRANSPLANTATION

According to the Open Procurement and Transplantation Network (OPTN, 2006), 16,000 kidney transplants will be performed in 2006. Transplants are either from a live donor (usually a relative) or a cadaver. There are approximately 76,000 persons on the waiting list for a kidney transplant (United Network for Organ Sharing, 2008).

Before being placed on the nationwide donor waiting list, the client with ESRD must be tissue- and blood-typed to determine a compatible donor. Insurance coverage varies for this procedure. Lack of funds does not exclude anyone from needed care. Since 1973, an amendment to the Social Security Act allows Medicare to pay 80% of the cost for treating ESRD clients, regardless of age, including dialysis and kidney transplantation.

When a donor kidney becomes available, the client is transported to the transplant medical center. The donor kidney can be preserved for 36 hours in solution or up to 72 hours if it is attached to an irrigating pump with perfusion maintained while en route to the recipient. Through a lower abdominal incision, the surgeon attaches the donor kidney to the client's blood supply. The donor kidney is usually placed in the iliac fossa anterior to the iliac crest. The donor ureter is anastomosed (surgical connection of tubular structure) to the client's ureter or surgically implanted into the client's urinary bladder (Figure 8-16). Generally, the client's nonfunctioning kidney is left in place to reduce the postoperative risk of hemorrhage.

After a couple days of bed rest, the client is allowed increasing activities and, if no complications occur, is discharged in 1 to 3 weeks. Routine nursing care includes monitoring urine output, blood tests, vital signs, and level of consciousness. Encourage turning, coughing, and deep breathing. Assess the incision to ensure that wound closure is intact. In addition, assess for rejection.

Organ Rejection

Signs of rejection include generalized edema, tenderness over the graft site, fever, decreased urine output, hematuria, edema (extremities or eyes), weight gain, oliguria or anuria, and/or an increase in feeling tired. The BUN and creatinine will be elevated.

Immunosuppressive drug therapy is begun to decrease the chance of organ rejection. These drugs include azathioprine (Imuran), cyclophosphamide (Cytoxan), cyclosporine (Sandimmune), and corticosteroids such as prednisone (Meticorten). The scheduling and dosage of these drugs vary with acceptance of the donor kidney and the side effects exhibited by the client. People continue to survive many years with a kidney transplant and maintain a quality life.

Researchers at the University of Cincinnati have discovered a new therapy for transplant clients. The cancer drug, bortezomib, used for cancer of plasma cells, is effective in treating and/or reversing rejection episodes that do not respond to standard therapies (American Association of Kidney Patients, 2009).

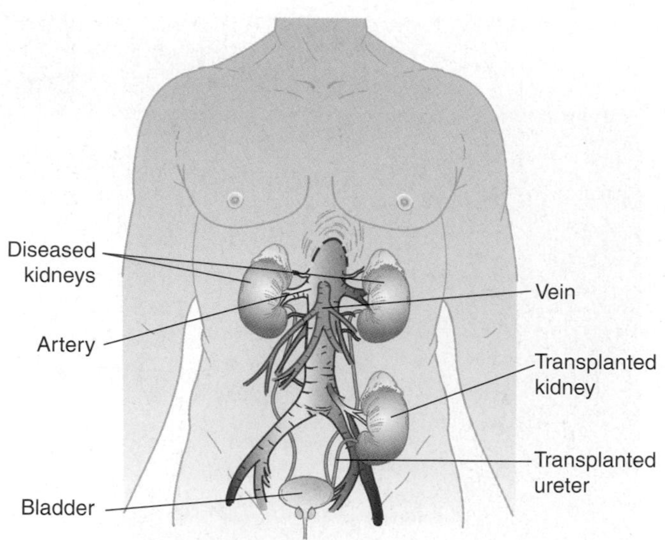

FIGURE 8-16 **Kidney Transplantation** (*Adapted from National Institute of Diabetes and Digestive and Kidney Diseases, 2006, Treatment Methods for Kidney Failure: Transplantation.*)

Complications

The greatest complication in renal transplantation is infection. The immunosuppressive therapy to prevent rejection of the kidney increases the risk and masks the usual signs of infection. The client and family must learn how to recognize these signs of infection. There will be only a slight increase in temperature, development of a cough, low back pain, cloudy urine, or wound drainage. The client must always monitor urine output.

CASE STUDY

A.R., 56, is a client in the extended care facility. She has amyotrophic lateral sclerosis (ALS) with muscle weakness that has progressed and involves her legs and arms. A hydraulic lift is used to transfer her out of bed. A student nurse and a classmate enter with the lift to assist A.R. OOB, when she asks to use the bedpan. As they help her onto the bedpan, they recall that the staff nurse gave A.R. the bedpan about a half hour ago. Returning in a few minutes, they help A.R. off the bedpan and notice the urine is cloudy with a foul odor. A.R. is not on I&O; however, they notice that there is a very small amount of urine. She tells them that she does not know why she is going to the bathroom so often and why her urine smells bad.

The following questions will guide your development of a nursing care plan for the case study.

1. What subjective data should be gathered? What objective data should be gathered?
2. List diagnostic tests that may be ordered.
3. Write two nursing diagnoses for A.R., related to her cystitis/UTI.
4. Write a goal related to each of A.R.'s nursing diagnoses.
5. List pertinent nursing actions for the care of A.R. for each of the following areas as they relate to the cystitis/UTI:
   - elimination—bladder
   - diet and fluids
   - safety, comfort, and rest
   - teaching (client and nursing staff)
6. List two classifications of medications used for the treatment of an UTI.
7. List two successful client outcomes for A.R.

SUMMARY

- The functions of the urinary system are reflected in their relationship with nearly all of the systems in the body.
- Accurate intake and output is imperative for every client with a urinary system disorder.
- Teach proper perineal care, especially to female clients of all ages, about cleansing from front to back.
- Diet management is important for clients with renal calculi, glomerulonephritis, renal failure, and dialysis.
- Encourage an adequate intake of fluids for clients unless fluids are restricted.
- Monitor laboratory test results for BUN, creatinine, and electrolytes.
- Level of consciousness, vital signs, lung sounds, edema, and urine characteristics are important to monitor.
- Strict aseptic care is mandatory for dialysis clients.

REVIEW QUESTIONS

1. A client has been admitted for chronic pyelonephritis. She is jittery and states she is concerned. Which of the following signs would indicate potential kidney damage?
   1. Urine output is 100 mL on your shift.
   2. Blood pressure is decreased with a rapid pulse.
   3. Blood pressure is elevated with a decreased pulse.
   4. BUN and creatinine clearance are within normal limits.
2. A male client, age 64, has had hematuria for several years. He is admitted to your same-day surgical unit scheduled for cystoscopic fulguration. Postoperatively, which of the following would you anticipate?
   1. Blood in the urine.
   2. An elevated temperature.
   3. Hypotension.
   4. Smoky urine.
3. A male client, age 29, had impetigo 2 weeks before his noting a decrease in urine output and urine that "did not look right." His admission diagnosis is acute glomerulonephritis. He is on intake and output with fluid restriction. Which of the following comments indicates knowledge of his nursing care?
   1. "I had my wife empty my urinal."
   2. "My urine still looks pretty bad."
   3. "I put my call light on so you can empty my urinal."
   4. "My wife helped me out of bed, so I urinated in the bathroom."
4. A client with chronic glomerulonephritis is discharged home with home health care. As the LP/VN assigned to her case, you are planning her a.m. care. While preparing the bath supplies, she says, "Please do not use any soap. My skin is so dry and flaky." The rationale for this would be:
   1. kidney failure leads to uremia.
   2. the bladder does not concentrate urine.
   3. her blood sugar is elevated.
   4. confusion leads to comments of this nature.
5. A client is attending classes to be able to do his own peritoneal dialysis. He states he feels well and is eager to continue to learn. He asks if washing his hands before the procedure is important. The best response is:
   1. "Yes, only if you have not done so today."
   2. "Yes, as you want to keep the procedure as clean as possible."
   3. "No, since you just went to the bathroom."
   4. "No, because all the equipment is sterile."
6. A client has been diagnosed with renal carcinoma. The client states, "My husband will leave me if I lose my hair from chemotherapy." What would be the most appropriate answer for this client?
   1. "You seem to be concerned that your relationship with your husband might change."
   2. "You should focus on your disease and not your hair."
   3. "Why don't you wait and see if your husband leaves you before you get too upset."
   4. "Everything is going to be fine. Don't worry about your hair loss."
7. A client has an order for a throat and skin culture; what might the physician be testing for?
   1. Nephrolithiasis.
   2. Glomerulonephritis.
   3. Nephrotic syndrome.
   4. Chronic renal failure.
8. The nurse is teaching a new hemodialysis client about dietary restrictions. Which of the following client statements indicates that further teaching is needed?
   1. "Peeling, dicing up, and boiling potatoes in fresh water when cooking helps to lower the amount of potassium."
   2. "I need to eat high quality protein in my diet."
   3. "Drinking several glasses of orange juice each day will keep me healthy."
   4. "I should only take vitamin supplements prescribed by my physician."
9. A client is scheduled for hemodialysis today and has called to see if she should take her blood pressure pills prior to coming in for the procedure. The nurse should inform the client:
   1. "Take your pills after your procedure is completed."
   2. "It is ok to take your pills prior to coming in for your procedure."

3. "No, do not take your blood pressure pills at all, today."
4. "You can take your blood pressure pills after we get your treatment started. I want to check your blood pressure first."

10. A women presents to the urgent care center with dysuria and hematuria, and states that she has a history of cystitis. The nurse assesses for which of the following symptoms that are indicative of cystitis?

1. Frequency and urgency of urination, flank pain, nausea, and vomiting.
2. Chills and flank pain.
3. Fever, nausea, vomiting and flank pain.
4. Frequency and urgency of urination, suprapubic pain, and foul smelling urine.

REFERENCES/SUGGESTED READINGS

American Association of Kidney Patients. (2009). Cancer drug may treat rejection. Retrieved April 18, 2009 from http://www.aakp.org/newsletters/Kidney-Transplant/January-2009/Drug-May-Treat-Rejection/

American Cancer Society. (2008). Cancer facts and figures 2008. Retrieved April 18, 2009 from http://www.cancer.org/downloads/STT/2008CAFFfinalsecured.pdf

American Cancer Society. (2009a). Detailed guide: Bladder cancer surgery. Retrieved July 25, 2009 from http://www.cancer.org/docroot/CRI/content/CRI_2_4_4X_Surgery_44.asp?rnav=cri

American Cancer Society. (2009b). What are the key statistics for bladder cancer? Retrieved July 25, 2009 from http://www.cancer.org/docroot/CRI/content/CRI_2_4_1X_What_are_the_key_statistics_for_bladder_cancer_44.asp?sitearea=

American Cancer Society. (2009c) What are the key statistics for kidney cancer? Retrieved July 25, 2009 from http://www.cancer.org/docroot/CRI/content/CRI_2_4_1X_What_are_the_key_statistics_for_kidney_cancer_22.asp?sitearea=

American Cancer Society. (2009d). What are the risk factors for bladder cancer? Retrieved July 25, 2009 from http://www.cancer.org/docroot/CRI/content/CRI_2_4_2X_What_are_the_risk_factors_for_bladder_cancer_44.asp?rnav=cri

American Cancer Society. (2009e). What are the risk factors for kidney cancer? Retrieved July 25, 2009 from http://www.cancer.org/docroot/CRI/content/CRI_2_4_2X_What_are_the_risk_factors_for_kidney_cancer_22.asp?rnav=cri

Arbique, J. (2003). Stop UTIs in their tracts. *Nursing2003, 33*(6), 32hn1–32hn4.

Bulechek, G., Butcher, H., McCloskey, J., & Dochterman, J., eds. (2008). *Nursing Interventions Classification (NIC)* (5th ed.). St. Louis, MO: Mosby/Elsevier.

Campbell, D. (2003). How acute renal failure puts the brakes on kidney function. *Nursing2003, 33*(1), 59–63.

Castner, D., & Douglas, C. (2005). Now onstage: Chronic kidney disease. *Nursing2005, 35*(12), 58–63.

Castina, S., Boyington, A., & Dougherty, M. (2002). Urinary incontinence. *AJN, 102*(8), 85–87.

Dowling-Castronovo, A., & Specht, J. (2009). Assessment of transient urinary incontinence in older adults. *American Journal of Nursing, 109*(2), 62–71.

Gray, M., Ratliff, C., & Donovan, A. (2002). Tender mercies: Providing skin care for an incontinent patient. *Nursing2002, 32*(7), 51–54.

Growe, S. (2009). Manuscript submitted for publication. Henderson, NV.

Hayes, D. (2003). Performing peritoneal dialysis. *Nursing2003, 33*(3), 17.

Kaplow, R., & Barry, R. (2002). Continuous renal replacement therapies. *AJN, 102*(11), 26–33.

Kobayashi, M., Nomura, M., Yamada, Y., Fujimoto, N., & Matsumoto, T. (2005). Bladder-sparing surgery and continent urinary diversion using the appendix (Mitrofanoff procedure) for urethral cancer. *International Journal of Urology, 12*(6), 581–584.

Lynch, D. (2004). Cranberry for preventions of urinary tract infections. *American Family Physician, 70*, 2175–2177.

Martchev, D. (2008). Improving quality of life for patients with kidney failure. *RN 71*(4), 31–36.

Martin, C. (2009). Unpublished manuscript. Denver, PA.

Mason, D., Newman, D., & Palmer, M. (2003). Changing UI practice: People have the right to be continent. *AJN, 103*(3), 129.

Mayo Clinic. (2009). Glomerulonephritis treatments and drugs. Retrieved July 24, 2009 from http://www.mayoclinic.com/health/glomerulonephritis/DS00503/DSECTION=treatments-and-drugs

McConnell, E. (2002). Protecting a hemodialysis fistula. *Nursing2002, 32*(11), 18.

Moorhead, S., Johnson, M., Maas, M., & Swanson, E. (2007). *Nursing Outcomes Classification (NOC)* (4th ed.). St. Louis, MO: Mosby.

National Association for Continence (NAFC). (2008). Prevalence. Retrieved from http://www.nafc.org/media/statistics/prevalence-2/

National Institute of Diabetes and Digestive and Kidney Diseases (NIDDK). (2006a). Glomerular Diseases. Retrieved April 18, 2009 from http://kidney.niddk.nih.gov/kudiseases/pubs/glomerular/index.htm

National Institute of Diabetes and Digestive and Kidney Diseases (NIDDK). (2006b). Treatment methods for kidney failure: hemodialysis. Retrieved July 26, 2009 from http://kidney.niddk.nih.gov/kudiseases/pubs/hemodialysis/index.htm

National Institute of Diabetes and Digestive and Kidney Diseases (NIDDK). (2006c). Treatment methods for kidney failure: transplantation. Retrieved July 26, 2009 from http://kidney.niddk.nih.gov/kudiseases/pubs/transplant/index.htm

National Institute of Diabetes and Digestive and Kidney Diseases (NIDDK). (2007a). Kidney stones in adults. Retrieved April 18, 2009, from http://kidney.niddk.nih.gov/kudiseases/pubs/stonesadults/index.htm

National Institute of Diabetes and Digestive and Kidney Diseases (NIDDK). (2007b). Kidney stones: what you need to know. Retrieved April 18, 2009 from http://kidney.niddk.nih.gov/kudiseases/pubs/stones_ES/index.htm

National Institute of Diabetes and Digestive and Kidney Diseases (NIDDK). (2007c). Polycystic kidney disease. Retrieved April 18, 2009 from http://kidney.niddk.nih.gov/kudiseases/pubs/polycystic/index.htm

National Institute of Diabetes and Digestive and Kidney Diseases (NIDDK). (2008). Eat right to feel right on hemodialysis. Retrieved July 26, 2009 from http://kidney.niddk.nih.gov/kudiseases/pubs/eatright/index.htm

National Institutes of Health (NIH). (2006). Kidney infection (pyelonephritis). Retrieved April 18, 2009 from http://www.nlm.nih.gov/medlineplus/ency/article/000522.htm

National Kidney Foundation (NKF). (2003). About kidney disease. Retrieved from www.kidney.org/general/aboutdisease/index.cfm

National Kidney Foundation (NKF). (2008). The problem of kidney and urologic disease. Retrieved April 18, 2009 from www.kidney.org/news/newsroom/fs_new/prblmkd&urologd.cfm

National Kidney Foundation (NKF). (2009a). Diet and kidney stones. Retrieved April 18, 2009 from http://www.kidney.org/atoz/atozItem.cfm?id=41

National Kidney Foundation (NKF). (2009b). How your kidneys work. Retrieved April 18, 2009 from http://www.kidney.org/kidneydisease/howkidneyswrk.cfm#whatare

National Kidney Foundation (NKF). (2009c). Kidney stones. Retrieved April 18, 2009 from http://www.kidney.org/atoz/atozItem.cfm?id=84

National Kidney Foundation (NKF). (2009d). Polycystic kidney disease. Retrieved April 18, 2009 from http://www.kidney.org/atoz/atozItem.cfm?id=102

National Kidney Foundation (NKF). (2009e). Use of herbal supplements in chronic kidney disease. Retrieved April 18, 2009 from http://www.kidney.org/news/newsroom/fs_new/herbalsuppckd.cfm

Newman, D. (2003). Stress urinary incontinence in women. *AJN, 103*(8), 46–55.

Newman, D., & Giovannini, D. (2002). The overactive bladder: A nursing perspective. *AJN, 102*(6), 36–45.

North American Nursing Diagnosis Association International. (2010). *NANDA-I nursing diagnoses: Definitions and classification 2009–2011*. Ames, IA: Wiley Blackwell.

Organ Procurement and Transplantation Network (OPTN). (2006). Scientific registry of transplant recipients annual report. Retrieved April 19, 2009 from www.ustransplant.org/annual_reports/current/107_dh.htm

Paton, M. (2003). Continuous renal replacement therapy. *Nursing2003, 33*(6), 48–50.

Patraca, K. (2005). Measure bladder volume without catheterization. *Nursing 2005, 35*(4), 46–47.

Polt, C. (2006). Taking the pressure off for women with stress incontinence. *Nursing2006, 36*(2), 49–51.

Rice, J. (2002). *Medications and mathematics for the nurse* (9th ed.). Clifton Park, NY: Delmar Cengage Learning.

Roth, R., & Townsend, C. (2002). *Nutrition and diet therapy* (8th ed.). Clifton Park, NY: Delmar Cengage Learning.

Scherer, J., & Timby, B. (2002). *Introductory medical–surgical nursing* (8th ed.). Philadelphia: Lippincott Williams & Wilkins.

Schofield, C. (2002). Patient may have a UTI—What next? *Nursing2002, 32*(10), 17.

Schultz, J. (2002). Urinary incontinence: Solving a secret problem. *Nursing2002, 32*(11), 53–55.

Smith, D. (1999). Gauging bladder volume without a catheter. *Nursing99, 29*(12), 52–53.

Stockert, P. (1999). Getting UTI patients back on track. *RN, 62*(3), 49–52.

Stothers, L. (2002). A randomized trial to evaluate effectiveness and cost effectiveness of naturopathic cranberry products as prophylaxis against urinary tract infection in women. *Canadian Journal of Urology,* (9), 1558–1562.

United Network for Organ Sharing (UNOS). (2008). U.S. transplant waiting list passes *100,000*. Retrieved April 18, 2009 from http://www.unos.org/news/newsDetail.asp?id=1165

Van Snell, S., & Miller-Anderson, M. (2007). Stress incontinence: It's no laughing matter. *RN, 70*(4), 25–29.

Wetherbee, S. (2006). New weapons to snuff out kidney cancer. *Nursing2006 36*(12), 58–63.

Williams, L., & Hopper, P. (2003). *Understanding medical surgical nursing*. (2nd ed.). Philadelphia: F. A. Davis.

Zabat, E. (2003). When your patient needs peritoneal dialysis. *Nursing2003, 33*(8), 52–54.

RESOURCES

American Association of Kidney Patients, http://www.aakp.org

American Foundation for Urologic Disease, http://www.afud.org

American Society of Nephrology, http://www.asn-online.org

Bard, C.R. Bard, Inc., http://www.crbard.com

Interstitial Cystitis Association, http://www.ichelp.org

Medic Alert® Foundation, http://www.medicalert.org

National Association for Continence (NAFC), http://www.nafc.org

National Kidney and Urologic Diseases Information Clearinghouse, http://www.kidney.niddk.nih.gov

National Kidney Foundation, http://www.kidney.org

Polycystic Kidney Disease Foundation, http://www.pkdcure.org

The Simon Foundation for Continence, http://www.simonfoundation.org

UNIT 4 Nursing Care of the Client: Mobility, Coordination, and Regulation

CHAPTER 9
Musculoskeletal System

MAKING THE CONNECTION

Refer to the following chapters to increase your understanding of the musculoskeletal system:

Adult Health Nursing

- ***Oncology***
- ***Cardiovascular System***
- ***Immune System***
- ***The Older Adult***

LEARNING OBJECTIVES

Upon completion of this chapter, you should be able to:

- Define key terms.
- List the diagnostic tests used in the evaluation of orthopedic disorders and diseases.
- Describe preventive nursing care of the orthopedic client (e.g., positioning, mobility).
- Identify the various types of casts used in the treatment of orthopedic disorders.
- Describe nursing care of clients with orthopedic devices.
- List four types of fractures and their related treatment.
- Discuss the nursing care of the client undergoing a total hip replacement.
- Utilize the nursing process to plan nursing care including physical and emotional needs of the orthopedic client.

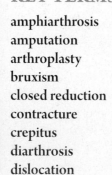

KEY TERMS

amphiarthrosis
amputation
arthroplasty
bruxism
closed reduction
contracture
crepitus
diarthrosis
dislocation
fracture
Heberden's nodes
internal fixation
kyphosis
locomotor
lordosis
open reduction
orthopedics
osteoporosis
paresthesia
phantom limb pain
scoliosis
sprain
strain
subluxation
synarthrosis
tophi
windowing

INTRODUCTION

Orthopedics, also spelled orthopaedics, is the branch of medicine that deals with the prevention or correction of the disorders and diseases of the musculoskeletal system. It involves the muscles, skeleton, joints, and supporting structures such as ligaments and tendons.

The prime concern of the nurse caring for a client with **locomotor** (pertaining to movement or the ability to move) disorders is the prevention of **contractures** (permanent shortening of a muscle) or deformities. The objective of all caregivers is to maintain good body alignment, preserve muscle tone, prevent disuse, and continue joint motion for the client with acute or long-term therapeutic or rehabilitative needs. Caring for orthopedic clients also requires an understanding of basic principles that apply to all clients whether they are in traction, casts, or recovering from surgery.

ANATOMY AND PHYSIOLOGY REVIEW

The musculoskeletal system consists of bones, muscles, tendons, ligaments, cartilage, and joints. When it is functioning properly, the musculoskeletal system allows an individual to stand erect and ambulate. Figure 9-1 identifies the bones of the skeleton.

The skeletal system consists of bones attached to each other by cartilage and strong ligaments. The functions of the skeleton are to:

- Provide the body with structural framework
- Act as a protective casing for internal organs such as the brain, heart, and lungs
- Allow movement by muscles attached to the skeleton
- Store calcium, phosphorus and magnesium and release these minerals when the body requires them
- Manufacture blood cells in the red bone marrow

Bones in the skeletal system are classified as long, short, flat, or irregular. Examples include the humerus, a long bone; the phalanges of the finger, short bone; occiput, flat bone; and the vertebrae, irregular bone. Figure 9-2 illustrates these bones.

There are two types of bone. One type of bone is *cancellous*, which resembles a sponge with spaces and is found in the epiphysis or end of the long bones as well as in all other bones. The other type is *cortical* bone, which is compact bone and is found in the diaphysis or shaft of the long bones. Short bones consist of cancellous bone covered by a layer of compact bone. Flat bones are made of cancellous bone layered between

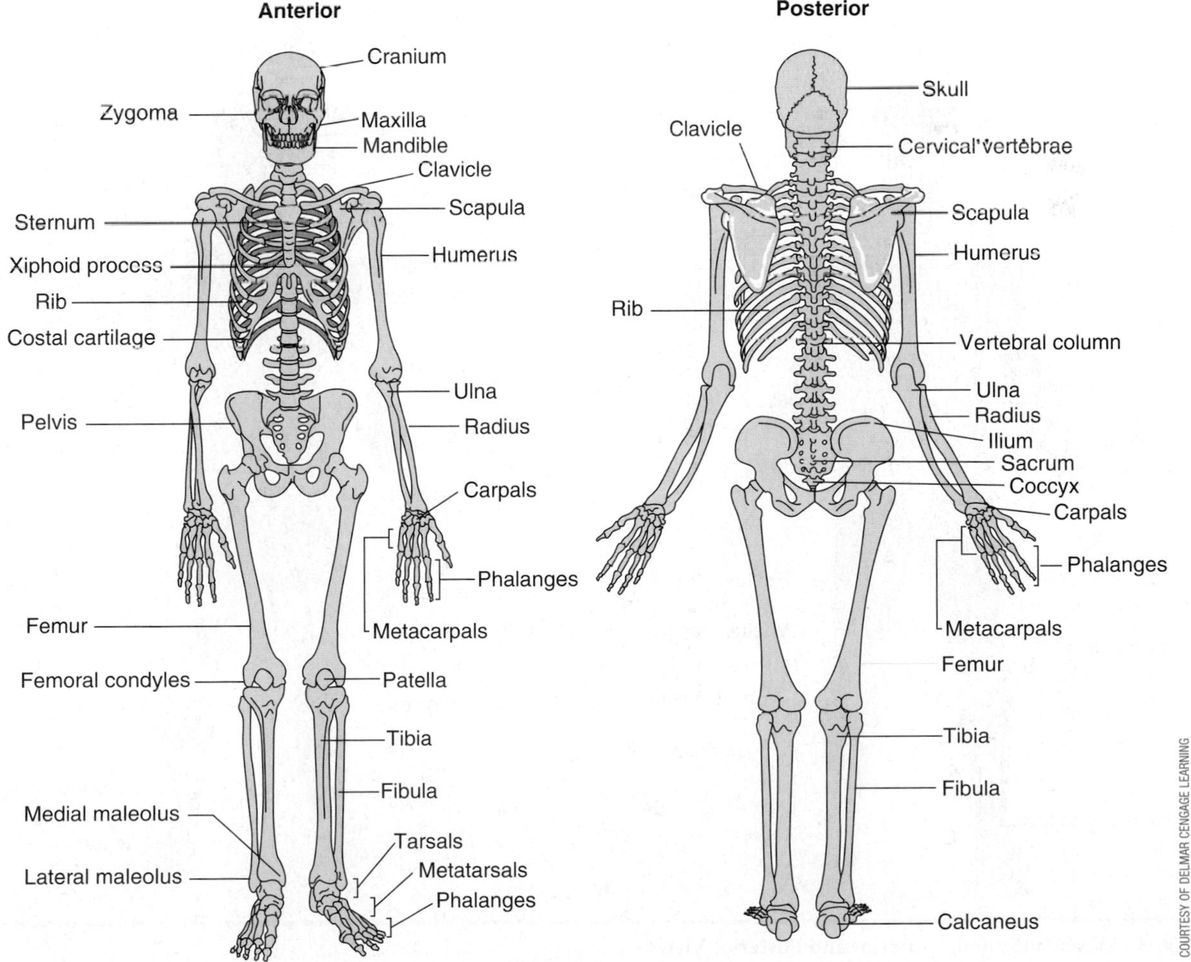

FIGURE 9-1 Anterior and Posterior Views of the Adult Human Skeleton

compact bone. Generally, the makeup of irregular bones is similar to that of flat bones.

The muscular system is composed of muscle fibers and tendons innervated by nerves (Figure 9-3). The muscle fibers vary in size and shape and are arranged according to a muscle's function. The muscles act as motors controlled by nerve impulses from the cerebral cortex. The muscles and the skeleton work together to permit body movement. Muscles are attached to bones by tendons.

The action of muscles is to contract or shorten. Muscles are arranged within the body as opposing pairs to act as antagonists to each other. For example, the biceps flex the forearm and the triceps extend it.

Muscles are surrounded and divided by fibrous envelopes called fascia. In the extremities, the muscles surround and give support to main blood vessels and nerves. Muscles also give support to and keep the body erect as well as give shape to the body.

Movement of the muscles may be either voluntary or involuntary. Muscles attached to bone can function at the will of the person (voluntary). Involuntary muscles, found within body organs, regulate the physical activity of the organs so the organs can perform their functions. These actions are not under the person's control. Involuntary muscles are located in the intestinal tract, the pupil of the eye, and in the heart and blood vessels.

A joint is a junction of two or more bones. There are three types of joints: diarthrosis, synarthrosis, and amphiarthrosis. **Diarthrosis** joints are freely movable, such as the hinge (elbow, knee), ball and socket (hip and shoulder), pivot (skull and first vertebrae), gliding (wrist), and saddle (thumb). **Synarthrosis** joints are immovable, such as the

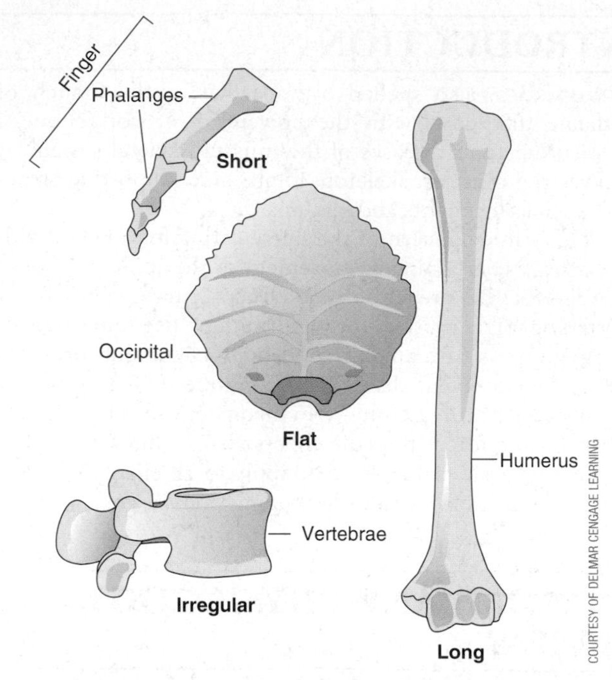

FIGURE 9-2 Bone Shape Classification

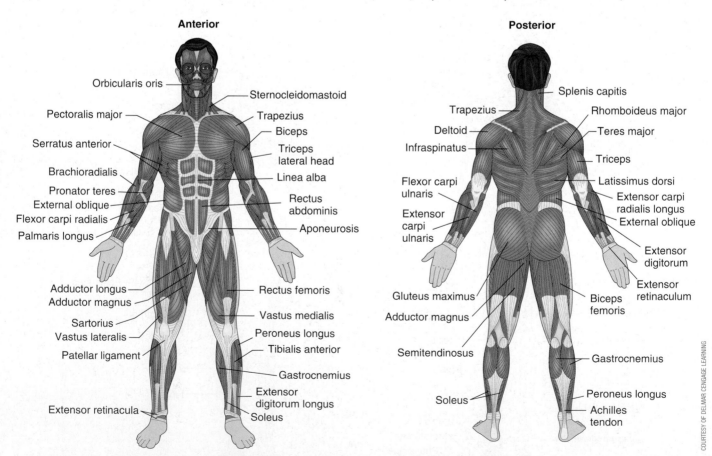

FIGURE 9-3 Muscular System: Anterior and Posterior Views

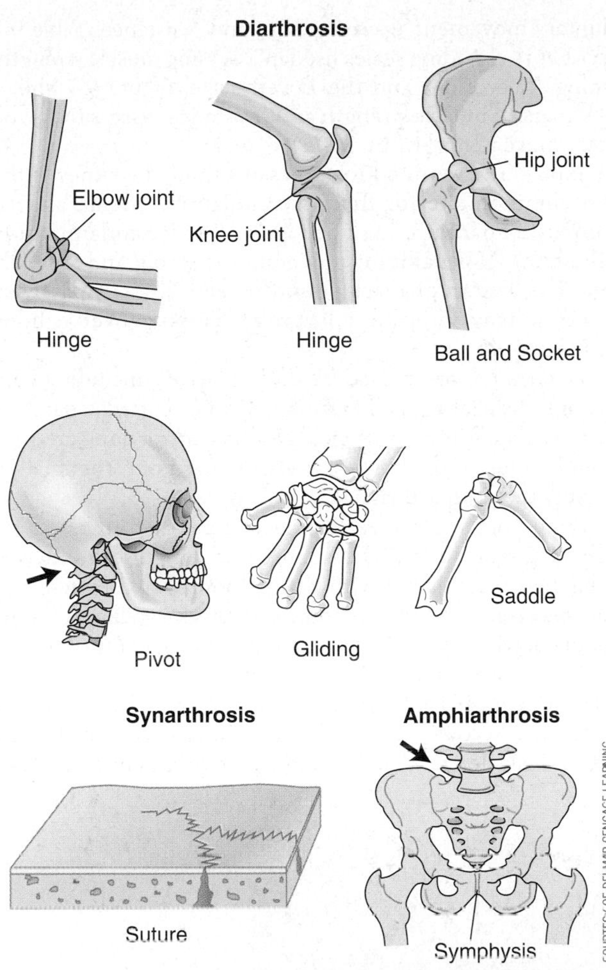

FIGURE 9-4 Joints Classified by the Degree of Movement Permitted

suture line between the temporal and occipital bones of the skull. **Amphiarthrosis** joints are slightly movable, such as the vertebrae and pelvic bones separated by fibrous cartilage. Figure 9-4 illustrates types of joints.

The ends of articulating joints are covered with a smooth articular cartilage. The joint capsule is composed of an outer fibrous layer and an inner synovial layer that secretes synovial fluid. This clear fluid acts as a lubricating fluid for the joints.

Other structures related to the musculoskeletal system include bursa, fascia, tendons, and ligaments. Bursae are sacs filled with fluid that facilitate joint movement by making it possible for muscles and tendons to move or glide over ligaments or bones. Fascia is connective tissue that covers a muscle. Tendons are strong fibrous tissue attaching muscle to bones, providing mobility. Ligaments grow out of the periosteum and lash bones together more firmly.

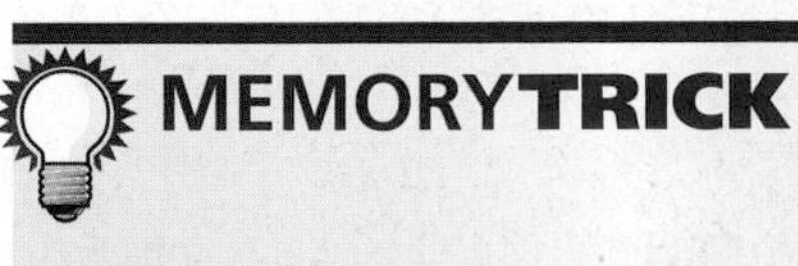

MEMORYTRICK

Tendons **tend** to bind muscles to bones, and ligaments bind bone to bone.

ASSESSMENT

Assessment of the musculoskeletal system ranges from a basic assessment of functional abilities done by the nurse to a complete physical exam by the physician for diagnosis of specific muscle and joint disorders. The extent of the physical exam depends on the client's symptoms, health history, and any other physical signs.

Inspect and palpate to evaluate bone integrity, posture, joint function, muscle strength, and gait. Also assess the client's ability to perform basic activities of daily living.

The medical history includes information on any past medical or surgical disorders and any symptoms relative to onset, duration, or location of discomfort or pain. Ask if activity makes symptoms better or worse. A family medical history should also be obtained.

Assessment of the bony skeleton includes notation of deformities, body alignment, abnormal growths, shortened extremities, amputations, abnormal angulation other than at the joints, and **crepitus**, a grating or crackling sensation or sound.

Assessment of the spine necessitates exposure of the client's back, buttocks, and legs for adequate visualization. Note differences in the height of the shoulders or iliac crests. Gluteal folds should appear symmetrical. The vertebral column should be straight and perpendicular to the floor, with the spine convex through the thoracic portion and concave through the cervical/lumbar portion.

Three common spinal curvatures are scoliosis, kyphosis, and lordosis. A lateral curving deviation is known as **scoliosis**. Scoliosis is seen most frequently in school-age children and adolescents. **Kyphosis** (hump back) is seen as an increased roundness of the thoracic spinal curve. This condition is frequently seen in older persons with osteoporosis. **Lordosis** (sway back) is an exaggeration of the lumbar spine curvature as seen in pregnancy as a woman's body adjusts its center of gravity. These three curvatures are illustrated in Figure 9-5.

Assessment of the articular system includes range of motion (limited, active, and passive), stability of joints, deformities and any nodular formation, and pulses in the extremities. Normal ranges of motion (ROM) are shown in Figure 9-6. Assess for the angle of the joint movement; presence of pain, tenderness, and crepitus; and client's ability to move joint by self through full range of motion (active), with limited movement (limited), or with assistance only (passive) (Estes, 2006). When assessing passive ROM, remember to keep the motion steady and avoid causing any pain.

ROM includes assessment of the client's ability to change position, muscle strength and coordination, and the size of individual muscles. Assess muscle groups for strength and equality with the client using the movements of ROM. Compare the right and left muscles in strength and size. Normal muscle strength is equal bilaterally. Assess if the client has

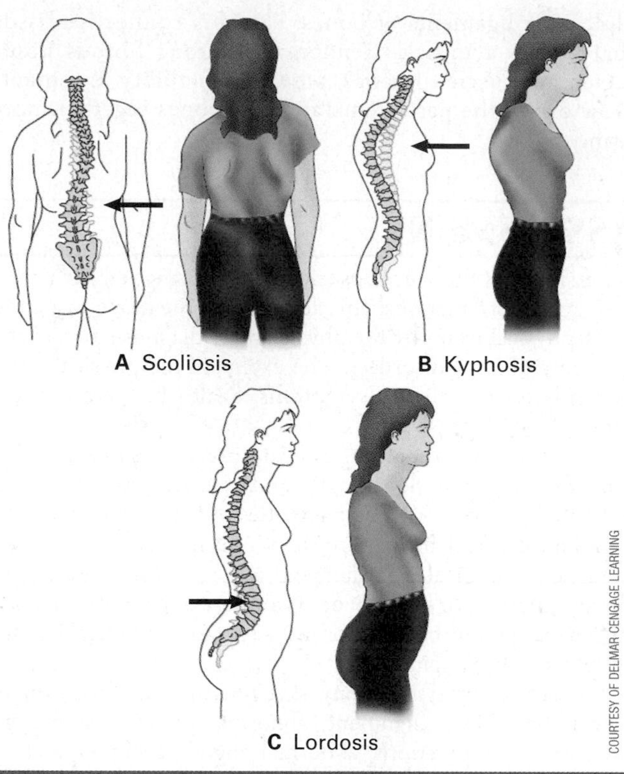

FIGURE 9-5 Curvatures of the Spine

voluntary movement against gravity and resistance. Table 9-1 describes two grading scales used in assessing muscle strength; grading scale of 0-5 and the Lovett scale. Figure 9-7 shows assessment of muscle strength and resistance. Assess for involuntary movements (Estes, 2006).

Joints are examined for excessive fluid. The knee is the most common site for fluid accumulation. Edema and an elevated temperature may be signs of active inflammation in the joint. Normal joint movement is stable and smooth. If there is a snap or crack sound when a joint is passively moved, it may indicate a ligament slipping over a bony prominence.

Deformities are caused by several factors, including contractures, dislocations, and **subluxation** (a partial separation of an articular [joint] surface). Nodular formations are produced by musculoskeletal diseases such as gout, rheumatoid arthritis, and osteoarthritis.

Pulse points in the extremities are palpated to assess for weak or absent pulses. The strength of the pulse in affected extremities is compared with that of nonaffected extremities. Note skin color and temperature and check capillary refill by pressing down on the client's fingernail or toenail for a few seconds, then release and note the time it takes for the client's nail to return to normal color. The color should return immediately (less than 2 seconds); if a client has an arterial disorder, the color will take longer than 2 seconds to return to normal. Refer

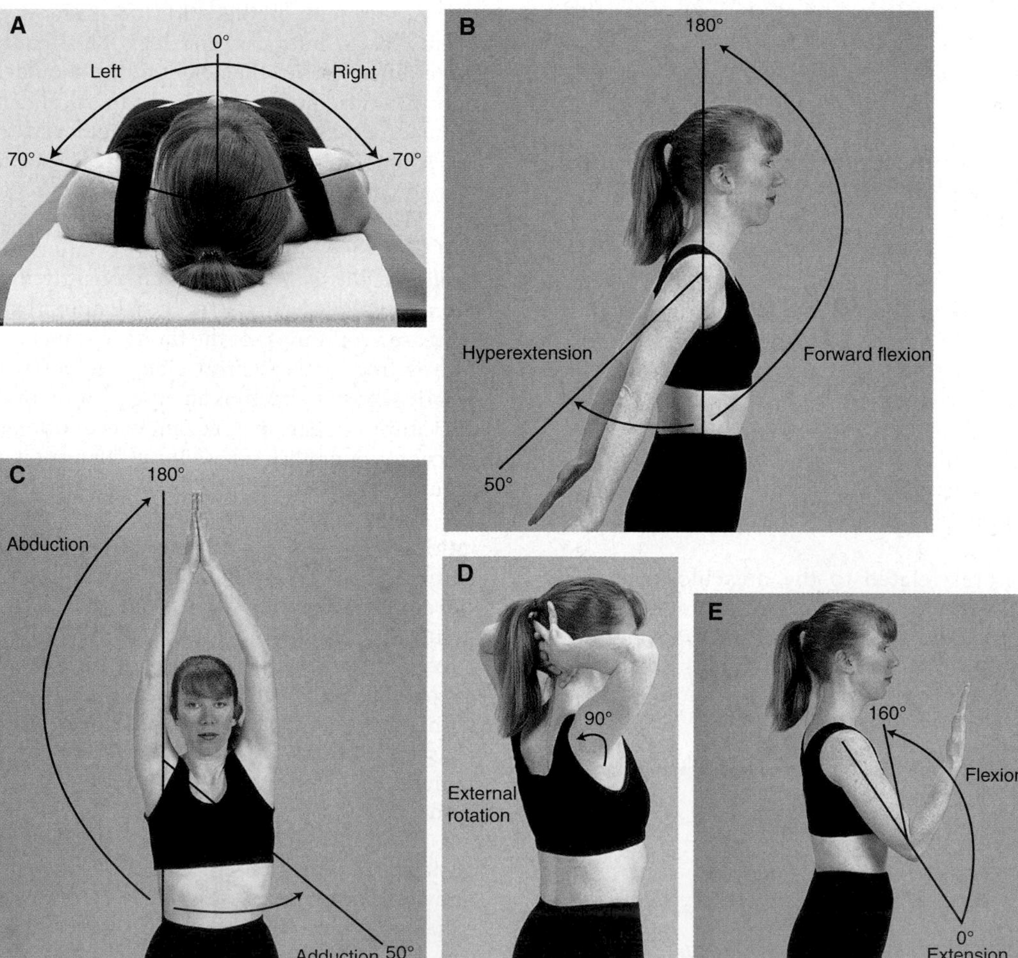

FIGURE 9-6 Range of Joint Motion; *A*, Cervical Spine Rotation; *B*, Shoulder Flexion and Hyperextension; *C*, Shoulder Abduction and Adduction; *D*, Shoulder Rotation; *E*, Elbow Flexion and Extension (*Continues*)

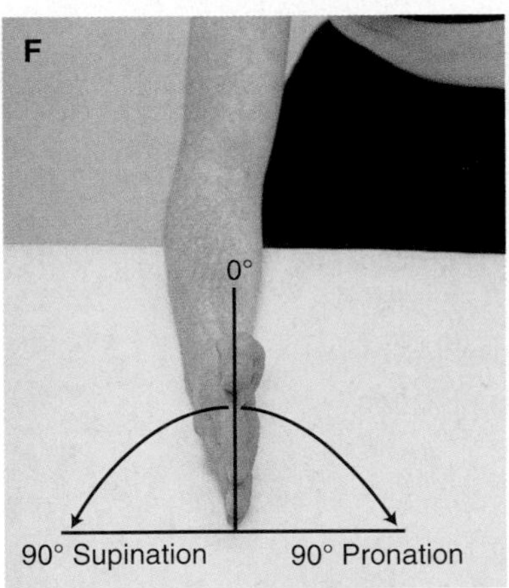

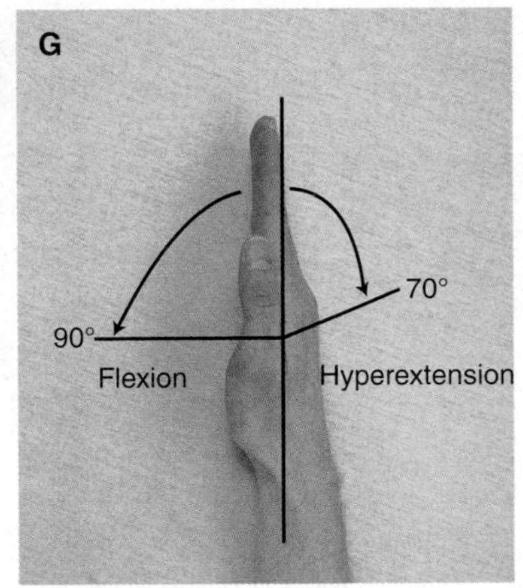

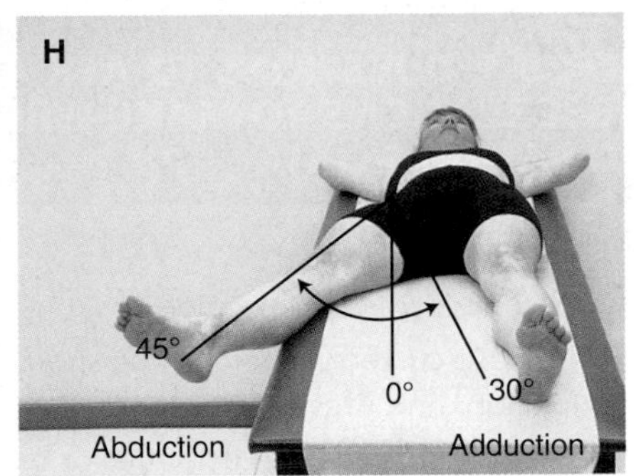

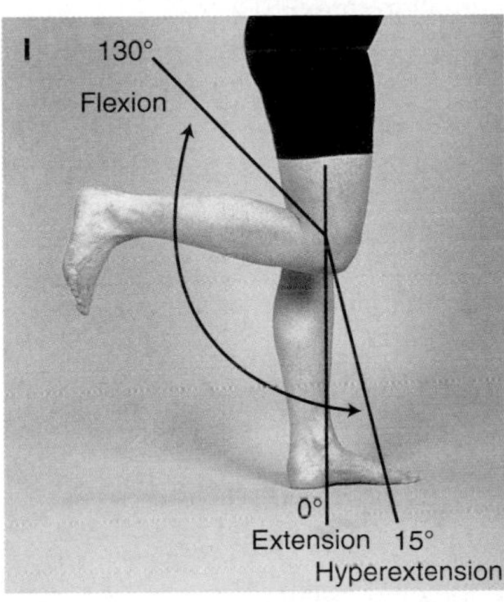

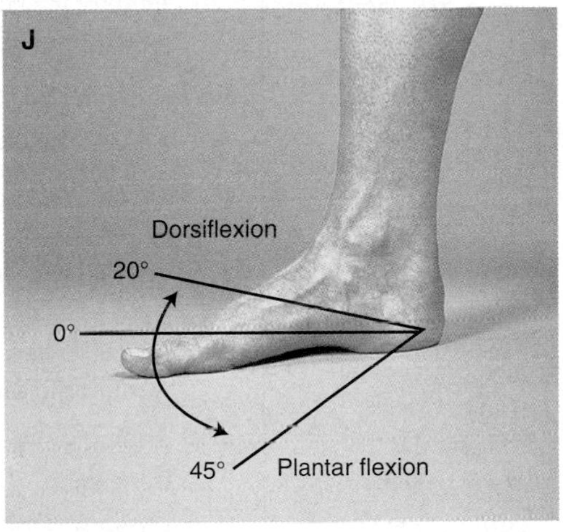

PHOTOS COURTESY OF DELMAR CENGAGE LEARNING

FIGURE 9-6 (Continued) *F,* Elbow Supination and Pronation; *G,* Wrist Flexion and Hyperextension; *H,* Hip Abduction and Adduction; *I,* Knee Flexion, Extension, and Hyperextension; *J,* Dorsiflexion and Plantar Flexion

TABLE 9-1 Assessing Muscle Strength

GRADING	DESCRIPTION	LOVETT SCALE
0	No contraction	Zero (0)
1	Slight contraction	Trace (T)
2	Full ROM with gravity eliminated (passive motion)	Poor (P)
3	Full ROM with gravity	Fair (F)
4	Full ROM against gravity, some resistance	Good (G)
5	Full ROM against gravity, full resistance	Normal (N)

Adapted from Assessing the Musculoskeletal System, by S. Wise, in press, and Caring and Clinical Decision Making (2nd ed.). Clifton Park, NY: Delmar Cengage Learning.

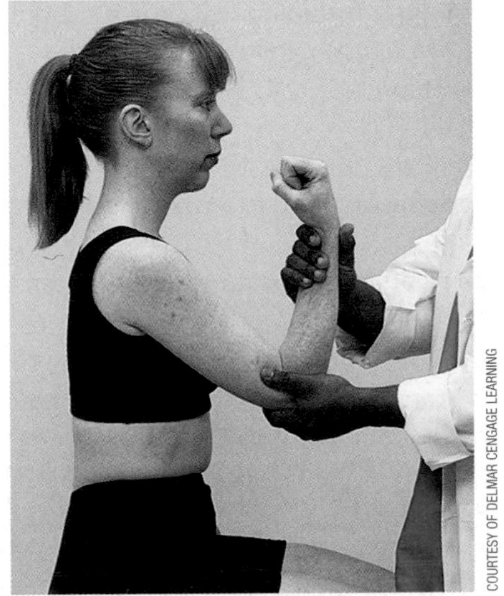

COURTESY OF DELMAR CENGAGE LEARNING

FIGURE 9-7 Assessment of Muscle Strength

to Box 9-1 for guidance in completing client musculoskeletal assessments.

BOX 9-1 QUESTIONS TO ASK AND OBSERVATIONS TO MAKE WHEN COLLECTING DATA

Subjective Data

What is your current occupation?

Describe your current activity level, sport participation, and lifestyle.

What leisure or recreation activities or exercise regimen do you enjoy?

Have you gained or lost any weight over the last few months?

Describe a typical 3-day diet.

Do you need assistance to care for yourself? Assistance to the bathroom? Assistance cleaning house? If the answer is yes, ask: Who is available to assist you with mobility or self-care activities?

Do you have any pain?

Do you take any medication for pain?

Have you ever broken any bones?

Have you gone to a chiropractor or masseuse for treatment?

Does muscle or joint pain or discomfort have an adverse impact on your ability to sleep and rest?

Tell me how you feel about yourself.

Do you feel in control of your life?

Tell me about your relationship with your spouse and family

Objective Data

Obtain vital signs, including height and weight. Compare to ideal body weight chart.

Assess the volume (1+, 2+, 3+, 4+) of peripheral pulses.

Observe the gait, use of assistive devices, and range of motion. Is the ability to transfer or ambulate limited?

Observe body build and posture. Visually scan the body for deformities.

Assess muscle strength according to grading scale.

Visually scan the body for symmetry, contour, and size of muscles, and muscle atrophy. Clients must be assessed bilaterally to compare one extremity or muscle group with the other side.

Assess for crepitus.

Assess for swelling and tenderness.

Assess for pain on a scale of 1–10, with 0 being no pain and 10 being the worst pain ever felt.

Assess ROM of joints.

Adapted from Wise (2008).

TABLE 9-2 Common Diagnostic Tests for Clients with Musculoskeletal Disorders

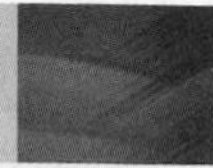

Laboratory Tests

Alkaline phosphatase (ALP)
Aspartate aminotransferase (AST)
Aldolase (ALD)
Antinuclear antibodies (ANA)
Complete blood count (CBC)

- WBC
- Hg

C-reactive protein (CRP)
Creatine kinase (CK-MM)
Erythrocyte sedimentation rate (ESR)
Lactate dehydrogenase (LDH)
Rheumatoid factor (RF)
Serum calcium
Serum phosphorus
Uric acid

- serum
- urine

Radiologic Studies

Arthrogram/graphy
Bone scan
Computed tomography (CT scan)
Dual energy x-ray absorptiometry scan (DEXA)
Electromyography (EMG)
Indium (white blood cell) scan
Magnetic resonance imaging (MRI)
Myelogram
Radiography (x-ray)

Other Tests

Arthrocentesis
Arthroscopy
Joint aspiration
Somatosensory evoked potentials (Evoked potentials)

COMMON DIAGNOSTIC TESTS

Commonly used diagnostic tests for clients with symptoms of musculoskeletal system disorders are listed in Table 9-2.

MUSCULOSKELETAL TRAUMA

Trauma to the musculoskeletal system causes a variety of injuries to clients of all ages. Such injuries include strains, sprains, dislocations, fractures, and compartment syndrome.

CRITICAL THINKING

Client Assessment

After reading the anatomy and physiology and assessment sections of the text, examine the accompanying photo of a client.

1. Identify the anatomical abnormality.
2. List the variations from the norm that you identify.

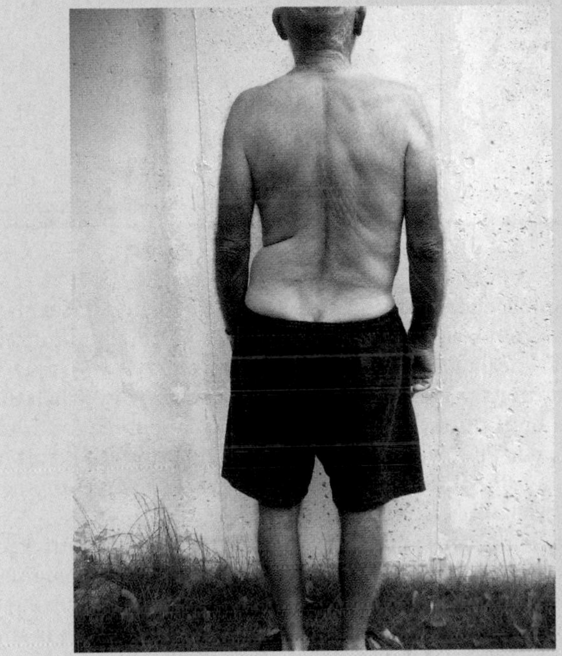

(Courtesy of Dick Hill. Photo by Susan Hill.)

STRAIN

A **strain** is an injury to a muscle or tendon caused by overuse or overstretching. A strain may be either acute or chronic. An acute strain may be caused when an individual performs unaccustomed exercises vigorously. A chronic strain may develop after repeated overuse of certain muscles. Individuals with acute strains experience sudden severe pain, whereas the onset is gradual in chronic strains, with the affected part feeling only stiff and sore.

Chronic strains require no specific treatment, but acute strains require rest and possibly immobilization. Immediately after injury, apply cold packs for 20- to 30-minute periods, and then remove for 1 hour during a 24-hour period to reduce any edema. Then apply heat for the client's comfort. In the case of a severe strain when the muscle may be completely ruptured, surgical repair may be necessary.

SPRAIN

A **sprain** is an injury to ligaments surrounding a joint caused by a sudden twist, wrench, or fall. Symptoms include pain, edema, loss of motion, and ecchymosis. X-ray will reveal soft tissue edema but no evidence of joint or bone injury. Immediate treatment is RICE (rest, ice, compression, and elevation). The client rests and ice is applied to the injured area. The part may then be immobilized with an elastic compression bandage or a brace and elevated. After the edema has decreased significantly, a cast may be applied.

DISLOCATION

Dislocation occurs when articular surfaces of a joint are no longer in contact. The bones are literally "out of joint." The displaced bone may hinder the blood supply, damage nerves, tear ligaments, or rupture muscle attachments. Traumatic dislocations are considered orthopedic emergencies. Congenital dislocations are present at birth, whereas spontaneous or pathologic dislocations are caused by diseases affecting joints.

Symptoms of a dislocation include localized joint pain, loss of function of the joint, and a change in the length of the extremity and contour of the joint. Diagnosis is based on the symptoms, physical exam, and x-rays. X-rays reveal either a complete or partial separation of the articulating surfaces.

FRACTURE

A **fracture** is a break in the continuity of a bone. Fractures occur when the forces from outside the body are greater than the strength of the bone, causing the bone to break. Fractures usually involve soft tissue (edema and bleeding), damaged nerves, and tendons. Most fractures are caused by accidents. These may be the result of direct force, torsion or twisting, or violent contractions of highly developed muscles. Other fractures may be the result of a disease process that weakens the bone. This type of fracture is known as *pathologic* or *spontaneous*. Individuals considered at high risk for fractures include those who have predisposing bone conditions such as metastatic or primary bone tumors or osteoporosis, poor coordination, diminished vision, dizzy spells, or general weakness.

There are more than 90 different classifications of fractures. Some of the more common types include greenstick or incomplete, simple or closed, compound or open, impacted or telescoped, spiral, comminuted, compression, and stress or fatigue.

In a *greenstick* fracture, the continuity of the bone is not completely disrupted but has splintering on one side and bending on the other. This fracture is seen most frequently in children. An uncomplicated (clean) fracture in which the skin remains intact is called a *closed or simple* fracture; the fractured surfaces are not contaminated by outside air. In a *compound or open* fracture, the bone is broken and the skin is also broken, allowing the bone to protrude and be susceptible to a greater chance for infection. An *impacted* fracture is also called a telescoped fracture; one portion of a bone fragment is forcibly driven into another. A *spiral* fracture twists around the shaft of the bone. This type of fracture may occur from a twisting force. In a *comminuted* fracture, the bone is splintered into many unaligned fragments. A *compression* fracture usually occurs when a bone, such as a vertebra, becomes weakened from osteoporosis. A fall or lifting excess weight causes a compression or crushing of the vertebral body (Zdeblick, 2009). *Stress or fatigue* fractures occur from repetitive overuse of a bone and are one of the five most common injuries of runners (Reeser, 2007). Various types of fractures are shown in Figure 9-8.

Healing time for fractures is affected by the age of the client and the type of injury or any underlying disease process, and may take weeks, months, or even years before healing is complete. The average healing time for an uncomplicated fracture is 6 to 8 weeks. The sequence of healing takes place

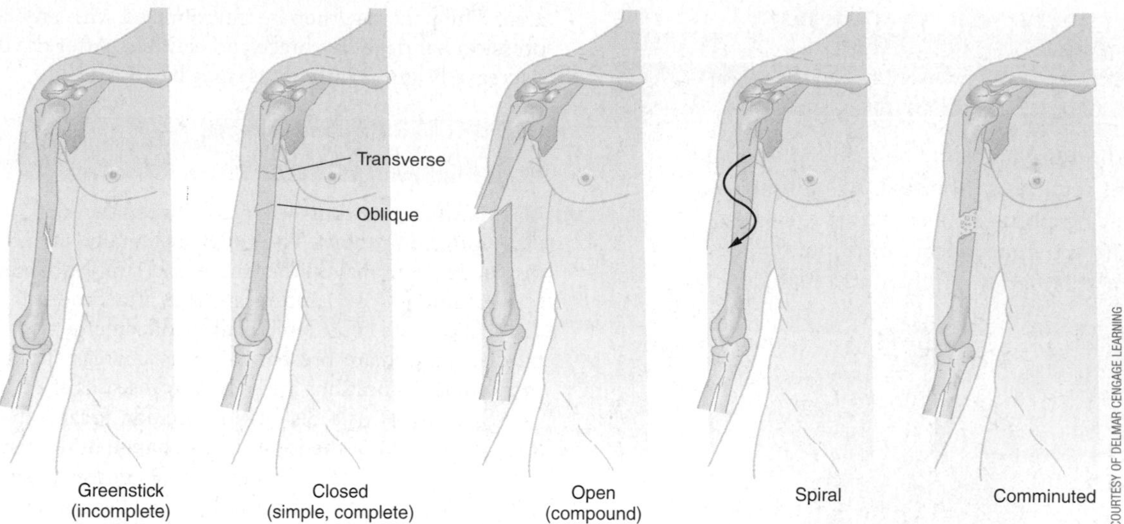

FIGURE 9-8 Classifications of Common Bone Fractures

beginning with the formation of a hematoma, then granulation tissue formation, callus formation, callus ossification, and ultimately remodeling.

Hematoma formation begins with the formation of a clot that serves as a fibrin network. Bleeding comes from ruptured vessels within the bone as well as from tears in the periosteum and adjacent tissues. The hematoma is not absorbed but develops into granulation tissue. Granulation tissue forms a soft tissue callus that surrounds the fracture site and serves as a temporary splint. Callus ossification is the result of deposits of calcium salts in the callus forming rigid bone in excess as a protective measure. The formation of bone binds the bone ends together. Remodeling is completed by osteoclastic activity, whereby excess bone is gradually reduced and removed by absorption until the original shape and outline of the fractured bone is reestablished. Figure 9-9 outlines the healing sequence.

Complications of a fracture include infection, fat embolism syndrome, and compartment syndrome. Complications may delay healing or be life threatening.

Infections may result from an open fracture in which the bone extends through the skin, allowing contamination from the outside. They may also occur following surgical repair of a fracture using an internal fixation device. Any infection may lead to a delayed union of the bone.

Fat embolism syndrome is usually associated with fractures of the long bones, multiple fractures, or crushing injuries. An embolus usually occurs within 24 to 72 hours following a fracture but may occur up to a week after injury. Much is still unclear about how a fat embolism occurs (Walls, 2002). When a small area of the lungs is involved, the symptoms are pain, tachycardia, and dyspnea. Larger areas of lung involvement produce more pronounced symptoms, including severe pain, dyspnea,

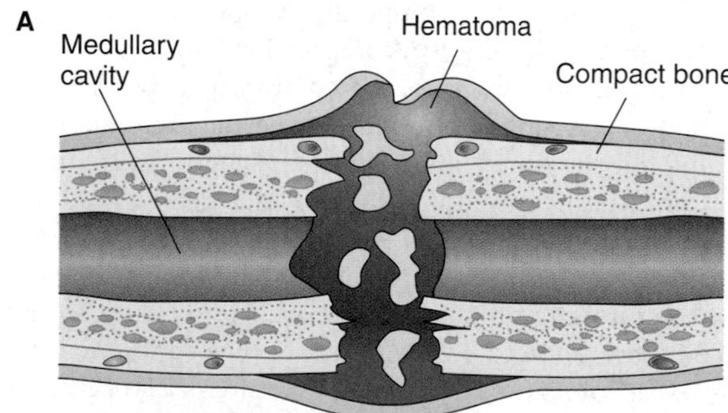

A hematoma forms from blood from ruptured vessels.

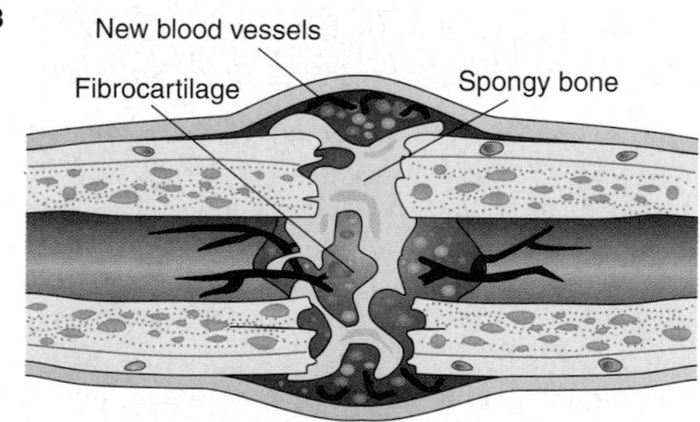

Spongy bone forms close to developing blood vessels; fibrocartilage forms away from new blood vessels.

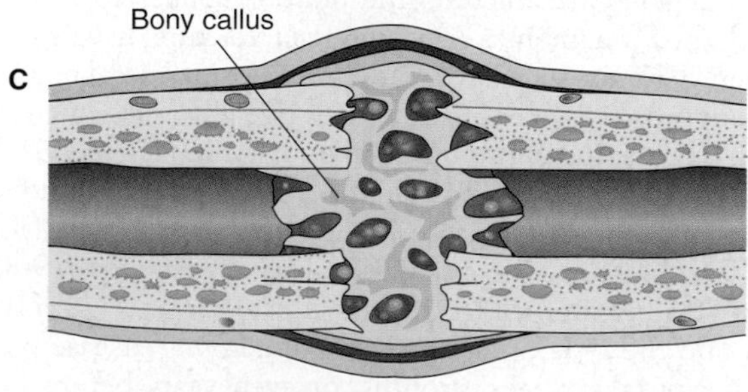

Bony callus replaces fibrocartilage.

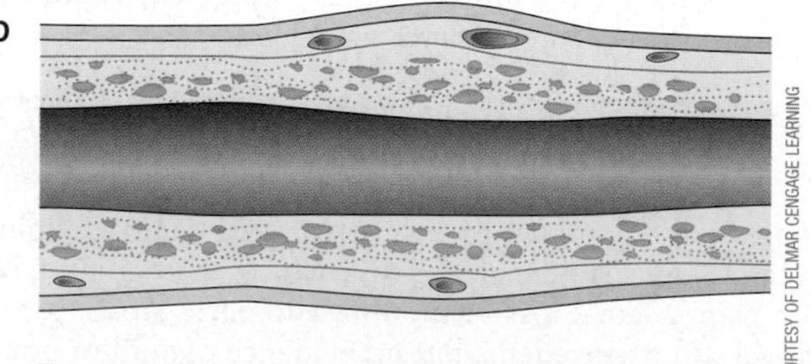

Excess bony tissue is removed by osteoclasts.

FIGURE 9-9 Steps of Bone Repair

cyanosis, restlessness, and shock. Petechiae may appear over the neck, upper arms, chest, or abdomen. Treatment consists of bed rest, respiratory support, oxygen, and IV fluids.

MEDICAL–SURGICAL MANAGEMENT

Medical

The treatment of a fracture requires immediate attention. The most important objectives are to (1) realign the fracture, (2) maintain the alignment, (3) regain the function of the injured part, and (4) prevent complications. The method of treatment depends on the first aid given; the site, severity, and type of the fracture; and the age and condition of the client.

Closed Reduction Repair of a fracture accomplished without surgical intervention is called **closed reduction**. External manipulation is used to correct bone position. This manipulation requires three maneuvers: traction and countertraction, angulation, and rotation. Following the reduction, x-rays are taken to visualize the fracture alignment. The part is then immobilized by using a cast, bandage, or traction. Local or general anesthesia may be used to make the reduction easier and less painful to the client.

Casts Casts are made either from plaster bandages or synthetic materials such as fiberglass. The cast should include the joint above and below the affected part. The major purposes of casts are immobilization, support and protection of the affected part, prevention of deformities resulting from conditions such as arthritis, and the correction of deformities such as scoliosis.

A fiberglass cast weighs less, wears longer, breathes better, and is more penetrable to x-rays than plaster casts (AAOS, 2007a). A dry cast should be odorless, shiny in appearance, resonant (produces vibrating sound on percussion) when percussed, and have a temperature similar to the room air. Moisture occurring from any underlying drainage gives the cast a musty smell, dullness on percussion, a lusterless color, and cool temperature.

Numerous types of casts exist. Long and short arm casts allow the fingers to be visible; long and short leg casts allow the toes to be visible. A spica cast is used for hip, shoulder, and thumb dislocations or injuries. The hip spica has an abduction bar that keeps the cast in the correct position. A walking cast with a cast shoe facilitates client ambulation. Body casts are used to immobilize the spine following surgical spinal fusions, unstable spinal injuries, or for degenerative disorders. Figure 9-10 shows different types of casts.

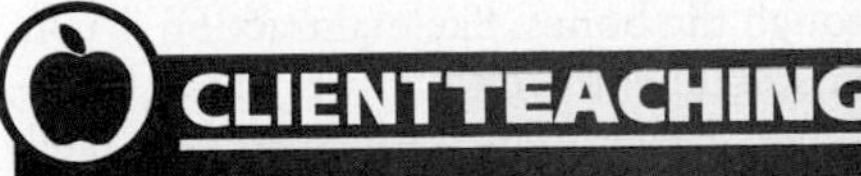

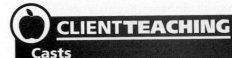

CLIENTTEACHING

Casts

Because plaster casts dry from the inside out, they should not be covered or dried with a hairdryer or heat lamp. Allow moisture and heat from the drying cast to evaporate naturally. Inform clients that the heat they feel during the application, drying, and setting process is normal and should subside in 10 to 15 minutes. To avoid indentation, a drying cast is placed on pillows and not on a hard surface. For the same reason, when handling the cast, only the palms of the hands are used. Plaster casts cause clients to feel cold when they are drying. Apply blankets only to body areas that are not covered with the cast. Synthetic casts dry in minutes to a couple of hours. Teach the client not to insert any objects such as rulers or hangers into the cast to relieve itching as the skin is soft and can be damaged. After the cast has dried, use a hairdryer to blow cool air inside the cast to alleviate itching.

Keep the plaster cast dry because the cast weakens if it gets wet. Sometimes a waterproof cast is applied so the client can shower or possibly swim. Obtain physician approval for swimming with a cast.

After the application and drying of a cast, the doctor may order a cast cut to allow visualization of a body area or to relieve pressure. This procedure is known as **windowing**. A cast is also split in half or bivalved to relieve pressure.

When a cast is removed, the client becomes conscious of aches and discomforts caused by the constricted joint structures and immobilized muscles. Minimize the client's discomfort by supporting the joint and maintaining the part in the same position as it was in the cast. The skin is cool and pale with mottling and edema present. A yellow exudate, which is part dead skin and part secretions from oil sacs, is on the skin. This exudate is not rubbed or forced off.

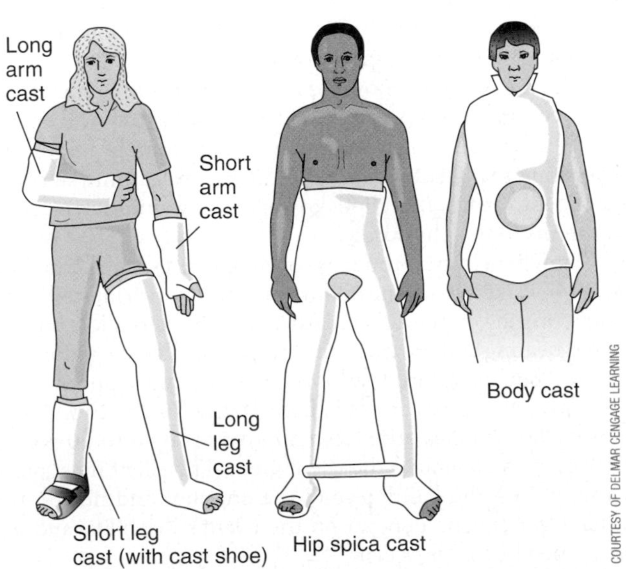

FIGURE 9-10 Casts Used to Correct Musculoskeletal Disorders

Traction The principle of traction is to have two forces pulling in opposite directions. Traction consists of weights and counterweights. Countertraction forces are provided by the weight of the client's body or other weight such as elevating the foot of the bed. Traction is used to reduce a fracture, immobilize an extremity, lessen muscle spasms, or correct or prevent a deformity.

Types of traction are skeletal, skin, and manual. Skeletal traction requires the surgical insertion of pins (Steinmann) or

LIFE SPAN DEVELOPMENT

Cast Removal

Children often are afraid when a cast is removed. Letting the child feel and see the cast cutter before starting to remove the cast alleviates fear.

wires (Kirschner) through the bones. Skeletal traction is continuous and is used most frequently for fractures of the femur, tibia, and cervical spine. Head tongs (e.g., Gardner-Wells tongs) are fixed in the skull to apply traction that immobilizes cervical fractures. An external fixation (fixator) is applied outside of the body to stabilize a break. Two or more pins are placed on either side of the fracture and attached to the fixator. The pins or screws remain in place with the fixator for 6 weeks or until the fracture heals, which may take up to a year or longer if complicated (The Ohio State University Medical Center, 2008). Figure 9-11 shows examples of traction devices.

Skin traction is a nonsurgical method of providing necessary pull for shorter periods, such as Buck's traction (Figure 9-11).

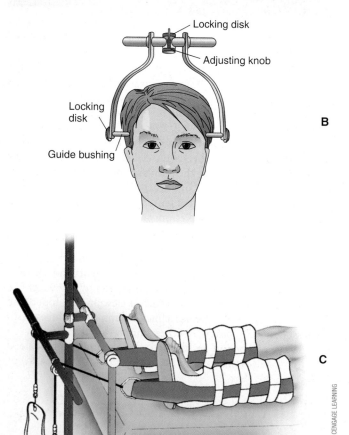

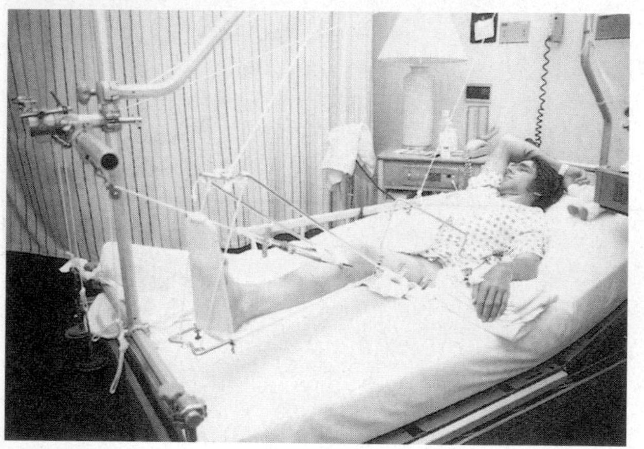

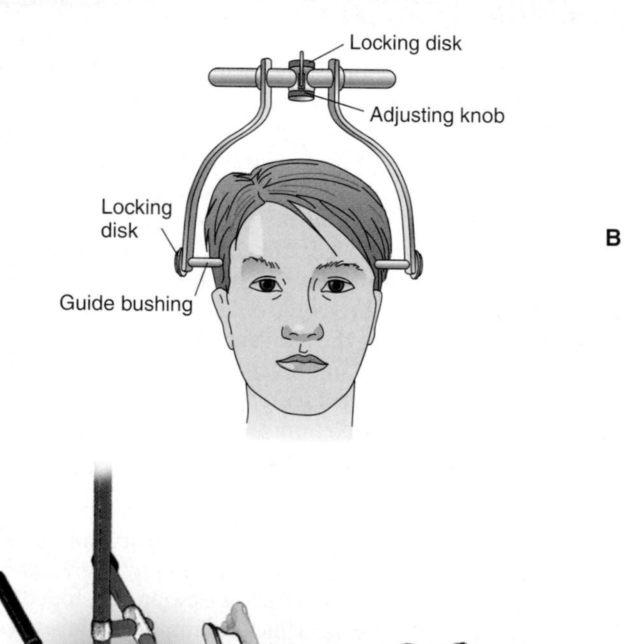

FIGURE 9-11 Types of Traction Devices; *A*, Skeletal Traction; *B*, Head Tongs; *C*, Buck's Traction, a Type of Skin Traction

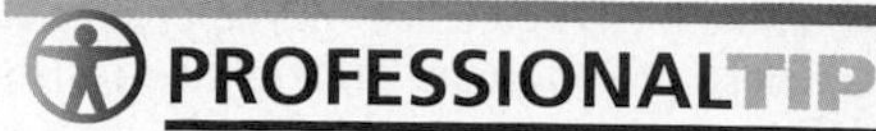

Pin Care

Pin care varies with health-care providers' orders and hospital protocol, therefore, basic guidelines are provided.

- Keep the pin site clean and dry.
- Cleanse the pin site with prescribed solution and a gauze pad using sterile technique.
- Use a new gauze pad for each pin.
- Remove any crust from the pin site.
- Remove all drainage from the pin site.
- Notify the health care provider if there is redness, swelling, purulent drainage, or pain at the pin site or if the pin becomes loose.
- Notify the health care provider if the client develops a fever of 101.5°F.

(The Ohio State University Medical Center, 2008)

Materials used include tapes, traction strips, cervical halters, pelvic belts, and lower extremity boots. Skin traction is frequently used to temporarily immobilize a part or stabilize a fracture. The disadvantage of skin traction for adult use is that it does not adequately control rotation and cannot be maintained for the length of time necessary for adult healing. Tapes and bandages are applied smoothly to prevent any pressure areas.

A nurse caring for a client in traction knows the purpose of the traction, how it accomplishes its purpose, and any complications associated with the use of the traction. It is also important to know the extent of the injury and the movements and positions allowed. Care of the client includes maintenance of the injured part, general body alignment, the alignment of the traction apparatus, and range of motion in as many joints as possible.

Rehabilitation The physician determines when the bone has healed sufficiently for rehabilitation. Healing is monitored by periodic x-rays and physical examinations. The major objective of rehabilitation is to assist the client to return to the former level of functioning. Rehabilitation programs vary depending on the injury and the client.

The nurse has a major role in client education reinforcing the directions of both the physician and the physical therapist. Patience and encouragement are extremely important in assisting the client to feel comfortable in learning self-care techniques. Teach the client to report any unusual signs or symptoms to the physician.

The client learns proper use of equipment such as crutches, canes, or walkers. Crutches allow ambulation with limited or no weight bearing on the affected extremity. Walkers allow limited weight bearing and provide stability when the client ambulates. Canes allow the client to walk with balance and support.

The tripod position is the basic stance for crutch walking. Tips of the crutches are placed approximately 8 to 10 inches in front of and lateral to the client's feet. The client must place his weight on the handpiece of the crutches and not on the axilla. Crutch gaits depend on the client's disability and are prescribed by the physician.

Canes are held in the hand *opposite* the affected extremity. In normal walking, the opposite arm and leg move together.

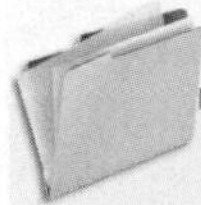

COLLABORATIVECARE

Use of Crutches, Canes, and Walkers

Nurses collaborate with physical therapists to assist clients in the use of crutches, canes, and walkers. Clients generally go to physical therapy to learn how to use the walking aid, and nurses reinforce the teaching when they see clients using their walking aid.

This same action is done when walking with a cane. Walkers provide more support than canes or crutches. They are especially useful for clients who have poor balance. The client places the walker 12 to 18 inches in front and walks toward the walker holding onto the hand grips.

Surgical

Open reduction is a surgical procedure that enables the surgeon to reduce (repair) the fracture under direct visualization. When an open reduction/**internal fixation** (ORIF) is done, orthopedic devices are used to maintain the reduction. Some of the devices used include pins, screws, nails, plates, wires, and rods. These internal fixation devices are inserted through bone fragments or fixed to the sides of the bones.

The major disadvantage of the open reduction is the possibility of introducing infection into the bone. Possible complications include impaired circulation and accidental injury to major nerves, blood vessels, and bone caused by the fixation devices. X-rays are taken during and after the open reduction to evaluate the alignment of the fracture.

Pharmacological

Analgesics are given to relieve pain. Muscle relaxants, such as cyclobenzaprine hydrochloride (Flexeril), also are prescribed for muscle spasms. Severe or continued pain indicates complications and is given immediate attention. Stool softeners, such as docusate sodium (Colace), are given to prevent constipation in the immobilized client.

Diet

The client is encouraged to eat regular meals with foods that provide fiber, protein, calcium, phosphorus, and fluids. For the client whose dietary intake is inadequate, vitamin and mineral supplements, especially calcium and phosphorus, are included. Consultation with a dietitian regarding client food preferences may be necessary.

Activity

Client activity and exercise are important in maintaining muscle strength and tone and minimizing cardiovascular problems. Joints that are not immobilized are exercised either actively or passively to maintain function. *Isometric* (maintaining constant resistive force) exercises help maintain muscle strength of immobilized muscles.

NURSING MANAGEMENT

Frequent and accurate assessment of the musculoskeletal trauma area includes circulation (color), movement, and sensation (CMS). CMS is very important. Provide comfort measures and administer analgesia as ordered. An important nursing responsibility is the prevention of constipation, skin breakdown, urinary calculi, and respiratory complications from immobility.

NURSING PROCESS

ASSESSMENT

Subjective Data

The neurovascular assessment of a client with a fracture may reveal subjective data of pain, especially on movement; muscle spasms; and paresthesia.

Objective Data

Assess for edema, shortening and deformity of the affected limb, hematoma, and pallor. Check pulses in the affected and unaffected extremity and compare with each other. Take the client's vital signs routinely, and note the client's general physical and mental condition. Check the skin, especially over bony prominences, for color and temperature.

When the client has a cast applied, check all cast edges for smoothness. Also check the cast for spots indicating wound drainage, including the color and amount. Mark the size of the drainage spot on the cast with a ballpoint pen and indicate the date and time. Then an increase in the size of the drainage spot can easily be identified. Assess extremities including fingers, toes, hands, and feet for changes in skin color, pulse, or temperature. Check all traction wires, pulleys, and weights. Weights should hang free and are not removed unless a health-care provider writes specific orders for removal. When providing pin care, nurses use sterile technique according to health-care facility guidelines. Observe for drainage and infection at the pin sites.

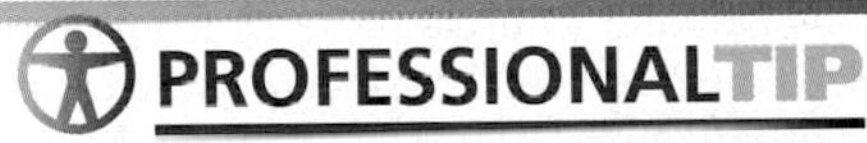

Neurovascular Assessment

- CMS assessments are performed on clients following musculoskeletal trauma; after surgery, if nerve or blood vessel damage is possible; and following casting, splinting, and bandaging.
- The CMS assessment is performed every 15 to 30 minutes for several hours, and then every 3 to 4 hours.
- All findings are documented.
- Tingling and numbness are relieved by flexing fingers or toes or repositioning extremity.
- Remember 6 Ps when performing a CMS assessment:
  1. Paresthesia (unrelieved tingling or numbness)
  2. Pain
  3. Pallor (Assessment may reveal a slow capillary return. Normal capillary refill is 2 to 4 seconds.)
  4. Paralysis
  5. Puffiness (edema)
  6. Pulselessness

Nursing diagnoses for a client with musculoskeletal trauma include the following:

NURSING DIAGNOSES	PLANNING/OUTCOMES	NURSING INTERVENTIONS
*Acute **P**ain* related to fracture	The client will have relief of pain with medication.	Assess for pain and swelling. Provide comfort measures. Administer medications for pain as ordered.
*Risk for Impaired **S**kin Integrity* related to immobility	The client's skin remains intact.	Change client position, if allowed, maintaining correct body alignment. Check bony prominences and keep the client's skin clean and dry. For the client in a cast, check the edges of the cast for roughness, keep the exposed skin next to the cast clean and dry. Inspect all body pressure points including the head, ears, and heels; turn the client as orders direct; and check for friction rubs. Instruct clients not to place anything inside the cast or use objects to scratch, causing skin breakdown or infections. Avoid getting the cast wet.
*Impaired Physical **M**obility* related to loss of integrity of bone structures	The client will perform range-of-motion exercises in unaffected joints. The client will demonstrate use of adaptive devices to improve mobility.	If the client in a cast is allowed to turn, use an overhead trapeze. Assist client in performing ROM exercises. Assist client in use of adaptive devices.

Evaluation: Evaluate each outcome to determine how it has been met by the client.

RHABDOMYOLYSIS

Crushing injuries most commonly cause rhabdomyolysis, the release of myoglobulin (muscle protein) from damaged muscle cells (MedlinePlus®, 2007). Myoglobin, creatine kinase (CK), and other inflammatory mediators escape from the injured muscle tissue into the circulation. The circulating myoglobin, filtered by the kidneys, can precipitate, causing renal tubular obstruction. About 15% of rhabdomyolysis cases will have acute renal failure (Walls, 2002). Two other major problems are respiratory distress from muscle weakness and fluid and electrolyte imbalance. Standard treatment includes IV fluids to maintain circulating blood volume and renal perfusion so the myoglobin is flushed from the kidneys.

COMPARTMENT SYNDROME

Compartment syndrome is a form of neurovascular impairment that may lead to permanent injury of an affected limb caused by progressive constriction of blood vessels and nerves. It occurs with any orthopedic injury as a result of bleeding into the tissue, tissue edema, or prolonged external pressure (cast or tight dressing). If untreated, in 4 to 6 hours it leads to irreversible damage to nerves and muscles, and within 24 to 48 hours permanent loss of normal limb function. Accurate, regular assessments and early detection are the best ways to avoid permanent disability. A neurovascular assessment that reveals throbbing pain not relieved by narcotic analgesics or greater in comparison with the injury, greater pain with passive motion than active, diminished capillary refill, weak or unequal pulses, **paresthesia** (numbness or tingling), and paralysis indicates this orthopedic emergency. Treatment consists of relieving pressure by removing the cast or dressing or by performing a fasciotomy. A surgical fasciotomy is an incision into the fascia to relieve pressure on the nerves and blood vessels.

CRITICAL THINKING

Immobility Complications

Prepare a teaching plan for an immobile client to prevent constipation, skin breakdown, urinary calculi, and respiratory complications.

INFLAMMATORY DISORDERS

Inflammatory disorders involve inflammation of the joints and include conditions such as rheumatoid arthritis, bursitis, and osteomyelitis.

RHEUMATOID ARTHRITIS

Rheumatoid arthritis is an autoimmune disease of unknown etiology, with recurring inflammation involving the synovium or lining of the joints. It can also affect the lungs, heart, blood vessels, muscles, eyes, and skin. Rheumatoid arthritis is a potentially destructive and disabling disease. The course is variable with either slow or rapid progress and/or periods of remissions. Women are affected more often than men. Rheumatoid arthritis occurs at any age; however, it most commonly affects young adults. In children, it occurs in a form known as juvenile rheumatoid arthritis (Still's disease). See the immune system chapter for more information on rheumatoid arthritis.

BURSITIS

Bursitis is inflammation of the bursa, a sac filled with synovial fluid that facilitates joint movement. Major bursae are found in the shoulder, knee, hip, and elbow. The inflammation is usually the result of trauma or repetitive movements. The client experiences painful joint movement. Diagnosis is made from the client's symptoms and x-ray, which shows a calcified bursa. Treatment includes rest of the joint and the administration of anti-inflammatory drugs including salicylates and nonsteroidal anti-inflammatory drugs (NSAIDs). For some clients, corticosteroids may be injected into the bursa.

OSTEOMYELITIS

Osteomyelitis is the inflammation of the bone and bone marrow. The most common cause of osteomyelitis is the introduction of pathogenic bacteria into a penetrating injury such as an open fracture. Bone infections may also result from the spread of infection from another site such as infected teeth, tonsils, or an upper respiratory infection. The most common pathogen causing osteomyelitis is *Staphylococcus aureus*. Other organisms found in osteomyelitis are *Pseudomonas* and *Escherichia coli*. Osteomyelitis may become a chronic disabling problem affecting the quality of life. The affected bone may have spontaneous fractures.

Local symptoms of an acute infection are sudden pain and tenderness of the affected bone, warmth, redness, edema, and pain on movement. General symptoms with acute severe bone infections include chills, elevated temperature, rapid pulse, and marked leukocytosis.

MEDICAL–SURGICAL MANAGEMENT

Medical

The client is placed on bed rest, and the infected bone is kept at rest with the use of sandbags or casts. Antibiotics are given IV as soon as osteomyelitis is suspected. Unless the infective process is controlled early, a bone abscess forms (Figure 9-12). Cultures of the abscess may indicate a need for change in the antibiotic therapy. The abscess may drain naturally; however, it usually requires an incision, allowing it to drain. The abscess cavity of dead bone tissue does not liquefy easily, drain, and heal as in soft tissue abscesses. A bone sheath forms around the sequestrum (dead bone), giving the appearance of healing; however, chronically infected sequestrum has the tendency to produce recurrent abscesses throughout the life of the individual.

Surgical

A sequestrectomy to remove the dead bone tissue may need to be performed. Strict aseptic technique is maintained when changing any dressings. Because infected bone is extremely painful, unnecessary movement is avoided and the affected extremity handled very gently.

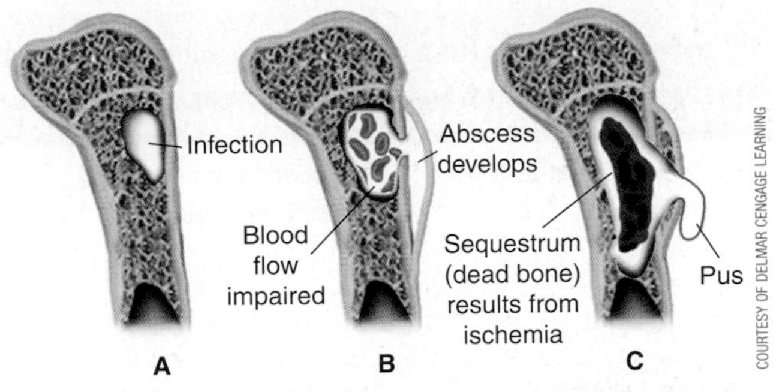

FIGURE 9-12 ***A***, **Osteomyelitis;** ***B***, **Without early treatment, an abscess forms;** ***C***, **Bone dies (sequestrum) and pus forms.**

Pharmacological

Osteomyelitis is treated with vigorous antibiotic therapy and analgesics. Wound irrigations with antiseptics or antibiotics are often prescribed by the physician. Specific drugs given are determined by the causative organism.

Diet

A high-calorie, high-protein diet is generally ordered for the client with osteomyelitis. Dietary supplements of vitamins and calcium are also given. Fluids are increased as tolerated, and a high-fiber diet is encouraged due to analgesic use and immobilization.

Activity

Absolute rest of the affected extremity is needed. Avoid excessive handling of the extremity because it is very painful. The extremity is handled in a smooth, unhurried manner, supporting the joints above and below the affected area.

NURSING MANAGEMENT

Maintain the client on bed rest and the infected bone at absolute rest. Avoid excessive handling of the affected extremity. Administer IV antibiotics, analgesics, and dietary supplements (vitamins and calcium) as ordered. Maintain strict asepsis if wound irrigations are ordered. Encourage the client to drink more fluids and to eat the high-calorie, high-protein diet ordered. Provide for diversional activities.

NURSING PROCESS

ASSESSMENT

Subjective Data

Inquire about pain, muscle spasms, and tenderness in the bone. Ask about any traumas, surgeries, and other diseases.

Objective Data

Observe the client for signs of infection, including chills, elevated temperature, pain, redness, and edema of the affected extremity. The client may also experience headaches, restlessness, and irritability.

Nursing diagnoses for a client with osteomyelitis include the following:

NURSING DIAGNOSES	PLANNING/OUTCOMES	NURSING INTERVENTIONS
*Acute **P**ain* related to inflammation	The client will verbalize reduction of pain.	Protect client from jerky movements and falls. Assess wound appearance and new sites of pain. Provide diet high in protein and vitamin C. Administer pain medications as ordered.
*Impaired Physical **M**obility* related to pain	The client will maintain movement of unaffected extremities.	Encourage and assist client to maintain active ROM or perform passive ROM to unaffected extremities.
*Risk for Impaired **S**kin Integrity* related to immobility	The client will maintain skin integrity.	Handle the affected extremity gently, protect it from injury, keep it in good body alignment and level with the body. Irrigate wound as ordered. Use aseptic technique when irrigating the affected area and when changing the dressing. Assess skin and bony prominences for reddened areas. Encourage adequate fluid intake.

Evaluation: Evaluate each outcome to determine how it has been met by the client.

DEGENERATIVE DISORDERS

Degenerative disorders include osteoporosis, degenerative joint disease, and total joint arthroplasty.

OSTEOPOROSIS

Osteoporosis is an increase in the porosity of bone. It is a common disorder in bone metabolism in which both mineral and protein matrix components are diminished and the bone becomes brittle and fragile. There is an increased susceptibility to fractures of the hip, spine, and wrist.

Ten million individuals in the United States have osteoporosis, and another 34 million have low bone mineral density, which places them at risk for osteoporosis (NOF, 2008d). Of those affected by osteoporosis, 80% are women (NOF, 2008d). In 2005, more than 2 million osteoporosis related fractures occured, including 297,000 hip fractures, 547,000 vertebral fractures, 397,000 wrist fractures, 135,000 pelvic fractures, and 675,000 fractures of other types (NOF, 2008d).

PROFESSIONALTIP

Absolute Fracture Risk

A DXA machine is in development that reports an *absolute fracture risk*. The report uses a client's bone mineral density results, age, risk factors for osteoporosis, and fractures to determine the client's risk of a fracture in the next 10 years. The information enables health care providers to determine appropriate osteoporosis treatment (NOF, 2008d).

Osteoporosis has been called the "silent disease" because there are no symptoms of bone loss. As the bone tissue loses density, fractures and kyphosis occur. Very slight trauma fractures the brittle bones. With multiple vertebral fractures, the individual experiences a loss of height.

The only way to determine whether an individual has osteoporosis is to measure bone mineral density (BMD). The recommended type of BMD test is the dual-energy x-ray absorptiometry (DXA or DEXA) that identifies low bone density prior to a fracture and predicts the chances of a person having a fracture in the future (NOF, 2008a, 2008c, 2008d). The test measures the bone density of the spine, hip, or total body and is painless, noninvasive, and safe.

MEDICAL–SURGICAL MANAGEMENT

There is no cure for osteoporosis. Prevention through diet, regular exercise, eliminating tobacco and alcohol use, having BMD testing, and taking medication is possible for most people (NOF, 2002e).

PROFESSIONALTIP

Osteoporosis

Risk factors for osteoporosis include being female, having thin or small bones, history of fractures, advanced age, family history of osteoporosis, postmenopause without estrogen replacement therapy, amenorrhea, eating disorders, low calcium intake, inactive lifestyle, smoking, excessive alcohol intake, use of corticosteroids or anticonvulsant medications, and low testosterone level in men.

Pharmacological

Several medications are approved for the prevention and treatment of osteoporosis. Alendronate sodium (Fosamax) and alendronate plus vitamin D3 (Fosamax plus D™), risedronate (Actonel®) and risedronate with calcium (Actonel® with calcium), and zoledronic acid (Reclast®) are used for prevention and treatment of osteoporosis in postmenopausal men and women. Ibandronate (Boniva®) is used for prevention and treatment of postmenopausal women only. Calcitonin (Forical® and Miacalcin®) is used in treatment of osteoporosis in women at least 5 years beyond menopause. Raloxifen (Evista®), an estrogen agonists/antagonists or selective estrogen receptor modulators (SERMs), is used for the prevention and treatment of osteroporosis in postmenopausal women. Estrogen is used both for prevention and treatment, but according to the FDA, other medications should be used first (NOF, 2008c). Estrogen is used both for prevention and treatment, but according to the FDA, other medications should be used first (NOF, 2008c). Teriparatide (Forteo®), a parathyroid hormone, is used in the treatment of postmenopausal men and women with very low BMD and at risk of a fracture. The FDA recommends the client take teriparatide for no more than 2 years (NOF, 2008c).

Testosterone-replacement therapy may be used for men with low testosterone levels.

Nonnarcotic analgesics are prescribed for relief of pain. The client also is advised to take supplemental vitamin D with calcium.

Diet

Encourage the client to maintain an adequate balanced diet rich in calcium and vitamin D. A reduction in the consumption of caffeine, alcohol, excess protein, and smoking cessation is recommended.

Activity

Encourage the client to practice good body mechanics and posture and to walk, preferably outdoors for the benefits of sunshine (vitamin D). This is effective in preventing further bone loss and stimulating new bone formation.

Nursing Management

Encourage clients to prevent osteoporosis through a diet adequate in calcium and vitamin D, regular exercise, and eliminating tobacco and alcohol use. Teach correct body mechanics and encourage good posture.

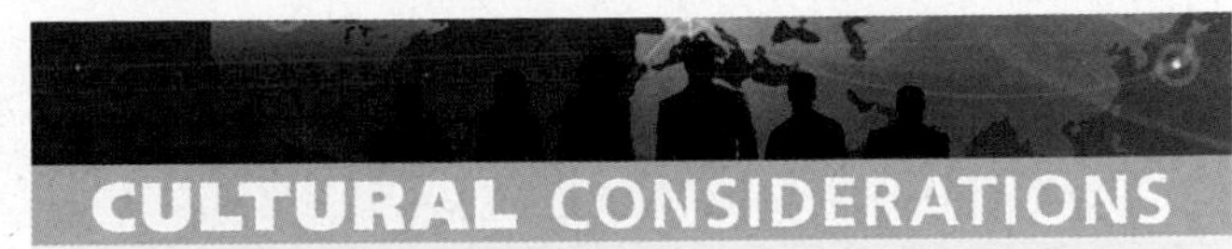

CULTURAL CONSIDERATIONS

Osteoporosis

- Significant risk has been reported in persons of all ethnic backgrounds.
- White women older than age 65 have twice as many fractures as African American women (NOF, 2002c).
- White men are at greater risk for osteoporosis, but osteoporosis is found in men from all ethnic groups (NOF, 2002d).

COMMUNITY/HOME HEALTH CARE

Osteoporosis

- Maintain physical activity—walking, isometric exercises.
- Remove potential hazards, such as throw rugs.
- Eat a diet high in calcium and vitamin D.
- Be out in the sun 10 to 15 minutes a day.
- Move items down from top shelves of cupboards because it is difficult to see or reach the items as a result of curvature changes in the spine.
- Wear sturdy shoes.

NURSING PROCESS

Assessment

Subjective Data

This includes the client's gender, age, and family health history. Note any symptoms the client expresses regarding altered body image or back or neck pain that worsens when coughing, sneezing, straining, or standing. Take a nutritional history. Note lifestyle patterns such as smoking, inactivity, or immobilization. A medical history regarding any medications is also important.

Objective Data

Kyphosis, gait impairment, and poor posture are noted.

Nursing diagnoses for a client with osteoporosis include the following:

NURSING DIAGNOSES	PLANNING/OUTCOMES	NURSING INTERVENTIONS
Chronic ***Pain*** *related to disease process*	The client will express minimal discomfort.	Administer analgesics as ordered; teach client about the medications.
		Handle client carefully; instruct client to avoid any twisting movements.
		The bed should have a firm mattress or bed board for support.

(*Continues*)

Nursing diagnoses for a client with osteoporosis include the following: (Continued)

NURSING DIAGNOSES	PLANNING/OUTCOMES	NURSING INTERVENTIONS
*Risk for **I**njury* related to disease process	The client will practice correct body mechanics.	Teach client correct body mechanics.
*Impaired Physical **M**obility* related to disease process	The client will maintain physical activity.	Teach client about types of exercises and physical activities that help maintain bone mass and isometric exercises to strengthen muscles. Encourage ambulation with the client using a walker or cane if necessary.

Evaluation: Evaluate each outcome to determine how it has been met by the client.

OSTEOARTHRITIS (DEGENERATIVE JOINT DISEASE)

Osteoarthritis (OA) is considered a "wear-and-tear" disease and is characterized by slow and steady progressive breakdown of cartilage. It is a nonsystemic, noninflammatory disorder causing bones and joints to degenerate. It is the most common type of arthritis. The etiology is unknown, but predisposing factors include increased age, obesity, an injury to a joint, poor posture, or occupations that put strain on joints. Genetics plays a role in OA, especially in the hands (Arthritis Foundation, 2002b). The weight-bearing joints of the lower extremities as well as the hands and cervical and lumbar vertebrae are the joints most frequently affected. The cartilage covering the bone becomes thin and then wears off. The synovial membrane thickens and fibrous tissue around the joint ossifies. The effects of degenerative changes on the knee joint are shown in Figure 9-13.

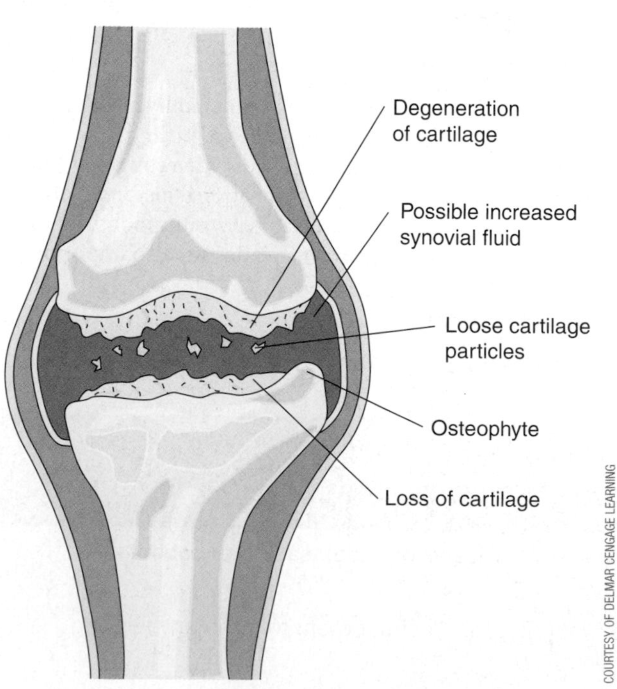

FIGURE 9-13 Degenerative Changes in the Cartilage of the Knee Due to Osteoarthritis

The onset of osteoarthritis begins during middle age, and by age 65 most people have some degeneration. Symptoms include early morning stiffness and pain after physical activity. There is joint enlargement and characteristic hypertrophic spurs, called **Heberden's nodes**, in the terminal interphalangeal finger joints. More women are affected with OA, especially in the hands. The hips are more affected in men.

Diagnosis is made from the client's symptoms and examination of the joints that are enlarged and tender. X-ray shows a narrowing of joint spaces and gross irregularities of joint structure. A CT scan or MRI shows vertebral joint involvement.

MEDICAL–SURGICAL MANAGEMENT

Medical

No treatment exists to stop the degenerative process; therefore, treatment focuses on relief of the client's discomfort. Medical management includes local heat and rest for the affected joint, weight reduction for obese clients to relieve strain on affected joints, and orthotic devices (braces, canes, crutches) to support the joints. Physical therapy can provide exercises to strengthen muscles and keep joints flexible and teach self-management skills.

Surgical

Surgical procedures such as total hip or knee replacement may be recommended for clients with severe osteoarthritis. Osteotomy may help correct malalignment situations. Refer to the section on total joint arthroplasty in this chapter.

Pharmacological

Pharmacological treatment includes the use of aspirin or NSAIDs. Narcotics are avoided because of the chronic nature of the disease. Steroids may be used and are sometimes injected into a joint to provide immediate relief of pain and to stop the degenerative process temporarily. If the client has vertebral involvement with muscle spasms, cyclobenzaprine hydrochloride (Flexeril) may be given to relax the muscles.

CLIENT TEACHING

Osteoarthritis

- Set priorities each day, and do the most important activities first.
- Do not plan too many activities for one day.
- Plan rest periods during the day between activities.
- Prevent rushing and stressful situations by planning ahead.
- Lose weight, if necessary.
- When knees or hips are affected, avoid climbing stairs, bending, stooping, or squatting.

NURSING MANAGEMENT

Encourage clients to maintain a proper weight for height and to practice good posture. Provide rest and heat for the affected joint. Collaborate with physical therapy for muscle-strengthening exercises and self-management skills.

NURSING PROCESS

ASSESSMENT

Subjective Data

The client describes nonspecific symptoms such as general musculoskeletal pain, joint stiffness especially on rising, and joint pain or tenderness. Note weight gain, occupation, and any conditions or situations that exacerbate the client's joint pain. Some of these situations include cold weather, overexercising, or extreme fatigue. Assess the client's understanding of the disease and its effect on lifestyle and ability to perform activities of daily and social living.

Objective Data

This includes edema and tenderness around the joints and bony enlargements of distal interphalangeal joints (Heberden's nodes).

Nursing diagnoses for a client with osteoarthritis include the following:

NURSING DIAGNOSES	PLANNING/OUTCOMES	NURSING INTERVENTIONS
*Chronic **Pain*** related to joint tenderness and edema	The client will express minimal discomfort.	Handle the affected extremity gently and apply heat as ordered. Administer prescribed analgesic and evaluate its effectiveness.
*Impaired Physical **Mobility*** related to joint deterioration	The client will maintain mobility within the parameters of the disease process.	Coordinate with physical therapy and assist in a planned exercise program as ordered. Advise client to plan rest periods during the day.

Evaluation: Evaluate each outcome to determine how it has been met by the client.

TOTAL JOINT ARTHROPLASTY

Joint replacement or **arthroplasty** is the replacement of both articular surfaces within a joint capsule. The hip, knee, shoulder, and fingers are the joints most frequently replaced. Replacements consist of metal and polyethylene and may be cemented in the prepared bone with methyl methacrylate, which has properties similar to bone. See Figure 9-14 for knee- and hip-replacement components.

Newer techniques use porous-coated cementless artificial joint components. These allow bone to grow into the joint component and securely fix the prosthesis. This reduces the incidence of prosthesis failure. Joint replacement is usually an elective procedure, and clients may wish to have autologous blood transfusions whereby they predonate their own blood in case a blood transfusion is needed.

TOTAL HIP REPLACEMENT

Total hip replacement is the replacement of a damaged hip with an artificial joint. The hip is replaced with a traditional procedure or a minimally invasive procedure. The minimally invasive method has less pain, less muscle injury, shorter hospitalization, and a faster rehabilitation. The incisions are 2 to 3 inches or less, whereas the traditional method has a 10- to 12-inch incision on the side of the hip and possibly with a portable suction device in place (AAOS, 2007c). The traditional method has more drainage and the drain is removed when the drainage is 30 mL or less. The hip prosthesis by either method can be cemented in place or be coated with a special textured metal or bone-like substance that is not cemented into the joint. A cemented ball and a noncemented socket are sometimes used (AAOS, 2007d).

Surgical complications are venous thrombosis, bleeding, respiratory problems, and, after several years, the hip prosthesis may loosen or need replacing. Potential problems with the hip replacement include dislocation of the prosthesis, excessive wound drainage, and infection. To prevent venous thrombosis, antiembolism stockings are worn. They are removed twice daily to inspect the skin.

After a total hip replacement, the client's hip and leg are kept in a position of abduction and extension. The knees are kept apart by using a foam V-wedge, several pillows, or an abductor pillow. When the client turns from the back to a side-lying position, the entire leg is supported with pillows to keep the hip abducted. The client usually prefers to lie on the unaffected side. Instruct the client to avoid acute hip flexion of greater than 90 degrees. The legs should not

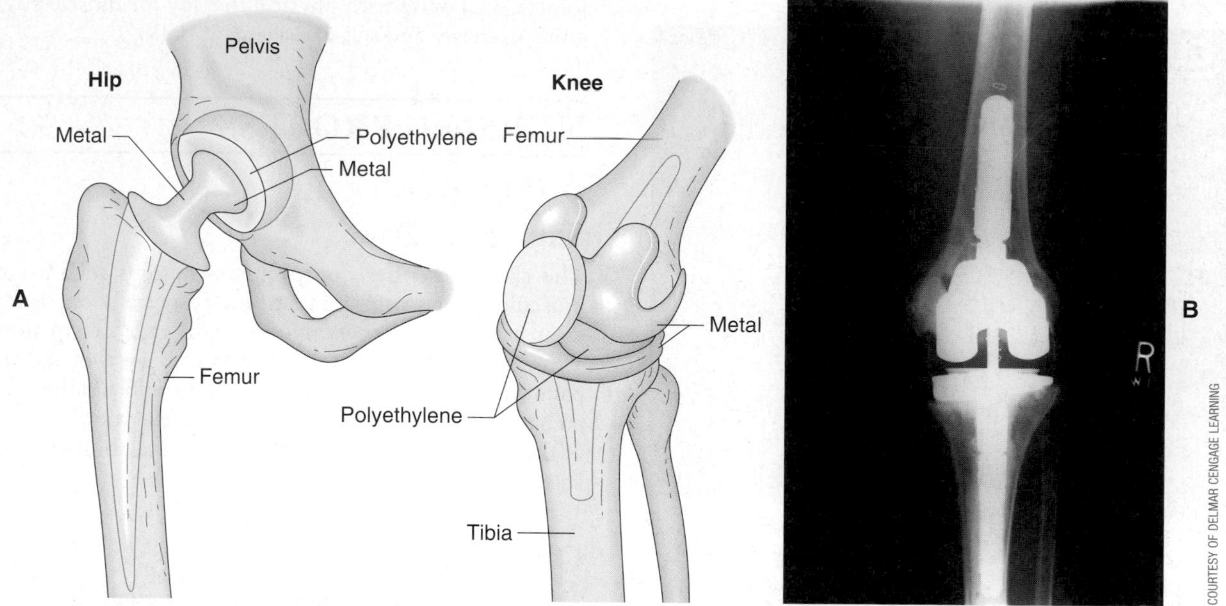

FIGURE 9-14 ***A,*** **Total Hip and Knee Replacement;** ***B,*** **Radiograph of a Total Knee Replacement (Anterior-Posterior View). The patella is plastic, and, therefore, it is not visible here.**

be crossed nor the hips flexed to pull up a blanket or sheet. A fracture bedpan is used until the client can ambulate to the bathroom. Use a raised toilet seat in the bathroom or a bedside commode. Any specific client turning, movement, and positioning are ordered by the physician. Vital signs and CMS checks are performed routinely. Encourage the client to cough and deep breathe or use an incentive spirometer after surgery to prevent respiratory problems. Inspect the dressings frequently.

The goal for clients who have total hip or knee joint replacement is to ambulate independently. Ambulatory activity progresses rapidly for clients with joint replacement. Clients who have total hip replacement are usually out of bed the night of surgery or early the next day. Physical therapy teaches exercises to strengthen the hip muscles. Gait training begins with the use of a walker and progresses to the use of crutches or a cane. The client avoids hip flexion of more than 90 degrees and stair climbing for at least 3 months.

Total Knee Replacement

Total knee replacement, like hip replacement, is considered for clients experiencing severe pain and functional disability related to joint destruction. The prosthesis chosen for the replacement provides the client with a painless, stable, and functional joint.

Immediately after surgery a firm compression dressing is applied to the operative site. The physician may order a special ice machine applied to circulate ice water around the knee. The cold water decreases pain and swelling. After the dressing is removed, a CPM machine helps increase circulation to the operative area and promotes flexibility within the knee joint. The surgeon orders the frequency of use and the amount of tension, flexion, and extension produced by the machine. A sequential compression device (SCD) is used or antiembolism stockings worn to minimize the development of thrombophlebitis. After the arthroplasty, the client wears an adjustable soft knee immobilizer to stabilize the leg when walking. The client may transfer out of bed to a wheelchair with the immobilizer in place. No weight bearing is allowed on the knee until it is prescribed by the surgeon.

The most common complication after total knee replacement is blood clots in the leg veins. The orthopedic surgeon may order periodic elevation of legs, leg exercises to improve circulation, support hose, and an anticoagulant (AAOS, 2007e).

Nursing Management

Perform neurovascular assessment of the affected extremity as well as incision assessment, vital signs, lung sounds, pedal pulses, and I&O. Maintain the client's hip in a position of abduction and extension for 6 to 10 days as ordered. Keep client's skin and bed dry and clean. Encourage the client to cough and deep breathe and to use the trapeze to raise hips off the bed for bedpan use.

NURSING PROCESS

Assessment

Subjective Data

Assess for irritability, restlessness, orientation, and neurovascular assessment of the affected extremity for pain, numbness, tingling, and paresthesia.

Objective Data

Assess the incision for approximation, redness, and drainage and the skin over all bony prominences. Assess for tachypnea, dyspnea, hypoxemia, and crackles and wheezes in the lungs (signs of fat embolism). Vital signs, pedal pulses, and I&O are also assessed.

The client with a total hip replacement is assessed for position of the affected hip. The hip should be maintained in a position of abduction and extension. The most prominent symptom of a dislocation is a clicking, popping sound. Other symptoms are a sudden sharp pain that is unrelieved by narcotic analgesics, loss of leg motion, and edema of the affected hip. The client is not moved, and the physician is notified immediately.

Assessment of the client with a total knee replacement includes the neurovascular status of the leg and the dressing and drainage device. Vital signs, intake and output, and the color and temperature of the extremity are also assessed. The knee is elevated and the nurse monitors the ice machine and CPM machine.

Nursing diagnoses for a client undergoing arthroplasty surgery include the following:

NURSING DIAGNOSES	PLANNING/OUTCOMES	NURSING INTERVENTIONS
*Impaired **S**kin Integrity* related to immobility and surgical incision	The client's skin will remain free from redness or any other signs of breakdown.	Maintain a clean and dry dressing. If a drainage device is used, assess functioning. Keep client's skin and bed clean and dry. Assess bony prominences for redness. Provide high-protein diet with dairy products and vitamin C.
*Impaired Physical **M**obility* related to surgery	The client will ambulate following physician's direction.	Keep hip in a position of abduction. Use an abductor pillow or wedge to maintain the position when turning the client. Encourage client to use the trapeze to raise hips off the bed to use the bedpan. Assist client in accomplishing activities of daily living.
*Ineffective Peripheral **T**issue Perfusion* related to surgery and immobility	The client will have adequate circulation of extremity.	Encourage client to cough and deep breathe. Monitor vital signs until stable. Assess pedal pulses and capillary refill in both extremities.

Evaluation: Evaluate each outcome to determine how it has been met by the client.

MUSCULOSKELETAL DISORDERS

Musculoskeletal disorders discussed include amputations, temporomandibular joint disease/disorder, and carpal tunnel syndrome.

AMPUTATIONS

An **amputation** is the removal of all or part of an extremity. Amputations are done in response to injuries resulting in extensive laceration of arteries or nerves, or diseases such as malignant tumors, infections, and peripheral vascular disorders. Other disease conditions that may require amputation include extensive osteomyelitis or congenital disorders. In severe trauma situations, an amputation may be done to save the client's life.

Recent advances in microsurgical techniques have allowed replantation (limb reattachment) in some injuries. These procedures involve the use of microscopes and highly specialized instruments to reconnect severed nerves and blood vessels. Amputations involving the hand or wrist are more likely considered for replantation rather than an injury involving a large muscle mass because of extensive tissue, bone, and muscle damage. Any amputation creates a major physical and psychological adjustment for the client.

MEDICAL–SURGICAL MANAGEMENT

Medical

Rehabilitation for the client with an amputation requires the effort of the entire rehabilitation team. The client's physical and psychological responses to the amputation are monitored by all members of the team. If appropriate, counseling and job training will enable many clients to return to their jobs.

Surgical

Before surgery, the surgeon evaluates the client and makes several decisions. These decisions include necessity of an amputation, type of amputation (open or closed), level of amputation, potential for rehabilitation, and type of prosthesis and rehabilitation program.

The surgeon attempts to save as much of the limb as possible. A closed amputation is done by using skin flaps to cover the bone end of the extremity. This type of amputation is done when there is no evidence of infection. Sometimes a Guillotine (open) amputation is necessary. This amputation requires a straight cut and allows for free drainage of infectious material. Tissue, bone, and vessels are severed at the same level without skin flaps. The major indication for doing an open amputation is infection.

The level of an amputation is determined by the vascular supply and is never higher than absolutely necessary. If the blood flow at the site of the incision is normal, the amputation is performed at that level. If the bleeding is scant, a higher level

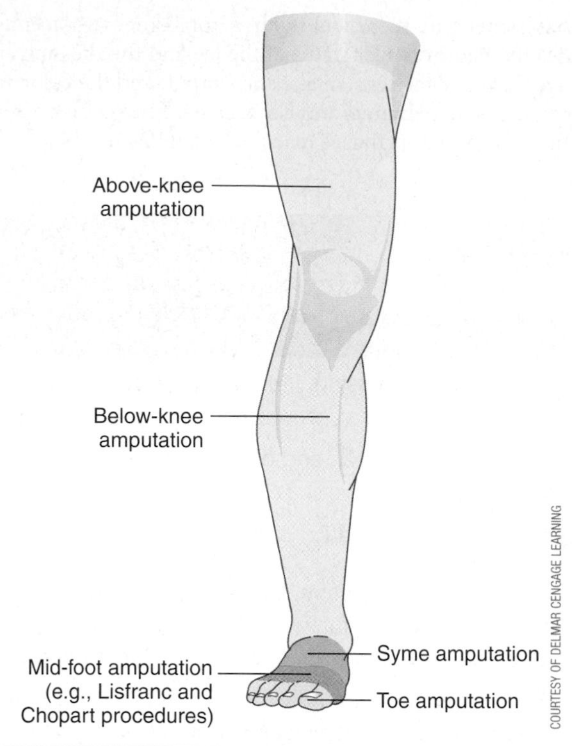

FIGURE 9-15 Different Amputation Levels

of amputation is performed to ensure adequate postoperative healing. See Figure 9-15 for different lower-extremity amputation levels.

Pharmacological

Narcotic analgesics are required immediately after surgery. After several days, pain is controlled with nonnarcotic analgesics. If infection exists, appropriate antibiotic therapy is ordered.

Diet

A balanced diet with adequate vitamins and protein is essential for adequate wound healing. Many elderly clients are poorly nourished or require special diets. Nutritional care plans are discussed with the physician and a dietitian.

Activity

The surgeon determines postoperative positioning of the stump. The stump is alternately placed in an extended position or elevated on pillows for short periods. Encourage the client to spend some time in the prone position. This position helps stretch the flexor muscles and prevents contractions of the hip. Physical therapy starts exercises to prevent contractures and increase muscle strength and assists with ambulation as soon after surgery as possible.

CRITICAL THINKING

Phantom Limb Pain

How would you explain phantom limb pain to a client?

Nursing Management

Perform routine postoperative care by encouraging deep breathing, coughing, and turning; assessing pain on a 1 to 10 scale; and administering analgesics as ordered. The residual limb is shaped for prosthesis by using a figure-8 wrapping of wide elastic bandages. Some physicians prefer a two-way elastic compression shrinker that forms the residual limb to the prosthesis. Other more rigid dressings are also used.

Encourage client to eat a balanced diet with extra protein for wound healing. Collaborate with physical therapy regarding bed exercises, transfer techniques, and later ambulation.

NURSING PROCESS

Assessment

Subjective Data

Subjective assessment data include pain, sensations felt on the extremity to be amputated, and the emotional status of the client. If a client has experienced chronic pain before the amputation, pain may seem mild following the surgery. Severe pain may indicate a hematoma or excessive pressure from a cast or elastic bandage on a bony prominence. Sometimes the client confuses **phantom limb pain** with the incisional pain. Phantom limb pain is the sensation that there is pain, soreness, tingling, burning, and stiffness in the amputated limb. The sensory sensations of the missing limb remain in the brain causing the feelings of phantom pain. Phantom pain decreases as inflammation subsides at the incisional site.

Objective Data

Objective assessment data include the color and temperature of the skin, pulse, and responses to limb movement. The unaffected extremity also is assessed for function and circulation.

PROFESSIONALTIP

Robotic Ankle

Hugh Herr developed a robotic ankle that simulates the action of the human ankle-foot. The prosthesis is made with springs and an electric motor so it propels the person with each step, giving the person a natural appearing gait. The robotic ankle makes one less tired when walking and improves balance (MIT, 2007).

Nursing diagnoses for a client who has an amputation include the following:

NURSING DIAGNOSES	PLANNING/OUTCOMES	NURSING INTERVENTIONS
*Impaired **S**kin Integrity* related to amputation	The client will remain free from infection.	Inspect the incision for any inflammation, excessive drainage, edema, increased pain, and hypersensitivity to touch. Use aseptic technique for all dressing changes. Monitor vital signs.
*Disturbed **B**ody Image* related to loss of limb	The client will participate in the care of the residual limb.	Handle the residual limb gently and treat it as though a prosthesis will be worn. Encourage client to watch dressing change and eventually assist with and do the dressing changes. Encourage client to express feelings and concerns about the amputation.
*Impaired Physical **M**obility* related to loss of limb	The client will demonstrate improved physical mobility.	Encourage client to participate in physical therapy and to perform ROM exercises. Assist client when ambulating with assistive devices.

Evaluation: Evaluate each outcome to determine how it has been met by the client.

SAMPLE NURSING CARE PLAN

The Client with a Below-the-Knee Amputation

R.S. is a 76-year-old resident in a retirement home. She has remained active since her retirement from the secretarial job she held for 20 years. Her health history indicates she has had circulatory problems with inadequate peripheral circulation resulting from atherosclerosis. Her physician hospitalized her for a planned below-the-knee amputation on the left leg and has ordered an arteriogram to assist in determining the site for the amputation. The arteriogram determines the point of adequate circulatory status to promote wound healing after the limb is amputated.

The nurse's assessment of R.S.'s vital signs are blood pressure 120/68 mm Hg, pulse 72 beats/minute, and respirations 18 breaths/minute. Femoral pulses are present in both extremities; however, the pedal pulse in her left foot is barely palpable, and the skin is cool and pale. She stated that lately her left foot is always cold and is a bluish-black color. R.S. expresses concern about her ability to take care of herself after she loses her foot.

NURSING DIAGNOSIS 1 *Disturbed **B**ody Image* related to scheduled amputation as evidenced by statement of concern over losing foot

Nursing Outcomes Classification (NOC)
Psychosocial Adjustment: Life Change
Grief Resolution

Nursing Interventions Classification (NIC)
Body Image Enhancement
Grief Work Facilitation

PLANNING/OUTCOMES	NURSING INTERVENTIONS	RATIONALE
R.S. will communicate her concerns and feelings about the changes in her body image.	Involve R.S. in participating in her daily care.	Gives sense of independence.
	Encourage R.S. to voice her concerns.	Helps resolve concerns.

(Continues)

SAMPLE NURSING CARE PLAN (Continued)

PLANNING/OUTCOMES	NURSING INTERVENTIONS	RATIONALE
	Provide positive reinforcement when R.S. attempts to adapt to body changes.	Encourages client to continue adapting.

EVALUATION

R.S. has demonstrated beginning acceptance of body changes by taking an active interest in her appearance.

NURSING DIAGNOSIS 2 *Situational Low **S**elf-Esteem* related to loss of body part as evidenced by expression of concern about ability to care for self

Nursing Outcomes Classification (NOC)
Psychosocial Adjustment: Life Change
Decision Making

Nursing Interventions Classification (NIC)
Coping Enhancement
Support Group
Cognitive Restructuring

PLANNING/OUTCOMES	NURSING INTERVENTIONS	RATIONALE
R.S. will identify at least two positive qualities about herself.	Encourage R.S. to express her feelings about herself.	Helps identify positive qualities.
	Involve R.S. in decision making regarding her care.	Helps maintain a sense of control over her life.
	Provide R.S. with positive feedback.	Gives a feeling of acceptance and approval.

EVALUATION

R.S. has voiced two positive qualities about herself.

NURSING DIAGNOSIS 3 *Deficient **K**nowledge* related to postoperative care and activity as evidenced by concern about ability to care for self

Nursing Outcomes Classification (NOC)
Knowledge: Treatment Regimen

Nursing Interventions Classification (NIC)
Teaching: Procedure/Treatment

PLANNING/OUTCOMES	NURSING INTERVENTIONS	RATIONALE
R.S. swill perform stump wrapping correctly.	Encourage R.S. to participate in the care of the residual limb.	Helps client adjust to body changes.
	Demonstrate how to wrap her stump, then allow her to do it several times.	Helps client to know how to care for self.

EVALUATION

R.S. demonstrated the ability to care for the residual limb by wrapping the stump correctly.

NURSING DIAGNOSIS

Anticipatory Grieving related to loss associated with amputation as evidenced by her expression of concern

NOC: *Coping, Grief Resolution*
NIC: *Coping Enhancement, Grief Work Facilitation, Emotional Support, Anticipatory Guidance*

NURSING GOAL

R.S. will express her feelings about the loss of her foot.

NURSING INTERVENTIONS

1. Encourage R.S. to express her feelings by talking, crying, writing.
2. Spend quality time each shift with R.S. to let her share her thoughts and feelings.
3. Inform R.S. and her family about support groups and organizations in the community.

SCIENTIFIC RATIONALES

1. Gives several options for expression.
2. Allows.expression of feelings and shows concern and understanding.
3. May help R.S. find new ways of adapting to loss.

EVALUATION

Is R.S. expressing feelings about her potential loss?

CONCEPT CARE MAP 9-1

TEMPOROMANDIBULAR JOINT DISEASE/DISORDER

Temporomandibular joint disease/disorder (TMD) is commonly referred to as TMJ. It is a collection of conditions affecting the temporomandibular joint and/or the muscles of mastication. More than 10 million people in the United States have TMD. It affects both males and females, but 90% of those seeking treatment are females between puberty and menopause (The TMJ Association, 2002).

The temporomandibular joint is the articular surface between the mandible and temporal bone of the skull. It is a combined hinge and gliding joint. Normally, the mandible moves smoothly, appears symmetrical, and is without deformity. Causes for TMD include trauma, stress, teeth clenching, or grinding (**bruxism**), and joint diseases such as rheumatoid arthritis or osteoarthritis. Common symptoms of TMD include limited jaw movement, clicking or crepitus when the jaw moves, popping when chewing or talking, and radiating pain in the face, neck, or shoulders. The clicking is caused by displaced cartilage. The jaw may lock as a result of muscle spasms.

Diagnosis of TMD may include an x-ray to evaluate the bony structure, a CT scan to evaluate any degenerative changes, an MRI or arthrography, and an evaluation of the teeth and jaw in a bite position. Nursing assessment of the joint includes movement and appearance. If the mandible protrudes, it may indicate a mandibular dislocation.

Medical–Surgical Management

Medical

Medical management consists of moist heat to promote muscle relaxation, cold therapy to reduce muscle spasms, and analgesics or nonsteroidal anti-inflammatory drugs. Clients may be fitted with a dental retainer or bite plate to prevent teeth clenching or grinding, or splints to help realign malocclusions.

Surgical

Procedures such as arthroscopy or surgery to reshape the joint may be done in some cases that do not respond to medical treatment.

Diet

A soft diet allows the jaw and muscles to relax. Clients are advised against chewing gum.

Nursing Management

Encourage clients to practice relaxation techniques. Advise client to see a dentist for an evaluation of the teeth and jaw and to use the dental retainer or bite plate if given one.

CARPAL TUNNEL SYNDROME

Carpal tunnel syndrome occurs when the median nerve in the wrist is compressed by inflamed, edematous flexor tendons and tenosynovium (Figure 9-16). Symptoms include pain, paresthesia, and weakness of the thumb, index, middle and part of ring fingers, but never the little finger. Persons performing assembly line work or extensive keyboarding are especially at risk. Assemblers are three times more likely to have carpal tunnel than data-entry personnel (NINDS, 2002). Arthritis or fractures may also be a cause. Diagnosis is based on a physical examination and the subjective symptoms of the client and may be confirmed by motor nerve velocity studies.

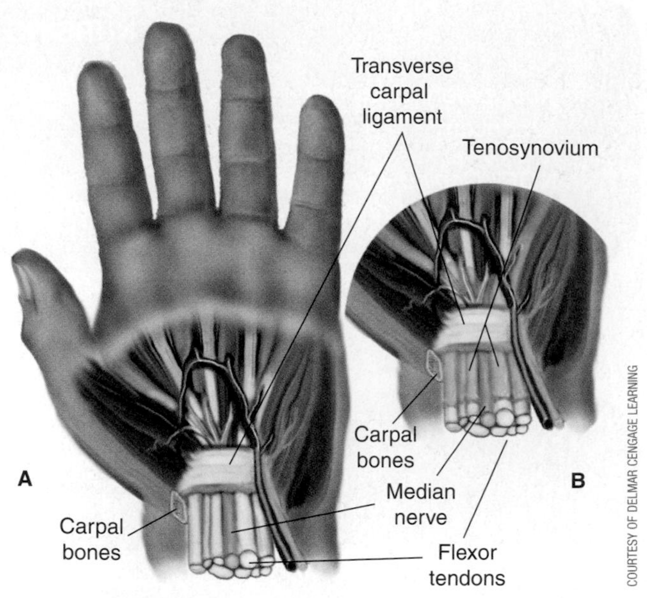

Figure 9-16 Carpal Tunnel Syndrome; *A,* Cross-section of carpal tunnel shows nerves and tendons; *B,* Inflamed flexor tendons and tenosynovium put pressure on the median nerve.

Medical–Surgical Management

Medical

Treatment consists of rest for the hands. Splints to immobilize the hand and wrist also are used to help relieve some of the discomfort.

Surgical

If conservative treatment does not control the symptoms, surgery is necessary to relieve the pressure on the median nerve. After surgery, the hand is elevated and may be in a splint for up to 2 weeks. Lifting is restricted for several weeks.

Pharmacological

Anti-inflammatory drugs may decrease inflammation and edema and reduce symptoms. NSAIDs may provide pain relief. If symptoms are not controlled with these measures, cortisone is injected into the carpal tunnel.

Nursing Management

Encourage clients performing repetitive hand movements to take rest periods from the task.

NURSING PROCESS

Assessment

Subjective Data

Subjective assessment data consist of the client's description of tingling in the hands and numbness in the thumb, index, middle and part of the ring fingers. The client may also state that there is a feeling of "puffiness" in the affected hand and that the client is unable to grasp or hold small objects. Waking in the middle of the night with pain and a feeling that the entire hand is asleep is very common.

Objective Data

Objective assessment data include atrophy of the padded area at the base of the thumb.

Nursing diagnoses for a client with carpal tunnel syndrome include the following:

NURSING DIAGNOSES	PLANNING/OUTCOMES	NURSING INTERVENTIONS
*Acute **P**ain* related to inflammation and swelling causing pressure on the median nerve	The client will have less discomfort.	Administer analgesics as ordered and teach client about use, side effects, and dosage. Encourage client to wear wrist brace. Encourage client to refrain from repetitive hand movements.
*Risk for **D**isuse Syndrome* related to tingling and numbness of hand and wrist	The client will use fingers and hand.	Teach client to do ROM exercises, and to prevent twisting and turning of wrist.

Evaluation: Evaluate each outcome to determine how it has been met by the client.

SYSTEMIC DISORDERS WITH MUSCULOSKELETAL MANIFESTATIONS

Systemic disorders that result in musculoskeletal symptoms include gout and Lyme disease.

GOUT

Gout is a metabolic disease of ineffective purine metabolism resulting in deposits of needlelike crystals of uric acid in connective tissue, joint spaces, or both. Middle-aged men are most commonly affected, but it may occur in women after menopause. Gout may be primary (an inherited problem with purine metabolism), secondary (complication from another disease or from use of certain drugs), or idiopathic (unknown cause). Up to 18% of clients with gout have a family history of the disease (NIAMS, 2002b). The excessive use of alcohol interferes with uric acid removal from the body and may contribute to or exacerbate symptoms.

The acute gout attack begins abruptly with severe constant pain. The joint becomes swollen, red, and tender. The great toe is the joint most frequently involved; however, any joint may be affected. The course of gout is variable, with one to two attacks being severe. If the disease is untreated, the attacks may occur with increasing frequency. Clients with symptoms of gout develop **tophi**, which are subcutaneous nodular deposits of sodium urate crystals appearing in various parts of the body, including the rim of the ears, the knuckles, and great toe. Diagnosis is made from the client's health history and an examination of the affected joint. Aspiration of the joint synovial fluid may show urate crystals. The client should be instructed to avoid foods high in purine, such as liver, sardines, sweetbreads, anchovies, gravies, and asparagus. Avoid excessive use of alcohol. Oral fluid intake is increased to 3,000 mL per day to reduce the possibility of urate stone formation in the kidneys.

To reduce inflammation, NSAIDs are given, especially indomethacin (Indocin) and ibuprofen (Motrin). Colchicine (Colsalide) is added in acute cases. When tophi develop, medicine to reduce hyperuricemia is used, such as allopurinol (Zyloprim) and probenecid (Benemid).

LYME DISEASE

Lyme disease is caused by a spirochete, *Borrelia burgdorferi*, carried by deer ticks. In the United States, it has been reported in nearly all states, but Lyme disease is endemic in Connecticut, Delaware, Maryland, Massachusetts, Minnesota, New Jersey, New York, Pennsylvania, Rhode Island, and Wisconsin. The onset of the disease is most prevalent in May (7%), June (25%), July (29%), and August (13%) (MMWR, 2005).

These ticks should be removed by using a tweezers. Early manifestations occur from spring through late fall. People living in states with a high incidence of Lyme disease should wear protective clothing and check for ticks frequently. Insect repellent containing 20% to 30% DEET is applied to exposed parts of the body and to clothing (CDC, 2008). For preventive protection, household pets wear a flea and tick collar, are given monthly preventive medication, and also are checked frequently for ticks.

For most individuals, the first symptom is a red rash called erythema migrans. It starts as a red spot at the site of the tick bite and expands, resembling a bull's eye. Other symptoms are headache, neck stiffness, fever, swelling in the knees and other large joints, and muscle pain. For those individuals untreated with antibiotics, arthritis (joint swelling and pain), fatigue, and neurological abnormalities such as facial palsy, meningitis, and encephalitis become evident. The antibody test ELISA is used to identify antibodies to *B. burgdorferi* in blood or spinal fluid specimens. Antibiotics such as doxycycline (Vibramycin), cefuroxime exetil (Ceftin), or amoxicillin (Amoxil) speed healing of the rash and may prevent arthritis and neurologic symptoms.

CASE STUDY

G.E., a 40-year-old truck driver, was getting ready to help unload his cargo. He was climbing into the truck when he lost his balance and fell to the ground, twisting his left leg. He stated he was in severe pain and was unable to stand. His coworkers called the emergency ambulance service to transport him to the hospital. Upon arrival in the emergency department, the nurse immediately took G.E.'s vital signs, which were temperature 98.6°F, pulse 92 beats/minute, respirations 24 breaths/minute, and blood pressure 158/90 mm Hg. The nurse also noted that G.E.'s face was flushed and his left leg was shorter than his right.

The following questions will guide your development of a nursing care plan for the case study:

1. List five types of fractures.
2. Based on the action of the fall, what type of fracture do you think G.E. sustained?
3. What diagnostic measures will determine whether or not G.E. has a fracture of his left leg?
4. What would be the best immediate care for G.E.?
5. List four nursing interventions for clients in traction.
6. What possible treatment options are best for G.E.'s injury?
7. What objective and subjective data are important for the nurse to obtain regarding G.E.'s injury?

SUMMARY

- When assessing the client with a musculoskeletal disorder, the nurse evaluates any changes in appearance, including alignment, loss of motion, and any signs of circulatory impairment.
- Treatment of a fracture includes any one or more of the following methods: closed reduction, open reduction that may include internal fixation, casts, and traction.
- Compartment syndrome is a serious form of neurovascular impairment. Symptoms include severe pain that is not relieved with narcotic analgesics, sluggish capillary refill, weak pulses, numbness, and paralysis.
- When a client is in traction, it is important to remember to preserve body alignment, maintain continuous pull and countertraction, keep the ropes moving freely through the pulleys, use the prescribed amount of weights, and keep the weights hanging freely.
- Osteoarthritis is characterized by slow progressive degeneration of joint articular cartilage.
- Hips, knees, and fingers are the joints most frequently considered for replacement.
- After total hip replacement, the hip is kept in a position of abduction and extension.
- After total knee replacement surgery, some clients use a CPM machine that promotes knee joint flexibility and increased circulation to the operative area.
- Individuals at greatest risk for developing osteoporosis are postmenopausal women and older adults who are generally inactive.

REVIEW QUESTIONS

1. A client is admitted to the hospital and expresses concerns for his job. This information will become what part of his nursing care plan?
   1. Nursing diagnosis.
   2. Goal.
   3. Validating data.
   4. Evaluation.
2. A client returned from surgery with an internal fixation of the right femur. The nursing primary treatment goal of the repaired fracture is:
   1. aid in the formation of osteoclasts.
   2. establish a callus between the broken ends of bone.
   3. aid in the formation of granulation tissue.
   4. prevent further injury to the fractured limb.
3. A nurse enters the room and notices a client in skeletal traction is lying with poor positioning and alignment. The nurse repositions the client in good alignment to prevent the possible deformity of:
   1. scoliosis.
   2. lordosis.
   3. contracture.
   4. muscle atony.
4. A client is admitted to the hospital with osteoarthritis (degenerative joint disease). Upon assessing the client, the nurse expects to find: (Select all that apply.)
   1. nausea after each meal.
   2. joint stiffness especially on arising.
   3. an increased appetite.
   4. muscle spasms after exercising.
   5. Heberden's nodes.
   6. pain after physical exercise.
5. A 48-year-old man has suffered low-back pain and sciatica for over 2 years. He is admitted to the hospital for evaluation and treatment of this problem. A thorough assessment of his level of discomfort from low-back pain is important primarily because:

1. this will provide a baseline for later comparison.
2. this is a method for identifying clients with "low back neurosis."
3. clients who have pain localized to the back and radiating to one extremity are probably not candidates for surgery.
4. surgery is contraindicated for clients who have had pain for less than 2 years.

6. In preparing a teaching plan for an adult who has had an arthroscopy, what following information will the nurse include?
   1. Client should check extremity for color, mobility, and sensation at least every 2 hours after the procedure.
   2. Client may return to regular activities immediately after procedure.
   3. Remove compression dressing 6 to 8 hours after procedure.
   4. Keep extremity in flexion for 24 hours after procedure.
7. A client just returned from surgery for the repair of a right fractured tibia and fibula and has a cast applied to the extremity. The nurse first:
   1. listens to the breath sounds for respiratory complications.
   2. listens to the abdomen for bowel sounds.
   3. covers the client with a warm blanket.
   4. checks the right toes for circulation, sensation, and movement.
8. A client was admitted to the hospital following a motorcycle accident with multiple fractures to the left leg. A long leg cast was applied and 6 hours after surgery the client is expressing extreme pain in his left leg after receiving medication by a PCA. The nurse suspects compartment syndrome. If the nurse is correct, what other symptoms would the client have? (Select all that apply.)
   1. Sluggish capillary refill.
   2. Pain from the lower spine down the back of the leg.
   3. Numbness or tingling in the leg.
   4. Weak pulse in the left toes and strong pulse in the right toes.
   5. Increased length of the right leg.
   6. Foul odor from the cast.
9. An appropriate nursing diagnosis for a client with a recent amputation is:
   1. *Ineffective Peripheral **T**issue Perfusion.*
   2. *Risk for **I**njury.*
   3. ***N**ausea.*
   4. *Disturbed **B**ody Image.*
10. A client was admitted to the hospital with a fracture after a skiing accident. One of the most common fractures from this type of accident is:
    1. comminuted.
    2. greenstick.
    3. spiral.
    4. impacted.

REFERENCES/SUGGESTED READINGS

American Academy of Orthopaedic Surgeons (AAOS). (2007a). Care of casts and splints. Retrieved April 8, 2009, from http://orthoinfo.aaos.org/topic.cfm?topic=a00204

American Academy of Orthopaedic Surgeons (AAOS). (2007b). Compartment syndrome. Retrieved April 8, 2009, from http://orthoinfo.aaos.org/topic.cfm?topic=a00204

American Academy of Orthopaedic Surgeons (AAOS). (2007c). Minimally invasive total hip replacement. Retrieved April 8, 2009, from http://orthoinfo.aaos.org/topic.cfm?topic=A00404

American Academy of Orthopaedic Surgeons (AAOS). (2007d). Total hip replacement. Retrieved April 8, 2009, from http://orthoinfo.aaos.org/topic.cfm?topic=A00377

American Academy of Orthopaedic Surgeons (AAOS). (2007e). Total knee replacement. Retrieved April 8, 2009, from http://orthoinfo.aaos.org/topic.cfm?topic=A00389

Arthritis Foundation. (2002a). Gout. Retrieved April 9, 2009, from http://ww2.arthritis.org/conditions/diseaseCenter/gout.asp

Arthritis Foundation. (2002b). Osteoarthritis. Retrieved April 9, 2009, from http://ww2.arthritis.org/conditions/DiseaseCenter/oa.asp

Bailey J. (2003). Getting a fix on orthopedic care. *Nursing2003, 33*(6), 58–63.

Bryant, G. (2001). Stump care. *AJN, 101*(2), 67–71.

Bulechek, G., Butcher, H., McCloskey, J., & Dochterman, J., eds. (2008). *Nursing Interventions Classification (NIC)* (5th ed.). St. Louis, MO: Mosby/Elsevier.

Burke, S. (2001). Boning up on osteoporosis. *Nursing2001, 31*(10), 36–42.

Centers for Disease Control (CDC). (2008). Lyme disease. Retrieved April 9, 2009, from http://www.cdc.gov/ncidid.dvbid/lyme?prevention/ld_Prevention_Avoid.htm

Curry, L., & Hogstel, M. (2002). Osteoporosis. *AJN, 102*(1), 26–32.

D'Arcy, Y. (2002). How to treat arthritis pain. *Nursing2002, 32*(7), 30–31.

Daniels, R. (2009). *Delmar's guide to laboratory and diagnostic tests.* Clifton Park, NY: Delmar Cengage Learning.

Daniels, R., Grendell, R., & Wilkins, F. (2010). *Nursing fundamentals: Caring & clinical decision making* (2nd ed.). Clifton Park, NY: Delmar Cengage Learning.

Estes, M. (2010). *Health assessment & physical examination* (4th ed.). Clifton Park, NY: Delmar Cengage Learning.

Fort, C. (2002). Getting a fix on long-bone fracture. *Nursing2002, 32*(6), 32hn1–32hn6.

Fort, C. (2003). How to combat 3 deadly trauma complications. *Nursing2003, 33*(5), 58–63.

Hayes, D. (2003a). How to wrap an above-the-knee amputation stump. *Nursing2003, 33*(1), 70.

Hayes, D. (2003b). How to wrap a below-the-knee amputation stump. *Nursing2003, 33*(2), 28.

Ignatavicius, D. (2002). Catching compartment syndrome early. *Nursing2002, 32*(11), 10.

Infectious Disease Society of America (IDSA). (2007). Updated guidelines on diagnosis, treatment of Lyme disease. Retrieved April 9, 2009, from http://www.idsociety.org/Content.aspx?id=3744

Ingham Regional Orthopedic Hospital, A McLaren Health Service. (2004). Regaining an active lifestyle: A helpful guide for patient undergoing knee replacement surgery. Retrieved April 10, 2009, from http://www.irmc.org/documents/Health%20Articles/KNEE%20 REPLACEMENT%20BROCHURE.pdf

Lawrence, B., & Tasota, F. (2003). Detecting neuromuscular problems with electromyography. *Nursing2003, 33*(4), 82.

Leslie, M. (2000). When the ache is not arthritis. *RN, 63*(3), 38–40.

Lewis, A. (1999). Orthopedic and vascular emergencies. *Nursing99, 29*(12), 54–56.

Lindgren, V. (2003). When to suspect this bone disorder. *RN, 66*(6), 32–36.

Maher, A. (2002). Assessment of the musculoskeletal system. In A. B. Maher, S. W. Salmond, & T. A. Pellino (eds.), Orthopaedic nursing (3rd ed., pp. 189–210). Philadelphia: W. B. Saunders Company.

McClung, B. (2001). Reducing your risk of osteoporosis. A Guide to Women's Health (supplement to *Nursing2001)*, April, 4–8.

McConnell, E. (2001). Myth & facts . . . about gout. *Nursing2001, 31*(5), 73.

McConnell, E. (2002a). Assessing neurovascular status in a casted limb. *Nursing2002, 32*(9), 20.

McConnell, E. (2002b). Myths & facts . . . about compartment syndrome. *Nursing2002, 32*(2), 92.

MedlinePlus®. (2007). Rhabdomyolysis. Retrieved April 7, 2009, from http://www.nlm.nih.gov/medlineplus/ency/article/000473.htm

MedlinePlus®. (2009). Lyme disease. Retrieved April 7, 2009, from http://www.nlm.nih.gov/medlineplus/print/lymedisease.html

MMWR Weekly. (June 15, 2005). Lyme disease—United States, 2003–2005. Retrieved April 7, 2009, from http://www.cd.gov/mmwr/preview/mmwrhtml/mm5623al.htm

Moorhead, S., Johnson, M., Maas, M., & Swanson, E. (2007). *Nursing Outcomes Classification (NOC)* (4th ed). St. Louis, MO: Elsevier–Health Sciences Division.

National Institute of Allergies and Infectious Diseases (NIAID). (2008). Lyme disease. Retrieved April 9, 2009, from http://www3.niaid.nih.gov/topics/lymeDisease/

National Institute of Arthritis and Musculoskeletal and Skin Diseases (NIAMS). (2006a). Osteoarthritis. Retrieved April 9, 2009, from http://www.niams.nih.gov/Health_Info/Osteoarthritis/default.asp

National Institute of Arthritis and Musculoskeletal and Skin Diseases (NIAMS). (2006b). Questions and answers about gout. Retrieved April 9, 2009, from http://www.niams.nih.gov/Health_Info/Gout/default.asp

National Institute of Neurological Disorders and Stroke (NINDS). (2008). Carpal tunnel syndrome fact sheet. Retrieved April 9, 2009, from http://www.ninds.nih.gov/disorders/carpal_tunnel/detail_carpal_tunnel.htm

National Osteoporosis Foundation (NOF). (2008a). Osteoporosis bone density. Retrieved April 9, 2009, from http://www.nof.org/osteoporosis/bonemass.htm

National Osteoporosis Foundation (NOF). (2008b). Osteoporosis: men. Retrieved April 9, 2009, from http://www.nof.org/men/index.htm

National Osteoporosis Foundation (NOF). (2008c). Prevention: Five steps to prevention. Retrieved April 9, 2009, from http://www.nof.org/prevention/index.htm

National Osteoporosis Foundation (NOF). (2008d). Fast facts on osteoporosis. Retrieved April 8, 2009, from http://www.nof.org/osteoporosis/diseasefacts.htm

North American Nursing Diagnosis Association International. (2010). *NANDA-I nursing diagnoses: Definitions and classification 2009-2011*. Ames, IA: Wiley-Blackwell.

O'Hanlon-Nichols, T. (1998). Basic assessment series: Musculoskeletal system. *AJN, 98*(6), 48–52.

Overdorf, J., Pachuki-Hyde, L., Kressenick, C., McClung, B., & Lucasey, C. (2001). Osteoporosis: There's so much we can do. *RN, 64*(12), 30–34.

Pauldine, E. (2003). Taking a bite out of Lyme disease. *Nursing2003, 33*(4), 49–52.

Preboth, M. (2001). Lyme disease: New guidelines. *American Family Physician, 63*(10), 2065–2067.

Queensland Government. (2009). Introduction to stump care. Retrieved April 8, 2009, from http://www.health.qld.gov.au/qals/docs/stump_care.pdf

Reeser, J. (2007). Stress fractures. Retrieved April 7, 2009, from http://emedicine.medscape.com/article/309106-overview

Rogers, D. (2003). New meaning for safe sex. *RN, 66*(1), 38–41.

Rupert, S. (2002). Pathogenesis and treatment of rhabdomyolysis. *Journal of the American Academy of Nurse Practitioners, 14*(2), 82.

Sauret, J. M., Marinides, G., & Wang, G. K. (2002). Rhabdomyolysis. *American Family Physician, 65*(1), 907.

Spratto, G., & Woods, A. (2009). *2009 PDR nurse's drug handbook*. Clifton Park, NY: Delmar Cengage Learning.

Sullivan, M., & Sharts-Hopko, N. (2000). Preventing the downward spiral. *AJN, 100*(8), 26–31.

The Ohio State University Medical Center. (2008). External fixator. Retrieved July 27, 2009 from http://medicalcenter.osu.edu/PatientEd/Materials/PDFDocs/surgery/ortho/externalfixation.pdf

The TMJ Association. (2009). Changing the face of TMJ. Retrieved April 9, 2009, from http://www.tmj.org/

University of Iowa Health Care. (2008). Cast care. Retrieved April 8, 2009, from http://www.uihealthcare.com/topics/bonesjointsmuscles/bone3418.html

Wade, C. (2000). Keeping lyme disease at bay. *AJN, 100*(7), 26–31.

Walls, M. (2002). Orthopedic trauma. *RN, 65*(7), 52–56.

Wise, S. (in press). Assessing the musculoskeletal system.

Yarnold, B. (1999). Hip fracture. *AJN, 99*(2), 36–40.

Zdeblick, T. (2009) Compression and wedge fractures. Retrieved April 7, 2009, from http://www.spineuniverse.com/displayarticle.php/article1441.html

RESOURCES

American Occupational Therapy Association, Inc., http://www.aota.org

American Physical Therapy Association, http://www.apta.org

Arthritis Foundation, http://www.arthritis.org

National Amputation Foundation, http://www.nationalamputation.org

National Institute of Arthritis and Musculoskeletal and Skin Diseases (NIAMS), http://www.niams.nih.gov

National Osteoporosis Foundation, http://www.nof.org

OrthoIllustrated Orthopaedic Surgery Patient Education, http://www.orthoillustrated.com

Osteoporosis and Related Bone Diseases, http://www.osteo.org

The TMJ Association, Ltd., http://www.tmj.org

CHAPTER 10
Neurological System

MAKING THE CONNECTION

Refer to the following chapters to increase your understanding of the neurological system:

Adult Health Nursing
- ***Oncology***
- ***Cardiovascular System***
- ***Musculoskeletal System***
- ***Endocrine System***
- ***The Older Adult***

LEARNING OBJECTIVES

Upon completion of this chapter, you should be able to:
- Define key terms.
- Identify basic functional areas of the human neurological system.
- Perform a neurological screening and a basic neurological examination.
- Prepare a client for common neurological diagnostic examinations.
- Derive a Glasgow Coma Scale score for a client.
- Recognize common symptoms of neurological disorders.
- Plan interventions for a client with a neurological disorder.

KEY TERMS

affect
agnosia
anosognosia
aphasia
areflexia
ataxia
aura
automatism
autonomic nervous system(ANS)
awareness
bradykinesia
central nervous system (CNS)
cephalalgia
chorea
coprolalia
decerebration
dysarthria
dysphagia
emotional lability
encephalitis
fasciculation
Glasgow Coma Scale
graphesthesia
hemiparesis
hemiplegia
homonymous hemianopia
Lasegue's sign
meningitis
mentation
neuralgia
neurogenic shock
neurotransmitter
nuchal rigidity
nystagmus
orientation
paraplegia
peripheral nervous system (PNS)
postictal
quadriplegia

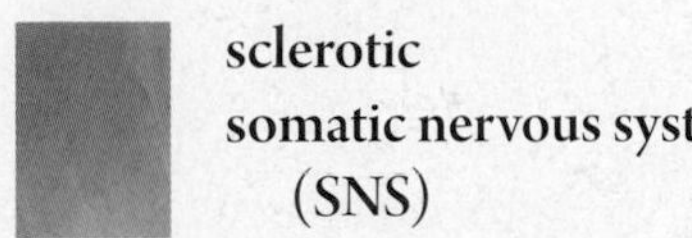

sclerotic
somatic nervous system (SNS)
spinal shock
status epilepticus
stereognosis
tetraplegia
unilateral neglect
vertigo

INTRODUCTION

The human neurological system (called nervous system) is highly complex, controlling and integrating all other body systems. This system controls motor, sensory, and autonomic functions of the body. This is accomplished by coordination and initiation of cellular activity through the transmission of electrical impulses and various hormones.

ANATOMY AND PHYSIOLOGY REVIEW

The nervous system is divided into the **central nervous system (CNS)**, consisting of the brain and spinal cord; the **peripheral nervous system (PNS)**, which consists of the cranial nerves and spinal nerves; and the **autonomic nervous system (ANS)**, which is part of the peripheral nervous system and consists of the sympathetic and parasympathetic systems.

Central Nervous System

The CNS comprises the brain and the spinal cord (Figure 10-1).

The Brain

The brain, composed of gray matter and white matter, controls, initiates, and integrates body functions through the use of electrical impulses and complex molecules. The gray matter, on the outer part of the brain, contains billions of neurons. Neurons, the basic cells of the nervous system, have three major components: the cell body, the axon, and the dendrites (Figure 10-2). The axon carries impulses away from the cell body, and the dendrites carry impulses toward the cell body. The cell body controls the function of the neuron. Functions include the conduction of impulses and the release of neurotransmitters. **Neurotransmitters** are chemical substances that excite, inhibit, or modify the response of another neuron (Hickey, 2008). Neuroglial cells are in the central and peripheral nervous systems and are not neurons. They protect, support, and nourish the neurons.

The white matter of the inner structures of the brain contains association and projection pathways that transmit nerve impulses to communicate information to the different areas of the brain. These communication pathways are necessary for integration of brain activity (Hickey, 2008).

The brain is contained within the skull, or cranium, which is a bony, rigid box that protects the brain tissue. There are three coverings of the brain, called meninges. They are the *dura mater, arachnoid mater,* and *pia mater* (Figure 10-1A). These coverings provide protection, support, and small amounts of nourishment.

The brain is divided into two hemispheres. The right side of the brain receives information from and controls the left side of the body. The left hemisphere receives information from and controls the right side of the body. Both hemispheres of the brain communicate through nerve fibers in the corpus callosum. A predominate hemisphere exists for special tasks so that confusion does not occur. The right side specializes in the perception of physical environment, art, nonverbal communication, music, and spiritual aspects. The left hemisphere generally specializes in analysis, calculation, problem solving, verbal communication, interpretation, language, reading, and writing.

The Spinal Cord

The spinal cord is a continuation of the brainstem. It exits the skull through the *foramen magnum,* an opening in the base of the skull. The spinal cord is approximately 45 centimeters, or 18 inches, in length and is the thickness of one finger. The cord is divided into right and left halves and has a shallow groove, called the posterior median sulcus, on the dorsal side and a deep groove, called the anterior median fissure, on the ventral side (Figure 10-3A). The cord tapers to a thin tip, called the conus medullaris, at the first lumbar vertebrae, and terminates as a thin cord of connective tissue, called the filum terminale, which continues as far as the second sacral vertebrae (Figure 10-3A and B). The vertebral column provides vertical support for the cord. The meninges cover the spinal cord, providing protection. Reflex activity is initiated within the spinal cord.

There are 31 pairs of spinal nerves originating from the spinal cord. Each pair contains a dorsal, or posterior, nerve root and a ventral, or anterior, nerve root (Figure 10-3C). The dorsal nerve roots carry sensory impulses from the body to the brain; the ventral nerve roots carry motor impulses from the spinal cord to the body. The spinal cord has an H-shaped appearance of gray matter within the white matter (Figure 10-3D). The horns forming the H shape are referred to as the anterior (ventral) horns, the posterior (dorsal) horns, and the lateral horns. These horns contain the cell bodies of neurons that innervate the skeletal muscles.

Cerebrospinal Fluid

Cerebrospinal fluid (CSF) is produced primarily in the choroid plexus. Five hundred milliliters of CSF are produced daily, with excess being reabsorbed by the arachnoid villi in the subarachnoid space. The circulation of CSF is from the lateral ventricles to the third and fourth ventricles. From there, it enters the subarachnoid space to flow around the spinal cord and the brain.

Cerebrospinal fluid absorbs shock and bathes the brain and spinal cord. It contains glucose, protein, urea, and salts. These nutritive substances are delivered to the CNS cells, and the waste and toxic substances are removed.

Peripheral Nervous System

All of the nerve tissue outside of the CNS is part of the peripheral nervous system (PNS). The PNS consists of the cranial nerves and the spinal nerves and has both sensory and motor

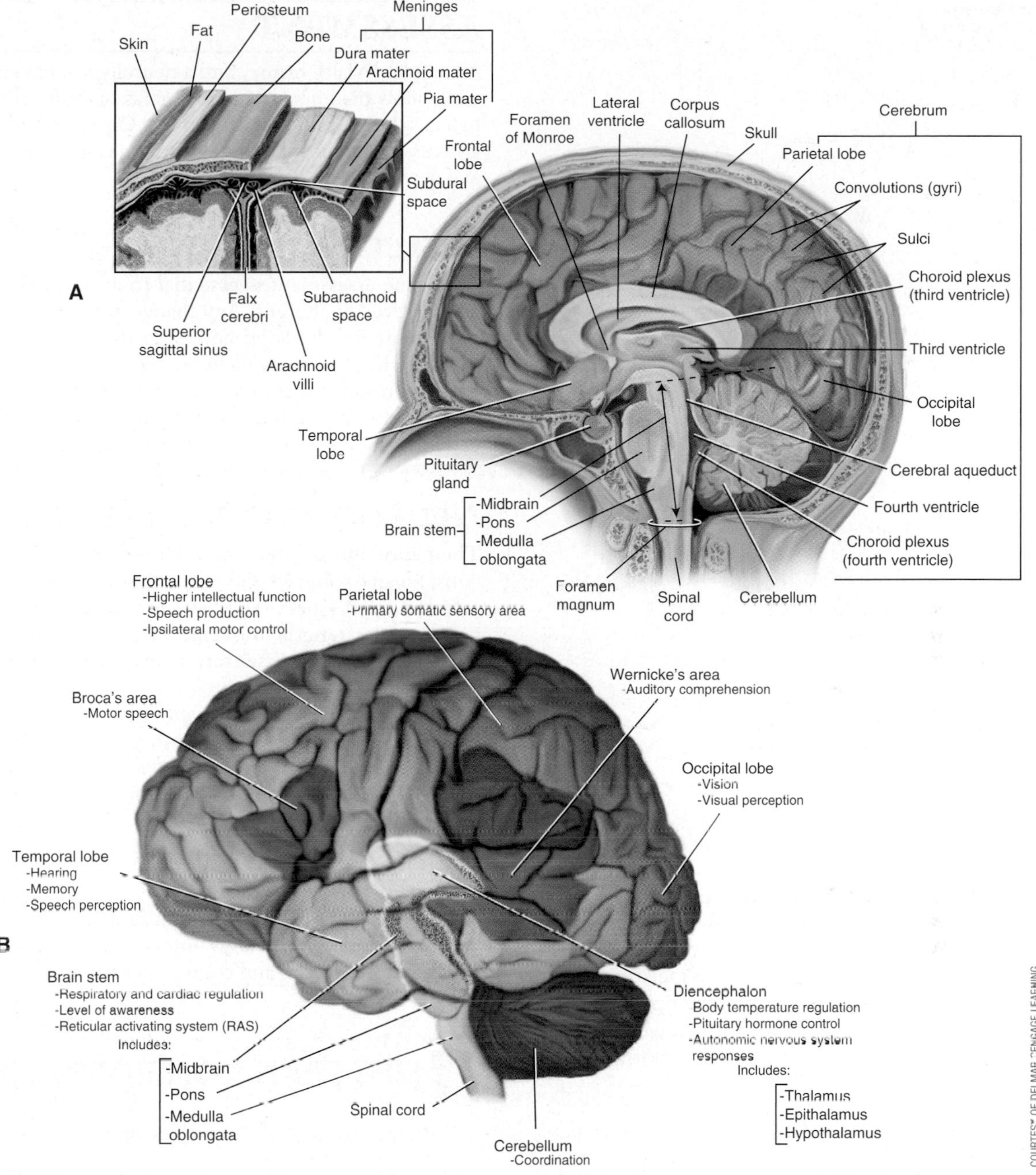

FIGURE 10-1 **The central nervous system includes the brain, spinal cord, and meninges. *A*, Structures of the Brain; *B*, Functional Area of the Brain.**

components. The PNS can be divided into the **somatic nervous system** and the ANS. The somatic portion connects the CNS to the skin and skeletal muscles. It is involved in conscious activities, such as walking. The autonomic portion connects the CNS to visceral organs such as the heart, stomach, intestines, and various glands. It is involved in unconscious activities, such as breathing.

Cranial Nerves

The 12 pairs of cranial nerves have sensory, motor, or mixed functions. Table 10-1 lists functions and describes assessment of cranial nerves. The cranial nerves originate from the brain or brainstem, with most originating from the brainstem. Although always identified by Roman numerals, the cranial nerves also have names.

Spinal Nerves

Thirty-one pairs of spinal nerves exit from the spinal cord through the vertebral column: cervical, 8 pairs; thoracic, 12 pairs; lumbar, 5 pairs; sacral, 5 pairs; and coccyx, 1 pair. The dorsal, or posterior, nerve roots carry sensory impulses to the brain. The ventral, or anterior, nerve roots carry motor impulses from the spinal cord and brain to the muscles. Motor and sensory impulses are transmitted from the body and internal organs.

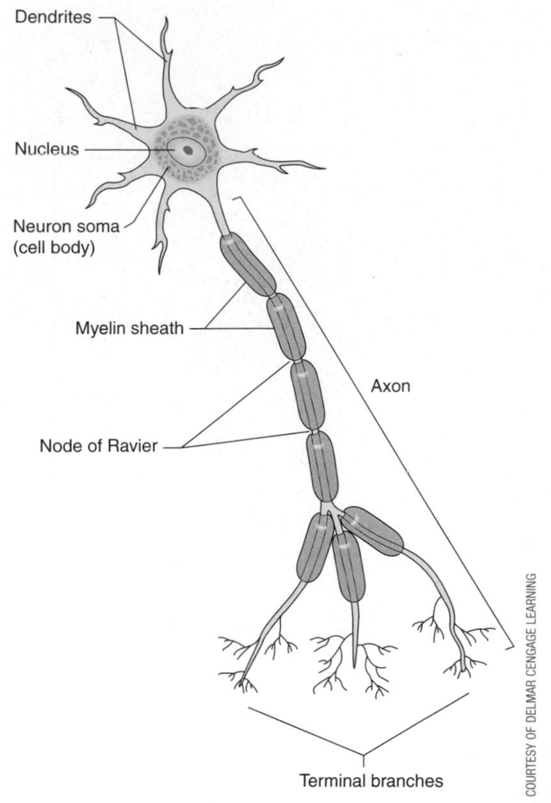

FIGURE 10-2 Neuron (Nerve Cell) Structure

Reflex activity is a stereotypical response to a stimulus that is initiated by the nervous system (Hickey, 2008). The three classifications of reflexes are muscle stretch, or deep tendon; superficial, or cutaneous; and pathological (see section on assessment of reflexes). Reflex activity requires the function of five areas in the nervous system: the sensory fibers, the neuron relaying the impulse, the association center in the brain, the neuron relaying the motor impulse from the brain to the body, and the specific organ involved. Disease processes at any of these areas can cause an abnormal reflex response.

Autonomic Nervous System

The main function of the ANS is to maintain internal homeostasis. There are two subdivisions of the ANS: the sympathetic system and the parasympathetic system. The sympathetic system, activated by stress, prepares the body for the "fight-or-flight" response. The sympathetic system causes increased heart rate, increased blood pressure, vasoconstriction, decreased peristalsis, dilated pupils, increased secretions of epinephrine and sweat, and decreased secretions of digestive juices and saliva (Table 10-2).

The parasympathetic system conserves, restores, and maintains vital body functions, slowing heart rate, increasing gastrointestinal activity, and activating bowel and bladder evacuation.

The sympathetic and parasympathetic systems work antagonistically to regulate the smooth muscles, the heart, and the glands of the body. When one system increases an action, the other system decreases the action. Thus, when one stimulates, the other inhibits; when one dilates, the other one constricts, and so forth. Both systems function simultaneously, but one can dominate the other as needed.

ASSESSMENT

A complete health history and a neurological screening assessment allow the nurse to identify areas of dysfunction in order to focus the neurological assessment. Observation (inspection) is necessary for most of the assessment; palpation, auscultation, and percussion are also used.

Health History

A baseline assessment is essential to ascertaining changes in neurological functioning. Any change from the baseline assessment must be identified and early intervention initiated. A thorough health history includes asking the client about headaches, clumsiness, loss of or change in function of an extremity, seizure activity, numbness or tingling, change in vision, pain, extreme fatigue, personality changes, and mood swings.

Neurological Assessment

The neurological screening involves assessment of level of consciousness and verbal responses to specific questions; selected cranial nerves for eye movement and visual acuity; muscle strength; movement; gait for motor function; and tactile and pain sensation of extremities for sensory screening.

A complete nursing assessment of neurological function includes assessment of the following areas: cerebral function, cranial nerve function, motor function, sensory function, and reflexes. Neurological nursing assessment is discussed in more detail in the next section.

Cerebral Function

Areas of assessment of cerebral function include level of consciousness, mental status, intellectual function, emotional status, pupil reaction, and communication.

LIFE SPAN CONSIDERATIONS

Neurological Changes with Aging

Remember the following with regard to the elderly client:

- Nerve impulse transmission slows.
- Cardiovascular system changes that lead to a decreased oxygen supply to the brain affect mental acuity, sensory interpretation, and motor ability.
- The amount of neurotransmitters produced diminishes, and the enzyme activity that degrades neurotransmitters increases.
- Changes in neurotransmitters affect sleep, temperature control, and mood.
- The brain tends to atrophy, leaving the cortical bridging veins, which connect the brain to the meninges, vulnerable to trauma and bleeding.

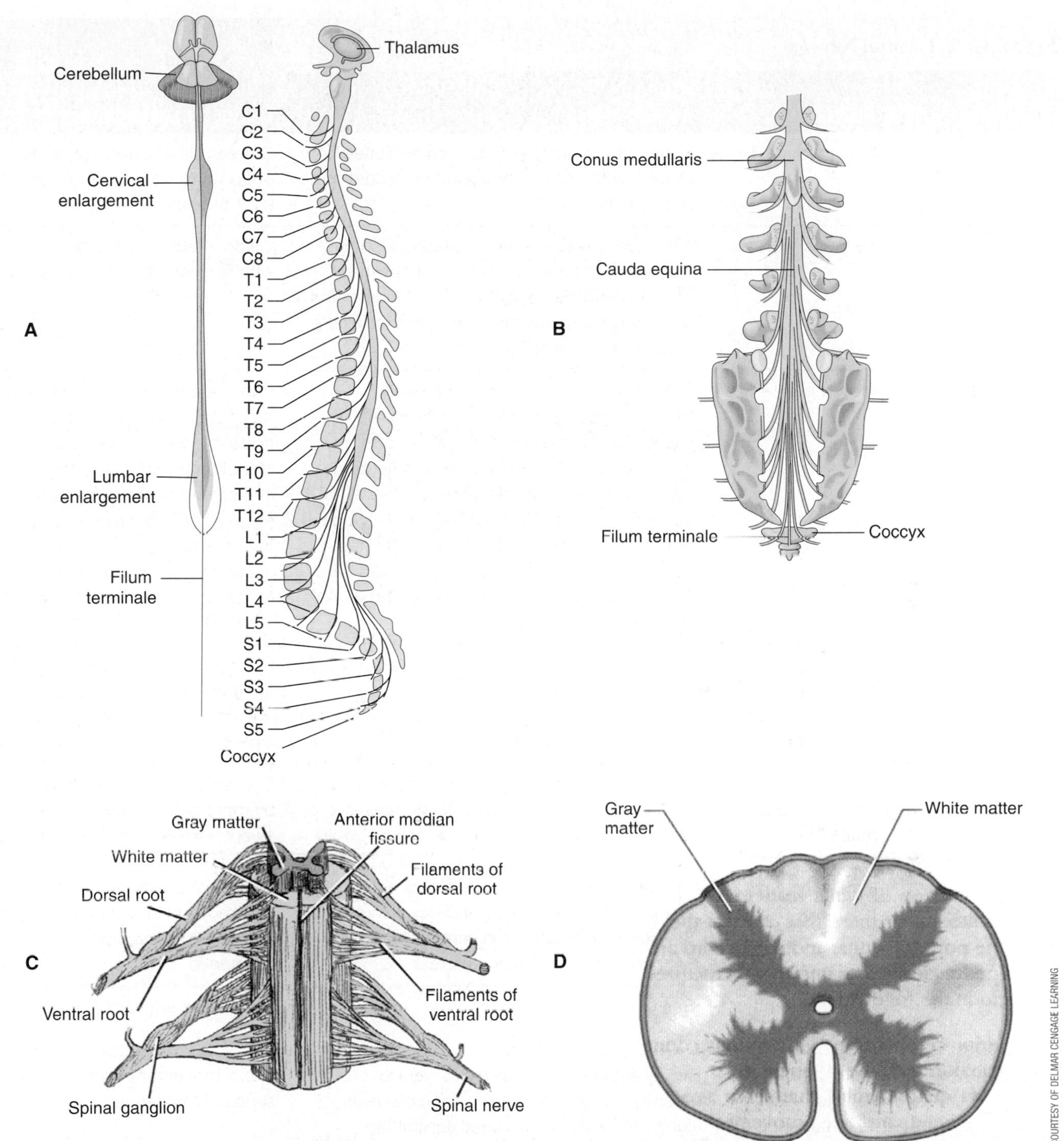

FIGURE 10-3 ***A*, Spinal Cord and Spinal Nerves; *B*, Conus Medullaris and Filum Terminale; *C*, Anterior View of Spinal Cord; *D*, H-Shaped Appearance of Gray Matter and White Matter in the Spinal Cord**

Level of Consciousness Level of consciousness is assessed by determining the client's awareness and orientation and is the most important indicator of change in neurological status. **Awareness** is the person's ability to perceive environmental stimuli and body reactions and then respond with thought and action. The client's awareness is assessed through four components: orientation, memory, calculation, and fund of knowledge (Lower, 2002).

A more objective assessment is made using the **Glasgow Coma Scale**, an objective tool for assessing consciousness in clients, most frequently in clients with head injuries. With the Glasgow Coma Scale, eye opening, verbal response, and motor response are scored using measurable criteria (Table 10-3). The totaled scores indicate coma severity. A score of 15 indicates a fully oriented person. A score of 3 is the lowest possible score, indicating deep coma. A score of 7 or less is considered a state of coma.

Changes in the Glasgow Coma Scale indicate changes in client condition. To prevent further damage to the brain in instances of decreasing scores, the nurse acts quickly. The physician must be notified immediately and measures taken to decrease intracranial pressure (see section on increased intracranial pressure).

TABLE 10-1 Cranial Nerves

CRANIAL NERVE	FUNCTION	ASSESSMENT	EXPECTED FINDINGS
Olfactory (I)	Sensory: smell	Have client identify smells such as coffee or alcohol with one nostril occluded; repeat for opposite nostril.	Correct identification of smell or ability to choose smell from a list of choices.
Optic (II)	Sensory: vision	Ask client to read printed material, identify number of fingers held in front of client, or read from Snellen eye chart. Test visual fields by having client identify when the examiner's finger enters visual field.	Vision intact or correctable with lenses; visual field intact.
Oculomotor (III)	Motor: pupil constriction	Cranial nerves III, IV, and VI are tested together. Inspect for ptosis, or drooping of eyelid. Assess extraocular eye muscles by having client follow the examiner's finger to each quadrant of the visual field. Assess for accommodation by asking the client to look at the examiner's finger held 4 to 6 inches from the client's nose, and then to follow the finger to 18 inches from the client's nose. Ask client about double vision.	Pupils are equal and round and react equally to light. No ptosis or double vision. Eyes move smoothly and consensually inward and downward. As the examiner's finger moves away from the client, the pupil will accommodate by dilating; as the finger moves closer; the pupil will normally constrict.
Trochlear (IV)	Motor: upper eyelid elevation, extraocular eye movement	See oculomotor (III).	Eyes should move smoothly and consensually upward and outward without nystagmus or diplopia.
Trigeminal (V)	Sensory: cornea, nose, and oral mucosa Motor: mastication	Test corneal reflex by lightly touching cornea with a small piece of cotton. Check sensation of face by touching lightly with a cotton ball while the client's eyes are closed and asking the client whether sensation is present. Check motor function by having client clench jaws shut while the examiner palpates the contraction of the temporalis and masseter muscles.	Corneal reflex as evidenced by rapid blinking when cotton swept across cornea. Feeling cotton ball on face indicates that facial sensation is intact. Jaw movement symmetrical and able to overcome resistance.
Abducens (VI)	Motor: extraocular eye movement	See oculomotor (III).	Eyes move outward.
Facial (VII)	Motor: facial muscles; Sensory: taste (anterior two-thirds of tongue)	Ask client to smile, show teeth, wrinkle forehead, or whistle. Have client close eyes lightly and keep them closed against the examiner's trying to open them. Have client identify salt and sugar when dabbed on tongue.	Facial movement symmetrical, sense of taste intact.
Acoustic (VIII)	Sensory: hearing, equilibrium	Assess ability to hear ticking watch or whispered voice. Observe gait for swaying. Perform Romberg test (refer to assessment of motor function).	Sense of hearing intact; no swaying or loss of balance.
Glossopharyngeal (IX)	Sensory: sensation to throat and taste (posterior one-third of tongue) Motor: swallowing	Have client identify taste of salt and sugar on back of tongue. Have client say "ah" and assess for symmetrical position of uvula. Test gag reflex by touching back of pharynx with tongue depressor. Observe swallowing ability and speech patterns.	Taste sensation intact; uvula raises symmetrically; gag reflex intact; swallowing and speech intact.

Table 10-1 Cranial Nerves (Continued)

CRANIAL NERVE	FUNCTION	ASSESSMENT	EXPECTED FINDINGS
Vagus (X)	Motor and sensory	Test along with glossopharyngeal nerve.	
Spinal accessory (XI)	Motor: movement of uvula, soft palate, sternocleidomastoid muscle, trapezius muscle	Place examiner's hand on side of client's face and ask client to turn head against resistance; have client shrug shoulders against resistance of the examiner's hand.	Ability to move shoulder and head against resistance.
Hypoglossal (XII)	Motor: tongue movement	Ask client to stick out tongue and observe for symmetry, deviation to side; have client push tongue against tongue depressor and move tongue from side to side.	Tongue should be centrally aligned, able to push against resistance of tongue depressor; no fasciculations (involuntary twitching of muscle fibers) should be present.

Table 10-2 Sympathetic and Parasympathetic Responses

SYSTEM	SYMPATHETIC RESPONSE	PARASYMPATHETIC RESPONSE
Neurological	Pupils dilated Heightened awareness	Pupils normal size
Cardiovascular	Increased heart rate Increased myocardial contractility Increased blood pressure	Decreased heart rate Decreased myocardial contractility Vasodilation
Respiratory	Increased respiratory rate Increased respiratory depth Bronchial constriction	Bronchial relaxation
Gastrointestinal	Decreased gastric motility Decreased gastric secretions Increased glycogenolysis Decreased insulin production Sphincter contraction	Increased gastric motility Increased gastric secretions Sphincter dilatation
Genitourinary	Decreased urine output Decreased renal blood flow	Normal urine output

Orientation is the person's awareness of self in relation to person, place, and time. Using open-ended communication techniques, instruct the client to "tell me your first and last name and age," "tell me the month, day, year, and day of the week," "tell me where you are (city, state, hospital)," in order to ascertain the client's level of orientation. The client also is asked to open and close his eyes or open and close his fist.

Mental Status Assessment of mental status requires observation of the client's appearance, behavior, posture, mood, gestures, movements, and facial expressions. The nurse compares these behaviors to expected behaviors based on the client's age, health status, educational level, and social position. Mood is assessed by observation and asking the client about moods and feelings.

Intellectual Function Intellectual function is the ability of the brain to perform thought processes. Ability to concentrate, memory function (both long-term and short-term), recall, calculation activities, and fund of knowledge are all aspects of intellectual function.

Nursing assessment of intellectual function involves asking individuals to perform certain tasks, such as the following:

- Repeating a series of numbers, such as 1, 3, 7, 1
- Telling what the individual ate for breakfast

TABLE 10-3 Glasgow Coma Scale

BEHAVIOR	RESPONSE	SCORE
Eye opening response	Spontaneous	4
	To verbal command	3
	To pain	2
	No response	1
Best verbal response	Oriented, conversing	5
	Disoriented, conversing	4
	Use of inappropriate words	3
	Incomprehensible sounds	2
	No response	1
Best motor response	Obeys verbal commands	6
	Moves to localized pain	5
	Flexion withdrawal to pain	4
	Abnormal posturing—decorticate	3
	Abnormal posturing—decerebrate	2
	No response	1
Total		3 to 15

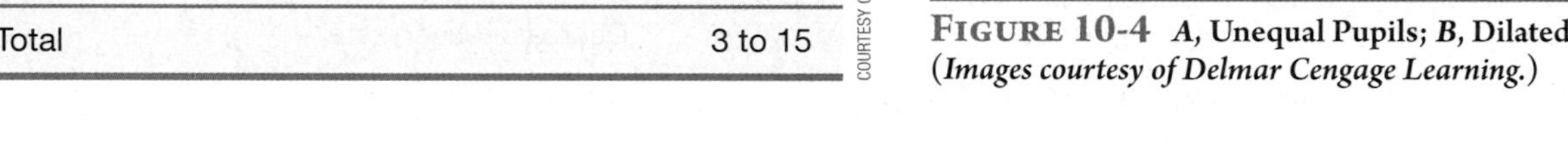

FIGURE 10-4 ***A*, Unequal Pupils; *B*, Dilated, Fixed Pupils** (*Images courtesy of Delmar Cengage Learning.*)

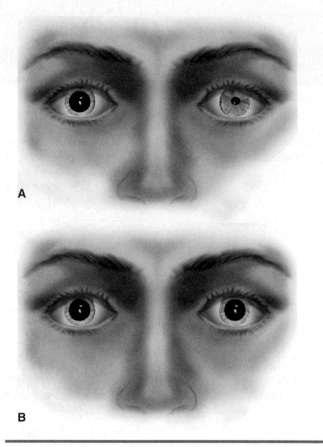

- Adding two numbers, for example, 2 + 6
- Reporting what is on the national news

The nurse determines the client's ability to process thoughts by evaluating the responses to questions such as these. For purposes of comparison, the client's ability to perform these tasks before assessment should be ascertained by asking the family. For example, if the client was math illiterate before the nursing assessment, the client will still not be able to add or subtract.

Emotional Status Emotional status is assessed by observation of the client's **affect** (emotional response or mood). Is affect appropriate for the situation? Is affect labile (prone to rapid change)? Is affect consistent with verbal communication?

Pupil Reaction Size, equality, and roundness of pupils are assessed (Figure 10-4). Size is measured in millimeters. Pupils are evaluated for symmetry of size and for reaction to light. The nurse briefly shines a penlight into the client's eye by passing the light from the outer edge of the eye toward the center of the eye (Figure 10-5). Reaction is assessed as being brisk, sluggish, or nonreactive; consensual reaction (the opposite pupil responding at the same time) is also noted. Accommodation is assessed as described in Table 10-1 under cranial nerve III.

The abbreviation PERRLA is used for documenting pupils that are equal, round, and reactive to light and that demonstrate accommodation. This abbreviation is used only when pupil reaction is normal. If any part of the assessment is abnormal in one or both eyes, the assessment findings are written out for clarity.

Communication Both written and oral communication are assessed. Various specialized areas of the nervous system are involved in communication. The inability to communicate verbally, termed **aphasia**, is caused by the inability to form words or the inability to understand written or spoken words. To assess communication function, various approaches are necessary. Ask the client to follow a simple command such as "Close your eyes." Also use a written card instructing the client to complete a simple task such as "Touch your nose." Note the ability to form words; appropriate use of words; speech patterns, clarity, rate, and flow; and voice modulation. During the health history, ask the client about health care expectations to evaluate the client's ability for verbal expression. Have the client write his name and address on paper to evaluate the ability to write.

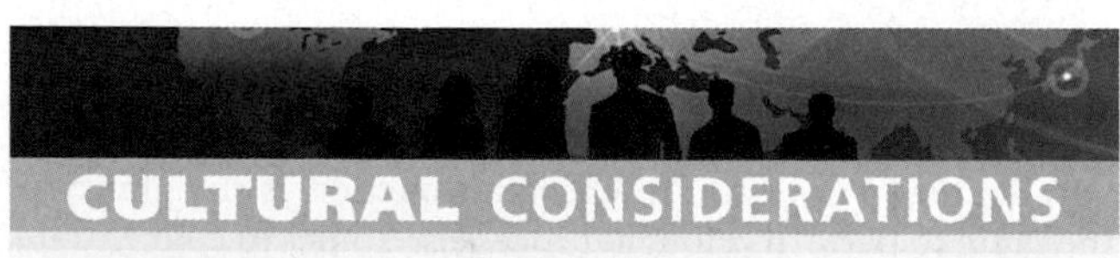

CULTURAL CONSIDERATIONS

Neurological Assessment

- Consider language and cultural norms when performing the mental status assessment.
- An interpreter may be required to ensure that the client understands the questions or directions.

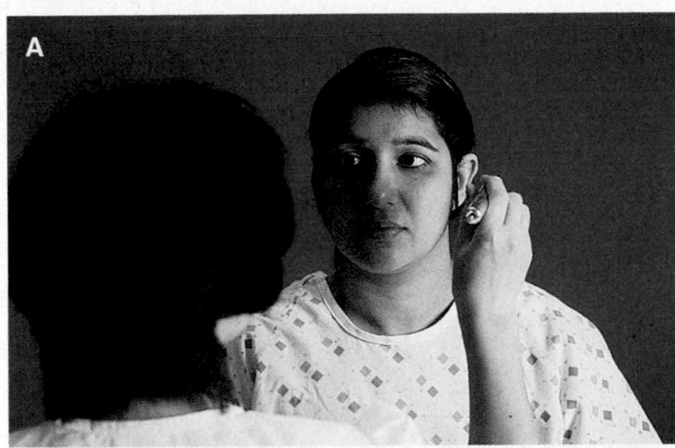

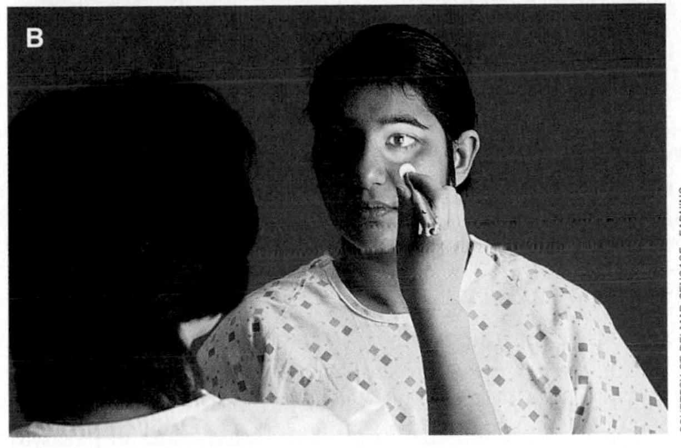

COURTESY OF DELMAR CENGAGE LEARNING

FIGURE 10-5 **Pupil Assessment; *A*, Starting Position, with Penlight to Side of Pupil; *B*, Moving Penlight Directly in Front of Pupil**

Cranial Nerve Function

Cranial nerve function essentially reflects brainstem activity. A complete cranial nerve examination, if required, is usually performed by the physician or advanced-practice nurse.

Motor Function

The neurological screening includes assessment of muscle strength, arm and leg movement, and gait. A complete motor function assessment is performed if a deficit is identified. A complete motor function assessment includes evaluating muscle size, symmetry, tone, and strength; coordination; balance; and posturing.

Muscle Size and Symmetry Muscle size and symmetry are assessed by palpating major muscle groups of the arms and legs and then comparing them to the muscle groups of the opposite side of the body. Unilateral atrophy indicates a nervous system problem.

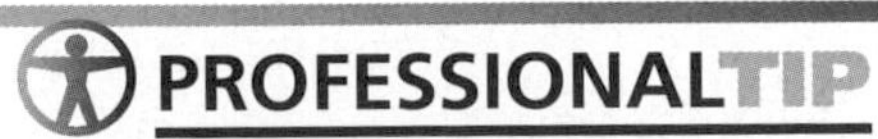

PROFESSIONALTIP

Assessment of Pupils

To ensure accuracy in assessing direct light reflex and consensual light reflex, the beginning examiner focuses the beam of light a total of four times, twice in each eye.

Muscle Tone Muscle tone is assessed during palpation of major muscle groups for size and symmetry, while at rest and during passive movement. Muscle tone is described as normal, flaccid, spastic, or rigid. Flaccid muscles are hypotonic, or soft and flabby. Spastic muscles are at first resistant to passive movement, but then release resistance. Rigid muscles may have tremors but are constantly rigid. Rigidity is a more constant state of spasticity, with fewer periods of release of resistance.

Muscle Strength To assess muscle strength, each extremity is placed through passive movement. The client is then asked to move the extremity, first against gravity, by lifting the extremity off the bed, then against resistance, by lifting against slight resistance exerted by the nurse's hand pushing on the extremity. Strength is graded on a scale of 0 to 5 (Table 10-4).

Coordination Coordination, a function of the cerebellum, is assessed by asking the client to perform repetitious movement. The client should close her eyes and repeatedly, rapidly touch her own nose with alternate index fingers (Figure 10-6). Lower extremity coordination is assessed by asking the client to run the heel of one foot down the opposite shin, and then repeat with the other heel (Figure 10-7). Inability to perform these movements is termed **ataxia**, incoordination of voluntary muscle action.

Balance Balance is evaluated by using the Romberg test. The client stands with the feet together, arms extended in front, and eyes closed. Balance is observed; a slight swaying is normal.

Posturing Abnormal posturing occurs with injury to the motor tract. Two types for which to observe are flexion

TABLE 10-4 Muscle Strength

SCORE	DEFINITION
5/5	Full power of contraction
4/5	Fair or moderate power of contraction
3/5	Just able to overcome force of gravity
2/5	Can move, but cannot overcome power of gravity
1/5	Minimal contractile power
0/5	No movement

COURTESY OF DELMAR CENGAGE LEARNING

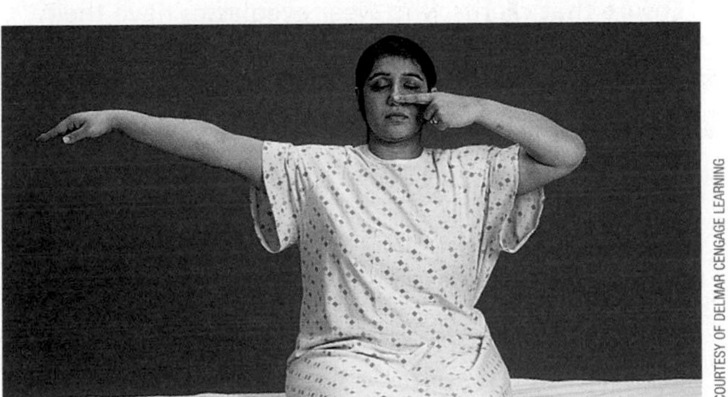

COURTESY OF DELMAR CENGAGE LEARNING

FIGURE 10-6 **Assessment of Coordination: Fingertip-to-Nose Touch**

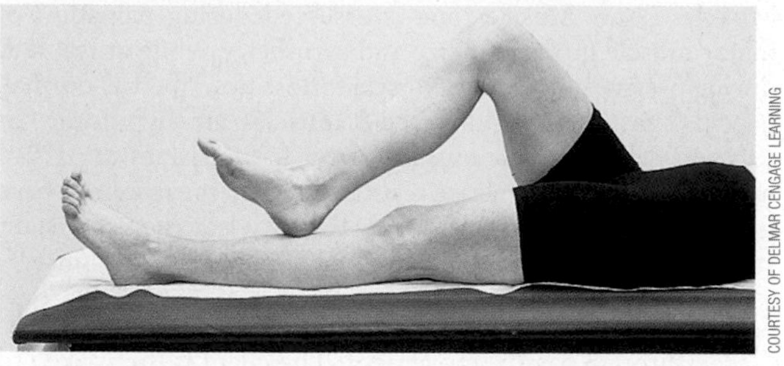

FIGURE 10-7 Assessment of Coordination: Heel Slide

(formerly decorticate) and extension (formerly decerebrate) posturing (Lower, 2002). Flexion posturing is characterized by flexion of the arms, adduction of the upper extremities, and extension of the lower extremities. Lesions of the cerebral hemispheres or internal structures of the brain cause flexion posturing. Extension posturing is caused by brainstem injury and is characterized by an arcing of the back, backward flexion of the head, adduction and hyperpronation of the arms, and extension of the feet (Figure 10-8).

Abnormal posturing may be present either at all times or in response to stimuli such as loud noises, bright lights, or painful stimuli. The nurse notes whether bilateral or unilateral posturing is present, and, if intermittent, the cause of the posturing. The presence of either type of posturing is reported at once, because either represents an ominous sign of cerebral dysfunction. Extension posturing represents greater dysfunction than does flexion posturing, and any change from flexion to extension posturing indicates a worsening of condition.

SAFETY

Romberg Test

Always stand in front of the client during the Romberg test, anticipating that the client might fall.

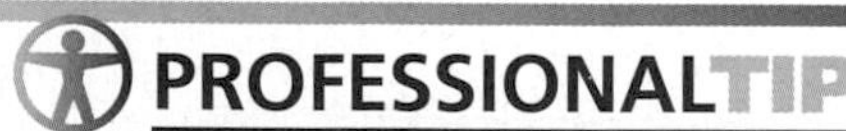

PROFESSIONALTIP

Assessing Coordination

Ensure that clients who wear eyeglasses have their glasses on before the assessment is performed.

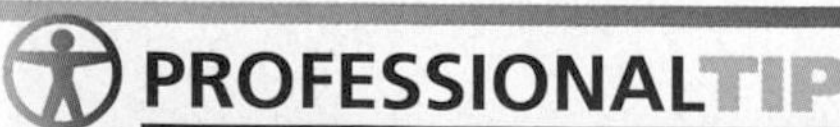

PROFESSIONALTIP

Assessing Pain and Temperature Sensory Function

- Test upper and lower extremities
- Begin with the upper arms, moving down to the hands; then work from thighs to feet (proximodistal)

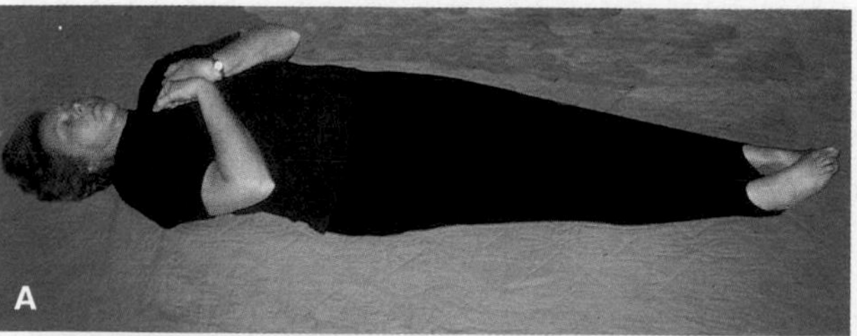

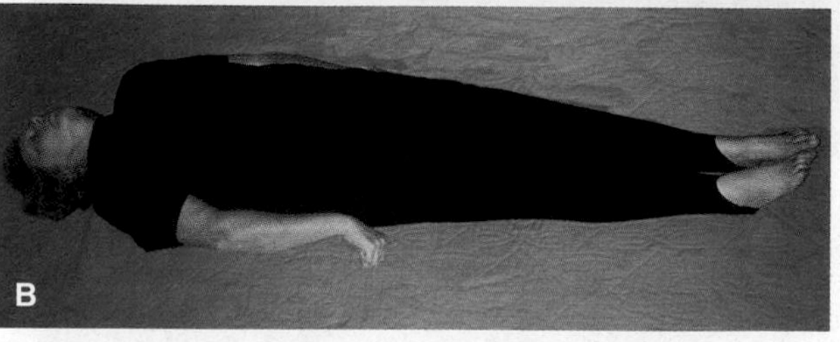

FIGURE 10-8 Abnormal Posturing; *A*, Flexion Posturing; *B*, Extension Posturing (*Photos courtesy of John White, Corpus Christi, TX.*)

Sensory Function

A subjective examination of sensory function, performed with the client's eyes closed, is generally done only when a dysfunction is suspected. Different pathways are used to transmit different sensory impulses. To evaluate all pathways, the examiner must test tactile sensation, pain and temperature, vibration, proprioception, stereognosis, graphesthesia, and integration of sensations.

Tactile Sensation Tactile sensation is tested by using a cotton ball to lightly touch the client's arms, hands, upper legs, and feet. Comparison is done side to side. The client, with eyes closed, indicates whether the cotton ball is felt.

Pain and Temperature Sensations of pain and temperature are transmitted along the same pathways and are evaluated using a sharp and dull touch. A paper clip or cotton-tipped applicator is used.

Touch the client with the rounded end of a paper clip or cotton-tipped applicator to test for dull sensation, and the pointed end of a paper clip or uncovered end of the applicator to test for sharp sensation. The client's ability to distinguish sharp and dull is noted, again comparing both sides of the body.

Vibration Vibration is tested using a tuning fork. Strike the tuning fork on the palm, holding only the handle, then place the end of the handle first on the client's wrists and then on the ankles and ask whether vibrations are felt (Figure 10-9). The client's eyes should be closed during the test.

SAFETY

Sensation

Do not use a safety pin to test pain because skin integrity may be compromised.

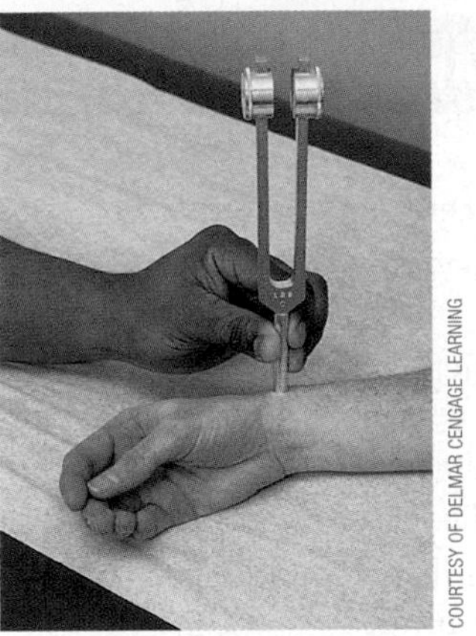

FIGURE 10-9 Assessment of Vibration

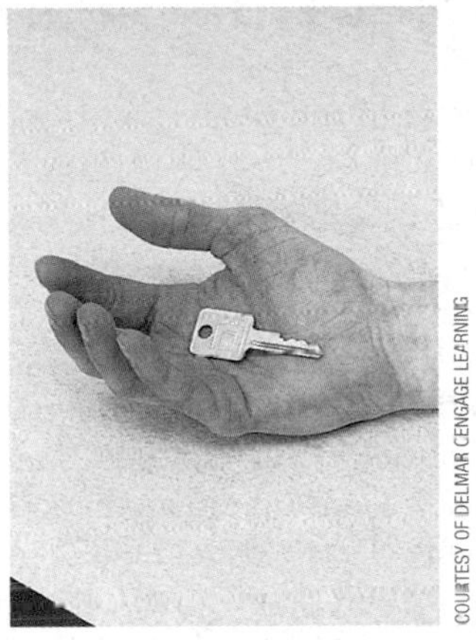

FIGURE 10-10 Assessment of Stereognosis

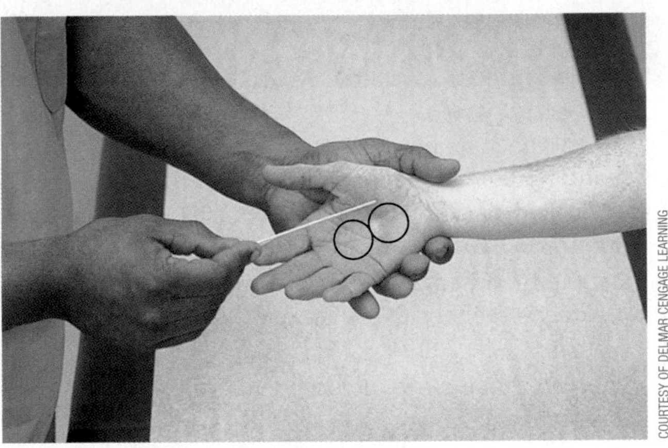

FIGURE 10-11 Assessment of Graphesthesia

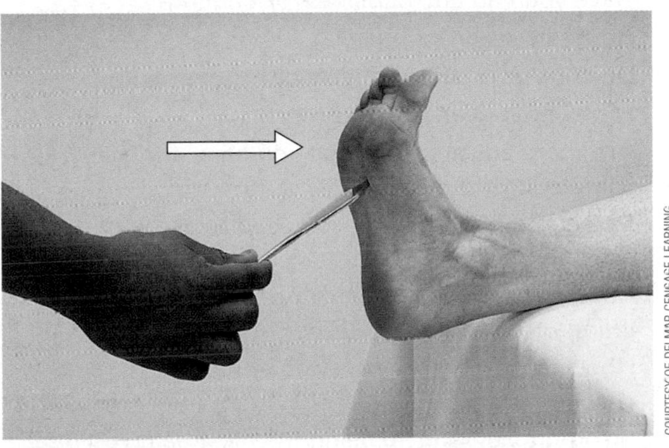

FIGURE 10-12 Pathologic Reflex: Babinski

Proprioception Proprioception is the sense of joint position in space. With the client's eyes remaining closed, move a joint of the client's finger or extremity up or down in space and ask the client to distinguish the direction of movement of the digit or extremity as being either up or down.

Stereognosis **Stereognosis** is the ability to recognize an object by feel. Place a familiar object such as a coin or key in the client's hand and ask what the object is. The sensation is a function of the brain, not of the spinal pathways (Figure 10-10).

Graphesthesia **Graphesthesia** is the ability to identify letters, numbers, or shapes drawn on the skin. Hold the client's hand and, with the stick end of a cotton-tipped applicator or a closed pen, trace an outline on the open palm, ensuring that the letter, number, or shape is right side up for the client (Figure 10-11).

Integration of Sensation Integration of sensation is a higher cortical function. A two-point discrimination test is performed by touching the client simultaneously on opposite sides of the body with a sharp object and asking the client to ascertain the number of objects felt. The normal response is two. If only one is felt, the brain function of integration is abnormal.

Reflexes

Both deep tendon reflexes and superficial reflexes are assessed. Deep tendon reflexes are involuntary contractions of muscles or muscle groups responding to brisk stretching near the insertion site of the muscle (Smeltzer & Bare, 2008). Testing these reflexes is generally the responsibility of the physician or registered nurse, although the LP/VN should be familiar with these assessments, as abnormal reflex responses are an early indicator of motor or sensory dysfunction.

Superficial, or cutaneous, reflexes are elicited by irritating the skin on the area assessed. They are diminished or absent with dysfunction of the reflex arc.

The superficial reflex generally assessed is the plantar. To assess the plantar reflex, the handle of the reflex hammer is used to stroke the outer aspect of the sole of the foot from the heel and across the ball of the foot to just below the big toe. Plantar flexion, or curling under of the toes, should occur.

Abnormal Reflexes The absence of deep tendon reflexes in clients is considered an abnormal finding. A fanning of the toes and dorsiflexion of the big toe in response to the assessment of the plantar reflex is called a positive Babinksi's reflex (Figure 10-12). This abnormal response indicates corticospinal disease and is the most important abnormal superficial reflex.

Refer to Box 10-1, "Questions to Ask and Observations to Make When Collecting Data," for guidance in completing client neurological assessments.

BOX 10-1 QUESTIONS TO ASK AND OBSERVATIONS TO MAKE WHEN COLLECTING DATA

Subjective Data

Do you have headaches? On a scale of 0 to 10, with 0 being no pain and 10 being the most pain you have experienced, rate your headaches. How long have you had these headaches?

Describe the headache to me. What makes the headache feel better? What make the headache feel worse?

Point to the area of your head where you have headaches.

Have you had a seizure?

If you have seizures, do you have an aura?

What precipitates (causes) your seizures?

Have you had any numbness or tingling?

Have you fallen recently?

Describe your sense of balance.

Have you had any vision problems?

Are there any activities that you have difficulty completing?

Do you have the energy you need to accomplish daily activities?

Have you or your family members noticed any mood swings or changes in your personality?

How many hours do you sleep at night?

Do you have back pain? On a scale of 0 to 10, with 0 being no pain and 10 being the most pain you have experienced, rate your back pain. How long have you had the back pain?

Describe the pain to me. What makes the back pain feel better? What make the back pain feel worse?

Have you had any difficulty with any of your extremities? Weakness? Lack of function?

How does the condition affect your life?

Has this condition affected your sexual relationships?

What do you do to cope with your condition?

Does the client answer questions appropriately?

During the subjective data assessment, determine if the client answers questions appropriately.

Objective Data

Assess client's orientation to person, place, and time.

Assess level of consciousness.

Is the client clean and neatly groomed?

Assess client's intellectual function by asking the client to:

Repeat a series of numbers, such as 6, 3, 7, 9.

Tell me what you had for breakfast.

Add 8 + 9.

Tell me a recent news event.

Assess appropriateness of verbal responses to questions.

Does the client have the expected behaviors based on the client's age, health status, educational level, and social position?

Have the client write a complete sentence.

Ask the client to complete a verbal request, such as "Cross your arms."

Check coordination by asking the client to touch his own nose with alternate index fingers.

Ask the client to close his eyes, then place a common object in the client's hand and ask him to identify the object.

Draw a number in the clients palm, and ask him to identify the number.

Asses the client's visual field. As the examiner's finger moves away from the client, does the pupil accommodate by dilating? Constrict as the finger moves closer to the client? Do the eyes move smoothly and consensually upward, downward, inward and outward? As the client's eyes follow your finger as you move it up, down, back, and forth in the path of the client's visual field, does the client see the finger at all times? Check the size, roundness, equality, reaction, and accommodation of the client's pupils.

Assess the client's sense of smell by introducing nonoffensive odors to the client.

Do the client's facial expressions match the conversation?

Check trigeminal nerve by swiping a piece of cotton over the client's check area.

Can the client smile? Frown?

Observe the client's posture. Does the client slump or sit erect?

Note the client's gait and ability to balance. Is the gait symmetrical, and how does the client approach you?

Assess muscle strength in all extremities. Do all extremities have full range of motion?

Assess superficial reflexes.

Does the client have a gag reflex?

Can the client stick out his tongue?

Complete the Glasgow Coma Scale.

COMMON DIAGNOSTIC TESTS

Commonly used diagnostic tests for clients with symptoms of nervous system disorders are listed in Table 10-5.

HEAD INJURY

Head injuries involve trauma to the scalp, skull, or brain.

SCALP

Scalp injuries bleed profusely because of the abundance of blood vessels in the scalp. As with any break in skin integrity, infection is of major concern. The wound is cleansed and irrigated to remove foreign matter before closing the wound with sutures or butterfly dressings.

SKULL

Skull injuries and fractures of the skull may occur with or without brain injury. A fracture is usually caused by extreme force. Skull fractures are considered closed if the dura mater is intact and open if the dura mater is torn. The clinical manifestation of skull fracture is localized pain. If the brain is injured, other symptoms occur.

Types of skull fractures are linear fracture, comminuted fracture, depressed fracture, and basilar fracture. Linear fractures are nondisplaced cracks in the bone. Comminuted fractures occur when the bone is broken into fragments. Depressed fractures have bone fragments pressing into the intracranial cavity. Basilar skull fractures are of the bones in the base of the skull.

Basilar fractures are of particular concern because of the proximity of the fragile sinus bones and the adhesion of the dura mater to this area. The dura mater can easily tear, and CSF can leak from the ears or nose. Two tests determine if the drainage is CSF; a dextrostick dipped in the liquid and the halo test. Because CSF has a high glucose level, a dextrostick is placed in the liquid. If the dextrostick reveals the presence of glucose, the liquid is CSF. The drainage can also be checked, by placing a drop on a white sheet. When the liquid dries, a yellow halo appears around the edges of the pink or bloody drainage if it is CSF (halo test). The internal carotid artery and cranial nerves can also be damaged easily with a basilar skull fracture.

Table 10-5 Common Diagnostic Tests for Nervous System Disorders

- Lumbar puncture (LP)
- Electroencephalogram (EEG)
- Electromyogram (EMG)
- Imaging procedures: computerized tomography (CT), positron emission tomography (PET), single-photon emission computed tomography (SPECT), magnetic resonance imaging (MRI)
- Cerebral angiography
- Brain scan
- Myelogram

LIFE SPAN CONSIDERATIONS

Reflexes

The absence of the Achilles reflex in the elderly client is not considered abnormal.

BRAIN

Brain injuries are caused by primary injuries of acceleration–deceleration force, rotational force, or penetrating missile. Acceleration injuries are caused by moving objects striking the head, such as a baseball bat. Deceleration injuries result when the head is moving and strikes a solid object such as a car dashboard. Rotational injuries are hyperextension, hyperflexion, or lateral flexion of the head, which cause twisting of the cerebrum on the brainstem, such as a whiplash injury. Penetrating missile injuries are a direct penetration of an object, such as a bullet, into brain tissue (Urden, Stacy, & Lough, 2009).

Open Injury

Skull fractures and penetrating injuries are referred to as open head injuries. Hemorrhaging from the nose, pharynx, or ears; ecchymosis over the mastoid area (Battle's sign); or blood in the conjunctiva may occur in conjunction with open head injuries. Raccoon eyes (ecchymosis around both eyes) indicates a basilar skull fracture. Cerebrospinal fluid may leak from the ears or nose. A computed tomography (CT) scan or magnetic resonance imaging (MRI) determines the extent of injury. Neurological deficits depend on the extent and area of injury.

Closed Injury

Closed head injuries are caused by blunt force to the head. Coup injuries are caused by the impact of the head against an object. Contrecoup injuries are caused by the impact of the brain against the opposite side of the skull (Figure 10-13).

Types of closed head injuries are concussion, contusion, and laceration. Concussions are transient neurological deficits caused by shaking the brain. Clinical manifestations may include immediate loss of consciousness lasting from minutes to hours, momentary loss of reflexes, respiratory arrest for several seconds, and amnesia for the period immediately before and after the event. Headaches, drowsiness, confusion, dizziness, irritability, visual disturbances, and unsteady gait may also occur (Hickey, 2008).

Post-concussion syndrome may develop after the injury, as manifested by headache and dizziness. Nervousness, irritability, emotional lability, fatigue, insomnia, loss of **mentation** (ability to concentrate, remember, or think abstractly), and sometimes other neurological deficits occur. This syndrome may last from several weeks up to a year (Hickey, 2008).

Contusions are surface bruises of the brain. Symptoms depend on the area of injury. Frequently, the client is unconscious for a longer period than with a concussion. The client becomes conscious only to drift back into unconsciousness. Pulse, blood pressure, and respirations are below normal. Skin is cool and pale. Cerebral edema occurs with widespread injury (see section on cerebral edema).

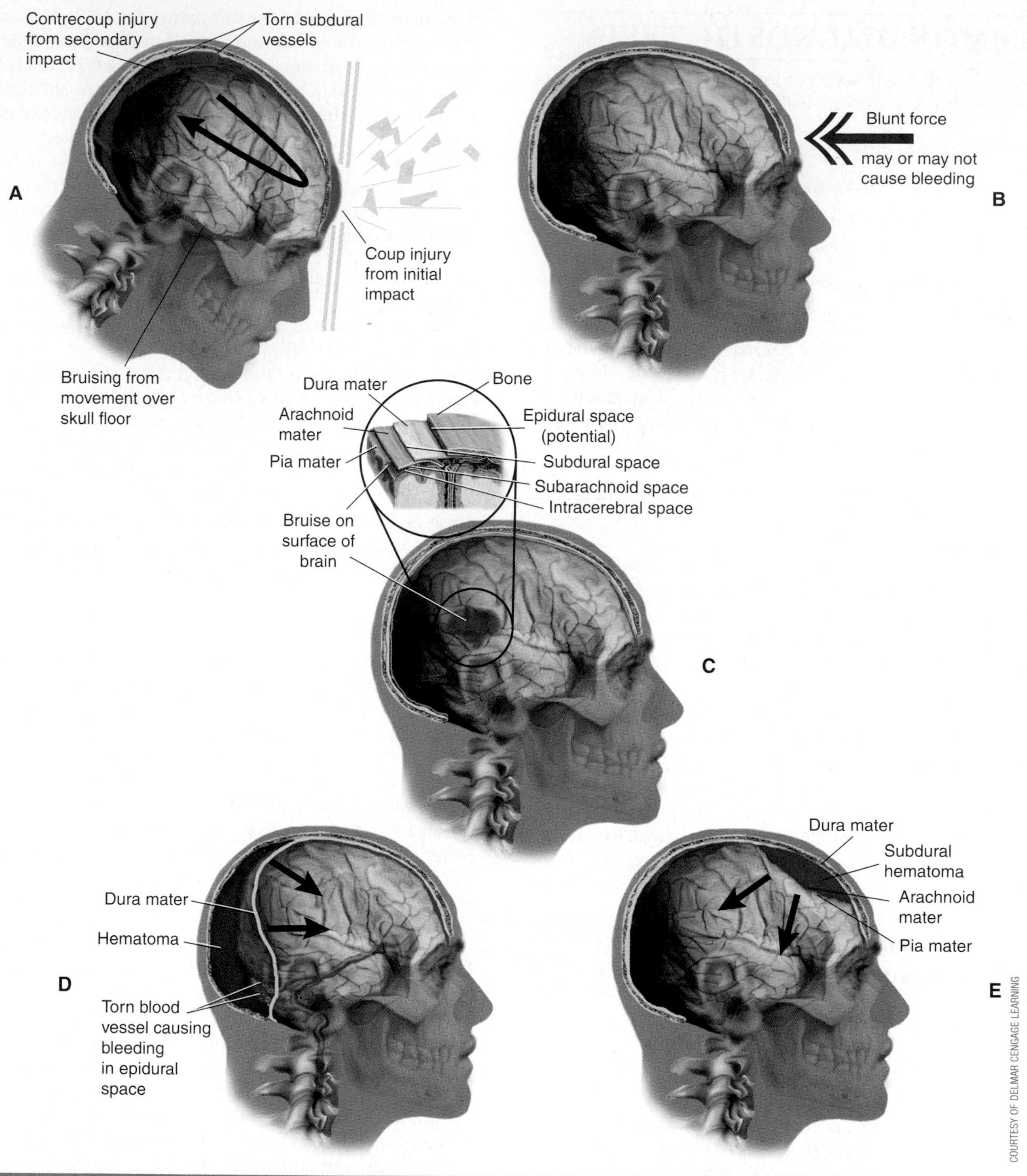

FIGURE 10-13 **Brain Injuries; *A*, Coup/Contrecoup; *B*, Concussion; *C*, Contusion; *D*, Epidural Hematoma; *E*, Subdural Hematoma**

Return of consciousness may be followed by cerebral irritability to stimuli. Headache and dizziness may be present for an indefinite period. Permanent damage causes either changes in mental function or seizure disorders. Prognosis ranges from full recovery to death.

Cerebral laceration is the tearing of cortical tissue. Symptoms of brainstem injury include deep coma from time of impact, extension posturing, autonomic dysfunction, nonreactive pupils, and respiratory difficulty. The ability to relay nerve impulses from high levels in the brain is lost. Diffuse axonal injury (DAI) usually occurs in conjunction with brainstem injuries. This widespread damage to nerve cells in the white matter of the brain causes immediate coma, extension posturing, and increased intracranial pressure (ICP).

Hemorrhage

Intracranial hemorrhage, usually due to an arterial bleed, is a common complication of any head injury. Bleeding occurs in the epidural space, subdural space, subarachnoid space, ventricles, or intracerebrally. Neurological change is caused by pressure on the brain resulting from the space-occupying hemorrhage. With epidural hematoma (bleeding in the epidural space), momentary unconsciousness is followed by a conscious state of a few hours within that day, depending on the rapidity of the bleeding. As the bleeding continues, neurological status begins to deteriorate, with decreasing level of consciousness; headache; seizures; hemiparesis; **decerebration** (severing spinal cord); and dilated, fixed pupils. This is a medical emergency, and the treatment is surgery to evacuate the hematoma, stop the bleeding, and relieve pressure on the brain.

Subdural hematomas (bleeding in the subdural space) cause immediate pressure on the brain. Subdural hematomas are acute (within 48 hours of injury), subacute (from 2 to 14 days after injury), or chronic (from 2 weeks to months after injury). Common symptoms are headache, drowsiness, slow mentation, and confusion. The symptoms slowly progress as the size of the subdural clot increases, causing increased pressure on the brain. Small hematomas are usually reabsorbed. Large hematomas require surgical removal.

Subarachnoid (below the arachnoid) and intraventricular (within the ventricles of the brain) hemorrhages are common in severe head injury. The symptoms include those listed for hematoma, as well as **nuchal rigidity**, stiffness or inability to bend the neck. Blood in the subarachnoid space interferes with the reabsorption of CSF, further increasing intracranial pressure.

Intracranial hematomas from contusions usually occur in the temporal or frontal lobes; from shearing forces, they usually occur deep in the brain. The hematoma usually expands rapidly. The injury usually causes immediate unconsciousness. Headache, deteriorating level of consciousness, hemiplegia, and dilated pupils are initial signs of an internal hematoma. As intracranial pressure increases, herniation of the brainstem occurs, causing changes in pupils, respirations, and vital signs. Craniotomy along with evacuation and control of bleeding may be performed depending on the condition of the client, extent of cerebral contusion, and accessibility of the bleeding site.

Signs and symptoms of increased intracranial pressure include deterioration in level of consciousness; confusion; difficulty in rousing; and, initially, restlessness. Other signs and symptoms are changes in pupil size or reaction to light. The pupil gradually dilates and becomes less responsive to light. Muscle weakness progressing to **hemiplegia** (paralysis of one side of the body) or **paraplegia** (paralysis of lower extremities), and abnormal posturing occurs. Headache and vomiting are experienced by some clients. Vital sign changes generally do not occur until the increased intracranial pressure has progressed to the point of involving the brainstem. An increase in systolic blood pressure and a widening pulse pressure accompanied by a slowing pulse are the effects of pressure on the brainstem.

Cerebral Edema and Increased Intracranial Pressure

The brain is contained in a rigid container, the skull. The only normal opening to the adult skull is the foramen magnum at the base of the skull. Intracranial pressure is a result of the pressure exerted by the contents of the skull, which are the brain, blood, and CSF.

Regulatory mechanisms maintain intracranial pressure between 0 and 15 mm Hg. The Monroe-Kellie hypothesis states that when one component of the cranial contents increases in volume, the volumes of the other components decrease in order to compensate and maintain intracranial pressure between 0 and 15 mm Hg. As long as this ability to compensate remains effective, no neurological changes occur.

In decompensation, the volume increase is so excessive that intracranial pressure cannot be maintained below 15 mm Hg by decreasing the volume of the remaining components. Neurological changes are exhibited because of cellular hypoxia and displacement of the brain, which compresses neurons, especially in the brainstem. These changes include deteriorating level of consciousness; decreased motor response to commands; fixed, dilated pupils; and vital sign changes known as Cushing's triad or reflex. Cushing's triad refers to bradycardia, widening pulse pressure along with increasing systolic pressure, and respiratory irregularities. Respiratory changes include periods of apnea, decreased respiratory rate and depth, and irregular respirations.

Causes of increased intracranial pressure are increased blood volume resulting from vascular vasodilation; increased volume of brain tissue resulting from edema, infection, tumor, or hemorrhage; or increased volume of CSF resulting from overproduction, decreased reabsorption, or interruption of CSF circulation. If intracranial pressure continues to increase, brain herniation will occur at the tentorial notch or through the foramen magnum, resulting in death.

Medical–Surgical Management

Management of head injury is focused on early recognition and treatment of increasing intracranial pressure and maintenance of normal body functions.

Medical

Intracranial pressure is monitored with an ICP device that has a small tube placed in the ventricles of the brain. CSF is drained through a ventricular drain (ventriculostomy) if the intracranial pressure increases (Daniels, 2007). Suctioning may be necessary but is *never* done through the nose on a head injury client because of the possibility of CSF leakage. Oxygen is given to maintain cerebral perfusion. Pulse oximetry and arterial blood gases (ABGs) are checked.

If the client has an endotracheal tube in place, the $PaCO_2$ level can drop below normal. This decrease causes a slightly alkaline pH, which decreases vasodilation and, thus, intracranial pressure.

Surgical

Decompression is performed surgically by placing burr holes in the skull to allow room for the expansion of the brain. A space-occupying lesion such as a tumor, hematoma, or abscess is surgically removed. Excess CSF is drained from the ventricles.

Pharmacological

Corticosteroids, such as dexamethasone (Decadron), are given to reduce cerebral edema. Antacids, such as Mylanta or

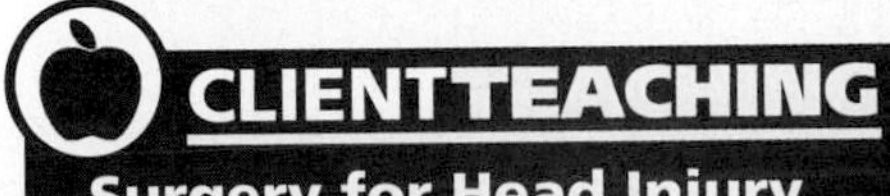

Surgery for Head Injury

Inform the client of the following:

- The head is shaved in the area of the incision.
- Edema of the head and face are present after surgery but will gradually disappear.
- A mechanical ventilator is used for a day or two after surgery.

Maalox, or histamine receptor antagonists, such as ranitidine (Zantac), are given to decrease both the side effects of corticosteroids and stress-induced gastric acidity. Osmotic diuretics, such as mannitol (Osmitrol), are administered to rapidly reduce fluid in the brain tissue; muscle relaxants, sedatives, barbiturates, or muscle-paralyzing agents are administered to decrease activity and reduce the oxygen need of the brain.

Antipyretic drugs are used to decrease body temperature and the metabolic needs of the brain, thereby reducing the volume of blood sent to the brain to supply oxygen and glucose. Anticonvulsants are given to prevent or treat seizure activity.

Activity

Activity is limited to keep the metabolic needs of the brain to a minimum. Increased metabolic needs require more oxygen and glucose supplied by increases in blood volume in the cranium, which further increases intracranial pressure.

Nursing Management

Frequently monitor level of consciousness, eye movements, pupil changes, vital signs, I&O, pulse oximetry and Glasgow Coma Scale score. Monitor the ICP if a device is in place. Maintain airway patency and administer oxygen as ordered. Keep head of bed at 30 to 40 degrees and client's head positioned at midline. Watch for signs of arm/leg muscle weakness, muscle twitching, nausea or vomiting, and visual or hearing disturbance. Fluids often are restricted.

NURSING PROCESS

Assessment

Nursing assessment for any head injury is focused on neurological status. At the nursing shift change, nurses may complete a neurologic assessment together for consistency in assessing the neuropathy.

Subjective Data

Subjective data includes a history of what happened, including type of trauma (acceleration, deceleration, or missile), site of blow, and any loss of consciousness, including timing, length, and ability to be roused.

Objective Data

A neurological screening is done to obtain a baseline neurological status; then, a more in-depth neurological exam is performed to identify any early signs of increasing intracranial pressure.

Frequent assessment of neurological status, including level of consciousness, motor function, eye movement, pupil size and reaction, protective reflexes, and vital signs, allows for early recognition of and intervention for increasing intracranial pressure. Nursing observation also includes assessing for double vision, headache, nausea, and bleeding from any orifice. Ipsilateral pupil reaction (reaction of the pupil on the same side as the injury or lesion) occurs as a result of pressure on the oculomotor nerve caused by increased intracranial pressure or cerebral edema. Assess for factors that cause increased intracranial pressure.

If a client is undergoing intracranial surgery, assess the teaching needs of the client and family. Also assess the emotional and psychosocial needs and support systems.

Longer-term care involves assessment of bowel elimination status to prevent the need for straining, skin assessment to prevent skin breakdown, and assessment for complications of immobility.

Nursing diagnoses for a client with a head injury include the following:

NURSING DIAGNOSES	PLANNING/OUTCOMES	NURSING INTERVENTIONS
*Ineffective **T**issue/ Perfusion (Cerebral)* related to disruption in cerebral blood flow	The client will demonstrate improvement or maintenance on Glasgow Coma Scale.	Assess neurological status of client every 15 to 60 minutes. Note findings on Glasgow Coma Scale. Compare findings to previous assessments to uncover changes in condition. Administer oxygen as ordered to supply a high concentration of oxygen to the brain. Position client with head of the bed at 30 to 40 degrees and client's head at midline to promote venous drainage from the head. Minimize physical activity to prevent increasing metabolic demands.
*Ineffective **B**reathing Pattern* related to neurological impairment of respiratory status or mechanical ventilation	The client will have an effective breathing pattern.	Assess respiratory status every 15 to 60 minutes. Administer oxygen as ordered to maintain blood oxygen concentration. Provide mechanical ventilation if necessary. Continually assess ABG levels or pulse oximeter readings to identify need for assisting respirations to prevent vasodilation in the brain and increasing intracranial pressure.

Nursing diagnoses for a client with a head injury include the following: (Continued)

NURSING DIAGNOSES	PLANNING/OUTCOMES	NURSING INTERVENTIONS
Interrupted Family Processes related to sudden crisis	The client and/or family will demonstrate effective coping mechanisms.	Assess family's coping mechanisms. Involve the family in client care as appropriate. Provide information about the client in an ongoing fashion. Provide teaching about the injury and pathophysiology involved. Prepare family for possible outcomes of the injury, such as paralysis or death. Collaborate with clergy, social services, mental health counselors, and support groups. Teach the family to report increased drowsiness, arm/leg weakness, muscle twitching, nausea or vomiting, visual or hearing disturbances, and so on. Inform the family that the client is not aware of the symptoms and that signs and symptoms of the head injury are not immediately apparent.

Evaluation: Evaluate each outcome to determine how it has been met by the client.

BRAIN TUMOR

Brain tumors are space-occupying intracranial lesions, either benign or malignant. Brain tumors are classified by location or tissue type. Intracranial lesions are primary lesions, which develop initially in brain tissue; extensions of tumors of the meninges, cranial nerves, or pituitary gland; or metastatic lesions from tumors originating in other body systems.

The etiology of primary lesions is unknown. Clinical manifestations differ according to the area of the lesion and the rate of growth. Intracranial pressure increases as compensatory mechanisms are no longer able to balance tumor growth. Clinical manifestations commonly include alteration in consciousness, decreased mental functioning, headaches, seizures, or vomiting (sometimes sudden and projectile). Other signs and symptoms are relative to the functions of areas involved, such as visual problems resulting from occipital lobe tumors.

Diagnostic evaluation is by CT scan, MRI, or electroencephalogram (EEG). Total body scans, chest x-rays, and needle biopsies of the tumor are performed to identify the type of tumor and, thus, serve as a basis for medical treatment.

MEDICAL–SURGICAL MANAGEMENT

Medical

Medical management is based on tumor type, growth rate, and assessment of the client. Radiation therapy is used for specific tumor types or for inoperable tumors. The goal is to destroy the tumor cells that are more susceptible to radiation than are normal cells. Radiation is used with surgery and chemotherapy.

Surgical

Surgical intervention removes tumors (benign or malignant) to decrease the space occupied by the lesion or obtains tissue for biopsy. Some CSF is removed to relieve increased pressure.

Pharmacological

Dexamethasone (Decadron) is given to decrease cerebral edema. Phenytoin (Dilantin) is given to prevent seizure activity. Antacids and H_2 blockers, such as cimetidine (Tagamet) or ranitidine (Zantac), are given to prevent gastric irritation. Analgesics, nonsteroidal anti-inflammatory drugs (NSAIDs), or codeine are used for headaches, and stool softeners are administered to prevent straining. A protective mechanism called the blood–brain barrier prevents many potentially harmful substances from reaching the brain tissue or CSF. It prevents chemotherapeutic agents from reaching the brain except in very large doses that are not well tolerated by other body systems. Antineoplastic agents are administered on the basis of tumor type and whether the client meets the requirements for receiving the drug. Antineoplastic alkylating agents (carmustine [BICNU, Gliadel], lomustine [CCNU], and semustube [Methyl-CCNU]) inhibit cell division in rapidly replicating cells. Temozolomide (Temodar) crosses the blood–brain barrier and is used for clients with glioablastoma multiforme.

Another alternative way of administering chemotherapeutics is to use the intrathecal (directly into the spinal canal) route. Sometimes chemotherapy disk-shaped wafers are left in the cavity after tumor removal. The wafers release the chemotherapy drug over the next few days (Mayo Clinic, 2008). The surgical insertion of an Ommaya reservoir under the scalp can also allow direct insertion of chemotherapy into the CNS.

NURSING MANAGEMENT

Prepare client and family for surgery in a caring, compassionate manner. Explain procedures, including shaving the head. The client generally will stay in the ICU for several days.

NURSING PROCESS

ASSESSMENT

Subjective Data

Ask the client about fatigue, pain, headache, weakness, and ability to perform daily activities. Note sensory/perceptual alterations such as hearing, visual, tactile, kinesthetic, or olfactory changes. Assess the client's pain and evaluate effectiveness of interventions. A thorough psychosocial assessment, including changes in personality or judgment, serves as the basis for providing emotional support.

Objective Data

Assess functional ability, mobility, and mental status, including motor strength, gait, ability to perform activities of daily living (ADLs), and level of consciousness. Note signs of neurological changes, deficits, or increased intracranial pressure, such as restlessness, changes in logic, changes in vital signs, pupil responses, speech abnormalities, seizure activity, or changes in respiratory patterns.

Nursing diagnoses for a client with a brain tumor include the following:

NURSING DIAGNOSES	PLANNING/OUTCOMES	NURSING INTERVENTIONS
Anxiety related to fear of unknown and treatment plans	The client will demonstrate effective use of coping mechanisms.	Allow client to verbalize feeling of anxiety and discuss coping patterns previously used. Observe for verbal and nonverbal cues of anxiety. Provide emotional support by listening and guiding client to explore feelings of helplessness, fear of the unknown, and potential impending death. Maintain a calm demeanor. Teach client and family about diagnostic tests, treatments, and expected outcomes. Collaborate with pastoral care, physician, social services, and family to provide emotional support. Teach relaxation exercises and techniques such as slow, deep breathing and progressive muscle relaxation. Administer tranquilizers and sedatives as ordered.
*Disturbed **S**ensory Perception* (visual, auditory, kinesthetic, tactile) related to displacement/ compression of brain tissue	The client will maintain sensory perceptions.	Maintain communication. Provide a safe environment. Provide orientation and appropriate stimuli. Encourage some social interaction.
*Imbalanced **N**utrition: Less than Body Requirements* related to side effects of treatment and disease process	The client will maintain weight within 5 pounds of initial weight.	Assess client's weight every other day. Provide frequent small feedings of high-calorie and high-protein foods. Offer foods of client's choice. Use nutritional supplements to maintain weight. Offer fluids frequently.

Evaluation: Evaluate each outcome to determine how it has been met by the client.

CEREBROVASCULAR ACCIDENT/TRANSIENT ISCHEMIC ATTACKS

Cerebrovascular accident (CVA), or stroke, is a "brain attack." It happens in the brain rather than the heart and causes a sudden loss of brain function accompanied by neurological deficit. It is a medical emergency and immediate treatment is crucial for the best outcome just as it is for a heart attack (NSA, 2002c). Stroke is the third leading cause of death in the United States, with nearly 144,000 deaths each year (NSA, 2009a). Approximately 795,000 strokes will occur in 2009 (NSA, 2009a). Refer to Figure 10-14 and complete the Stroke Risk Scorecard to evaluate your stroke risk (NSA, 2009b).

Strokes are caused by ischemia (oxygen deprivation) resulting from a thrombus, embolus, severe vasospasm, or cerebral hemorrhage. Blood supply to the brain is interrupted, causing neurological deficits of sensation, movement, thought, memory, or speech. The loss of function can be temporary or permanent.

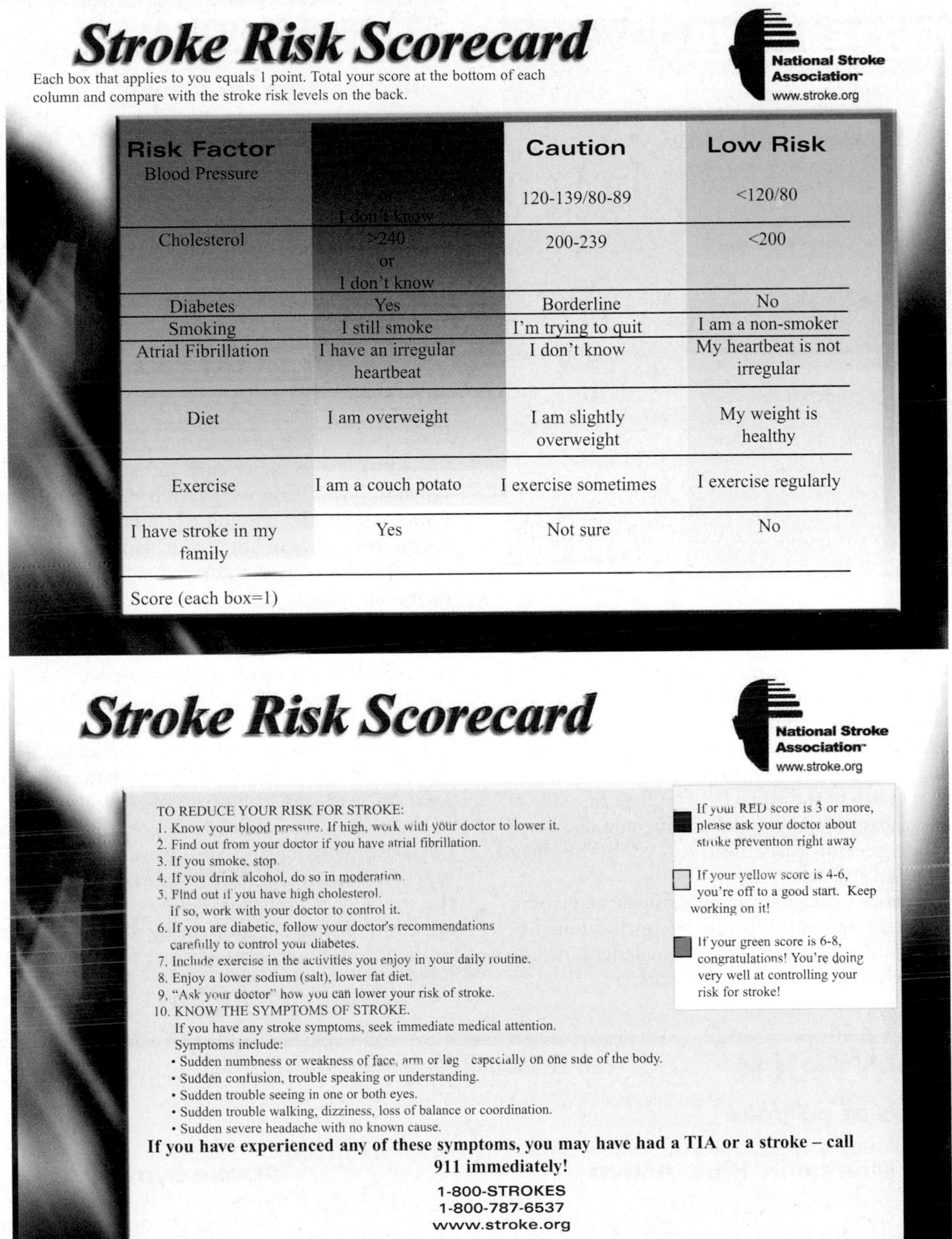

Stroke Risk Scorecard

National Stroke Association
www.stroke.org

Each box that applies to you equals 1 point. Total your score at the bottom of each column and compare with the stroke risk levels on the back.

Risk Factor		Caution	Low Risk
Blood Pressure	I don't know	120-139/80-89	<120/80
Cholesterol	>240 or I don't know	200-239	<200
Diabetes	Yes	Borderline	No
Smoking	I still smoke	I'm trying to quit	I am a non-smoker
Atrial Fibrillation	I have an irregular heartbeat	I don't know	My heartbeat is not irregular
Diet	I am overweight	I am slightly overweight	My weight is healthy
Exercise	I am a couch potato	I exercise sometimes	I exercise regularly
I have stroke in my family	Yes	Not sure	No
Score (each box=1)			

Stroke Risk Scorecard

National Stroke Association
www.stroke.org

TO REDUCE YOUR RISK FOR STROKE:

1. Know your blood pressure. If high, work with your doctor to lower it.
2. Find out from your doctor if you have atrial fibrillation.
3. If you smoke, stop.
4. If you drink alcohol, do so in moderation.
5. Find out if you have high cholesterol. If so, work with your doctor to control it.
6. If you are diabetic, follow your doctor's recommendations carefully to control your diabetes.
7. Include exercise in the activities you enjoy in your daily routine.
8. Enjoy a lower sodium (salt), lower fat diet.
9. "Ask your doctor" how you can lower your risk of stroke.
10. KNOW THE SYMPTOMS OF STROKE.
    If you have any stroke symptoms, seek immediate medical attention.
    Symptoms include:
    - Sudden numbness or weakness of face, arm or leg especially on one side of the body.
    - Sudden confusion, trouble speaking or understanding.
    - Sudden trouble seeing in one or both eyes.
    - Sudden trouble walking, dizziness, loss of balance or coordination.
    - Sudden severe headache with no known cause.

If your RED score is 3 or more, please ask your doctor about stroke prevention right away

If your yellow score is 4-6, you're off to a good start. Keep working on it!

If your green score is 6-8, congratulations! You're doing very well at controlling your risk for stroke!

If you have experienced any of these symptoms, you may have had a TIA or a stroke – call 911 immediately!

1-800-STROKES
1-800-787-6537
www.stroke.org

FIGURE 10-14 Stroke Risk Scorecard (*© 2009 National Stroke Association. National Stroke Association holds copyright to all of its educational publications and materials. In addition, National Stroke Association is the sole distributor of those publications and materials.*)

Transient ischemic attacks (TIAs) are mini-strokes and frequently precede a stroke. A TIA is a temporary or transient episode of neurological dysfunction caused by temporary impairment of blood flow to the brain. The loss of motor or sensory function may last from a few seconds to minutes to 24 hours. The classic symptoms are sudden blurring of vision or blindness, loss of balance or coordination, difficulty speaking or understanding simple statements, and weakness/numbness/paralysis in the face, arm, or leg (NSA, 2002b, 2008).

Clinical manifestations of TIA or CVA vary according to the location of interrupted blood supply in the brain. As with head injury, the specific functions of the involved area of the brain are interrupted, causing the symptoms. Common neurological deficits are motor deficits of hemiplegia (paralysis of one side of the body on the side opposite of the brain lesion), **hemiparesis** (weakness of one side of the body), **dysarthria** (impairment of speech caused by muscle dysfunction), and dysphagia (impairment of swallowing muscles). **Emotional**

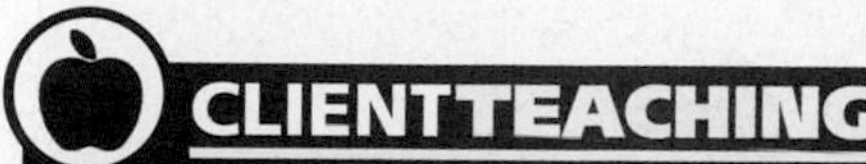

Stroke-Prevention Guidelines

- Have an annual blood pressure check.
- Be aware of cholesterol level.
- Consume lesser amounts of sodium (salt) and fat.
- Exercise daily.
- Do not smoke.
- If you drink alcohol, do so in moderation.
- Check with a doctor for symptoms of atrial fibrillation.
- Check cholesterol level.
- Control diabetes.
- Check with a doctor for circulation problems.
- See a doctor immediately with any stroke-like symptoms.

(National Stroke Association, 2009)

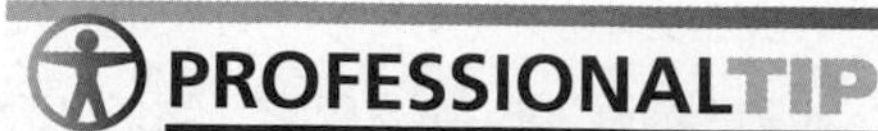

Risk Factors for Stroke

- The major risk factor for stroke is hypertension.
- Other risk factors are diabetes mellitus, atherosclerosis, aneurysm, cardiac disease, high blood cholesterol, obesity, sedentary lifestyle, smoking, stress, drug abuse (especially of cocaine), and use of oral contraceptives. Clients with more than one risk factor are at even greater risk.
- One in twenty people who have a TIA will have a stroke within 2 days (NSA, 2009b)

lability (loss of emotional control), inability to control behavior, and inability to process multiple pieces of information are also common manifestations of a stroke.

Sensory deficits include visual deficits of double vision, decreased visual acuity, and **homonymous hemianopia**, the loss of vision in half of the visual field on the same side of both eyes. Other possible sensory deficits include decreased sensation to touch, pressure, pain, heat, and cold. The client also may be confused and disoriented.

Intellectual deficits include memory impairment, poor judgment, short attention span, difficulty organizing thoughts, and inability to reason or calculate. Emotional deficits include depression and decreased tolerance to stressors.

Most clients experience initial bowel and bladder dysfunction. With early recognition of the problem and use of bowel and bladder retraining programs, however, most clients regain continence of bowel and bladder.

Differences in the affected side of the brain have been identified. Clients with left-side CVA tend to have communication deficits of aphasia, or inability to communicate. These clients tend to be slow and cautious in behavior and have intellectual impairments such as memory deficits or loss of problem-solving skills. Defects in the right visual field occur, and hemiplegia occurs on the right side.

Clients with right-side CVA have left-sided paralysis and defects in the left visual field. Spatial–perceptual defects, called **agnosia**, cause the inability to recognize familiar objects such as a hairbrush. These clients demonstrate poor judgment and impulsive behavior and are unaware of the deficits. This is called **anosognosia**, which is gross or unconscious denial of the stroke or neurological deficit. Furthermore, these clients are easily distracted and usually show **unilateral neglect**, or the failure to recognize or care for the affected side of the body.

MEMORY TRICK

Indicators of a Stroke

Mnemonic	Mnemonic Hint	Action	Stroke Symptom
S	Smile	Ask the client to smile.	One side of the face may droop.
T	Talk or speak	Ask the client to say a simple sentence, e.g., The grass is green.	The speech is slurred or garbled.
R	Raise both arms	Ask the client to raise both arms.	One arm is weak and falls downward.
T	Tongue	Ask the client to stick his tongue out.	Tongue moves to one side.
T	Time	If any of these signs are present in a nonhospitalized client, call 911 to transport the client to an acute facility	

Adapted from National Stroke Association (NSA). (2009a). Stroke 101. Retrieved on June 3, 2009 at http://www.stroke.org/site/DocServer/STROKE_101_Fact_Sheet.pdf?docID=454; and Santa Rosa County Citizen Service Center. (2009) Blood Clots/Stroke – They now have a fourth indicator, the tongue. Retrieved on June 3, 2009 at http://www.santarosa.fl.gov/hr/documents/identiyastroke.pdf

PROFESSIONALTIP

Medication and Cerebrovascular Accident

Calcium channel blockers should not be used for the client with CVA because they dilate blood vessels and increase cerebral perfusion.

Cerebral edema and increased intracranial pressure may further complicate neurological status. Cerebral edema maximizes in 3 to 5 days following CVA. Neurological deficits begin to resolve within 2 days as cerebral edema decreases. Gradual progression in the return of various functions from proximal to distal can occur for 1 to 2 years.

Medical–Surgical Management

Medical

Medical management of the client with CVA is directed toward airway maintenance and supportive therapy during the first 24 to 48 hours. Early diagnosis of the cause and type of stroke is necessary to determine the appropriate treatment. Maintaining adequate cerebral perfusion and preventing cerebral edema reduce neurological deficit. Respiratory failure is treated with mechanical ventilation; temperature is regulated, with the help of a hypothermia blanket if necessary. (See the section on increased intracranial pressure for information on prevention and treatment.)

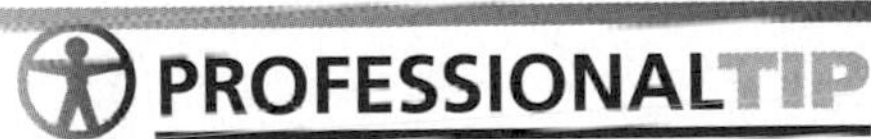

Caregivers for Client with CVA

- Give the CVA client ample time to process and then answer the question before proceeding with more conversation.
- To provide consistency in understanding the needs of a client with a CVA, assign the same caregiver to the client whenever possible.

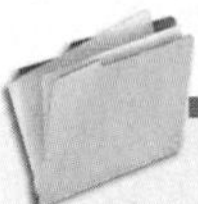

COLLABORATIVECARE

Post-CVA Care

Depending on the location of the CVA and the extent of neurologic deficit, collaboration with physical, occupational, and speech therapists is necessary for the client to reach the optimal functional level of recovery.

COMMUNITY/HOME HEALTH CARE

Post-CVA Care

- Consult with the family to evaluate the home for safety and use of wheelchair or walker, if needed.
- Evaluate the client's ability to perform self-care so that assistive devices or personal assistance is obtained.
- Determine whether a hospital bed or other medical equipment will need to be rented.

To prevent further loss of function, a focus on rehabilitation begins on admission. After a stroke, all effort is made to maintain self-care and mobility.

Surgical

Surgical removal of the thrombus (thrombolectomy) or embolus (embolectomy) may be necessary to relieve pressure on the brain.

Pharmacological

Antihypertensive agents are used to control blood pressure. Anticoagulants, aspirin, heparin, or Coumadin are used to prevent further clot formation in cases of stroke caused by thrombi. To dissolve the clot, thrombolytic agents such as alteplase (Activase), anistreplase (Eminase), streptokinase (Streptase), or urokinase (Abbokinase) are given within 3 hours of the stroke. A stroke caused by bleeding would not be treated with thrombolytic agents. Dexamethasone (Decadron) is be used to reduce intracranial pressure. Anticonvulsants such as phenytoin (Dilantin) is used if convulsions are present.

Diet

Fluid is restricted for a few days after a CVA. The client will, however, be given intravenous fluids or tube feedings. The gag reflex is assessed to identify choking risk and food restrictions implemented accordingly.

Activity

In cases of an embolic or thrombolic stroke, the client's bed is kept flat with the head midline to increase cerebral perfusion. In the event of a hemorrhagic stroke, the head of the bed is elevated to decrease cerebral perfusion. The type of CVA and the physician's judgment determines the length of time the client stays in bed.

Nursing Management

Maintain a patent airway and fluid and electrolyte balance. Administer oxygen and medications as ordered. Monitor vital signs, neurologic status, I&O, pulse oximetry, and ABGs. Ensure adequate nutrition. Provide careful mouth and eye care. Keep client's body in correct alignment, using a footboard to prevent foot drop and contractures. Turn client at least every 2 hours to prevent pneumonia. Perform and assist client to perform range of motion (ROM) exercises using the unaffected side to exercise the affected side. Communicate with the client; often an unresponsive client can hear. Set realistic short-term goals. Involve the client's family in client care when possible.

NURSING PROCESS

Assessment

Subjective Data

Subjective data include client statements regarding how the client is feeling, frustration level with limitations, reports of pain, numbness, tingling, and sensory deficits of vision or hearing.

Objective Data

Give specific attention to the objective assessment findings of level of consciousness, respiratory status, hemiparesis, hemiplegia, mobility, and cognitive perceptual functioning, including the inability to think clearly and the ability to understand the condition.

Nursing diagnoses for a client with a CVA include the following:

NURSING DIAGNOSES	PLANNING/OUTCOMES	NURSING INTERVENTIONS
*Deficient **K**nowledge* related to home care	The client and/or family will verbalize or demonstrate home health care management.	Assess client's and family's needs for discharge teaching and knowledge level about necessary home care. Develop a multidisciplinary plan for client and family teaching. Provide education in verbal, written, and picture forms to accommodate the varying possible impairments from the stroke. Teach small segments of information at a time and reinforce teaching, then, to ascertain effectiveness of teaching, have client and family return demonstrate or verbalize knowledge. Primary areas of teaching are medication administration; dosages, actions, and side effects to report to the physician; mobility needs; self-care needs; safety factors; communication; swallowing; elimination; and skin care.
*Impaired Verbal **C**ommunication* related to neuromuscular impairment	The client will communicate needs to the caregiver.	Assess communication deficits and consult a speech therapist to determine a method of communication, if deficits are apparent. Allow time for the client to attempt to communicate needs; anticipate needs to prevent client frustration in trying to communicate. Use gestures, pictures, and closed questions (those requiring only a "yes" or "no" answer). Provide paper and pencil if dominant side is unaffected.
*Unilateral **N**eglect* related to neuromuscular impairment	The client will move paralyzed extremities with assistance from functioning extremities.	Adapt environment to prevent injury of the client with unilateral neglect by positioning water and personal items on the unaffected or unneglected side. Approach the client from the unneglected side. Gradually cue client to remind to tend to the neglected side. Remind client of safety factors such as arm trailing over edge of wheelchair or close proximity of a wall on the neglected side. Teach client and family to place small bites of food on unaffected side and to check for food in the cheek on the affected side after meals. Instruct client to scan environment for safety factors at all times. Teach client how to dress and tend to neglected side. Place arm either in a sling if client is ambulatory, or on a wheelchair tray if client is in a wheelchair.

Evaluation: Evaluate each outcome to determine how it has been met by the client.

EPILEPSY/SEIZURE DISORDER

Epilepsy is a disorder of cerebral function in which the client experiences sudden attacks of altered consciousness, motor activity, or sensory phenomenon. Convulsive seizures are the most common type. Most recurrent seizure patterns are caused by epilepsy. Most clinicians and authors use the term "seizure disorder" for epilepsy or seizures (Hickey, 2008).

A seizure is initiated by an electrical disturbance in the neurons, which, in turn, causes an aberrant discharge of electrical activity from any part of the cerebral cortex and possibly from other areas of the brain (Samuels, 2004). This electrical discharge may cause involuntary episodes of loss of consciousness, excessive muscular movement or loss of muscle tone, and changes in behavior, mood, sensation, and/or perception (Smeltzer, Bare, Hinkle, & Cheever, 2008).

The etiology of the electrical disturbance may be birth trauma, hypoxia, infection, tumor, alcohol toxicity, drugs, drug withdrawal, carbon monoxide or lead poisoning, vascular abnormalities such as CVA, hypoglycemia electrolyte imbalance, or fever. Often, the cause is idiopathic, or unknown.

Seizures are classified as generalized or partial. In generalized seizures, the entire brain is affected simultaneously, causing bilateral, symmetrical reactions. Generalized seizures are classified as tonic and/or clonic (grand mal), absence (petit mal), or myoclonic.

Tonic–clonic seizures involve rigid tonic contractions of muscles and loss of postural control followed by a clonic stage of intermittent contraction and relaxation. Incontinence of stool or urine is common. Absence seizures involve loss of conscious activity without the muscular involvement of tonic–clonic seizures. Myoclonic seizures are very mild, sudden, involuntary contractions of a muscle group or rapid, forceful movements. They usually occur in the trunk or extremities and involve no loss of consciousness.

Partial seizures initiate in a focal point in the brain and involve the function of those specific neurons. Partial seizures are either simple or complex. In simple partial seizures, the area affected may be a hand, a finger, the ability to talk, or a sense such as smell. Consciousness is not lost.

Complex partial seizures generally involve loss of consciousness and produce cognitive, affective, psychosensory, or psychomotor symptoms. The client performs inappropriate purposive behaviors, called **automatisms**, or mechanical, repetitive motor behaviors performed unconsciously, such as lip-smacking. **Auras**, peculiar sensations that precede a seizure, may take the form of a taste, smell, sight, or sound; dizziness; or a "funny" feeling. After the seizure, the client typically cannot remember the episode.

Diagnostic testing to determine the type of seizure activity includes an EEG to identify abnormal electrical activity and/or the focal point of the seizure. Sleep and video EEGs document changes in electrical activity of the brain. CT scans identify or rule out lesions, degenerative changes, or vascular abnormalities.

MEDICAL–SURGICAL MANAGEMENT

Surgical

Surgical intervention is indicated for a very small percentage of clients; those for whom pharmacological treatment has not been effective and when the focal points are identified. Microsurgery is used to irradiate focal points of abnormal electrical discharge caused by tumor, vascular abnormality, or abscess.

Pharmacological

The primary method of controlling seizure activity is pharmacological. Seizure activity is controlled with an anticonvulsant agent or a combination of anticonvulsants in 75% of clients (Hickey, 2008). Phenytoin (Dilantin), phenobarbital (Phenobarbital), carbamazepine (Tegretol), valproic acid (Depakene), and primidone (Mysoline) are often used. Anticonvulsant agents are started one at a time in gradually increasing doses. The client's blood level is monitored for therapeutic range, and the client is assessed for side effects of the drug and signs of drug toxicity, such as drowsiness, dizziness, gastric distress, rash, blood dyscrasias, and ataxia.

The goal is to obtain seizure control with minimal side effects. Any anticonvulsant is gradually discontinued. Abrupt

SAFETY

Precautions During a Seizure

If the client is in bed:

- Be sure the side rails are up.
- Put padding (blankets) on the side rails to prevent injury.

If the client is out of bed:

- Carefully ease the client to the floor.
- Move nearby objects so that the client will not be injured.
- Place a soft item beneath the client's head.

Whether the client is in or out of bed:

- Never leave the client alone.
- Do not restrain the client.
- Do not attempt to put anything in the client's mouth after the seizure has begun.
- Loosen any restrictive clothing around the client's neck.
- Turn the client's head to the side.
- Monitor seizure activity carefully, noting the exact time that the seizure began and ended.

After the seizure:

- Call the client by name and ask to perform a simple command.
- Test the client's memory by asking to remember two words.
- Ask the client whether an aura was experienced before the seizure.
- Check the oral cavity—especially the tongue—for injury.
- Offer comfort and reassurance, as the client is frightened and embarrassed.
- Document everything observed.
- Keep the client in a side-lying position if the client remains lethargic.

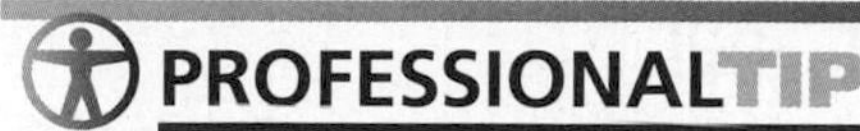

Long-Term Use of Dilantin

The client on Dilantin requires good oral hygiene because of hyperplasia of the gums, which become edematous and enlarged.

withdrawal can cause **status epilepticus**, an acute prolonged episode of seizure activity lasting at least 30 minutes with or without loss of consciousness (Smeltzer, Bare, Hinkle, & Cheever, 2008). Status epilepticus is a medical emergency that results in respiratory arrest and irreversible brain damage.

Diet

Nutritionally balanced meals are required. The client should not consume alcohol.

Activity

Adequate rest is required. Driving, operating machinery, and swimming are not allowed until seizures are controlled.

Nursing Management

Monitor for toxic signs of anticonvulsant medications. Stress importance for compliance with prescribed medication schedule. Encourage scrupulous oral hygiene. Warn client not to drink alcoholic beverages. Encourage client to have anticonvulsant medication blood level checked regularly.

NURSING PROCESS

Assessment

Subjective Data

Include client statements of experiences before the seizure and activity the client was performing when the seizure occurred. Determine whether an aura was experienced and the sensations that were manifested, and ascertain if the client has a prior history of seizure disorder.

Objective Data

Assessment of the nature of the seizure and sequencing of events is important in determining cause and management of seizure activity. During the seizure, assess the client's respiratory status and observe for muscular stiffness or flaccidity, the position of the eyes and head, the size and equality of the pupils, automatism, any cry or sounds made, and incontinence of urine or stool. Note the duration of the phases of the seizure, total duration, and whether unconsciousness occurred. Note if the onset of seizure activity was observed, along with what the client was doing when the seizure began.

After the seizure, assess airway and observe the client for **postictal** (after a seizure) signs of paralysis of arms or legs, inability to speak, sleep following seizure, difficulty in awakening from sleep, confusion, or general dazed affect (Smeltzer, Bare, Hinkle, & Cheever, 2008; Hickey, 2008). The postictal phase lasts from several minutes to hours. Assess the client for signs of injury and vital signs. Clients on anticonvulsant therapy are assessed thoroughly because of the wide variety of side effects involving multiple body systems.

Nursing diagnoses for a client with a seizure include the following:

NURSING DIAGNOSES	PLANNING/OUTCOMES	NURSING INTERVENTIONS
*Ineffective **A**irway Clearance* related to mucus accumulation during the seizure and uncontrollable tonic–clonic muscle contractions involving the respiratory muscles	The client will maintain an effective airway during seizure activity.	Following tonic–clonic activity, turn client to the side to allow secretions to drain from the airway. Prepare to suction oropharynx if necessary to clear airway. Assess skin color and respiratory rate and depth during and following seizure. Administer oxygen as needed. Insert oral airway or epistick if client's jaw is not clenched. Never insert an object if the jaw is already clenched. Do not place fingers between client's teeth. Loosen restrictive clothing.
*Risk for **I**njury* related to seizure activity	The client will be free of injury related to seizure activity.	During seizures in bed, use blankets or protective pads to pad side rails. If client is standing or sitting, ease client to the floor when seizure activity begins. Place client in a supine position, but do not physically restrain client. Remove objects from around client so that he will not hit them. After the seizure, assess airway and turn client to the side to allow secretions to drain from the mouth. Observe client for injuries (e.g., tongue lacerations; broken bones; body lacerations or bruising). Maintain a low-stimulus environment to prevent further seizure activity.

Nursing diagnoses for a client with a seizure include the following: (Continued)

NURSING DIAGNOSES	PLANNING/OUTCOMES	NURSING INTERVENTIONS
		Teach client about ways of maintaining a safe environment, including driving restrictions; lying down in a safe area if an aura is experienced; showering instead of tub bathing; either avoiding swimming or swimming with a partner if the physician allows; and wearing a medical identification tag.
*Ineffective **Coping*** related to anxiety secondary to seizure disorder and altered self-concept	The client will verbalize fears and concerns about seizure activity; and will use effective coping methods.	Allow client to verbalize fears and concerns. Explore coping mechanisms with client. Collaborate with mental health counselor or clergy to assist client in development of coping mechanisms.

Evaluation: Evaluate each outcome to determine how it has been met by the client.

HERNIATED INTERVERTEBRAL DISK

Herniated intervertebral disks are a major cause of chronic back pain. Most clients with herniated disks are 30 to 50 years of age. Most herniated disks occur in the lumbar or cervical spine because of the flexibility of these regions (Hickey, 2008). This can occur either suddenly from trauma, lifting, or twisting or gradually from aging, osteoporosis, or degenerative changes. Most herniated disks are caused by trauma, such as falls, accidents, or repeated lifting. Degenerative changes related to arthritis, aging, or repeated minor injuries predispose the client to herniated intervertebral disks.

The intervertebral disk is a cartilaginous cushion between vertebral bodies (Figure 10-15). In herniation, or rupture of the disk, the nucleus pulposus protrudes into the fibrous ring, the annulus fibrosus. This protrusion presses on the spinal cord and nerve roots, causing pain, motor changes, sensory changes, and alterations in reflexes.

The nerve root affected and the degree of compression leads to specific symptoms. Ninety percent to 95% of lumbar herniations occur at the L-4 to L-5 and S-1 levels (Hickey, 2008). Low-back pain that radiates across the buttock and down the leg along the path of the sciatic nerve is the most common symptom. The affected leg tingles and is numb. Sneezing, straining, stooping, standing, sitting, blowing the nose, and jarring movements aggravate the pain. Positions of comfort are lying on the back, with knees flexed and a small pillow under the head, or lying on the unaffected side, with the affected knee flexed.

Motor weakness is experienced. Paresthesia and numbness of the leg and foot occur. Knee and ankle reflexes are diminished or absent. **Lasegue's sign**, pain experienced upon gentle raising of the fully extended leg of the supine-positioned client to 20 to 60 degrees, stems from stretching of the inflamed sciatic nerve. With a low-back herniated disk, however, the client is unable to extend the knee because of severe pain radiating down the hip and leg. Symptoms vary with the area and degree of nerve root compression.

Cervical herniation commonly occurs at levels C-5 to C-6 or C-6 to C-7. Symptoms of lateral herniation include pain and paresthesia in the neck, arms, and shoulders. Loss of muscle strength and reflexes also occur, as does muscle atrophy.

Because of anatomic position, cervical disks herniate centrally more frequently than do lumbar disks, thereby compressing the spinal cord. Symptoms are weakness of the lower extremities and unsteady gait. Spasticity and hyperactive reflexes develop in the lower extremities. Difficulty in voiding and sexual dysfunction occur.

Degenerative spinal cord disease can follow compression from a herniated disk. Spinal cord tumors and herniated lumbar disk are differential diagnoses that are ruled out through the use of MRI or CT scans.

MEDICAL–SURGICAL MANAGEMENT

Medical

Conservative medical treatment, i.e., providing rest, stress reduction and immobility of the spine, and pain relief, often is tried for several weeks. Physical therapy is ordered, with exercises to strengthen back muscles and possibly ultrasound treatments.

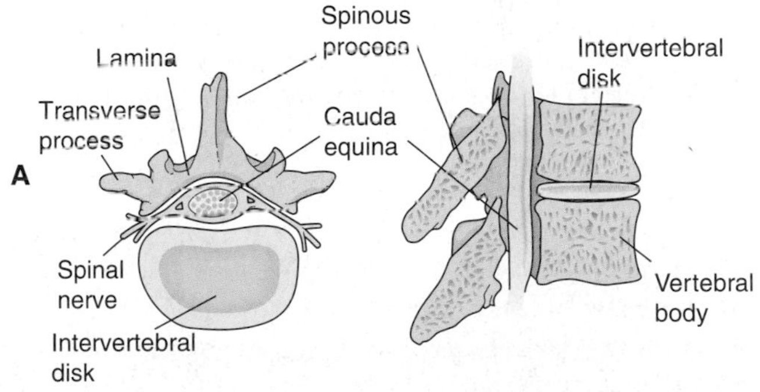

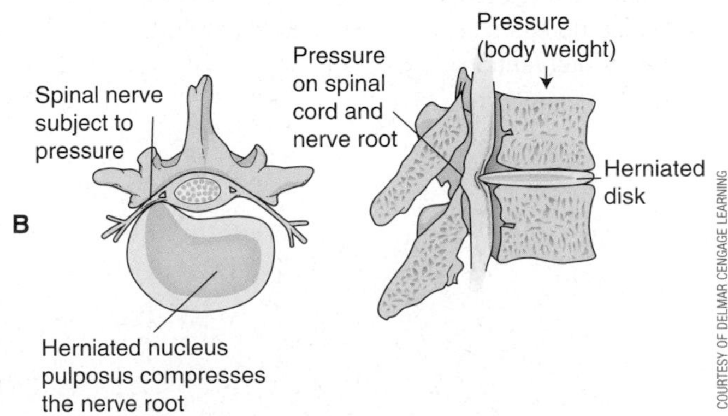

FIGURE 10-15 ***A*, Normal Intravertebral Disk; *B*, Herniated Disk**

A transcutaneous electrical nerve stimulation (TNS) unit may also be used to decrease pain.

Surgical

Surgery to remove the herniated disk is performed when neurological deficit or pain are not responsive to conservative treatment or when symptoms require immediate surgical intervention.

Pharmacological

Narcotic analgesics, such as hydrocodone bitartrate with acetaminophen (Vicodin), and nonnarcotic analgesics, such as tramadol hydrochloride (Ultram), are ordered for pain control. Antiinflammatory drugs, steroids, or NSAIDs, such as ibuprofen (Motrin) or naproxen (Anaprox), are prescribed to reduce the inflammatory response. Clients in chronic pain sometimes benefit from an antiepileptic drug, e.g., gabapentin (Neurontin), because it treats neuropathic pain. Muscle relaxants, such as methocarbamol (Robaxin), are given to reduce spasms of surrounding muscles, which decreases the pain. Antianxiety medications, such as diazepam (Valium), are given to decrease muscle tension and promote rest. Short-term oral corticosteroids may be ordered, or local or epidural corticosteroid injections may be used

Diet

To decrease the workload on the involved muscles, weight reduction is advocated if the client is overweight. A high-protein diet with calcium, vitamin D, and phosphorus is necessary for bone repair and prevention of osteoporosis. Fiber is necessary for bowel function because constipation is a common side effect of analgesics.

Activity

Bed rest, a support garment (back brace) or cervical collar, a firm mattress, and traction are used to decrease stress on the affected vertebrae. Postoperatively, log-roll turning prevents injury to the vertebrae and spine.

The client may not lift or carry more than 5 pounds for at least 8 weeks. Twisting movements are avoided. The client cannot drive a car until the surgeon permits. Sitting is limited during the early postoperative period; the client either stands or lies down. Physical therapy is focused on muscle strengthening and client comfort. Heat therapy, ultrasound, and exercises promote comfort and healing.

Nursing Management

Preoperatively, monitor neurological status and vital signs. Encourage client to cough, deep breathe, use incentive spirometer, and move legs as allowed. Provide adequate fluids to prevent renal stasis and constipation.

Postoperatively, monitor vital signs, neurovascular status of legs, and check dressing for any bleeding. If drain is in place (e.g., Hemovac or Jackson-Pratt drain), check frequently and empty at end of shift and record on I&O sheet. Use the log-rolling technique for turning the client.

NURSING PROCESS

Assessment

Subjective Data

Assessment includes eliciting client statements about motor and sensory function, pain, and effectiveness of comfort measures.

Objective Data

Assessment entails a neurological evaluation of motor and sensory function of the extremities innervated below the herniated area. Reflex testing is a part of the nursing assessment in some facilities. Assess range of motion (ROM) of the affected extremity. Assess the client's knowledge about the disease process, the planned treatment including pain management and surgery, and the postsurgical care. Assess bowel and bladder elimination for potential nerve involvement or effects of immobility. Note gait alteration and bending limitations.

Nursing diagnoses for a client with a herniated intervertebral disk include the following:

NURSING DIAGNOSES	PLANNING/OUTCOMES	NURSING INTERVENTIONS
Chronic **Pain** related to nerve compression or surgical intervention	The client will experience increased comfort.	Assess pain intensity and location, as well as activities or position when pain began. Have the client rate pain on a scale of 1 to 10.
		Maintain activity level as ordered by physician. Provide diversional activities.
		Place client in position of comfort, usually on back, with knees slightly flexed and a small pillow beneath head, or on unaffected side, with affected extremity flexed and a pillow between the legs.
		Maintain immobility of vertebrae with corset, brace, or traction.
		Apply moist heat as prescribed and administer medications to relieve pain, relax muscles, and relieve inflammation and anxiety, as ordered. Document effectiveness.

Nursing diagnoses for a client with a herniated intervertebral disk include the following: (Continued)

NURSING DIAGNOSES	PLANNING/OUTCOMES	NURSING INTERVENTIONS
Impaired Physical Mobility related to nerve compression or surgical intervention	The client will have no complications of immobility.	Assess for complications of immobility. Turn client every 1 to 2 hours. The client tends to limit position to one of comfort. Assist the client to log roll, that is, move the body as a unit without twisting the back. Ambulate as ordered by the physician.

Evaluation: Evaluate each outcome to determine how it has been met by the client.

SPINAL CORD INJURY

Spinal cord injury (SCI) occurs from trauma to the spinal cord or from compression of the spinal cord caused by injury to the supporting structures. Each year, almost 12,000 new spinal cord injuries occur. Most of the victims are males between the ages of 16 and 30 years. Leading causes of injury in the order of prevalence are motor vehicle accidents; falls; acts of violence; and sporting accidents (Spinal Cord Injury Information Network, 2009).

Numerous classification systems exist for SCIs. Spinal cord injuries are classified by level of injury, mechanism of injury, or neurological or functional level (Figure 10-16). The injury may be considered complete or incomplete. When injury is complete, no impulses are carried below the level of injury. There is complete disruption of the spinal cord functions, including motor (voluntary) movement, sensation, and reflexes to areas innervated by the spinal nerves at and below the level of the injury. In an incomplete injury, some of the spinal cord tracts are affected while others are able to carry impulses normally.

The mechanism of injury is usually an acceleration-deceleration event that causes hyperflexion, hyperextension, axial loading, or excessive rotation injury (Hickey, 2008). Hyperflexion is the extreme forward movement of the head, which causes compression of the vertebral bodies and damage to the posterior ligaments and intervertebral disks, as shown in Figure 10-17A. Hyperextension is the extreme backward movement of the head, causing injury to the posterior vertebral structures and the anterior ligaments, as shown in Figure 10-17B. Axial loading or compression occurs when extreme pressure is placed on the spinal column, such as in diving accidents or falls landed on feet or buttocks (Figure 10-17C). Compression of the vertebrae shatters the vertebral body. Compression fractures and posterior ligament injury can also be caused by excessive rotation, or turning the head beyond the normal range.

Classification of injury by cause includes concussion, contusion, laceration, transection, hemorrhage, or damage to blood vessels supplying the spinal cord. Immediately after injury to the spinal cord, an autodestructive process begins, with chemical and vascular changes that lead to ischemia and necrosis of the spinal cord.

Spinal shock (cessation of motor, sensory, autonomic, and reflex impulses) and **areflexia** (the absence of reflexes) occur immediately upon transection of the spinal cord or upon injury to the spinal cord. Flaccid paralysis of all skeletal muscles, loss of spinal reflexes, loss of sensation, and absence of autonomic function below the level of injury also occur. The diaphragm is innervated at levels C3 through C5. Injuries in this area cause partial or complete disruption of respiratory function. The client does not perspire below the level of the injury. Bowel and bladder function is lost either for a few days to months, or permanently, although this loss generally lasts from 1 to 6 weeks.

As spinal shock resolves, reflex activity returns below the level of injury. The client with a lower motor neuron injury continues to experience flaccid paralysis, areflexia, hypotonic bowel and bladder function, and sexual dysfunction. Lower motor neuron injury causes paraplegia, or paralysis of lower extremities.

Neurogenic shock, a hypotensive situation resulting from the loss of sympathetic control of vital functions from the brain, may occur during spinal shock. This happens in clients with injury above the sixth thoracic vertebra. The client develops orthostatic hypotension, bradycardia, decreased cardiac output, loss of ability to sweat below the level of injury, and poikilothermia (body temperature adjusts to room temperature).

Upper motor neuron injury results in spastic paralysis, loss of voluntary skeletal muscle movement, and reflexive bowel, bladder, and sexual responses. Complete upper motor neuron injury results in **quadriplegia (tetraplegia)**, or dysfunction or paralysis of both arms, both legs, bowel, and bladder. Injuries above C5 affect respiratory function because of innervation of the diaphragm and accessory respiratory muscles. Mechanical ventilation is required to keep the client alive. Fractures below the cervical vertebrae result in diaphragmatic breathing, if the phrenic nerve is functioning.

Once spinal shock has passed, the client with an injury above the sixth thoracic vertebra is at risk for developing *autonomic dysreflexia* or *autonomic hyperreflexia*. Autonomic dysreflexia is an emergency situation resulting in a hypertensive crisis (elevated systolic pressures of 260 to 300 mm Hg), bradycardia, severe headache, and possibly stroke or seizure activity. The cause is noxious stimuli such as a full bladder, a fecal impaction, a wrinkle in clothing, menstrual cramps, an erection, an ingrown toenail, a bladder infection, or sitting on catheter tubing. Autonomic reflexes below the level of the injury cause vasoconstriction in this area. The controlling impulses from the higher cortical levels do not transmit past the level of injury but cause bradycardia and vasodilation above the level of injury. Skin above the level of injury is warm and moist, but skin below the level of injury is cold, with goose flesh (Beare & Meyers, 1998; Hickey, 2008).

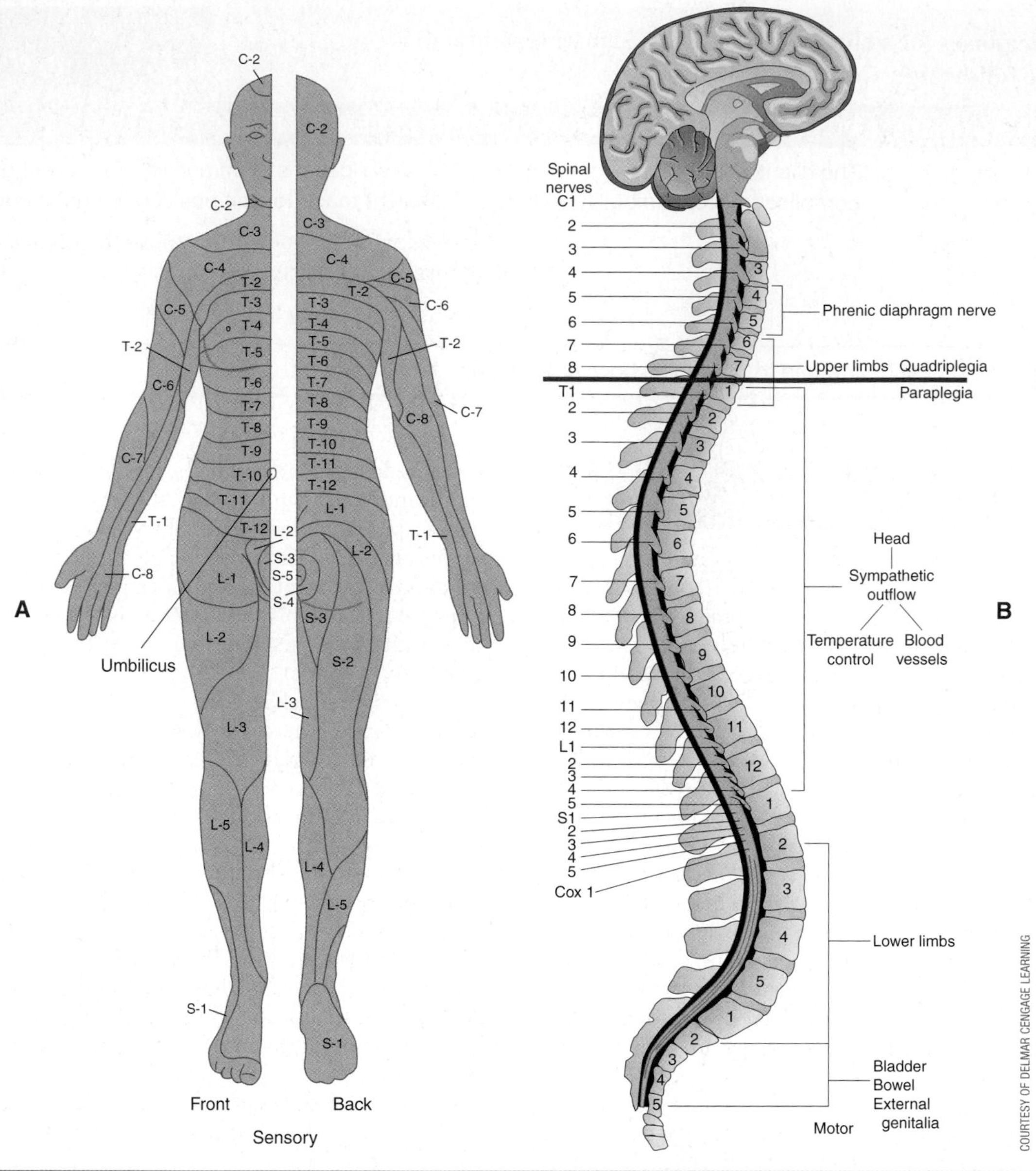

FIGURE 10-16 Spinal Cord—Levels of Injury; *A*, Areas of Sensory Function (Dermatomes); *B*, Areas of Motor Function

The noxious stimuli must be removed, if possible, and the client placed in a sitting position immediately. Assess blood pressure immediately and monitor every few minutes until within normal limits (Huston & Boelman, 1995). The drug of choice, nitroprusside sodium (Nipride), is given if the conservative measure does not work. Nifedipine (Procardia) is also used. Prevent autonomic dysreflexia when possible, recognize when it develops, and treat immediately. Once autonomic dysreflexia is relieved, the client may develop hypotension from the decreased sympathetic response and the residual effects of medication and positioning changes. A pattern of individual response to stimuli and of sympathetic response is soon identified for the client; however, the client with an upper motor neuron injury above T-6 is always at risk for developing autonomic dysreflexia. Some clients experience the first episode years after the injury.

The extent of permanent injury cannot be determined immediately because of necrosis, edema, and spinal shock. Functional loss depends on the level, degree, and type of injury.

MEDICAL–SURGICAL MANAGEMENT

Medical

Medical management of the client with spinal cord injury begins before reaching the hospital. Further damage to the spinal cord is prevented by immobilizing the head, neck, and vertebral column with devices such as rigid cervical collars and splinting backboards. All trauma clients are treated as potential spinal cord injuries. When the client reaches the emergency room, x-rays of the spine are taken before removing the immobilizing devices.

Respiratory function is continuously assessed, and ventilatory support is provided as necessary. The client may have multiple injuries, necessitating astute diagnostic skills by the emergency room physician. Assessment of the trauma client involves evaluating for internal hemorrhaging, cardiac contusion, head injury, hemorrhagic shock, and spinal shock resulting from the spinal cord injury. A thorough assessment is done to specifically evaluate the degree of deficit and to establish the level or degree of injury.

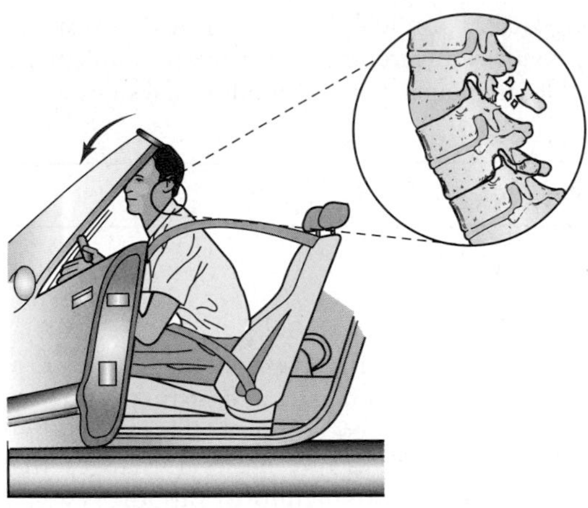
A

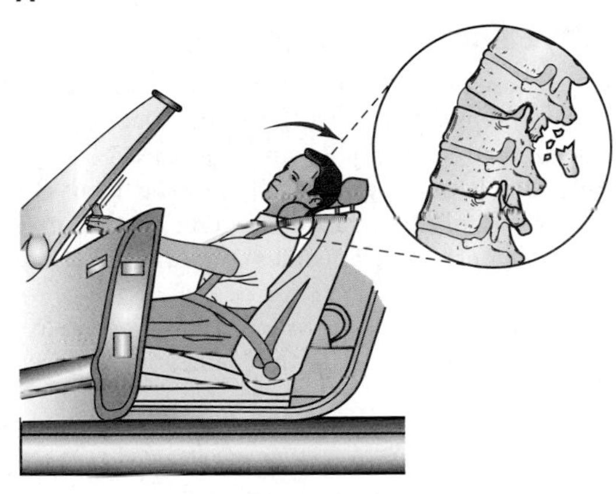
B

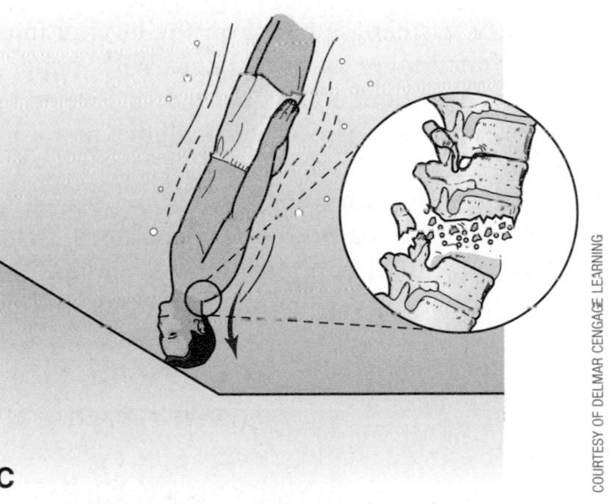

C

FIGURE 10-17 Acceleration/Deceleration Injuries; *A*, Hyperflexion: The extreme forward movement of the head causes compression of the vertebral bodies and damage to the posterior ligaments and intervertebral disks; *B*, Hyperextension: Extreme backward movement of the head causes injury to the posterior vertebral structures and the anterior ligaments; *C*, Axial loading or compression: Extreme pressure is placed on the spinal column, such as in diving accidents or falls landing on feet or buttocks

Blood pressure monitoring is crucial. A systolic BP below 90 mm Hg should be avoided or corrected as soon as possible because one episode can send the client into shock and cause permanent damage (Baker & Saulino, 2002).

Immobilization of the spinal cord continues to be the focus of care during early medical management of the client. Traction is used to maintain alignment of the spinal column. Cervical tongs and halo devices are used to apply traction and to immobilize the cervical spine (Figure 10-18). Under local anesthesia, cervical tongs and halo rings are applied with spring-loaded pins that are embedded into the scalp. Antiseptic solution is used to cleanse the scalp, and a local anesthetic is injected into the insertion sites. Traction weights are applied to the cervical tongs or halo rings after the insertion pins are firmly embedded. Body casts, jackets, vests, or braces are used to immobilize thoracic and lumbar fractures.

Surgical

Surgical interventions are performed for decompression, realignment, and stabilization of the vertebral column, depending on the nature of the injury. A laminectomy is performed to decompress the spinal cord with fusion or placement of Harrington rods to stabilize the vertebral column. Realignment is maintained by surgical manipulation of the vertebral column.

If the client has respiratory involvement, an endotracheal tube is put in place to provide mechanical ventilatory support. Following urgent treatment, a tracheostomy is performed to continue ventilation.

Pharmacological

Nitroprusside sodium (Nipride) and nifedipine (Prodardia) are ordered to reduce blood pressure in cases of autonomic dysreflexia.

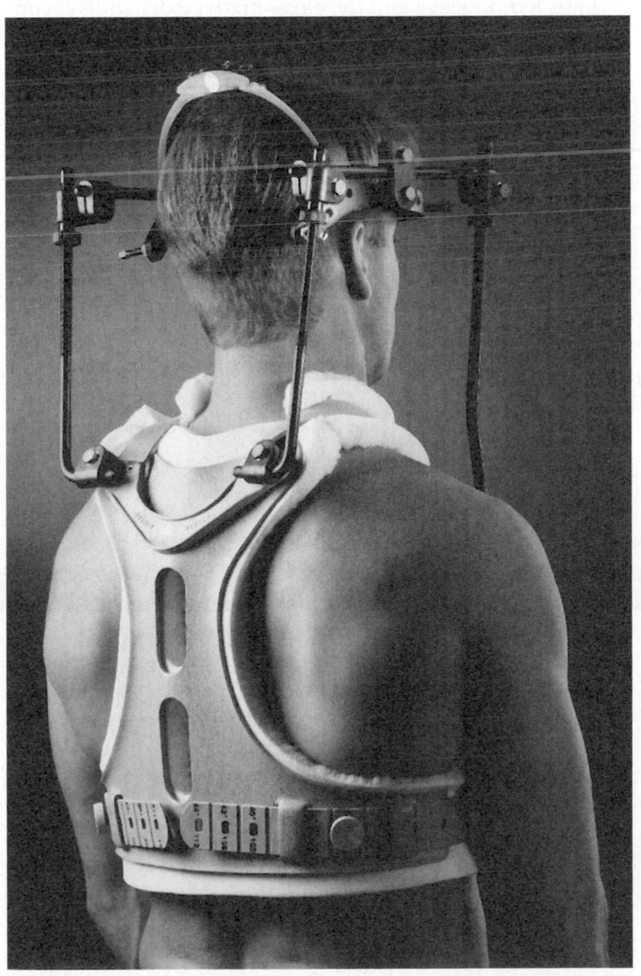

FIGURE 10-18 **Halo Vest (*Courtesy of DePuy AcroMed.*)**

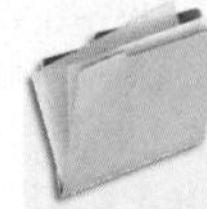

COLLABORATIVE**CARE**

After a Spinal Cord Injury

The interdisciplinary team works together to optimize the functional capabilities of the client. The physical therapist works on activity level, the occupational therapist on ADLs, the speech therapist on swallowing and communication, and nursing coordinates the team and reinforces what the client has been taught. The focus is to prevent disabilities and maximize and strengthen functional ability.

Activity

Initially, immobilization of the spinal column is necessary. In the acute phase, ROM for all joints is performed to prevent mobility loss and muscle contracture. As the spine is stabilized, the client's activity progresses to sitting up in a chair, performing strengthening exercises, and increasing endurance. The nurse observes for the complication of orthostatic hypotension.

Orthostatic hypotension is caused by the venous pooling of blood in the lower body and extremities resulting from impairment of the sympathetic nervous system. The client becomes hypotensive and develops bradycardia and syncope. Asystole may even occur. Prevention of orthostatic hypotension also requires the application of full leg support stockings and pneumatic boots and the gradual lowering of the lower extremities. Monitor the client's vital signs throughout the mobilization process to ascertain tolerance to the procedure. After spinal shock has subsided, active rehabilitation begins.

Nursing Management

After stabilization, turn client frequently to prevent embolism, pneumonia, and skin breakdown. Use log-rolling technique. Keep call light within client's reach. Provide passive and active ROM exercises as allowed. Maintain adequate nutrition and fluid intake. If client has a halo device, perform pin-site care following facility protocol. For a client with a vest, jacket, or brace, provide skin care under the device. Implement bowel and bladder training regimen. Monitor vital signs.

NURSING PROCESS

Assessment

Subjective Data

Subjective assessment involves eliciting input from the client regarding sensation, pain, and history of the accident. Note how the client is coping with the injury, the resulting disability, and the major lifestyle changes that have occurred. Evaluate how the family or support system is coping with the changes.

Objective Data

In the acute phase of care of the client with a spinal cord injury, nursing assessment focuses on the critical factors of airway, breathing, circulation, disability, and exposure.

Assess circulatory status by monitoring vital signs and observing for complications of neurogenic shock; orthostatic hypotension; hypertensive episodes of autonomic dysreflexia; and hemorrhaging.

Assess disability by performing a baseline neurological assessment (as described under the Neurological Assessment section in this chapter).

Exposure refers to removing the client's clothing to perform a thorough assessment of the client's body for skin condition and for entrance and exit wounds. Monitor body temperature because of the neurological deficit in temperature regulation caused by dysfunction of the ANS.

Subacute assessment is based on the level of injury and neurological functioning of the client. With upper motor neuron injuries, the client is at higher risk of developing autonomic dysreflexia; thus, assessment includes monitoring for these signs.

Assess all clients with spinal cord injury for skin condition, bowel and bladder function, respiratory status, and signs and symptoms of complications of immobility. Psychosocial assessment is very important to the well-being of the client.

Nursing diagnoses for a client with a spinal cord injury in the subacute phase of care include the following:

NURSING DIAGNOSES	PLANNING/OUTCOMES	NURSING INTERVENTIONS
Risk for Injury related to motor and sensory deficits secondary to spinal fractures	The client will not experience additional injury.	Assess the client's risk factors for additional injury. Monitor skin condition for pressure areas or shearing injuries from sliding across sheets or the mats in physical therapy. Turn client frequently to prevent pressure areas. Use enough personnel to turn client correctly to maintain alignment of client's spinal column. Provide a call light that the client can operate; teach to call nurse for assistance as necessary. Reinforce wheelchair safety factors and observe client for use of wheelchair.

Nursing diagnoses for a client with a spinal cord injury in the subacute phase of care include the following: (Continued)

NURSING DIAGNOSES	PLANNING/OUTCOMES	NURSING INTERVENTIONS
		Prevent falls when transferring client to wheelchair. Prevent foot drop. Provide passive and active ROM exercises. Maintain adequate fluid intake and nutrition. Provide routine care for halo device by opening vest on one side to cleanse skin under vest at least daily and to assess for skin breakdown. Repeat procedure on the other side. Monitor pin sites of halo device every shift for placement. Perform pin site care using facility protocol.
Powerlessness related to changes in motor and sensory function and in lifestyle	The client will make decisions regarding care, treatment, and future.	Explain all procedures and care options. Allow client to participate in care decisions. Establish an open, trusting relationship with client to foster therapeutic communication. Allow time for client to express concerns, anger, and fears. Foster a positive environment for client to explore feelings and accept disability. Assess for signs and symptoms of depression. Collaborate with mental health professional to provide assistance in coping with lifestyle changes. Collaborate with family and support people to include them in the plan of care
Autonomic Dysreflexia related to noxious stimulation secondary to overstimulation of ANS	The client will state factors that cause autonomic dysreflexia, describe treatment, and notify the nurse if experiencing symptoms of dysreflexia.	Teach client causes and symptoms of autonomic dysreflexia: increased blood pressure, sudden throbbing headache, chills, pallor, goose flesh, nausea, and/or metallic taste in mouth. Prevent bladder distention and fecal impaction by implementing a bowel and bladder training program. Observe for bradycardia, vasodilatation, flushing, and diaphoresis above the level of spinal cord injury. If these symptoms occur, immediately notify the physician and administer medications as ordered to decrease blood pressure. Raise head of bed and lower legs to reduce blood pressure. Then, remove the noxious stimuli, which may include constrictive clothing, shoes, splints, or linens. Assess client for a distended bladder and empty the bladder if distended. Observe urine for signs of infection and obtain a urine specimen for culture, if needed to identify the cause of the reaction. Check for fecal impaction using xylocaine viscous per physician's order to decrease stimulation. Monitor blood pressure every few minutes.

Evaluation: Evaluate each outcome to determine how it has been met by the client.

PARKINSON'S DISEASE

Parkinson's disease (PD) is a chronic, progressive, degenerative disease affecting the area of the brain controlling movement. The cause is unknown in most cases, but toxicity, hypoxia, or encephalitis may precede the onset of PD. Vascular and genetic factors have been implicated. Drugs such as cocaine, haloperidol (Haldol), and chlorpromazine (Thorazine) may cause a parkinsonian syndrome. The theory is that these drugs interfere with the synthesis or storage of dopamine.

Typical signs and symptoms of PD are muscular rigidity, **bradykinesia** (slowness of voluntary movement and speech), resting tremors, muscular weakness, and loss of postural reflexes. Muscular rigidity along with bradykinesia impairs the person's ability to perform daily activities and speech.

Rigidity is noted along with increased muscle tone when the client is at rest. Stiffness of the trunk, head, and shoulders is present. The rigidity causes loss of arm swing when walking. A cogwheel phenomenon results from the muscle contractions breaking through the muscular rigidity. The alternating rigidity and rhythmic contractions causes a jerking-like movement. Motor impairment progressively affects facial expressions, eye blink, and voice, causing a typical presentation of a mask-like face and a monotone voice.

Resting tremors, usually in the upper extremities, are present when the hand is motionless. The hand moves in a "pill-rolling" motion. When the client is moving or sleeping, the tremors are usually absent. Tremors also occur in other areas, including the feet, lips, tongue, or jaw. The tremors usually begin unilaterally in one area and progress to other areas and then to the opposite side of the body. Anxiety and concentration tend to increase the degree of tremors.

The posture and gait of people with PD is characterized by bowed head, forward-bent trunk, drooped shoulders, and flexed arms. The gait is characterized by shuffling movement and small steps. Balance is affected, resulting in a tendency to fall forward. Figure 10-19 shows the classic posture of a client with PD.

Autonomic dysfunction includes drooling, **dysphagia** (difficulty swallowing), excessive sweating, hyperactivity of oil glands, and constipation. Orthostatic hypotension may occur from loss of the peripheral autonomic response. Urinary incontinence and frequency occur.

Mental changes may also occur. Intelligence is not impaired, but problems with judgment and emotional stability may occur. Dementia, depression, cognitive, perceptual, or memory deficits may occur. The major cause of death is from the complications of immobility or injury. Fatigue increases all signs and symptoms. There is no definitive diagnostic procedure for PD. The diagnosis is based on history, physical, and the client's response to anti-Parkinson's medications. Imaging studies and EEG are performed to rule out other neurological diseases. Position emission tomography (PET) scanning is performed as a way of researching information about the degeneration of the neurons that make dopamine (National Institute Neurological Disorders and Stroke, 2006c). In cases of early onset, it is important to differentiate from Wilson's disease, an increased absorption of copper, for which testing is available.

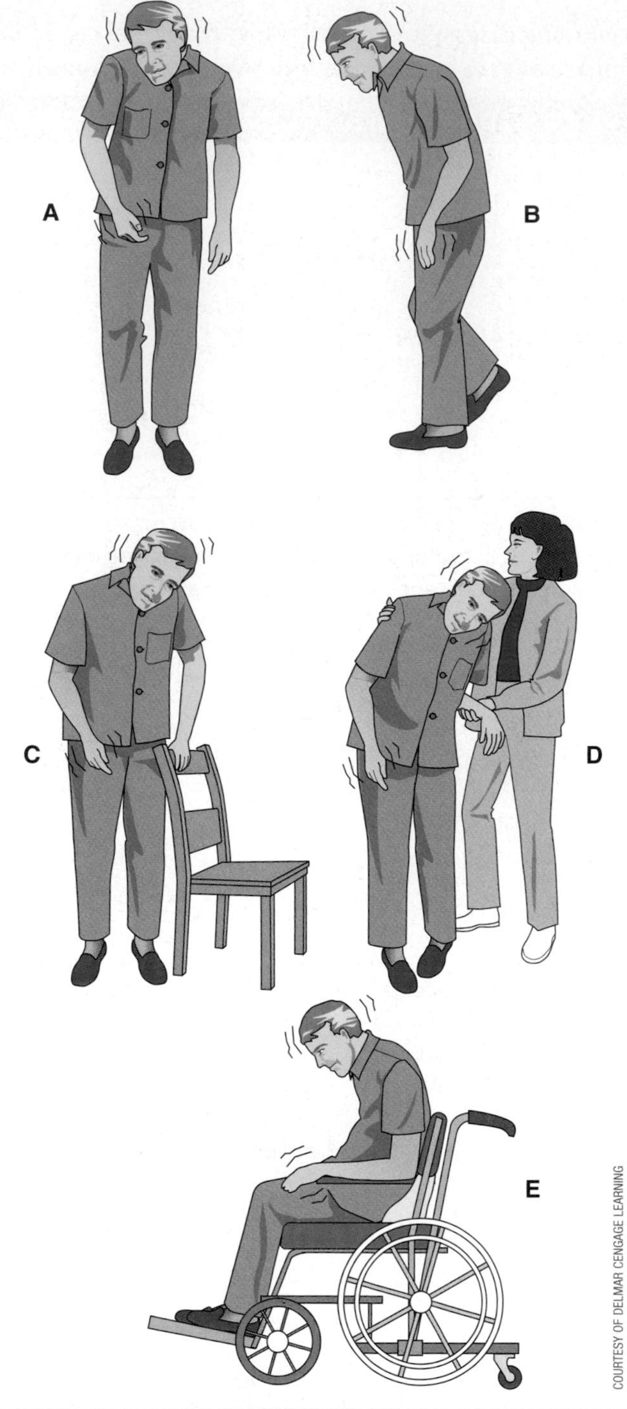

FIGURE 10-19 Progression of Parkinson's Disease; *A*, Flexion of Affected Arm; *B*, Shuffling Gait; *C*, Need for Sources of Support to Prevent Falling; *D*, Progression of Weakness to Point of Needing Assistance for Ambulation; *E*, Profound Weakness

MEDICAL–SURGICAL MANAGEMENT

Medical

The goals of medical management are to control the symptoms, provide supportive therapy and maintenance, maintain function via physiotherapy, and provide psychotherapy as necessary.

Surgical

Surgical procedures are usually only used in clients who are unresponsive to drug therapy. Ablation procedures (thalamotomy, pallidotomy, and subthalamic nucleotomy) destroy areas of the brain to control intractable tremors or akinesia. The risk of causing permanent neurological deficits is high. Deep brain stimulation has been approved by the U.S. Food and Drug Administration to reduce the severity of symptoms (National Institute of Neurological Disorders and Stroke, 2006c). In deep brain stimulation, an electrode is placed in the thalamus, globus pallidus, or subthalamic nucleus to deliver a specific current to the targeted brain location. These jolts of electricity counter balance the hyperactivity of these parts of the brain in clients with PD. Surgical interventions are believed to be most effective in relatively young clients with unilateral tremor. Still in the experimental stages are neural tissue transplants, gene therapy, and stem cell transplantation.

Pharmacological

Drug therapy is used to control the symptoms of PD. Levodopa (L-Dopa) is converted into dopamine in the basal ganglia to replace the deficit of dopamine. Dopamine is not given orally because it is metabolized before reaching the brain. L-Dopa, a precursor to dopamine, is given orally and reaches the brain to be converted into dopamine.

Dopadecarboxylase inhibitors such as carbidopa-levodopa (Sinemet) prevent the conversion of levodopa (L-Dopa) to dopamine in peripheral tissue. Dopamine in the peripheral tissue causes numerous side effects as well as decreases the amount of L-dopa available to the brain. Dopadecarboxylase inhibitors that do not cross the blood–brain barrier are used to inhibit the enzyme that changes L-dopa to dopamine so that the conversion in the brain is not inhibited.

Anticholinergic drugs, such as trihexyphenidyl hydrochloride (Artane), cycrimine hydrochloride (Pagitane hydrochloride), and benztropine mesylate (Cogentin), are administered to control tremors and rigidity. Anticholinergics are used alone for mild symptoms or if levodopa is contraindicated. In other instances, they may be administered in conjunction with levodopa.

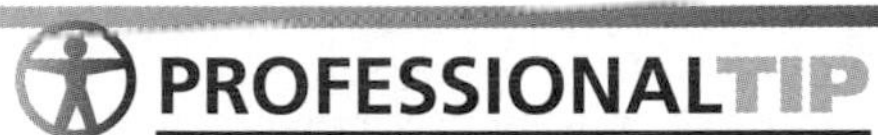

Pallidotomy

Pallidotomy, an operation of the 1950s for PD, is being used again. Improved surgical equipment and clients who no longer benefit from medications are causing a resurgence in the use of pallidotomy.

Using MRI and stereotactic equipment, the physician can pinpoint the area of the brain that is causing the unwanted symptoms. A probe is then inserted into the brain through a small hole in the client's head. A small lesion is made deep in the brain to interrupt the electrical pathways that cause the rigidity and tremors. The surgery relieves symptoms but does not cure PD. Furthermore, associated risks such as paralysis and bleeding must be considered (PDF, 2002).

COMMUNITY/HOME HEALTH CARE

Adaptations for the Client with Parkinson's Disease

- Arrange for bathroom facilities and bedroom on first floor.
- Remove crepe- or rubber-soled shoes from the client because they may drag on the floor, especially on carpeting.
- Remove throw rugs or other obstacles over which the client may trip.
- Install handrails at steps, hallways, and bathroom.
- Have no highly waxed floors.
- Provide assistance to client as needed.

CLIENTTEACHING

Parkinson's Disease

Advise caregivers to:

- Encourage the client to be as independent as possible.
- Protect the client from injury and unnecessary stress and fatigue.

Advise the client to:

- Use adaptive devices (e.g., cane, walker, feeding utensils).
- Take medications at scheduled times to maintain level in the body.
- Avoid taking multivitamins, foods high in vitamin B_6, and high-protein foods when taking levodopa.
- Prevent constipation by drinking plenty of water and, possibly, using a stool softener.
- Have intraocular pressure measured frequently if client has glaucoma.

Amantadine hydrochloride (Symmetrel), an antiviral agent, is effective in treating parkinsonian symptoms. The mechanism by which the drug works is not known, but the theory is that it either releases dopamine storage areas or delays the reuptake of dopamine.

Ethopropazine hydrochloride (Parsidol), a phenothiazine derivative, is used in combination with other anti-Parkinson drugs to alleviate symptoms. Dopamine agonist-ergot derivatives, such as pergolide mesylate (Permax), directly stimulate the dopamine receptors to improve the use of available dopamine. The monoamine oxidase inhibitor (MAOI), selegiline hydrochloride (Eldepryl), inhibits dopamine breakdown. The tricyclic antidepressants, amitriptyline hydrochloride (Elavil) and imipramine hydrochloride (Tofranil), alleviate depression as well as other symptoms.

Diet

Puréed foods or tube feedings are required because of dysphagia. Maintenance of weight may require high- or low-calorie diets. In the early stages of PD, a diet high in antioxidants may alleviate some symptoms. Free-radicals are attracted to cells that produce dopamine. Antioxidants are chemicals that destroy free radicals, thus allowing the release of dopamine. A diet that discourages the formation of free radicals is high in complex carbohydrates (such as those found in whole-grain breads and lentils), low in fat, and high in vitamins A and E. See Box 10-2 for foods high in antioxidants. Large doses of supplemental vitamins A and E are also given. A high-fiber diet helps prevent constipation.

SAFETY

Mealtime

The client with PD must be monitored for choking while eating because of dysphagia.

BOX 10-2 FOOD HIGH IN ANTIOXIDANTS

Dark-colored fruits and vegetables:
Leafy green vegetables
Broccoli
Tomatoes
Carrots
Garlic
Red kidney beans
Pinto beans
Blueberries
Cranberries
Strawberries
Plums
Apples

Teas:
Green tea
Black tea

Activity

Ambulation with assistance is necessary to maintain joint mobility and prevent injury. Ambulate at the client's pace because the bradykinesia becomes worse when the client attempts to hurry.

Other Therapies

Physical therapy is directed toward maintaining joint mobility, posture, and gait. Occupational therapy focuses on maintaining optimal functioning in achieving ADL. Speech therapy is used to promote communication and maintain swallowing function. Psychotherapy addresses the implications of living with a chronic disease, depression, and the possible psychiatric side effects of the medication regimen.

Nursing Management

Encourage independence. Fatigue may cause more dependence. Assist to establish a regular bowel routine by encouraging the client to drink at least 2,000 mL of liquids daily and eat high-fiber foods. Provide an elevated toilet seat. Assist client and family to express feelings and frustrations.

NURSING PROCESS

Assessment

Subjective Data

Nursing assessment focuses on functional ability and activities. It includes eliciting client statements about symptom control and emotional status. Ascertain bowel and bladder elimination patterns.

Objective Data

Objective assessment involves evaluation of tremors, muscular rigidity, movement, posture, and gait for degree of impairment. Assessment of swallowing ability is necessary to maintain adequate nutrition and prevent aspiration. Evaluate mental/emotional status for signs and symptoms of depression or dementia.

Assess skin for diaphoresis, or excessive oil production; skin integrity; and signs of injury from falls. Obtain supine, sitting, and standing blood pressures to assess for orthostatic hypotension.

Nursing diagnoses for a client with Parkinson's disease include the following:

NURSING DIAGNOSES	PLANNING/OUTCOMES	NURSING INTERVENTIONS
Impaired Physical Mobility related to muscle rigidity, gait disturbance, and bradykinesia	The client will maintain optimal mobility.	Assess degree of muscle involvement by testing ROM, muscular rigidity, tremors, and gait. Perform passive and active ROM exercises to maintain function. Administer medications within the time window that provides a constant therapeutic level for symptom control. Ambulate, as client is able to tolerate. Frequently turn client when in bed.
Bathing/Hygiene and Dressing/Grooming Self-care Deficit related to immobility, tremors, and bradykinesia	The client will maintain optimal independence in self-care.	Assess client's ability to perform self-care. Encourage client to perform as much self-care as possible. Consult with occupational therapy for methods to increase the ability to perform self-care. Assist with daily care that the client is unable to perform alone.
Impaired Swallowing related to neuromuscular Impairment	The client will swallow with minimal choking and coughing and no aspiration.	Position client sitting upright when eating with client's head slightly forward and never extended to facilitate swallowing. Encourage client to take small bites. Provide small bites of food or pureed foods to prevent client from choking. Have suction equipment available during meals.

Evaluation: Evaluate each outcome to determine how it has been met by the client.

MULTIPLE SCLEROSIS

Multiple sclerosis (MS) is a chronic, progressive, degenerative disease of the CNS characterized by a loss of myelin in the brain, spinal cord, or both and by the occurrence of **sclerotic** (hardened) patches (Figure 10-20). The disease interferes with the conduction of impulses. The neurological deficit that occurs depends on which nerve cells are affected. The cause of MS is unclear, but research suggests that it is an abnormal response to the body's immune system. The disease is more prevalent among people of Northern European ancestry (NMSS, 2003). Diagnosis is usually made between the ages of 20 and 50 years. Women are affected two to three times more often than are men (NMSS, 2003).

The white matter of the brain and spinal cord consists of axons covered by a white, lipid substance called myelin. This myelin sheath is an insulator that is involved in the conduction of impulses.

As sclerotic tissue replaces the myelin, neurological function returns. Nerve fibers begin to degenerate as periods of exacerbation become more frequent. Degeneration of the nerve fibers leads to permanent neurological deficits.

Signs and symptoms of MS vary according to the areas of demyelination. The client may have one symptom or a combination of symptoms. Periods of exacerbation and remission also make diagnosis difficult. Symptoms may vary from hour-to-hour or day-to-day. Medical diagnosis is generally based on history and on elimination of other possible diagnoses. Magnetic resonance imaging and CT scan can be used to identify lesions of sclerotic tissue as the disease progresses. Cerebrospinal fluid reveals increased white blood cells, protein, and immunoglobulin (IgG), a diagnostic indicator.

Client symptoms may be sensory, motor, or other disturbances. Sensory symptoms include visual disturbances, numbness, paresthesia (burning, prickling, tingling), pain, and decreased sense of temperature. Motor symptoms include decreased muscle strength, spasticity, paralysis, or bowel and bladder incontinence or retention.

Ataxia (loss of balance or coordination), **nystagmus** (constant, involuntary eye movements in any direction), speech disturbances, tremors, and **vertigo** (dizziness) occur. Other possible symptoms are sexual dysfunction and mood changes ranging from depression to euphoria. Profound fatigue is common.

Exacerbations are frequently precipitated by periods of emotional or physical stress, such as infections, pregnancy, trauma, or fatigue. Hot baths or strenuous exercise may aggravate motor symptoms. Periods of exacerbation last hours to months. Commonly, the periods of exacerbation become more frequent as the disease progresses. Complications such as urinary tract infection, pneumonia, pressure ulcers, contractures, and depression frequently occur. As the disease progresses and permanent neurological deficits occur, the client becomes bedridden, has difficulty speaking and handling oral secretions, and/or develops emotional and intellectual disturbances.

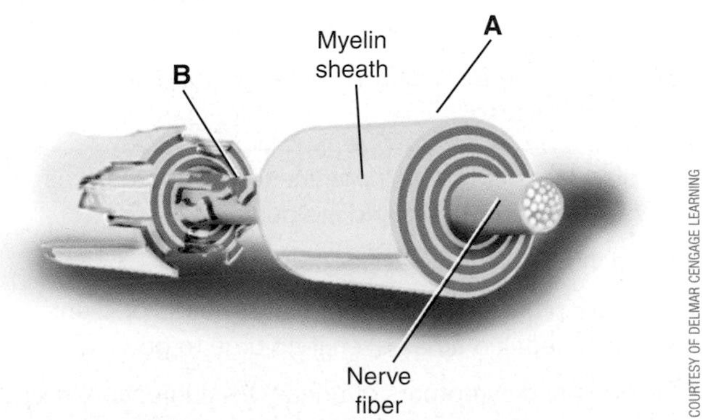

FIGURE 10-20 ***A*, Normal Nerve Fiber and Myelin Sheath; *B*, Multiple Sclerosis Destruction of Myelin Sheath**

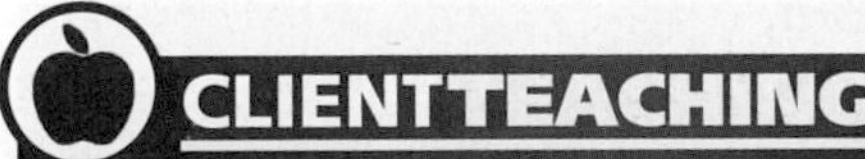

CLIENT TEACHING

Temperature Sensation

Because the client with MS has a decreased sense of temperature, advise to:

- Be careful when cooking or otherwise around the kitchen stove.
- Use a bath thermometer to test bath or shower water so as to prevent burning.
- Use only the low setting on a heating pad.

MEDICAL–SURGICAL MANAGEMENT

There is no cure or specific treatment for MS. Treatment goals are to limit exacerbations, prevent complications, and maintain functional level.

Pharmacological

The treatment of choice for relapsing–remitting MS is interferon beta (Avonex, Betaseron). For 2 or 3 months, clients usually experience flu-like symptoms after each injection. For clients who cannot take either of these two drugs, glatiramer acetate (Copaxone) is an option. The steroids adrenocorticotropic hormone (ACTH) or prednisone (Delasone) are used to decrease periods of exacerbation. Muscle relaxants such as dantrolene sodium (Dantrium) or baclofen (Lioresal) are used for muscle spasticity.

The immunosuppressive agents azathioprine (Imuran), cyclophosphamide (Cytoxan), or cyclosporine (Sandimmune) are administered to decrease immune response. Propantheline bromide (ProBanthine) is often used for urinary frequency and urgency. Bethanechol chloride (Urecholine) may be helpful for the client with a neurogenic bladder. Trimethoprim sulfamethoxazole (Bactrim or Septra) or nitrofurantoin macrocrystals (Macrodantin) is given prophylactically when urinary tract infections are a problem.

CRITICAL THINKING

Multiple Sclerosis

What are the most important things to teach a client with multiple sclerosis?

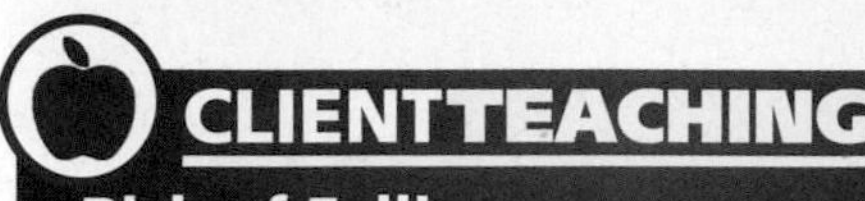

COMMUNITY/HOME HEALTH CARE

Adaptive Devices

To assist the client with MS in self-care:

- Purchase a raised toilet seat.
- Use a long-handled comb and shoe horn.
- Modify clothing so that the client can dress self.

CLIENTTEACHING

Risk of Falling

Advise the client with MS to:

- Use assistive devices such as a walker or cane.
- Wear high-topped (above the ankles) shoes, with laces.
- Watch feet when walking to know where they are stepping.

Diet

A well-balanced diet complete with roughage is necessary to promote bowel elimination. Plenty of fluids are also necessary. If the client is obese, a dietitian should be consulted for meal planning to help the client lose weight while maintaining adequate nutrition.

Activity

The goal of maintaining the highest possible functional level must be individualized to each client. Daily exercise is necessary for clients with limited motor involvement. Physical therapy may be necessary to prevent contractures, maintain muscle strength, or prevent loss of function from spasticity, or for gait training. Passive/active ROM exercises should be done several times per day. Occupational therapy may be used to maintain or attain self-care. Daily skills of cooking, doing laundry, or maintaining a job may also be encouraged.

Nursing Management

Emphasize avoiding stress, infections, and fatigue. Encourage independence and individualized ways of performing daily activities. Stress the importance of a well-balanced diet, high in fiber to prevent constipation. Encourage adequate fluid intake and regular urination.

NURSING PROCESS

Assessment

Subjective Data

Subjective assessment includes eliciting client statements of symptoms and an historical accounting of exacerbations and remissions. Subjective data should include incidence of visual disturbances, hazy vision, loss of central vision, or diplopia (double vision). Note symptoms of weakness, numbness, fatigue, bowel or bladder problems, sexual dysfunction, emotional instability, vertigo, changes in gait, urinary incontinence or retention, constipation, or difficulty swallowing. Pain is not common.

Objective Data

Objective assessment includes observation of gait for spastic or ataxic gait and a complete neurological examination.

Nursing diagnoses for a client with MS include the following:

NURSING DIAGNOSES	PLANNING/OUTCOMES	NURSING INTERVENTIONS
*Impaired **P**hysical Mobility* related to muscle weakness, ataxia, spasticity, or perceptual impairment	The client will maintain optimal mobility within physical limitations.	Assess motor status every 4 to 24 hours. Provide active and passive ROM every 8 hours. Ambulate client four times daily with use of assistive devices as necessary. Turn bedridden clients every 2 hours. Use pillows, splints, high-topped (above the ankles) shoes with laces to maintain proper body alignment. Encourage client to perform daily activities as able given the limitations of the disease.
*Impaired **U**rinary Elimination* related to changes in innervation of the bladder	The client will have adequate bladder elimination with minimal postvoid residual, urinary tract infections, and episodes of incontinence.	Assess for bladder retention or incontinence. Catheterize as necessary for retention or postvoid residual. Maintain fluid intake of 1,000 cc per day. Develop bladder program to meet individual needs of client. Toilet client at scheduled times even if no urge to go. Assess for signs and symptoms of urinary tract infection, such as elevated temperature and burning on urination.

Nursing diagnoses for a client with MS include the following: (Continued)

NURSING DIAGNOSES	PLANNING/OUTCOMES	NURSING INTERVENTIONS
Situational Low ***S****elf-esteem* related to neuromuscular and perceptual impairment	The client will verbalize positive statements of self-esteem.	Assess client's concept of self in relation to changes brought about by the disease process. Teach client about the disease process. Allow client to verbalize feelings. Assist client in methods of adapting to change. Collaborate with other health care providers, such as mental health counselors and physicians. Refer client to local support groups (see Resources).
S*exual Dysfunction* related to changes in sensation, genitalia, and musculature, and psychological response to diagnosis	The client will seek counseling concerning sexual dysfunction.	Allow client to verbalize concerns. Suggest adaptations (planning time for sexual contact so as to conserve energy; alternatives to sexual intercourse, such as touching or holding). Refer client to appropriate health care providers.

Evaluation: Evaluate each outcome to determine how it has been met by the client.

SAMPLE NURSING CARE PLAN

The Client with MS

D.B., a 37-year-old wife and the mother of two children, ages 3 years and 5 years, was diagnosed with MS 2 days ago. She presents with decreased sensation (paresthesia) in the lower extremities and muscle weakness of the right lower extremity. She has also experienced episodes of loss of central vision. Fatigue has affected her ability to care for her children and perform household tasks. She states, "I do not know what is going to happen to me." She is crying and states, "I do not know about MS or how I am going to take care of my children," and "I cannot get my housework done, and my children need more from me than I can give right now."

Her employer is concerned about her ability to perform her teaching responsibilities, but because he values her excellence as a teacher, he is willing to give her a few weeks off. She has bruises on her thigh, face, and arm from a fall that she experienced several days ago. The client presents in an outpatient clinic for follow-up care.

NURSING DIAGNOSIS 1 *Deficient* ***K****nowledge* related to disease process and lifestyle changes as evidenced by client statements, "I do not know what is going to happen to me, I do not know about multiple sclerosis or how I am going to take care of my children."

Nursing Outcomes Classification (NOC)
Knowledge: Disease Process

Nursing Interventions Classification (NIC)
Teaching: Disease Process

PLANNING/OUTCOMES	NURSING INTERVENTIONS	RATIONALE
D.B. will verbalize knowledge of the disease process, pathophysiology,	Assess D.B.'s knowledge of diagnosis, treatment regimen, and lifestyle changes. Ask specific questions.	Provides a frame of reference for D.B., helping her to relate new information and integrate it into her behavior.

(*Continues*)

SAMPLE NURSING CARE PLAN (Continued)

PLANNING/OUTCOMES	NURSING INTERVENTIONS	RATIONALE
prognosis, and treatment, including the need to reduce stressors in her life, eat a balanced diet, drink adequate fluids, and get adequate rest.	Begin teaching information about the pathophysiology and signs and symptoms of MS.	Assists understanding about the disease.
	Discuss needed lifestyle changes, such as planning rest periods, avoiding stressors, eating a balanced diet, and drinking plenty of fluids.	Helps understanding of necessary changes in life.
	Emphasize the importance of keeping a diary of symptoms, activities, and feelings to identify stressors that exacerbate symptoms.	Helps identify activities that exacerbate the symptoms.
	Provide information about the Multiple Sclerosis Society and offer available pamphlets.	Provides resources to strengthen D.B.'s knowledge base.
	Provide the name and telephone number of a contact from the local MS support group or of another client who is willing to share.	Provides a great deal of emotional support as well as practical solutions to problems.

EVALUATION

D.B. verbalizes accurate information regarding the disease process, prognosis, and treatment. She states that by reducing stressors, maintaining a balanced diet, taking in adequate fluids, and obtaining plenty of rest, she can prevent exacerbations of MS.

NURSING DIAGNOSIS 2 *Impaired **H**ome Maintenance* related to fatigue, neuromuscular impairment, and difficulty in performing child care and household tasks as evidenced by client statements, "I cannot keep my housework done, my children need more from me than I can give right now" and by objective data including decreased sensation in lower extremities, muscle weakness, and fatigue

Nursing Outcomes Classification (NOC)
Family Functioning

Nursing Interventions Classification (NIC)
Home Maintenance Assistance

PLANNING/OUTCOMES	NURSING INTERVENTIONS	RATIONALE
By the next appointment, D.B. will identify concerns and solutions to accomplishing home maintenance management.	Allow D.B. to verbalize concerns about home maintenance management.	Gives D.B. time to plan and organize tasks and responsibilities within her ability to perform home maintenance management.
	Assist D.B. in identifying areas of concern, items that can be delegated, and possible solutions.	Can then investigate methods of solving her home maintenance problems.
	Assess the extended family's ability to assist with home maintenance management.	May uncover opportunities that she had not considered.

SAMPLE NURSING CARE PLAN (Continued)

PLANNING/OUTCOMES	NURSING INTERVENTIONS	RATIONALE
	Ask D.B. to start identifying ways to decrease workload and to set priorities for expending energy.	Helps focus on needed changes.
	Collaborate with social services to identify social agencies that can be of assistance.	Gives other possible solutions to achieving home maintenance management.
	Plan activities around rest periods.	Conserves strength and prevents fatigue.
	Identify peak energy times and plan activities with peak energy in mind.	Allows more to be accomplished.

EVALUATION

D.B. identifies that she is able to care for her children with the assistance of her husband and her mother, but that she does not have the strength to maintain the housekeeping responsibilities. Following further discussion of family commitments and availability of social supports, D.B. agrees to request weekly assistance from the women's group at her church.

NURSING DIAGNOSIS 3

Risk for Injury related to muscle weakness, decreased sensory perception (vision, tactile, kinesthetic), and fatigue as evidenced by recent falls

NOC: *Risk Control, Falls Occurrence, Safety Behavior: Home Physical Environment, Safety Behavior: Personal*
NIC: *Fall Prevention, Environmental Management: Safety, Surveillance: Risk Identification*

CLIENT GOAL

D.B. will remain free of injury.

NURSING INTERVENTIONS	SCIENTIFIC RATIONALES
1. Teach D.B. to identify risk-factors in the environment.	1. Avoids injury.
2. Teach D.B. to identify risk factors of the disease process.	2. Reduces her risk of injury.
3. Teach D.B. to avoid hot baths, hot tubs, and saunas because muscle weakness and paresthesia is exacerbated by the heat.	3. Prevents exacerbation of weakness and decreased sensation, thereby reducing her risk of injury.
4. Teach safety factors of wearing well-fitting, oxford-style shoes.	4. Decreases the risk of falling by providing support for feet.

EVALUATION

Have injuries been prevented by increasing D.B.'s awareness of the risks involved with the disease process?

AMYOTROPHIC LATERAL SCLEROSIS (LOU GEHRIG'S DISEASE)

Amyotrophic lateral sclerosis (ALS) is a progressive, fatal disease characterized by the degeneration of motor neurons in the cortex, medulla, and spinal cord. The cause of the disease is not known, but a viral immune response or genetic defect are suggested by current research. Age at onset is 40 to 70 years; men are affected two to three times more often than are women. Average time from onset to death is 3 years, but some clients with ALS have remained active 10 to 20 years after diagnosis.

The upper and lower motor neurons degenerate and deteriorate, causing atrophy of the muscles innervated by those neurons. The involved motor neurons are in the anterior horns of the spinal cord and lower brainstem. The muscles of the hands, forearms, and legs usually atrophy first. As the disease progresses, most body muscles are affected. Muscle spasticity and reduced muscle strength result when upper motor neurons are involved. Lower motor neuron involvement causes muscle flaccidity, paralysis, and muscle atrophy. Sensory and intellectual function are not affected. Respiratory function, ability to communicate, and emotional lability are affected as the disease progresses. Drooling, inability to handle oral secretions, and impaired swallowing occur.

MEDICAL–SURGICAL MANAGEMENT

There is no known cure for ALS. The focus of medical management is to treat the symptoms and to promote independence for as long as possible.

Pharmacological

Muscle relaxants including diazepam (Valium), baclofen (Lioresal), and dantrolene sodium (Dantrium) are used to reduce spasticity. Quinidine is prescribed for muscle cramping. Increased salivation is treated with trihexyphenidyl hydrochloride (Artane), clonidine hydrochloride (Catapres), or amitriptyline hydrochloride (Elavil).

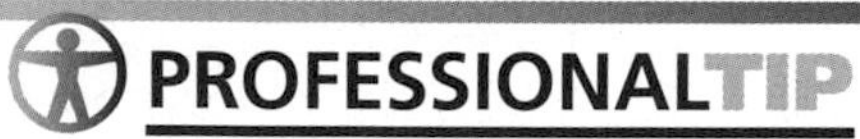

Advance Directives

Before the client with ALS becomes unable to communicate, suggest some advantages of drawing up a living will or giving someone power of attorney for health care.

Riluzole (Rilutek) is the only drug currently approved for use in ALS treatment. Riluzole is believed to reduce damage to motor neurons by decreasing the release of glutamate. Clinical trials with ALS clients showed that riluzole prolongs survival by several months, mainly in those with difficulty swallowing. The drug also extends the time before a client needs ventilation support. Riluzole does not reverse the damage already done to motor neurons, and clients taking the drug must be monitored for liver damage and other possible side effects.

Diet

A regular diet adapted to provide soft, easily chewed food is maintained as long as the client can swallow. Tube feeding is required to prevent aspiration as chewing and swallowing difficulties arise.

Activity

Ambulation and other activities are encouraged as long as possible.

Other Therapies

Physical and occupational therapy are used to maintain ROM and independence as much as possible. Speech therapy promotes maintenance of communication skills. Mental health counseling assists individual and family coping with the fatal disease.

NURSING MANAGEMENT

Encourage independence as long as possible. Assist with personal hygiene and getting in and out of bed. Provide good skin care, turn client often, keep the bed dry, and use pressure-relieving devices. Position client upright for meals and offer soft, solid foods. When gastrostomy feedings are needed, teach client or family how to administer them.

NURSING PROCESS

ASSESSMENT

Subjective Data

Subjective data gathered include the client's and family's emotional status and knowledge status. The client may also indicate chewing or swallowing difficulties as well as dyspnea and fatigue.

Objective Data

Objective assessment includes evaluation of muscle weakness, muscle atrophy, spasticity of upper extremities, flaccid paralysis, difficulty chewing and swallowing, and respiratory status.

Nursing diagnoses for a client with ALS include the following:

NURSING DIAGNOSES	PLANNING/OUTCOMES	NURSING INTERVENTIONS
Impaired Physical Mobility related to muscle atrophy, weakness, and spasticity	The client will maintain the highest possible functional ability within limitations of the disease.	Provide active and passive ROM at least twice daily. Use assistive devices to prevent contractures, for ambulation, and for muscle strengthening.

Nursing diagnoses for a client with ALS include the following: (Continued)

NURSING DIAGNOSES	PLANNING/OUTCOMES	NURSING INTERVENTIONS
		Assess breath sounds for presence of congestion; skin for pressure areas; and legs for thrombophlebitis. Turn every 2 hours.
Impaired Verbal ***C****ommunication* related to weakness of muscles used for speech	The client will communicate verbally or through an alternate communication method as speech muscles deteriorate.	Prolong verbal communication with speech therapy interventions consisting of voice projection and speech devices. Develop alternate methods of communicating prior to the loss of verbal skills, e.g., eye-blinking for "yes" and "no"; communication boards, if any arm movement remains; and computer programs can be used.
Ineffective ***B****reathing Pattern* related to weakness of respiratory muscles and to fatigue	The client will maintain an adequate PaO_2 level.	Assess breathing patterns frequently and observe for aspiration and the loss of the swallow reflex. Assess breath sounds every 4 to 8 hours, depending on the progress of the disease. Provide good pulmonary hygiene to prevent aspiration and pneumonia by liquefying secretions and suctioning. Turn from side to side to allow oral secretions to drain from mouth; suction oral pharynx, as necessary. Provide ventilation support, as ordered.
P*owerlessness* related to loss of control over life; physical dependence; and presence of a fatal disease	The client will inform significant others of wishes while still able to communicate, so as to maintain some control over decisions.	Explore client and family emotional status and coping abilities. Allow client to verbalize feelings while still able to communicate and make decisions in daily care. Promote discussion of client's wishes with family, health care team, and legal representative while client is still able to speak. Provide client education about the disease process, support groups, and counseling to provide support.

Evaluation: Evaluate each outcome to determine how it has been met by the client.

ALZHEIMER'S DISEASE

Alzheimer's disease (AD) is a progressive, degenerative neurological disease wherein brain cells are destroyed. The cerebral cortex atrophies, and neuron loss and changes within the brain cells occur. The neurons of the frontal and medial temporal lobes are affected, with resultant biochemical and structural changes. Characteristic physiologic changes are neurofibrillary tangles and amyloid plaques (deposits of protein), which interfere with the cells' ability to transmit impulses. These changes are found in the association areas and scattered throughout the cortex. The hippocampus, that part of the limbic system responsible for learning, memory, and emotions, is affected. The cells most affected are neurons that use acetylcholine as the neurotransmitter. The size of the brain and the

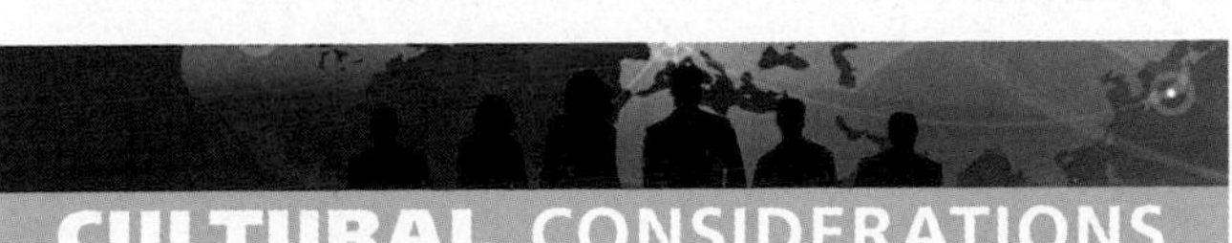

CULTURAL CONSIDERATIONS

African Americans show a greater incidence rate of AD than the Caucasian population. Latinos appear to develop the symptoms almost 7 years earlier on average than non-Latino Americans (Alzheimer's Association, 2008).

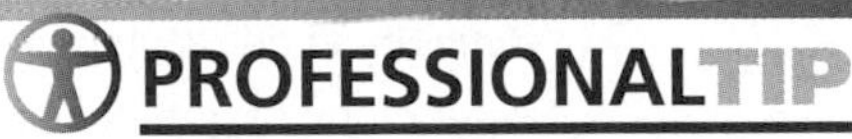

PROFESSIONAL TIP

Sniff Test to Diagnose AD

A new way to diagnose AD, PD, and other neurodegenerative disorders may be through evaluating the client's sense of smell. Measuring how deeply clients inhale a strong or unpleasant odor may be an early warning of brain dysfunction. A device known as a Sniff Magnitude test may be able to identify one of the earliest symptoms of some neurodegenerative diseases, the loss of the sense of smell. Clients with a normal sense of smell take only a small inhalation before detecting strong or unpleasant odors, while those with a damaged sense of smell will inhalation longer and deeper. The test is portable and can be administered to clients with decreased intellectual and language abilities (Hally, 2007; Frank, Gesteland, Bailie, Rybalsky, Seiden, & Dulay, 2006).

amount of acetylcholine both decrease. An increased amount of aluminum is found in the brain tissue on autopsy (Hickey, 2008; Smeltzer, Bare, Hinkle, & Cheever, 2008).

The cause of AD is unknown. Identified risk factors are advanced age, female gender, head injury, a history of thyroid disorders, and chromosomal abnormalities. More than five million Americans have AD, a 10% increase from the last official tally in 2002, and a number expected to more than triple by 2050 as the elderly population increases (Alzheimer's Association, 2008).

Diagnosis is difficult because of the variety in clinical manifestations and the lack of a test specific to AD. Diagnosis is thus based on the clinical picture and the exclusion of other conditions that cause similar clinical patterns, such as overmedication, metabolic disorders, depression, thyroid imbalance, or brain tumors. Neuropsychological tests measuring memory, problem solving, attention, counting, and language assist physicians in diagnosing AD (Alzheimer's Disease Education and Referral Center, 2002). A CT scan may show evidence of brain atrophy, and a PET scan will show changes in the metabolism of the cerebral cortex.

The stages of AD are scaled from early to late. Different authors identify from three to six stages of the disease. The time frame for each stage varies from person to person. Table 10-6 lists clinical manifestations of early, middle, and late stages of AD.

In late stages of the disease, an EEG may indicate general slowing of brain waves. Definitive diagnosis is determined on autopsy with a brain biopsy. Although generally a disease of older people, AD occurs in people ages 40 to 50.

The personal freedom of the family caring for a member who has AD becomes more limited as the disease progresses. Many clients with advanced AD cannot be left alone. Respite care is important for the physical and mental health of the caregiver. With respite care, someone else (e.g., another family member, a friend, or a hired professional licensed

TABLE 10-6 Stages of Alzheimer's Disease

STAGE	CLINICAL MANIFESTATIONS
Stage 1: Early	Forgetfulness, often subtle and masked by client Indecisiveness Increasing self-centeredness; decreasing interest in others, environment, social activities Difficulty in learning new information Slowed reaction time Beginnings of compromised performance at home and at work
Stage 2: Middle	Progressing forgetfulness, inability to remember names of family members or close friends Tendency to lose things Confusion Fearfulness Easily induced frustration and irritability; sometimes, angry outbursts Repetitive storytelling Beginnings of communication problems (inability to remember words, apparent aphasia) Inability to follow simple directions Difficulty in calculating numbers Beginnings of getting lost in familiar places Evasive or anxious interactions with others Physical activity (pacing, wandering) Changes in sleep–rest cycle (with frequent activity at night) Changes in eating patterns (possible constant hunger or none at all) Neglect of ADL and personal hygiene, changes in bowel and bladder continence, and dressing difficulties Inability to maintain safety without supervision Losses of social behaviors Paranoia
Stage 3: Late	Inability to communicate Inability to eat Incontinence (urine and feces) Inability to recognize family or friends Confinement to bed Total dependence relative to care

COMMUNITY/HOME HEALTH CARE

Safe Environment for the Client with AD

- Keep furniture in the same place.
- Orient client to surroundings and reorient as necessary.
- Keep floors free of clutter.
- Provide adequate lighting.
- Monitor temperature of hot water and food.
- Maintain monitoring system to prevent outside wandering.
- Prevent access to sharp items such as knives and razors; hot items such as coffee pot and heaters; poisonous solutions such as cleaning supplies, paints, medications, and insecticides; and hazardous items such as power tools, guns, and electric fans.

practical/vocational nurse or registered nurse) comes in to care for the client with Alzheimer's while the primary caregiver gets away for a time. Respite care should be provided on a routine basis, such as every 2 or 3 weeks or as often as is feasible.

MEDICAL–SURGICAL MANAGEMENT

There is no curative treatment for AD. Management of the client is geared toward controlling undesirable symptoms and behaviors.

Pharmacological

No drug can stop the progression of AD. Cholinesterase inhibitors (galantamine hydrobromide [Razadyne], rivastigmine tartrate [Exelon], and donepezil hydrocholoride [Aricept]) slow the progression of the disease and enhance cognition in early to middle stage AD. N-methyl-D-asparate (NMDA) Receptor Antagonist, memantine hydrocholoride (Namenda), delays progression of symptoms in moderate-to-severe AD. Other medications treat symptoms such as anxiety, depression, and insomnia.

CRITICAL THINKING

Parkinson's and Alzheimer's

What are the similarities between Parkinson's disease and AD?
What distinguishes Parkinson's disease from AD?

Diet

A high-fiber diet is used to prevent constipation. A high-calorie diet is needed for hyperactive clients. Frequent feedings of high nutritive value are preferable to three meals a day.

NURSING MANAGEMENT

Maintain a safe, structured environment and a consistent daily schedule for the client. Develop memory aids and cues to help the client remember. Support family in adjusting to the client's altered cognitive ability.

NURSING PROCESS

ASSESSMENT

Subjective Data

Data about sleeping and eating habits is collected. Each client is assessed for individual signs and symptoms. The client is an expert at hiding these deficits in the early stages of the disease. A family interview is helpful in ascertaining health and personal history.

Objective Data

An objective neurological examination with particular attention to memory loss and gradual loss of thought processes and impaired judgment is important. Eating patterns, bowel and bladder control, aggressiveness, depression, ambulation, agitation, restlessness, sleep patterns, vision, and hearing are assessed. The client's ability to provide self-care, manage finances, drive, prepare meals, use the telephone, perform housekeeping, communicate needs, and perceive the environment also are assessed. Attention is directed to assessing the support system, the family caregiver, support groups, and availability of respite care for the caregiver. The care of the caregiver is often the focus of nursing care of the AD client.

Nursing diagnoses for the client with Alzheimer's include the following:

NURSING DIAGNOSES	PLANNING/OUTCOMES	NURSING INTERVENTIONS
Risk for Injury related to inability to perceive danger in the environment, confusion, impaired judgment, and weakness	The client will not experience injury.	Assess client's ability to perceive environmental hazards. Teach family to provide a safe home environment.
		Maintain a safe environment: eliminate clutter, position furniture/equipment in same place, monitor temperature of hot water and food, maintain monitoring system to prevent wandering into adverse climate or into traffic, provide adequate lighting, orient client and family to surroundings and reorient as necessary.
		Ensure that the client wears well-fitting, tied shoes to reduce risk of falls.

(Continues)

Nursing diagnoses for the client with Alzheimer's include the following: (Continued)

NURSING DIAGNOSES	PLANNING/OUTCOMES	NURSING INTERVENTIONS
*Disturbed **T**hought Processes* related to neuron degeneration, sleep deprivation	The client will maintain optimal cognitive ability.	Assess for cognitive, memory, and communication deficits. Develop memory aids and cues to help client remember. Maintain a consistent environment and daily schedule. Approach client in a quiet, nonthreatening manner. Do not confront client with reality if it will only upset and agitate him. For example, do not tell a 90-year-old client who wants his mother that she is dead. Attend to nonverbal cues for unmet needs (e.g., pacing, grimacing, crying, agitation). The client may be hungry, have a full bladder, or be unable to ask to be repositioned. Obtain a photo of client that can be recognized by the client. A current photo of client may appear as a stranger to the client, but a photo of the client at age 20 or 30 may be remembered. Give simple, single instructions.
*Disturbed **S**leep Pattern* related to disorientation or irritability	The client will sleep 4 to 5 hours each night.	Advise the client to avoid caffeine. Maintain a quiet environment. Provide comfort measures. Provide a night light. Increase daytime activities to tolerance, and use exercise to tire client.

Evaluation: Evaluate each outcome to determine how it has been met by the client.

CRITICAL THINKING

Alzheimer's Disease

V. A. is a 73-year-old male client diagnosed 5 years ago with AD. He has been married for 52 years and owns a hardware store now managed by his son. Spanish is his native language, but he is fluent in English. At this time he is having significant word-finding difficulties and is unable to name common objects in both English and Spanish. He requires his wife's assistance to eat, bathe, toilet, dress, and take medications. He is able to walk independently. Until 2 weeks ago, his wife drove him to the hardware store daily, where he would interact with customers and restock nails, screws, and other small items. The last day at the store, though, he wandered out when his son was occupied with customers and became lost. He was found by the police 2 miles from the store. His son now wants V.A. placed in a nursing home, but his wife feels that he should remain at home until he "no longer knows who I am."

1. Identify V.A.'s stage of Alzheimer's disease and explain the rationale.
2. Identify safety issues and appropriate nursing interventions.
3. How can the nurse help the family reach consensus on appropriate placement and care for V.A.?

GUILLAIN-BARRÉ SYNDROME

Guillain-Barré syndrome (GBS) is an acute inflammatory process involving the motor and sensory neurons of the peripheral nervous system. The cause of Guillain-Barré syndrome is not known, but most cases are preceded by a nonspecific infection. There may be an autoimmune or viral basis for this syndrome. Both spinal and cranial motor nerves are involved. The demyelination process begins in distal nerves and ascends symmetrically. Remyelination occurs from proximal to distal (Hickey, 2008).

Clinical manifestations occur in differing patterns but include motor weakness and areflexia, or absence of reflexes. Characteristically, motor weakness begins in the legs and progresses up the body. Respiratory failure results from loss of respiratory muscle function. Cranial nerve involvement results in facial muscle deficits, difficulty in swallowing, and autonomic dysfunctions. Autonomic functions possibly affected are cardiac rhythm, blood pressure regulation, gastrointestinal mobility, and urine elimination.

Sensory involvement causes paresthesia and pain in the hands and feet. The pain progresses up the body and may interfere with sleep.

The three stages of Guillain-Barré syndrome are acute onset, lasting 1 to 3 weeks, the plateau period, lasting several days to 2 weeks, and the recovery phase, which involves remyelination and may last up to 2 years.

Diagnosis is based on the clinical picture of a recent viral infection and motor and possibly sensory deficits, along with characteristic diagnostic results. These results include both an elevated protein level in CSF without elevation of red blood cells or white blood cells and EMG showing slowed nerve conduction velocity of paralyzed muscles.

MEDICAL–SURGICAL MANAGEMENT

Medical

The goal of medical management is prevention and treatment of complications such as immobility, infection, and respiratory failure.

Plasma exchanges decrease the severity and duration of symptoms. Plasmapheresis is performed in severe cases. Complete plasma exchange removes the antibodies affecting the myelin sheath. Three to four exchanges 1 to 2 days apart are initiated within the first 2 weeks of diagnosis of Guillain-Barré. Plasmapheresis also is used late in the disease process for continued demyelination or lack of progress in remyelination. Mechanical ventilatory support may be required. Blood gas monitoring is used to assess respiratory function.

Surgical

Those who develop respiratory failure require a tracheostomy along with mechanical ventilation.

Pharmacological

Steroids, such as adrenocorticotropic hormone (ACTH) and prednisone (Detasone), and immunosuppressive agents, such as azathioprine (Imuran) or cyclophosphamide (Cytoxan), slow the demyelination process. Low doses of anticoagulants, such as heparin, prevent thrombophlebitis.

Diet

A balanced diet is necessary to prevent tissue and muscle breakdown and to promote healing. If severe paralysis is present, a gastrostomy tube is used to provide adequate nutrition.

Activity

Physical therapy maintains range of motion and muscle strength. Occupational therapy activities teach the client to maintain optional self-care within the limitation of the disease process. Pool therapy, or exercising in a swimming pool, maintains and strengthens muscles.

NURSING MANAGEMENT

Monitor vital signs, LOC, pulse oximetry, ABGs, and for ascending sensory loss, which precedes motor loss. Turn client frequently and encourage coughing and deep breathing. Provide skin care to prevent skin breakdown and position client to prevent contractures. Perform passive ROM exercises. Apply antiembolism stockings and assess Homans' sign. Provide eye and mouth care every 4 hours if there is facial paralysis. Monitor I&O and encourage adequate fluid intake. Offer prune juice and high-fiber diet to prevent constipation.

NURSING PROCESS

ASSESSMENT

Subjective Data

Subjective data include client statements about return of sensation, pain, respiratory function, and knowledge.

Objective Data

Assessment includes the status of motor and sensory functions, which are monitored continuously in the acute phase of the illness. Monitor progression of loss of function from distal to proximal with particular emphasis on respiratory status. Decreased depth and quality of respirations and diminished breath sounds may be found. Monitor status of autonomic functions by assessing blood pressure, cardiac rhythm, urinary elimination, and bowel sounds. Assessment for complications of immobility includes breath sounds, signs of thrombophlebitis, loss of ROM, skin condition, and temperature.

Nursing diagnoses for a client with Guillain-Barré syndrome include the following:

NURSING DIAGNOSES	PLANNING/OUTCOMES	NURSING INTERVENTIONS
*Ineffective **Breathing** Pattern* related to loss of respiratory muscle function	The client will be adequately ventilated.	Monitor respiratory status of client by assessing breath sounds, respiratory rate, and respiratory quality. Position client to facilitate maximal expansion of the chest wall for optimal breathing. Monitor oxygenation by assessing skin color, mental status, pulse oximeter readings, and blood gas values. Administer oxygen as ordered. Report failing respiratory status to the physician. Provide mechanical ventilation for respiratory failure.
*Impaired **Physical** Mobility* related to progressive loss of motor function	The client will avoid complications of immobility (pneumonia, thrombophlebitis, pressure areas, and loss of ROM).	Monitor status of motor and sensory functions in an ongoing fashion. Have client turn, deep breathe, and cough every 2 hours. Suction client as necessary. Perform respiratory assessment for diminished breath sounds or congestion. Monitor vital signs (blood pressure, pulse, respiration, and temperature) every 4 to 8 hours. Assess for calf tenderness, redness, or increased warmth. Monitor for positive Homans' sign, indicative of deep vein thrombosis.

(*Continues*)

Nursing diagnoses for a client with Guillain-Barré syndrome include the following: (Continued)

NURSING DIAGNOSES	PLANNING/OUTCOMES	NURSING INTERVENTIONS
		Perform ROM to lower extremities every 2 to 4 hours. Use PlexiPulse boots, which are intermittent-pumping boots that promote return blood flow from the lower extremities. Administer low doses of heparin or other anticoagulants as prescribed. Apply antiembolism stockings or alternating compression devices. Assess condition of skin for pressure areas. Massage client's back and pressure points with lotion three times a day. Use specialty mattress. Assist client to sitting position in wheelchair two to three times daily. Progress to ambulation as motor function returns. Apply high-topped shoes to keep feet in correct alignment.
*Dressing/Grooming **S**elf-care Deficit* related to decreased motor function	The client will have self-care needs met.	Encourage self-care within the limitations of the neurological deficits. Provide daily care needs that client is unable to perform. Maintain muscle strength and ROM with physical therapy. Provide ROM to all extremities three to four times daily. Initiate rehabilitation following acute phase of illness with strengthening exercises, occupational therapy, and getting client out of bed several times per day to build strength and endurance.

Evaluation: Evaluate each outcome to determine how it has been met by the client.

HEADACHE

Headache, or **cephalalgia**, the condition of pain in the head, is caused by stimulation of pain-sensitive structures in the cranium, head, or neck. Headaches are symptoms rather than a disease.

The pain-sensitive areas of the intracranial structure include the peripheral nerves, cerebral vasculature, and parts of the dura mater. The external supporting structures of the skin, muscles, and nasal passages are also sensitive to pain. The skull, brain tissue, and most of the meninges are insensitive to pain.

More than 45 million people in the United States each year have chronic, recurring headaches (National Headache Foundation, 2002). Headaches are generally classified as either primary or secondary.

PRIMARY HEADACHES

Primary headaches are not caused by an underlying medical condition. They include tension-type, migraine, and cluster headaches (AHS, 2007) (Table 10-7).

Tension-Type Headache

The most common type of headache is the tension type (ACHE, 2007). The ache is steady rather than throbbing, affects both sides of the head, and occurs frequently, sometimes daily.

Migraine Headaches

Up to 18% of women experience migraine headaches each year, compared to 6% of men (AHS, 2007). Migraine headaches are vascular and recurrent. The initial vasoconstriction causes neurological symptoms or an aura before the vasodilation that causes the headache. The aura is a visual disturbance typically consisting of brightly colored or blinking lights or a pattern moving across the field of vision. When only the aura occurs, and there is no pain in the head, the migraine is termed "silent." Migraines generally are a throbbing on one side of the head. Other symptoms include irritability, anorexia, nausea, vomiting, and photophobia. Some migraine headaches are triggered by certain foods or chemicals.

Cluster Headaches

A cluster headache develops around or behind one eye and is very severe. Generally, it awakens the person from sleep. The affected eye may tear and the nose becomes congested on the same side. These headaches occur in clusters daily for weeks or months, and then disappear for a year or more. Most cluster headaches occur in men. Alcohol often triggers attacks.

SECONDARY HEADACHES

Secondary headaches are the result of pathological conditions such as aneurysm, brain tumor, or inflamed cranial nerves.

TABLE 10-7 Primary Headache Patterns

TYPE	AURA	PAIN	TYPICAL PATTERN	DURATION
Tension	None	Steady ache	Usually begins gradually in frontal or temporal areas; affects both sides of the head; occur frequently, maybe daily	Hours
Classic Migraine	Duration of 15 to 30 minutes; sensory, usually visual (bright spots, zig-zag lines), unilateral or bilateral numbness or tingling in lips, face, or hand; difficulty thinking; confusion or drowsiness; sometimes preceded by premonition 24 hours before	Throbbing, intense; unilateral; tenderness in scalp; muscle contractions in neck and scalp followed by feelings of exhaustion	Periodic, recurrent; usually begins on awakening; begins in childhood or early adolescence; tends to be familial; nausea and vomiting typical; sensitivity to light and sound	Hours to days
Cluster	None	Intense throbbing; unilateral pain in orbitotemporal area	Causes awakening two to three times during the night; accompanied by watering eyes, nasal congestion, runny nose, facial flushing over the throbbing area; after cluster headaches for days, weeks, or months may be free of symptoms for a year or more; same side of head usually involved; usually in men	30 minutes to 2 hours

The headache is caused by compression, inflammation, or hypoxia of pain-sensitive structures.

MEDICAL–SURGICAL MANAGEMENT

Medical

Medical management is based on the underlying cause of the headache. A thorough history of headache pattern, dietary pattern, and coping pattern is essential. Underlying pathology of brain tumor, aneurysm, and infection is ruled out. If pathology is identified, secondary headache is diagnosed and, therefore, treatment is based on findings. If no cause is found, management of primary headache is based on symptoms.

Surgical

Surgical management includes repair of an aneurysm or resection of a brain tumor.

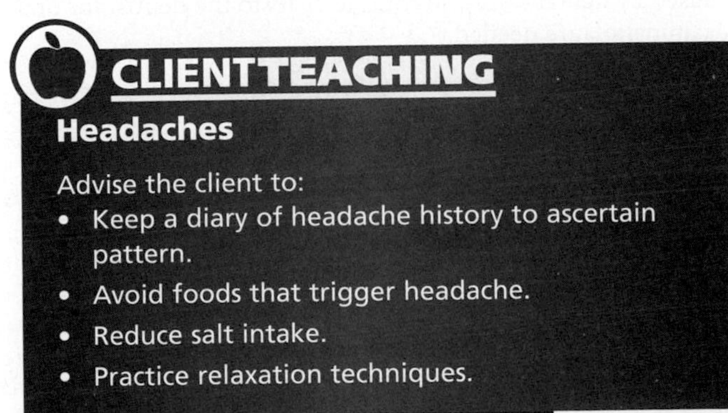

CLIENT TEACHING

Headaches

Advise the client to:

- Keep a diary of headache history to ascertain pattern.
- Avoid foods that trigger headache.
- Reduce salt intake.
- Practice relaxation techniques.

Pharmacological

Management is either abortive, to stop the headache, or prophylactic, to prevent reoccurrence or to decrease frequency of headaches. Abortive therapy for migraine headaches includes naproxen (Aleve), ibuprofen (Advil), sumatriptan (Imitrex), rizatriptan (Maxalt), zolmitriptan (Zomig), naratriptan (Amerge), almotriptan (Axert), and older drugs like cafergot, containing ergotamine and caffeine (McGuire, 2002). Promethazine hydrochloride (Phenergan) controls nausea and vomiting.

Prophylactic treatment includes the beta-blockers propranolol hydrochloride (Inderal) and methysergide maleate (Sansert), which prevent dilation of the blood vessels and interrupt the serotonin mechanism. Clonidine hydrochloride (Catapres) directly affects the ability of the blood vessels to constrict or dilate. Tricyclic antidepressants, such as amitriptyline hydrochloride (Elavil), block the uptake of serotonin.

Diet

A strict food diary is kept to identify precipitating foods. After all suspect foods are eliminated from the diet, skin testing for allergies is performed. Introduction of suspect foods is done one at a time to identify triggering foods. Alcohol, cured meats containing nitrates, aged cheeses, monosodium glutamate (MSG), citrus fruits, chocolate, and red wines are common precipitating foods.

Activity

Activities that precipitate headaches are identified and eliminated if possible. Stressful situations are frequently precipitating agents. Biofeedback, relaxation techniques, stress reduction, and development of coping mechanisms are useful in reducing the occurrence of headaches caused by stress and tension.

Nursing Management

Nursing interventions focus on relieving pain and assisting the client in managing the pain. Identifying methods of decreasing pain, such as effective use of medications and managing the environment to minimize stimulation from light, noise, and activity, are also nursing priorities.

Assist the client to develop a plan for accomplishing daily activities when incapacitated by a headache. Teach the client to keep a diary of headache history to determine patterns in headache development. Assist the client in changing lifestyle to decrease the incidence of headaches by minimizing stress, avoiding certain foods, reducing salt intake during premenstrual time frame, and using relaxation techniques.

TRIGEMINAL NEURALGIA (TIC DOULOUREUX)

Trigeminal neuralgia is a condition of cranial nerve V and is characterized by abrupt paroxysms of pain and facial muscle contractions. **Neuralgia** is nerve pain. The pain follows one of the three branches of the trigeminal nerve: the ophthalmic, maxillary, or mandibular. The last two branches are most commonly affected (Figure 10-21).

The etiology of trigeminal neuralgia is not known, but injury, dental caries, dental work, and anatomic position of the nerves have been identified as possible causes. Pain begins when trigger points are stimulated, causing periods of intense pain and facial twitching lasting from seconds to minutes. These periods may last several weeks to months. Periods of remission interspersed with exacerbations occur with increasing frequency with advancing age (Hickey, 2008).

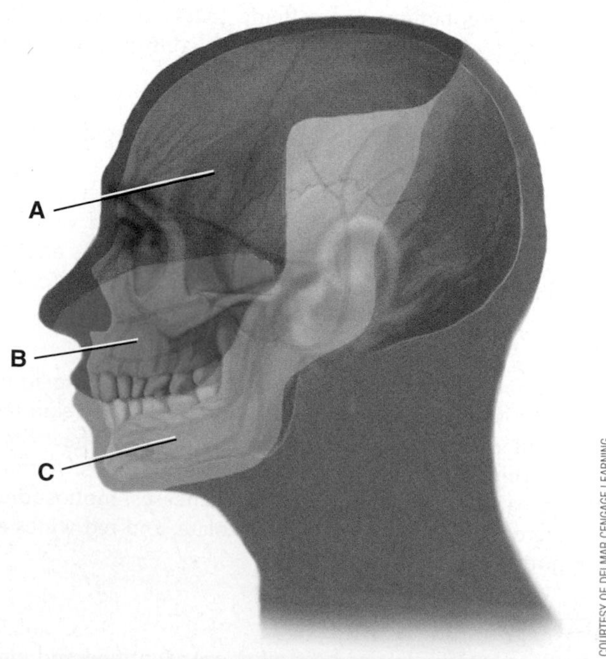

FIGURE 10-21 Areas of Face Innervated by the Trigeminal Nerve (CN-1); *A*, Ophthalmic; *B*, Maxillary; *C*, Mandibular

CLIENT TEACHING

Dental Work on the Client with Trigeminal Neuralgia

The client with trigeminal neuralgia should:

- Plan to have dental work done during a period of remission.
- Inform the dentist of the condition.
- Maintain good dental hygiene, especially during remission.

Medical–Surgical Management

Drug therapy, nerve blocks, and surgery are treatment modalities for trigeminal neuralgia.

Surgical

Surgical approaches to relieve pain include percutaneous electrocoagulation with radio frequency. This procedure affects the pain-sensory fibers but causes little damage to the touch, proprioception, and motor fibers. Longer-term relief or permanent relief may be obtained.

Pharmacological

Phenytoin (Dilantin) and carbamazepine (Tegretol) are used to shorten the length of the paroxysmal pain. Nerve blocks using alcohol and phenol injections into the nerve provide temporary relief for 8 to 16 months.

Nursing Management

Goals of nursing interventions are relief of pain, prevention of injury, prevention of self-care deficits, and promotion of social interaction. The client with trigeminal neuralgia frequently experiences such severe pain that grooming, talking, and eating are avoided. It is especially important to provide good oral hygiene if the client is on phenytoin (Dilantin) because the medication causes hyperplasia of the gums. Teach the client to identify both the trigger points that stimulate the pain and ways to avoid those areas without neglecting daily needs.

The client who has had surgery may have lost the mechanisms that protect the eye from injury, and is taught not to touch his eye and to observe for redness of the eye and conjunctiva. Following surgery, the client may not feel pain caused by dental caries, so routine visits to the dentist for oral examination are needed.

ENCEPHALITIS, MENINGITIS

Encephalitis is inflammation of the brain. **Meningitis** is inflammation of the meninges. The most common cause of encephalitis or meningitis is a virus. Bacteria, fungi, or parasites also are causative factors. Meningococcal meningitis is highly contagious. Contacts of the client are identified and prophylactic medication is recommended. The virus or other causative agent enters the brain either through the bloodstream as a direct extension of trauma or by nerve pathways.

The inflammatory process causes demyelination of white matter and degeneration of neurons. Cerebral edema, hemorrhage, and necrosis of brain tissue also occur. Clinical manifestations vary depending on the causative agent, area of involvement, and degree of damage to nerve tissue. Fever, headache, nuchal rigidity, photophobia, irritability, lethargy, nausea, and vomiting are typical signs and symptoms. As the disease progresses, level of consciousness decreases and other neurological dysfunctions occur, including motor weakness, aphasia, seizures, behavioral changes, or even death. A lumbar puncture is performed to test CSF for the causative agent, presence of white blood cells or red blood cells, and elevated protein level. A complete blood count identifies the presence of viral or bacterial infection.

Medical–Surgical Management

Medical

Treatment is supportive and based on presenting symptoms. The aim of treatment is to prevent or decrease increased intracranial pressure and to minimize neurological deficits. Intravenous fluids are given to rehydrate the client. Clients are placed in isolation until the cause of meningitis can be determined.

Pharmacological

Antibiotics or antiinfectives are administered in massive doses as appropriate for the causative agent. They are given intravenously or intrathecally into the spinal canal. Most viral agents do not respond to antibiotics or antiinfectives. Glucocorticosteroids are administered to prevent cerebral edema. Osmotic diuretics may be used to reduce cerebral edema. To prevent seizures, anticonvulsants are often ordered. Antipyretics are often given to reduce fever.

Diet

Optimal nutritional status is maintained to promote response to the infection.

Activity

A quiet environment with minimal stimulation from noise, light, or client activity is maintained. Routine turning, ROM exercises, pulmonary hygiene, and skin care are required to prevent the complications of immobility.

Nursing Management

In the acute stage, monitor the client for changes in neurological status, especially for changes in level of consciousness and for signs of increasing intracranial pressure. A quiet environment decreases external stimulation. Observe the client for seizure activity and protect from injury. Comfort measures such as oral hygiene, tepid baths, and administration of analgesics for relief of headaches are offered.

HUNTINGTON'S DISEASE

Huntington's disease (HD) is a chronic, progressive hereditary disease of the nervous system. It is characterized by a progressive involuntary choreiform movement and progressive dementia.

The cells of the basal ganglia, which control movement, die prematurely. Cells in the cerebral cortex also die, interfering with thought processes, memory, perception, and judgment. Age of onset is usually 35 to 45 years, with death occurring 10 to 15 years following onset of symptoms (Smeltzer, Bare, Hinkle, & Cheever, 2008). Each child of a person with Huntington's disease has a 50% chance of inheriting the fatal gene. Everyone who has the gene will develop the disease (HDSA, 2002). However, there is no cure for this devastating progressive disease.

Clinical manifestations are **chorea**, abnormal involuntary, purposeless movements of all musculature of the body. Facial tic, grimacing, difficulty in chewing and swallowing, speech impairment, disorganized gait, and bowel and bladder incontinence also occur. Mental or intellectual impairment progresses to dementia. The client may experience paranoia, hallucinations, or delusions. Emotions are labile, from outbursts of anger to profound depression, apathy, or euphoria. A ravenous appetite is usually present, but because of the constant movement, the client is often emaciated and exhausted. Death usually results from heart failure, pneumonia, infection, or choking (HDSA, 2002).

The entire family experiences this disease in an emotional, physical, social, and financial way. Supportive care is required as the family progresses through life with a loved one with Huntington's disease. Because of the hereditary factor, genetic counseling is suggested.

Medical–Surgical Management

Pharmacological

A medication that decreases choreiform movement is the benzodiazepine, clonazepam (Klonopin). Do not stop clonazepam abruptly but taper off medication to avoid symptoms of withdrawal, especially if client has epilepsy. Assess client for excessive fatigue. Antidepressants, such as desipramine hydrochloride (Norpramin) and fluoxetine hydrochloride (Prozac), and antipsychotics, such as fluphenazine hydrochloride (Prolixin), are used for emotional disturbances. Many people do better with minimal medication (HDSA, 2001).

Diet

The diet must be high in calories to provide for the high energy needs caused by the continuous movement. Chewing and swallowing difficulties necessitate foods that are easy to chew or foods cut into small pieces to prevent choking.

Activity

Ambulation is maintained as long as possible. A safe environment is maintained to prevent injury from falls or from sharp objects. Driving is usually restricted when choreiform movement or impaired judgment interferes with the ability to drive safely.

Nursing Management

Nursing interventions include a holistic approach to the client's care. Collaboration with the social worker, the chaplain, the physician, and the mental health worker is necessary.

Teach the client and family about the disease process, the progress of the disease, and the genetic factors involved.

Safety factors are considered. Fall prevention measures, such as removing throw rugs and small objects from the floor, and injury prevention measures, such as removing sharp or dangerous objects such as guns and knives from the home, are implemented. The hazard of choking also is addressed, by teaching the family to cut the client's food into small pieces, to serve soft foods, and by teaching the Heimlich maneuver.

GILLES DE LA TOURETTE'S SYNDROME

Gilles de la Tourette's syndrome is a neurological movement disorder that also has prominent behavioral manifestations. Clinical manifestations include motor tics and involuntary repetitive movements of the mouth, face, head, or neck muscles. The trunk and extremities may also be involved. Motor tics take the form of forceful eye blinking or toe touching. Vocal tics or repetitive involuntary vocalizations take the form of sniffing, grunting, throat clearing, or **coprolalia** (involuntary and inappropriate swearing). Other complex motor and vocal tics that also are present include copropraxia, involuntary and effectively appropriate use of obscene gestures; echolalia, involuntary repetition of the speech of others; and palilia, involuntary repetition of the person's own speech. The obsessive–compulsive symptoms of repetitive handwashing or checking rituals also are exhibited. Attention deficit hyperactivity disorder (ADHD) and obsessive–compulsive disorders may also coexist with Tourette's syndrome.

Onset is before age 18 years, with males being more commonly affected than females. Tourette's is an inherited disorder, with the affected individual having a 50% chance of passing the gene on to children.

MEDICAL–SURGICAL MANAGEMENT

Pharmacological

Tics are controlled with clonadine (Catapres), haloperidol (Haldol), or primozide (Orap). Coexisting ADHD is controlled with clonidine (Catapres), methylphenidate (Ritalin), or pemoline (Cylert). Clomypramine (Anafranil) or fluoxetine (Prozac) are used to keep obsessive–compulsive behaviors under control (Kurlan, 1998). Acetaminophen (Tylenol) may help the discomfort of muscle spasms.

Other Therapies

As they age, clients learn to suppress tics in social situations. Psychotherapy and family counseling are beneficial in coping with social stigma and adjustment problems.

NURSING MANAGEMENT

The client and the family with Tourette's syndrome need a great deal of emotional support and benefit from knowing about the availability of support groups for clients with Tourette's syndrome. The nurse instructs the client about the disease process and personal and behavioral expectations. Behavioral modification techniques are generally effective; the nurse must know which modification techniques are being used and must follow through with consistent responses.

CASE STUDY

D.O., a 76-year-old retired farmer, was admitted to the emergency department with left-sided hemiplegia, difficulty swallowing, and inability to speak. He was awake and watching the staff upon admission. He moved his right arm to indicate that M.O. was his wife but was unable to speak or form sounds. M.O. stated that her husband was working in the garden, picking tomatoes and cucumbers, when he fell to the ground 30 minutes before admission. The department room nurse administered oxygen through nasal cannula at 2 liters per minute and obtained vital signs. His blood pressure was 182/110 mm Hg, pulse was 88 beats per minute, respirations were 20 breaths per minute, and temperature was 100.5°F. The emergency department physician ordered an MRI scan of the head, a complete blood count, and prothrombin time (PT). The MRI indicated that D.O. experienced a CVA caused by bleeding into the brain.

The following questions will guide your development of a nursing care plan for the case study.

1. List clinical manifestations other than the symptoms D.O. experienced that can occur with a CVA.
2. List subjective and objective data that a nurse would obtain.
3. Identify three individualized nursing diagnoses and goals for D.O.
4. D.O. is transferred to a general medical unit for 3 days, and then is transferred to a rehabilitation center for intensive therapy. What pertinent nursing actions should a nurse perform in caring for D.O. in the acute setting and the rehabilitation setting related to:
   - Mobility
   - Safety
   - Elimination
   - Skin integrity
   - Comfort and rest
5. What teaching will D.O. need before discharge from the rehabilitation facility?
6. List at least three client outcomes for D.O.

SUMMARY

- The nervous system controls all bodily functions, from movement to thinking to processing information to autonomic responses.
- The frontal lobe of the cerebrum specializes in emotional attitudes and responses, formation of thought processes, motor function, judgment, personality, and inhibitions.
- The parietal lobe of the cerebrum is a purely sensory region for interpretation of all senses except smell; the purpose is to analyze sensations, including pain, touch, and temperature, from receptors in the skin.
- The temporal lobe of the cerebrum houses Wernicke's area, the primary auditory association area, where words that are heard are interpreted. Memory is also a function of the temporal lobe, especially memories that are highly detailed or involve multiple sensations.
- A special interpretive area located at the junction of the temporal, parietal, and occipital lobes integrates somatic, auditory, and visual sensory interpretations.
- The occipital lobe of the cerebrum is responsible for visual interpretation and visual association.
- Disorders of the nervous system cause complex dysfunctions; the nurse uses assessment skills and quickly recognizes changes in condition.
- Teaching about injury prevention and the effects and prognosis of the disorder are required to meet the physical and psychosocial needs of the client and family.
- Many neurological disorders potentiate injury. Nursing care includes providing the client and family with necessary safety information.
- To maintain and restore functional ability, rehabilitation is initiated from the first contact with the client.

REVIEW QUESTIONS

1. The most important indicator of change in neurological status is:
   1. level of consciousness.
   2. pupil reaction.
   3. vital signs.
   4. motor function.
2. Assessment of intellectual function requires that the nurse:
   1. have knowledge of the client's previous ability to function.
   2. administer a written test to determine the client's IQ level.
   3. utilize auscultation, percussion, and palpation skills.
   4. observe the client's behavior, posture, and facial expression.
3. Contusion of the brain is a (an):
   1. shaking of the brain.
   2. bleeding into the brain tissue.
   3. open head injury.
   4. bruising of the brain.
4. Benign brain tumors can be:
   1. more anxiety producing than are malignant tumors.
   2. more life threatening than are malignant tumors.
   3. treated with radiation therapy.
   4. the cause of increased intracranial pressure.
5. A nurse is teaching A.W., a 24-year-old client with Guillain-Barré syndrome, about her condition. What statement does the nurse include in her teaching?
   1. The nerve degeneration continues to slowly progress in this chronic degenerative nerve disease.
   2. The disease is an acute inflammatory process with most clients regaining complete function.
   3. Respiratory failure requiring chronic ventilatory support may occur.
   4. Motor function deficit will occur, but sensation will remain.
6. The client's wife asks the nurse what she thinks of memory training and reality orientation for a client with Stage 2 Alzheimer's disease. The nurse responds that those interventions should be used with caution because:
   1. reality is painful.
   2. they are very costly.
   3. they can accelerate the disease process.
   4. they might trigger anger and agitation.
7. A nurse is caring for a client with amyotrophic lateral sclerosis (ALS) who has the following symptoms. What symptom requires a prompt nursing intervention?
   1. Loss of bowel and urine control.
   2. Confusion.
   3. Tonic-clonic seizures.
   4. Shallow respirations.
8. What client response indicates he understands the nurse's instructions about taking carbidopa-levodopa (Sinemet)?
   1. "I will slowly rise from a sitting position to standing position."
   2. "I will limit my fluids to 1000 milliliters a day."
   3. "I will reduce my medication dosage by half when my symptoms improve."
   4. "I will have a diet high in protein and vitamin B_6 since I am taking Sinemet."
9. A nurse completes an assessment on her client. She finds that the client opens his eyes when she enters the room; answers questions but has incorrect answers about time, place, and events; and raises

right hand when requested. According to the Glasgow Coma Scale, what score does the nurse give the client?
1. 3
2. 6
3. 12
4. 14

10. What are expected findings when the nurse assesses the client's trigeminal nerve? (Select all that apply.)
1. Eye moves smoothly upward and outward.
2. Eye blinks rapidly when cotton ball sweeps across cornea.
3. Client tastes sweet sensation when given a piece of candy.
4. Jaw moves symmetrical and overcomes resistance.
5. Gag reflect is intact.
6. Client feels cotton ball when swiped across cheek.

REFERENCES/SUGGESTED READINGS

Agnew, T. (2006). Nurses out of step with Parkinson's patients. *Nursing Older People, 18*(6), 8–9.

Alzheimer's Association. (2002). Facts: About Alzheimer's disease. Retrieved from http://www.alz.org/Resource Center/FactSheets/FSAlzheimerdisease.pdf

Alzheimer's Disease Education and Referral Center. (2002). Alzheimer's disease fact sheet. Retrieved from http://www.alzheimers.org/pubs/adfact.html

Alzheimer's Organization. (2008). Alzheimer's disease prevalence rates rise to more than 5 million in the United States. Retrieved July 19, 2008 from http://www.alz.org/news_and_events_rates_rise.asp

American Headache Society (AHS). (2007). Types of headaches. Retrieved June 5, 2009 from http://www.achenet.org/education/patients/TypesofHeadaches.asp

Andersen, G. (1998). DX dementia: But what kind? *RN, 61*(6), 26–30.

Backer, J. (2006). The symptom experience of patients with Parkinson's disease. *Journal of Neuroscience Nursing, 38*(1), 51–57.

Barker, E. (1999). Brain attack! A call to action. *RN, 62*(5), 54–57.

Barker, E. (2001). What's your patient's stroke risk? *Nursing2001, 31*(4), 32hn1–32hn5.

Barker, E., & Saulino, M. (2002). First-ever guidelines for spinal cord injuries. *RN, 65*(10), 32–37.

Beare, P. & Myers, J. (Eds.). (1998). *Principles and practice of adult health nursing* (3rd ed.). St. Louis, MO: Mosby.

Best, J. (2001). Cauda equina syndrome. *Nursing2001, 31*(4), 43.

Bond, C. (2002). Traumatic brain injury: Help for the family. *RN, 65*(11), 60–66.

Bulechek, G., Butcher, H., McCloskey, J., & Dochterman, J., eds. (2008). *Nursing Interventions Classification (NIC)* (5th ed.). St. Louis, MO: Mosby/Elsevier.

Bunting-Perry, L. (2006). Palliative care in Parkinson's disease: Implications for neuroscience nursing. *Journal Neuroscience Nursing, 38*(2), 106–113.

Costa, M. (1998). Clinical snapshot: Trigeminal neuralgia. *AJN, 98*(6), 42–43.

Crigger, N., & Forbes, W. (1997). Assessing neurologic function in older patients. *AJN, 97*(3), 37–40.

Cross, C. (2002). Spotting concussions in children and in adults. *RN, 65*(7), 72.

Finesilver, C. (2003). Multiple sclerosis. *RN, 66*(4), 36–43.

Frank, R., Gesteland, R., Bailie, J., Rybalsky, K., Seiden, A., & Dulay, M. (2006). Characterization of the sniff magnitude test. *Archives of Otolaryngol Head Neck Surgery, 132*(5), 532–536.

Galvan, T. (2001). Dysphagia: Going down and staying down. *AJN, 101*(1), 37–42.

Gendreau-Webb, R. (2001). Acute ischemic stroke. *Nursing2001, 31*(11), 120.

Gray-Vickrey, P. (2002). Advances in Alzheimer's disease. *Nursing2002, 32*(11), 64.

Gumm, S. (2000). Straight talk about MS. *Nursing2000, 30*(1), 50–51.

Hally, Z. (2007). Simple sniff test could diagnose Alzheimer's and Parkinson's disease. Retrieved June 5, 2009 from http://www.associatedcontent.com/article/202499/simple_sniff_test_could_daignose_alzheimer?cat=5

Halper, J., & Holland, N. (1998a). Meeting the challenge of multiple sclerosis (Part I). *AJN, 98*(10), 26–31.

Halper, J., & Holland, N. (1998b). Meeting the challenge of multiple sclerosis (Part II). *AJN, 98*(11), 39–46.

Hickey, J. (2008). *The clinical practice of neurological and neurosurgical nursing* (6th ed.). Philadelphia: Lippincott Williams & Wilkins.

Hilgers, J. (2003). Comforting a confused patient. *Nursing2003, 33*(1), 48–50.

Hilton, G. (2001). Acute head injury: Distinguishing subdural from epidural hematoma. *AJN, 101*(9), 51–52.

Huntington's Disease Society of America (HDSA). (2002). *Huntington's disease.* Retrieved from http://www.hdsa.org/edu/HD_booklet.htm

Huston, C. (1998). Emergency! Cervical spine injury. *AJN, 98*(6), 33.

Huston, C., & Boelman, R. (1995). Autonomic dysreflexia. *AJN, 95*(6), 55.

Kurlan, R. (1998). Current pharmacology of Tourette's syndrome. Bayside, NY: Tourette Syndrome Association. Retrieved from http://www.2mgh.harvard.edu/lsa/medsci/medicationsanddosages.html

Lewis, A. (1999). Neurologic emergency! *Nursing99, 29*(10), 54–56.

Lower, J. (2002). Facing neuro assessment fearlessly. *Nursing2002, 32*(2), 58–64.

Lower, J. (2003). Using pain to assess neurologic response. *Nursing2003, 33*(6), 56–57.

MayoClinic.com. (2008). Brain tumor. Retrieved June 2, 2009 from http://www.mayoclinci.com/helath/brain-tumor/DS00281/METHOD=print&DSECTION-all

McCance, K., & Huether, S. (2001). *Pathophysiology: The biological basis for disease in adults and children* (4th ed.). St. Louis, MO: Mosby.

McGuire, L. (2002). How to treat a migraine. *Nursing2002, 32*(12), 76–77.

McNamara, P. (2009). Parkinson's disease: Diet in early stages of PD. Retrieved June 4, 2009 from http://parkinsons.about.com/od/livingwithpd/a/foods_to_eat.htm?p=1

Monlus-Swift, C. (2002). Neurological disorders. In P. L. Swearingen (Ed.), *Manual of medical–surgical nursing care: Nursing interventions and collaborative management* (5th ed.). St. Louis, MO: Mosby.

Moorhead, S., Johnson, M., Maas, M., & Swanson, E. (2007). *Nursing Outcomes Classification (NOC)* (4th ed.). St. Louis, MO: Mosby.

Morgan, J., & Sethi, K. (2005). Treatment of early Parkinson's disease. In M. Ebadi & R. E. Pfeiffer (Eds.), *Parkinson's disease* (pp. 839–849). New York: CRC Press.

Mower-Wade, D., Cavanaugh, M., & Bush, D. (2001). Protecting a patient with ruptured cerebral aneurysm. *Nursing2001, 31*(2), 52–57.

Nadler-Moodie, M., & Wilson, M. (1998). Latest approaches in Alzheimer's care. *RN, 61*(7), 42–46.

National Headache Foundation (NHF). (2002). Fact sheet. Retrieved from http://www.headaches.org/consumer/generalinfo/factsheet.html

National Institute of Neurological Disorders and Stroke. (2006). Hope through research. Retrieved July 17, 2008 from http://www.ninds.nih.gov/disorders/parkinsons_disease/detail_parkinsons_disease.htm#120463159

National Multiple Sclerosis Society (NMSS). (2003). *What is multiple sclerosis?* Retrieved from http://www.nationalmssociety.org/What%20is%20MS.asp

National Parkinson's Foundation. (2000). Parkinson's and B_6: What's the connection. Retrieved July 20, 2008 from http://www.parkinson.org/NETCOMMUNITY/Page.aspx?pid=458&srcid=377

National Parkinson Foundation. (2008). About Parkinson disease. Retrieved July 17, 2008 from http://www.parkinson.org?NETCOMMUNITY/Page.aspx?pid=225&srcid=210

National Stroke Association (NSA). (1999). *Stroke prevention guidelines.* Retrieved from http://www.stroke.org/pages/ prev_guide.cfm

National Stroke Association (NSA). (2002a). *Stroke in America campaign.* Retrieved from http://www.stroke.org/pages/america_main.cfm

National Stroke Association (NSA). (2002b). *Stroke statistics.* Retrieved from http://www.stroke.org/brain_stat.cfm

National Stroke Association (NSA). (2002c). *Stroke: What it is.* Retrieved from http://www.stroke.org/whats.cfm

National Stroke Association (NSA). (2008). Talk about TIA! Retrieved June 3, 2009 at http://www.stroke.org/site/PageNavigator/HOME

National Stroke Association (NSA). (2009a). Stroke 101. Retrieved June 3, 2009 at http://www.stroke.org/site/DocServer/STROKE_101_Fact_Sheet.pdf?docID=454

National Stroke Association (NSA). (2009b). Stroke risk factors. Retrieved June 3, 2009 from http://www.stroke.org/site/PageServer?pagename=RISK

North American Nursing Diagnosis Association International. (2010). *NANDA-I nursing diagnoses: Definitions and classification 2009–2011.* Ames, IA: Wiley-Blackwell.

O'Hanlon-Nichols, T. (1999). Neurologic assessment. *AJN, 99*(6), 44–50.

Parini, S. (2001). 8 faces of meningitis. *Nursing2001, 31*(8), 51–53.

Parkinson's Disease Foundation (PDF). (2002). *Parkinson's disease.* Retrieved from http://www.pdf.org/aboutdisease/overview.html

Parkinson's Disease Foundation.(2008). Ten frequently asked questions about Parkinson's disease. Retrieved July 19, 2008 from http://www.pdf.org/Publications/factsheets/PDF_Fact_Sheet_1.0_Final.pdf

Pullen, R. (2003). Protecting your patient during a seizure. *Nursing2003, 33*(4), 78.

Rudick, R. (1997). New approaches to multiple sclerosis. *Health News, 3*(17), 1–2. Waltham, MA: Massachusetts Medical Society.

Samuels, M. (Ed.). (2004). *Manual of neurological therapeutics* (7th ed.). Philadelphia: Lippincott Williams & Wilkins.

Santa Rosa County Citizen Service Center. (2009) Blood clots/stroke–They now have a fourth indicator, the tongue. Retrieved June 3, 2009 from http://www.santarosa.fl.gov/hr/documents/identiyastroke.pdf

Schweiger, J. (1999). Alzheimer's disease. *Nursing99, 29*(6), 34–41.

Smeltzer, S., Bare, B., Hinkle, J., & Cheever, K. (2008). *Brunner & Suddarth's textbook of medical-surgical nursing* (11th ed.). Philadelphia: Lippincott Williams & Wilkins.

Smith, L. (2002). Steady the course of Parkinson's disease. *Nursing2002, 32*(3), 43–45.

Son, G., Therrien, B., & Whall, A. (2002). Implicit memory and familiarity among elders with dementia. *Journal of Nursing Scholarship, 34*(3), 263–267.

Spinal Cord Injury Information Network. (2009). Facts and figures at a glance. Retrieved June 4, 2009 from http://www.spinalcord.uab.edu/show.asp?durki=119513&site=4716&return=19775

Taggart, H.(1998). Multiple sclerosis update. *Orthopaedic Nursing (March/April),* 23–29.

The American Association of Neurological Surgeons & The Congress of Neurological Surgeons. (2002). Guidelines for the management of acute cervical spine and spinal cord injuries. *Neurosurgery, 50*(3), S1.

Thomure, A. (2006). Helping your patient manage Parkinson's disease. *Nursing 2006, 6*(8), 20–21.

Urden, L., Stacy, K., & Lough, M. (2009). *Critical care nursing: Diagnosis and management* (6th ed.). St. Louis: Mosby.

Weintraub, D., & Stern, M. (2005). Psychiatric complications in Parkinson's disease. *American Journal of Geriatric Psychiatry, 13,* 844–851.

Williams, M., Wood H., & Waxman, J. (2002). How to assess swallowing after a stroke. *Nursing2002, 32*(8), 32hn5–32hn6.

Wilson, R., Mendes de Leon, C., Barnes, L., et al. (2002). Participation in cognitively stimulating activities and risk of incident Alzheimer's disease. *JAMA, 287*(6), 742.

RESOURCES

Alzheimer's Association, http://www.alz.org

American Academy of Neurology, http://www.aan.com

American Association of Spinal Cord Injury Professionals, http://nurses.ascipro.org

American Headache Society, http://www.achenet.org/

American Spinal Injury Association, http://www.asia-spinal injury.org

Brain Injury Association of America, http://www.biausa.org

Coma/Traumatic Brain Injury Recovery Association, Inc., http://www.comarecovery.org

Epilepsy Foundation of America, http://www.epilepsyfoundation.org/

Guillain-Barré Syndrome/Chronic Inflammatory Demyelinating Polyneuropathy Foundation International, http://www.gbs-cidp.org/

Huntington's Disease Society of America, http://www.hdsa.org/

National Headache Foundation, http://www.headaches.org

National Institute of Neurological Disorders and Stroke, http://www.ninds.nih.gov

National Multiple Sclerosis Society,
http://www.nationalmssociety.org/index.aspx

National Parkinson's Foundation, Inc.,
http://www.parkinson.org

National Spinal Cord Injury Association,
http://www.spinalcord.org

National Stroke Association, http://www.stroke.org

Parkinson's Disease Foundation, http://www.pdf.org

Tourette Syndrome Association, Inc.,
http://www.tsa-usa.org

CHAPTER 11
Sensory System

MAKING THE CONNECTION

Refer to the following chapters to increase your understanding of the sensory system:

Adult Health Nursing
- ***Surgery***
- ***Neurological System***
- ***The Older Adult***

LEARNING OBJECTIVES

Upon completion of this chapter, you should be able to:

- Define key terms.
- Compare and differentiate common disorders of the special senses.
- Identify the structure and function of the major parts of the eye and ear.
- Explain the purpose of the common diagnostic tests for sensory problems.
- List the nursing assessments and common nursing diagnoses related to sensory impairment.
- Assist in planning nursing care for clients with sensory disorders.
- List some of the common sensory aids for the visual and hearing impaired.

KEY TERMS

affect
afferent nerve pathway
arousal
astigmatism
awareness
cerumen
chalazion
cognition
conductive hearing loss
conjunctivitis
consciousness
disorientation
efferent nerve pathway
hallucination
hyperopia
illusion
judgment
keratitis
myopia
nystagmus
orientation
perception
presbycusis
presbyopia
sensation
sensorineural hearing loss
sensory deficit
sensory deprivation
sensory overload
sensory perception
strabismus
stye
tinnitus
vertigo

INTRODUCTION

From the moment we wake in the morning until we fall asleep at night, we are inundated with information from the outside world through our senses. We depend on visual and auditory alarms to keep us from harm. This chapter reviews the structure and function, identifies appropriate nursing diagnoses, and presents the medical and nursing management for hearing and vision with some discussion of taste, smell, and touch.

SENSATION, PERCEPTION, AND COGNITION

Sensation is the ability to receive and process stimuli through the sensory organs. There are two types of stimuli: external and internal. External stimuli are received and processed through the senses of sight (visual), hearing (auditory), smell (olfactory), taste (gustatory), and touch (tactile). Internal stimuli are received and processed through kinesthetic (an awareness of the position of the body) and visceral (feelings originating from large organs within the body) modes.

Perception is the ability to experience, recognize, organize, and interpret sensory stimuli. **Sensory perception** is the ability to receive sensory impressions and, through cortical association, relate the stimuli to past experiences and form an impression of the nature of the stimulus.

Perception is closely associated with **cognition**, the intellectual ability to think. The processes of organizing and interpreting stimuli depend on a person's level of intellectual functioning. Cognition includes the elements of memory, judgment, and orientation. The well-being of an individual depends on the functions of sensation, perception, and cognition because the person fully experiences and interacts with the environment through these mechanisms.

Sensory, perceptual, and cognitive alterations are either temporary or progressive in their manifestations and result from disease or trauma. Whatever the status or cause of the alterations, these conditions usually lead to social isolation and increased dependence on others. In addition, impairment in sensory, perceptual, and cognitive functions place the individual at risk for injury to self or others.

ANATOMY AND PHYSIOLOGY REVIEW

Sensation, perception, and cognition are neurological functions. The nervous system is composed of two major subsystems: the central nervous system (CNS) and the peripheral nervous system (PNS), which consists of the somatic and autonomic nervous systems. The CNS and PNS act in unison to accomplish three purposes: (1) collection of stimuli from the receptors at the end of the peripheral nerves; (2) transportation of the stimuli to the brain for integration and cognition processing; and (3) conduction of responses to the stimuli from the brain to responsive motor centers in the body.

Sensory perception involves the function of both the cranial and peripheral nerves. The cranial nerves arise from the brain and govern the movement and function of various muscles and nerves throughout the body. The peripheral nerves connect the CNS to other parts of the body.

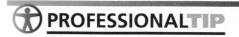

PROFESSIONALTIP

CNS Deficits and Illness

Specific conditions, such as diabetes mellitus and atherosclerosis, can impair neurosensory pathways and result in deficits in sensation, perception, and cognition. Diseases of the CNS can result in loss of sensory function and paralysis.

COMPONENTS OF SENSATION AND PERCEPTION

The sensory system is a complex network that consists of **afferent nerve pathways** (ascending pathways that transmit sensory impulses to the brain), **efferent nerve pathways** (descending pathways that send sensory impulses from the brain), the spinal cord, the brainstem, and the cerebrum.

COMPONENTS OF COGNITION

Cognition includes the cerebral functions of memory, affect, judgment, perception, and language. In order for these higher functions to occur, consciousness must be present.

Consciousness

Consciousness is a state of awareness of self, others, and the surrounding environment. It affects both cognitive (intellectual) and affective (emotional) functions. An alert individual (one who is aware of self and stimuli) is able to perceive reality accurately and to base behavior on those perceptions. The components of consciousness provide a foundation for behavior and emotional expression, thereby contributing to the uniqueness of each individual's personality. Consciousness may be altered by various metabolic, traumatic, or other factors, such as the pharmacological actions of drugs that affect mental status. The primary components of consciousness are arousal and awareness, both of which must be present before higher cognitive functioning occurs.

Arousal The degree of **arousal** (state of wakefulness and alertness) is indicated by a person's general response and reaction to the environment. People exhibit arousal by behaving in an alert and aware manner and by experiencing periods of wakefulness. The degree of an individual's arousal is indicated by the general response and reaction to the environment. Impaired arousal can exist when a sleep pattern deficit is

PROFESSIONALTIP

Effects of Medications on Sensation

Certain medications have the potential to alter or depress the neurosensory system. For example, sedatives and narcotics alter the perception of sensory stimuli. Medications such as analgesics alter the level of consciousness.

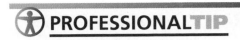

Remote Memory

Remote memory is accurately assessed only when client responses about past events can be validated, either by others or by written account.

experienced. There may be an inability to take advantage of opportunities for activity because of inadequate periods of rest.

Awareness Awareness is the capacity to perceive sensory impressions and react appropriately through thoughts and actions. An essential element in awareness is **orientation** (perception of self in relation to the surrounding environment). When awareness is impaired, orientation to time is frequently the first area affected. The degree of disorientation is worse when the individual loses awareness of place, self (person), and purpose/situation.

Memory

There are three types of memory: immediate, recent, and remote. Immediate memory is the retention of information for a specified and usually short period of time. The recall of a telephone number long enough to dial it is an example of immediate memory. Recent memory is the ability to recall events that have occurred over the past 24 hours, such as remembering the foods eaten for dinner the previous night. Remote memory is the retention of experiences that occurred during earlier periods of life, such as an adult's memories of childhood or school days. The ability to learn depends on remote memory.

Affect

Affect (expression of mood or feeling) is an important component of cognition in that variations of mood can affect one's thinking ability. For example, a client with a flat affect caused by depression may have difficulty sustaining concentration or attention.

Judgment

Judgment is the ability to compare or evaluate alternatives to arrive at a conclusion based on sound reasoning and supported by evidence. Judgment is closely related to reality testing and depends on effective cognitive functioning. Behaviors indicating impaired judgment include impulsiveness, unrealistic decision making, and inadequate problem-solving ability.

Perception

Perceptions are considered in the context of the individual's awareness of reality. Misperceptions of reality can occur in the form of an **illusion** (an inaccurate perception or misinterpretation of sensory stimuli) or a **hallucination** (a sensory perception that occurs in the absence of external stimuli and is not based on reality).

Clients who are anxious and fearful or who are on therapeutic regimens involving the use of certain medications may experience misperceptions of environmental stimuli. For example, a postoperative client, after receiving analgesic medication for pain, may see the belt from his bathrobe lying on the floor and become terrified because he thinks there is a snake in the room. Once the nurse determines that the client is experiencing an illusion, appropriate reassurance and reality orientation is implemented to reduce the client's anxiety.

Language

Language is one of the most complex of cognitive functions, involving not only the spoken word but also reading, writing, and comprehension. Characteristics of speech are fluency (ability to talk in a steady manner), prosody (melody of speech that conveys meaning through changes in the tempo, rhythm, and intonation), and content.

ASSESSMENT

When caring for clients with sensory, perceptual, and cognitive alterations, the nurse obtains a health history and performs a physical examination to identify existing or potential problems in this area of functioning. The physical examination focuses specifically on the client's ability to hear, see, taste, smell, and touch. For hearing (auditory): Ask about hearing problems, ability to distinguish sounds, buzzing or ringing noises, recent changes in hearing ability, and use of a hearing aid. For seeing (visual): Ask about blurred vision, double vision, blind spots, photosensitivity, rainbows or halos around objects, difficulty seeing far or near, family history of visual problems, use of glasses or contact lenses, and date of last eye examination. For tasting (gustatory): Ask about changes in tasting ability or appetite and ability to differentiate sweet, sour, salty, and bitter tastes. For smelling (olfactory): Ask about changes in the ability to smell and the ability to distinguish common smells. For touch (tactile): Ask about ability to feel temperature changes and pain perception in extremities and the presence of unusual sensations in extremities (tingling or numbness). Refer to the neurologic system chapter for assessment of cranial nerves.

When assessing clients for sensory, perceptual, and cognitive alterations, the level of consciousness (LOC) also is evaluated. Refer to the neurologic system chapter for the Glasgow Coma Scale, developed to assess LOC objectively.

SAFETY

Sensory Impairments

Vision—Risk of tripping, falling

Hearing—Lack of awareness of warning sounds such as automobile horns, sirens, smoke alarms

Olfactory—Inability to perceive warning odors such as burning food, escaping gas

Gustatory—Inability to recognize spoiled or contaminated food or beverages

Tactile—Lack of awareness of excessive pressure on a body part; at risk for exposure to extreme temperatures (frostbite, burns)

The Ear

The human ear is divided into three main anatomical components: the outer ear, middle ear, and inner ear (Figure 11-1). Each part plays a major role in hearing. Similar to other paired organs in the body, dysfunction of part or all of one ear does not affect the function of the other.

Outer Ear

The outer ear is composed of the auricle (pinna), a cartilaginous flap on the temporal sides of the head, and the external ear canal, or external auditory meatus. The outer ear is responsible for collecting, conducting, and amplifying sound waves. The auricle directs sounds through the external ear canal to the tympanic membrane (eardrum). This canal is lined with ceruminous glands that secrete **cerumen** (ear wax), a yellowish brown protective substance that guards against certain bacteria and small insects, and traps dust and debris that may damage the inner ear. Normally, the cerumen works its way out of the ear as we eat, chew, or speak; however, cerumen can build up and actually cause significant hearing loss in the affected ear.

The tympanic membrane (TM) serves as a boundary between the outer and middle ear. As sound waves vibrate against the membrane, the motion is transmitted to the bones of the inner ear. In an acute ear infection, fluid fills the middle ear, creating significant pressure on the tympanic membrane.

Middle Ear

The three bones of the middle ear are collectively referred to as the ossicles and include the *malleus* (hammer), *incus* (anvil), and *stapes* (stirrup), so named because they resemble the tools of a blacksmith's trade. The malleus is attached to the upper, inner portion of the tympanic membrane. The head of the malleus connects with the incus, which then joins the stapes. The flat oval bone of the stapes, called the footplate, rests on the oval window (part of the inner ear). The vibration created by sound waves passes through the outer ear canal to the tympanic membrane and then to these three bones.

The eustachian tube opens into the pharynx from the middle ear. It is approximately 3 to 4 cm long, and its primary function is to equalize pressure on both sides of the eardrum by providing a path (via the nasal passages) to relieve the pressure. In addition to pressure equalization, the functions of the middle ear include amplification of the sound waves and stimulation of the oval window to move the fluids of the inner ear.

LIFE SPAN CONSIDERATIONS

Sensory Changes in the Elderly

- When the eye lens yellows and becomes cloudy, the ability to discern colors, especially greens and blues, is impaired.
- The elderly need more light to see because the pupils become smaller, letting in less light.
- It takes the elderly longer to accommodate (adjust) to darkness and glare.
- Tear production decreases with age, predisposing to dry eye syndrome and corneal irritation.
- The most common hearing loss is sensorineural, which can be helped by a hearing aid.
- Taste sensation may be dulled with age.

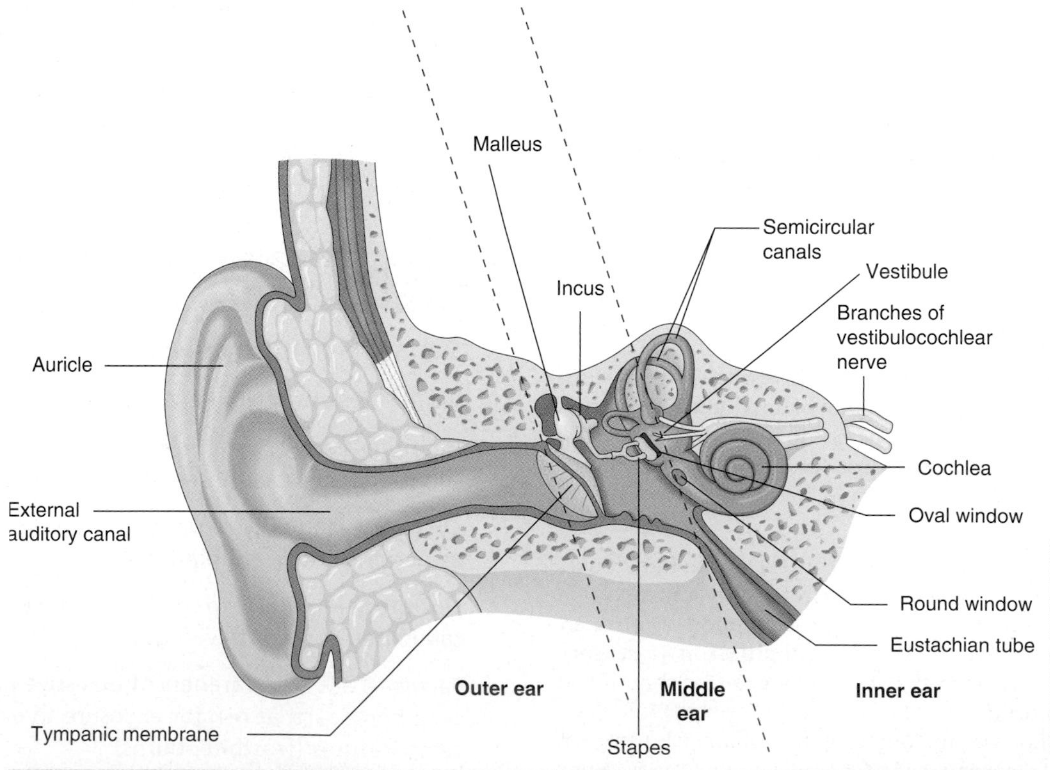

Figure 11-1 Structures of the Ear

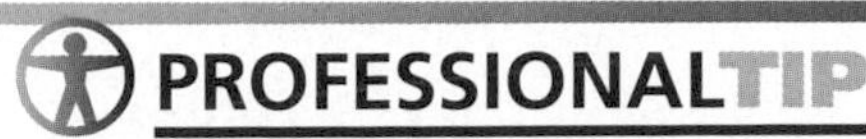

Tympanic Membrane

The tympanic membrane is normally concave on otoscopic exam, so a convex or bulging tympanic membrane is an important sign of an acute infectious process.

Inner Ear

The inner ear has two main functions: hearing and equilibrium. It consists of a complex series of interconnected, fluid-filled chambers and tubes called the labyrinth. It is divided into three main parts: the semicircular canals, the vestibule, and the cochlea, all located in the temporal bone. The semicircular canals, which function in providing the sense of balance, open into the vestibule. The vestibule is the central chamber of the inner ear. The cochlea is a snail-shaped structure that contains the auditory organ for the sense of hearing.

Vibration of the stapes creates pressure and causes the nerves to respond to different sounds and initiate neural responses that are sent along the auditory nerve (cranial nerve VIII) to the brain. Thus mechanical information is translated into nerve impulses and sent to the brain, which translates the sound into meaningful impressions and language.

THE EYE

The eyes are a pair of spherical organs located in bony orbital cavities in the front of the skull. They are the sensory receptor organs of the visual system that transduce light from the environment into electrical impulses, which the optic nerve (cranial nerve II) then transmits to the brain, where they are interpreted as the sensation of vision. The adult eyeball measures about 1 inch in diameter. Of its total surface area, only the anterior one-sixth is exposed. The remainder is recessed and protected by the bony orbit into which it fits. Anatomically, the eye is divided into three separate coats, or "tunics": the outer fibrous tunic, the middle vascular tunic, and the inner nervous tunic.

Fibrous Tunic

The fibrous tunic is the outer coat of the eyeball and is composed posteriorly of the sclera and anteriorly of the transparent cornea. The sclera, or "white of the eye," is leathery, white, and relatively thick and is composed of connective tissue. The cornea, or "window of the eye," is a continuation of the sclera and forms a transparent rounded bulge through which light passes.

Vascular Tunic

The vascular tunic is the eye's middle layer and is composed of three portions: the posterior choroid, the anterior ciliary body, and the iris. Collectively, these three structures are called the uveal tract. The choroid carries the blood vessels for the eyeball and contains a large amount of pigment, thus preventing internal reflection of light. Around the edge of the cornea the choroid forms the ciliary body, a thickened structure containing smooth muscle. A thin diaphragm of mostly connective tissue and smooth muscle fibers with an opening in the center is attached around the anterior margin of the ciliary body. The muscles of the ciliary body serve to change the shape of the lens, allowing changes in the focal distance of the eye. The third portion of the vascular tunic is known as the iris and contains the pigment responsible for the color of the eye. The hole in the iris is the pupil, which permits light to enter the eye. Some of the smooth muscle fibers in the iris encircle the pupil and others radiate from it. Contraction of the radial muscle dilates the pupil and contraction of the circular muscle constricts the pupil. By their control of pupil diameter, these muscles regulate the amount of light entering the eye.

Nervous Tunic

The third and innermost tunic of the eye, the retina, translates light waves into neural impulses. An extremely complex structure, the retina contains several layers of nerve cells and their processes, including two types of receptors, the rods for vision in dim light, and the cones for daytime or color vision. Cones are most densely concentrated in the central fovea, a small depression in the center of the macula lutea. The macula lutea, or yellow spot, is in the central part of the retina. The fovea is the area of sharpest vision because the highest concentration of cones is located there. Rods are absent from the fovea and macula, but they increase in density toward the periphery of the retina. The optic disk, where the optic nerve exits the eye, is a weak spot in the fundus (posterior wall) of the eye because it is not reinforced by the sclera. The optic disk is also called the blind spot because it lacks photoreceptors and light focused on it is not detected.

The interior of the eyeball contains an anterior and posterior chamber separated by the lens. The anterior chamber is filled with a watery fluid, called the aqueous humor, that maintains intraocular pressure, provides nourishment, and helps maintain the shape of the eyeball. The posterior chamber is filled with a jelly-like substance, called the vitreous humor, that maintains the spherical shape of the eye and supports the inner structures. Both substances are transparent, thus allowing light to pass through the eye to the retina (Figure 11-2).

The lens, located in the anterior chamber of the eye, is a transparent biconvex crystalline body enclosed in an elastic capsule held by suspensory ligaments. The shape of the lens changes to focus the image.

External Structures

The eyeball is protected from the external world by the eyelid, which contains a thin protective layer of epithelium, the conjunctiva (Figure 11-3). The conjunctiva covers the anterior portion of the eyeball and lines the eyelid. Projecting from the border of each eyelid is a row of eyelashes that protect the eye from foreign particles. The lacrimal gland produces a secretion called tears that contains a lysozyme, muramidase, to destroy pathogens.

COMMON DIAGNOSTIC TESTS

Commonly used diagnostic tests for clients with problems in hearing and vision are listed in Table 11-1.

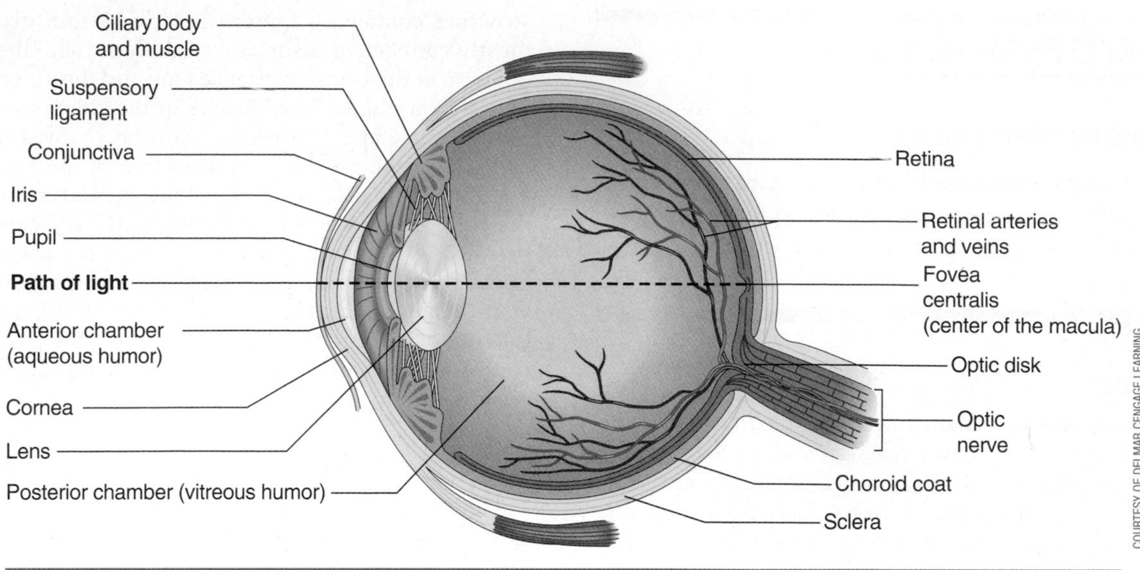

FIGURE 11-2 Lateral View of the Interior Eyeball

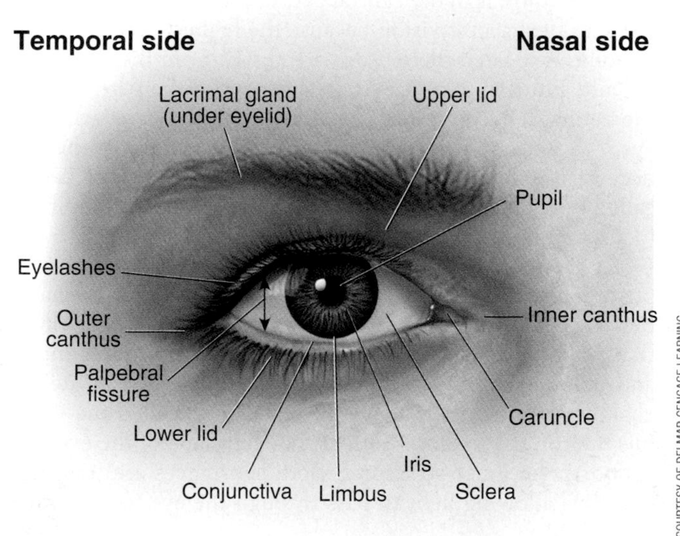

FIGURE 11-3 External View of the Right Eye

TABLE 11-1 Common Diagnostic Tests for Sensory Alterations

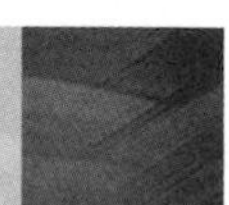

- Weber test (tuning fork)
- Rinne test (tuning fork)
- Audiometric testing (audiogram)
- Speech audiometry (Spondee threshold)
- Caloric test
- Brainstem auditory evoked response (ErA and BAER)
- Tympanometry
- Computed tomography (CT)
- Magnetic resonance imaging (MRI)
- Romberg test
- Otoscopic exam
- Past-point testing
- Color vision tests
- Tonometry
- Slit lamp examination
- Perimetry
- Visual acuity
- Electroretinogram (ERG)
- Ocular ultrasonography
- Ophthalmoscopic examination
- Orbital computerized tomography
- Fluoresce in angiography

SENSORY, PERCEPTUAL, AND COGNITIVE ALTERATIONS

An individual usually experiences discomfort and/or anxiety when subjected to a change in the type or amount of incoming stimuli. A person can become confused as a result of either overstimulation or understimulation. According to the individual's ability to process the stimuli, confusion (or disorientation) may occur. **Disorientation** is a mentally confused state in which the person's awareness of time, place, self, and/or situation is impaired. When awareness of these four factors is accurate, a person is said to be "oriented × 4."

A person admitted to a health-care agency experiences stimuli that are different from those usually encountered. A change in environment can overwhelm one's ability to perceive and interpret sensory input. As a result, the treatment setting becomes a stressor that negatively affects sensory, perceptual, and cognitive functions. If one or more of the factors just discussed causes an alteration in sensation, perception, or cognition, the client experiences problems with perceiving and interpreting stimuli. These problems are manifested by three types of alterations: sensory deficit, sensory deprivation, and sensory overload.

SENSORY DEFICIT

A **sensory deficit** is a change in the perception of sensory stimuli. This deficit affects all five senses. Examples of sensory deficit are vision and hearing losses such as those caused by cataracts, glaucoma, and presbycusis (steady loss of hearing acuity that occurs with aging).

The client's response to these losses usually depends on the time of onset and the severity of the condition. If the problem occurs suddenly and without warning, the client has difficulty adjusting to the loss of sensory and perceptual function. If these alterations occur gradually, the client may be able to accommodate the change and actually compensate for it by strengthening one or more of the other senses.

The effects of hospitalization or intensive medical treatments exacerbate the problems related to sensory deficit. For example, a client with acute hearing loss can feel alone and vulnerable. Clients with sensory deficit are at serious risk of experiencing either sensory deprivation or sensory overload.

SENSORY DEPRIVATION

Sensory deprivation is a state of reduced sensory input from the internal or external environment, manifested by alterations in sensory perception. Individuals experience sensory deprivation as a result of illness, trauma, or isolation. A person experiencing sensory deprivation misinterprets the limited stimuli with a resultant impairment of thoughts and feelings. Factors that contribute to sensory deprivation include:

- Visual or auditory impairments that limit or prohibit perception of stimuli
- Drugs that produce a sedative effect on the CNS and interfere with the interpretation of stimuli
- Trauma that results in brain damage and decreased cognitive function
- Isolation (either physical or social) that results in a nonstimulating environment

Some contributing factors (such as brain damage or blindness) result in chronic sensory deprivation. Other factors lead to acute, transient states of deprivation (such as receiving analgesic medications).

Individuals who are sensory-deprived may exhibit any of the following characteristics:

- Inability to concentrate
- Poor memory
- Impaired problem-solving ability
- Confusion
- Irritability
- Emotional lability (mood swings)
- Hallucinations
- Depression
- Boredom and apathy
- Drowsiness

SENSORY OVERLOAD

Sensory overload is a state of excessive and sustained multisensory stimulation manifested by behavior change and perceptual distortion. The individual experiencing this alteration is unable to process the amount or intensity of stimuli received. Factors contributing to sensory overload are:

- Pain originating from a heightened quality or quantity of internal stimuli
- Invasive procedures that result in an increased amount of external stimuli
- Activity-filled, busy environment that contributes to the amount of stimuli perceived
- Medications that stimulate the CNS and prohibit the client from ignoring selective stimuli
- Presence of strangers (both health care professionals and others) who contribute to the quantity of stimuli
- Diseases that affect the CNS and maximize the perception of stimuli

DISORDERS OF THE EAR

Disorders of the ear include impaired hearing, Ménière's disease, otosclerosis, acoustic neuroma, otitis media, otitis externa, and mastoiditis.

IMPAIRED HEARING

According to a study by Agrawal, Platz, and Niparko (2008), an estimated 55 million Americans have high-frequency hearing loss. Men were 5.5 times more likely to have hearing loss than women (Crosta, 2008). It can be seriously debilitating by limiting the ability to socialize and work, or respond to the telephone or alarms, yet relatively few individuals who experience impaired hearing actually seek help. Some may deny the problem and others may feel that a hearing aid is a sign of old age. Family members are often the first to be aware of a hearing deficit.

TYPES OF HEARING LOSS

Hearing loss is generally categorized in two ways: conductive and sensorineural. Mixed hearing loss, both conductive and

> **LIFE SPAN CONSIDERATIONS**
>
> **Effects of Aging**
>
> Sensory, perceptual, and cognitive function begin to diminish with aging. Decreased visual or auditory senses or impairments in memory are experienced. These changes can have a profound effect on a client's self-esteem and response to life.

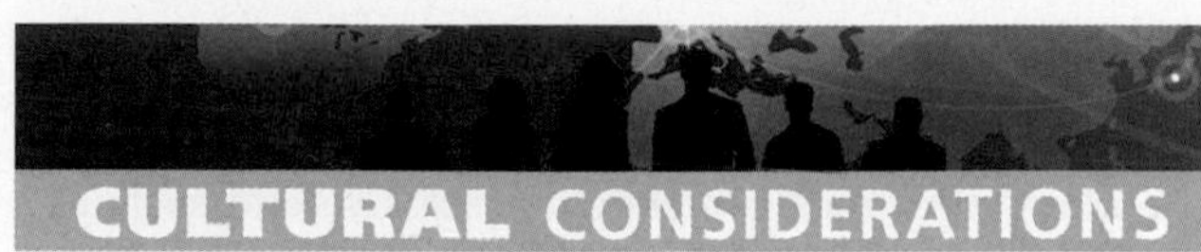

CULTURAL CONSIDERATIONS

Hearing Loss

Caucasian and Mexican-American men had the greatest incidence of both high-frequency hearing loss and hearing loss in both ears. African-American clients were 70% less likely to have hearing loss than Caucasian clients. Hearing loss is preventable by reducing risk factors and by screening for hearing loss in young adulthood, especially in Caucasian and Mexican-American men (Agrawal, Platz, & Niparko, 2008).

sensorineural, is possible but far less likely. Either may occur at birth (congenital), develop later in life, be genetic, or be caused by injury or trauma.

Conductive hearing loss indicates an inability of the sound waves to reach the inner ear. This is caused by cerumen buildup or blockage, perforated tympanic membrane, or fixation of one or all of the ossicles.

In **sensorineural hearing loss**, the inner ear or cochlear portion of cranial nerve VIII is abnormal or diseased. A tumor, infection, trauma, or exposure to loud noises may cause destruction of the nerve and result in sensorineural hearing loss.

Sensorineural hearing loss associated with aging is termed **presbycusis**. Higher frequency sounds such as women's voices become especially difficult to hear, and distinguishing words may be a problem. People with sensorineural hearing loss can be helped by hearing aids or cochlear implants (Ruben, 2007).

Behaviors Indicating Hearing Loss

A hearing impairment is a serious disorder that is often debilitating and embarrassing to the client. Hearing is part of the communication process, so the inability to hear may cause the person to do or say the wrong thing in response to a question or command. Persons with hearing impairment may withdraw from conversation or seem indifferent to their surroundings or to those around them.

Alterations in hearing are often manifested by changes in speech habits and patterns. Individuals with hearing impairments may not notice the changes in their own speech pattern until someone constantly asks them to repeat themselves or to speak clearly. Indifference and withdrawal are common behaviors in response to hearing loss. If left undiagnosed and untreated, the person may truly regress, become unhappy, lonely, and possibly even paranoid. Some individuals overcompensate for the hearing loss by becoming very loud and aggressive.

Research on hearing impairment has created many devices to aid speech and sound discrimination. Early diagnosis, treatment, and rehabilitation are essential to help hearing-impaired persons enjoy and appreciate the world in which they live.

Hearing Aids/Assistive Devices

Hearing aids today come in a variety of designs and sizes. Some are quite small and tinted to a person's skin color so as to be virtually unnoticeable. Some are worn in the ear, behind the ear, or are part of eyeglasses frames. Persons with bilateral hearing loss may need *binaural* (worn in both ears) hearing aids.

A hearing aid converts environmental sound and speech into electronic signals that are amplified and converted to acoustic signals. It makes speech and sound louder but not necessarily clearer. Depending on the extent of hearing impairment and preference, the client may need to experiment with several different types of hearing aids. In addition, speech therapy, lip reading, and auditory training may be necessary to help discriminate speech and develop better listening skills.

Many other assistive hearing devices are available for the hearing impaired. Numerous television programs are closed-caption. Advanced technology allows telecommunication through a device called the Telecommunication Device for the Deaf (TDD), also called TTY Typewriter, which sends a printed message onto a small screen. Both sender and receiver must have the typewriter/telephone device. Many hospitals have these to comply with ADA requirements.

Alarm clocks offer strobe lights or vibrators to awaken clients. State-of-the-art receivers give instant access to radio, television, computer, and stereos to enhance receiving and listening systems. For travelers, complete kits are available to provide ready access for smoke alarm, clock, TDD, and door-knock alert in hotels or inns.

Hearing guide dogs are also available. The animals are specially trained to meet the needs of the hearing impaired. At home, the dog responds to alarms, knocking on doors, and babies crying. In public, the dog takes a position between owner and a potential threat. Special identifiers, such as a collar for the dog and ID card for the owner, are available. The dogs are trained to go wherever their master goes, including restaurants, grocery stores, and on public transportation.

PROFESSIONAL TIP

Hearing Specialists

An audiologist evaluates hearing and determines the extent and type of hearing loss, and provides nonmedical treatment such as fitting hearing aids, advice about assistive listening devices, and communication/aural rehabilitative training. An otolaryngologist (ear, nose, and throat physician) provides medical evaluation of hearing disorders and medical and surgical interventions. A hearing aid specialist is licensed to dispense hearing aids but is not a medical doctor.

Medical–Surgical Management

Medical

The type of hearing loss and underlying etiology determines the best medical or surgical management. The client undergoes a complete physical examination as well as thorough diagnostic hearing tests to determine the etiology. The client and doctor together decide on the best course of therapy.

Surgical

The cochlear implant is a possible treatment for persons with profound deafness. In this procedure, a receiver/stimulator is implanted in the skull and a group of electrodes are planted in front of the round window in the inner ear. The client wears a microphone near the ear that picks up and translates sound into electrical signals. These signals are then transmitted to the brain via the cochlear implant and cranial nerve VIII.

Nursing Management

If the client uses a sign language interpreter, arrange for one to assist with communication. Writing notes, using a TDD, or a computer may be helpful. Approach the client and elicit the client's attention by waving. Make sure all personnel know the client is hearing impaired as well as the client's preferred method of communication. The publication *Pictograms for Hospital Communication* is available from the U.S. Department of Justice.

NURSING PROCESS

Assessment

Subjective Data

Ask the client to describe the initial onset of symptoms and possible familial traits, recent infections of the ears, nose, or upper respiratory system. Determine recent trauma and past surgery as well as medical history such as diabetes, heart disease, or cancer. Ask about allergies to food, drugs, or environmental factors, associated symptoms such as **tinnitus** (ringing sound in the ear), **vertigo** (dizziness), nausea, and vomiting. The client's work history may reveal exposure to loud noises.

Objective Data

Listen closely to the client and note any deterioration of speech, slurring, or dropping of word endings. Document current and recent medications used.

Inspect the outer ear for abnormalities, lesions, or cerumen. Palpate the mastoid process, neck, jaw, and temporal regions of the head for swelling or tenderness to touch. Note the degree of hearing loss as reported by the client and compare it to the diagnostic tests such as the speech audiogram. The client's perception of hearing loss may be significantly different from the diagnostic findings.

A nursing diagnosis for a client with impaired hearing is:

NURSING DIAGNOSES	PLANNING/OUTCOMES	NURSING INTERVENTIONS
Social Isolation related to hearing impairment	The client will participate in conversations and other social situations.	Take time to engage client in conversation. Make sure you have the client's attention and be at eye level.
		Speak slowly and distinctly.
		Give the client time to respond.
		Provide the client and family members written information regarding the availability, variety, and quality of assistive hearing devices.
		Encourage client to participate in social situations.

Evaluation: Evaluate each outcome to determine how it has been met by the client.

MÉNIÈRE'S DISEASE

Ménière's disease, also known as endolymphatic hydrops, is a state of hearing loss characterized by tinnitus and vertigo. Although the exact etiology is unknown, it is thought to be an excessive accumulation of endolymph in the cochlear duct and possible leakage of endolymph into the perilymph caused by increased capillary permeability. Mixing of the two fluids chemically alters the homeostasis of the perilymph and endolymph and could be responsible for the symptoms associated with Ménière's disease.

The major symptoms are the classic triad of vertigo, tinnitus, and unilateral fluctuating hearing loss. The vertigo is often associated with nausea and vomiting. Tinnitus may either be a preceding aura or occur simultaneously with the vertigo. Initially, tinnitus is intermittent, but as the disease progresses, it may be a constant, low-pitched roaring sound. The fluctuating, unilateral hearing loss becomes more profound with each attack.

The symptoms are frequently at their worst during the first attack, which may last from a few minutes to six hours. **Nystagmus**, repetitive and involuntary movement of the eyeballs, and diaphoresis may occur during an attack. Subsequent attacks are less severe, but over time may involve both ears and cause permanent bilateral hearing loss. Clients report many different precipitating events, such as stress, weather changes, menstruation, or pregnancy, and various dietary influences, including caffeine, alcohol, and salt. Smoking has also been implicated.

Medical–Surgical Management

Medical

Medical management is the preferred treatment and most helpful to 80% to 85% of persons with this disease. Diagnosis is not difficult and is usually made based on the client's report of symptoms. Diagnosis may also be confirmed with caloric stimulation (although this test is primarily conducted on comatose clients) and magnetic resonance imaging to rule out a tumor. Medical management is symptomatic.

Surgical

Surgical intervention is needed only when the attacks are frequent and debilitating, or when the disease severely affects the quality of life and the ability for self-care. Surgical treatment includes endolymphatic, subarachnoid shunt placement to drain excessive endolymph. With this procedure, hearing is preserved in 60% to 70% of the clients. With a vestibular neurectomy, the vestibular portion of cranial nerve VIII is severed; hearing is preserved in 90% of clients having this procedure. In surgical destruction of the labyrinth, hearing is destroyed but the incapacitating vertigo is completely relieved.

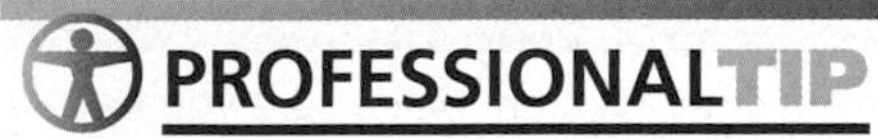

Assisting the Hearing-Impaired Client

- Speak slowly and distinctly after getting the client's attention.
- Face the client and sit or stand to be at eye level with the client.
- Use short, simple sentences and give the client time to respond. Repeat or rephrase if necessary.
- Use written materials when possible to communicate information.
- Keep a notepad and pen or pencil available to write down new or unfamiliar words and concepts.
- If sign language is the client's preferred method of communication, locate a person who understands sign language.
- If the client wears a hearing aid, make sure that the battery is functional, it is turned on, and is adjusted to a comfortable level.

Pharmacological

Several medications are useful to help control the symptoms, such as antihistamines, antiemetics, benzodiazepines, diuretics, tranquilizers, vasoactive agents, and oral niacin. The medications are prescribed for long-term use or at the onset of symptoms. Because the cause of Ménière's disease is unknown, there is no cure.

Diet

Dietary interventions include strict salt restriction and avoidance of those foods or beverages that precipitate or aggravate an attack. Examples are beer, wine, soda, salty food or snacks, chocolate, and caffeinated coffee and tea.

Activity

Activity is not limited except during or after an attack, when clients require prolonged bed rest and restriction of activities that are unsafe, such as driving or operating heavy equipment.

Nursing Management

Advise client against reading and use of glaring lights. Instruct client to avoid sudden position changes and have assistance when getting out of bed or ambulating. Keep side rails up and the call light within the client's reach.

NURSING PROCESS

Assessment

Subjective Data

The history begins with identifying significant contributory data. Ask the client to describe the initial onset of symptoms including, but not limited to, the classic triad of tinnitus, vertigo, and fluctuating unilateral hearing loss.

Relate questions to recent viral illness; upper respiratory infections; past medical, surgical, and dental history; and any problems related to the neck and face. Document food, drug, or environmental allergies. Record current or recent long-term medications. Identify the client's occupation and hobbies that contribute to hearing loss.

Objective Data

A thorough physical examination includes looking at the ear for abnormalities, lesions and cerumen blockage, or unusual drainage. Palpate the neck, jaw, and mastoid process for possible lymph node enlargement and tenderness. The nurse assists with the otologic examination as needed. Audiologic testing determines unilateral or bilateral hearing loss.

Nursing diagnoses for a client with Ménière's disease include the following:

NURSING DIAGNOSES	PLANNING/OUTCOMES	NURSING INTERVENTIONS
Activity Intolerance related to severe vertigo	The client will be able to tolerate activities of daily living.	Provide adequate periods of bed rest. Provide assistance with ambulation and encourage increased activity as tolerated. Keep the room dim and quiet when possible. Avoid jarring the bed and caution client to avoid sudden movements. Administer antiemetic before symptoms become too severe.
Deficient Knowledge related to abrupt onset and unknown progression of the disease	The client will verbalize understanding of the disease process and potential precipitating factors and how to manage or control the symptoms.	Assess the client's current knowledge of the disease process. Review the disease process and underlying etiology of Ménière's disease with the client. Ask the client to identify possible precipitating factors such as stress or dietary habits. Discuss health promotion programs for stress management and healthy cooking classes. Suggest consultations with dietary and social services. Review follow-up appointments, medications, dietary management, activity, and rest parameters. Evaluate client's readiness to discuss progressive hearing loss and current assistive hearing devices available.
Risk for Injury related to vertigo	The client will not fall or be injured because of vertigo.	Keep side rails up. Teach client to move or turn slowly. Instruct client to sit or lie down when vertigo occurs. Reiterate need to call for assistance when ambulating. Keep call bell within client's reach. Administer medications for vertigo prior to worsening of symptoms. Avoid glaring, bright lights.

Evaluation: Evaluate each outcome to determine how it has been met by the client.

CRITICAL THINKING

Hearing Impaired

How can nurses assist the hearing impaired during a hospitalization?

OTOSCLEROSIS

Otosclerosis, the most common conductive hearing loss, is secondary to a pathologic change of the bones in the middle ear. The exact cause is unknown. The ossicles are normally hard, but over time and without warning, the bone becomes softened, spongy, highly vascular, and partially or totally fixed. This fixation reduces or prevents transmission of source waves to inner ear fluids. Although all three bones may be affected, the stapes, which must vibrate on the oval window in order to transmit sound waves, is most commonly afflicted.

Otosclerosis is more common in adults, more often in women, and it is familial in some cases. The primary clinical manifestations are subtle changes in hearing and low-pitched tinnitus. It becomes more difficult to distinguish a whisper, or to hear in crowded places or understand conversation. Individuals affected by otosclerosis often blame others for speaking too softly or mumbling. Frequently, rather than asking others to speak up or to repeat themselves, the person will be irritable and withdrawn.

Diagnostic testing begins with the Weber and Rinne tuning fork tests. In addition, audiometric testing should be performed. Schwartz's sign, a pink blush, is seen on otoscopic examination. Tympanometry shows stiffness in the sound conduction system.

Medical–Surgical Management

Medical

Treatment for otosclerosis is limited to three options. The individual may choose to do nothing and obtain periodic audiometry to evaluate progression of the disease. The second choice is to use a hearing aid, and the third choice is surgical management with an outpatient procedure known as a stapedectomy.

Surgical

A stapedectomy is the preferred surgical technique for improving hearing loss caused by otosclerosis. A stapedectomy is done under local or general anesthesia and routinely requires a surgical incision in the posterior ear canal, removal of the stapes, and implantation of a plastic prosthesis. Laser stapedectomy is performed through the ear canal without an incision. The stapes tendon is vaporized, chards are removed with delicate micro instruments, and an opening is made allowing the surgeon to implant a prosthetic piston. This restores normal vibration against the inner ear.

Nursing Management

Postoperatively, instruct the client to turn or move slowly, not to blow the nose for 10 days, to avoid lifting for 1 month, and if sneezing occurs, to keep the mouth open. Administer antibiotics as ordered. Advise the client that hearing is decreased for 3 to 4 weeks until gel-foam packing dissolves.

NURSING PROCESS

Assessment

Subjective Data

A careful history discovers possible hereditary traits or acquired disease. Ask about recent infections of the ears, nose, or upper respiratory system, and also about past surgery, trauma, or other illnesses such as diabetes, heart disease, or cancer. Identify associated symptoms, such as dizziness, tinnitus, vertigo, and nausea.

Note allergies to foods, drugs, or any environmental factors, such as exposure to loud noises. Record current and recent medications, especially those known to be ototoxic.

Objective Data

Objective data include a thorough physical examination. Inspect the outer ear for abnormalities, lesions, or impacted ear wax and palpate the mastoid process, neck, jaw, and temporal regions of the head for pain or swelling. Assess the degree of hearing loss. The client may experience vomiting.

Nursing diagnoses for the client with otosclerosis include the following:

NURSING DIAGNOSES	PLANNING/OUTCOMES	NURSING INTERVENTIONS
Anxiety related to decrease or loss in hearing	The client will show evidence of reduced anxiety and verbalize understanding of the disease process and treatment regimen.	Encourage the client to explore feelings of anxiety and to ask questions to clarify concerns. Provide honest and realistic feedback. Collaborate with the physician to provide thorough and clear explanations of the disease process, treatment options, and anticipated results.
*Risk for **Injury*** related to vertigo	The client will not fall or be injured because of vertigo.	Keep side rails up. Reiterate need to call for assistance when ambulating and keep call bell within client's reach. Instruct the client to move or turn slowly. Administer medications for vertigo prior to worsening of symptoms. Keep room well lit when client is ambulating.
*Deficient **Knowledge*** related to activities after surgery	The client will demonstrate the ability to change dressing correctly and verbalize knowledge of self-care and follow-up.	Teach client how and when to perform dressing change and have client demonstrate the procedure. Instruct client to avoid pressure changes (such as flying in an unpressurized aircraft), avoid heavy lifting (60 lbs) for 1 month, avoid nose blowing for 10 days, and if sneezing occurs, keep mouth open. Advise client to keep water out of the ear and keep the ear exposed to air as much as possible for one month. There will be some drainage which is initially red, then pink, and then brownish. Tell client to report any greenish, yellowish, or foul-smelling drainage.

Nursing diagnoses for the client with otosclerosis include the following: (Continued)

NURSING DIAGNOSES	PLANNING/OUTCOMES	NURSING INTERVENTIONS
		Instruct client to take all antibiotics as prescribed and complete the full course of treatment. Advise client there should be very little pain or discomfort but if there is, take prescribed analgesics and notify doctor if pain is prolonged or intense. Warn client that hearing is decreased for 3 to 4 weeks after surgery until gel-foam packing dissolves. Inform client that audiometric testing will be conducted 1 month after surgery. Instruct client to schedule an appointment with the physician in 1 month but call physician if uncontrolled pain is experienced or a malodorous, greenish discharge comes from the ear.

Evaluation: Evaluate each outcome to determine how it has been met by the client.

ACOUSTIC NEUROMA

Acoustic neuroma is a slow-growing and usually benign tumor of the vestibular portion of the inner ear (cranial nerve VIII). Detection at the onset of symptoms is essential and is accomplished with magnetic resonance imaging. Presenting symptoms of dizziness, tinnitus, and hearing loss are common to many dysfunctions of the ear, and the possibility of acoustic neuroma must not be overlooked.

Clients who present with dizziness, tinnitus, and hearing loss have a complete workup for auditory and vestibular (balance) function. Facial weakness is caused by compression of the tumor on cranial nerve VII. Cranial nerve V may also be affected as the tumor grows, causing paresthesia of the face and loss of the corneal reflex. Large neuromas cause increased intracranial pressure, papilledema, vomiting, and headache.

Medical–Surgical Management

Treatment is almost always surgical excision of the tumor. Although antihistamines may reduce the dizziness, pharmacologic treatment is only temporary until diagnostic tests are completed and surgery is planned.

Nursing Management

Assist client to express feelings about progressive hearing loss and the changes in activities of daily living, employment, and quality of life issues. Note the family's feelings and ability to cope. Perform postoperative care as ordered.

NURSING PROCESS

Assessment

Subjective Data

Obtain through the client history signs and symptoms and all contributing data.

Objective Data

Obtain with the physical examination a complete cranial nerve evaluation performed by the physician or audiologist to determine the extent of cranial nerve involvement.

A nursing diagnosis for a client with acoustic neuroma is:

NURSING DIAGNOSES	PLANNING/OUTCOMES	NURSING INTERVENTIONS
*Anticipatory **Grieving*** related to diminished quality of life, loss of ability for self-care, or possible loss of life	The client will express feelings of grief and demonstrate adaptive coping mechanisms.	Assist the client to express feelings about progressive hearing loss and changes in activities of daily living, employment, and quality of life issues. Collaborate with physician and other members of the health care team to provide thorough and clear explanations of the disease process, treatment options, and anticipated results.

(Continues)

A nursing diagnosis for a client with acoustic neuroma is: (Continued)

NURSING DIAGNOSES	PLANNING/OUTCOMES	NURSING INTERVENTIONS
		Observe the client's coping styles. Support those that the client finds helpful and explore other coping mechanisms that may prove useful in time (e.g., hobbies and other diversional activities, prayer, reading, and so on).
		Include the family in all interventions that the client desires. Examine the family's feelings and ability to cope.
		Consult social services, pastoral care, or other hospital and community resources when appropriate.

Evaluation: Evaluate each outcome to determine how it has been met by the client.

OTITIS MEDIA

Otitis media is an inflammation of the middle ear and a common cause of conductive hearing loss, although usually temporary. Symptoms include ear pain, fever, redness of auricle and ear canal, and sometimes enlarged lymph nodes over the mastoid process, parotids, and upper neck. Otitis media occurs more frequently in children than in adults.

Fluid accumulates behind the eardrum because of blockage of the eustachian tube. This is secondary to an upper respiratory infection, allergies, or acute bacterial infection. On physical examination, the tympanic membrane is retracted, normal, or bulging. A pneumatic otoscope allows the practitioner to blow soft puffs of air against the tympanic membrane to assess movement. A stiff, nonmoving, or bulging tympanic membrane indicates inflammation or fluid accumulation in the middle ear (Figure 11-4A-C). Visualization of the normal landmarks may be obscured. The Rinne tuning fork test and audiometry confirm a conductive hearing loss.

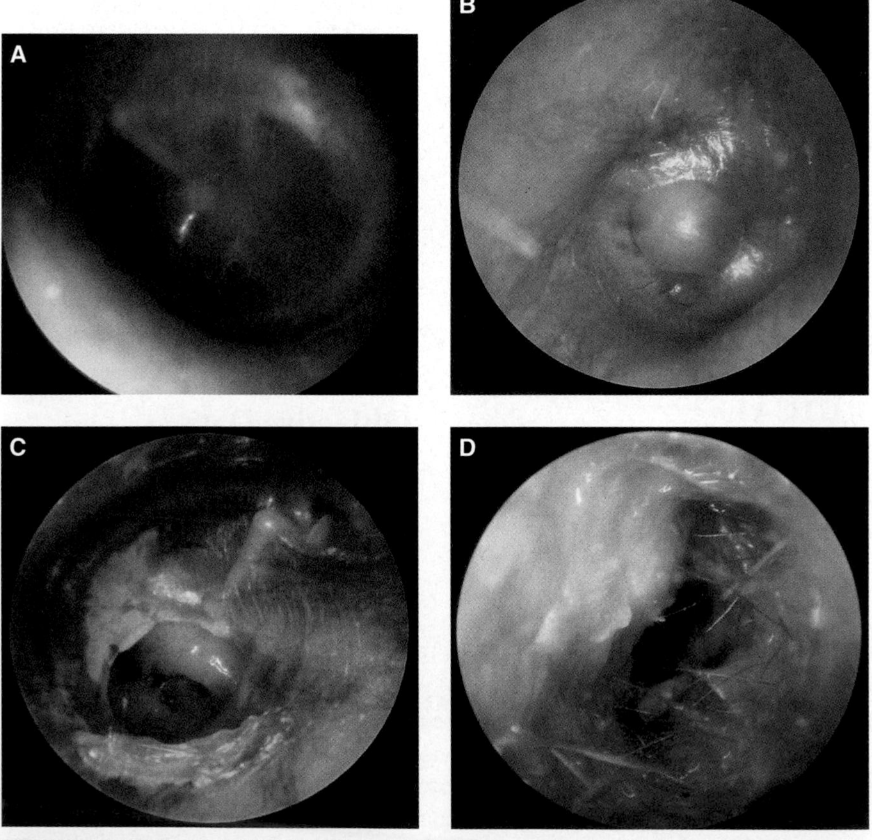

FIGURE 11-4 *A,* **Normal Tympanic Membrane;** *B,* **Bulging Tympanic Membrane;** *C,* **Tympanic Membrane Perforation;** *D,* **Acute Otitis Externa** *(Images A and C courtesy of Dr. Andrew B. Silva, Pediatric Otolaryngology; images B and D courtesy of Bruce Black, MD, Brisbane, Australia.)*

CRITICAL THINKING

Hearing Impairment

What modifications would need to be made in the life of a person who could suddenly no longer hear?

MEDICAL–SURGICAL MANAGEMENT

Medical

Topical heat and systemic analgesics may be used to control pain. The client should lie on the affected side to facilitate drainage.

Surgical

Surgical management may be necessary for diagnostic or therapeutic reasons. A myringotomy may be performed, in which an incision is made in the eardrum and fluid is aspirated. A polyethylene tube may be placed in the eardrum to equalize pressure and allow drainage of fluid.

A tympanoplasty may be needed if the tympanic membrane is ruptured. If there is a large tympanic membrane perforation, the malleus, which is connected to the tympanic membrane, or other ossicles may be damaged. Ossicular chain reconstruction typically refers to the removal of the actual bones and replacement with a plastic prosthesis. The prosthesis and the tympanic membrane reconstruction often result in a significant improvement in hearing.

Pharmacological

Medications used include decongestants, such as pseudoephedrine hydrochloride (Sudafed); antihistamines, such as diphenhydramine hydrochloride (Benadryl); and systemic antibiotics, such as ampicillin (Omnipen).

Activity

Activity is not restricted unless surgical management is indicated.

NURSING MANAGEMENT

After myringotomy, maintain drainage flow. Sterile cotton may be loosely placed in the external ear to absorb drainage. Change cotton whenever it is damp. Perform hand hygiene before and after ear care. Monitor vital signs. Warn client against blowing nose or getting ear wet when bathing. Encourage client to complete prescribed antibiotics.

NURSING PROCESS

ASSESSMENT

Subjective Data

Ask about the onset, duration, and severity of pain and what home remedies have been used. Hearing loss and/or tinnitus and a deep throbbing pain in the ear may be reported.

Objective Data

A watery or yellow discharge may be seen. It may have a foul odor. The client may have a fever.

A nursing diagnosis for a client with otitis media is:

NURSING DIAGNOSES	PLANNING/OUTCOMES	NURSING INTERVENTIONS
*Acute **Pain*** related to inflammation in the middle ear	The client will experience pain relief.	Administer antibiotics and analgesics as ordered. Teach client and family the importance of administering medications as ordered and to complete full course of prescription. Apply heating pad, set on low, for 20 minutes every 2 hours. Do not use on small children. Teach client if pain is unrelieved in 48 hours, to contact physician.

Evaluation: Evaluate each outcome to determine how it has been met by the client.

OTITIS EXTERNA

Otitis externa, or "swimmer's ear," typically involves a bacterial infection of the external ear canal skin. The canal skin becomes red and edematous. If the swelling is severe enough, it will block the ear passage and cause a mild conductive hearing loss (Figure 11-4D). Also, in most cases, there is a discharge. If the discharge is copious and the canal size is constricted, a mild conductive hearing loss results.

MASTOIDITIS

Mastoiditis (inflammation of the mastoid) is most often the direct result of chronic or recurrent bacterial otitis media. The recurrent infection may find its way into the bone and structures surrounding the middle ear and, if left untreated, causes severe damage, sensorineural deafness, facial weakness, brain abscess, and meningitis. Symptoms include earache, fever, headache, and malaise. Antibiotics are given for a trial period. If symptoms do not resolve, surgical intervention such as mastoidectomy or meatoplasty may be necessary.

DISORDERS OF THE EYE

Disorders of the eye include cataracts, glaucoma, retinal detachment, infections, refractive errors, injuries, impaired vision, and macular degeneration.

CATARACTS

A cataract is a disorder that causes the lens or its capsule to lose its transparency and/or become opaque (Figure 11-5). The lens is normally clear and transparent and allows light to pass through to the retina. As clouding develops, visual impairment occurs. Cataracts usually affect both eyes; however, the degree of visual impairment is often different in each eye.

Cataracts are typically associated with aging; however, they may be congenital, caused by severe eye injury, or secondary to certain systemic diseases, such as metabolic problems (diabetes mellitus) and chronic eye disease (uveitis). Ophthalmoscopic examination is the primary method of evaluation.

MEDICAL–SURGICAL MANAGEMENT

Surgical

The only treatment for a cataract is surgical removal of the lens; however, the mere finding of a cataract is not an indication for surgery. Surgery is indicated when significant vision loss has occurred. The lens are removed by the intracapsular or extracapsular approach. During the intracapsular cataract extraction, the ophthalmologist removes the lens within its capsule.

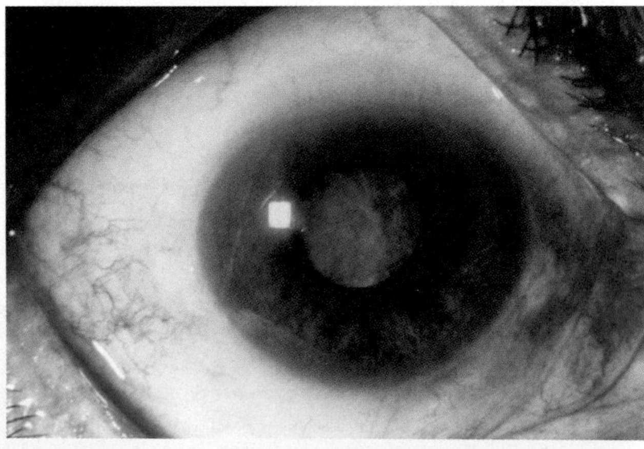

FIGURE 11-5 A cataract results in the loss of transparency of the lens of the eye. (*Courtesy of the National Eye Institute, Bethesda, MD.*)

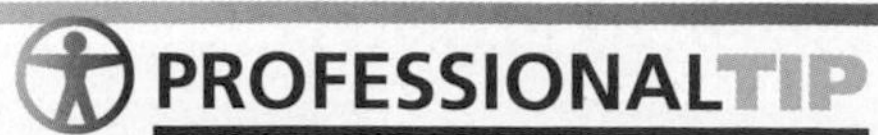

Eye Specialists

An ophthalmologist is a medical doctor who specializes in the diagnosis and treatment, medical and surgical, of diseases of the eye, visual disorders, and eye injuries. An optometrist is a doctor of optometry and is licensed to examine, diagnose, manage and treat vision problems, diseases, and other abnormalities of the eyes and related structures.

Extracapsular cataract extraction is the procedure most commonly used (Figure 11-6). The ophthalmologist removes the anterior portion of the capsule and then expresses, or removes, the lens. An intraocular lens (IOL) is generally implanted. Glasses or special contact lenses also are used.

Most eye surgery is done on an outpatient basis under local anesthesia. General anesthesia is used at the client's request and for clients who are extremely anxious, deaf, or mentally retarded. A tranquilizer such as diazepam (Valium) or midazolam (Versed) is often given to reduce anxiety when receiving injections on the face and around the eye.

Preoperatively, the client can receive several types of eye medications to prepare the eye for surgery: mydriatic (makes pupil dilate) and cycloplegic (paralyzes ciliary muscle) eyedrops, antibiotic eyedrops as a prophylaxis against infection, and an intravenous infusion of an agent

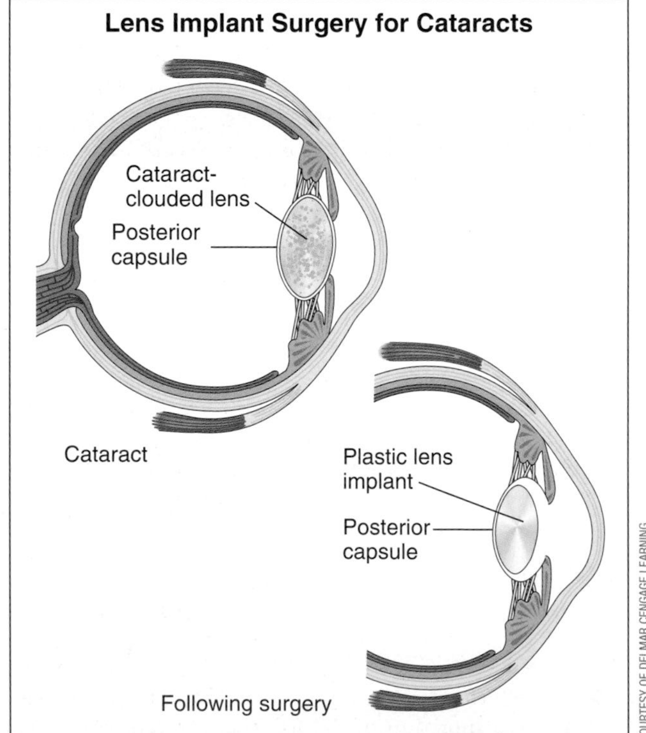

FIGURE 11-6 To correct cataracts with an extracapsular extraction, the lens is removed, the posterior lens capsule is left intact, and a plastic IOL is placed.

to lower intraocular pressure (mannitol or a carbonic anhydrase inhibitor).

After the anesthesia wears off, the client is discharged. The client is instructed to have a driver available for the trip home. Driving is restricted for a few days.

Postoperatively, the client has a patch over the eye. The patch is removed and reapplied on the first postoperative day, when miotic (makes pupil contract) eye drops are begun. Mild discomfort and scratchiness are expected. Atropine sulfate eyedrops and cold compresses are ordered to relieve these discomforts.

Nursing Management

Assist with ambulation because depth perception has changed. Maintain eye patch on affected eye. Advise client to sleep with eye patch on as ordered. Teach client or family to administer eyedrops and ointments. Client should avoid heavy lifting, straining during defecation, and vigorous coughing and sneezing. Dark glasses will relieve glare. Encourage client to keep all follow-up appointments.

NURSING PROCESS

Assessment

Subjective Data

A general medical history as well as a history of symptoms is obtained. Symptoms may include haziness, cloudiness, blurred vision, double vision, altered color perception, and glare when looking at lights, especially with night driving. Fear of losing one's eyesight is very devastating. There is often a great deal of anxiety when the client seeks an eye examination.

Objective Data

Upon inspection of the eye, the usual black pupil appears clouded, progressing to a milky white appearance, which is a characteristic finding of a mature cataract and indicates significant vision loss.

Nursing diagnoses for a client with cataracts include the following:

NURSING DIAGNOSES	PLANNING/OUTCOMES	NURSING INTERVENTIONS
Disturbed ***S****ensory Perception* (Visual) related to ocular lens opacity	The client will demonstrate improved ability to process visual stimuli and communicate visual limitations.	Assess and document baseline visual acuity. Elicit functional description of what the client can and cannot see.
Risk for ***I****njury* related to difficulty in processing visual images and altered depth perception	The client will avoid activities associated with increased potential for injury.	Teach the client to change position slowly. Teach the client to avoid reaching for objects to maintain stability when ambulating, as depth perception is altered.
Impaired ***H****ome Maintenance* related to age, limited vision or activity restrictions imposed by surgery	The client will perform self-care activities in home environment.	Discuss the client's ability to meet self-care needs and activities of daily living. Evaluate how the client's current functional abilities are affected by activity restrictions and postoperative care needs. Help the client decide on a realistic site for postoperative care needs.

Evaluation: Evaluate each outcome to determine how it has been met by the client.

GLAUCOMA

Glaucoma is a disorder characterized by an abnormally high pressure of fluid inside the eyeball (intraocular pressure, IOP). The aqueous humor does not return into the bloodstream through the canal of Schlemm as quickly as it is formed. The fluid accumulates and, by compressing the lens into the vitreous humor, puts pressure on the neurons of the retina. If the pressure continues over a long period, it destroys the neurons and brings about blindness.

There are two primary forms of glaucoma: open-angle glaucoma and closed-angle glaucoma. In open-angle glaucoma (chronic simple glaucoma) there is a gradual rise in IOP, a slowly progressive loss of peripheral vision, and, if not controlled, a late loss of central vision and ultimate blindness. This is the most prevalent form of glaucoma and is usually bilateral. Closed-angle glaucoma (acute glaucoma) is characterized by attacks of suddenly increased IOP, exhibited clinically by a bulging iris, which is an emergency situation. Closed-angle glaucoma is usually unilateral with severe pain and loss of vision caused by acute obstruction of aqueous humor drainage within the eye.

Secondary glaucoma results from ocular or systemic disorders that elevate the IOP. These disorders indirectly disrupt the activity of the structures involved in circulation and/or reabsorption of aqueous humor. This can happen suddenly and without warning.

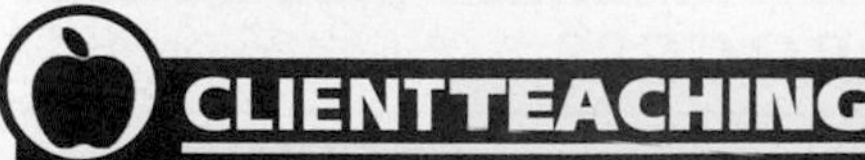

CLIENT TEACHING

Glaucoma Care

- Continue the use of eye medications as ordered.
- Continue to receive medical supervision for observation of intraocular pressure to ensure control of the disorder.
- Avoid exertion, stooping, heavy lifting, or wearing constrictive clothing because these actions increase intra-ocular pressure.

MEDICAL–SURGICAL MANAGEMENT

Medical

Medical management for glaucoma is focused on drug therapy, and the main objective is to reduce intraocular pressure. Two mechanisms for reducing this pressure are (1) physically constricting the pupil so that the ciliary muscle is contracted, which allows better circulation of the aqueous humor to the site of absorption, and (2) inhibiting the production of aqueous humor.

Surgical

Surgical intervention to facilitate drainage of the aqueous humor is called an iridectomy. A surgical incision is made through the cornea to remove a portion of the iris to facilitate aqueous drainage.

A laser also is used to treat various eye disorders. In open-angle glaucoma, a laser is used to create multiple scars around the trabecular meshwork (a supporting or anchoring strand that allows increased outflow of aqueous humor), thereby reducing intraocular pressure. In closed-angle glaucoma, laser energy is used to create a hole in the periphery of the iris, creating an opening between the anterior and posterior chambers for aqueous drainage.

Pharmacological

Drugs that enhance pupillary constriction are commonly used to treat glaucoma. Miotics and cholinesterase inhibitors such as pilocarpine hydrochloride (Isopto Carpine), carbachol (Carbacel), and demecarium bromide (Humorsol) are frequently used.

Beta-adrenergics such as timolol maleate (Timoptic Solution) are the drugs of choice for decreasing IOP. When used as eyedrops, beta-adrenergics reduce aqueous humor production without pupil constriction.

Carbonic anhydrase inhibitors, such as acetazolamide (Diamox), reduce production of aqueous humor to help maintain a lowered IOP. Side effects reported are numbness, weakness, tingling of extremities, and rashes. Adrenergics such as epinephrine bitartrate (Epitrate) also reduce aqueous humor production. Osmotic agents such as mannitol and glycerin (Osmoglyn) are administered systemically to the client with closed-angle glaucoma in an emergency as an effort to decrease IOP. The high osmolarity of these agents draws fluid into the intravascular space, which lowers the IOP.

NURSING MANAGEMENT

Administer medications as ordered. Stress client compliance with prescribed medication therapy. Encourage glaucoma screening for all persons older than age 35, especially if there is a family history of glaucoma.

NURSING PROCESS

ASSESSMENT

Subjective Data

Obtain a history, noting the presence of risk factors: positive family history (believed to be linked in open-angle glaucoma), eye tumor, intraocular hemorrhage, intraocular inflammation, or contusion of the eye from trauma during cataract surgery.

Symptoms of open-angle glaucoma include gradual loss of peripheral vision, eye pain, difficulty adjusting to darkness, halos around lights, and an inability to detect color. For closed-angle glaucoma, symptoms include sudden onset of severe pain in the eye often accompanied by headache, nausea, vomiting, malaise, rainbow halos around lights, and blurred vision.

Objective Data

Assessment reveals acute increased intraocular pressure (21 to 32 mm Hg) as measured with a tonometer (normal range is 12 to 22 mm Hg).

A nursing diagnosis for a client with glaucoma is:

NURSING DIAGNOSES	PLANNING/OUTCOMES	NURSING INTERVENTIONS
Acute ***Pain*** related to closed-angle glaucoma	The client will verbalize relief from discomfort.	Administer prescribed ophthalmic agent for glaucoma. Notify physician of the following: hypotension, urinary output less than 240 mL for 8 hours, no relief in eye pain within 30 minutes of drug therapy, and continual diminishing visual acuity. Monitor blood pressure, pulse, and respiration every 4 hours if not receiving osmotic agent intravenously and every 2 hours if receiving intravenous osmotic agent.

A nursing diagnosis for a client with glaucoma is: (Continued)

NURSING DIAGNOSES	PLANNING/OUTCOMES	NURSING INTERVENTIONS
		Monitor degree of eye pain every 30 minutes.
		Monitor intake and output every 8 hours while receiving intravenous osmotic agent.
		Monitor visual acuity before each instillation of prescribed ophthalmic agent by asking if objects are clear or blurred and if the client can read printed material held at arm's length.
		Remind the client that miotics may cause blurred vision for 1 to 2 hours after use and that adaptation to dark environments is difficult because of the pupillary constriction.

Evaluation: Evaluate each outcome to determine how it has been met by the client.

RETINAL DETACHMENT

In retinal detachment, the retina separates from the choroid (Figure 11-7). Partial separation becomes complete, if untreated, with the subsequent total loss of vision. A tear or hole in the retina can extend the separation as vitreous humor seeps through the opening and separates the retina from the choroid. The cause of retinal detachment is from severe trauma to the eye or from intraocular disorders such as cataract extraction, perforating injuries, or severe **myopia** (nearsightedness). This condition is painless because there are no pain receptors in the retina.

MEDICAL–SURGICAL MANAGEMENT

Medical

Early corrective intervention to reattach the retina uses one of several techniques. Two procedures are used to create an inflammatory reaction that, once healing and scarring occur, results in the retina reattaching to the choroid. Freezing (cryoplexy) is an intensely cold probe applied to the scleral surface directly over the hole in the retina. Laser photocoagulation also seals tears or holes in the retina.

Surgical

A surgical procedure called scleral buckling is sometimes used. This operation reduces the scleral surface and allows contact between the choroid and retina.

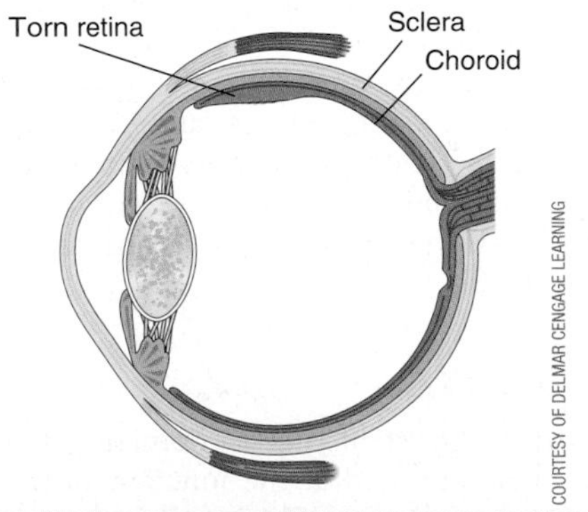

FIGURE 11-7 Retinal Detachment

Pneumatic retinopexy is used for an uncomplicated detachment. A small amount of fluid is withdrawn from the anterior chamber and an expandable gas is injected into the posterior chamber. The gas pushes against the retinal tear and seals it off. The fluid under the retinal tear is absorbed and the gas is released from the eye over several weeks (Mayo Clinic, 2008).

Sometimes when the surgeon cannot see the retinal tear because of vitreous cloudiness or retinal scarring that prevents a pneumatic retinopexy or scleral buckling, sections of the vitreous are removed (vitrectomy). Delicate instruments are inserted into the eye through incisions in the sclera. The surgeon removes scar tissue from the vitreous and infuses a salt solution into the eye to maintain the normal pressure and shape. A scleral buckling may be performed after the vitrectomy, and the posterior chamber is filled with air, gas, or silicone oil to hold the retina against the inside of the eye (Mayo Clinic, 2008).

Pharmacological

Cycloplegic-mydriatic and antiinfective eyedrops are often ordered following the attachment procedure.

Activity

Bed rest and a patch on one or both eyes restricts activity. If air is injected into the vitreous humor, the client either lies prone or sits forward with the unaffected eye upward.

NURSING MANAGEMENT

Explain surgery routines. *Preoperative*: Level of activity—ocular rest, which includes bilateral eye patching and bed rest to facilitate settling of the retina and prevent detachment from worsening. The affected eye is maximally dilated before surgery to permit adequate visualization of the fundus. *Intraoperative*: Client must lie still during surgery or give surgeon warning if needs to cough or change position. Face covered with drapes. Air and oxygen provided. Monitoring, including frequent blood pressure measurements. *Postoperative*: Positioning (supine with a small pillow under the head), bilateral eye patches, activity restrictions, and need to call for assistance with ambulation until stable and vision is adequate.

NURSING PROCESS

ASSESSMENT

Subjective Data

Obtain a medical history for presence of causative factors: trauma, recent cataract surgery, eye tumor, severe myopia, uveitis. The client may describe sudden flashes of light (photopsia), floating spots (caused by bleeding into the vitreous cavity), blurred vision that becomes progressively worse, or complaints of a sensation of a veil in the line of sight.

Objective Data

Ophthalmoscopic examination visualizes the detachment. An ultrasound is ordered if blood restricts ophthalmoscopic vision of the retina.

Nursing diagnoses for a client with retinal detachment include the following:

NURSING DIAGNOSES	PLANNING/OUTCOMES	NURSING INTERVENTIONS
Anxiety related to sensory visual impairment and lack of understanding about treatment	The client will demonstrate reduction of emotional stress, fear, and depression; and an acceptance of surgery	Assess degree and duration of visual impairment. Encourage conversation to determine client's concerns, feelings, and level of understanding. Answer questions, offer support, and assist client to devise methods for coping. Orient client to new surroundings. Explain interventions clearly. Announce yourself with each interaction; interpret unfamiliar sounds; use touch to assist with verbal communication. Encourage to carry out ADLs as ability allows. Order finger foods for those who cannot see well enough or do not have the coping skills to use implements. Encourage participation of family or significant others in client care. Encourage participation in social and diversional activities as allowed (visitor, radio, audio tapes, television, crafts, games).
Risk for Injury related to visual impairment or knowledge deficit	The client will not have injury caused by visual impairment.	Assist client when able to ambulate postoperatively until stable and has adequate vision or coping skills (remember that clients with bilateral eye patches are unable to see). Assist client in arranging environment and do not rearrange furnishings without reorienting client. Discuss importance of wearing metal shield or glasses as ordered. Apply no pressure to the affected eye. Use proper procedure to administer eye medications.

Evaluation: Evaluate each outcome to determine how it has been met by the client.

INFECTIONS

Infections of the eye include keratitis, stye, chalazion, and conjunctivitis.

KERATITIS

Keratitis is inflammation of the cornea that may be caused by infection, irritation, injury, or allergies. Symptoms associated with keratitis include severe eye pain, red watering eye, photophobia, sometimes reduced vision, and sometimes rash (e.g., herpes simplex, herpes zoster, or rosacea).

Treatment of keratitis includes optical anesthetics to relieve pain and mydriatics to dilate the pupil. Dark glasses should be worn to relieve the photophobia. Antibiotic solutions are prescribed for the specific type of infection.

STYE

A **stye** is also referred to as a hordeolum. It is a pustular inflammation of an eyelash follicle or sebaceous gland on the lid margin commonly caused by staphylococcal organisms. Symptoms include pain, redness, and swelling of a specific area of the eyelid. Treatment consists of warm compresses and topical antibiotic ointments. More severe cases may require incision and drainage. Once the pus drains, the pain is relieved and healing begins.

CHALAZION

A **chalazion** is a cyst of the meibomian glands, which are sebaceous glands located at the junction of the conjunctiva and inner eyelid margins (Figure 11-8A). The hard cyst is filled with fatty material from the chronically obstructed

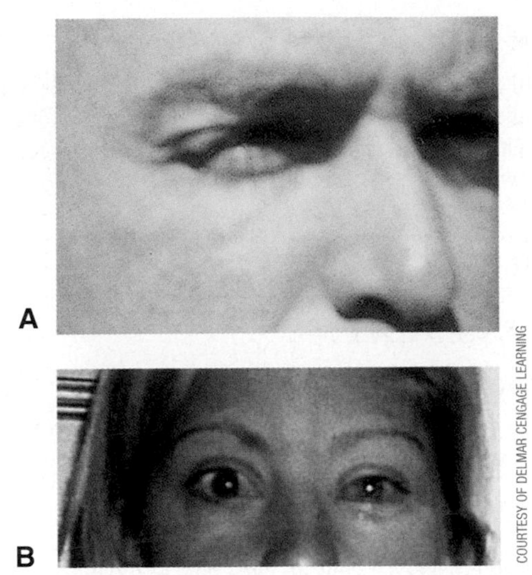

FIGURE 11-8 *A*, Chalazion; *B*, Bacterial Conjunctivitis

meibomian glands. The inherent feature of a chalazion is painless localized swelling that develops over a period of weeks. Treatment usually involves surgical excision if the cyst is large, becomes infected, or interferes with vision or closure of the eyelids. The cyst remains when the inflammation subsides.

CONJUNCTIVITIS (PINK EYE)

Conjunctivitis is an inflammation of the conjunctiva (a membrane that lines the inside of the eyelids and covers the cornea) that results from invasion by bacterial, viral, or rickettsial organisms, allergens, or irritants (Figure 11-8B). Symptoms include burning and itching of eyes, discharge, swelling, pain, and redness. Treatment consists of applying warm compresses using saline or boric acid solution and instilling antibiotic or antiviral ointments. When caused by allergens, treatment includes avoiding the allergen, taking antihistamines, or being desensitized.

Conjunctivitis is contagious. Proper hand hygiene is essential for the nurse and client. Gloves are worn when applying compresses or instilling ointment. The client's linen is disinfected to prevent spread of the infection.

REFRACTIVE ERRORS

Refraction is the deflection or bending of light rays when they pass from a medium of one density to a medium of another density. In the case of the eye, light waves pass through the air (less dense) into the fluids of the eye (more dense) and are brought to focus on the retina.

Refractive errors result in changes in visual acuity or vision that is not 20/20. Refractive errors include **myopia** (nearsightedness), **hyperopia** (farsightedness), **astigmatism** (asymmetric focus of light rays on the retina), **presbyopia** (inability of the lens to change curvature in order to focus on near objects), and **strabismus** (inability of the eyes to focus in the same direction) (Figure 11-9).

With myopia, parallel light rays come to focus in front of the retina because the refractive system is too strong or the eyeball is elongated. Near vision is normal, but distant vision is poor.

With hyperopia, parallel light rays come to focus behind the retina because the refractive system is too weak or the eyeball is flattened. Vision beyond 20 feet is normal, but near vision is poor. Figure 11-10 illustrates where light rays focus for myopia and hyperopia.

Astigmatism is a visual defect caused by unequal curvatures of the refractive surfaces of the eye. Light rays from a point do not come to focus on the retina, resulting in visual distortion.

Presbyopia is the loss of elasticity of the lens of the eye caused by aging that causes the near point of vision to recede.

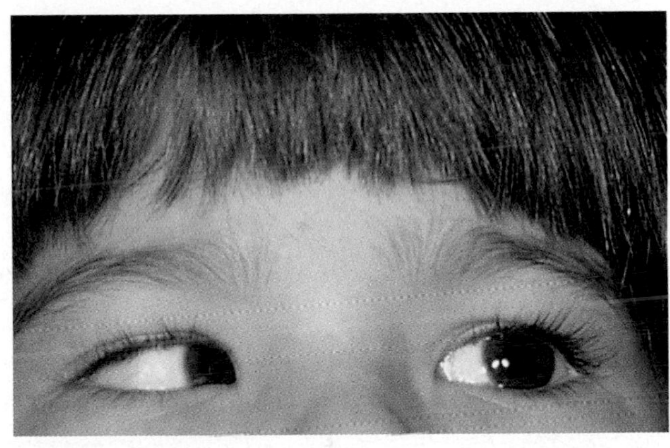

FIGURE 11-9 Strabismus (*Courtesy of the Armed Forces Institute of Pathology*)

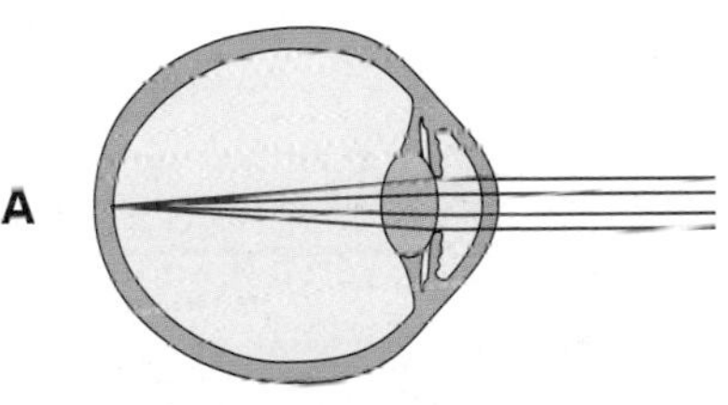

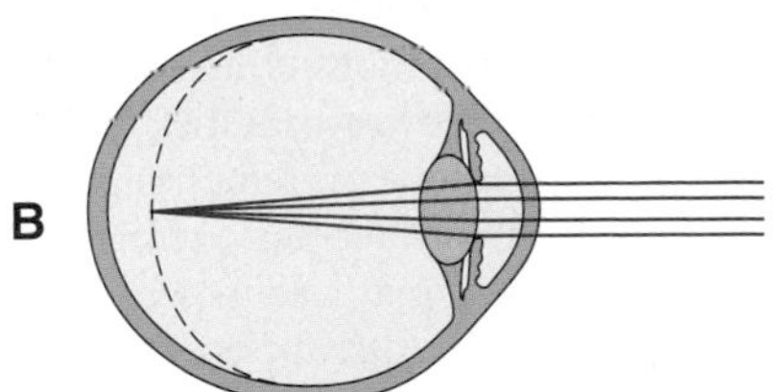

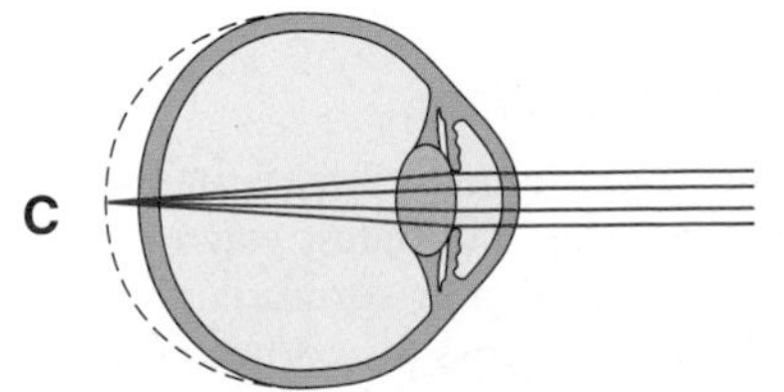

FIGURE 11-10 Refraction; *A*, Normal Eye; *B*, Myopia; *C*, Hyperopia

The eye loses the ability to accommodate to near objects but remains accommodated for far objects.

Strabismus occurs when one eye is constantly deviated to the side.

Medical–Surgical Management

Medical

Refractory errors are corrected by prescription glasses or contact lenses. The corrective lenses bend light rays to compensate for a client's refractive error.

Surgical

Radial keratotomy is a surgical procedure used to correct myopia and astigmatism. Under local anesthesia, incisions that resemble the spokes of a wheel are made in the cornea. After the cuts are made, pressure in the anterior chamber of the eye reshapes the cornea to a normal or near-normal curvature. Both LASIK (laser-assisted in-situ keratomileusis) and PRK (photo-refractive keratectomy) use laser to correct nearsightedness and astigmatism.

Nursing Management

Reassure client that refraction testing is painless and that dilating eyedrops are instilled. Advise client that it takes time to adjust to new glasses and not to wear old glasses after getting new ones.

NURSING PROCESS

Assessment

Subjective Data

Obtain a general medical history as well as a history of symptoms. Symptoms include blurred vision, headache, or eye fatigue.

Objective Data

The client is asked to view an eye chart while lenses of different strengths are systematically placed in front of the eye. The client is asked if the lenses sharpen or blur vision. The power or strength of the lens necessary to permit focusing of the image on the retina is expressed in measurements called diopters.

A nursing diagnosis for a client with refractive errors is:

NURSING DIAGNOSES	PLANNING/OUTCOMES	NURSING INTERVENTIONS
Anxiety related to impaired vision and having to wear glasses or contact lenses	The client will accept wearing glasses or contact lenses.	Allow client to discuss impact of wearing glasses or contact lenses. Encourage client to wear the glasses or contact lenses as prescribed.

Evaluation: Evaluate each outcome to determine how it has been met by the client.

INJURY

Injury to the eye or periorbital area results from a variety of things, such as chemical sprays, tree branches, slingshots, BB guns, flying debris from lawn mowers, and fireworks. Both children and adults are susceptible to eye injuries, and the importance of protecting the eyes cannot be overemphasized. Injuries to the eyes require immediate attention by an ophthalmologist. Even a few hours' delay in treatment may lead to permanent damage.

Corneal abrasion is the disruption of cells and the loss of the superficial epithelium. The outer surface is easily separated from the underlying layers and is injured or destroyed by exposure (lack of moisture), chemical irritants that dissolve in the protective tear film, and abrasion from foreign bodies.

SAFETY

Avoiding Eye Injury

The eyes are easily protected from injury by wearing protective goggles when performing tasks that are potentially hazardous to the eyes. Those who wear contact lenses should follow the manufacturer's recommendations for wearing them during certain activities, such as swimming or when sleeping.

Foreign Bodies

Foreign bodies in the conjunctiva or on the cornea cause excessive tearing and redness. The safest way to remove a foreign object from the conjunctiva or cornea is to flush sterile saline starting from the sclera across the cornea (Primary Care Ophthalmology, 2004). Foreign bodies often become embedded in the conjunctiva under the upper eyelid. The lid must be everted and the client instructed to look up to facilitate inspection and removal. If the particle is not located and removed, sterile fluorescein drops or strips are instilled to visualize minute foreign bodies that are not readily visible with the naked eye.

Chemical Burns

Emergency treatment of chemical burns to the conjunctiva or cornea includes immediate lavage of the eye with tap water and referral to an emergency room or ophthalmologist. In the emergency room, a specially made lid speculum is placed directly on the eyeball and connected to a minimum of 1 liter of isotonic saline solution for irrigation. A topical anesthetic may be instilled to minimize pain during irrigation. No attempt is made to neutralize the chemical because the heat generated by the chemical reaction may cause further injury. Both eyes are then patched to allow more comfort.

IMPAIRED VISION

The term *blindness* evokes an image of total darkness and is used for many legal purposes when central visual acuity is 20/200 or less with corrective lenses, in the better eye. Those who have visual acuity between 20/70 and 20/200 in the better eye, with the use of glasses, are often referred to as partially sighted.

The aids that follow are designed to make the most of the available vision (those in italics can also be used by persons who are blind): magnifying glasses; hand and stand magnifiers; telescopes; large-print books, newspapers, magazines; talking books; *Braille* books; closed-circuit television, which produces highly magnified images; *tactually marked watches and clocks; tactually modified tabletop games*; enlarged telephone dials, kitchen implements, tools, medication devices; talking clocks, timers, scales, calculators, computers; *text scanner, which converts text to audio mode or Braille*; speech synthesizer; flashlight eye sonar devices; canes, laser canes, and seeing eye dogs.

MACULAR DEGENERATION

Macular degeneration is atrophy or deterioration of the macula, the point on the retina where light rays meet as they are focused by the cornea and lens of the eye. The person loses central vision but still has peripheral vision.

The most common form of macular degeneration is associated with the aging process and is called age-related macular degeneration. Other forms of this disorder include exudative (wet) macular degeneration (sudden growth of new blood vessels in the area of the macula) and injury, infection, or inflammation that damages the macula.

MEDICAL–SURGICAL MANAGEMENT

Medical

The treatment of age-related macular degeneration is geared toward assisting the client to maximize the use of the remaining vision. The loss of central vision interferes with the client's ability to read, write, recognize safety hazards, and drive.

Management of clients with exudative macular degeneration is geared toward halting the initiating process and identifying further changes in visual perception. Fluid and blood may resorb in a small percentage of clients with exudative degeneration. Laser therapy to seal the leaking blood vessels in or near the macula may also limit the extent of the damage.

> **CRITICAL THINKING**
>
> **Visual Impairment**
>
> What modifications have to be made in the life of a person who can no longer see?

NURSING MANAGEMENT

Provide a safe environment. Announce your presence when entering the client's room and let the client know when you are leaving. Make sure all personnel know of the client's decreased vision. Respond to the client's call light quickly.

NURSING PROCESS

ASSESSMENT

Subjective Data

Obtain a general medical history and a history of symptoms. Symptoms include blurred vision, disturbance in color vision (colors become dim), difficulty in reading or doing close work, distortion of objects (especially those with lines), and an empty area within the central field of vision.

Objective Data

Note coping mechanisms such as turning the head to use peripheral vision.

A nursing diagnosis for the client with macular degeneration is:

NURSING DIAGNOSES	PLANNING/OUTCOMES	NURSING INTERVENTIONS
Disturbed **S**ensory *Perception (Visual)* related to macular degeneration	The client will discuss the impact of vision loss on lifestyle and use adaptive measures.	Allow client to express feelings about vision loss such as its impact on lifestyle. Convey a willingness to listen, but do not pressure client to talk.
		Provide a safe environment by removing excess furniture or equipment from client's surroundings.
		Orient client to surroundings and show how to use call light.
		Provide reality orientation if client is confused or disoriented.
		Always introduce yourself or announce your presence upon entering the client's room; let client know when you are leaving.
		Provide sensory stimulation by using tactile, auditory, and gustatory stimuli to help compensate for vision loss.
		Suggest large-print books, talking books, audiotapes, or radio as preferred by client.
		Give clear, concise explanations of treatments and procedures but avoid information overload.

(*Continues*)

A nursing diagnosis for the client with macular degeneration is: (Continued)

NURSING DIAGNOSES	PLANNING/OUTCOMES	NURSING INTERVENTIONS
		Make sure that health care personnel are aware of client's vision loss. Record information on the client's chart or post in room.
		Respond to call light quickly.
		Provide continuity by assigning same staff members to care for client when possible.
		Refer to appropriate community resources.

Evaluation: Evaluate each outcome to determine how it has been met by the client.

SAMPLE NURSING CARE PLAN

The Client with Macular Degeneration

J.R. is a 60-year-old high school Latin teacher. He describes having blurred vision in both eyes with a gradual loss of vision in only the right eye. He has trouble reading and is afraid to drive because he can no longer recognize safety hazards. He denies having pain. He also relates having fallen several times recently at home while going up and down the stairs. The family practitioner referred him to an ophthalmologist, who diagnosed J.R. as having macular degeneration in the right eye.

NURSING DIAGNOSIS 1 *Disturbed **S**ensory Perception (Visual)* related to macular degeneration as evidenced by his inability to recognize safety hazards when driving

Nursing Outcomes Classification (NOC)
Vision Compensation Behavior

Nursing Interventions Classification (NIC)
Environmental Management
Communication Enhancement: Visual Deficit

PLANNING/OUTCOMES	INTERVENTION	RATIONALE
J.R. will discuss impact of vision loss on lifestyle.	Encourage J.R. to express feelings about vision loss.	Aids in the acceptance of vision loss.
	Convey a willingness to listen, and discuss J.R.'s current ability to meet self-care needs and activities of daily living.	Determines J.R.'s awareness of his limitations.
	Educate J.R. in alternative ways of coping with vision loss; care of such adaptive devices as eyeglasses, magnifying glass, and contact lenses.	Client will be better able to cope with vision loss.
	Refer to appropriate community resources.	Helps J.R. and his family cope better with his vision loss.

EVALUATION

J.R. discussed the effects of vision loss on his lifestyle and contacted a local agency that provides assistance to the visually impaired.

NURSING DIAGNOSIS 2 *Risk for **I**njury* related to difficulty in processing visual images and altered depth perception as evidenced by recent falls

Nursing Outcomes Classification (NOC)
Risk Control: Visual Impairment

Nursing Interventions Classification (NIC)
Teaching: Disease Process
Fall Prevention

SAMPLE NURSING CARE PLAN (Continued)

PLANNING/OUTCOMES	NURSING INTERVENTIONS	RATIONALE
J.R. will not experience injury or visual compromise resulting from a fall.	Advise J.R. that depth perception is changed with macular degeneration.	Information promotes understanding.
	Teach J.R. to avoid reaching for objects for stability when ambulating.	Objects may not be where they are perceived. Excessive reaching alters the center of gravity which can precipitate a fall.
	Advise J.R. to go up and down steps one at a time.	Enhances the sense of balance.

EVALUATION

J.R. has not fallen in 2 weeks.

NURSING DIAGNOSIS

Impaired Home Maintenance related to limited vision, as evidenced by recent falls at home.

NOC: Family Functioning
NIC: Home Maintenance Assistance, Environmental Management: Safety

CLIENT GOAL

J.R. will develop a plan for self-care in the desired living environment.

NURSING INTERVENTIONS	SCIENTIFIC RATIONALES
1. Inform J.R. about required self-care activities: personal care, eyedrop instillation, activities permitted, activity restrictions, medications, and how to monitor for complications.	1. Knowing what self-care activities are needed helps J.R. plan for his care at home.
2. Assist J.R. to determine which activities will require assistance.	2. Helps J.R. to plan for his care at home.
3. Evaluate sources of assistance: friends/family, home health care (skilled nursing care), or home-care aids.	3. Determines availability of assistance.
4. Critique the safety of J.R.'s home: location of telephone, emergency plan, presence of loose rugs or carpets.	4. Changes are made to make J. R.'s home safer.

EVALUATION

Has J.R. developed a plan to care for himself at home?

OTHER SENSES

Other senses include taste, smell, and touch.

TASTE

The sense of taste (gustation) serves as a protector from rotten or putrid food and provides delightful sensations of creamy chocolate, crunchy carrots, chewy taffy, and fruitful pies. Taste sensors are most efficient at room temperature and respond only to substances in solution. The taste buds are located in four areas of the tongue that sense sweet, salt, bitter, and sour (as shown in Figure 11-11).

Taste sensations are altered secondary to neurological disorders or trauma. Assess clients who complain of food not "tasting good" for possible causes, including dietary habits, medication use, smoking and caffeine use, as well as olfactory disturbances. The sense of taste works very closely with the sense of smell for identification of the taste sensations.

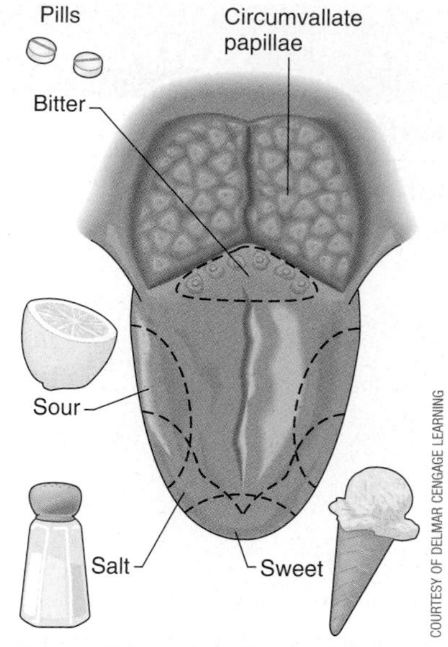

FIGURE 11-11 Taste Regions of the Tongue

SMELL

The sense of smell (olfaction) also serves as a guardian from danger. An individual's nose warns of impending danger from gas leaks, smoke, fires, rancid meat or fish, and sour dairy products. Body odors and halitosis are clues for personal hygiene and dental care.

Disorders of the olfactory sense often go unnoticed. Tests such as the University of Pennsylvania Smell Identification Test (UPSIT) allow self-testing of smelling deficiencies. Early identification of the loss of the sense of smell offers clues to alterations in dietary habits, weight loss or gain, anorexia, malnourishment, and changes in daily habits, such as bathing and brushing teeth. The receptors for the sense of smell are located in the roof of the nasal cavity. If these cells are damaged, the sense of smell is impaired. The body cannot regenerate the olfactory cells.

TOUCH

The sense of touch (tactile) includes sensations pertaining to the skin. The tactile receptors are located throughout the integumentary system. Cutaneous sensations of touch, pressure, vibration, cold, heat, and pain are examples. Clients who are unable to sense temperature variations are taught cautionary measures when applying heat or cold therapies, preparing bath water, cooking, or exposing self to hot or cold climates and environmental temperatures.

Clients with reduced or loss of tactile sensation risk injury when their condition confines them to bed. They are unable to sense pressure on bony prominences or the need to change position. The nurse's role in reducing or preventing impairment of skin integrity is crucial. Timely positioning, securing tubes or devices away from the client's body, and using products to minimize skin breakdown are a few of the interventions vital to excellent client care.

LIFE SPAN CONSIDERATIONS

Aging and Taste Sensation

The ability to taste sweetness remains as one ages, but the ability to taste bitterness declines.

CASE STUDY

K.R. is a 34-year-old nurse who was diagnosed with a right ear hearing impairment during a routine physical examination. She admitted to her doctor that she noticed she would only use her left ear to talk on the phone and that she had particular difficulty hearing her family or friends in a crowded restaurant or other public settings. She also noted that her husband asked her why she played the television so loud, yet if he turned it down to his normal hearing level, she could not hear it clearly. Her physician ordered an audiogram, which showed a conductive hearing loss of 40% secondary to otosclerosis. Hearing in her left ear was normal.

K.R.'s doctor gave her three medical treatment options:

1. Do nothing and monitor her hearing impairment by audiogram every 6 months. If it were to worsen, other options would be considered.
2. Be fitted with a hearing aid.
3. Have a surgical procedure to correct the hearing loss.

CASE STUDY (Continued)

K.R. agreed to have surgery. She thought she would be too self-conscious to wear a hearing aid, after all she was only 34, but she simply could not ignore the problem by doing nothing. K.R. was scheduled for same-day surgery.

The following questions will guide your development of a nursing care plan for the case study.

1. How is a conductive hearing loss differentiated from a sensorineural hearing loss?
2. What does an audiogram reveal? What special things should K.R. know before she has the audiogram?
3. Describe the surgical procedure that will most likely be used to correct the conductive hearing loss.
4. What will the nurse teach K.R. before her surgery about the procedure and expected postoperative course?
5. List four individualized nursing diagnoses and expected outcomes for K.R., and nursing interventions for each diagnosis.
6. Describe the expected discharge instructions that K.R. must know related to diet, medications, activity restrictions, and follow-up care.

SUMMARY

- Hearing loss is conductive, sensorineural, or a combination of the two. It may also be congenital.
- Ménière's disease is a result of excessive accumulation of endolymph, causing severe vertigo, dizziness, and hearing loss. Treatment is primarily symptomatic.
- Otosclerosis is a conductive hearing loss that is treated medically with the use of a hearing aid or surgically with a stapedectomy
- Otitis media is inflammation of the middle ear. Treatment usually includes antibiotics, decongestants, and possibly a myringotomy.
- Cataract surgery is indicated when significant vision loss has occurred.
- Untreated retinal detachment results in total loss of vision.
- Many resources are available for the hearing impaired through community and national agencies.
- The senses of taste, smell, and touch are essential to our enjoyment of life and serve to protect us from danger or harm.

REVIEW QUESTIONS

1. In a conductive hearing loss:
   1. the endolymph may cross the capillary membrane and mix with the perilymph, resulting in severe vertigo.
   2. the ossicles of the middle ear fracture, resulting in a tear of the eighth cranial nerve.
   3. sound waves are not transmitted through the ear canal to inner ear fluid.
   4. a tumor in the inner ear blocks the flow of fluid through the bony and membranous labyrinths.
2. A possible nursing diagnosis for a client with Ménière's disease is:
   1. activity intolerance related to impaired hearing.
   2. knowledge deficit related to surgical shunt placement to drain excessive endolymph.
   3. communication, impaired, verbal, related to tinnitus.
   4. risk for injury related to vertigo.
3. Chemical burns of the eye are initially treated with:
   1. local anesthetics and antibacterial drops for 24 to 36 hours.
   2. hot compresses applied at 15-minute intervals.
   3. flushing of the lids, conjunctiva, and cornea with water.
   4. cleansing of the conjunctiva with a small, cotton-tipped applicator.
4. A clinical symptom of a detached retina is:
   1. an increase in tearing.
   2. an area of vague vision.
   3. momentary flashes of light.
   4. pain in the eye.
5. Macular degeneration is characterized by:
   1. purulent periorbital drainage.
   2. pupil dilation.
   3. loss of central vision.
   4. ptosis (droopy lid).
6. A client presents to the emergency room with symptoms of seeing several floaters with flashes of light in the affected eye and having blurred vision. The nurse recognizes these as symptoms of:
   1. macular degeneration, and it is not an emergency.
   2. glaucoma, and it is not an emergency.
   3. a cataract, and it is not an emergency.
   4. a retinal detachment, and it is an emergency.
7. A teenager arrives at the clinic with an inflamed conjunctiva of the right eye that burns and itches, is swollen and reddened, and has a discharge. The nursing interventions include: (Select all that apply.)
   1. washing his hands after examining the client's eye.
   2. teaching the client to wash her hands frequently and especially after touching her eye.
   3. teaching the client that conjunctivitis is contagious.

4. instilling an antibiotic in the eye without wearing gloves because he is going to wash his hands after the instillation.
5. teaching the client to wash linens to prevent spreading the conjunctivitis to others.
6. teaching the client to apply ice to the affected eye.

8. Nursing interventions for a client with glaucoma include: (Select all that apply.)
   1. applying warm compresses and topical antibiotic ointment.
   2. administering prescribed ophthalmic agent.
   3. teaching the client to avoid reaching for objects to maintain stability when ambulating, as depth perception is altered.
   4. monitoring blood pressure, pulse, and respiration every 4 hours if not receiving osmotic agent intravenously.
   5. reminding the client that miotics may cause blurred vision for 1 to 2 hours after use.
   6. immediately lavaging the eye with saline solution.
9. The nurse completed teaching postoperative stapedectomy care to a client. The nurse knows the client needs some reteaching when he states:
   1. "I will turn and move slowly."
   2. "I will sneeze with my mouth closed."
   3. "I will report any greenish, yellowish, or foul-smelling drainage."
   4. "I will keep water out of my ear and keep it exposed to air as much as possible."
10. Which of the following is an appropriate nursing diagnosis for a gradual hearing impaired client who is 80- years-old?
    1. *Activity Intolerance* related to severe vertigo.
    2. *Deficit **K**nowledge* related to abrupt onset and unknown progression of the disease.
    3. *Social **I**solation* related to hearing impairment.
    4. *Acute **P**ain* related to inflammation in the middle ear.

REFERENCES/SUGGESTED READINGS

Agrawal, Y., Platz, E., & Niparko, J. (2008). Prevalence of hearing loss and differences by demographic characteristics among US adults: Data from the national health and nutrition examination survey, 1999–2004. *Archives of Internal Medicine, 168*(14), pp. 1522–1530.

American Speech-Language-Hearing Association. (2002). Types of hearing loss. Retrieved December 27, 2004 from www.asha.org/hearing/disorders/types/cfm

Barnie, D. (2002). Restoring vision in older patients. *RN, 65*(1), 30–35.

Bulechek, G., Butcher, H., McCloskey, J., & Dochterman, J., eds. (2008). *Nursing Interventions Classification (NIC)* (5th ed.). St. Louis, MO: Mosby/Elsevier.

Crosta, P. (2008). Hearing loss affects millions of US adults. Medical News Today. Retrieved August 3, 2008 from http:www/medicalnewstoday.com/printerfriendlynews.php?newsid=116360

Cavendish, R. (1998). Clinical snapshot: Hearing loss. *AJN, 98*(8), 50–51.

Dana, R. (1998, January 27). Dry eye syndrome. *Health News 1*, 3.

Daniels, R. (2009). *Delmar's guide to laboratory and diagnostic tests* (2nd ed). Clifton Park, NY: Delmar Cengage Learning.

Estes, M. (2010). *Health assessment & physical examination* (4th ed.). Clifton Park, NY: Delmar Cengage Learning.

Kearney, K. (1997). Retinal detachment. *AJN, 97*(8), 50.

Lucas, L., & Matthews-Flint, L. (2001). Sound advice about hearing aids. *Nursing2001, 31*(2), 59–61.

McConnell, E. (2001a). Instilling ear drops. *Nursing2001, 31*(4), 17.

McConnell, E. (2001b). Myths & Facts . . . about macular degeneration. *Nursing2001, 31*(8), 30.

McConnell, E. (2002). How to converse with a hearing-impaired patient. *Nursing2002, 32*(8), 20.

Mayo Clinic. (2008). Retinal detachment. Retrieved August 3, 2009 from http://mayoclinic.com/health/retinal-detachment/DS00254/METHOD=print&DSECTION=all

Moorhead, S., Johnson, M., Maas, M., & Swanson, E. (2007). *Nursing Outcomes Classification (NOC)* (4th ed). St. Louis, MO: Elsevier - Health Sciences Division.

National Institute on Deafness and Other Communication Disorders. (2002). Cochlear implants. Retrieved October 4, 2004 from www.nidcd.nih.gov/health/pubs_hb/coch.htm

North American Nursing Diagnosis Association International. (2010). *NANDA-I nursing diagnoses: Definitions and classification 2009–2011.* Ames, IA: Wiley-Blackwell.

Primary Care Ophthalmology. (2004). Foreign body removal. Retrieved August 3, 2009 from http://www.med.uottawa.ca/procedures/slamp/body_removal.htm

Ralph, S. & Taylor, C. (2007). *Sparks and Taylor's nursing diagnosis reference manual* (7th ed.). Philadelphia: Lippincott Williams & Wilkins.

Ramponi, D. (2000). Go with the flow during an eye emergency. *Nursing2000, 30*(8), 54–56.

Ramponi, D. (2001). Contact lens removal. *Nursing2001, 31*(8), 56–57.

Ruben, R. (2007). Hearing loss and deafness. Retrieved August 3, 2009 from http://www.merck.com/mmhe/sec19/ch218/ch218a.html

Shelp, S. (1997). Your patient is deaf, now what? *RN, 60*(2), 37–40.

Smeltzer, S., Bare, B., Hinkle, J., & Cheever, K. (2008). *Brunner and Suddarth's textbook of medical surgical nursing* (11th ed.). Philadelphia: Lippincott Williams & Wilkins.

Sommer, S., & Sommer, N. (2002). When your patient is hearing impaired. *RN, 65*(12), 28–32.

Spencer, J. (1998, February 17). Coping with hearing loss. *Health News 2*, 1–2.

Spratto, G., & Woods, A. (2008). *2009 Delmar's (nurses drug handbook).* Clifton Park, NY: Delmar Cengage Learning.

Tupper, S. (1999). When the inner ear is out of balance. *RN, 62*(11), 36–40.

Walbecker, J. (1997). Knowing the signs. *RN, 60*(2), 40–41.

RESOURCES

Alexander Graham Bell Association for the Deaf, http://www.agbell.org

American Academy of Ophthalmology Head and Neck Surgery, http://www.aao.org

American Academy of Otolaryngology, http://www.entnet.org

American Council of the Blind, http://acb.org

American Foundation for the Blind, Inc., http://www.afb.org

American Speech-Language-Hearing Association, http://www.asha.org

American Tinnitus Association, http://www.ata.org

Better Hearing Institute, http://www.betterhearing.org/

Guide Dogs for the Blind, http://www.guidedogs.com

Guide Dog Users, Inc., http://www.gdui.org

Guiding Eyes for the Blind, http://www.guidingeyes.org

Hearing Loss Association of America, http://www.hearingloss.org/

International Hearing Dog Inc., http://www.hearinglossweb.com

Leader Dogs for the Blind, http://www.leaderdog.org/

Lion's Club International, http://www.lionsclubs.org

Prevent Blindness America, http://www.preventblindness.org

National Association for the Deaf, http://www.nad.org

National Association for Visually Handicapped, http://www.navh.org

Recording for the Blind & Dyslexic, Inc., http://www.rfbd.org

Self Help for the Hard of Hearing, http://www.shhh.org

The Vision Council/The Better Vision Institute, http://www.thevisioncouncil.org/bvi/

University of Ottawa – Canada's University, http://www.med.uottawa.ca

CHAPTER 12
Endocrine System

MAKING THE CONNECTION

Refer to the following chapters to increase your understanding of the endocrine system:

Adult Health Nursing

- *Oncology*
- *Cardiovascular System*
- *Hematologic and Lymphatic Systems*
- *Urinary System*
- *Musculoskeletal System*
- *Neurological System*
- *Sensory System*
- *Reproductive System*
- *Integumentary System*
- *Immune System*
- *The Older Adult*

LEARNING OBJECTIVES

Upon completion of this chapter, you should be able to:

- Define key terms.
- Identify and locate the endocrine glands and list function(s) and hormone(s) secreted by each.
- Differentiate between type 1 and type 2 diabetes in terms of pathophysiology, presenting symptoms and treatment.
- Discuss the roles of diet and exercise in the management of diabetes mellitus.
- Identify signs, causes, and treatment of acute complications of hypoglycemia, diabetic ketoacidosis, and hyperosmolar hyperglycemic nonketotic syndrome.
- Discuss the major long-term complications of diabetes.
- Discuss rationale for the pituitary gland being traditionally called the "master" gland.
- Compare symptoms of the disease process resulting from a hyper- or hyposecretion of an endocrine gland.
- Discuss assessment techniques for a client suspected of having an endocrine disorder.
- Formulate a nursing care plan for the client with an endocrine disorder.

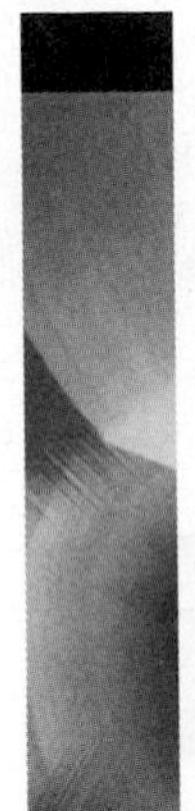

KEY TERMS

agranulocytosis
autosomal
Chvostek's sign
cretinism
dawn phenomenon
endocrine
exophthalmos
glucagon
glycosuria
goiter
gynecomastia
hirsutism
hormone
hyperglycemia
hypoglycemia
hypovolemia
iatrogenic
insulin
ketonuria
lipodystrophy
myxedema
paroxysmal
polydipsia
polyphagia
polyuria
Somogyi phenomenon
tetany
Trousseau's sign

INTRODUCTION

The endocrine system provides the same general functions as the nervous system: communication and control; however, the endocrine system is generally slower and has longer-lasting control over the various body activities and functions. It exerts this control through the secretion of hormones that circulate through the blood. A malfunction of any part of the endocrine system can result in a shift of homeostasis with far-reaching systemic reactions.

Assessment of the endocrine system is difficult. Not only are the components not in direct contact, but only the thyroid gland is close enough to the body surface for direct physical assessment. Still, the nurse needs to be familiar with the normal functioning of the endocrine system. In assessing the client for endocrine dysfunction, the nurse must note negative findings as well as positive ones. Assessment includes results of diagnostic tests as well as any precipitating or aggravating factors.

ANATOMY AND PHYSIOLOGY REVIEW

The endocrine system is unique in that it is composed of a group of various glands scattered throughout the body. The glands of the body have either exocrine or endocrine functions. Exocrine glands, including sweat glands and lacrimal glands, are responsible for secreting substances directly into ducts that lead to the target area. The term **endocrine** (*endo*—within, *crin*—secrete) indicates that the secretions formed by these glands directly enter the blood or lymph circulation, rather than being transported via tubes or ducts. These secretions, called **hormones**, are chemical substances that initiate or regulate activity of another organ, system, or gland in another part of the body. The level of hormone in the blood is regulated by the homeostasis mechanism called *negative feedback*. If the blood level for a specific hormone falls below normal, negative feedback causes the specific endocrine gland to produce more of the hormone, which when increased to the normal level causes a decrease in production.

The glands discussed in this chapter that make up the endocrine system are the pancreas, pituitary, hypothalamus, thyroid, parathyroid, and adrenals (Figure 12-1). Several endocrine glands such as the pineal, thymus, ovaries, and testes are of great importance; however, they are discussed in other chapters in connection with the organ system in which they function.

The pancreas lies horizontally behind the stomach at the level of the first and second lumbar vertebrae. The head of the pancreas is attached to the duodenum with the tail reaching to the spleen. It has both exocrine and endocrine functions.

The pituitary gland consists of an anterior and a posterior lobe. It has traditionally been called the "master" gland because so many of its secretions influence other endocrine glands and body systems. It is attached to the hypothalamus by a stalk called the *infundibulum*. The hypothalamus is located in the lower portion of the brain and produces secretions influencing the production and release of the anterior pituitary hormones as well as the posterior pituitary hormones. Both the pituitary and hypothalamus are located in the head. The pituitary, about the size of a pea, is located in the sella turcica, a small depression in the sphenoid bone. Refer to Table 12-1 for specific endocrine hormones and functions.

The thyroid gland is butterfly-shaped and lies in the neck. It consists of two lobes—one on each side of the trachea connected by an isthmus. The gland sits saddle-like starting on the anterior surface of the trachea just below the larynx and surrounds it partway. The thyroid gland stores iodine. The thyroid gland produces thyroid hormones including thyroxine,

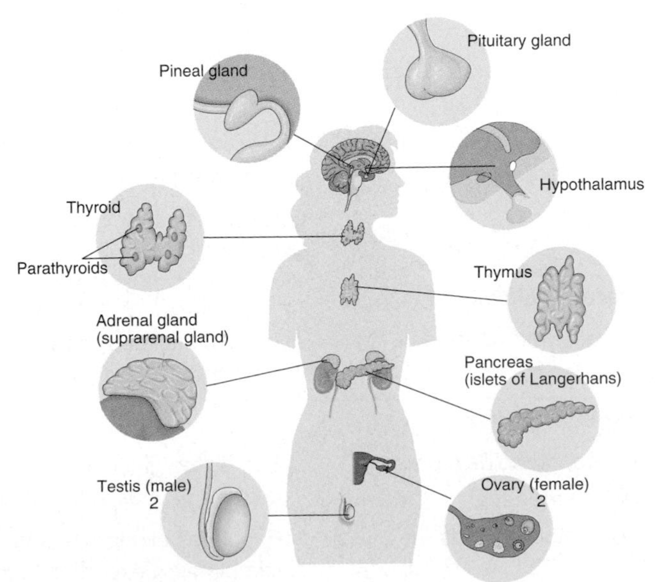

FIGURE 12-1 Structures of the Endocrine System

which is the most abundant, and triiodothyronine. It regulates the metabolic rate for carbohydrates, protein, and fats.

There are usually four parathyroid glands. Two glands are embedded in the posterior portion of each thyroid lobe. They produce parathyroid hormone, parathormone, which regulates the concentration of blood calcium and phosphorus.

The adrenal, or suprarenal, glands are located on top of each kidney. The adrenal cortex secretes mineralocorticoids including aldosterone, glucocorticoids including cortisol, and androgens, which are sex hormones. The adrenal medulla secretes epinephrine or adrenalin and norepinephrine or noradrenalin, which help the body function under stress.

TABLE 12-1 Endocrine Glands and Hormones

HORMONE	FUNCTION
Pancreas	
Glucagon	Released by alpha cells to increase the blood glucose level
Insulin	Released by beta cells to decrease blood sugar
Somatostatin	Inhibits secretion of insulin, glucagon, and growth hormone (GH) from the anterior pituitary and gastrin from the stomach
Anterior Pituitary	
Thyroid-stimulating hormone (TSH)	Stimulates thyroid growth and secretion of the thyroid hormone
Adrenocorticotropic hormone (ACTH)	Stimulates the growth and secretion of glucocorticoids from the adrenal cortex
Follicle-stimulating hormone (FSH)	Stimulates ovarian follicle to mature and produce estrogen; in the male, stimulates sperm production
Luteinizing hormone (LH)	Acts with FSH to stimulate estrogen production; causes ovulation; stimulates progesterone production by corpus luteum; in male, stimulates testes to produce testosterone
Melanocyte-stimulating hormone (MSH)	Causes increase in synthesis and spread of melanin (pigment) in skin
Growth hormone (GH)	Stimulates growth by stimulating the epiphyseal plates of long bones and by increasing protein production
Prolactin or lactogenic hormone	Stimulates breast development during pregnancy and milk secretion after delivery of baby
Posterior Pituitary	
Antidiuretic hormone (ADH)	Stimulates water retention by kidneys to decrease urine secretion
Oxytocin	Stimulates uterine contractions; causes breast to release milk into ducts
Thyroid Gland	
Thyroid hormone (thyroxine T_4 and triiodothyronine T_3)	Controls metabolic rate of all cells; aids in carbohydrate, fat, and protein metabolism Both released in response to TSH
Calcitonin	When stimulated, decreases blood calcium (Ca) by promoting excretion of Ca and phosphorus by the kidneys; also decreases bone resorption by maintaining adequate Ca levels
Parathyroid Gland	
Parathyroid hormone	When stimulated, increases blood calcium concentration by promoting resorption of Ca and phosphorus from the bones; by increasing blood calcium levels, bone formation is decreased
Adrenal Cortex	
Glucocorticoids (cortisol, hydrocortisone)	Stimulates gluconeogenesis and increases blood glucose; antiinflammatory; antiimmunity; antiallergy; aids in the metabolism of carbohydrates, fats, and proteins
Mineralocorticoids	Regulates electrolyte and fluid homeostasis by increasing sodium and water reabsorption; stimulates K excretion in the kidneys
Sex hormones (androgen)	Stimulates sexual drive in females; in males, negligible effect

Table 12-1 Endocrine Glands and Hormones (Continued)

HORMONE	FUNCTION
Adrenal Medulla	
Epinephrine (adrenalin)	Prolongs and intensifies sympathetic nervous response to stress, resulting in increased heart rate, constriction of blood vessels, dilation of bronchioles, and hyperglycemia
Norepinephrine	Prolongs and intensifies sympathetic nervous response to stress, resulting in increased heart rate, constriction of blood vessels, dilation of bronchioles, and hyperglycemia

COURTESY OF DELMAR CENGAGE LEARNING

It is important to understand the normal function of the endocrine glands and hormones. Most endocrine disorders are a result of either overactivity or underactivity of these glands.

COMMON DIAGNOSTIC TESTS

Commonly used diagnostic tests for clients with symptoms of endocrine system disorders are listed in Table 12-2.

DIABETES MELLITUS

Nearly 23.6 million Americans or approximately 7.8% of the American population have diabetes mellitus. Of the 23.6 million people, almost 1 in 4 cases are undiagnosed (CDC, 2007). Diabetes mellitus (DM) is a disorder of metabolism. When we eat, most of the food we eat is broken down by digestive juices. Of the food we eat, 100% of carbohydrate and approximately 58% of protein and 10% of fat is broken down to glucose. For the glucose to get into the cells, insulin must be present (Figure 12-2).

Insulin is a hormone produced and secreted by the beta cells of the islets of Langerhans in the pancreas. Insulin stimulates the active transport of glucose into muscle and adipose tissue cells, making it available for cell use. For glucose to cross the cell membrane, insulin must connect with a receptor on the cell membrane. Some clients with diabetes mellitus have enough insulin but too few functioning receptor sites. Others have inadequate or no insulin production. Blood glucose can

Table 12-2 Common Diagnostic Tests for Endocrine System Disorders

Pancreas Diagnostic Tests

- Blood glucose, Fasting blood sugar (FBS)
- 2-hour postprandial glucose (2hPPG) or 2-hour postprandial blood sugar (2hPPBS)
- Glucose tolerance test (GTT)

Pituitary Gland Diagnostic Tests

- Adrenocorticotropic hormone (ACTH), Corticotropin
- Antidiuretic hormone (ADH), Vasopressin
- Follicle-stimulating hormone (FSH)
- Growth hormone (GH), Human GH (HGH), Somatotropin hormone (SH)
- Growth hormone (GH) stimulation test, GH provocation test, Insulin tolerance test (ITT), Arginine test
- Luteinizing hormone (LH) assay
- Prolactin level (PRL)
- Thyrotropin-releasing hormone (TRH) test, Thyrotropin-releasing factor (TRF) test
- Urine specific gravity
- Long bone x-rays
- Sella turcica x-ray
- Computed tomography of head (CT scan of head), Computerized axial transverse tomography (CATT)

Thyroid Gland Diagnostic Tests

- Antithyroid microsomal antibody, Antimicrosomal antibody, Microsomal antibody, Thyroid autoantibody, Thyroid antimicrosomal antibody
- Calcitonin, HCT, Thyrocalcitonin
- Serum-free triiodothyronine (T_3)
- Thyroid-stimulating hormone (TSH), Thyrotropin
- Thyroid-stimulating hormone (TSH) stimulation test
- Thyroxine index free, FTI, FT_4 Index
- Thyroxine, T_4, Thyroxine screen
- Triiodothyronine, T_3 radioimmunoassay, T_3 by RIA
- Radioactive iodine uptake (RAIU), Iodine uptake test, ^{131}I uptake
- Thyroid scan, Thyroid scintiscan
- Thyroid ultrasound, Thyroid echogram, Thyroid sonogram
- Thyroid biopsy

Parathyroid Gland Diagnostic Tests

- Parathyroid hormone (PTH), Parathormone
- Calcium, total/ionized Ca^{++}
- Phosphorus

(Continues)

TABLE 12-2 Common Diagnostic Tests for Endocrine System Disorders (Continued)

Adrenal Glands Diagnostic Tests	17-Hydroxycorticosteroids (17-OHCS)
Adrenocorticotropic hormone (ACTH) stimulation test, Cortisol stimulation test, Cosyntropin test	17-Ketosteroids (17-KS)
Cortisol, Hydrocortisone	Urine cortisol, Hydrocortisone
Dexamethasone suppression test (DST), Prolonged/rapid DST, Cortisol suppression test, ACTH suppression test	Vanillylmandelic acid (VMA) and catecholamines, VMA and epinephrine, Norepinephrine, Metanephrine, Normetanephrine, Dopamine
Plasma renin assay, Plasma renin activity (PRA)	Adrenal angiography, Adrenal arteriogram
Progesterone assay	Adrenal venography
Aldosterone assay	Computed tomography of adrenals (CT scan of adrenals)

always be used by the brain and kidneys. Insulin is not needed for glucose to enter brain cells or cells of the glomeruli.

The amount of glucose in the blood regulates the rate of insulin secretion. When a meal is eaten, the blood glucose elevates and the beta cells of the islets of Langerhans release insulin. As the blood glucose level drops, insulin secretion diminishes. It is important to note that during times of fasting (overnight or between meals), a low level of insulin continues to be secreted along with **glucagon**. Glucagon secreted by the alpha cells of the pancreas stimulates release of glucose by the liver. The balance and interactions of insulin and glucagon maintain a constant serum glucose level.

Other functions of insulin include:

- Promoting conversion of glucose to glycogen for storage in the liver and inhibiting conversion of glycogen to glucose
- Promoting conversion of fatty acids into fat that can be stored as adipose tissue and preventing breakdown of adipose tissue and conversion of fat to ketone bodies
- Stimulating protein synthesis within tissues and inhibiting the breakdown of protein into amino acids

In summary, insulin actively promotes those processes that lower the blood glucose level and inhibits those processes that raise the blood glucose level. A deficiency of insulin results in **hyperglycemia**, or elevated blood glucose. Excess insulin results in **hypoglycemia** (low blood glucose). Diabetes mellitus is actually a group of disorders characterized by chronic hyperglycemia.

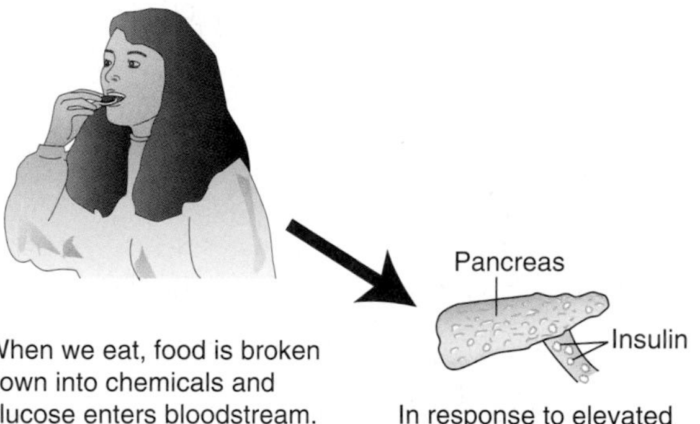
Pancreas
Insulin
When we eat, food is broken down into chemicals and glucose enters bloodstream.
In response to elevated serum glucose, beta cells of pancreas secrete insulin into bloodstream.

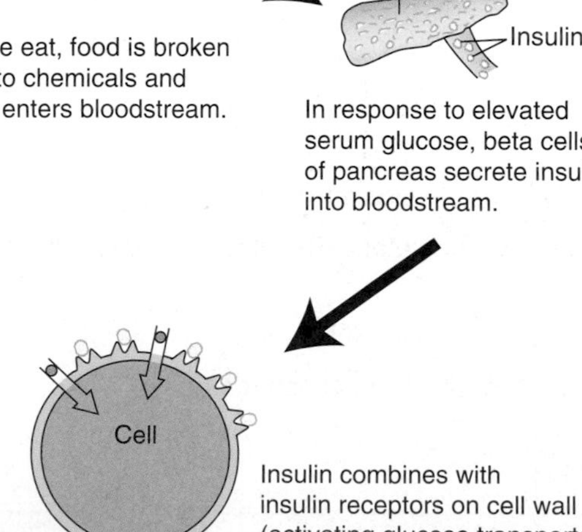
Cell
Insulin combines with insulin receptors on cell wall (activating glucose transporters), allowing glucose to enter cell.
= Glucose
= Insulin
= Insulin receptors

FIGURE 12-2 How Insulin Works

DIAGNOSIS AND CLASSIFICATION

The Expert Committee on the Diagnosis and Classification of Diabetes Mellitus (1997) presented to the American Diabetes Association (ADA) new criteria for diagnosis and new classifications for diabetes, which the ADA approved.

DIAGNOSIS

The Committee identified two precursors to diabetes, screening criteria, and diagnostic criteria.

The two precursors identified are:

1. Impaired glucose tolerance (IGT)—a glucose level of 140 to 199 mg/dL 2 hours after a glucose load
2. Impaired fasting glucose (IFG)—a fasting glucose of 110 to 125 mg/dL

The criteria for who should be screened for diabetes include:

1. Anyone age 45 and older
2. Anyone, regardless of age, with one of the following risk factors:
   - Obesity (body mass index of 27 or greater)
   - Immediate family member with diabetes
   - Member of high-risk ethnic group (African American, Hispanic American, some Native American groups)
   - Having a baby weighing more than 9 pounds
   - History of gestational diabetes mellitus (GDM)
   - Hypertension
   - High-density lipoprotein level of 35 mg/dL or less, or a triglyceride level of 250 mg/dL or more
   - Have either of the two precursors of diabetes

The diagnostic criteria identify when a physician can make a diagnosis of diabetes. The situations are:

- A random blood glucose of 200 mg/dL or greater with the classic symptoms of polyuria, polydipsia, and unexplained weight loss

  or

- A fasting blood sugar of 126 mg/dL or greater

  or

- The 2-hour sample of the oral glucose tolerance test is 200 mg/dL or greater using a load of 75 grams of anhydrous glucose
- In the absence of a definitive diagnosis, the testing should be repeated on an alternative date.

The committee also recommended not using glycosylated hemoglobin (HA1C) to diagnose diabetes since terminology is confusing, and many methods of measuring glycosylated hemoglobin are used. Glycosylated hemoglobin (HA1C) is primarily used to evaluate the effectiveness of the client's adherence to the treatment regimen.

Classification

Etiology, not insulin use, is used to classify diabetes into four categories: type 1 diabetes, type 2 diabetes, other specific types, and gestational diabetes mellitus.

Type 1 Diabetes

There are two forms of diabetes resulting from pancreatic beta-cell destruction or a primary defect in beta-cell function, resulting in no release of insulin and ineffective glucose transport. There is usually an absolute insulin deficiency so the clients are insulin-dependent. The two subdivisions of type 1 diabetes are:

> **PROFESSIONALTIP**
>
> **Diabetes**
>
> According to the Centers for Disease Control and Prevention (CDC, 2007), 17.9 million Americans are diagnosed as having diabetes mellitus. Another 5.7 million are estimated to be undiagnosed. Diabetes was the seventh-leading cause of death in the United States in 2006 and is associated with many serious complications (CDC, 2007). Diabetes is the leading cause of new blindness among adults and accounts for 44% of new cases of renal failure. The risk of heart disease and stroke is 2-4 times greater in clients with diabetes mellitus.
>
> Diabetes is seen in all age groups and races. About 33% of clients with diabetes are older than age 60. African American, Hispanic, and some Native American populations have a higher incidence of diabetes than the white population (CDC, 2002a).
>
> Direct and indirect medical costs (disability, lost work, health care costs) have risen to $174 billion annually (CDC, 2007).

- *Immune-mediated*—the body's immune system destroys the beta cells. These beta cells are the body's only mechanism to produce insulin to help control blood glucose levels. The rate of this destruction is usually higher in children than in adults. Children and adolescents may rapidly develop ketoacidosis. Adults seldom develop ketoacidosis unless they have an infection or other stressor. This is what used to be called insulin-dependent diabetes mellitus (IDDM), or juvenile-onset diabetes.
- *Idiopathic*—no evidence of autoimmunity; the individual just does not produce insulin and is prone to ketoacidosis.

In the absence of insulin, glucose from food eaten cannot be used or stored and remains in the bloodstream, resulting in hyperglycemia. In addition, glucose production from the liver goes unchecked, further elevating the blood glucose level.

As the blood glucose rises, the kidney begins to excrete excess glucose in the urine (**glycosuria**). Glucose eliminated in the urine pulls excessive amounts of water with it (osmotic diuresis), resulting in fluid volume deficit and producing symptoms of excessive thirst (**polydipsia**) and increased urination (**polyuria**).

Insulin deficiency also results in impaired metabolism of fats and proteins. Because of the impaired glucose, fat, and protein metabolism and the inability to store glucose, clients frequently experience protein wasting, weight loss, and increased hunger (**polyphagia**).

Metabolism of fat stores for energy leads to production of acid by-products called ketones, which can be detected in the urine (**ketonuria**). As ketones accumulate, the associated decrease in pH leads to metabolic acidosis, or more specifically a condition known as diabetic ketoacidosis, discussed later in this chapter.

Type 2 Diabetes

Type 2 diabetes mellitus initially begins with insulin resistance, where the cells are not able to use the insulin properly. Then, as the disease progresses, the pancreas gradually loses its ability to produce adequate quantities of insulin. Most of these clients are obese. When weight is lost, insulin resistance diminishes but reappears if the client regains weight. A strong family history of diabetes is often evident. Many clients do not require insulin, but eventually one-third will need insulin to maintain a normal glucose level. This is what used to be called noninsulin-dependent diabetes mellitus (NIDDM), or adult-onset diabetes.

Hyperglycemia results when the pancreas cannot match the body's need for insulin and/or when the number of insulin receptor sites are decreased or altered. Although available insulin may be insufficient to meet the body's metabolic needs and prevent hyperglycemia, there is a sufficient amount of insulin to prevent fat breakdown for energy and the resulting ketoacidosis. Extremely elevated glucose in the type 2 diabetic will result in development of hyperosmolar hyperglycemic nonketotic syndrome (HHNS), discussed later in this chapter. Table 12-3 compares the clinical manifestations of type 1 and type 2 diabetes.

Other Specific Types

This section includes conditions such as beta-cell genetic defects, endocrinopathies, and drug- or chemical-induced diabetes. These are in a separate category because there are different disease etiologies.

Gestational Diabetes Mellitus

Occurring during pregnancy, this may be controlled either with or without insulin. Generally, the client's glucose tolerance

TABLE 12-3 Comparison of the Clinical Manifestations of Type 1 Diabetes and Type 2 Diabetes

	TYPE 1 DIABETES	TYPE 2 DIABETES
Etiology	Autoimmune	Genetic susceptibility associated; usually associated with obesity.
Age of onset	Rare before age 1	Incidence increases with age
Percent of diabetics	5%–10%	90%–95%
Onset	Abrupt, rapid	Gradual, over years
Body weight at onset	Normal or thin	80% are overweight
Insulin production	None	Less than normal, normal, or greater than normal
Insulin injection	Always	Necessary for approximately 30%
Ketosis	Occurs mainly in children and adolescents	Unlikely
Management	Insulin, diet, exercise	Diet and weight loss, exercise, possibly oral hypoglycemics or insulin

returns to normal after the infant's birth. The client should be rechecked 6 weeks after the birth to see if the diabetes persists.

CONTRIBUTING FACTORS

Persons with a family history of diabetes are at greater risk for developing diabetes. Other factors associated with diabetes include obesity, lack of exercise, aging, and ethnicity. The most powerful risk factor for type 2 diabetes is obesity. For persons with a family history of type 2 diabetes, maintenance of an ideal body weight may delay or prevent the onset of diabetes. Aging can also be considered a contributing factor.

It is known that members of certain racial groups are more likely to develop diabetes. In the United States, there is a greater chance of developing type 2 diabetes for Hispanics, Latinos, certain Native American populations, African Americans, and Asian/Pacific Islanders. Other groups at risk for development of diabetes include those with a history of gestational diabetes or impaired glucose tolerance (IGT).

MEDICAL–SURGICAL MANAGEMENT

Medical

There is no known cure for diabetes. The goal of therapeutic management is aimed at the control of blood sugar and the prevention and early detection of the complications associated with diabetes. Diabetes is considered under control if the client maintains ideal body weight and enjoys good health, preprandial glucose levels are less than 140 mg/dL, and postprandial glucose levels do not rise above 180 mg/dL.

Treatment plans vary and are individualized for each client. Control of blood glucose generally involves a balance of a dietary prescription, an exercise plan, and medications. Ultimately, the client is the manager of the treatment plan and, therefore, must be very well informed about diabetes and involved in all aspects of care planning and decision making.

Since the advent of home glucose monitoring devices, urine testing for glucose is rarely used. Testing urine for ketone (product of fatty acid oxidation) production, however, continues to be recommended when the blood glucose level is consistently higher than 240 mg/dL or when any symptoms of ketoacidosis are present.

The client with type 1 diabetes will always require administration of insulin to lower the glucose level and prevent complications of diabetes. Diet and exercise regimens are also important to control the glucose level and maintain health.

Dietary management is the cornerstone of treatment for the person with type 2 diabetes. As the obese person loses weight, the body's insulin requirements decrease, resulting in improved glucose tolerance. Exercise plays an important role in losing weight and lowering the blood glucose level. Type 2 diabetes not controlled by diet and exercise may necessitate administration of medications. Oral hypoglycemic agents or parenteral administration of insulin may be required for optimal control.

Surgical

Pancreas transplantations have been performed and have successfully eliminated the need for exogenous insulin in some clients. At present, pancreas transplants are being performed primarily on clients with type 1 diabetes who also need kidney or other organ transplants because the serious side effects of the antirejection medications do not justify a pancreas transplant alone. Pancreatic islet cell transplants are also being done experimentally with limited success but hold much promise for the future.

Pharmacological

Various pharmacological treatments that are used in the management of type 1 and type 2 diabetes are discussed in the following text.

Insulin Persons with type 1 diabetes always require insulin administration. Persons with type 2 diabetes may not initially require insulin, but it may become necessary as endogenous insulin production decreases or during times of stress or illness.

COMMUNITY/HOME HEALTH CARE

Glucose Monitoring

The availability and use of home glucose monitoring equipment to evaluate serum (blood) glucose has revolutionized self-care for the diabetic client. Also called "fingerstick blood glucose" (FSBG), self-monitoring of blood glucose (SMBG) can be done quickly using capillary blood that provides fairly accurate reading of the current blood glucose. Most often, the glucose level is checked before meals and at bedtime so the client can adjust the treatment plan accordingly. Self-monitoring of blood glucose is recommended for all clients requiring insulin or those with a widely fluctuating glucose level. Symptoms of hypoglycemia at any time warrant immediate evaluation of the blood glucose level.

Historically, insulin has been obtained from beef or pork pancreas. Today, biosynthetic human insulin is used almost exclusively, but some clients still use pork or beef insulin. Human insulin is purer, more effective, and has a much lower incidence of causing insulin allergies and resistance. Insulin is available in very short-, short-, fast-, intermediate-, and long-acting forms that can be injected separately or mixed in the same syringe. Premixed insulins are also available. See Table 12-4 for descriptions of types of insulins and their actions. Insulin is routinely administered subcutaneously. Regular insulin (short-acting) may be administered intravenously when immediate response is desired, as in treatment of greatly elevated glucose levels occurring with diabetic ketoacidosis (DKA) or HHNS. Regular insulin is the *only* insulin that can be given intravenously (IV).

The strength of insulin correlates to the number of units of insulin per cubic centimeter. The most common concentrations of insulin used today are U-50 and U-100 insulin (50 and 100 units of insulin per 1 mL, respectively). U-500 insulin is available for clients who require very high doses.

Insulin should always be measured in an insulin syringe, which is marked in units (Figure 12-3). When mixing two types of insulin in the same syringe, it is important that the regular (clear, short-acting) insulin be drawn up first. The

TABLE 12-4 Types of Insulin and their Actions

TYPES OF INSULIN	APPEARANCE	ACTION IN HOURS			NURSING INTERVENTIONS
		ONSET	PEAK	DURATION	
Very short-acting					
Insulin lispro (Humalog)	Clear	¼	1–1½	5 or less	Eat meals 5 to 10 minutes after injection. Glulisine (Apidra) can be taken 15 minutes before or 20 minutes after the start of a meal. Medication can be mixed with NPH insulin.
Insulin aspart (Novolog)	Clear	¼	1–3	3–5	
Glulisine (Apidra)	Clear	⅓	½–1½	3–4	
Short-acting					
Humulin R	Clear	½–1	2–4	6–8	Available in U-100 and U-500 strengths. Eat meal 15 minutes following injection.
Intermediate-acting					
Humulin N	Cloudy	1–1½	4–12	Up to 24	Roll insulin vial between palms of hands to equally distribute.
Humulin L	Cloudy	1–2½	7–15	22	
Long-acting					
Humulin U	Cloudy	4–8	10–30	36+	Usually given once a day. Cannot be mixed with any other insulin preparations.
Insulin glargine (Lantus)	Clear	1	None	up to 24	
Detemir (Levimir)	Clear	1	None	24	
Premixed					
Humulin N/Reg	Cloudy	½–1	4–8	24	Roll insulin vial between palms of hands to equally distribute. Do not mix with any other insulin preparations. With Humalog 75/25, eat meal within 5 to 10 minutes of injection.
Humulin 70/30	Cloudy	½–60	Varies	10–16	
Humulin 50/50	Cloudy	½–1	Varies	10–16	
Humalog mix 75/25	Cloudy	¼	Varies	10–16	

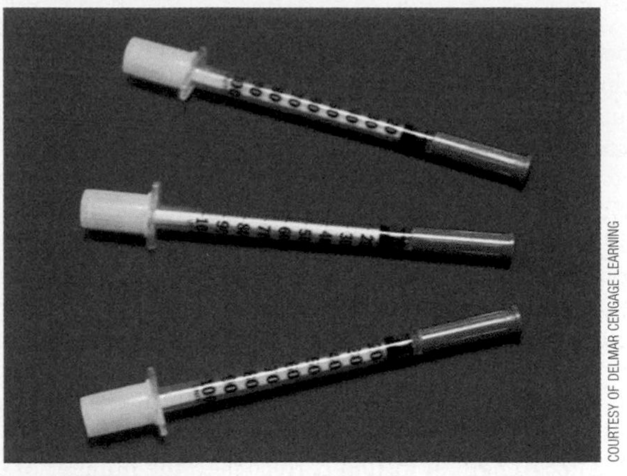

FIGURE 12-3 Insulin syringes are used to administer insulin subcutaneously.

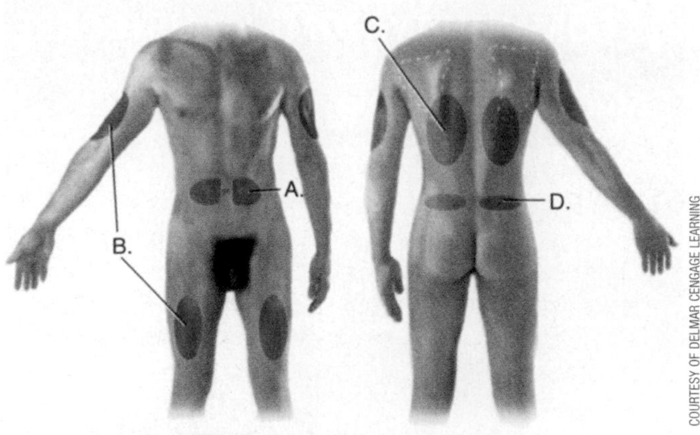

FIGURE 12-4 Subcutaneous Injection Sites; *A*, Abdomen; *B*, Lateral and Anterior Aspects of the Upper Arm and Thigh; *C*, Scapular Area of Back; *D*, Upper Ventrodorsal Gluteal Area

policy of many health care institutions requires that two nurses check insulin dosages before administration. Even if the facility does not have such a policy, checking the insulin dosage with another nurse will help protect against an adverse reaction resulting from error.

Insulin dosages are individually determined, usually requiring two or more injections per day and involving a combination of a short-acting and a longer-acting insulin. Various regimens of insulin administration can be used, each with its own advantages and disadvantages. In general, the more complex the regimen, the more normal the blood glucose level throughout the day. Clients can be taught to use the results of their self-monitoring blood glucose to adjust their insulin doses, allowing more flexibility in their meals and schedules. Recent studies strongly support the theory that intensive insulin regimens that tightly control the blood glucose level delay the onset and progression of complications of diabetic retinopathy, nephropathy, and neuropathy.

Sliding-Scale Insulin During times of surgery, illness, or stress, clients may have their glucose level managed with an insulin sliding scale in lieu of their regular regimen of insulin or oral hypoglycemics. A sliding scale determines insulin dosage based on fingerstick blood glucose level. Regular lispro (Humalog) or aspart (Novolog) insulin may be used, and a dose is administered every 4 or 6 hours based on the blood glucose level. The sliding scale allows for much flexibility and ensures frequent monitoring of and response to changes in the client's glucose level. An example sliding scale might be as follows:

- 4 units of Humulin R Insulin for glucose 151–200 mg/dL
- 6 units of Humulin R Insulin for glucose 201–250 mg/dL
- 8 units of Humulin R Insulin for glucose 251–300 mg/dL
- 10 units of Humulin R Insulin for glucose 301–350 mg/dL
- Call physician for glucose >350 mg/dL

Insulin Injections Insulin injections are administered into the subcutaneous tissue. If an inch of skin can be pinched, the needle is injected at a 90-degree angle, otherwise, at a 45-degree angle. The five main areas for injection are the abdomen, arms, thighs, hips, and subscapular regions (Figure 12-4). Factors affecting absorption should be considered when selecting an injection site. Absorption occurs most quickly in the abdomen, followed by the arms, thighs, hips, and subscapular regions.

Rotation of sites for injection has traditionally been recommended to prevent **lipodystrophy** (atrophy or hypertrophy in the subcutaneous fat). More recently, some authorities are recommending that the abdomen, which provides the most predictable absorption of insulin, be used exclusively for insulin administration.

If sites other than the abdomen are used, site rotation needs to be done systematically to prevent erratic absorption. Failure to rotate injection sites may cause a complication known as lipodystrophy; a change in the subcutaneous fat that decreases the absorption of the insulin. One system of rotation is to always use the same area of injection the same time each day (e.g., always using the abdomen in the morning and the thigh in the afternoon). Another system of rotation is to use all available injection sites in one area before moving to another.

Exercise will increase the rate of absorption, so diabetics planning to exercise should not inject insulin into the areas to be exercised.

Vials of insulin not being used should be refrigerated to prevent loss of potency. Vials in use may be kept at room temperature to decrease local irritation at the injection site, which can occur when cold insulin is used. When mixing a short-acting and a longer-acting insulin in the same syringe, the regular (clear) should always be drawn up into the syringe first, followed by the longer-acting (cloudy) insulin. Figure 12-5 illustrates mixing and administering insulin. It is recommended that insulin syringes be used only once and then discarded.

The visually and/or neurologically impaired diabetic client may benefit from assistive devices available to facilitate drawing up the insulin and administering it. Clients dependent on others for drawing up their insulin may benefit from prefilled syringes, which are considered stable for up to 3 weeks when stored in the refrigerator.

The nurse should keep in mind that the most important factor in the administration of insulin is consistency in technique. Also, simplification of the procedure may have a major impact on a client's ability to comply and to maintain independence. It is important that the nurse understand the basic principles of insulin administration and thereby remain flexible when teaching new clients or assessing the skills of experienced clients.

Insulin Pumps A portable insulin infusion pump delivers insulin continuously through a subcutaneous needle, usually anchored in the abdomen. A continuous, or basal, rate of regular

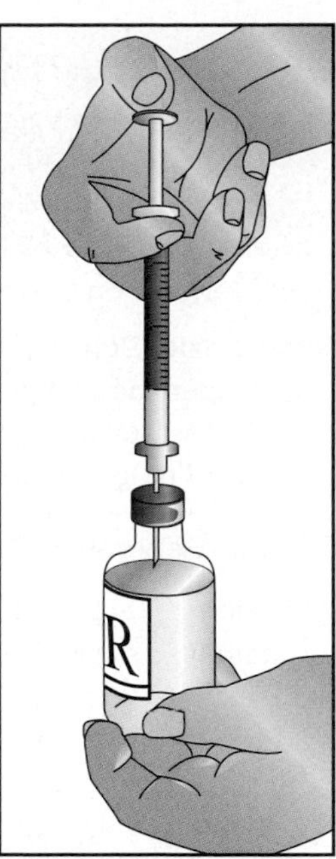

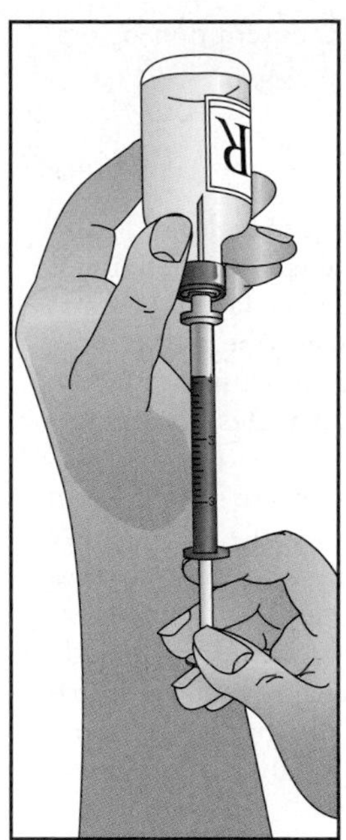

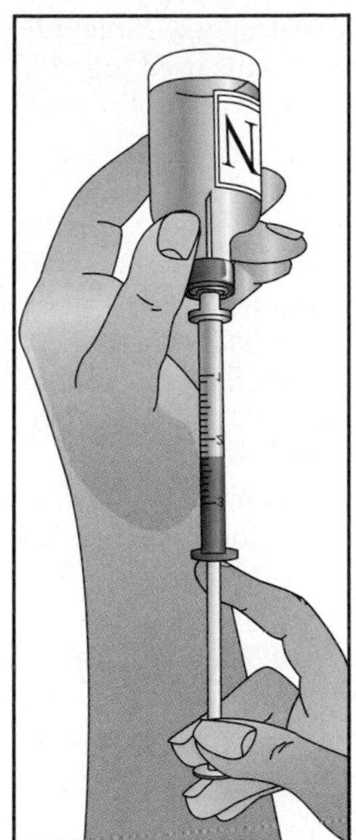

1. Cleanse the rubber stopper on both vials with an alcohol wipe, then inject the amount of air equal to the dose of the intermediate-acting insulin into the N vial.

2. Inject the amount of air equal to the dose of the rapid acting insulin into the R vial.

3. Withdraw the correct amount of rapid-acting insulin.

4. Withdraw the correct amount of intermediate-acting insulin by pulling the plunger down to the unit mark that equals the dose of rapid-acting insulin plus the dose of intermediate-acting insulin. The insulins mix immediately in the syringe. If too much intermediate-acting insulin is withdrawn, the entire contents of the syringe must be discarded.

FIGURE 12-5 How to Mix Insulin

aspart (Novolog) or lispro (Humalog) insulin is programmed and delivered to closely imitate the body's natural insulin secretion. Additional boluses can be manually administered to coordinate with meal times. The injection site is changed every 48 to 72 hours. The use of the insulin pump prevents multiple injections and allows flexibility in meal size and time. Use of the pump requires a motivated and educated client because intensive self-monitoring of blood glucose is essential.

Complications of Insulin Therapy Complications of insulin therapy include hypoglycemia (discussed later in this chapter), insulin resistance (requiring >200 units/day), lipodystrophy, Somogyi phenomenon, and the dawn phenomenon. Lipodystrophy can be minimized by using human insulin, using room temperature insulin, and by rotating sites of insulin injection.

The **Somogyi phenomenon** occurs when a rapid decrease in blood glucose (hypoglycemia) causes the release of glucose-elevating hormones (epinephrine, cortisol, glucagon). The hypoglycemia usually occurs during the night but manifests as an elevated glucose in the morning and may be inadvertently treated with an increase in insulin dosage. The Somogyi phenomenon can be diagnosed by checking the blood glucose during the night at about 3:00 a.m. Adjusting the insulin regimen to avoid the peaking of insulin during the night will correct this effect.

The **dawn phenomenon** is an early morning glucose elevation produced by the release of growth hormone. The release of the growth hormone decreases the peripheral uptake of the glucose resulting in elevated morning glucose levels. Administering the evening insulin dose at a later time will coordinate the insulin peak with the hormone release.

Oral Hypoglycemic Agents Oral hypoglycemic agents are used to treat persons with type 2 diabetes who are not controlled with exercise and diet. These agents are meant to supplement diet and exercise, not replace them. Oral hypoglycemics are not insulin and work by other mechanisms.

Sulfonylurea is the original class of oral hypoglycemic medications used for diabetes therapy. The sulfonylureas work primarily by increasing the ability of the islet cells of the pancreas to excrete insulin. To a lesser degree, they increase the cells' sensitivity to insulin and decrease glucose production by the liver.

Metformin (Glucophage), a biguanide, does not increase insulin release but works by making existing insulin more effective at the cellular level. Metformin decreases the amount of glucose produced by the liver. Muscle tissues become more sensitive to insulin and improve glucose absorption. Metformin may be given alone or in combination with other oral hypoglycemics. In some clients, Glucophage works more effectively if given with some dose of Diabeta. Because it does not stimulate increased insulin release, metformin is not associated with episodes of hypoglycemia. The major side effects of metformin are gastrointestinal and include anorexia, nausea, abdominal discomfort, and diarrhea.

Oral hypoglycemics require some production of insulin by the pancreas and, therefore, are not useful in the treatment of type 1 diabetes. See Table 12-5 for a description of oral hypoglycemic agents used today.

Diet

Medical nutrition therapy provides an individualized dietary prescription to meet client and family needs. Consideration is given to usual eating habits and other lifestyle factors, such as dietary likes and dislikes, cultural influences, who prepares the meals, and family finances. It is important that meals remain a social experience, and the person with diabetes not feel isolated or different.

The goals of medical nutrition therapy are (1) maintain as near-normal blood glucose level as possible, (2) achieve optimal serum lipid levels, (3) provide adequate calories to maintain or attain a reasonable weight, (4) prevent complications of diabetes, and (5) improve overall health. Because of the complexity of individualizing medical nutrition therapy, it is recommended that clients be referred early to a registered dietician (RD) for nutritional assessment and education.

Diabetes is a strong risk factor for atherosclerosis and cardiovascular disease. Therefore, reducing serum lipid levels is a goal of medical nutrition therapy. To reduce the risk of cardiovascular disease, the ADA recommendations incorporate a reduction in saturated fat and cholesterol consumption.

It is recommended that individuals taking insulin or oral hypoglycemic agents eat at consistent times synchronized with the actions of the medications used. Distribution of calories over 24 hours, with regular meals and snacks, helps prevent extreme highs and lows in blood glucose.

Consistent-Carbohydrate Meal Plan Current ADA nutrition guidelines suggest using a "consistent-carbohydrate meal plan." The client eats an individually prescribed amount of carbohydrates at each meal or snack. Carbohydrates determine premeal insulin requirements more than the amount of protein or fat in the meal, and they have the greatest effect on the postprandial blood glucose level. Protein and fat intake must be watched to avoid weight gain and increased serum lipid levels.

Protein intake of both animal and vegetable sources should make up 15% to 20% of the daily calorie intake. Cholesterol intake should not exceed 300 mg per day (Bartels, 2004). If nephropathy is present, protein should be 10% of the daily calorie intake.

Total fat intake depends on the goals set by the client and health care provider for desired levels of glucose, lipid, and weight. If lipid level is normal, 30% or less of calories should come from fat with less than 10% from saturated fat. If weight loss is a primary issue, reduction in fat intake is an efficient way to reduce calorie intake. When lipid level is a problem, a decrease of saturated fat intake to less than 7% of the total calories, total fat to less than 30% of total calories, and cholesterol to less than 300 mg per day is recommended.

The remainder of the calorie intake comes from carbohydrates. The amount consumed is more important than the source of the carbohydrate.

Persons with diabetes should follow the same precautions regarding the use of alcohol as applied to the general public. Alcohol may increase the risk for hypoglycemia in people treated with insulin or sulfonylureas, such as acetohexamide (Dymelor), chlorpropamide (Diabinese), or tolazamide (Tolinase).

TABLE 12-5 Oral Hypoglycemics

GENERIC (BRAND)	USUAL DOSE	ONSET TIME (HOURS)	DURATION (HOURS)
First-Generation Sulfonylureas			
Tolbutamide (Orinase), tolazamide, (Tolinase), and chlorpropamide (Diabinese) are seldom used because of their long action, higher incidence of adverse effects, and risk of drug interactions (Cincinnati & Veliko, 2001).			
Second-Generation Sulfonylureas			
glipizide (Glucatrol)	2.5–40 mg single or divided dose	1–1½	10–16
glimepride (Amaryl)	1–4 mg single dose	1	24
glyburide (Diabeta, Micronase)	1.25–20 mg single or divided dose	2–4	24
Biguanides			
metformin HCl (Glucophage)	500–2,500 mg two or three divided doses	24–48	6–12
Alpha-Glucosidase Inhibitors			
acarbose (Precose)	25–100 mg with meals (tid)	1	No data
miglitol (Glyset)	25–100 mg with meals (tid)	2–3	4–6
Thiazolidenediones			
rosiglitazone maleate (Avandia)	4 mg daily	1	
Combinations			
glyburide and metformin HCl (Glucovance)	1.25 mg/250 mg 2.5 mg/500 mg once or twice a day		
rosiglitazone maleate and metformin HCl (Avandamet)	1 mg/500 mg 2 mg/500 mg 4 mg/500 mg		

Activity

The beneficial effects of regular exercise for the diabetic are multiple. Exercise decreases the blood glucose by increasing the uptake of glucose by muscles and improving insulin usage. Exercise also increases circulation, improves cardiovascular status, decreases stress, and assists with weight loss.

Before starting an exercise program, the person with diabetes should have a complete physical and review the exercise plan with the physician or primary health care provider. Regular daily exercise rather than sporadic exercise should be encouraged.

Persons with diabetes need to correlate exercise with their blood glucose, taking care to avoid periods of hypoglycemia or exercising when blood glucose is too high. Exercise potentiates the action of insulin, resulting in lower insulin requirements and an increased risk of hypoglycemia during and after exercise. On the other hand, in the person with diabetes who is insulin-deficient, exercise may cause a further rise in blood glucose and rapid development of ketosis. Diabetics should not exercise at the peak of insulin activity, when their blood glucose is greater than 250 mg/dL, or if they have ketones in their urine.

Health Promotion

The diabetic educator plays a pivotal role in assisting the diabetic client/family to understand diabetes and the necessary lifestyle changes. Some teaching is unique to an individual client and is done one-to-one, whereas some teaching applies to all clients with diabetes and is often done in a class setting. This also allows clients with diabetes to meet each other and share concerns, information, and ideas that have worked for them.

The diabetic educator nurse is part of a team, including the client/family, physician, dietician, and pharmacist, who all work together to help the client understand and comply with the treatment plan.

Sick-Day Management It is important that persons with diabetes have a plan for managing their diabetes in the event of illness. It is important that they continue taking their insulin or oral hypoglycemic medication when they are experiencing illness because illness and fever can increase blood glucose and the need for insulin. Some persons with diabetes who do not normally take short-acting insulin may require it during times of fever or illness. Blood glucose should be monitored 4 to 6 times per day (Figure 12-6), and urine should be checked for ketones. Blood glucose greater than 300 mg/dL or ketones in the urine should be reported to the physician.

If the client cannot ingest the planned meal, carbohydrates in the form of soft foods and liquids can be substituted. Extreme nausea and vomiting or diarrhea should be reported to the physician because extreme fluid loss can be dangerous. Clients with type 1 diabetes who are unable to retain fluids may need to be hospitalized to avoid ketoacidosis.

Acute Complications of Diabetes

There are three major acute complications of diabetes related to blood glucose imbalance: hypoglycemia, diabetic ketoacidosis (DKA), and HHNS (Table 12-6).

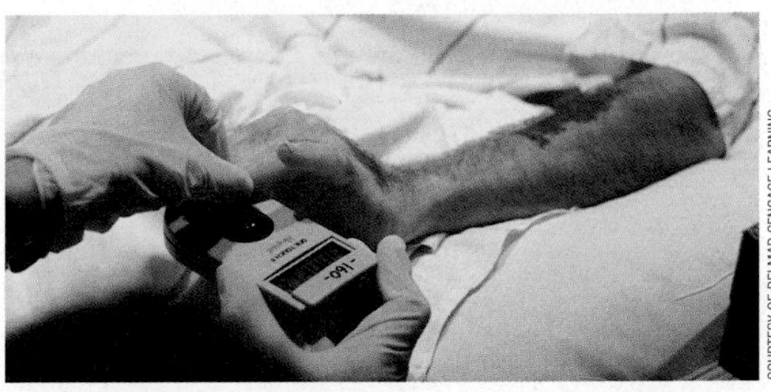

Figure 12-6 The nurse measures a client's blood glucose level.

Hypoglycemia (Insulin Reaction)

Hypoglycemia (low blood glucose) occurs when a client's glucose level decreases to less than 70 mg/dL, with the most severe reactions occurring when it decreases to less than 50 mg/dL. Hypoglycemia can occur any time of the day, but most often will occur before meals or when insulin action is peaking. Factors that can contribute to the development of a hypoglycemic reaction are skipping meals or eating late, unplanned exercise, and administration of excess insulin.

Hypoglycemic symptoms can occur suddenly and unexpectedly and vary from client to client. The cardinal rule is: *Always believe clients who tell you they are having an insulin reaction.* Most persons with diabetes have had hypoglycemic reactions before, so they know the symptoms that precede an insulin reaction. Hypoglycemia unawareness occurs when the client experiences an inability to recognize the warning symptoms of hypoglycemia. It is usually a complication of type 1 diabetes but can occur in type 2.

When a hypoglycemic reaction is suspected, the nurse must respond immediately according to the institution's protocol. Treatment involves assessing the client, checking blood glucose level, and administering glucose in the most appropriate form. Daniels (2007) recommends providing

LIFE SPAN CONSIDERATIONS

Hybrid or Mixed Diabetes

Usually a child or teenager develops either type 1 or type 2 diabetes. Some teenagers have elements of both kinds of diabetes. This phenomenon is referred to as "hybrid" or "mixed" diabetes. Given the fact that more children and teenagers are becoming overweight and obese, it is not surprising that these age groups have elements of both types of diabetes. Youth with "hybrid" or "mixed" diabetes typically have:

- insulin resistance associated with obesity and type 2 diabetes, and
- antibodies against the pancreatic islet cells that are associated with autoimmunity and type 1 diabetes.

(National Diabetes Education Program, 2008; Lorenz & Silverstein, 2005)

CLIENT TEACHING

Guidelines for Exercising

- Try to exercise at the same time and in the same amount each day.
- Test blood glucose level before, during, and after exercise.
- Do not inject insulin into a limb that you will be exercising.
- Do not exercise at the peak of insulin activity.
- Do not exercise before meals unless trying to lower blood glucose level.
- Do not exercise with a blood glucose level over 250 mg/dL or with ketones in the urine. This indicates severe insulin deficiency and may predispose to hyperglycemia.
- Eat a snack (15 g of carbohydrates) before or during exercise if appropriate, based on blood glucose level.
- Always carry a source of carbohydrates and emergency cash, if away from home, in case hypoglycemia occurs while exercising.
- Always carry personal and medical alert identification.
- Watch for post-exercise hypoglycemia. Individuals who have more than usual exercise during the day should increase their carbohydrate intake and test their glucose during the night to detect nocturnal hypoglycemia. (Hypoglycemia can occur 8 to 15 hours after exercise.)

CLIENT TEACHING

Fingersticks

- Use shallow skin penetration, just to get enough blood for the meter.
- Rotate sites; use sides of fingertips and thumb.
- Use alcohol sparingly or wash hands with warm soapy water before fingerstick *instead* of using alcohol. The warm water brings more blood into the fingers.
- Apply firm pressure *directly* over the puncture for 10 to 15 seconds; if area is still bleeding, apply pressure until it stops.

the client with 10–15 grams of simple carbohydrates, for example 8 oz of low-fat milk or 4 oz of fruit juice. The client taking acarbose (Precose), which slows digestion and absorption of most carbohydrates—including hard candies and many fruit juices—but not glucose, will not have the rapid response to fruit juice or sugar that other clients will

TABLE 12-6 Symptoms of Acute Complications of Diabetes

Symptoms of Hypoglycemia (Insulin Reaction)

Mild hypoglycemia
- Diaphoresis; cold, clammy skin
- Palpitations
- Pallor
- Tremors
- Excess hunger
- Anxious but alert

Moderate hypoglycemia
- Confusion, vertigo
- Behavior changes
- Slurred speech
- Irritability
- Paresthesia

Severe hypoglycemia
- Seizures
- Loss of consciousness
- Shallow respirations
- Nursing Alert: Severe hypoglycemia is a medical emergency. Administer some form of glucose immediately.

Symptoms of Diabetic Ketoacidosis (DKA)
- Same as HHNS plus symptoms of acidosis:
  - "Fruity" odor to breath
  - Kussmaul's respirations (deep, nonlabored)

Symptoms of Hyperosmolar Hyperglycemic Nonketotic Syndrome (HHNS)
- Polyuria
- Polydipsia
- Skin hot, dry, decreased turgor
- Dehydration—hypotension, increased pulse
- Blurred vision
- Weakness
- Mental status changes, confusion to coma

have. Hypoglycemic reactions can be fatal, *so leaving the client untreated is more dangerous than causing mild hyperglycemia with overtreatment.* Figure 12-7 provides a sample hypoglycemic protocol.

Persons with diabetes and their families must know the symptoms and treatment for hypoglycemia. Hypoglycemic episodes can be prevented by following a regular pattern of eating, exercise, and insulin administration. Between-meal and bedtime snacks can be used to cover times of peak insulin action. Additional food should be eaten when engaging in greater than usual exercise. Blood glucose level should be checked at the first suspicion of hypoglycemia. All clients should wear an identification bracelet or tag indicating that they have diabetes because hypoglycemic reactions can occur unexpectedly.

Diabetic Ketoacidosis

Diabetic ketoacidosis (DKA) is one of the most serious complications of hyperglycemia. Glucose is a hyperosmolar

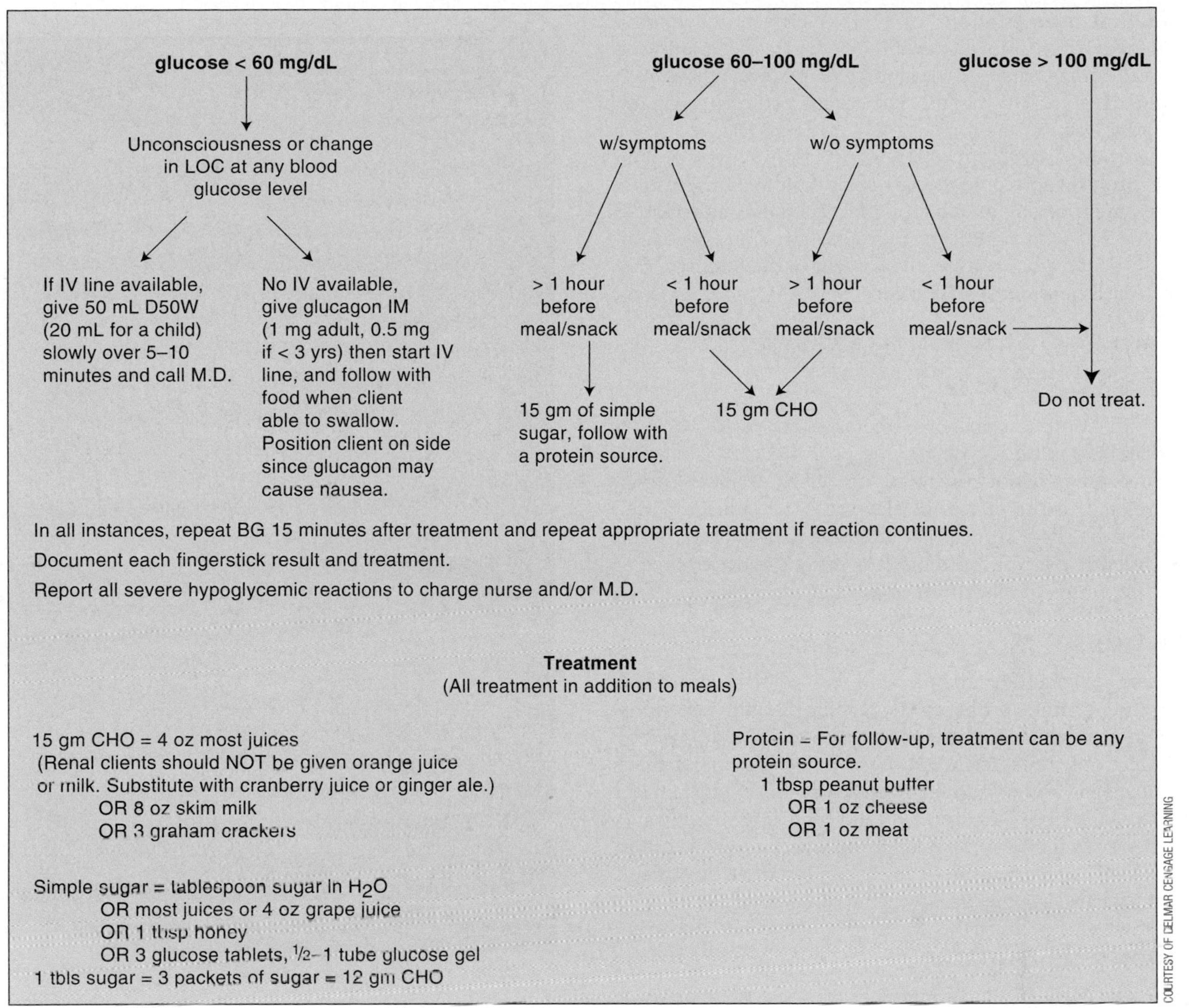

FIGURE 12-7 Sample Hypoglycemic Protocol

substance drawing fluid out of the cell and into the circulation, where it is excreted by the kidneys. This oncotic diuresis results in polyuria (increased urine output), dehydration, and electrolyte imbalances. Increased fat metabolism results in accumulation of ketones, resulting in metabolic acidosis. Surgery, stress, or illness may trigger DKA, which usually develops in clients with immune-mediated type 1 diabetes, although it can occur in clients with type 2 diabetes. The client with undiagnosed immune-mediated type 1 diabetes may also present with DKA.

The onset of DKA may be gradual or sudden. Classic symptoms of hyperglycemia (polyuria, polyphagia, polydipsia) usually precede DKA. Other symptoms include nausea and vomiting, abdominal pain from acidosis, headache, weakness, fatigue, and blurred vision. Assessment may reveal hot, flushed skin and signs of hypovolemia or shock. Acidosis will produce signs of hyperpnea (Kussmaul's breathing), fruity odor to breath from respiratory elimination of acetone, and decreased level of consciousness ranging from lethargy to coma.

Laboratory values will reveal blood glucose from 300 mg/dL to 800 mg/dL and metabolic acidosis. Urine will be positive for glucose and ketones.

Treatment regimen must be initiated immediately with clients experiencing DKA. Fluid replacement consists of NS intravenously to improve blood pressure. Regular insulin may be provided intravenously to assist in decreasing the blood glucose levels. Potassium replacement is also necessary to prevent any additional complication associated with fluid replacement (Daniels, 2007).

Hyperosmolar Hyperglycemic Nonketotic Syndrome

HHNS occurs when there is insufficient insulin to prevent hyperglycemia but enough insulin to prevent ketoacidosis. HHNS occurs in persons with type 2 diabetes. Because symptoms of acidosis do not occur, no symptoms may be noticed until the glucose level is dangerously high.

HHNS occurs most often in the elderly client with undiagnosed type 2 diabetes. HHNS can also occur in the poorly controlled client and is usually precipitated by illness or another stressor. The onset of symptoms of HHNS is lower than DKA, often taking days to weeks to display clinical symptoms.

Clinical manifestations of HHNS reflect dehydration and shock. Hyperosmolality eventually results in lethargy, seizures, and coma (Table 12-6). Blood glucose level ranges from 600 mg/dL to 2,000 mg/dL and serum osmolality greater than 350 mOsm/L.

Medical management of DKA and HHNS involves fluid and electrolyte replacement (particularly potassium), insulin, and treatment of any precipitating factors. DKA and HHNS are associated with significant mortality rates, and the client is usually acutely ill. Treatment will occur in the intensive care setting until the client is stabilized.

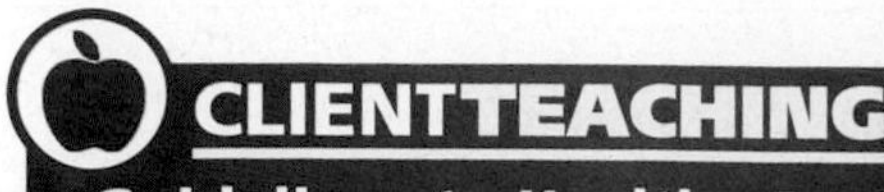

CLIENTTEACHING

Guidelines to Healthy Feet

- Wash feet daily and dry them carefully, especially between the toes.
- Inspect feet and between toes for blisters, cuts, and infections. Use a mirror to see the bottoms of the feet. If your vision is impaired, have a family member examine your feet. Remember, because of decreased feeling in your feet, you may have an infection and not know it.
- Avoid activities that restrict blood flow to the feet, especially smoking and sitting with legs crossed.
- Wear shoes that are comfortable, well-fitting, and closed toed. Wear new shoes for short intervals until broken in. Do not walk barefoot.
- Prevent cuts and irritations. Always wear stockings. Look inside shoes for rough edges, nail points, foreign objects.
- Avoid temperature extremes. Test bath water with hands before getting in. Do not use water bottles or heating pads on feet.
- See your physician regularly and make sure that your feet are examined each visit.
- When toenails are trimmed, cut them straight across. When corns or calluses are present, see a physician or podiatrist. *Do not* cut them yourself.

Chronic Complications of Diabetes

Long-term complications of diabetes occur 5 to 10 years after diagnosis in both type 1 and type 2 diabetes. The exact pathophysiology is not completely understood but is known to be related to the effects of elevated blood glucose level. Recent studies have shown that intensive insulin therapy and tight glycemic control can reduce or delay the occurrence of many long-term complications associated with diabetes.

Infections

Diabetics, particularly clients who are poorly controlled, appear to be more prone to developing certain infections. Infections of particular concern to diabetics include diabetic foot infections, boils, cellulitis, necrotizing fasciitis, urinary tract infections, and yeast infections. Small cuts on the feet can become gangrenous (Figure 12-8) and require amputation.

Infections increase the need for insulin and can result in ketoacidosis. Infections, once they occur, can often be difficult to treat and heal slowly because of impaired circulation.

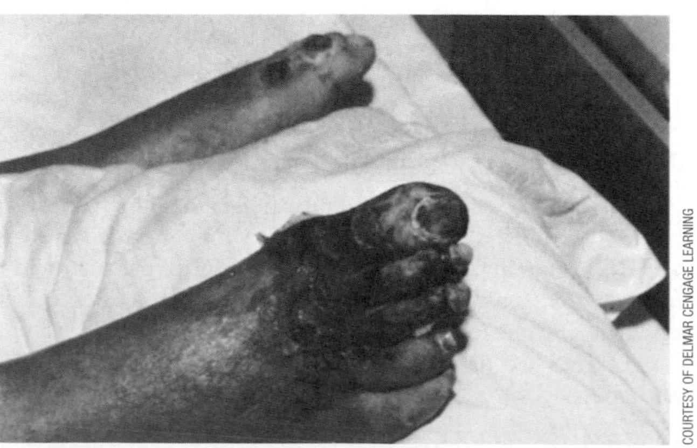

COURTESY OF DELMAR CENGAGE LEARNING

FIGURE 12-8 Gangrene of the toes and foot as a result of an infection often means eventual amputation.

Diabetic Neuropathy

Neuropathy is the most common chronic complication associated with diabetes. The incidence of neuropathy increases with age and duration of disease and is related to elevated blood glucose level. Neuropathy can affect all types of nerves, but the two most common types of diabetic neuropathy are peripheral neuropathy and autonomic neuropathy.

Peripheral neuropathy causes paresthesias and burning sensations, primarily in the lower extremities. Decreased sensations of pain and temperature coupled with decreased peripheral circulation place the client at risk for undetected foot injury.

Autonomic neuropathy can affect almost any organ system, including gastrointestinal (delayed gastric emptying, constipation, diarrhea), urinary (retention, neurogenic bladder), and reproductive (male impotence).

Nephropathy (Chronic Renal Failure)

Diabetic nephropathy develops slowly over many years, progressing eventually to kidney failure. Elevated blood glucose level causes a decrease in the glomerular filtration rate resulting in fluid retention. Prolonged injury to the nephron may eventually lead to renal failure. Controlling hypertension and blood glucose level is the key to delaying renal damage. Good hydration before and diuresis following any dye study is valuable in preventing renal damage. Diligent monitoring of a

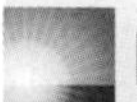

LIFE SPAN CONSIDERATIONS

Diabetic Neuropathy

Advancing age is the strongest risk factor regardless of disease duration and blood sugar control.

client's urinary output is essential. Clients may be required to adhere to a low protein, low salt diet.

Retinopathy

Changes in the small vessels of the retina result in diabetic retinopathy, which is a major cause of blindness among persons with diabetes (Figure 12-9). Because of the insidious onset of type 2 diabetes, retinopathy is often present at diagnosis. The severity and progression of retinopathy appear to be closely related to glucose and blood pressure control. Persons with diabetes also develop cataracts at an earlier age. Although most clients develop some degree of retinopathy, most do not develop visual impairment. To facilitate early detection, diabetics should have ophthalmologic evaluations every 6 to 12 months.

Vascular Changes

Diabetes is an independent risk factor for atherosclerotic vessel disease. Atherosclerotic changes that occur in persons with diabetes are similar to those that occur in nondiabetics, but they occur at earlier ages and progress at a more rapid rate.

Cardiovascular Hypertension is twice as common in persons with diabetes and is an important factor in the progression of retinopathy, nephropathy, and vascular (large vessel) disease. The incidence of coronary artery disease, angina, and myocardial infarction is higher when compared to the nondiabetic population. Cerebral vascular disease and cerebral vascular accident are also more common in persons with diabetes. Therapies aimed at lowering risk factors and effects of atherosclerosis include weight control, low-fat diet, treatment of hypertension and hyperlipidemia, regular exercise, and control of blood glucose level.

Peripheral Vascular Disease Peripheral vascular disease occurs most commonly in diabetics with hypertension or hyperlipidemia and in diabetics who smoke. Diabetics have two to three times the incidence of occlusive peripheral arterial disease when compared to the nondiabetic population. Diabetes is present in more than half of persons experiencing nontraumatic lower extremity amputations.

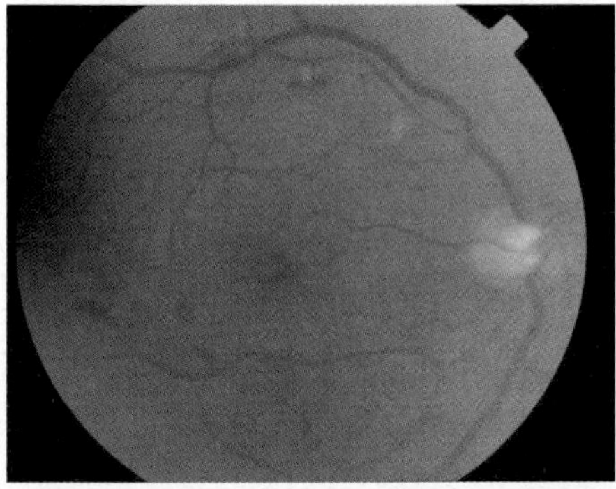

FIGURE 12-9 Microaneurysms in Diabetic Retinopathy *(Courtesy of Salim I. Butrus, M.D., Senior Attending, Department of Opthalmology, Washington Hospital Center, Washington, D.C., and Associate Clinical Professor, Georgetown University Medical Center, Washington, D.C.)*

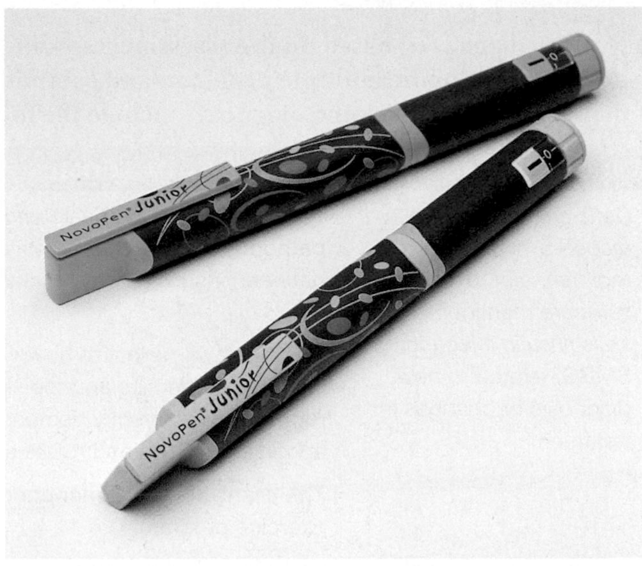

FIGURE 12-10 NovoPen Junior insulin pens are used by younger children and adolescents. *(Courtesy of Novo Nordisk.)*

Nursing Management

Monitor vital signs and serum electrolytes. Record I&O, administer fluids as ordered, and encourage oral fluid intake. Teach client about diabetes, use of insulin or oral hypoglycemics, methods of insulin administration (syringe, pen injector [Figure 12-10], and pump), relationship of exercise to diabetes management, and how to perform SMBG. Provide a list of symptoms and treatment for hypoglycemia.

NURSING PROCESS

Assessment

Subjective Data

This includes assessment of the health history, family history, diet, activity regimen, and the understanding of the disease and medical therapies. The client may describe fatigue, weakness, weight changes, mental status changes, polyuria, polyphagia, polydipsia, numbness or tingling of the extremities, blurred vision, and increased appetite.

Objective Data

Objective data should focus on the symptoms of diabetes, the common acute and chronic complications, and the results of diagnostic tests. There may be dependent redness or cyanosis of the lower extremities as well as the absence of hair. A fasting

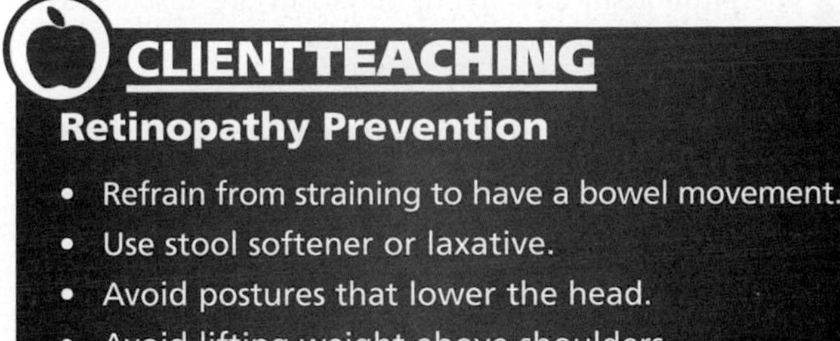

CLIENTTEACHING

Retinopathy Prevention

- Refrain from straining to have a bowel movement.
- Use stool softener or laxative.
- Avoid postures that lower the head.
- Avoid lifting weight above shoulders.

Nursing diagnoses, based on the assessment findings, may be varied and extensive due to the multiple problems and complications caused by diabetes mellitus. Nursing diagnoses include the following:

NURSING DIAGNOSES	PLANNING/OUTCOMES	NURSING INTERVENTIONS
*Deficient **K**nowledge diabetes, medical regimen, diet, exercise, self-care management skills (insulin injection, SMBG)* related to new diagnosis or changes in treatment	The client will relate basic understanding of pathophysiology of diabetes, and relationship between insulin and hyper-/hypoglycemia.	Teach client about diabetes and the use of insulin to prevent hyper-/hypoglycemia or assist client to enroll in a formal diabetic education program.
	The client will verbalize how/when to take oral hypoglycemics and the side effects to report or will correctly demonstrate how to administer insulin and rotate sites.	Teach client about oral hypoglycemics or insulin, whichever the client will be using.
	The client will relate importance of an exercise program.	Discuss how exercise is related to diabetes management.
	The client will describe the relationship between dietary management and glycemic control; choose foods that comply with diet prescription.	Discuss how dietary management is related to the control of blood glucose and provide an exchange list of foods.
	The client will correctly demonstrate how to use SMBG to determine blood glucose level.	Teach client how to perform SMBG and have client return demonstration.
	The client will verbalize symptoms and treatment of hypoglycemia.	Provide client with a list of symptoms and treatment for hypoglycemia.
*Risk for Deficient **F**luid Volume* related to hyperglycemia, polyuria, and dehydration	The client will exhibit normal skin turgor, moist mucous membranes, and maintain oral fluid intake of 2,500–3,000 mL/day.	Measure client's intake and output, administer intravenous fluids as ordered, and encourage oral fluids.
	The client will have vital signs within normal limits.	Monitor vital signs and serum electrolytes.
*Imbalanced **N**utrition: Less than Body Requirements* related to imbalance between insulin, diet, and activity	The client will have weight within normal range for height and age.	Refer client to dietician to adjust dietary intake in order to maintain weight in normal range.

Evaluation: Evaluate each outcome to determine how it has been met by the client.

glucose level greater than 126 mg/dL or a nonfasting (random) level greater than 200 mg/dL on two separate occasions is diagnostic of diabetes.

PITUITARY DISORDERS

Hyperpituitarism and hypopituitarism are discussed in this section.

HYPERPITUITARISM

Hyperpituitarism is most commonly diagnosed between the second and fourth decade of life but can appear in infancy and childhood. Although other pituitary hormones may be affected, the most common are the GH and antidiuretic hormone.

Excess secretion of GH produces different changes depending on the client's age when it occurs. When the excess secretion occurs in childhood before the epiphyses close, gigantism is the result; in adults, acromegaly is the result.

Syndrome of inappropriate antidiuretic hormone and pituitary tumors are also discussed.

GIGANTISM

Gigantism affects infants and children, causing proportional overgrowth of all body tissues. By the time these children reach adulthood, they may be more than 8 feet tall.

Hyperplasia of the anterior pituitary is usually the cause of GH oversecretion. The oversecretion of GH is often caused by benign tumors of the pituitary gland. Clients with gigantism do not have the strength their size implies. Additional signs and symptoms often experienced by clients with gigantism include delayed puberty, double vision, increased sweating, large hands and feet with thick fingers and toes, and weakness.

Medical–Surgical Management

Medical

Irradiation of the anterior pituitary may be the treatment chosen. The child must then be observed for heart failure, hypertension, thickened bones, osteoporosis, and delayed sexual development.

Surgical

If the cause is a tumor, surgery may be performed to remove the tumor (explained under the section "Acromegaly"). If surgery cannot completely remove the tumor, medication management including somatostatin analogs may be used.

Pharmacological

When the pituitary is either destroyed by irradiation or removed by surgery, pituitary hormone replacement is necessary.

Nursing Management

Monitor children's growth for early identification of a problem. Be understanding and emphasize the positive aspects of being tall.

NURSING PROCESS

Assessment

Subjective Data

Listening to the child's description of the disease process may provide insight into the child's emotional responses.

Objective Data

Frequent measurements of growth indicate a more rapid rate of growth than expected.

ACROMEGALY

Acromegaly affects nearly 60 of every 1 million Americans (NIDDK, 2008a). Because acromegaly occurs after epiphyseal closure of bones, there is bone thickening with transverse growth and tissue enlargement. This occurs between 30 and 50 years of age. Photographs over years will reveal a progressive enlargement of the face and hands.

Acromegaly involves a gradual onset of clinical manifestations, including visual defects from pressure of the pituitary tumor on the optic nerve, soft tissue swelling, or hypertrophy of the face and extremities. The cartilaginous and connective tissue overgrowths result in a characteristic hulking appearance with thickened ears and nose, and marked projection of the jaw. The jaw can appear enlarged and the tongue may also thicken. The paranasal sinuses can become enlarged. Also laryngeal hypertrophy can occur. The client has thick fingers with tips that appear "tufted" (shaped like arrowheads on x-rays). The client exhibits a characteristic moist, weak, doughy handshake. The heart, liver, and spleen may enlarge. Some other characteristics are diaphoresis (profuse perspiration), oily or leathery skin, fatigue, heat intolerance, weight gain, headache, joint pain, hirsutism (excessive hairiness especially in females), and sleep disturbance. The client may experience decreased libido or impotence, oligomenorrhea (scanty or infrequent menstruation), and infertility.

The client's history and clinical manifestations along with cranial x-rays and a CT scan make a diagnosis of acromegaly. Serum GH level is elevated.

Prognosis depends on the causative factor, hyperplasia or a tumor; however, there is generally a reduced life span. Diabetes mellitus, hypertension, and a higher risk of cardiovascular disease are the most serious health consequences (NIDDK, 2009).

Medical–Surgical Management

Medical

Medical treatment consists of either medication that affects the GH or irradiation of the pituitary gland. Proton beam therapy uses a very low dose of radiation and is much less destructive to nearby tissue than conventional radiation therapy.

Surgical

Surgical treatment for hyperpituitarism is to remove the pituitary gland. Two surgical approaches to remove the pituitary are transfrontal or transsphenoid hypophysectomy. The transfrontal approach is rarely used because it has a high risk of mortality as well as permanent loss of smell and taste and causes severe diabetes insipidus. The transsphenoid approach (Figure 12-11) involves an incision in the superior maxillary gingiva. Surgery may be the treatment of choice or used after attempting medical treatment.

Postoperatively, nasal packing should be checked for clear, colorless drainage. If it occurs, the drainage must be documented and reported to the physician. If this drainage is suspected of being cerebrospinal fluid, it should be checked for glucose, which is found in cerebrospinal fluid. The nurse should observe for meningitis infection, which includes elevated leukocytes, sudden temperature elevation, or complaint of headache or nuchal rigidity. Analgesics are administered as needed. The client should avoid activities such as coughing,

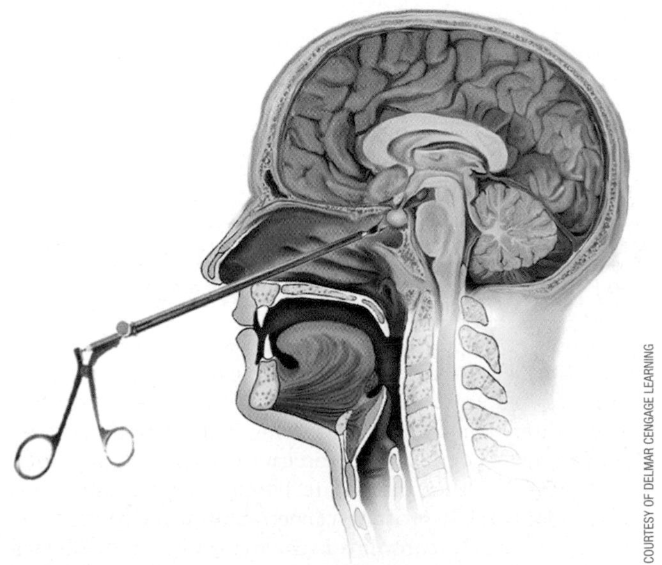

Figure 12-11 Transsphenoidal Approach to Hypophysectomy

straining, vomiting, or sneezing. The client should be encouraged to use an incentive spirometer instead of coughing. The client should not brush teeth for 2 weeks to avoid problems with the incision. Mouthwash can be used. The client should be instructed to avoid lifting and bending at the waist for 2 to 3 months after surgery.

Pharmacological

Two drugs may be prescribed for acromegaly. Bromocriptine mesylate (Parlodel) is a nonhormonal drug that activates dopamine receptors to inhibit the release of the GH and prolactin. Bromocriptine mesylate (Parlodel) should be given with food to decrease gastric upset. Because this drug can cause drowsiness or dizziness, the client should be instructed to avoid activities that require mental alertness. If the client is on oral contraceptives, alternate contraceptive measures should also be used because bromocriptine can stimulate ovulation.

The other drug, octreotide acetate (Sandostatin), inhibits the GH. Although octreotide is given by injection, it can still cause gastric distress. The injections should be given between meals and at bedtime. Clients with diabetes mellitus should closely monitor their blood sugar level.

Nursing Management

Be supportive. Show respect and acceptance. Assess ability to perform ADLs. Provide soft diet and encourage client to thoroughly chew food and drink fluids often.

NURSING PROCESS

Assessment

Subjective Data

Obtain a thorough nursing history, asking about vision impairment, headache, muscular weakness, menstrual irregularities, fatigue, sleep pattern changes, and sexual and psychological disturbances.

Objective Data

Objective data includes gait changes, vital sign changes (tachycardia or hypotension, which may indicate congestive heart failure), dyspnea, thick oily skin, and a deepening of the voice. The jaw is enlarged and projected, so the client may have difficulty in chewing.

Nursing diagnoses for a client with gigantism or acromegaly include the following:

NURSING DIAGNOSES	PLANNING/OUTCOMES	NURSING INTERVENTIONS
*Risk for Disproportionate **Growth** related to increased level of GH*	The client will comply with treatment to minimize hyperpituitarism and stop excessive growth with treatment.	Assist client with activities of daily living and range-of-motion exercises. Administer medications as ordered. Remind client to carry medications on person.
*Disturbed **Body** Image related to irreversible physical changes*	The client will acknowledge physical changes, express positive feelings about self, and exhibit ability to cope with altered body.	Encourage client to verbalize feelings. Assist client in setting achievable short-term goals. Offer emotional support and help client to develop coping strategies. Show respect and acceptance of the client as a person. Provide a positive but realistic assessment of the situation. Refer to professional counseling as needed. Provide education to client and family members concerning disease process.

Evaluation: Evaluate each outcome to determine how it has been met by the client.

SYNDROME OF INAPPROPRIATE ANTIDIURETIC HORMONE

Syndrome of inappropriate antidiuretic hormone (SIADH) results from an excess of ADH. The posterior pituitary gland continues to release ADH, causing the kidneys to reabsorb excess water, which decreases urine output and increases fluid volume. The most common cause is oat-cell lung cancer (NIH, 2007). Other causes are lymphoid pancreatic, duodenal, thymus, and prostate cancer; central nervous system trauma; infection; chronic obstructive pulmonary disease; acute respiratory failure; mechanical ventilation; and medications such as antineoplastic agents, tricyclic antidepressants, anesthetics, thiazides, and opioids.

The client will have hyponatremia (<130 mEq/L), water retention, weight gain, concentrated urine (urine osmolality >1,200 mOsm/L; specific gravity >1.020), muscle cramps, and weakness. The low osmolality of the blood allows fluid to leak out of vessels and causes brain swelling. If untreated, lethargy, seizures, coma, and death will result.

Medical–Surgical Management

Medical

The underlying disorder must be treated or medications stopped that may be contributing to SIADH. Fluid restriction will be implemented to prevent further hemodilution. Serious hyponatremia (<120 mEq/L) usually is treated with intravenous administration of 3% NaCl. The serum sodium level should be increased by 12 mEq/L or less per day. If the Na level is increased too rapidly, the client may experience fluid volume overload and congestive heart failure.

Pharmacological

Furosemide (Lasix) is given to increase urine output, while demeclocycline hydrochloride (Declomycin) and fludrocortisone (Florinef) are given to enhance sodium retention.

Diet

Fluid restriction is determined by the serum sodium level. Fluid restrictions of 1–1.5 liters/day are often implemented for the client with SIADH (Goh, 2004).

NURSING MANAGEMENT

Assess client's hydration and neurologic status every 3 to 4 hours. Provide a safe environment for the client. Accurately record I&O. Auscultate lungs every 2 to 4 hours. Explain why fluid intake is restricted. Weigh client daily. Provide frequent mouth care and apply lubricant to lips.

NURSING PROCESS

ASSESSMENT

Subjective Data

The client may describe muscle cramps, weakness, anorexia, nausea, and headache.

Objective Data

The client will have weight gain and fluid intake greater than output, may be irritable and disoriented, become progressively lethargic, and have seizures and diminished or absent deep tendon reflexes. Serum sodium and osmolality will be decreased. Urine osmolality and specific gravity will be increased.

Nursing diagnoses for a client with SIADH include the following:

NURSING DIAGNOSES	PLANNING/OUTCOMES	NURSING INTERVENTIONS
*Excess **Fluid** Volume* related to decreased urine output	The client will have increased urine output.	Assess client's weight daily on same scale at same time and vital signs. Accurately record I&O. Maintain fluid restrictions. Monitor laboratory reports, including Na, serum osmolality, urine Na, and urine osmolality. Administer medications as ordered.
*Impaired **Oral** Mucous Membrane* related to restriction of fluid intake	The client will have moist, intact oral mucous membranes.	Provide frequent oral care, avoiding alcohol-based mouth washes and lemon-glycerine swabs. Allow client to rinse mouth with water, but not swallow any. Provide lubricant for client's lips. Allow client to choose fluids and times to drink them.

Evaluation: Evaluate each outcome to determine how it has been met by the client.

PITUITARY TUMORS

Pituitary tumors more often affect the anterior pituitary rather than the posterior portion. Adenomas of the pituitary, which are rarely malignant, replace glandular tissue and enlarge the sella turcica. The cause is unknown, but there may be a predisposition toward tumor formation from an inherited **autosomal** dominant trait, meaning it is a dominant characteristic carried on any chromosome other than the one determining sex.

Clinical manifestations frequently start with a headache unrelated to stress or other factors. The next obvious manifestation is visual problems caused by the tumor putting pressure on the optic nerve. Others include personality changes, dementia, amenorrhea, impotence, lethargy, and weakness. The client may complain of cold intolerance, increased fatigue, constipation, and may have seizures. Although the tumor is not malignant, damage is done by tumor invasion of normal tissue.

Treatment is removal of the tumor. Complications of pituitary tumors are endocrine abnormalities if there is no replacement therapy after removal of the tumor. If the hypothalamus is compressed, diabetes insipidus can result. If the tumor has eroded the base of the skull, the client may have rhinorrhea (thin watery nasal discharge). Prognosis depends on the extent of invasion. In most cases, the tumor causes excessive secretion of the anterior pituitary hormones. Diagnostic testing includes dexamethasone suppression test, urine cortisol, FSH, LH, free T_4, TSH, and MRI of the head.

MEDICAL–SURGICAL MANAGEMENT

Medical

Medical treatment of a pituitary tumor often includes radiation therapy. This can be used for small tumors or if the client is a poor surgical risk. Radiation can also be used after surgery to shrink tissue remaining after surgical excision. Another alternative to surgery is cryohypophysectomy. This involves freezing the area with a probe inserted via the transsphenoidal approach.

Surgical

Large tumors, especially those impinging on the optic nerve, are generally removed by using the transfrontal approach. Smaller tumors can be resected via the transsphenoidal approach.

Pharmacological

Permanent hormone imbalances frequently result from surgical removal of the tumor. Consequently, long term hormone replacement therapy is necessary.

Nursing Management

Provide a safe, clutter-free environment. Keep a call light within the client's reach. Provide periods of rest after activity. Adjust room temperature for client's comfort or provide extra blankets. The client will be in ICU for several days if surgery is performed.

After a transphenoid approach to removal of the tumor, prohibit the client from sneezing, coughing or brushing the teeth. Monitor dressing for clear leakage which may indicate CSF leakage.

NURSING PROCESS

Assessment

Subjective Data

Obtain a thorough client history and assess for manifestations of a tumor, such as visual problems, headache, impotence, lethargy, cold intolerance, fatigue, or constipation. The family may provide insight into any personality changes.

Objective Data

Assess the client for tilting of the head to compensate for visual disturbances, axillary and pubic hair loss, a waxy appearance to the skin, and few wrinkles.

Nursing diagnoses for a client with a pituitary tumor include the following:

NURSING DIAGNOSES	PLANNING/OUTCOMES	NURSING INTERVENTIONS
Fatigue related to decreased ACTH and TSH levels	The client will verbalize an understanding of the relationship between fatigue, the disease, and activity level, and express feeling of increasing energy as treatment progresses.	Explain relationship between pituitary tumor, fatigue, and activity level. Suggest alternating periods of activity with periods of rest. Administer medications as ordered. Encourage completion of all treatments.
*Disturbed **S**ensory Perception (Visual)* related to altered sensory reception, transmission, and/or integration due to pressure on optic nerve by the pituitary tumor	The client will use adaptive devices and appropriate resources to compensate for visual changes, and regain normal vision with treatment.	Provide information about adaptive devices and resources for visual changes. Provide a safe clutter-free environment. Make certain that the bed is in the low position and the call signal is in reach of the client. Use side rails as needed.

Evaluation: Evaluate each outcome to determine how it has been met by the client.

HYPOPITUITARISM

Hypopituitarism is a complex syndrome marked by metabolic dysfunction, sexual immaturity, and growth retardation when it occurs in childhood; Simmonds' disease and diabetes insipidus are examples of hypopituitarism. The most common cause of hypopituitarism is a tumor. Other causes are congenital defects (hypoplasia or aplasia), pituitary infarction (from postpartum hemorrhage), pituitary surgery or irradiation, or chemical agents. Hypopituitarism can be primary (meaning there is no known cause) or secondary. Secondary hypopituitarism can be a result of a deficiency of hypothalamic-releasing hormones. This deficiency can be idiopathic (without a known cause) or a result of infection, trauma, or tumor.

Clinical manifestations develop slowly and generally are not apparent until 75% of the pituitary is destroyed. Specific manifestations will vary with the specific hormone that is deficient.

Deficiency of the GH results in dwarfism, which becomes apparent by 6 months of age as the infant exhibits growth retardation, with chubbiness in the lower trunk and a short stature. As it progresses, secondary tooth eruption is delayed, and later there is a delay in puberty. Growth continues at about half the normal rate until the child reaches about 4 feet in height. Body proportions are normal, as is mental development. Frequently in adulthood, sex organs may not develop normally unless treated with hormones. Clients experience an accelerated pattern of aging, resulting in the life span being shortened by as much as 20 years. If the deficiency occurs in adults, manifestations are not as apparent. There are subtle signs such as wrinkles near the mouth and eyes.

Deficiencies of follicle-stimulating hormone and LH cause differences in clinical manifestations between female and male clients. In the female, symptoms include amenorrhea, dyspareunia, infertility, decreased libido, breast atrophy, sparse or absent axillary and pubic hair, and dry skin. In the male, symptoms include weakness, impotence, decreased libido, decreased muscle strength, testicular softening and shrinkage, and retarded secondary sexual hair growth.

In a child, a deficiency of TSH will result in severe growth retardation even with treatment. Other deficiency manifestations include cold intolerance; constipation; increased or decreased menstrual flow; lethargy; dry, pale puffy skin, and bradycardia. Thought processes may also be slowed.

A deficiency of adrenocorticotrophic hormone (ACTH) results in fatigue, nausea, vomiting, anorexia, weight loss, and depigmentation of the skin and nipples. Vital signs taken during periods of stress would show fever and hypotension.

Prolactin deficiency results in absent postpartum lactation, amenorrhea, and sparse or absent axillary and pubic hair. There may also be manifestations of thyroid or adrenal cortex failure.

Findings of hypopituitarism depend on the specific hormone, client's age, and severity of condition when detected. X-rays of the wrist determine bone age, and a skull series will rule out a pituitary tumor. Total failure of the pituitary without treatment is fatal; however, prognosis is good with treatment by the appropriate hormone(s). Treatment is primarily replacement therapy for the deficient hormone(s).

SIMMONDS' DISEASE

Simmonds' disease is defined as a total absence of all pituitary secretions. This is also called *panhypopituitarism*. This disease results from surgery, infection, injury, or tumor. It may also occur after a difficult labor in childbirth because of thrombosis formation during or after delivery.

Clinical manifestations, which vary in intensity, include extreme weight loss, general debility, lethargy, pallor, dry yellowish skin, loss of libido, amenorrhea, and intolerance to cold. The disease leads to loss of axillary and pubic hair and atrophy of genitalia and breasts. It progresses to bradycardia (slow pulse), hypotension, premature wrinkling of the skin, and atrophy of the thyroid and adrenal glands.

Treatment consists of administration of ACTH, TSH, or thyroid, adrenal, and sex hormones for a lifetime.

DIABETES INSIPIDUS

Diabetes insipidus (DI) is a deficiency of ADH, causing a metabolic disorder characterized by severe polyuria and polydipsia. Diabetes insipidus generally starts in childhood or early adulthood, with a median onset of 21 years. It affects males more often than females. Although a deficiency of ADH is the most common cause (central), diabetes insipidus can also be caused by failure of the kidneys to respond to ADH (nephrogenic), a defect in or damage to the thirst mechanism (dipsogenic), or during pregnancy (gestational) (NIDDK, 2008b).

Neurogenic diabetes insipidus may be caused by injury or ischemia to the hypothalamus or pituitary gland, CNS infections, head injuries, neurosurgery, or sickle-cell disease. Nephrogenic diabetes insipidus may be caused by pyelonephritis, chronic renal failure, polycystic disease, or medications such as lithium carbonate (Carbolith), amphotericin B (Fungizone), furosemide (Lasix), or ethycrynic acid (Edecrin). Dipsogenic diabetes insipidus results in an extreme increase in thirst and then fluid intake, which suppresses ADH secretion, increasing urine output. Often dypsogenic DI is caused by damage to the hypothalamus. Gestational diabetes insipidus is caused by a placenta enzyme that destroys ADH in the mother (NIDDK, 2008b).

Clinical manifestations have an abrupt onset. The client experiences extreme polyuria of 4–16 L of dilute urine daily. In some cases, there can be up to 30 L of urine per day. Serum osmolality is >295 mOsm/L and urine osmolality is <150 mOsm/L. Urine specific gravity is <1.005 and serum sodium is 145–150 mEq/L. The client has extreme thirst, preferring cold beverages. Even though there is an extraordinary volume of fluid intake, weight is lost. Other manifestations include dizziness, weakness, bed wetting, constipation, nocturia, and fatigue that may be a result of inadequate rest because of frequent nighttime voiding and excess thirst. Diagnostic tests used to diagnose DI include measurement of ADH, MRI (brain), a trail of DDAVP (synthetic ADH), and water deprivation test.

Complications of untreated diabetes insipidus are **hypovolemia** (abnormally low circulatory blood volume), circulatory collapse, unconsciousness, and central nervous system damage. Prolonged urine flow can cause chronic urinary system conditions such as bladder distension, enlarged calyces, and hydronephrosis.

Prognosis is generally good with fluid replacement in uncomplicated cases. Prognosis also depends on the underlying cause of diabetes insipidus.

MEDICAL–SURGICAL MANAGEMENT

Pharmacological

In addition to intravenous fluids, several medications can be used to treat diabetes insipidus. For neurogenic and gestational diabetes insipidus, desmopressin acetate (DDAVP), a synthetic antidiuretic hormone that can be given parenterally or nasally, is the drug of choice. Also, vasopressin (Pitressin Synthetic) may be given parenterally or nasally. Make certain that the nasal passage is clear before administering the medication. Monitor intake and output and assess for hypovolemia and electrolyte imbalance. The client should drink fluids or water only when thirsty (NIDDK, 2008b).

For nephrogenic diabetes insipidus, a diuretic such as hydrochlorothiazide (HydroDiuril) may be given alone or with amiloride (NIDDK, 2008b).

NURSING MANAGEMENT

Carefully and accurately monitor and record the client's I&O. Assess skin turgor and condition of oral mucous membranes. Weigh client daily. Oral fluids are often restricted and provided only in amounts equal to the client's urine output. Assess skin on each shift. Apply moisturizing lotion to skin. Provide egg-crate mattress or sheepskin.

NURSING PROCESS

ASSESSMENT

Subjective Data

Obtain a thorough client history, including severity of thirst, weakness, fatigue, lethargy, bed wetting, dizziness, constipation, and nocturia.

Objective Data

Assess for weight loss, constipation, and signs of fluid volume deficit, such as dry skin and mucous membranes, fever, dyspnea, and poor skin turgor. Check urine for color, amount, and specific gravity. Assess weight daily. Figure 12-12 illustrates the comparison of assessment findings between SIADH and DI.

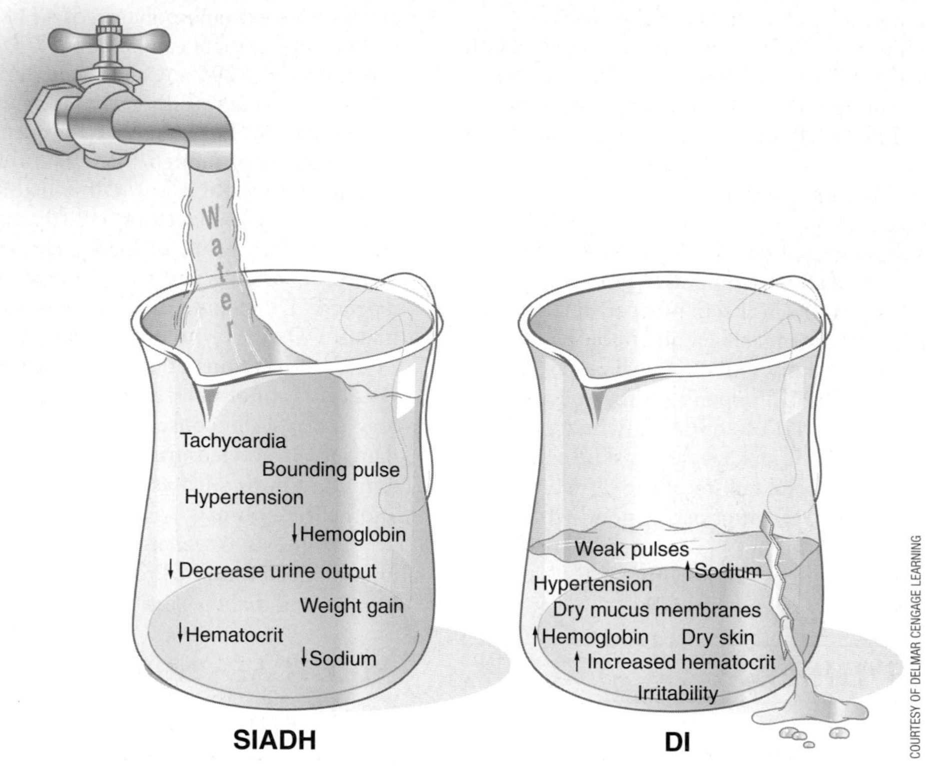

FIGURE 12-12 Comparison of Assessment Findings between SIADH and DI

Nursing diagnoses for a client with diabetes insipidus include the following:

NURSING DIAGNOSES	PLANNING/OUTCOMES	NURSING INTERVENTIONS
*Risk for Imbalanced **F**luid Volume* related to polyuria	The client will have sufficient fluid intake to prevent dehydration.	Provide easy access to bedpan/bathroom. Answer call signal promptly. Monitor the client for dizziness and weakness. Record client intake and output. Teach client and family how to record intake and output. Provide fluids as ordered to cover output. Monitor weight daily. Use same scale, same amount of clothing, at the same time daily. Provide oral care. Use a soft toothbrush, mild mouthwash, and lubricant for the lips. Assess condition of oral mucous membranes. Administer medications via intranasal or subcutaneous routes.
*Risk for Impaired **S**kin Integrity* related to altered hydration	The client will maintain skin integrity.	Assess skin, especially pressure points, 3 times a day. Apply moisturizing lotion to skin. Prevent pressure on skin by turning or ambulating client. Use egg-crate mattress or sheepskin. Encourage adequate intake of fluids, protein, vitamin C, and calories. Monitor for incontinence and nocturia. Thoroughly clean and dry area following episodes of incontinence.

Evaluation: Evaluate each outcome to determine how it has been met by the client.

THYROID DISORDERS

Worldwide, a deficiency of iodine is the most likely cause of thyroid disorders; however, in countries where iodine in food is plentiful, autoimmune thyroid disease is the most common thyroid disorder (Walpert, 1998). The thyroid gland is a butterfly shaped gland located anteriorly to the trachea. The purpose of the thyroid gland is to produce, store, and release hormones into the bloodstream. The hormones, T_3 and T_4, are responsible for the regulation of body metabolism (brain development, breathing, heart rate, temperature, and the nervous system) (NIDDK, 2008c). The production of T_3 and T_4 is regulated by the release of TSH from the anterior pituitary gland. Thyroid disorders are classified as hyperthyroidism, hypothyroidism, tumors, cancer, or goiter.

HYPERTHYROIDISM

Hyperthyroidism is a collective term for a condition marked by increased thyroid activity and overproduction of thyroid hormones thyroxine (T_4) and triiodothyronine (T_3). The thyroid gland may be enlarged. Different forms of hyperthyroidism are Graves' disease, Basedow's disease, Parry's disease, or thyrotoxicosis. Graves' disease is the most common cause of hyperthyroidism and occurs more frequently in women over age 20 (NIH, 2009).

In this autoimmune disorder, the immune system triggers the formation of thyroid-stimulating immunoglobulins (TSIs). The TSIs bind with TSH receptors, causing an overproduction of thyroid hormone.

Clinical manifestations include two obvious physical changes. The thyroid, palpated for asymmetry and size, may be enlarged 3 to 4 times its normal size. The enlargement of the thyroid gland is called **goiter**. This is generally a result of overactivity of the thyroid gland. The accumulation of orbital fluid behind the eyeball, forcing it to protrude, is called **exophthalmos**. This occurs in about half the cases of hyperthyroidism. It produces a characteristic stare.

The increased thyroid hormone production causes an increased metabolic rate. This leads to weight loss despite increased appetite, fatigue, poor tolerance to heat, and profuse perspiration. The client is very nervous, restless, irritable, has difficulty concentrating, is emotionally labile, has mood swings, possible personality changes, and sleep disturbances. The client may have fine tremors of the fingers and tongue, shaky handwriting, clumsiness, trouble climbing stairs, or dyspnea on exertion and possibly at rest. The skin is warm and moist with a velvety texture. The skin may be a characteristic salmon color. The hair is fine and soft with premature graying and increased hair loss. The nails appear fragile with distal nail separation from the nail bed (onycholysis). There may be general or local muscle atrophy and acropachy (soft tissue swelling with underlying bone changes where new bone forms). There is a tachycardia with bounding pulse up to 160 beats per minute and down to 80 beats per minute during sleep. Pulse pressure is widened. There can be muscular weakness and atrophy; osteoporosis; paralysis; vitiligo, milky-white patches on the skin surrounded by areas of normal pigmentation; decreased libido; impaired fertility; and **gynecomastia** (abnormal enlargement of one or both breasts in males).

> ### LIFE SPAN CONSIDERATIONS
> #### Hyperthyroid Complications
> The older client in particular develops cardiovascular problems such as arrhythmias (atrial fibrillation), cardiac insufficiency leading to cardiac decompensation, and resistance to the usual dose of digoxin.

Diagnostic tests generally include TSH, T_3, T_4, radioactive iodine uptake, and a thyroid scan.

One major complication is thyrotoxic crisis, also called *thyroid storm*. This is a medical emergency that can lead to cardiac, hepatic, or renal failure. Undiagnosed or inadequately treated hyperthyroid clients often experience thyroid storm. Thyroid storm can be precipitated by stressful situations such as surgery, infection, or trauma. Less common causes are cerebrovascular accident (CVA), myocardial infarction, sudden discontinuing of antithyroid medications, subtotal thyroidectomy with excess intake of synthetic thyroid hormone, toxemia, or diabetic ketoacidosis. Any of these events can lead to overproduction of thyroid hormone, causing an increase in systemic adrenergic activity. This causes an overproduction of epinephrine and severe hypermetabolism, leading to rapid cardiac, gastrointestinal, and sympathetic nervous system decompensation. The client will rapidly exhibit severe clinical manifestations of hyperthyroidism, including extreme high fever, restlessness, agitation, coma, heart failure, and angina.

If the nurse suspects that the client is experiencing thyrotoxic crisis, inform the physician immediately. The client will be transferred to intensive care for closer monitoring of vital signs, EKG pattern, and cardiopulmonary status. Priority treatment includes respiratory support and hemodynamic stability. Antithyroid therapy is initiated immediately. Adrenergic blocking agents are administered to decrease the sympathetic nervous system stimulation. The client's temperature is monitored and cooling measures initiated as needed. Acetaminophen is administered to lower the temperature, but aspirin is not given because it can increase the free T_4 level. Supportive care is given until the client is out of the thyrotoxic crisis.

MEDICAL–SURGICAL MANAGEMENT

Medical

The goal of managing hyperthyroidism is to decrease excessive thyroid hormone production. With treatment to decrease the thyroid production of the thyroid's hormone, the prognosis is good. The client can live a normal life. There can be a combination of treatment methods. The first method is to administer antithyroid medications. This is usually a temporary solution.

Radiation therapy of the thyroid gland could be external radiation to the neck; however, the more accepted method is the oral administration of radioactive iodine, either liquid or capsule, that targets the thyroid tissue. Radioactive iodine acts on the thyroid tissue to destroy thyroid cells, potentially leading to hypothyroidism (NIDDK, 2008c). It is most commonly used for women past the reproductive years or clients not planning to have children. The client of reproductive age must sign an informed consent form because small amounts of the radioactive iodine could lodge in the gonads.

Antithyroid medications are stopped 4 to 7 days before treatment. The physician must know if the client is receiving amiodarone hydrochloride (Cordarone), an antiarrhythmic, because it contains large amounts of iodine. The oral ^{131}I should not be given to the client with severe vomiting or diarrhea.

A single dose of oral ^{131}I will destroy some iodine concentrating cells that produce the thyroxine. Clinical manifestations decrease in about 3 weeks, with the full effect in about 3 months. Some clients require a second or third dose.

The client usually resumes the thyroid hormone antagonist 3 to 5 days after ^{131}I therapy until the physician determines the thyroid to be atrophic (decreased in size). The client may continue to take propranolol hydrochloride (Inderal) for tachycardia, tremor, and diaphoresis. Continued monitoring of thyroid hormone blood levels and physical condition is necessary.

The most common complication is hypothyroidism, which occurs about 2 to 4 months after treatment. The client is then placed on thyroid replacement therapy, generally for life.

Surgical

Generally just a portion of the thyroid gland is removed, but a total thyroidectomy may be performed. This is the most expensive option and has the most risks. A thyroidectomy may also be done for respiratory obstruction by a goiter or thyroid cancer. If a partial thyroidectomy is done, the remaining thyroid tissue should provide adequate amounts of thyroid hormones. If a complete thyroidectomy is done, the client will require thyroid hormone replacement for life.

Clients usually take propylthiouracil (PTU) for 4 to 6 weeks before surgery and iodine preparations may be prescribed 10 to 14 days before surgery to decrease thyroid vascularity and decrease bleeding. Depending on the symptoms, the client may also be taking propranolol hydrochloride (Inderal). Thyroid function tests and an EKG are performed before surgery to provide baseline information. Informed consent must be obtained.

Preoperatively, the client should be told about activities after surgery. There will be a neck incision, generally with some type of drain. The client may experience a sore throat and hoarseness. The client is kept in high-Fowler's position to promote venous drainage. The client should support the head with a hand when moving the head to prevent strain on the incision. Respiratory problems may occur, such as tracheal collapse, tracheal mucous accumulation, or laryngeal or local tissue edema.

> **▼ SAFETY ▼**
>
> **Radioactive Iodine**
>
> No pregnant nurse should care for the client. The client should expectorate carefully for the first day because the saliva is radioactive. The client should drink plenty of fluids for 2 days to help circulate and eliminate the radioactive iodine. The toilet should be flushed twice after each use for at least 2 days or throughout the hospitalization. Disposable eating utensils should be used by the client. Close contact with children or pregnant females should be avoided for a week after the administration. Females should avoid pregnancy for 6 months after treatment.

Laryngeal spasms may occur following injury to the parathyroid glands resulting in hypocalcemia and tetany. *A tracheotomy tray or endotracheal tubes and insertion tray are kept readily available at the client's bedside in case of a respiratory emergency.*

Because the thyroid is so vascular, the dressing must be checked frequently for drainage, especially at the back of the neck. If there is a drain, approximately 50 mL of drainage is expected the first day. If there is no drainage, the drain must be checked for kinks or obstruction. Voice rest is encouraged for 48 hours, with voice checks every 2 to 4 hours as ordered to make certain there is no laryngeal nerve damage.

Because the parathyroid glands could be accidentally removed during the thyroidectomy, the client's blood calcium level is monitored. The client is checked for Chvostek's sign or Trousseau's sign. (These are discussed under hypoparathyroidism.) Analgesics are administered as needed.

Complications of thyroidectomy are respiratory distress and hemorrhage. There can be damage to the laryngeal nerves, affecting the voice. Manipulation of the thyroid gland during surgery can cause a release of large amounts of thyroid hormone causing thyroid storm, which is rare but may occur. Thyroid crisis usually occurs within the first 12 hours postoperative. Hyperthyroid signs and symptoms are exaggerated, plus the client may vomit, have severe hypertension and tachycardia, and sometimes have hyperthermia up to 106°F (41°C). The client may develop congestive heart failure and die. The client must be advised that tetany can occur up to 10 days after surgery. **Tetany** is sharp flexion of the wrist and ankle joints, muscle twitchings, or cramps caused by decreased blood calcium level.

Pharmacological

Antithyroid therapy is used for children, younger adults, pregnant females, the client who refuses surgery, or clients after surgery. The goal of pharmaceutical management includes the client reaching a euthroid state (Daniels, 2007). Several drugs can be used for antithyroid therapy. PTU is used frequently, especially in cases of thyroid storm. It reduces the production of the thyroid hormones. It should be given with food. The client must be instructed to avoid foods high in iodine such as shellfish and iodized salt. Over-the-counter preparations must be checked to see if they contain iodine. This drug requires several weeks to exert the full effect, and it may be administered up to 2 years. This drug may cause **agranulocytosis** (a decreased number of granulocytes), so it is important to report signs and symptoms of infection immediately to the physician.

Methimazole (Tapazole) is another antithyroid preparation that interferes with thyroid hormone synthesis. It has a more rapid onset than PTU; however, it does not have as much consistency in effect. It should be administered at evenly spaced intervals with food to prevent gastric upset. This drug can also cause agranulocytosis, particularly in the client older than age 40.

Iodide preparations may be given to the client with hyperthyroidism. Because iodides inhibit the release of thyroid hormones rather than the synthesis, they take effect in 2 days. Two common preparations are saturated solution potassium iodide (SSKI) and a solution of iodine and potassium iodide that is called Lugol's solution. When iodide preparations are administered orally, they should be mixed with milk, juice, or water and given after meals to decrease gastric upset. Drinking

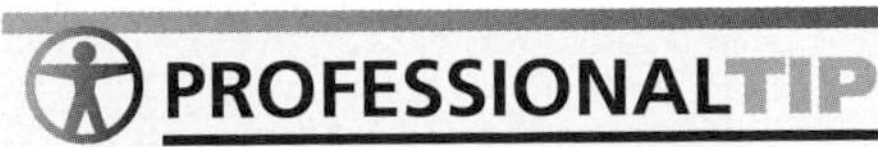

Hypersensitivity to Iodides

The first signs of hypersensitivity reactions caused by iodides are irritation and swollen eyelids.

the preparations through a straw will decrease discoloration of the teeth. These drugs are contraindicated in the client with acute bronchitis or a known hypersensitivity to iodine and shellfish.

Clients may be prescribed propranolol hydrochloride (Inderal) to counteract tachycardia and peripheral effects of hyperthyroidism. Clients should not smoke while taking this medication. Abrupt withdrawal of the drug can cause hypertension, myocardial ischemia, or cardiac arrhythmias. Clients should rise slowly from a sitting or lying position in order to prevent orthostatic hypotension.

Topical medications such as isotonic eyedrops may be ordered to protect the eyes of the client with exophthalmos. Care must be taken that the eyes are not injured or infected, including the use of tinted eye glasses, artificial tears, ointments and protective shields. Some physicians may order high doses of corticosteroids to help reduce exophthalmos.

During a thyrotoxic crisis, antithyroid drugs are given. Other medications that may be used are propranolol, corticosteroids, and iodine preparations. Individual client needs could indicate a need for vitamins, nutrients, fluids, or sedation.

Diet

Because the client has a greatly increased metabolic rate as well as weight loss, diet is important. The client may require between 4,000 to 6,000 calories per day. There is a need for increased protein, vitamins (especially vitamins B and C), and minerals. In addition to 3 meals per day, the client needs additional meals or snacks. Fluids should be encouraged, but caffeine should be avoided. Clients also may experience extreme fatigue due to the increased metabolism.

NURSING MANAGEMENT

Provide a high-calorie diet and snacks throughout the day. Encourage fluids, but avoid caffeine. Keep client's skin dry and clean and change gown and linens as needed. Preoperatively, teach the client how to support his head while turning or rising to a sitting or standing position. Inform client that "voice rest" may be enforced for 48 hours and provide paper and pencil for writing notes.

Postoperatively, keep bed in semi-Fowler's position with head and shoulders supported by pillows. Keep suction equipment and tracheotomy tray in the client's room. Monitor vital signs. Inspect dressing, sides and back of neck, and shoulders frequently for bleeding. Watch for signs of internal bleeding (apprehension, restlessness, increased pulse, decreased blood pressure, and fullness feeling in the neck). Watch for signs of tetany and for signs of edema in the operative area.

NURSING PROCESS

ASSESSMENT

Subjective Data

Obtain a thorough client history and ask about the ability to concentrate, nervousness, insomnia, jitteriness, excitability, emotional lability, dysphagia, weight loss, personality changes, or sleep disturbances.

Objective Data

Assess for rapid pulse, elevated blood pressure, warm skin, elevated temperature, diaphoresis, or hand tremors. Female clients may cease to menstruate. Hair is fine and soft.

Nursing diagnoses for a client with hyperthyroidism include the following:

NURSING DIAGNOSES	PLANNING/OUTCOMES	NURSING INTERVENTIONS
Preoperative		
*Imbalanced **N**utrition: Less than Body Requirements* related to increased metabolism	The client will eat a nutritionally balanced diet with enough calories to prevent weight loss.	Monitor weight daily. Use same scale, same amount of clothing, at the same time daily. Encourage 6 meals per day with adequate protein, carbohydrate, and caloric intake. Arrange a consultation with the dietitian to assist in determining the client's increased nutritional needs. Encourage client to eat a well-balanced diet. Provide snacks throughout the day. Complete pre-albumin test to determine protein reserve.
*Risk for **I**njury* related to exophthalmos	The client's eyes will not be injured from exophthalmos.	Administer isotonic solutions or eye lubricants to keep the eye moist. At night, elevate head of the bed which may assist in keeping the eyelids closed, or cover the eyes with eye guards to prevent drying.

(*Continues*)

Nursing diagnoses for a client with hyperthyroidism include the following: (Continued)

NURSING DIAGNOSES	PLANNING/OUTCOMES	NURSING INTERVENTIONS
		Suggest to client that dark or tinted wraparound glasses may protect the eyes from wind and airborne particles.
Postoperative		
*Impaired **S**wallowing* related to mechanical obstruction (edema)	The client will have diminished problems with swallowing.	Ensure gag, cough, and swallowing reflexes are present before offering oral fluids. Maintain client in Fowler's position when drinking or eating. Encourage client to drink slowly and chew thoroughly.
*Ineffective **A**irway Clearance* related to edema and pain	The client will be able to clear airway.	Keep intubation and tracheostomy kits readily available. Keep suctioning equipment ready. Administer analgesic as ordered. Complete respiratory assessment frequently and monitor for respiratory distress and laryngeal spasms.

Evaluation: Evaluate each outcome to determine how it has been met by the client.

SAMPLE NURSING CARE PLAN

The Client with Hyperthyroidism

A.J., 33 years old, has returned to her physician's office to find out results of her tests for hyperthyroidism. She continues to have multiple complaints. "I have lost 15 pounds in the last month despite eating all the time. I am restless and can't sleep. I feel jittery and irritable. My family says my moods change so rapidly they don't know what to expect from me. I feel so hot most of the time and sweat a lot."

During assessment, the client appears flushed and her eyes protrude slightly. Her vital signs are temperature 100.6°F orally, pulse 120 beats/min, respiration 26 breaths/min, and blood pressure 140/88 mm Hg, which are slightly elevated from her previous office visit. Test results confirm the presence of hyperthyroidism.

NURSING DIAGNOSIS 1 *Imbalanced **N**utrition: Less than Body Requirements* related to increased metabolism as evidenced by weight loss despite eating

Nursing Outcomes Classification (NOC)
Nutritional Status: Food & Fluid Intake
Nutritional Status: Nutrient Intake

Nursing Interventions Classification (NIC)
Fluid Management
Nutrition Management

PLANNING/OUTCOMES	NURSING INTERVENTIONS	RATIONALE
A.J. will eat a nutritionally balanced diet with enough calories to prevent weight loss.	Monitor amount of food ingested and caloric intake.	Provides data to determine if diet is adequate to prevent weight loss.
	Monitor weight daily.	Determines weight gains or losses.
	Provide a diet high in calories, protein, and carbohydrates.	Maintains or increases weight while preventing muscle mass breakdown.
	Advise A.J. to avoid highly seasoned or fibrous foods or foods causing flatulence.	Prevents increased peristalsis resulting in diarrhea.

SAMPLE NURSING CARE PLAN (Continued)

PLANNING/OUTCOMES	NURSING INTERVENTIONS	RATIONALE
	Provide small frequent meals spread over waking hours, up to 6 meals per day.	Provides calories without extremely large meals.
	Obtain nutritional consult as needed.	Ensures nutritional status.

EVALUATION

A.J. gained or maintained weight.

NURSING DIAGNOSIS 2 *Hyperthermia* related to increased metabolic rate as evidenced by complaints of feeling hot, flushing, and elevated temperature

Nursing Outcomes Classification (NOC)
Hydration
Thermoregulation

Nursing Interventions Classification (NIC)
Fluid Management

PLANNING/OUTCOMES	NURSING INTERVENTIONS	RATIONALE
A.J.'s body temperature will be within normal range.	Assess for elevated temperature, heat intolerance, and diaphoresis.	Indicates increased heat production from increased metabolic rate.
	Provide a well-ventilated room with temperature control.	Promotes comfort if heat intolerant.
	Suggest wearing cool, loose-fitting, lightweight clothing.	Provides comfort and prevents overheating.
	Provide frequent bathing and changes in linens or clothing.	Promotes comfort if diaphoretic.
	Provide fluids up to 3 L per day.	Replaces fluid if diaphoretic.

EVALUATION

A.J. maintained her temperature in a normal range.

NURSING DIAGNOSIS 3 *Risk for Impaired Skin Integrity* related to diaphoresis as evidenced by excessive sweating

Nursing Outcomes Classification (NOC)
Nutritional Status
Tissue Integrity: Skin & Mucous Membranes

Nursing Interventions Classification (NIC)
Fluid/Electrolyte Management
Nutrition Management

PLANNING/OUTCOMES	NURSING INTERVENTIONS	RATIONALE
A.J.'s skin will remain intact and free of injury.	Complete Braden Scale.	Indentifies risk level of skin breakdown.
	Assess skin for flushing and moisture.	Indicates heat intolerance.
	Assess skin for redness, especially bony prominences.	Indicates potential for breakdown.
	Keep skin clean and dry.	Prevents skin breakdown.

EVALUATION

A.J. maintained intact skin without impairment.

HYPOTHYROIDISM

Hypothyroidism is a condition in which the metabolic processes are decreased because of a deficiency of thyroid hormones. It is termed primary if the problem arises from a dysfunction solely of the thyroid. It is secondary if the thyroid gland is not stimulated to produce normally or if the target cells fail to respond to normal thyroid functioning. This condition is more common in females than males. There is a significant increase in incidence between the ages of 30 to 60. Hypothyroid conditions include cretinism, myxedema, and Hashimoto's thyroiditis.

CRETINISM

A congenital condition with decreased thyroid hormone production causes defective physical development and mental retardation. This is called **cretinism** and occurs in about 1 of 3,000 live births (NIH, 2007). Female clients are two times more likely to be affected than male clients. The child generally has a large head, short limbs, puffy eyes, thick and protruding tongue, excessively dry skin, and a lack of coordination. If untreated, the child will be permanently dwarfed, mentally retarded, and sterile. This condition is rare in the United States and is diagnosed by the T_4, serum TSH, x-ray of long bones, and thyroid scan.

MYXEDEMA

Myxedema is the term for severe hypothyroidism in adults. A variety of abnormalities lead to decreased thyroid hormone production. The obvious ones are thyroid gland surgery such as thyroidectomy or irradiation of the thyroid gland. Some other causes are chronic autoimmune Hashimoto's thyroiditis, inflammatory conditions (sarcoidosis), pituitary failure to produce TSH, or hypothalamus failure to produce thyrotropin-releasing hormone. There may be an inability to synthesize thyroid hormones related to iodine deficiency (rarely from general diet deficiency) or as a result of taking antithyroid medications.

Clinical manifestations are vague and varied, developing slowly over a period of time, but are primarily related to the reduced metabolic rate. These include an energy loss, fatigue, forgetfulness, sensitivity to cold, unexplained weight gain, hypoventilation, and constipation. As the condition progresses, manifestations include reduced libido, menorrhagia, paresthesias, joint stiffness, and muscle cramping. There is a characteristic alteration in overall appearance and behavior, including decreased mental stability and a thick and dry tongue, causing hoarseness and slow, slurred speech. The skin is flaky and inelastic, and feels cool, dry, rough, and doughy. There is edema of the face, hands, and feet. The hair is dry and sparse, with patchy hair loss including loss of the outer third of the eyebrow. The nails are thick and brittle with visible transverse and longitudinal grooves. The pulse is weak and bradycardic because of the decreased pumping strength of the heart. The thyroid gland may be so small that it may not be palpated unless there is a goiter. The blood pressure is generally lower than normal for the client.

Diagnostic tests generally include TSH, T_3, T_4, radioactive iodine uptake, and a thyroid scan.

Complications affect almost every system. Cardiovascular complications include ischemic heart disease, poor peripheral circulation, enlarged heart, or pleural or pericardial effusion. Gastrointestinal complications include adynamic colon (decreased functioning of the colon), megacolon (massive and abnormal dilation of the colon), or intestinal obstruction. Other complications include conductive or sensorineural deafness, psychiatric disorders, carpal tunnel syndrome, or impotence or infertility. Prognosis depends on the organs involved, duration, and severity of condition.

Myxedema coma or hypothyroid crisis is a rare but serious complication of extreme hypothyroidism. It is life threatening, with symptoms of unresponsiveness, hypothermia, decreased respirations, low blood pressure, and low blood sugar. It has a gradual onset but is triggered by severe stress such as infection, exposure to cold, or trauma. Abrupt withdrawal of thyroid medication or the use of narcotics, sedatives, or anesthetics can also cause myxedema coma. If myxedema coma occurs, it must be reported to the physician immediately. The client is moved to the ICU, where intubation and mechanical ventilation are instituted. The client is monitored closely for vital signs, EKG changes, and cardiopulmonary status. Wrapping the client in blankets will warm the client, but a warming blanket should not be used because it could cause peripheral vasodilation and shock. Thyroid medications and possibly corticosteroids are administered. Supportive care is given until the client comes out of the myxedema coma. Myxedema coma is often fatal.

MEDICAL–SURGICAL MANAGEMENT

Pharmacological

Thyroid replacement therapy is lifelong. Thyroid (Armour Thyroid) is a natural form, whereas levothyroxine sodium (Levothroid, Synthroid) is a synthetic. The physician orders thyroid hormone to begin slowly and increases the dosage every 2 to 3 weeks until the desired response is achieved. Medication should be administered 1 hour prior to or 2 hours after meals to improve absorption. The medication should be given in the morning to prevent insomnia.

If the client has diabetes mellitus, insulin or oral hypoglycemic dosage might have to be adjusted. The blood sugar level must be monitored closely. If the client is on anticoagulant therapy, thyroid potentiates the anticoagulant action. The client should be taught to watch for excessive bleeding or bruising. Digitalis preparations are also potentiated by thyroid.

Because hypothyroidism impairs the metabolic rate, the client may have difficulty metabolizing medications. The client may have an increased sensitivity to hypnotics, sedatives, or opiates. Dosage may have to be adjusted appropriately. Synthesis of the thyroid hormone can be impaired by drugs such as lithium carbonate (Lithotabs) or aminoglutethimide (Cytadren).

Diet

The client is instructed to avoid foods high in iodine and foods that interfere with thyroid hormone replacement, such as dried kelp, shellfish, iodized salt, saltwater fish, cabbage, turnips, pears, and peaches. The diet is designed for weight loss and to combat constipation. A high-fiber, high-protein, low-calorie diet is given. Sodium is decreased to prevent fluid retention. A dietary consultation for meal planning and a list of foods to avoid is provided to the client.

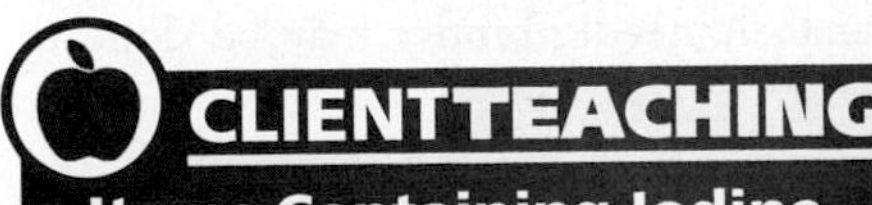

Items Containing Iodine

Check the labels on multivitamins, dentrifices, and nonprescription medications; they may contain iodine.

Nursing Management

Monitor vital signs, heart sounds, lung sounds, I&O, weight, and check for edema. Prevent client fatigue by providing rest periods between activities. Provide a high-fiber diet and encourage intake of oral fluids. Administer stool softener, bulk laxative, or enema as ordered.

NURSING PROCESS

Assessment

Subjective Data

Obtain a thorough client history, asking about lethargy, depression, irritability, impaired memory, and slowing of thought processes. The client may describe speech and hearing problems, anorexia, decreased libido, constipation, cold intolerance, and changes in menstruation.

Objective Data

Assess for hearing and speech deficits, thin hair, dry and thickened skin, enlarged facial features, masklike expression, low and hoarse voice, bradycardia, decreased blood pressure and respirations, and exercise intolerance.

Nursing diagnoses for a client with myxedema include the following:

NURSING DIAGNOSES	PLANNING/OUTCOMES	NURSING INTERVENTIONS
Activity Intolerance related to decreased metabolic and energy level	The client will express understanding to increase activity level gradually. The client will maintain blood pressure, pulse, and respirations within normal limits when active. The client will regain normal activity levels.	Assist client to gradually increase activity level but encourage rest between activities to avoid fatigue and decrease cardiac oxygen demands. Measure client's legs correctly so antiembolic hose, which help venous return, will fit properly when worn. Reposition client every 2 hours and encourage client to continue activity when normal activity level is achieved. Assess blood pressure, pulse, and respirations frequently and inform physician of abnormal results.
Ineffective Tissue Perfusion (Cardiopulmonary) related to decreased cardiac output	The client will not have chest pain at rest. The client will have a normal heart rate and rhythm. The client will avoid ischemic EKG changes. The client will maintain adequate cardiopulmonary perfusion.	Assess for chest pain and advise client to report any episodes of angina immediately. Monitor client's vital signs. Monitor cardiac status through EKG and assessment of heart and lung sounds plus checking for edema. Restrict fluid and sodium during the time of cardiac decompensation as ordered. Monitor intake and output and weight.
Constipation related to decreased motility of the gastrointestinal tract	The client will have regular bowel movements.	Provide high-fiber diet. Encourage intake of oral fluids. Assess frequency and character of stool. Administer stool softener, bulk laxative, or enema as ordered.

Evaluation: Evaluate each outcome to determine how it has been met by the client.

HASHIMOTO'S THYROIDITIS

Hashimoto's thyroiditis, the most common cause of hypothyroidism, is an autoimmune disease characterized by the production of antiperoxidase antibodies, which destroy an essential enzyme necessary for production of T_3 and T_4. The disease occurs more often in females than in males, between the ages of 30 and 50, and shows a marked hereditary pattern. There is an increased incidence in clients with Down syndrome and Turner's syndrome.

Clinical manifestations include a thyroid that is enlarged and has a lumpy surface. Generally, the goiter is asymptomatic, but it could cause dysphagia and a feeling of local pressure. The thymus gland is also enlarged. Other clinical manifestations are similar to hypothyroidism.

Treatment of Hashimoto's thyroiditis is similar to that of hypothyroidism. Thyroid hormone replacement is used. This chronic disorder can be treated but not cured. The client will be on lifetime thyroid hormone replacement.

THYROID TUMORS

There are several neoplasms of the thyroid gland. The benign thyroid cyst and adenoma are firm, encapsulated, noninvasive, slowly growing neoplasms of unknown etiology. Diagnosis of benign neoplasms is done by needle biopsy. These growths tend to be nonfunctioning (not affecting the functioning of the thyroid gland), so there is no treatment other than continued monitoring. If the adenoma is functioning (increasing the functioning of the thyroid gland), then it is treated by radioactive iodine or surgery.

CANCER OF THE THYROID

Cancer of the thyroid is rare and occurs in all age groups. Individuals who have had radiation therapy to the neck are more susceptible. There are four major types of thyroid cancer:

- Papillary carcinoma is the most common type. It can affect any age but is more common in females of childbearing age. It is well-differentiated, grows slowly, is usually contained, and does not spread beyond the adjacent lymph nodes. Cure rate after thyroidectomy is excellent.
- Follicular carcinoma metastasizes to the regional lymph nodes and spreads through the blood vessels to the bone, liver, and lungs. It has a very low cure rate.
- Medullary carcinoma is a solid carcinoma associated with pheochromocytoma. These tumors often secrete calcitonin, adrenocorticotropic hormone, serotonin, and prostaglandins. It is curable if detected before signs and symptoms occur. Without treatment, it grows rapidly, metastasizing to the bones, liver, and kidneys.
- Anaplastic or undifferentiated carcinoma resists radiation. It is almost never curable by resection. It metastasizes rapidly, generally causing death by invasion of the trachea and adjacent structures. It generally affects individuals older than age 60.

There are several risk factors, such as radiation exposure, especially in those children and adolescents who received radiation therapy to treat severe cases of acne vulgaris, or to shrink enlarged tonsils, adenoids, and thymus tissue; prolonged secretion of TSH resulting from radiation or heredity; familial disposition; or chronic goiter.

The first clinical manifestation is a painless lump. As it enlarges, it destroys the thyroid, which leads to clinical manifestations of hypothyroidism. Although rare, the tumor could trigger excessive thyroid hormone production, causing the client to display the clinical manifestations of hyperthyroidism. There can be dysphagia, hoarseness, and vocal stridor. There may be a detectable, disfiguring thyroid mass with a firm nodule on palpation.

The thyroid scan shows a "cold" nodule (decreased uptake of ^{131}I) for papillary carcinoma. Follicular carcinoma and benign adenomas show a "hot" nodule. Thyroid function tests are usually normal. A needle biopsy may be done to confirm diagnosis.

MEDICAL–SURGICAL MANAGEMENT

Surgical

All carcinomas can be treated with surgery (discussed previously). Radioactive iodine or external radiation therapy may also be used. Radioiodine ablation may be used to destroy any remaining thyroid tissue. Response of the tumor will depend on early diagnosis and treatment. These methods of treatment may be used individually or in combination. Client care is the same as for hyperthyroidism.

Pharmacological

Exogenous thyroid hormone may suppress thyroid activity. To increase tolerance to surgery or radiation therapy, the physician may prescribe simultaneous exogenous thyroid hormone and adrenergic blocker such as propranolol hydrochloride (Inderal). If there is widespread metastasis, the cancers will be treated with neoplastic chemotherapy.

NURSING MANAGEMENT

The nurse monitors the client's level of anxiety and encourages the client to discuss feelings about the diagnosis and possible surgery. The nurse also assists the client in identifying previously successful coping methods and teaches new coping methods if needed. After surgical intervention, the nurse must monitor the client for signs and symptoms of airway obstruction. Clients will also require education regarding long-term medical management of the disease.

GOITER

A goiter is an enlargement of the thyroid unrelated to inflammation or neoplasm. There are three types of goiter. One type is a diffuse toxic goiter found in hyperthyroidism. The body's immune system creates an antibody known as thyroid-stimulating immunoglobin that mimics TSH, creating an overproduction of thyroid hormone. This type of goiter may be moderate to massively enlarged. The consistency varies from soft to firm and rubbery. It generally feels smooth. It is often associated with exophthalmos.

Another type of goiter is a simple nontoxic goiter. It develops when the thyroid is unable to use iodine properly or in response to a low iodine level in the blood. These goiters are more common in females. They develop during times of great metabolic demands such as adolescence or pregnancy. A deficiency of iodine can cause goiter formation. Clinical manifestations depend on the size of the goiter. There is an obvious enlargement of the thyroid gland. A large goiter can compress the esophagus or trachea, causing dysphagia, a choking sensation, or respiratory difficulty. If the goiter impairs venous return from the head and neck, the client may experience dizziness and syncope.

Diagnosis is based on history, clinical manifestations, and results of thyroid function tests. T_3 is generally very low. Treatment concentrates on the underlying cause and may involve thyroid hormone replacement therapy, iodine supplements, or increasing dietary iodine sources. Surgery is done when respiration or swallowing is impaired or for cosmetic effect.

The third type of goiter is the nodular goiter. It is similar to the simple goiter except that palpation reveals multiple nodules causing the enlargement. It is found frequently in females older than 40. It usually is asymptomatic. Treatment varies with the client's age and clinical manifestations.

PARATHYROID DISORDERS

Disorders discussed include hyperparathyroidism and hypoparathyroidism.

HYPERPARATHYROIDISM

Hyperparathyroidism is a condition resulting from overactivity of one or more of the parathyroid glands. It results in increased secretion of parathyroid hormone (PTH), which causes calcium to leave the bones and accumulate in the blood. This cannot be compensated by renal excretion or uptake into the soft tissues. It occurs twice as often in postmenopausal females than males. It occurs frequently between the ages of 35 and 65. Hypercalcemia may also be caused by excessive intake of thiazide diuretics, vitamin D, or calcium supplements.

X-rays will show skeletal decalcification. Blood PTH and alkaline phosphate levels are increased. Serum calcium level is elevated. As the result of calcium loss from the bones, a bone density test may be completed to assess the risk for fractures.

Hyperparathyroidism is termed primary if there is an enlargement of one or more of the parathyroid glands, increasing secretion of PTH and thus increasing the blood calcium level. The most common cause is adenoma, but other primary causes include genetics, multiple endocrine neoplasms, or hyperplasia.

The condition is termed secondary if there is excess compensatory production of PTH stemming from a hypocalcemia-producing abnormality other than the parathyroid gland. Some of these abnormalities are rickets, chronic renal failure, vitamin D deficiency, or osteomalacia caused by laxative abuse or phenytoin (Dilantin).

Many clients are asymptomatic; however, there are several clinical manifestations. The client may have polyuria, chronic low-back pain, bone tenderness, or renal calculi. The client may also experience nausea, vomiting, anorexia, constipation, lethargy, or drowsiness. There can be changes in level of consciousness, disorientation, stupor, coma, or personality changes with a loss of initiative and memory. There may be marked muscle weakness and atrophy especially of the legs, joint hyperextensibility, long bone skeletal deformity, or hyporeflexia.

Without treatment, there can be permanent damage to the skeleton or kidneys. There can be bone and articular problems including pathologic fractures. Renal complications include colic, nephrolithiasis, urinary tract infection, and renal insufficiency leading to chronic renal failure. Other complications may be stone formation in various organs, cardiac or vascular problems, or central nervous system changes.

MEDICAL–SURGICAL MANAGEMENT

Medical

Medical management is aimed at decreasing overactivity of the parathyroid glands. This may be accomplished by medication or surgery. If there is severe renal involvement, the client may require dialysis.

Surgical

Primary hyperparathyroidism can be treated by surgical removal of three and one-half of the four parathyroid glands. Surgery can relieve bone pain in 3 days but may not reverse renal damage.

Preoperative care includes explanations, encouraging fluids, limiting calcium intake, and administering medications to lower the blood calcium level.

Postoperative care involves administration of magnesium or phosphate. The client may receive calcium supplements for several days. The nursing care is similar to that provided to the client with thyroidectomy (refer to hyperthyroidism). A major complication is airway obstruction.

Pharmacological

Pharmacological treatment is aimed toward correcting secondary hyperparathyroidism, which involves treating the underlying cause. Because hypercalcemia is a major manifestation, medications are geared to decrease the calcium level in the blood. This includes the use of diuretics such as furosemide (Lasix) and ethacrynic acid (Edecrin).

Other drugs that decrease the calcium level in the blood are calcitonin-human (Cibacalcin), plicamycin (Mithracin), and magnesium- or phosphate-based drugs. Phosphate-based drugs lower the calcium level based on the inverse relationship between phosphorus and calcium.

NURSING MANAGEMENT

Preoperatively, encourage oral fluid intake, monitor I&O, strain urine for calculi, and offer cranberry juice to acidify the urine. Postoperatively, carefully monitor I&O, and assess for signs of hypocalcemia (tetany, cardiac dysrhythmias, and carpopedal spasms). Teach client the principles of good body mechanics. Reassure client that bone pain will gradually disappear. Encourage mild exercise as ordered.

NURSING PROCESS

ASSESSMENT

Subjective Data

Obtain a thorough client history and ask about muscle weakness, apathy, nausea, mental status, and pain (low back or renal). Ask about increased calcium intake, either dietary or supplements.

Objective Data

Note fatigue, drowsiness, anorexia, constipation, personality changes, renal colic, skeletal deformity, output, hematuria, vomiting, weight loss, hypertension, bradycardia, or dysrhythmias.

Nursing diagnoses for a client with hyperparathyroidism include the following:

NURSING DIAGNOSES	PLANNING/OUTCOMES	NURSING INTERVENTIONS
Activity Intolerance related to generalized weakness caused by neuromuscular dysfunction	The client will regain and maintain normal muscle mass and strength, maintain maximum joint range of motion, and perform self-care activity as tolerated.	Alternate rest and activity periods. Assist client with prescribed, individualized activities. Assist client to identify factors that increase or decrease activity intolerance. Encourage client to perform self-care.
*Acute **Pain*** related to musculoskeletal changes resulting from persistently increased serum calcium level	The client will express relief after analgesics, use comfort measures to decrease pain, and be pain-free when serum calcium level reaches normal.	Administer analgesics as ordered. Provide comfort measures for bone pain, and include turning and repositioning every 2 hours. Assess pain level and compare to serum calcium level. Assess environment for hazards and eliminate them. Assist the client to ambulate. Maintain the bed in a low position with side rails up and call light in reach. Lift and move the client gently to prevent pathologic fractures. Provide a safe environment to prevent injuries associated with pain and weakness.

Evaluation: Evaluate each outcome to determine how it has been met by the client.

HYPOPARATHYROIDISM

Hypoparathyroidism is a condition resulting from a deficiency of PTH secretion by the parathyroids or the decreased action of peripheral PTH. Because the parathyroids normally regulate the serum calcium level, hypoparathyroidism will result in a decreased serum calcium level. PTH normally maintains the serum calcium level by increasing bone resorption and gastric reabsorption. It also maintains the inverse relationship between calcium and phosphorus levels. Hypoparathyroidism can be acute or chronic.

If hypoparathyroidism is idiopathic, it may be the result of an autoimmune disorder or congenital absence of parathyroid glands. Acquired hypoparathyroidism is generally irreversible. The most common cause is accidental removal of the parathyroid glands during thyroid or other neck surgery. It can also result from ischemic infarction during surgery, sarcoidosis, tuberculosis, neoplasms, trauma, or massive thyroid irradiation. Reversible hypoparathyroidism can result from hypomagnesemia-induced impairment of hormone synthesis, suppression of normal gland function because of hypercalcemia, or delayed maturation of the parathyroid glands.

The characteristic sign of hypoparathyroidism is tetany, which is muscle spasms and tremors caused by a lack of calcium. Other clinical manifestations include dry skin, brittle hair, alopecia (loss of hair or baldness), and loss of eyelashes and fingernails. The teeth are stained, cracked, and decayed because of weak enamel. The client may have altered level of consciousness, neuromuscular irritability, tingling and twitching of the face and hands, and increased deep tendon reflexes. There may be personality changes or EKG changes.

Two diagnostic assessment tests can be performed. One is the **Chvostek's sign**, which is an abnormal spasm of the facial muscles in response to a light tapping of the facial nerve. The other test is **Trousseau's sign**, which is a carpal spasm caused by inflating a blood pressure cuff above the client's systolic pressure and leaving it in place for 3 minutes (Figure 12-13).

Expected test results include decreased serum calcium, increased urinary calcium, increased serum phosphorus, and decreased urinary phosphorus.

Complications are related to long-standing hypocalcemia, which leads to decreased heart contractility leading to cardiac failure. There can be cataract formation or papillary edema from increased intracranial pressure. There may be bone deformity. In cases of severe tetany, the client can experience laryngospasm, respiratory stridor, anoxia, paralysis of vocal cords, and death.

MEDICAL–SURGICAL MANAGEMENT

Pharmacological

Calcium gluconate or calcium chloride may be given intravenously. Give very slowly because it is very irritating to the vessel wall. Too-rapid IV calcium infusion can cause cardiac arrest. Additional complications from IV administration of calcium gluconate include seizure activity and laryngeal spasms. After the initial IV dose, calcium may be given orally.

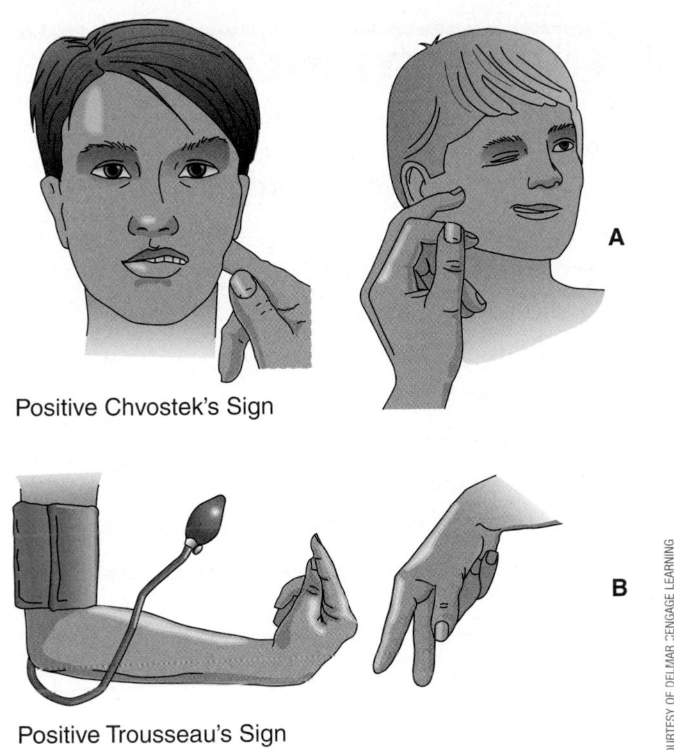

FIGURE 12-13 Signs of Hypocalcemia and Hypoparathyroidism; *A*, Chvostek's Sign; *B*, Trousseau's Sign

Unless the hypoparathyroidism is reversible, the client will require lifelong calcium replacement. Vitamin D may also be given to assist in the absorption of calcium. The calcium supplements should be given 1 to 1½ hours after meals to increase absorption. If the client cannot swallow the large tablets, they can be dissolved in hot water and the suspension cooled before administering to the client. The best sources of calcium are from the diet. The client needs to take calcium as ordered and not abruptly stop taking it. The client must be advised that calcium may cause digitalis toxicity. Cimetidine (Tagamet) interferes with normal parathyroid functioning.

Diet

The diet should be high in calcium and low in phosphorus-containing foods. Because many foods that are high in calcium are also high in phosphorus, the client should be given a list of foods that are high in calcium but lower in phosphorus. Foods on this list include vegetables such as asparagus, broccoli, collards, and tomatoes; fruits such as apricots, bananas, cantaloupe, and many berries; and other foods such as kidney beans, lima beans, and brown sugar. Foods that have a high phosphorus content and should be avoided include most legumes, nuts, cheeses, and seafood.

NURSING MANAGEMENT

Monitor vital signs and for signs of hypercalcemia (anorexia, vomiting, disorientation, abdominal pain, and weakness). Assess for respiratory distress. Provide a diet high in calcium-containing foods. Emphasize the importance of having the blood level of calcium and phosphorus checked.

NURSING PROCESS

ASSESSMENT

Subjective Data

Obtain a thorough client history, asking the client about recent surgery or irradiation, use of alcohol, numbness or tingling of the skin, anxiety, headache, irritability, depression, or nausea.

Objective Data

Assess for dysphagia, level of conscioiusness changes, laryngeal spasm, stridor, cyanosis, dysrhythmias, Chvostek's sign, and Trousseau's sign.

Nursing diagnoses for a client with hypoparathyroidism include the following:

NURSING DIAGNOSES	PLANNING/OUTCOMES	NURSING INTERVENTIONS
*Risk for **Injury*** related to calcium deficiency	The client will not exhibit signs and symptoms of tetany, and will prevent injury from hypocalcemia.	Monitor Chvostek's and Trousseau's signs, serum calcium and phosphorus levels, as well as EKG changes. Keep tracheotomy tray readily available and maintain seizure precautions. Support client while walking to prevent injury. Monitor client taking digoxin for toxicity.
*Imbalanced **Nutrition**: Less than Body Requirements,* related to calcium intake	The client will have adequate calcium intake.	Provide diet with calcium-rich foods. Give calcium replacement as ordered. The client who is taking digoxin must be monitored for toxicity. Give calcium supplement 1 to 1½ hours before or after meals to increase absorption.

Evaluation: Evaluate each outcome to determine how it has been met by the client.

ADRENAL DISORDERS

Disorders in this category include Cushing's disease/syndrome, Addison's disease, and pheochromocytoma.

CUSHING'S DISEASE SYNDROME (ADRENAL HYPERFUNCTION)

Cushing's *disease,* primary adrenal hyperfunction, is the result of increased pituitary secretion of ACTH, which causes an increased production of cortisol by the adrenal cortex. Cortisol, a stress hormone, regulates the body's metabolism of carbohydrates, fats, and proteins. Cushing's *syndrome* refers to symptoms of cortisol excess caused by other factors. One cause is a corticotropin-producing tumor in another organ, such as oat-cell carcinoma of the lung (secondary adrenal hyperfunction). The most common cause of Cushing's syndrome is prolonged use of glucocorticoid or corticotropin medications for chronic inflammatory disorders such as chronic obstructive pulmonary disease, Crohn's disease, and rheumatoid arthritis. This is **iatrogenic** (caused by treatment or diagnostic procedures) adrenal hyperfunction.

Cushing's syndrome occurs in females more than males, generally between 30 and 50 years of age.

Classic clinical manifestations are adiposity of the face, neck, and trunk, which give rise to the moon-shaped face and buffalo hump. Others include purple striae on the abdomen, hirsutism, and thin extremities caused by muscle wasting. Boys exhibit an early onset of puberty, whereas girls exhibit development of masculine characteristics. The client may complain of fatigue, muscle weakness, weight gain, sleep disturbances, water retention, amenorrhea, decreased libido, irritability, and emotional lability. There could be petechiae, ecchymoses, decreased wound healing, or swollen ankles.

There are multiple complications of Cushing's syndrome, most of which are produced by the stimulating and catabolic effects of cortisol. There can be increased calcium resorption from the bone, leading to osteoporosis and pathologic fractures. It can cause increased hepatic gluconeogenesis and insulin resistance, causing glucose intolerance and diabetes mellitus. The client may have frequent infections and slowed wound healing. There is a suppressed inflammatory response that can mask severe infections. The client may have decreased ability to handle stress, which can lead to psychological problems from mood swings to psychosis. Other complications include hypertension, ischemic heart disease, congestive heart failure, menstrual disturbances, and sexual dysfunction.

Plasma cortisol level is elevated. Plasma ACTH level may be elevated or low. Adrenalangiography is done for adrenal tumor. Twenty-four-hour urine tests for 17-ketosteroids, 17-hydroxysteroids, and free cortisol are elevated. A dexamethasone suppression test may also be completed. If the client's blood and urine cortisol levels do not decrease, then Cushing's disease is suspected.

Prognosis depends on early diagnosis, identifying the underlying cause, and effective treatment. Without treatment, about half of these clients will die within 5 years.

MEMORYTRICK

The following is a memory trick to remember the signs and symptoms of **CUSHING'S** Disease:

- **C** = Cortisol
- **U** = Unusually high ACTH
- **S** = Sleep disturbances
- **H** = Hirsutism
- **I** = Infection
- **N** = Non-healing wounds
- **G** = Gain weight
- **S** = Striae

MEDICAL–SURGICAL MANAGEMENT

Medical

The major goal is to restore hormone balance. Treatment is based on the causative factor. This is accomplished primarily by medications. If there is adrenal cancer, the client may have either radiation therapy to the adrenal gland or surgery on either the pituitary gland or the adrenal glands, or all three treatments.

Surgical

If the underlying cause of Cushing's syndrome is related to the pituitary gland, the client may have a hypophysectomy done. (Refer to hypophysectomy in the section on hyperpituitarism.)

For an adrenal tumor, an adrenalectomy is performed to decrease the high levels of circulating cortisol. This could be unilateral or bilateral. During the first 24 to 48 hours after surgery, the client is observed closely for hemorrhage and shock. Vital signs and urine output are monitored. Glucocorticoids are administered with changing dosage until a maintenance dose is established. The client's blood glucose level must be monitored, especially for hypoglycemia.

COMMUNITY/HOME HEALTH CARE

Cushing's Syndrome

- Carry Medic Alert tag, indicating Cushing's syndrome.
- Avoid extreme temperature changes, activities that could result in trauma, and people with infections.
- Wash hands often and protect skin with good care.
- Maintain medication regimen.
- Notify physician if weakness, fainting, fever, nausea, or vomiting occur.

Pharmacological

Aminoglutethimide (Cytadren) inhibits synthesis of adrenal steroids. It can cause dizziness or drowsiness. The client should be instructed to avoid activities requiring mental alertness or manual dexterity.

Ketoconazole (Nizoral), while classified as an antifungal, inhibits adrenal steroidogenesis and is used to treat Cushing's syndrome.

Mitotane (Lysodren) directly suppresses the activity of the adrenal cortex. This cytotoxic agent is generally used for inoperable adrenal cortex cancer. It is given for at least 3 months. The client should avoid situations that cause injury or exposure to infections.

If the client had pituitary or adrenal surgery, cortisol therapy may be given before and after surgery to decrease physical stress. The client may need to adhere to lifetime treatment with steroids. The client should take the drug with food or antacids to decrease gastric distress. Two-thirds dose of the steroids should be taken in the morning, with the remaining one-third in the early evening to mimic the body's diurnal schedule. Steroids can lead to osteoporosis and the possibility of pathologic fractures. Females should be warned that steroid use can interfere with oral contraceptive effectiveness. There may be an adverse effect on the male's sperm production and count.

The client with diabetes mellitus may have to adjust insulin dosage because the steroids can affect the glucose level. Steroids can mask severe infections and cause some immunosuppression. Wounds are slower to heal. The client should be instructed to contact a physician before using over-the-counter preparations. The client should not abruptly discontinue the steroid drug; dosage must be tapered before discontinuing.

Diet

The diet should be high in protein and potassium but low in sodium. Foods high in protein include eggs, milk, whole grains, legumes, and meat; however, milk, cheeses, and whole grains are also high in sodium, depending on processing. Many foods high in potassium are also low in sodium. These foods are legumes; fruits such as figs, oranges, bananas, prunes, and raisins; and vegetables such as avocado, potato, and spinach. The client should be advised to read labels for sodium content. Processed foods and many preservatives have high sodium content and should be avoided. Reduced carbohydrates and calories help control hyperglycemia.

NURSING MANAGEMENT

Encourage client to turn frequently and ambulate to prevent pressure on bony prominences. Gently handle client to prevent ecchymosis. Provide elbow and heel protectors and an egg-crate mattress. Provide rest periods during personal hygiene activities.

NURSING PROCESS

ASSESSMENT

Subjective Data

Obtain a thorough client history, asking about the use of steroids, stress, methods of coping with stress, irritability, depression, mood swings, loss of libido, and the possibility of suicide.

Objective Data

Assess for thin and fragile skin, petechiae, ecchymoses, delayed wound healing, weight gain, increased abdominal girth, thin extremities with muscle wasting, purple striae, hyperglycemia, and hypokalemia. Women may have **hirsutism** (excessive body hair in a masculine distribution), deepening of the voice, and menstrual irregularities.

Nursing diagnoses for a client with Cushing's syndrome include the following:

NURSING DIAGNOSES	PLANNING/OUTCOMES	NURSING INTERVENTIONS
*Disturbed **B**ody Image* related to changes in physical appearance	The client will verbalize feelings about changed appearance.	Encourage client to verbalize feelings about changed body image. Offer emotional support and a positive realistic assessment of the condition.
*Risk for **I**nfection* related to suppressed inflammatory response from excessive corticosteroid production	The client will take precautions to avoid or decrease exposure to infection.	Advise client to avoid people with infections. Provide a private room with reverse or protective isolation as indicated. Monitor client's vital signs, intake and output, and weight.

Evaluation: Evaluate each outcome to determine how it has been met by the client.

ADDISON'S DISEASE (ADRENAL HYPOFUNCTION)

Addison's disease, primary hypofunctioning of the adrenals, involves decreased functioning of the adrenal cortex and its secretions—mineralocorticoids, glucocorticoids, and androgens. It can also be called *adrenal hypofunction* or *insufficiency*. It is fairly uncommon, occurring in 5 per 100,000 people in the United States (Daniels, 2007). Although it affects all ages and both sexes, it is less common among the elderly.

Addison's disease occurs when more than 90% of the adrenal gland is destroyed. It is an autoimmune disease in response to conditions such as tuberculosis, histoplasmosis, HIV, and meningococcal pneumonia. It can be caused by bilateral adrenalectomy, hemorrhage into the adrenal gland related to anticoagulant therapy, or cancer of the adrenal gland. It is termed secondary if it results from decreased pituitary or hypothalamus function or abrupt withdrawal of long-term steroid therapy.

A classical clinical manifestation of Addison's disease is a bronze coloration of the skin resembling a deep suntan, especially in the creases on the hands, elbows, and knees. There may be some areas of vitiligo. The client may complain of fatigue, muscle weakness, lightheadedness upon rising, weight loss, and craving for salty foods. The client may have decreased tolerance even to minor stress. The client is anxious, irritable, and may become confused. The pulse may be weak and irregular. There is hypotension and a variety of gastrointestinal complaints. The client is also at risk for orthostatic hypotension.

The acute form is called adrenal crisis. It may occur when there is trauma, surgery, other physiologic stress, or abrupt withdrawal of steroids. The clinical manifestations are the same, only more severe with a rapid onset. The crisis requires immediate treatment. The client will be placed on intravenous therapy and IV administration of hydrocortisone (Cortef, Hydrocortone). Measures to maintain a stable blood pressure and normal water and sodium levels are instituted. EKG monitoring is needed to assess for complications associated with elevated K and Ca levels. After the crisis, the client will be placed on a maintenance dose of hydrocortisone.

Expected test results include low serum sodium, high serum potassium, low serum glucose, low cortisol and aldosterone serum levels, and decreased urinary 17-ketosteroid and 17-hydroxysteroid levels.

Medical–Surgical Management

Medical

Treatment is geared toward prompt restoration of fluid and electrolyte balance and replacement of deficient adrenal hormones.

Pharmacological

The client will require lifetime maintenance of steroids. Administration of glucocorticoids such as hydrocortisone (Hydrocortone) and mineralocorticoids such as fludrocortisone acetate (Florinef) are given two-thirds of the daily dose in the morning and one-third in the evening. In times of stress, the dose may need to be doubled or tripled.

Diet

The diet should be high in sodium and low in potassium. It should contain adequate calories and protein. If the client is anorexic, six small meals may increase caloric intake. A late afternoon or evening snack should be available if the client's blood glucose level drops.

Nursing Management

Carefully assess the client's circulatory status. Weigh client daily. Accurately record I&O. Monitor vital signs and skin turgor. Provide a private room and screen visitors for infections. Teach importance of taking medications as prescribed, wearing a Medic Alert bracelet, reporting any illness to the physician, and having regular checkups. A kit including injectable hydrocortisone should be available when oral intake is not feasible.

NURSING PROCESS

Assessment

Subjective Data

Obtain a thorough client history, asking about recent synthetic steroid use, adrenal surgery, infection, salt craving, nausea, weakness, vertigo, headache, disorientation, emotional status, anxiety, and apprehension.

Objective Data

Assess for postural hypotension, inability to perform normal activities, syncope, dark pigmented areas on skin and mucous membrane, weight loss, vomiting, diarrhea, and very low or very high temperature.

Nursing diagnoses for a client with Addison's disease include the following:

NURSING DIAGNOSES	PLANNING/OUTCOMES	NURSING INTERVENTIONS
*Deficient **F**luid Volume* related to low sodium level, vomiting, diarrhea, and increased renal losses	The client will regain normal fluid and electrolyte balance.	Monitor client's vital signs, level of consciousness, intake and output, and weight. Administer IV fluids as ordered and encourage fluid intake.
*Risk for **I**nfection* related to suppressed inflammatory response	The client will maintain normal temperature and leukocyte count and differential, and use precautions to avoid or reduce risks of infection.	Monitor temperature every 4 hours unless elevated, then every 2 hours. Provide a private room with reverse or protective isolation as needed. Screen personnel and visitors for infection. Teach proper hand hygiene. Monitor laboratory test results for WBC and differential.

Evaluation: Evaluate each outcome to determine how it has been met by the client.

LIFE SPAN CONSIDERATIONS

Pheochromocytoma

Pheochromocytoma is frequently diagnosed during pregnancy when the enlarged uterus puts pressure on the tumor, causing more frequent attacks. The attacks could prove fatal to both mother and fetus. Although there is an increased risk of spontaneous abortion, most fetal deaths occur during labor or immediately after delivery.

PHEOCHROMOCYTOMA

Pheochromocytoma, sometimes known as *chromaffin cell tumor*, is a rare disease characterized by **paroxysmal** (a symptom that begins and ends abruptly) or sustained hypertension caused by excessive secretion of epinephrine and norepinephrine. The excessive secretion of epinephrine and norepinephrine stimulates the sympathetic nervous system leading to hypertension and tachycardia. Some medical experts estimate that about 0.5% of clients newly diagnosed with hypertension have pheochromocytoma. Although the tumor is generally benign, it can be malignant in 5% to 10% of the cases. It affects all races and both sexes. It is most common in women ages 20 to 50 years.

It is caused by a chromaffin cell tumor of the adrenal medulla, more commonly on the right side. Extraadrenal pheochromocytomas can also occur. Epinephrine overproduction occurs with the adrenal pheochromocytoma; however, norepinephrine overproduction is associated with both adrenal and extraadrenal pheochromocytoma. It is associated with a family history of pheochromocytoma or endocrine gland cancer. It is considered to be inherited on the autosomal-dominant gene in about 5% of the cases.

The classic triad of clinical manifestations is hypertension with diastolic pressure above 115 mm Hg, unrelenting headache, and profuse diaphoresis. Other clinical manifestations include palpitations, visual disturbances, nausea, or vomiting. These attacks may be triggered by activities or conditions that displace the abdominal contents, such as heavy lifting, exercise, bladder distention, or pregnancy. Severe attacks can be precipitated by administration of opiates, histamine, glucagon, and corticotropin. Some attacks may have no precipitating factor. Some other clinical manifestations are mild to moderate weight loss caused by increased metabolism and orthostatic hypotension when rising to an upright position. The client will have tachycardia. The actual tumor is rarely palpable; however, palpation could trigger a hypertensive attack.

The complications are similar to those of severe and persistent hypertension. These complications are stroke, retinopathy, heart disease, or irreversible kidney disease. The client with pheochromocytoma has an increased risk of severe complications or death during invasive diagnostic tests or surgery.

Although pheochromocytoma can be potentially fatal, the prognosis is good with treatment. About 90% of the clients are cured.

MEDICAL–SURGICAL MANAGEMENT

Surgical

The treatment of choice is surgical removal of the tumor. Sometimes the adrenal gland is also removed. The blood pressure is monitored closely during the immediate postoperative period. The client may have hypotension, but hypertension is more common. About 10% of the clients are not candidates for surgery. They are treated with medications to lower the blood pressure.

Pharmacological

During acute hypertensive attacks, the drugs of choice are phentolamine mesylate (Regitine) or nitroprusside sodium (Nipride). Phentolamine mesylate (Regitine) and phenoxybenzamine HCl (Dibenzyline) are alpha-adrenergic blocking agents. They are used to control hypertension before surgery or when surgery is contraindicated. The client should be warned about orthostatic hypotension and rise slowly from a supine position to an upright position. The client should not take over-the-counter drugs or alcohol.

Nitroprusside sodium (Nipride, Nitropress) acts on the vascular smooth muscle to cause peripheral vasodilation. The drug is given in an intravenous infusion. An electronic infusion device must be used to monitor the infusion rate. The client's blood pressure is used to titrate the infusion rate per the physician's orders.

Metyrosine (Demser) is used to block catecholamine synthesis. This drug must be continued for life if the tumor is inoperable. Ongoing medications include adrenergic blockers such as propranolol hydrochloride (Inderal), atenolol (Tenormin), prazosin HCl (Minipress), labetalol HCl (Normodyne), or nifedipine (Procardia), a calcium channel blocker. The client's blood pressure must be monitored frequently to determine the effectiveness of the medication.

Propranolol hydrochloride (Inderal) should not be stopped abruptly. The client should not smoke while taking this medication. Atenolol (Tenormin) may enhance the client's sensitivity to cold. Prazosin HCl (Minipress) should be taken on an empty stomach. The initial dose should be given at bedtime. The client should not use cough, cold, or allergy medications without the physician's knowledge. If the client is given parenteral labetalol HCl (Normodyne, Trandate), the client should remain supine for 3 hours to decrease the possibility of orthostatic hypotension. Nifedipine (Adalat, Procardia) should be protected from light and moisture and stored at room temperature. Over-the-counter medications should not be taken.

Diet

The diet should be high in protein with adequate calories. Stimulating foods such as aged cheeses and yogurt; caffeine-containing beverages such as coffee, tea, and soft drinks; and beer and red wine should be avoided (Smeltzer & Bare, 2006).

NURSING MANAGEMENT

The nurse should ask about heat intolerance, severe headaches during hypertensive crisis, anxiety, trouble sleeping, palpitations, nervousness, dizziness, paresthesias, and nausea. The client is assessed for dyspnea, tremors, diaphoresis, glycosuria, hyperglycemia, or dilated pupils. Frequently assess blood pressure, pulse, and respirations for elevations, and observe for signs of anxiety.

CASE STUDY

A.F., a 44-year-old African-American man, is admitted to the medical unit from his physician's office. He reports that he has lost 18 pounds over the last month and has been very tired. He also reports symptoms of thirst, frequent urination, and blurred vision. His vital signs are blood pressure 166/92 mm Hg, pulse 88 beats/min, respiration 16 breaths/min, and temperature 99.2°F. Physical assessment reveals hot, dry, flushed skin. Laboratory exams reveal a blood glucose 490 mg/dL and urine negative for ketones. A.F. is a truck driver and leads a fairly sedentary lifestyle. History reveals that he is usually 30 to 35 pounds overweight but has otherwise been in good health. He reports that his mother died from diabetes and renal failure, and an older brother was diagnosed as having type 2 diabetes 3 years ago.

The following questions will guide your development of a nursing care plan for this case study:

1. List physical symptoms that A.F. is experiencing that are suggestive of diabetes.
2. On the basis of the client's history and laboratory values, would you expect A.F. to be diagnosed with type 1 or type 2 diabetes?
3. Which nursing diagnoses would you identify as priorities for A.F. right now? List two.
4. A.F. is treated with IV fluids and insulin sliding scale until his blood glucose is stabilized. Describe what an insulin sliding scale is, and when it is used.
5. A 2,000-calorie ADA diet is ordered for A.F. He does not care to eat the apple that came on his breakfast tray and asks if he can exchange it for another serving of scrambled eggs. How would you respond to Mr. Carnes?
6. A.F. is being discharged and will continue to attend diabetic education classes at a local diabetic treatment center. Assuming A.F. is to continue on a diabetic diet and will be receiving mixed insulin injections, list the pertinent information A.F. will need to know about his disease and therapies related to:
   - Diabetes and symptoms of hyperglycemia
   - Role of exercise
   - Effects of diet
   - Self-monitoring blood glucose
   - Insulin injections/technique
   - Symptoms of hypoglycemia
   - Sick-day care
   - Long-term complications

SUMMARY

- The endocrine system is composed of glands at various body locations producing secretions (hormones) that directly enter the blood or lymph circulation.
- The endocrine system provides slower and longer-lasting control over various body activities and functions.
- A malfunction of any part of the endocrine system can result in a shift of homeostasis with far-reaching systemic reactions.
- Assessment of the endocrine system can be challenging because the glands are scattered. Negative findings are as important as positive findings.
- Diabetes is a complex chronic disease with multiple acute and chronic complications. It is a systemic disease caused by an imbalance between insulin supply and demand.
- A coordinated program of exercise, diet, and medications is used to achieve diabetic control. Persons with type 1 diabetes always require insulin therapy in addition to dietary control and an exercise program. Persons with type 2 diabetes are managed through diet and exercise and may or may not require oral hypoglycemic agents or insulin.
- The goal of diabetes management is enabling the diabetic to manage the disease by maintaining a blood glucose level within an acceptable range and thereby minimizing the incidence of acute and chronic complications.
- Regardless of disorder, the client should wear a Medic Alert bracelet and be aware that the treatment generally lasts a lifetime.

REVIEW QUESTIONS

1. A client tells the nurse that she is surprised that she developed diabetes at 40 years of age. The nurse knows that the development of diabetes in middle-aged people is most directly the result of:

1. atherosclerosis.
2. eating too much sugar.
3. obesity.
4. viral infection.

2. Which of the following principles is used when planning for a client with diabetes who is to undergo surgery?
   1. All insulin is withheld until surgery is over and the client is eating.
   2. Insulin or oral hypoglycemics are given as usual.
   3. Sliding-scale insulin is used to regulate glucose levels during the operative period.
   4. Hyperglycemia poses the most serious danger to the client during surgery.
3. Which of the following nursing diagnoses would be most appropriate for the client with diabetes insipidus?
   1. Alteration in growth and development related to increased growth hormone production.
   2. Alteration in thought processes related to decreased neurologic function.
   3. Fluid volume deficit related to polyuria.
   4. Hypothermia related to decreased metabolic rate.
4. Meticulous skin care is especially important for the client with hyperthyroidism because of:
   1. diaphoresis from heat intolerance.
   2. edema from sodium and water retention.
   3. poor nutrition due to nausea and vomiting.
   4. pressure from immobility due to paralysis.
5. The nurse is caring for a client immediately after surgery for a complete thyroidectomy. Which of the following signs/symptoms would alert the nurse to a life threatening complication of the surgery?
   1. Urine output of 30 mL/hour.
   2. Laryngeal stridor.
   3. Neck stiffness.
   4. Sinus tachycardia 110 beats/min.
6. Which of the following statements made by a client indicates the need for further teaching regarding foot care associated with diabetes mellitus?
   1. "I will contact my podiatrist to have callouses and corns removed."
   2. "I will use a mirror to inspect my feet for bruises, cuts, and abrasions."
   3. "Walking barefoot is advised. It will improve the circulation in my feet."
   4. "I will check the temperature of my bath water before entering the tub."
7. A client with SIADH has been admitted to the hospital. Which of the lab values listed below is congruent with this diagnosis?
   1. Serum Na 124 meq/L.
   2. Urine osmolality <300 mOsm/L.
   3. Urine specific gravity 1.010.
   4. Hemoglobin A1C 4.7.
8. Which of the following nursing diagnoses would the nurse plan to institute on a client suffering from SIADH?
   1. *Fluid **V**olume Excess* related to decreased urine output.
   2. *Ineffective **C**oping Mechanism* related to disease process progression.
   3. *Risk for **H**yperthermia* related to alteration in temperature regulation control.
   4. *Fluid **V**olume Deficit* related to excessive urine output.
9. A client with suspected Addison's disease is admitted to the hospital. Which diagnostic tests indicate a positive diagnosis of Addison's disease?
   1. Elevated blood sugar.
   2. Decreased cortisol.
   3. Decreased potassium.
   4. Elevated sodium.
10. Which of the following nursing diagnoses would the nurse question when caring for a client with Cushing's disease?
    1. *Risk for Disturbed **B**ody Image* related to disease process.
    2. *Risk for **I**nfection* related to immunological changes.
    3. *Risk for **I**njury* related to muscle weakness and wasting.
    4. *Risk for Deficient **F**luid Volume* related to excessive excretion of water and sodium.

REFERENCES/SUGGESTED READINGS

Alexander, I. (2008). *PDR nurses drug handbook.* Clifton Park, NY: Delmar Cengage Learning.

American Diabetes Association. (2009). Diagnosis and classification of diabetes mellitus. *Diabetes Care 32,* S62–S67.

American Thyroid Association. (2004). Severe mental impairment and poor physiological status predict mortality in patients with myxedema coma. Retreived from www.thyroid.org/patients/notes/july4/04_07_28.html

Anthony, M. (2003). Hypoglycemia. *Nursing2003, 33*(2), 88.

Bacoka, J. (2001). Thyroid storm. *Nursing2001, 31*(12), 88.

Bartels, D. (2004). Adherence to oral therapy for type 2 diabetes: Opportunities for enhancing glycemic control. *Journal of American Academy of Nurse Practitioners, 16*(1), 8–16.

Bartol, T. (2002). Putting a patient with diabetes in the driver's seat. *Nursing2002, 32*(2), 53–55.

Bulechek, G., Butcher, H., McCloskey, J., & Dochterman, J., eds. (2008). *Nursing Interventions Classification (NIC)* (5th ed.). St. Louis, MO: Mosby/Elsevier.

Caffrey, R. (2003). Are all syringes created equal? *AJN, 103*(6), 46–49.

Cameron, B. (2002). Making diabetes management routine. *AJN, 102*(2), 26–32.

Centers for Disease Control and Prevention. (2007). National diabetes fact sheet, 2007. Retrieved May 2009 from http://www.cdc.gov/diabetes/pubs/general.htm

Centers for Disease Control and Prevention. (2008). Frequently asked questions: Groups especially affected by diabetes. Retrieved August 2, 2009 from http://www.cdc.gov/diabetes/faq/groups.htm#9

Cincinnati, R., & Veliko, J. (2001). Oral medications. *RN, 64*(8), 30–36.

Clarke, K. (2002). No needles needed. *Nursing2002, 32*(5), 49–51.

Cypress, M. (2001). Acute complications. *RN, 64*(4), 26–31.

Daniels, R. (2009). *Delmar's guide to laboratory and diagnostic tests* (2nd ed.) Clifton Park, NY: Delmar Cengage Learning.

Diabetes Insipidus Foundation Inc. (2003–Update 2006). Available from http://www.diabetesinsipidus.org/whatisdi.htm

Estes, M. E. Z. (2010). *Health assessment & physical examination* (4th ed.). Clifton Park, NY: Delmar Cengage Learning.

Fain, J. (2001). Lowering the boom on hyperglycemia. *Nursing2001, 31*(8), 49–50.

Fain, J. (2003). Pump up your knowledge of insulin pumps. *Nursing2003, 33*(6), 51–53.

Flood, L., & Constance, A. (2002). Diabetes & exercise safety. *AJN, 102*(6), 47–55.

Goh, K. (2004). Management of hyponatremia. *American Family Physician*, 69(10), 2387–94, 2303–5, 2480.

Goldberg, J. (2001). Nutrition and exercise. *RN, 64*(7), 34–39.

Halpin-Landry, J., & Goldsmith, S. (1999). Feet first: Diabetes care. *AJN, 99*(2), 26–33.

Hardman, L., & Young, F. (2001). Combating hyperosmolar hyperglycemic nonketotic syndrome. *Nursing2001, 31*(3), 32hn1–32hn4.

Holcomb, S. (2003). Detecting thyroid disease, part 1. *Nursing2003, 33*(8), 32cc1–32cc4.

Ignatavicius, D., & Workman, L. (2006). *Medical surgical nursing – critical thinking for collaborative care* (5th ed.). St. Louis, MO: Saunders/Elsevier.

LeMone, P., & Burke, K. (2008). *Medical-surgical nursing: Critical thinking in client care* (4th ed.). New York, NY: Prentice Hall.

Lorenz, R., & Silverstein, J. (2005). *Managing insulin requirements at school.* Retrieved August 2, 2009 from http://ndep.nih.gov/media/SNN_March_2005.pdf

Malchiodi, L. (2002). Thyroid storm. *AJN, 102*(5), 33–35.

McCance, K., & Huether, S. (2005). *Pathophysiology: The biologic basis for disease in adults and children* (5th ed.). St. Louis, MO: Mosby.

McConnell, E. (2002). Myths & facts . . . about Addison's disease. *Nursing2002, 32*(8), 79.

McConnell, E. (2003). Myths & facts . . . about diabetes insipidus. *Nursing2003, 33*(6), 84.

Melmed, S., Kleinberg, D., et al. (2008) *Williams textbook of endocrinology* (11th ed.). Philadelphia, PA: Saunders/Elsevier

Moorhead, S., Johnson, M., Maas, M., & Swanson, E. (2007). *Nursing Outcomes Classification (NOC)* (4th ed.). St. Louis, MO: Mosby.

National Cancer Institute. (2009). Retrieved from http://www.cancer.gov/cancertopics/pdq/treatment/pheochromocytoma/patient

National Diabetes Education Program. (2008). Overview of diabetes in children and adolescents. Retrieved August 2, 2009 from http://ndep.nih.gov/media/diabetes/youth/youth_FS.htm#Diabetes

National Institutes of Health. (2009). Graves disease. Retrieved August 3, 2009 from http://www.nlm.nih.gov/medlineplus/ency/article/000358.htm

National Institution of Diabetes and Digestive and Kidney Diseases (NIDDK). (2008a). Acromegaly. Retrieved from http://www.nlm.nih.gov/medlineplus/encyc/article/00321.htm

National Institution of Diabetes and Digestive and Kidney Diseases (NIDDK). (2008b). Diabetes insipidus. Retrieved October 18, 2009 from http://www.nlm.nih.gov/medlineplus/ency/article/000377.htm

National Institution of Diabetes and Digestive and Kidney Diseases (NIDDK). (2008c). Hyperthyroidism. Retrieved from http://www.nlm.nih.gov/hyperthyroidism.htm

National Institution of Diabetes and Digestive and Kidney Diseases (NIDDK). (2008d). Hypoparathyroidism. Retrieved from http://www.nlm.nih.gov/medlineplus/encyc/article/00385.htm

National Institution of Diabetes and Digestive and Kidney Diseases (NIDDK). (2008e). Pheochromocytoma. Retrieved from http://www.nlm.nih.gov/medlineplus/pheochromocytoma.htm

Norris, J. (senior ed.). (1998). *Handbook of medical–surgical nursing* (2d ed.). Springhouse, PA: Springhouse Corp.

North American Nursing Diagnosis Association International. (2010). *NANDA-I nursing diagnoses: Definitions and classification* 2009–2011. Ames, IA: Wiley-Blackwell.

Olohan, K., & Zappitelli, D. (2003). The insulin pump. *AJN, 103*(4), 48–56.

Plummer, E. (2001). Chronic complications. *RN, 64*(5), 34–40.

Robertson, C. (2001). The untold story of disease progression. *RN, 64*(3), 60–64.

Ruiz, E. (2001). Type 2 disease in children. *RN, 64*(10), 44–48.

Sachse, D. (2001). Acromegaly. *AJN, 101*(1), 69–77.

Sammer, C. (2001). How should you respond to hypoglycemia? *Nursing2001, 31*(7), 48–50.

Schori-Ahmed, D. (2003). Thyroid disease, *RN, 66*(6), 38–43.

Seley, J. (2003). Giving the fingers a rest. *AJN, 103*(3), 73–77.

Shelly, A. (2002). Elderly patients with diabetes. *AJN, 102*(2), 15–16.

Smeltzer, S., & Bare, B. (2006). *Brunner & Suddarth's textbook of medical–surgical nursing* (11th ed.). Philadelphia: Lippincott Williams & Wilkins.

Spratto, G., & Woods, A. (2009). *2009 PDR nurse's drug handbook.* Clifton Park, NY: Delmar Cengage Learning.

Strowig, S., (2001). Insulin therapy. *RN,* 64(9), 38–44.

The Expert Committee on the Diagnosis and Classification of Diabetes Mellitus. (1997). Report of the expert committee on the diagnosis and classification of diabetes mellitus. *Diabetes Care, 20*(7), 1183–1197.

Thibodeau, G., & Patton, K. (2009). *The human body in health & disease* (4th ed.). St. Louis, MO: Mosby.

Tkacs, N. (2002). Hypoglycemia unawareness. *AJN, 102*(2), 34–39.

U.S. Department of Health and Human Services, National Center for Chronic Disease Control and Prevention, Division of Diabetes Translation. (1992). *Diabetes in the United States: A strategy for prevention.* Washington, DC: U.S. Public Health Service.

Valentine, V. (2002). Using a laser to make a point. *Nursing2002, 32*(10), 56–57.

Watts, S., Anselmo, J., & Smith, M. (2003). Combating hypoglycemia in the hospital and at home. *Nursing2003, 33*(3), 32hn1–32hn5.

Williams, J. (2001). We make foot exams a priority. *RN, 64*(5), 40–41.

RESOURCES

American Association of Diabetes Educators, http://www.aadenet.org

American Diabetes Association, http://www.diabetes.org

American Dietetic Association, http://www.eatright.org

Juvenile Diabetes Foundation International, http:// www.jdrf.org

National Institutes of Health, http://www.nih.gov/science/campus

National Organization for Rare Disorders, Inc. (NORD), http://www.rarediseases.org

The Diabetes Insipidus Foundation, Inc., http://www.diabetesinsipidus.org

UNIT 5 Nursing Care of the Client: Reproductive and Sexual Health

CHAPTER 13
Reproductive System

MAKING THE CONNECTION

Refer to the following chapters to increase your understanding of the female and male reproductive systems:

Adult Health Nursing

- ***Oncology***
- ***Cardiovascular System***
- ***Urinary System***
- ***Endocrine System***
- ***Sexually Transmitted Infections***
- ***The Older Adult***

LEARNING OBJECTIVES

Upon completion of this chapter, you should be able to:

- Define key terms.
- Identify the anatomy of the reproductive systems.
- Describe the hormonal mechanisms that regulate the reproductive functions, including the menstrual cycle.
- Interpret diagnostic tests for disorders of the reproductive systems.
- List the changes in the reproductive systems that occur with aging.
- Discuss common problems of the reproductive system.
- Differentiate between impotence and infertility.
- Discuss contraceptive methods, including actions, side effects, and client teaching.
- Utilize the nursing process to develop a care plan for a client with a reproductive system disorder.

KEY TERMS

abortion
amenorrhea
contraception
cystocele
dysmenorrhea
dyspareunia
endometriosis
hematuria
hesitancy

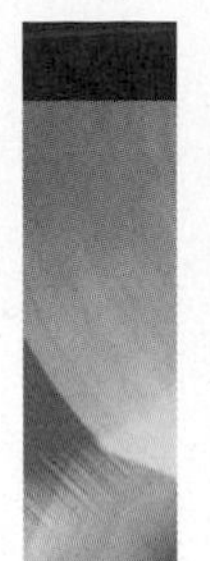

impotence
infertility
menopause
menorrhagia
metrorrhagia
nocturia
oligomenorrhea
orchiectomy
polymenorrhea
postvoid residual
priapism
prolapsed uterus
rectocele
spermatogenesis
stent
tenesmus
urethrocele
urethrostomy
vasectomy

INTRODUCTION

Through modern technology, current medical and nursing knowledge, and health education programs, laypersons have access to much information about their bodies and their reproductive systems. Yet, individuals continue to be seriously affected by health disorders. In some instances they may lack knowledge of how to detect signs and symptoms of these disorders. Often, they simply delay routine medical examinations or avoid seeking medical treatment. In addition, individuals may have difficulty discussing symptoms related to their reproductive system.

Routine health care must be maintained and early diagnosis made in order to reduce the incidence and seriousness of reproductive health disorders. These goals can be facilitated with skilled nursing assessment and client education.

For most people, the reproductive system functions without problems throughout life. For others, minor and major disorders require treatment. Some of the problems are related to alterations in structure; others are related more to altered physiology of the reproductive system. This chapter discusses disorders of the reproductive systems by applying the steps of the nursing process.

ANATOMY AND PHYSIOLOGY REVIEW

The female and male reproductive systems consist of external and internal structures and organs.

EXTERNAL FEMALE STRUCTURES

The area known as the vulva includes the external female structures, such as the mons pubis, labia majora, labia minora, and clitoris. The Bartholin glands and Skene's glands, located proximal to the vaginal opening, produce and secrete lubricating fluids. The labia majora and minora serve as protective barriers for the softer internal structures. The clitoris, located proximal to the mons pubis and superior to the urinary meatus, plays a role in sexual arousal in the female and is considered analogous to the male penis. During foreplay, the clitoris engorges and stimulates orgasm or climax in the female. It is covered by a small hood called the prepuce. The perineum is the distal portion of the vulva, located below the vaginal opening and superior to the anus.

The breasts are also a part of the external female reproductive system (Figure 13-1). Their external structures include the nipple, areola, and Montgomery tubercles. The nipples have several openings, or ducts, that lead from the lactiferous glands inside the breast. Milk is ejected through the ducts when the infant sucks on the breast. The areola, or the darker area around the nipple, becomes darker in response to the increased hormone levels during pregnancy. Small, mole-like, raised areas around the areola are the Montgomery tubercles. These glands produce a lubricant that keeps the nipple soft and supple.

INTERNAL FEMALE STRUCTURES

The vagina is an elastic, tube-like structure leading from the outside of the female body to the cervix. Approximately 2 to 3 inches long, it contains many rugae that allow it to stretch during intercourse and also permit the passage of the baby during delivery. The pH environment of the vagina is normally acidic, providing protection from microorganisms that could cause infections.

The uterus is a 3-inch-long, 2-inch-wide, 1-inch-thick hollow, muscular structure, as seen in Figure 13-2. The top is the fundus, the middle is the body (corpus), and the lower

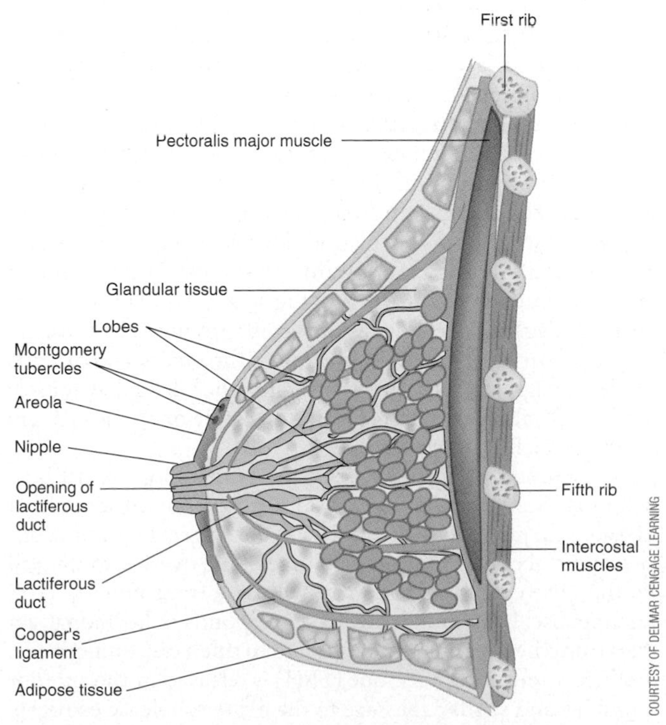

FIGURE 13-1 Cross Section of the Female Breast

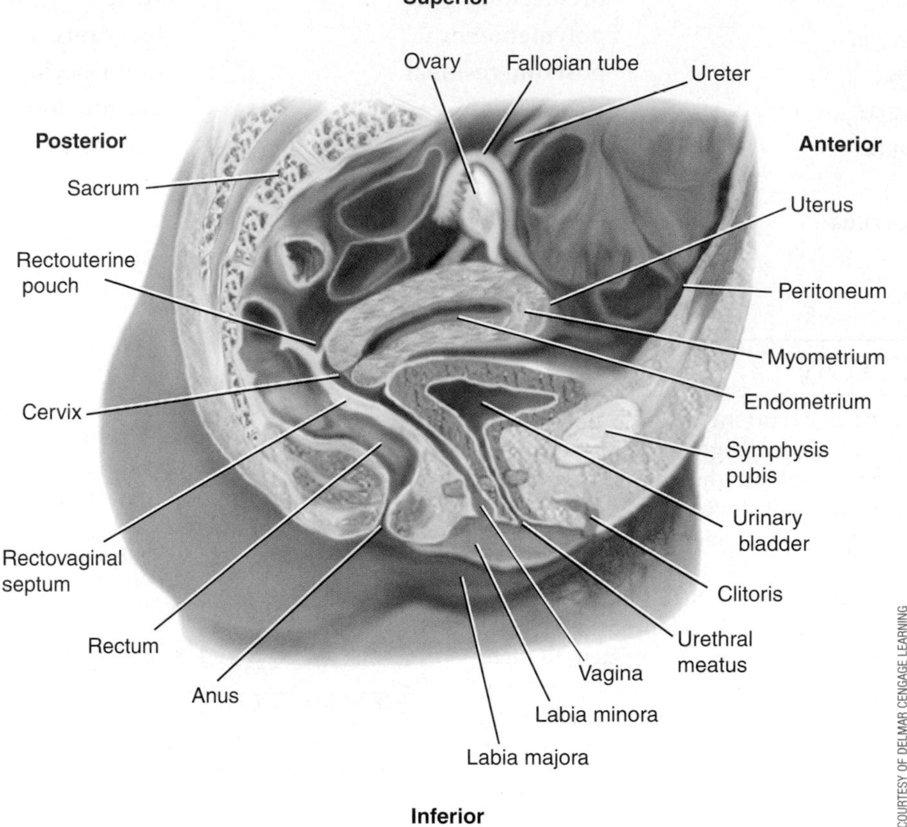

FIGURE 13-2 The Female Reproductive System

portion is the cervix. Four sets of ligaments hold the uterus in its normal anteverted (forward) position and permit it the freedom to grow and move during pregnancy. The uterus has three distinct layers. The innermost layer is the endometrium, which sloughs with menstruation each month. The middle layer is the myometrium, which is constructed of many muscle fibers that are interwoven for strength, stretch, and contractility. The outer layer is the perimetrium, which is an external serous membrane covering.

The fallopian tubes are connected to the uterus on either side. They are continuous with the mucous membrane lining of the endometrium on the inside. Billions of cilia line each fallopian tube and make a sweeping motion toward the uterus, especially at the time of ovulation. This sweeping action moves the ovum along the path toward the uterus. The movement may also impede the progress of the sperm, which must swim upstream against the downward current produced by the cilia.

The cervix is the lower portion of the uterus and extends into the vaginal vault. Like the vagina, the cervix has muscle layers that allow it to stretch to a diameter of at least 10 cm (about 4 inches) during delivery.

An almond-shaped ovary, about 2 inches long and 1 inch wide, is located within the broad ligament on either side of the uterus, just below the fimbriae, the fingerlike projections at the distal end of the fallopian tubes. The ovaries contain all of the ova (eggs) that a woman will have from puberty until menopause. Each month, the ovary responds to hormonal signals from the anterior pituitary gland to ripen one or more ova. Follicle-stimulating hormone (FSH) is released by the anterior pituitary and sends a message to the ovary to release estrogen, which causes the ovum to ripen and enlarge. The entire first part of the cycle is known as the proliferative phase.

Luteinizing hormone (LH) is then released. LH triggers a chain of events that stimulates the ovary to release the ovum. This point in the menstrual cycle is called ovulation. Another hormone, progesterone, causes the glands and blood vessels of the endometrial lining to grow and thicken in preparation for implantation of a fertilized ovum. If fertilization does not occur, the progesterone level decreases, the endometrium sloughs off, and the woman experiences menstruation. If fertilization does occur, the progesterone level remains elevated to ensure the optimal environment for implantation of the zygote about 6 to 8 days after fertilization. Figure 13-3 illustrates the menstrual cycle.

MALE REPRODUCTIVE STRUCTURES

The male reproductive organs and associated structures are illustrated in Figure 13-4. The scrotum is a fleshy structure suspended below the perineum, anterior to the anus. It is divided into two parts, each of which contains a testis, an epididymis, and a portion of the spermatic cord (vas deferens). The left side of the scrotum is usually lower than the right because the left spermatic cord is often longer.

The testes, two smooth, oval endocrine glands, are suspended in the scrotum. This location helps maintain proper temperature and also protects the testes from trauma. Certain cells of the epithelium lining the seminiferous tubules of the testes produce half a billion sperm each day (**spermatogenesis**). They also secrete the androgenic (causing masculinization) hormone testosterone. Spermatogenesis is regulated by follicle-stimulating hormone (FSH), produced by the anterior pituitary gland. The production of testosterone

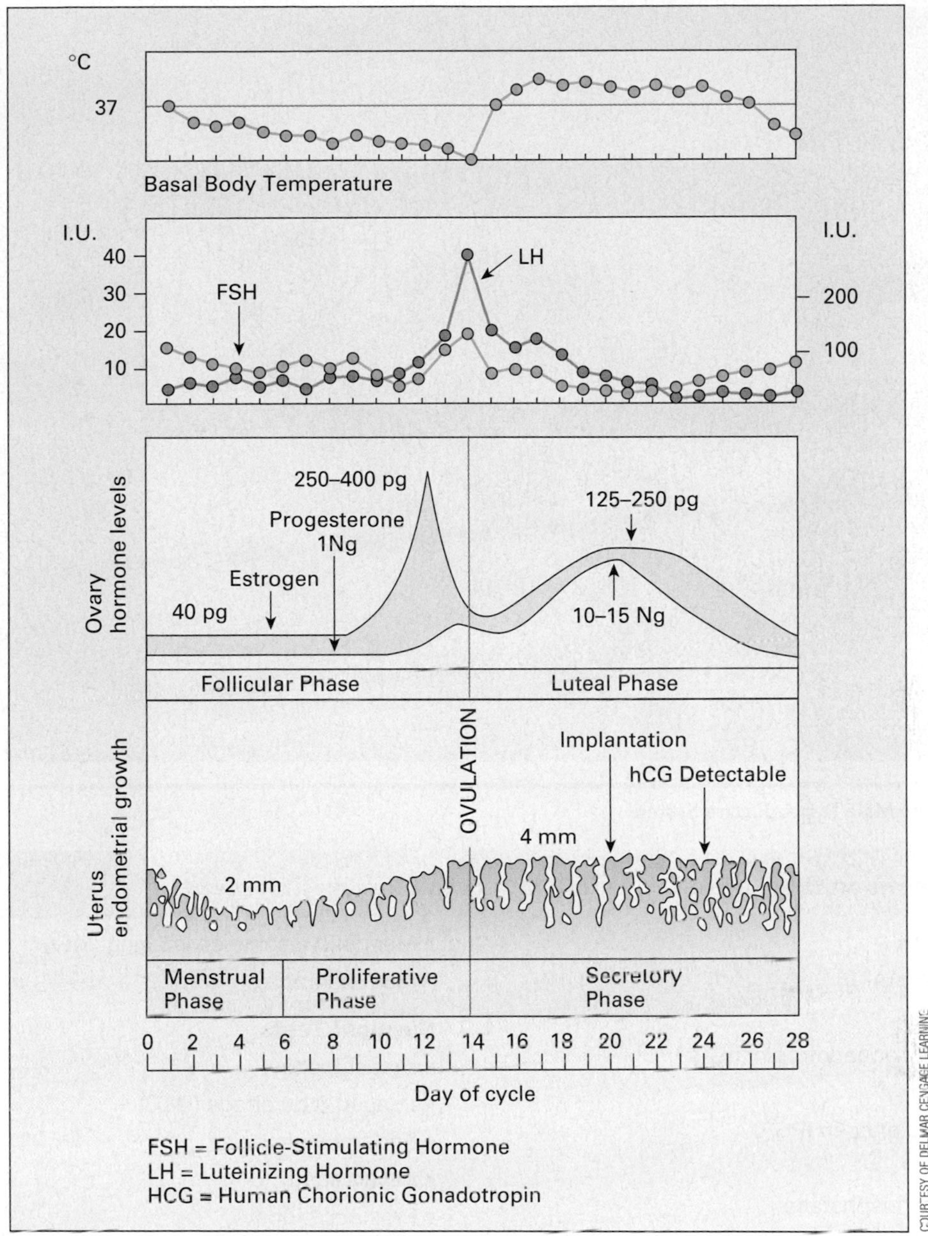

FIGURE 13-3 Cyclic Changes Associated with the Menstrual Cycle

is regulated by luteinizing hormone (LH), also produced by the anterior pituitary gland. After the sperm mature in the epididymis, they travel through the vas (ductus) deferens, a long tube attached to the epididymis. The vas deferens, along with associated nerves and blood vessels, forms the spermatic cord.

The vas deferens travels up and around the bladder and carries sperm from the epididymis to the seminal vesicle, a small pouch that produces secretions that, when mixed with sperm and prostatic fluid, form semen.

The prostate is an encapsulated gland that encircles the proximal portion of the urethra. The prostatic fossa, a depression on the cranial border of the prostate, allows entry of the ejaculatory ducts. Within the prostate is a cluster of 30 to 50 tubuloalveolar glands that secrete prostatic fluid. The prostate gland is of clinical significance because as men age, it is a common site for malignant disease or benign enlargement that can cause urethral obstruction.

The penis is a cylindrical organ through which urine is passed and semen is ejaculated. Half of the penis is located within the body. The external half of the penis is flaccid, unless the male is sexually aroused, at which time it becomes erect because of engorgement with blood. A fold of skin, the prepuce, surrounds the tip of the penis in the uncircumcised male.

COMMON DIAGNOSTIC TESTS

Commonly used diagnostic tests for clients with symptoms of reproductive system disorders are listed in Table 13-1.

INFLAMMATORY DISORDERS

Inflammatory disorders discussed include pelvic inflammatory disease, endometriosis, vaginitis, toxic shock syndrome, and epididymitis/orchitis/prostatitis.

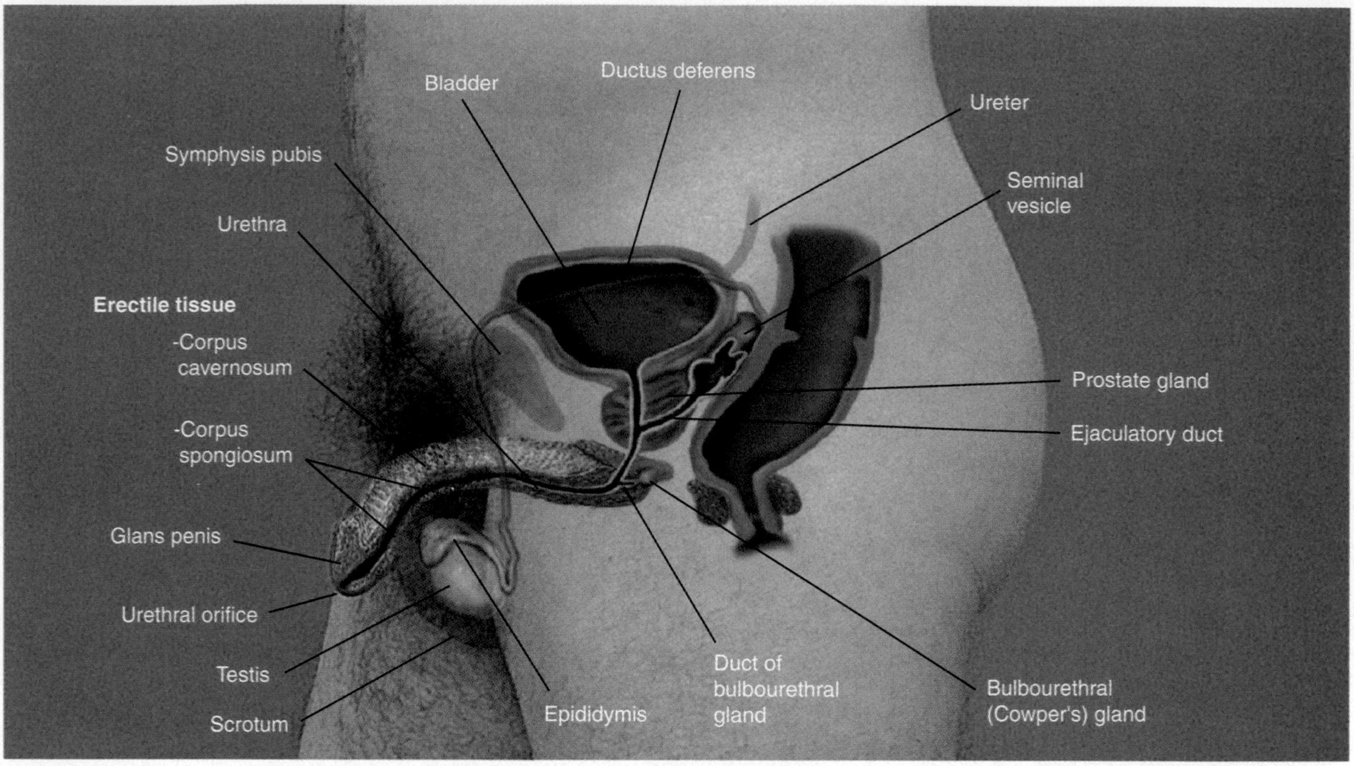

COURTESY OF DELMAR CENGAGE LEARNING

FIGURE 13-4 The Male Reproductive System

TABLE 13-1 Common Diagnostic Tests for Reproductive System Disorders

Laboratory Tests
- Alpha-fetoprotein (AFP)
- Cultures
- Human chorionic gonadotropin (hCG)
- Pap smear
- Prostate-specific antigen (PSA)
- Prostatic smear
- Serum alkaline phosphatase
- Serum calcium
- Semen analysis
- Segmented bacteriologic localization culture

Radiologic Tests
- Computed tomography (CT) scan
- Dynamic infusion cavernosometry and cavernosography (DICC)
- Hysterosalpingogram
- Magnetic resonance imaging (MRI)
- Mammography

Surgical Tests
- Breast biopsy
- Dilation & curettage (D&C)
- Endometrial biopsy
- Laparoscopy
- Prostatic biopsy
- Testicular biopsy

Other Tests
- Colposcopy
- Nocturnal tumescence penile monitoring
- Pelvic examination
- Schiller test
- Ultrasound

COURTESY OF DELMAR CENGAGE LEARNING

PELVIC INFLAMMATORY DISEASE

Pelvic inflammatory disease (PID) is an inflammatory process involving pathogenic invasion of the uterus, fallopian tubes (salpingitis), and ovaries (oophoritis), along with vascular and supporting structures within the pelvis. Pathogenic microorganisms such as chlamydia, gonococcus, streptococcus, staphylococcus, and herpes simplex virus II, may cause PID. The CDC estimates that each year more than 1 million American women will experience an episode of acute PID, and more than 100,000 women will become infertile as a result (CDC, 2008). Infections are usually ascending by nature; that is, the pathogens are introduced into the reproductive system from outside and travel upward from the vagina to the fallopian tubes and then out into the pelvis. Risk factors associated with the incidence of PID include multiple sexual partners, frequent intercourse, IUDs (intrauterine contraceptive devices), douching, and childbirth.

The symptoms of PID include a low-grade fever, pelvic pain, abdominal pain, a "bearing down" backache, a foul-smelling vaginal discharge, nausea and vomiting, abnormal uterine bleeding, **dysmenorrhea** (painful menstruation), **dyspareunia** (painful intercourse), and intense pelvic tenderness upon examination. Peritonitis or pelvic abscesses may develop as complications of PID if the pathogens spread into the pelvic cavity. Future **infertility** (inability or diminished ability to produce offspring) can be related to scarring and strictures of the fallopian tubes, which develop from the chronic inflammatory process within the pelvis. These problems have been associated with ectopic pregnancies because the fertilized ovum becomes trapped inside the fallopian tube before it can complete its trip to the uterus.

PID is often diagnosed during a pelvic examination. Vaginal and cervical cultures are obtained at the time of the exam to determine the causative agent. A pelvic ultrasound may be ordered to rule out other causes of pelvic pain. Instruct the client on the purpose of the procedures and any special preparations that may be required, such as having a full bladder.

MEDICAL–SURGICAL MANAGEMENT

Medical

The client who is not acutely ill from PID may be treated as an outpatient at home with oral antibiotics and bed rest, unless the infection is herpes simplex virus II. Clients with herpes simplex II infections may require more intensive care in the hospital with IV antibiotic therapy. The physician may also order medicated vaginal suppositories for the vaginal discharge. The acutely ill client may require hospitalization for IV antibiotic therapy.

Surgical

If the inflammation is extensive, or if medical treatment is not successful, the client may require a hysterectomy.

Pharmacological

Antibiotics used may include doxycycline monohydrate (Vibramycin), metronidazole (Flagyl), cefoxitin (Mefoxin), clindamycin (Cleocin), and gentamicin (Garamycin). IV fluids are frequently administered to promote adequate hydration, and analgesics are given for pain management.

Activity

During hospitalization, the client is placed on bed rest with bathroom privileges. A semi-Fowler's position is preferred because it will facilitate drainage of the pelvis. If vaginal suppositories are used, the client should lie in a supine position for 30 minutes.

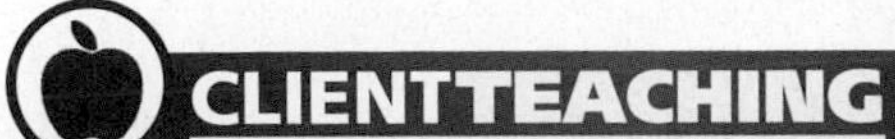

CLIENT TEACHING

Inserting Vaginal Suppositories

- Have the client wash her hands, then cleanse the vulva with a mild soap and warm water to remove any external discharge.
- Client should lie down in a supine position with her knees flexed.
- With one hand, the client can separate the labia and gently insert the suppository high inside the vagina.
- The client should remain supine for a minimum of 30 minutes to ensure adequate absorption of the medication through the vaginal mucosa.

NURSING MANAGEMENT

Support the client with a nonjudgmental attitude. Maintain client in semi-Fowler's position to facilitate drainage. Monitor vital signs and I&O. Teach client proper pericare, hygiene, and hand hygiene. Administer antibiotic therapy as ordered.

NURSING PROCESS

ASSESSMENT

Subjective Data

Obtain information about the client's sexual activity, including the number of partners. Unprotected intercourse is the most frequent method of entry for the microorganisms that cause PID. Also include the client's history of **contraception** (measures taken to prevent pregnancy), previous vaginal infections and treatments, obstetrical history, and normal hygiene practices such as douching and tampon use. Description of nagging pelvic pain and a low-grade fever are often expressed.

Objective Data

Assess for an elevated temperature, flushed, dry skin, the presence of a malodorous vaginal discharge, and positive vaginal or cervical cultures.

Nursing diagnoses for a client with pelvic inflammatory disease include the following:

NURSING DIAGNOSES	PLANNING/OUTCOMES	NURSING INTERVENTIONS
*Acute **Pain** related to inflammation of the pelvic structures caused by invasion of pathogens*	Using a pain rating scale of 0 to 10, the client will report that her pain has decreased.	Assess client's pain level every 4 hours, noting the location, duration, sensation, intensity, and factors that increase or decrease the pain. Administer analgesics as ordered.

(*Continues*)

Nursing diagnoses for a client with pelvic inflammatory disease include the following: (Continued)

NURSING DIAGNOSES	PLANNING/OUTCOMES	NURSING INTERVENTIONS
*Deficient **K**nowledge* related to the etiology of the pelvic inflammatory process, treatment regimen, self-care, and preventive measures	The client will follow prescribed treatment regimen, self-care, and preventive measures.	If suppositories are ordered, instruct the client in the proper method of insertion. Provide instructions to the client and partner (if available) about the causes of PID and ways to prevent the inflammation. Teach proper pericare and hygiene, especially hand hygiene before and after changing sanitary pads. Change sanitary pads every 3 to 4 hours. Encourage client to make time for rest periods during the acute phase of the inflammation and to avoid strenuous activities such as straining or heavy lifting. Instruct client about pelvic rest, which includes no douching, tampons, or intercourse. Recommend that the client wear underpants with a cotton crotch. Teach client to cleanse the perineal area from front to back after each voiding or bowel movement. Discuss and encourage the use of safe sexual practices and the use of barrier contraceptives to prevent recurrence of PID symptoms. Encourage client to make follow-up appointment.
	The client will contact her health care provider for follow-up and if her symptoms persist, worsen, or return.	Encourage client to notify the NP or physician at the first sign of PID symptoms. Recommend that the client monitor her own temperature, upon discharge, twice daily for 2 weeks and notify the physician or nurse practitioner (NP) if the temperature increases or remains elevated.
***H**yperthermia* related to physiologic responses to the inflammatory or infectious process	The client's temperature will return to normal range after the initiation of therapy.	Monitor client's vital signs every 4 hours. Administer antipyretic and antibiotic as ordered by the physician.

Evaluation: Evaluate each outcome to determine how it has been met by the client.

ENDOMETRIOSIS

Endometriosis is the growth of endometrial tissue, the normal lining of the uterus, outside of the uterus within the pelvic cavity. It occurs most frequently in women 30 years and older and tends to be familial. It predominantly affects Caucasian females who have not given birth and is most common among the higher socioeconomic population. Endometriosis has been called the "career woman's disorder," because it is often diagnosed in the late twenties or thirties when the working woman makes plans for childbearing.

The endometrial tissue implants itself on other pelvic structures (Figure 13-5). Two of the most common areas for endometrial implants are the pouch of Douglas and the ovaries. The tissue implants respond to the monthly hormonal changes in the same way as the endometrial tissue inside the uterus does. Bleeding of the implants during the menses results in the formation of adhesions and scar tissue. The endometriosis appears as brownish or black "powder burns" or larger lesions. If the endometriosis becomes encapsulated in an ovarian cyst it is called a "chocolate cyst."

The disease appears to be progressive and has a tendency to be recurrent. Some women with minimal endometriosis experience severe monthly symptoms, such as lower backache, painful intercourse, a feeling of heaviness on the pelvis, and spotting. Other women have a more extensive disease but have minimal symptoms. Thus the amount of endometriosis present may or may not be correlated with the severity of the client's symptoms.

Endometriosis is one cause of female infertility because of the amount of scar tissue and adhesions around the pelvic organs, ligaments, and fallopian tubes. Pregnancy inhibits the growth and bleeding of the endometrial implants because ovulation and menstruation are suppressed.

MEDICAL–SURGICAL MANAGEMENT

Medical

Endometriosis may be tentatively diagnosed by palpation of endometrial implants within the pelvis or a pelvic ultrasound

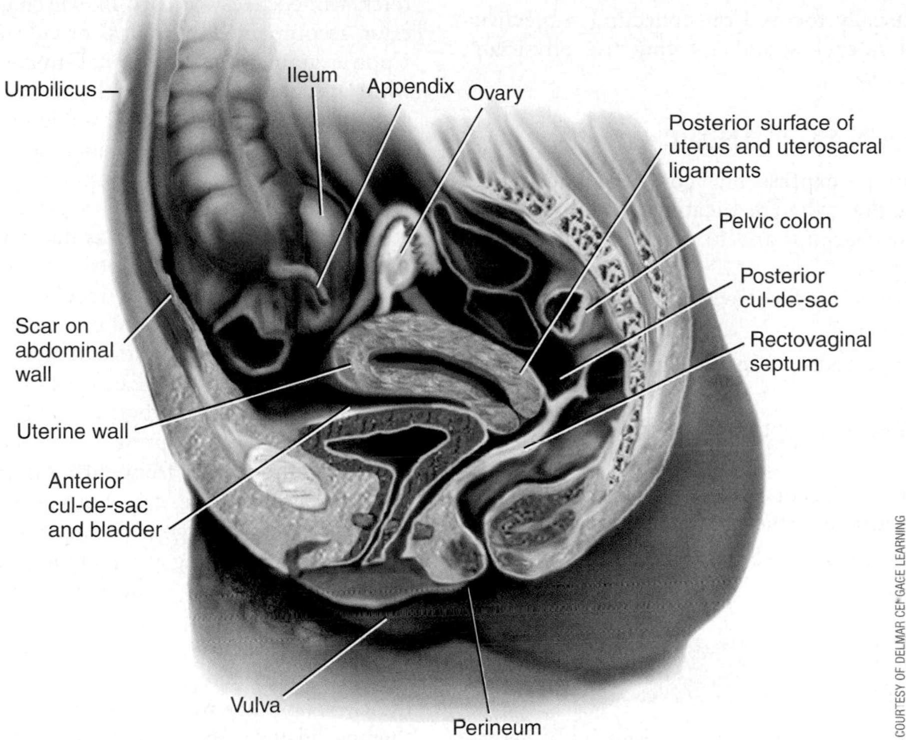

FIGURE 13-5 Common Areas of Endometriosis

may be ordered. To confirm the diagnosis, laparoscopy, performed under general anesthesia is the best method of diagnosis by direct visualization of the pelvic structures. Consideration for treatment depends on the client's age and desire for future childbearing. Sometimes pregnancy relieves the symptoms even after delivery.

Surgical

The older multigravida who is experiencing severe, debilitating symptoms that affect her lifestyle and normal functions, role, or activity may desire a hysterectomy. If the lesions are large or extensive, a laparotomy may be performed for adequate removal; however, if the implants are small and scattered, laparoscopic cauterization or laser ablation may be most desirable. Lysis of pelvic adhesions is performed at the same time.

Pharmacological

The goals of pharmacological therapy are to suppress ovulation and menstruation, reduce symptoms, and cause the implants to shrink. Medications used in the treatment of endometriosis must effectively suppress the monthly hypothalamic-pituitary-ovarian hormonal stimulation of ovulation. Some medications act on the body as "pseudopregnancy" agents that produce anovulation, breast tenderness, nausea, weight gain, and hirsutism. Other hormonal therapies cause a temporary medically induced menopause state. Hormonal treatments include contraceptives (pills, patches, vaginal rings), medroxyprogesterone (Depo-Provera), gonadotropin-releasing hormone (Gn-RH) agonists and antagonists, and aromatase inhibitors (CDC, 2008). Nafarelin acetate (Synarel) is a nasally administered gonadotropin analog that inhibits cyclic hormone release. Danazol (Danocrine) is an androgen hormone that must be taken continuously for at least 6 to 8 months. This medication inhibits the release of gonadotropin. The resulting **amenorrhea** (absence of menstruation) will suppress the growth of the endometrial tissue and is used in moderate to severe cases of endometriosis. Occasionally, Danocrine is given after surgical removal or cauterization of the endometriosis to relieve symptoms from residual disease.

All medications used to treat endometriosis cause mild to moderate side effects that may affect the client's desire to take them or her compliance with continuous usage. Examples of problems that may be experienced include oily skin, fluid retention, weight gain, acne, hot flashes, metrorrhagia, mastalgia, depression, and masculization.

NURSING PROCESS

ASSESSMENT

Subjective Data

Obtain a description of the pelvic pain, which increases at the time of menstruation. The client may voice concerns about dyspareunia, pelvic discomfort with intercourse. This may result in marital tension if the client avoids sexual intimacy to reduce her pain. Be alert to what the client says as well as what is left unsaid. The client may describe prolonged, excessive menstrual periods that are getting closer and closer together. Another sign, although not as significant, is pain with defecation during the menstrual period.

Also note the onset of menses, regularity of cycles, and any changes that client has noted in the frequency, comfort, duration, and amount of menstrual flow. Note the onset of the client's symptoms in relationship to the menstrual cycle, the severity as reported by the client, any alterations in lifestyle related to the pain or other symptoms, and the client's future plans for childbearing.

Objective Data

The nurse's role is usually focused on collecting subjective data from the client interview and assisting the physician during actual procedures.

NURSING MANAGEMENT

Encourage the client to express her concerns and fears. Teach the client about prescribed medications. Emphasize the importance of regular checkups and to report any abnormal vaginal bleeding.

Nursing diagnoses for a client with endometriosis may include the following:

- *Acute* ***Pain*** related to bleeding from endometrial implants in the pelvic cavity
- ***Anxiety*** related to treatment options, possible side effects, and infertility
- *Ineffective* ***Sexuality*** *Patterns,* or ***Sexual*** *Dysfunction,* related to altered body function or structure (painful intercourse)
- *Situational Low* ***Self****-Esteem,* related to the inability to conceive

VAGINITIS

Several common types of vaginitis are caused by bacteria, protozoa, viruses, and yeasts. The vaginal mucosa is normally protected by an acid mantle. The acidic (pH less than 5.0) environment inhibits the growth of many pathogenic microorganisms. Because the vaginal opening is close to the external environment, microorganisms have an opportunity to invade the reproductive tract. Some organisms that cause vaginitis are transmitted to the female from the male partner during sexual contact. Natural protective barriers may vary with the fluctuating hormonal levels during the woman's monthly cycle because the hormones affect the vaginal pH. At ovulation, the vaginal pH becomes slightly less acidic because of the high level of estrogen. Times when the woman's system has a lower estrogen level, such as immediately after the menses and after menopause, are times when there is a higher risk for infection because the epithelium is less active, no glycogen is present, and the pH may be as high as 7.0.

Diagnosis is made after performing a vaginal examination and obtaining a cervical culture and a sample of the vaginal discharge. When the client contacts the physician or nurse practitioner to report symptoms of vaginitis, the nurse should instruct her to avoid douching or using tampons before being examined because douching will wash away the discharge needed to be examined and tampons will absorb it.

Common types of vaginitis include candidiasis caused by *Candida albicans* (yeast infection), trichomoniasis caused by *Trichomonas vaginalis* (a protozoan), *Gardnerella vaginalis* (a bacterium), and *Chlamydia trachomatis* (a parasite). Other causes of vaginitis may include streptococcus, staphylococcus, gonococcus, and herpes simplex II. Usually the symptoms depend on the causative agent. The client's description of her symptoms along with the examination of the discharge help confirm the diagnosis. Most infections have a characteristic discharge and irritation with burning or itching that may be internal, external, or both.

Predisposing factors for candidiasis, also called monilia, may include obesity, diabetes, pregnancy, oral contraceptives, antibiotics, bubble baths, and frequent douching. Many of these factors alter the pH of the vagina. Symptoms include a thick, white, cheesy or curd-like discharge with a musty, sweet odor, accompanied by vaginal or vulvar itching and irritation. Upon examination, the vaginal mucosa will have patches of white discharge present. If the patches are scraped off, the tissue underneath will appear reddened and may bleed. Externally, the vulva may be reddened and edematous. The client may have scratches from attempting to ease the itching.

The preferred treatment is vaginal application of antifungal creams or suppositories such as miconazole (Monistat), clotrimazole (Mycelex-G, Gyne-Lotrimin), or nystatin (Mycostatin). Alternative therapies include douching with white vinegar solution (1 tablespoon per 1 pint of water) twice a day for a week. This treatment restores the acid balance of the vagina and washes away the *Candida albicans*. Eating cultured yogurt with active acidophilus or applying the yogurt directly to the labia helps restore the normal bacteria and protective mechanisms in the vagina.

Trichomoniasis is frequently passed from partner to partner during intercourse. A copious green-yellow, foul-smelling, frothy vaginal discharge is characteristic. It may produce itching or external burning and irritation. Metronidazole (Flagyl) should be taken orally by both partners.

Flagyl is normally contraindicated in the first trimester of pregnancy, so obtaining a menstrual history or a pregnancy test may be needed before administering this medication. Inform the client and her partner to avoid any alcohol intake during therapy. Flagyl causes a strong antabuse-like effect, which results in severe nausea and vomiting. Clients should read labels on over-the-counter medications being taken concurrently with the Flagyl because many preparations contain alcohol bases.

Instruct the client and her partner to abstain from intercourse during therapy and to finish all of the medication.

Gardnerella vaginalis often produces a gray-white vaginal discharge with a strong fishy odor or is asymptomatic. If itching or burning is present, it may suggest another microorganism. For the treatment of *Gardnerella,* and other bacterial vaginitis, the physician may order Flagyl or an oral antibiotic such as tetracycline hydrochloride (Achromycin) or ampicillin (Omnipen). Sulfa-based creams such as Sultrin, Triple Sulfa, and AVC may be used vaginally in conjunction with the oral medications once or twice a day for 6 to 14 days to completely treat this type of infection.

Chlamydial vaginitis infections are often asymptomatic but have been associated with infertility problems. A culture of vaginal secretions is necessary to specifically identify the organism. The treatment is usually oral antibiotics for at least 7 days. A repeat culture is recommended following treatment to ensure that the parasites have been eradicated.

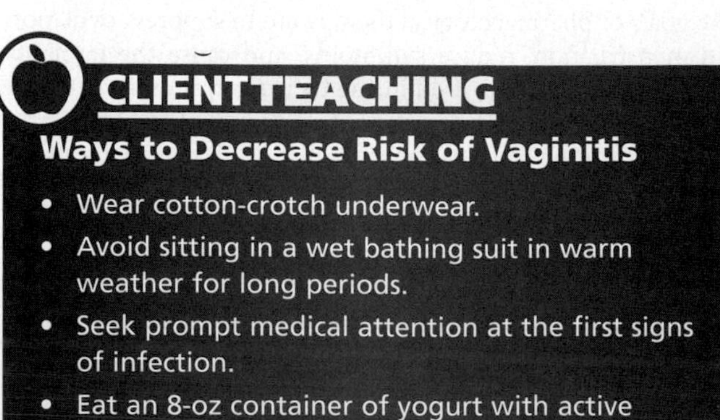

CLIENT TEACHING

Ways to Decrease Risk of Vaginitis

- Wear cotton-crotch underwear.
- Avoid sitting in a wet bathing suit in warm weather for long periods.
- Seek prompt medical attention at the first signs of infection.
- Eat an 8-oz container of yogurt with active cultures daily while taking antibiotics.

Postmenopausal vaginitis (atrophic) is caused by a decreased level of estrogen in the vaginal tissue. The client may describe painful intercourse (dyspareunia), itching, burning, or irritation. Estrogen replacement therapy often relieves the symptoms of this type of vaginitis. The medication may be administered orally, vaginally, or by transdermal patch.

NURSING PROCESS

ASSESSMENT

Subjective Data

Obtain information from the client regarding the nature of her symptoms, the onset, menstrual history, contraceptive methods, recent or current use of antibiotics or other medications, recent illness, diabetes mellitus, sexual history, pregnancy history, usual hygiene practices such as douching, deodorant sprays, bubble baths, wearing of pantyhose, type of underwear, and use of deodorized tampons or pads.

Objective Data

Observe the vaginal discharge and note any odor. Vaginal or vulvar irritation and possible scratches may be seen.

NURSING MANAGEMENT

Emphasize the significance of hand hygiene before and after applying vaginal medications. Notify client that her sexual partner should also be treated.

Nursing diagnoses for a client with vaginitis, regardless of the etiology, include the following:

- *Acute **Pain**,* related to irritation, excoriation, or ulceration of vaginal tissue
- *Deficient **Knowledge**,* related to the origin of the infection, prevention, and treatment options
- *Impaired **Tissue Integrity**,* related to the presence of vaginal discharge, itching, or irritation
- ***Sexual** Dysfunction,* related to discomfort during intercourse or fear of transmitting the infection to the sexual partner
- *Risk for Impaired **Skin** Integrity,* related to internal and external irritation from discharge and itching

TOXIC SHOCK SYNDROME

Toxic shock syndrome (TSS) is a rare, life-threatening condition most often associated with *Staphylococcus aureus*, which enters the bloodstream. Toxins produced by group A *streptococcus* have also been associated with causing TSS. A strong relationship has been found between the use of tampons (especially superabsorbent) during menstruation and the onset of TSS symptoms. It has been hypothesized that the fibers from the tampon lower the level of magnesium in the woman's body and, therefore, produce a favorable environment for the growth of pathogenic microorganisms. The condition was first diagnosed in the mid-1970s, and the incidence increased throughout the 1980s. A high percentage of women who are affected by TSS are younger than age 30. TSS can also occur in nonmenstruating women, men, and children.

The client presents with a sudden high temperature of 102°F or greater, vomiting, diarrhea, progressive hypotension, and flulike symptoms of malaise, muscle soreness, sore throat, and headache (Neighbors & Tannehill-Jones, 2006). There may be a macular erythematous (flat, red) rash followed in 1 to 2 weeks by peeling of the palms and soles. Disorientation may occur from the release of toxins and dehydration. Symptoms of TSS develop suddenly and can be fatal.

> **CLIENT TEACHING**
>
> **TSS and Tampon Use**
>
> Instruct client to avoid tampon use for several cycles. If she chooses to use tampons in the future, they should be changed every 2 to 3 hours. Avoid the superabsorbent types.

MEDICAL–SURGICAL MANAGEMENT

Medical

Blood, urine, genitourinary, and throat cultures may be obtained and are usually negative except for *Staphylococcus aureus*. The goals of treatment are focused on controlling the falling blood pressure, replacing fluid volume, halting the infectious process, and maintaining adequate ventilation efforts. IV fluids are administered per the physician's order. The client may require mechanical ventilation and CPAP (continuous positive airway pressure). Dialysis may be needed if kidney failure occurs.

Pharmacological

Broad-spectrum antibiotic therapy is recommended. Culture and sensitivity tests will indicate which type of antibiotic is best. Examples include dicloxacillin sodium (Dynapen), clexacillin sodium (Tegopen), nafcillin sodium (Nafcil), and methicillin sodium (Staphcillin). The medication regimen is continued for at least 2 weeks to ensure control of the pathogens.

Activity

Bed rest is usually prescribed.

NURSING MANAGEMENT

Maintain client on prescribed bed rest. Administer antipyretics and antibiotics as ordered. Monitor vital signs, I&O, and skin turgor. Encourage oral fluid intake.

NURSING PROCESS

ASSESSMENT

Subjective Data

Obtain information on recent use of tampons, length of time tampon is left in before changing, use of contraceptive sponges, sore throat, headache, myalgia, and fatigue.

Objective Data

Assess erythematous rash, edema, peeling of palms and soles, hypotension, fever, level of consciousness, nonpurulent conjunctivitis, and hyperemia of vagina and oropharynx.

Nursing diagnoses for a client with toxic shock syndrome include the following:

NURSING DIAGNOSES	PLANNING/OUTCOMES	NURSING INTERVENTIONS
***H**yperthermia* related to inflammatory process	The client will have normal-range temperature within 48 hours.	Administer antipyretics as ordered. Give cooling sponge bath. Encourage oral fluids as tolerated. Monitor body temperature.
*Deficient **F**luid Volume* related to diarrhea, vomiting, fever, and decreased intake	The client will have normal fluid and electrolyte balance within 24 hours.	Administer intravenous fluids as ordered. Encourage oral fluids if client is not vomiting. Monitor I&O. Monitor blood pressure. Administer antiemetic and antidiarrheal medications as ordered. Assess skin turgor and mucous membranes.
*Risk for Impaired **S**kin Integrity* related to dehydration and effects of circulating toxins	The client will maintain skin integrity.	Encourage or assist with position change every 2 hours. Provide or assist with personal hygiene, especially after diarrhea. Assess bony prominences for reddened areas.

Evaluation: Evaluate each outcome to determine how it has been met by the client.

EPIDIDYMITIS/ORCHITIS/ PROSTATITIS

Epididymitis can be a sterile or nonsterile inflammation of the epididymis. A sterile inflammation is caused by direct injury or reflux of urine down the vas deferens. Urinary reflux that is related to strain exerted by a male while his bladder is full can be caused by lifting heavy objects or doing strenuous exercises. Nonsterile inflammation may occur as a complication of gonorrhea, chlamydia, mumps, tuberculosis, prostatitis, or urethritis. Prolonged use of an indwelling catheter or an invasive procedure can also lead to nonsterile inflammation.

Signs and symptoms of epididymitis include sudden severe scrotal pain, warmth, redness and swelling, testicular tenderness usually on one side that worsens when having a bowel movement, dysuria, pyuria, chills, fever, penile discharge, and blood in the semen. Treatment includes bed rest, antibiotics, scrotal support (Figure 13-6), and ice compresses to the area. Bilateral epididymitis can cause sterility. Untreated epididymitis leads quickly to testicular tissue necrosis, septicemia, and death.

Orchitis is an inflammation of the testes that most often occurs as a complication of a bloodborne infection originating in the epididymis. Other causes of orchitis include gonorrhea, trauma, surgical manipulation, and tuberculosis and mumps that occur after puberty. In most instances, both testes are involved, and often sterility results. In orchitis, unilateral involvement does not cause sterility. Signs and symptoms of orchitis include sudden scrotal pain with pain radiating to the inguinal canal, scrotal edema, chills, fever, nausea, and vomiting. Treatment includes bed rest, scrotal support, and ice to the area.

Prostatitis, an inflammation of the prostate, is a common complication of urethritis caused by chlamydia or gonorrhea. Infecting organisms may reach the genital tract by direct spread through the urethra or may be borne by blood or lymph. The condition may be acute or chronic, with the chronic form leading to development of fibrotic tissue. This fibrotic tissue causes the prostate to harden, so prostatitis may be difficult to differentiate from prostate cancer. It may take 3 to 6 months for the granulomatous form to resolve. Signs and symptoms of prostatitis include perineal pain, fever, dysuria, and urethral discharge.

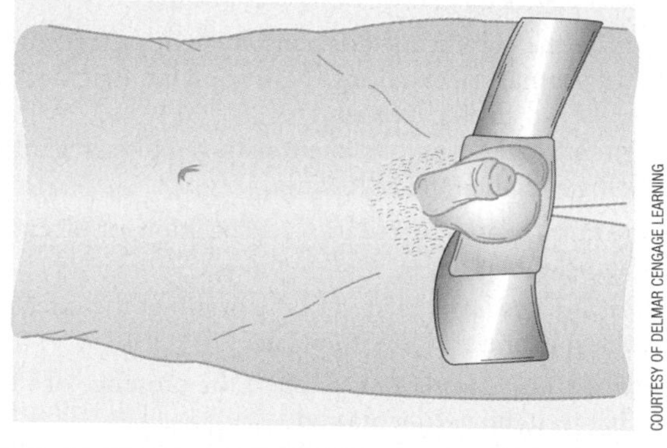

FIGURE 13-6 Bellevue Bridge for Scrotal Support

MEDICAL–SURGICAL MANAGEMENT

Medical

When it is suspected that the client currently has urethritis, he should not be catheterized. The infection spreads rapidly to the genital organs because of the trauma of catheterization and the possible spread of bacteria from the nonsterile distal part of the urethra. The physician may order that segmented bacteriologic localization cultures be obtained.

Pharmacological

Treatment of epididymitis and orchitis includes antibiotics and injection of procaine around the spermatic cord.

Pharmacological treatment of prostatitis includes antibiotics, analgesics, and stool softeners.

Activity

Treatment of prostatitis includes bed rest. While the client is in bed, his scrotum should be elevated and cold packs applied to the area. Encourage the client to drink a large amount of fluids and use sitz baths for comfort. These interventions are used to reduce inflammation, swelling, and discomfort. Periodic digital massage of the prostate by the physician increases the flow of infected prostatic secretions.

Nursing Management

Monitor vital signs, especially temperature and I&O. Encourage intake of oral fluids. Objectively assess client's pain and administer analgesics as ordered. Maintain client on bed rest. Keep scrotum elevated when the client is in bed and have client use an athletic support when ambulatory. Apply cold pack under scrotum as ordered.

NURSING PROCESS

Assessment

Subjective Data

Ask the client about the presence of urethral discharge or dysuria as well as the nature and location of the pain. A description of pain may include arthralgia, low-back pain, and myalgia. A positive history of recent bacterial or viral infection is of special significance. Ongoing nursing assessment includes monitoring of pain, using a pain scale to objectify data. Ask the client if he is experiencing nausea, because this could be a sign that his condition is deteriorating. Assess the client's educational and emotional needs because he may be worrying needlessly about possible sterility or impotence.

Objective Data

Assess vital signs, especially temperature. An increase in temperature may be an indication that the client's condition is worsening. Scrotal edema and purulent urethral discharge may be present. Monitor intake and output. Ask about constipation.

Nursing diagnoses for the male client with an inflammatory disorder include the following:

NURSING DIAGNOSES	PLANNING/OUTCOMES	NURSING INTERVENTIONS
Risk for Injury related to worsening of the inflammatory process	The client will not experience worsening of his condition.	Monitor client's vital signs, especially his temperature. Report hyperthermia, hypotension, nausea, and tachycardia to the physician immediately.
Deficient Fluid Volume related to nausea and vomiting	The client will maintain fluid balance.	Monitor client's I&O. Encourage him to drink plenty of fluids when not nauseated.
Acute Pain related to Inflammation	Using a pain scale of 0 to 10, the client will report pain has decreased to 2 or less within 48 hours after treatment initiation.	Assess client's pain level every 4 hours. Administer analgesics as ordered. Encourage client to maintain bed rest. Provide diversional activities to increase compliance. Encourage client with prostatitis to take a sitz bath, but never the client with epididymitis or orchitis as local heat may increase destruction of sperm cells. Fill a plastic glove with crushed ice and place it under the scrotum when heat is contraindicated. Remove the ice for short intervals every hour to prevent ice burns.
Anxiety related to concerns about possible sterility or impotence	The client will verbalize decreased anxiety.	Reassure client that with proper treatment, sterility and impotence are not likely complications of prostatitis.

Evaluation: Evaluate each outcome to determine how it has been met by the client.

BENIGN NEOPLASMS

Benign neoplasms include fibrocystic breast changes, fibroid tumors, and benign prostatic hyperplasia.

FIBROCYSTIC BREAST CHANGES

Fibrocystic breasts (formerly called fibrocystic breast disease) contain lumpy, nodular, glandular tissue. Fibrocystic breast changes are common between 30 and 50 years of age and occur in more than half of women at some point in their lifetime. Many cases will subside after menopause. The incidence of the potential for developing breast cancer is increased 3 to 4 times with fibrocystic breast changes. There appears to be a familial tendency toward the development of breast cancer.

Lumps may occur as single or multiple cysts that are frequently fluid-filled. It is difficult to differentiate fibrocystic tissue changes from other breast lesions because the dense fibrocystic areas may mask areas of breast cancer. Figure 13-7 shows the differences among cysts, fibroadenomas, and carcinomas of the breast.

The pathophysiology of a fibrocystic breast is found in the formation of fibrous tissue caused by hyperplasia of the epithelial cells in the breast lobules and ducts. The proliferation of the fibrous tissue deviates from the expected normal cyclic response to female hormone shifts during the menstrual cycle.

Routine mammograms provide baseline information and differentiate the palpable breast lumps between benign and malignant types. A computer-directed biopsy may also be performed.

Women should be taught breast self-examination (BSE) as adolescents and encouraged to practice it at the end of each menstrual cycle, when it is easier to palpate the breast tissue. Figure 13-8 provides specific information on how to perform a BSE.

A yellow-greenish, sticky discharge from the nipple is occasionally present with fibrocystic breasts. A Pap smear may be done on the discharge to rule out the presence of malignant cells. Note the presence of any breast discharge and report it to the health care provider as soon as possible. The physician or nurse practitioner (NP) may perform a biopsy or aspiration of the abnormal areas in the office. If fluid is obtained from the area, it is sent to pathology for examination. If no fluid is obtained, it may be a solid cyst or tumor, and biopsy may be required.

In the office, a breast biopsy may be performed with a local anesthetic. If there is any question of malignancy, or if the physician suspects that the lesion will be malignant on the basis of the mammography report, the biopsy may be performed in the hospital under general anesthetic so that additional tissue may be removed if necessary. A frozen section may be obtained and sent to the laboratory for a preliminary examination to rule out a malignant lesion.

MEDICAL–SURGICAL MANAGEMENT

Surgical

Aspiration or surgical excision may be indicated for diagnostic or therapeutic reasons. The cystic tissue may be aspirated with a small-gauge needle and syringe. The nurse prepares the client for the procedure and assists the doctor or NP with the procedure. The nurse assists the client into a supine position on the examination table and sets up the equipment and instruments needed. The area to be biopsied is cleansed. Upon completion of the aspiration or biopsy, the nurse labels the specimen and sends it to the pathology department.

If the areas of fibrocystic tissue are extensive and have not responded to conservative treatments and methods, or if the risk of cancer is high, the tissue may be excised completely. Removal of fibrocystic tissue does not guarantee that the client will not develop breast cancer in the remaining tissue, and she must continue to perform monthly BSE.

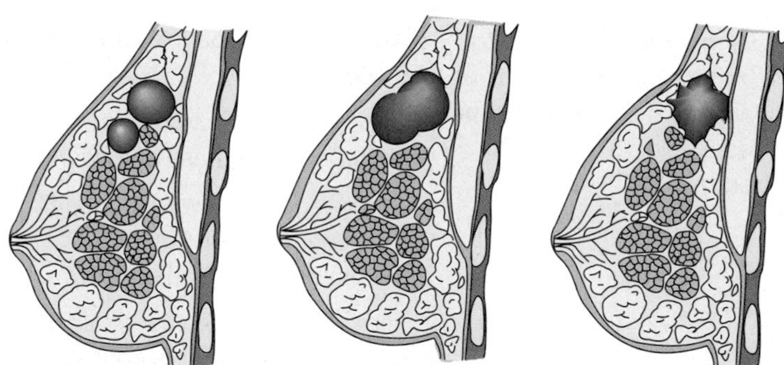

	GROSS CYST	FIBROADENOMA	CARCINOMA
Age	30–50; diminishes after menopause	Puberty to menopause; peaks between ages 20–30	Most common after 50 years
Shape	Round	Round, lobular, or ovoid	Irregular, stellate, or crab-like
Consistency	Soft to firm	Usually firm	Firm to hard
Discreteness	Well defined	Well defined	Not clearly defined
Number	Single or grouped	Most often single	Usually single
Mobility	Mobile	Very mobile	May be mobile or fixed to skin, underlying tissue, or chest wall
Tenderness	Tender	Nontender	Usually nontender
Erythema	No erythema	No erythema	May be present
Retraction/dimpling	Not present	Not present	Often present

FIGURE 13-7 Characteristics of Common Breast Masses

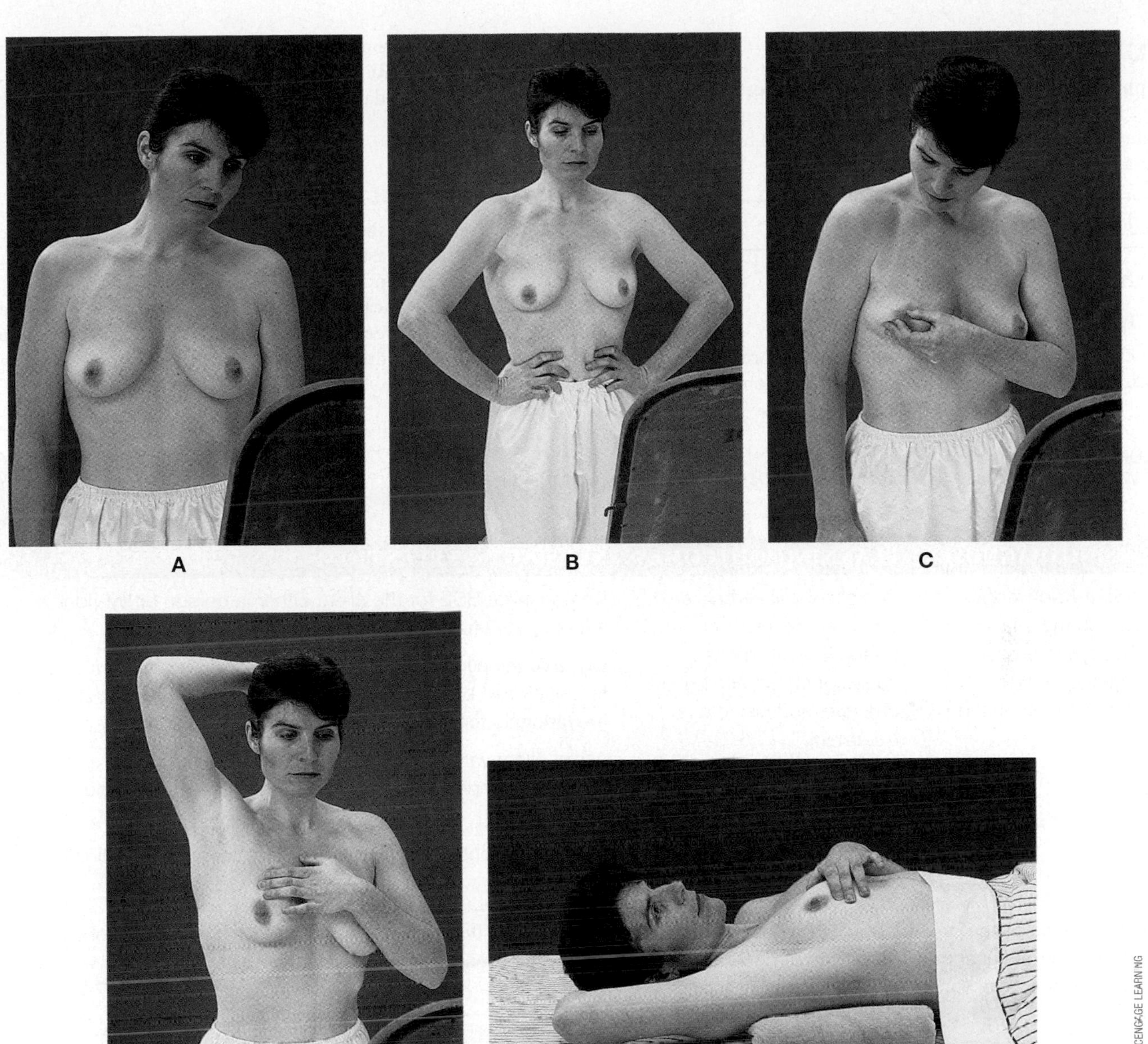

FIGURE 13-8 Performing a Breast Self-Examination; *A,* Standing in front of mirror, check breasts for puckering, dimpling, scaliness, or discharge from nipples; *B,* Clasp hands behind head and press hands forward, watching for changes in the shape or contour of breasts. Press hands on hips and bend toward mirror while pulling shoulders and elbows forward (shown); *C,* Gently squeeze each nipple, looking for discharge; *D,* Raise one arm and use fingers of other hand to check breast for lumps or masses under skin. Use a pattern of motion (circular, up-and-down, etc.) to cover entire breast; *E,* Repeat "D" while lying flat on back with one arm over head and a towel under the shoulder.

CRITICAL THINKING

Breast Self-Examination

How would you teach a client to do a breast self-examination? Make a teaching plan.

Pharmacological

Some physicians recommend up to 600 units of vitamin E daily. It is believed that the vitamin supplement helps break down the fibrocystic tissue because it reacts with the polyunsaturated fats in the cell membrane. It may also have some effect on the balance of female hormones.

Diet

Most health care providers recommend limiting or completely eliminating caffeine-containing products from the woman's diet. This would include teas, colas, coffee, and chocolate. These products are all available in caffeine-free forms. Dietary fat should be decreased to less than 20% of total calories (Mayo Clinic, 2008b).

Nursing Management

Emphasize the importance of the client performing BSE one week following menses and having a mammogram as appropriate for age and risk factors. Teach the client how to perform BSE and to wear a firm, supportive bra.

NURSING PROCESS

Assessment

Subjective Data

The client may report that the lumps are more tender as she approaches her menstrual period and that there is a greenish, sticky discharge from one or both breasts. Inquire about the client's dietary habits, especially caffeine intake, frequency of BSE, and the date of the most recent mammogram, if applicable.

Objective Data

When examined, single or multiple lumps may be palpated in one or both breasts. The lumps are not always discrete but should be freely movable. Because fibrocystic breast lumps are more tender near the menses, the client should be seen for an exam the week after her menstrual period. The tissue contains less fluid during that time and palpation is easier and less uncomfortable.

Nursing diagnoses for a client with fibrocystic breast changes include the following:

NURSING DIAGNOSES	PLANNING/OUTCOMES	NURSING INTERVENTIONS
*Deficient **K**nowledge* related to the cause of fibrocystic breast changes and method of breast self-examination	The client will verbalize and demonstrate her understanding of the cause of fibrocystic breast changes and her role in treatment.	Demonstrate BSE for the client either in person or by video with a follow-up return demonstration by the client. Observe the client as she performs the BSE so that immediate feedback can be given. Explain the best timing for the BSE and the rationale for performing the procedure after the menses. Assist client with mammogram. Encourage mammography at regular intervals dependent upon the client's age and risk factors. Teach the client about dietary modifications, such as limiting caffeine.
***A**nxiety* related to the underlying potential and risk of breast cancer	The client will display behaviors of decreased anxiety related to the potential for breast cancer.	Explain the differences between malignant breast lesions and fibrocystic breast changes to help alleviate the client's anxiety.

Evaluation: Evaluate each outcome to determine how it has been met by the client.

FIBROID TUMORS

Fibroids (leiomyomas) are benign tumors that grow in or on the uterus. A higher incidence is seen with nulliparous women and those who are more than 35 years old. The fibroids may appear below the serosal membrane or the mucosa. An early symptom is often **menorrhagia**, an excessively heavy menstrual flow. Later, the client may experience increasing pelvic pressure as the tumors grow, along with dysmenorrhea, abdominal enlargement, and constipation. Growth of the fibroids is usually slow but can be stimulated by estrogen. During pregnancy, when the estrogen and progesterone levels increase dramatically, the tumors grow much faster. Concern arises for the fetus when the fibroids begin to enlarge and crowd the uterus. Overcrowding may compress the fetus or initiate the onset of preterm labor. With either situation, the pregnancy must be monitored carefully.

A medical diagnosis of uterine fibroids may initially be based on the client's symptoms and the findings of the pelvic examination. If on palpation the uterus feels like an irregular mass or several masses, a pelvic ultrasound or a laparoscopy is ordered to confirm the diagnosis.

Medical–Surgical Management

Medical

The physician may opt to wait and observe the growth pattern of the fibroids before advising the client to have surgery. This

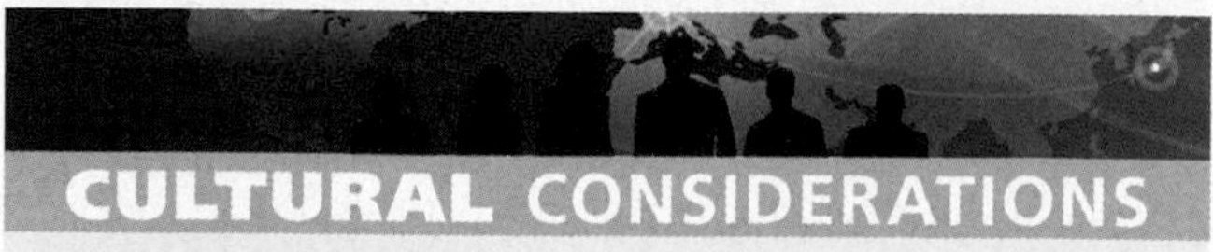

CULTURAL CONSIDERATIONS

Fibroid Tumors

Fibroid tumors are most prevalent in African-American and Mediterranean clients with dark skin.

"wait-and-see" attitude may be swayed by the significance of the client's symptoms, size of the fibroids, amount of discomfort the client is experiencing, and amount of menorrhagia and/or **metrorrhagia**, vaginal bleeding between menstrual periods. Reexamination is encouraged at least every 6 months.

Surgical

If the menorrhagia is significant with each menstrual cycle, a dilation and curettage (D&C) may be performed to determine the exact etiology of the bleeding. A myomectomy, a surgical procedure to remove the tumor, may be performed if the client desires future pregnancies. In the case of severe menorrhagia, with a dropping hemoglobin level or multiple tumors, the physician may recommend a hysterectomy as the option of choice.

Diet

A diet with many sources of iron helps prevent iron-deficiency anemia, which may result from the extra blood loss.

Nursing Management

Monitor vital signs and hemoglobin level. Assess client's blood loss for amount, color, and clots. Objectively assess pain with a 0 to 10 scale and administer analgesics as ordered. Encourage a diet high in iron-containing foods to prevent iron-deficiency anemia.

NURSING PROCESS

Assessment

Subjective Data

Obtain the client's description of menstrual flow, dysmenorrhea, and/or pelvic pain and pressure. The client may also report difficulty fitting into clothes because of abdominal enlargement, constipation, or urinary frequency or urgency.

Objective Data

Count the number of sanitary pads the client saturates in an hour; observe the presence or absence of clots in the blood, a hemoglobin level of less than 12 mg/dL, and the client's pale skin color. Her blood pressure may be slightly lower than normal and her pulse may be increased as a compensatory mechanism.

Nursing diagnoses for a client with fibroids include the following:

NURSING DIAGNOSES	PLANNING/OUTCOMES	NURSING INTERVENTIONS
*Risk for Deficient **Fluid** Volume* related to excessive blood losses	The client will have a hemoglobin above 12 mg/dL and will maintain fluid balance.	Assess client's blood loss for amount, color, and clots. Provide an accurate count of the saturated sanitary pads, along with the length of time taken to saturate a pad. Monitor vital signs at least every 4 hours, or more frequently if the client is having active blood loss. Monitor laboratory reports for Hgb level.
*Acute **Pain*** related to pressure on pelvic structures caused by growing tumors and cramping during the menses	The client will verbalize less discomfort and pelvic pressure.	Assess pain on 0 (least) to 10 (most) pain scale and note location, onset, and duration. Administer analgesics as ordered.

Evaluation: Evaluate each outcome to determine how it has been met by the client.

BENIGN PROSTATIC HYPERPLASIA

Benign prostatic hyperplasia (BPH) is a progressive adenomatous enlargement of the prostate gland that occurs with aging. More than 50% of men older than age 60 and 90% of men older than age 70 have some symptoms of BPH (National Institutes of Health, 2006). Although this disorder is not harmful, the urinary outlet obstruction that may be associated with the disorder is a problem.

Because the urethra is encircled by the prostate, common early symptoms of BPH are related to partial or complete obstruction of the urethra. Early symptoms include **hesitancy** (difficulty initiating the urinary stream), decreased force of stream, urinary frequency, and **nocturia** (awakening at night to void). However, a temporary reduction of these symptoms may occur as the bladder muscles hypertrophy in response to the increased work they must do to force the urinary stream past the obstruction.

Although this bladder muscle compensatory response may temporarily reduce symptoms, eventually the muscle decompensates, becoming noncompliant and hypotonic. This decompensation leads to atony of the mucous membranes between the muscle bands, which causes stagnant urine to collect in the small compartments (cellules) of the membranes. In addition, the man is unable to completely empty the bladder when voiding (**postvoid residual**). Because these changes in urinary function promote urinary alkalosis by increasing the urine pH, a perfect environment for bacterial growth is created. This bacterial growth can cause a urinary tract infection (UTI), which may eventually lead to kidney damage.

Medical–Surgical Management

Medical

The physician performs a digital rectal examination (DRE) to identify any enlargement of the lateral lobes or nodular lumps on the surface of the prostate gland. Diagnostic tests ordered to learn more about the client's condition may include a prostate-specific antigen (PSA), blood test, post-void bladder scan, cystoscopy, rectal ultrasonography, and prostate biopsy. The physician will carefully monitor the client's condition to detect any exacerbation of symptoms such as increased hesitancy, urgency, hematuria, or repeated UTI.

Many alternatives to surgical treatment of BPH have been introduced over the past several years, including balloon dilation of the prostate, a prostate urethral **stent**, as shown in Figure 13-9, and thermotherapy. Balloon dilation of the prostate during an endoscopic examination breaks the prostatic capsule and facilitates decompression of the prostate. A stent is material that is used to hold tissue in place or, in this instance, to provide support to the urethra, which is being compressed by the prostate. An alternative to a transurethral resection of the prostate (TURP) is a thermotherapy transurethral microwave procedure (TUMP) (Daniels, Nosek, & Nicoll, 2007). This outpatient procedure does not correct the problem of incomplete bladder emptying, but does reduce urinary flow symptoms. Another minimally invasive procedure is the transurethral needle ablation (TUNA) system that delivers low-level radiofrequency energy via twin needles to burn away enlarged prostate tissue and improve urine flow with fewer side effects than the TURP (NIH, 2006).

Surgical

The traditional surgical intervention for 90% of all prostate surgeries for BPH is a TURP. This surgery is performed via a resectoscope, an instrument that includes a cutting and cauterization device (Figure 13-10). The client receives either a general or a spinal anesthetic, and the resectoscope is passed through the urethra to remove small pieces of prostate tissue while controlling bleeding. The bladder is continuously irrigated with normal saline or another solution during the procedure. This irrigation is continued during the postoperative period to reduce clot formation that can interfere with urinary drainage.

The traditional surgical alternative to a TURP is open surgery. A suprapubic resection (Figure 13-11), in which the prostate is removed from around the urethra via the bladder, is performed when the prostate mass is large. In a retropubic prostatectomy, the bladder is not opened but instead is retracted and prostatic tissue is removed through an incision in the anterior prostatic capsule. Both of these alternatives involve an abdominal incision. In a perineal prostatectomy, a perineal incision is made and the prostatic tissue is removed through an incision in the posterior prostatic capsule.

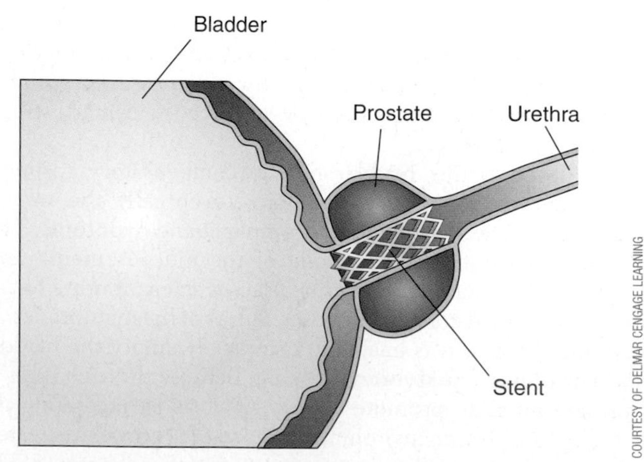

FIGURE 13-9 Urethral Stent

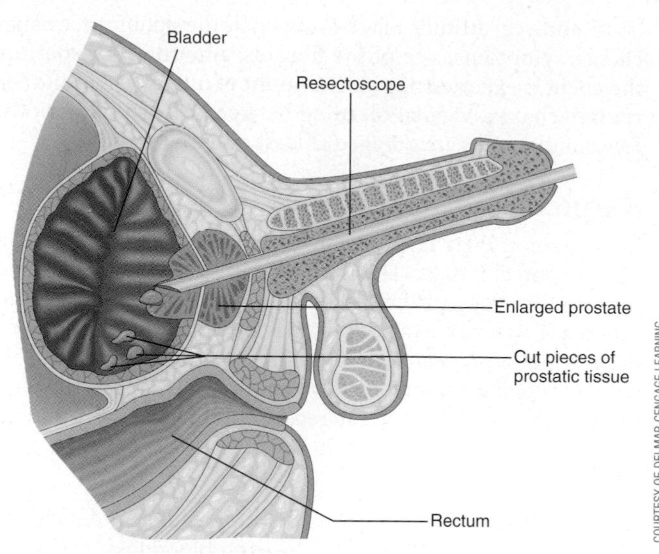

FIGURE 13-10 Transurethral Resection of the Prostate Gland via Resectoscope

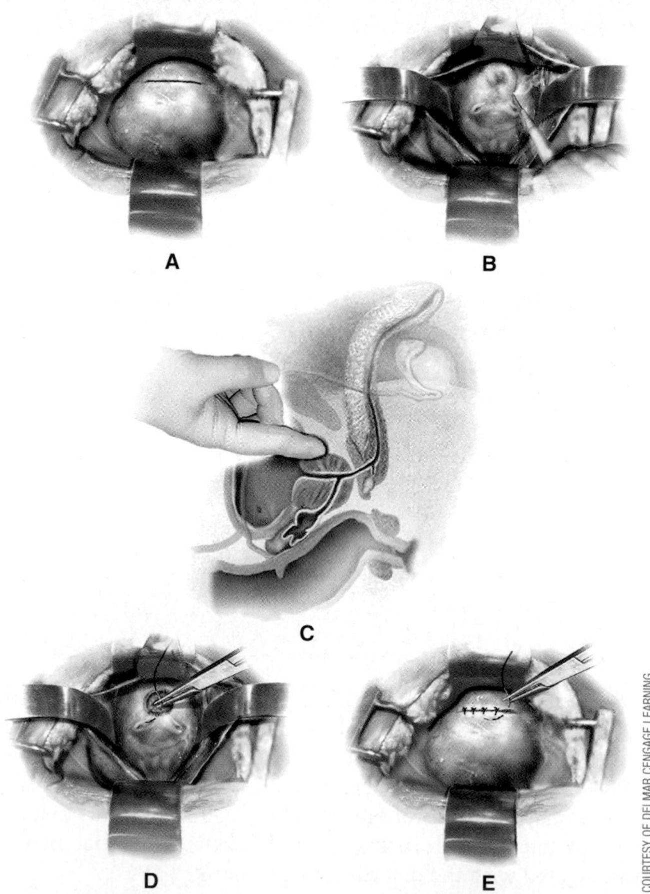

FIGURE 13-11 Suprapubic Prostatectomy; *A*, Bladder Exposed through Low Transverse Incision; *B*, Bladder Entered; *C*, Blunt Dissection of Prostate; *D*, Prostate Fossa Sutured to Bladder Mucosa

Although these traditional surgeries successfully relieve bladder obstruction, they are costly, and postoperative complications can endanger or seriously affect the quality of a man's life. These complications include hemorrhage, water intoxication, infection, thrombosis, damage to surrounding structures, sexual dysfunction, and urinary incontinence.

Laser prostatectomy is based on thermal action. The transurethral ultrasound-guided laser-induced prostatectomy (TULIP) is performed with a probe that is passed transurethrally into the prostatic urethra. While the adjacent prostate area is visualized by ultrasound, the laser energy is directed at the prostate tissue, resulting in tissue necrosis and sloughing. The client is less likely to experience water intoxication because this surgical method allows blood vessels to seal rapidly, keeping irrigant fluid from being forced into the circulation.

Pharmacological

Finasteride (Proscar) can shrink the prostate in some men. Alpha blockers relax the smooth muscles along the urinary tract without compromising normal urinary control reflexes. Examples are terazosin hydrochloride (Hytrin), doxazosin mesylate (Cardura), alfuzosin (Uroxatral), and tamsulosin Hcl (Flomax). They are also used to treat hypertension, so the side effect of orthostatic hypotension is possible. Belladonna and opium (B & O) suppositories are used to reduce postoperative bladder spasms, and narcotic analgesics are used to relieve postoperative pain.

NURSING MANAGEMENT

When inserting a Foley catheter, remove no more than 1,000 mL initially. Provide preoperative care as ordered. Monitor and accurately record I&O to prevent water intoxication; monitor vital signs and color of urine. Provide routine postoperative care. After catheter removal, encourage client to void with the first urge to prevent increased bladder pressure.

NURSING PROCESS

ASSESSMENT

Subjective Data

Ask the client about the presence of urinary frequency, hesitancy, dribbling, number of times he gets up at night to void, and the force of the urinary stream. In addition to a careful general medical history, any information pertaining to a history of chronic urinary tract infections needs to be noted.

Postoperative nursing assessment includes assessing for pain (on a 0 to 10 scale) related to bladder spasms. The client's emotional needs should also be assessed, especially for anticipatory grieving, body image disturbance, anxiety, incontinence, or concerns about alteration in sexuality patterns or possible sexual dysfunction. Observe for client behavioral or verbal cues indicating a need for further information or reassurance about his condition and treatment.

Objective Data

Monitor vital signs but *avoid* the use of a rectal thermometer. A bright red urine color persisting for more than a few hours after surgery may be a sign of hemorrhage. Report hemorrhage, hyperthermia, hypotension (low blood pressure), and tachycardia to the physician immediately.

After a TURP, the client will have a three-way Foley catheter and continuous bladder irrigation for at least 24 hours. Accurately record I&O to ensure that the client has adequate oral intake to promote urinary flow and reduce the infection risk. *In measuring output, the amount of irrigant must be subtracted from the total output in order to determine the actual urinary output.* After the catheter is removed, assess the client for postvoid residual and incontinence. Palpate the abdomen for bladder distention, check the bed linens and clothing for signs of incontinence, and ask the client if he is experiencing loss of urinary control.

Assess for water intoxication, which may be the result of absorbing irrigating fluid in addition to the IV fluids. The most common early symptoms of water intoxication are changes in the client's mental status. These may be manifested by agitation, confusion, and, later, convulsions. The client may also have a slow bounding pulse with an increase in systolic and decrease in diastolic blood pressure.

A suprapubic or retropubic prostatectomy does not require a three-way Foley. Instead, the client will have a urethral catheter, a tissue drain from the prostatic fossa, and an abdominal dressing. Assess for incisional pain and do a dressing check. Especially check the linens underneath the client's back for drainage.

Nursing diagnoses for a postoperative client having a TURP for benign prostatic hyperplasia include the following:

NURSING DIAGNOSES	PLANNING/OUTCOMES	NURSING INTERVENTIONS
*Acute **Pain*** related to bladder spasms or incision	The client will state that pain has decreased.	Assess for pain using a pain scale every 2 to 4 hours. Maintain traction on the urethral catheter by anchoring the catheter to the leg with tape, ensuring that accidental additional traction will not occur with leg movement. Monitor for signs of bladder spasm pain such as facial grimacing, nonflow of irrigating solution into bladder, and urinating around the catheter. Administer analgesics and antispasmodics as ordered. Teach deep breathing, relaxation techniques.

(Continues)

Nursing diagnoses for a postoperative client having a TURP for benign prostatic hyperplasia include the following: (Continued)

NURSING DIAGNOSES	PLANNING/OUTCOMES	NURSING INTERVENTIONS
Risk for Imbalanced Fluid Volume related to postoperative irrigation	The client will not experience water intoxication.	Accurately record I&O including irrigation fluid. Monitor for changes in the client's behavior, especially confusion and agitation, which may be the first signs of cerebral edema. Monitor for hypertension, bradycardia, weakness, and seizures.
Stress or Urge Urinary Incontinence related to poor sphincter control after catheter removal after surgery	The client will achieve urinary control after removal of the catheter.	Educate the client that temporary urinary incontinence frequently occurs after surgery, and reassure him that this is normal. Teach the client perineal exercises that will help him regain urinary control. These exercises consist of tightening and relaxing gluteal muscles and are to be used each time the client urinates.
Sexual Dysfunction related to surgery	The client will regain sexual function postoperatively.	Monitor client's statements to determine if he has any misunderstanding of the surgery and sexual function. Instruct client to avoid sexual intercourse until physician approval is given and that it may take time for his previous level of sexual function to return. Encourage client to use a variety of forms of sexual expression, such as kissing, stroking, and cuddling. Provide client with opportunities to voice his feelings and ask questions. Teach client that it is normal and not harmful if his urine has a milky appearance due to retrograde ejaculation.

Evaluation: Evaluate each outcome to determine how it has been met by the client.

MALIGNANT NEOPLASM

Malignant neoplasms include breast, cervical, endometrial, ovarian, prostate, testicular, and penile cancers.

BREAST CANCER

Breast cancer is the second major cause of cancer death among women. Statistics indicate that 1 woman in 8 will develop breast cancer some time during her life. The American Cancer Society (ACS) estimates that 192,370 new cases were diagnosed in the United States in 2009. The 5-year survival rate is 98% for localized stage and 89% for all stages combined (ACS, 2008). Older adult women (older than 61) have twice the incidence of breast cancer as do younger women. Less than 1% of all breast cancers occur in men; in 2008, approximately 1,990 new cases of breast cancer were diagnosed in men (ACS, 2008).

The key to cure is early detection by physical examination, mammography, and BSE. A new painless mass or lump is the most common presenting symptom.

Because it is so uncommon, breast cancer in men is all the more dangerous. Late diagnosis is quite common; therefore, males need to be educated in the technique of and encouraged to perform BSE. Signs and symptoms of breast cancer include breast masses, lumps, thickening, and generalized swelling of part of a breast; skin dimpling, redness, scaliness, and irritation; nipple pain, retraction (Figure 13-12), or discharge other than breast milk.

Women at greatest risk for developing breast cancer are those who:

- Had a mother or sibling with breast cancer
- Never had children or had their first child after the age of 30
- Never breast-fed
- Have a history of fibrocystic breast changes
- Started menstruating before age 10
- Are obese
- Consume a high-fat diet and a moderate amount of alcohol

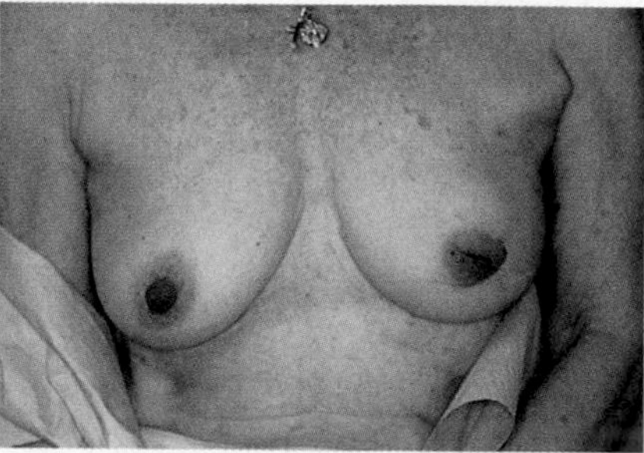

FIGURE 13-12 **Nipple Retraction of Left Breast** (*Courtesy of Steven M. Lynch, MD.*)

- Smoke
- Experienced a late menopause
- Are physically inactive
- Take postmenopausal hormone therapy
- Have had previous chest radiation to treat different cancer

A woman generally presents at the health-care office after the discovery of a lump in her breast. If she has been performing BE routinely each month, she is likely to be familiar with even minute changes in her breast tissue. Breast cancers often occur in the upper, outer quadrant of the breast and may extend into the tail of the breast and spread upward into the axilla (Figure 13-13). It is important to teach clients to examine the axillary region as well as the breast during BSE (Figure 13-8).

Women also seek medical advice because they notice a discharge from the breast, dimpling of the skin, retraction of the nipple, pain, a unilateral change in breast size, or an orange-peel appearance (peau d'orange) of the skin (Figure 13-14). Dimpling and puckering are usually associated with the breast tissue or tumor attaching to the skin or the underlying muscle mass, which does not permit movement. The nurse should not be misled by the client's report of a tender lump or mass and assume it is fibrocystic breast changes. All new or enlarged lumps or masses in the breast require immediate assessment.

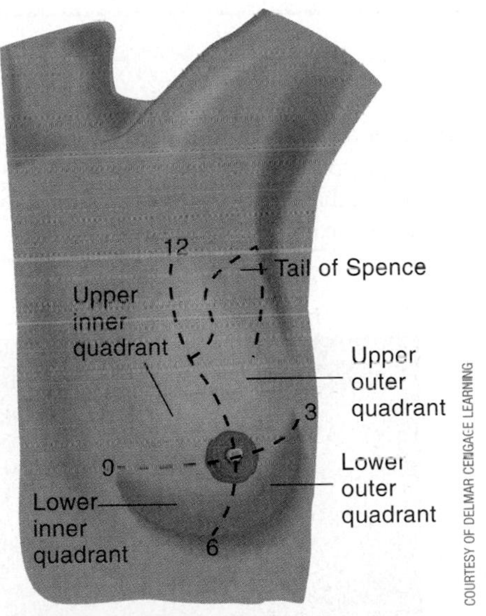

FIGURE 13-13 Quadrants of the Left Breast

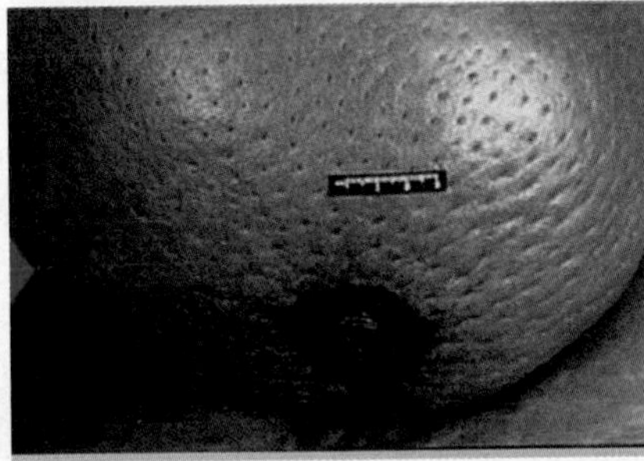

FIGURE 13-14 Peau d' Orange (*Courtesy of Dr. S. Eva Singletary, University of Texas, M.D. Anderson Cancer Center.*)

MEMORYTRICK

Staging Breast Cancer

Using a staging system provides a standardized method for health care providers to summarize how far the breast cancer has spread. The most common system used is the American Joint Committee on Cancer's **TNM** system. This staging system classifies cancers based on their **T**, **N**, and **M** stages:

T = Tumor (the size and how far has it spread within the breast and to nearby organs)

N = Nodes (spread to lymph nodes)

M = Metastasis (spread to distant organs)

(American Cancer Society, 2009b)

The presence of tiny, palpable clusters of calcium, or "microclusters," may be an early sign of breast cancer. These should be followed closely with mammography every 6 to 12 months to detect subtle changes in shape or size.

The American Cancer Society (2009) recommends that women ages 20 to 39 perform BSE each month and have a clinical breast examination every 3 years. For women age 40 and older, BSE should be performed monthly, a clinical examination every year, and a mammogram every year.

Mammography may be performed by the stereotactic computer-guided technique. This advanced method allows needle biopsies to be taken at the same time if necessary. The physician or nurse practitioner may recommend this method after an initial mammogram has shown suspicious areas. This technique is less costly than excisional biopsy and can be performed with little discomfort to the client. The client is placed in a prone position on the special examination table with the breast hanging down through the opening in the table. The operator moves the position of the table to visualize the entire breast area via computerized guidance.

After the breast has been biopsied and the tissue has been examined by the pathologist, if a malignancy is confirmed, the client may be advised to proceed with surgical removal (lumpectomy or mastectomy) of the affected tissue. Figure 13-15 shows the staging of breast cancer.

MEDICAL–SURGICAL MANAGEMENT

Medical

Radiation and chemotherapy are used as adjuvant therapy, but surgery is the primary treatment. Other types of treatment for breast cancer include targeted therapy, immunotherapy, photodynamic therapy, gene therapy, hyperthermia, and antiangiogenesis therapy. For more information about these treatments go to the American Cancer Society website at www.cancer.org.

Surgical

There is an abundance of lymphatic vessels proximal to the breast. Malignant cells can thus escape into the general lymphatic

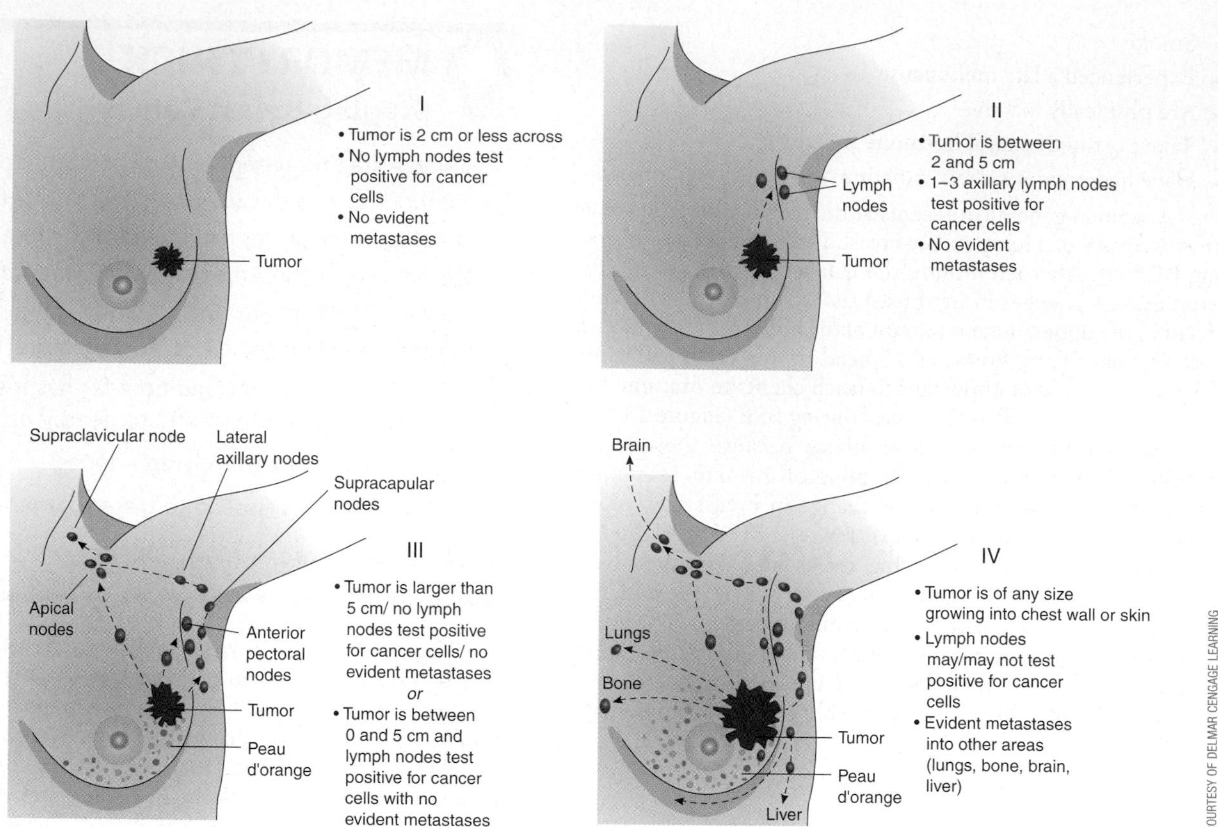

FIGURE 13-15 Breast Cancer Staging

system and be spread throughout the body. A lumpectomy is surgical removal of the cancerous mass. A simple mastectomy removes the tumor mass and only a small portion of the adjacent tissue. In the modified mastectomy, the entire breast tissue and nearby lymph nodes are removed; the muscles of the chest wall are left relatively intact (Figure 13-16A). With the radical mastectomy, the entire breast, lymph nodes, and underlying pectoralis muscle are removed (Figure 13-16B). Figure 13-17 shows the various options in the surgical management of breast cancer. The greater the extent of the surgical removal, the longer the client's recovery process and the greater the need for rehabilitation in using the upper extremity on the affected side.

The more lymph nodes that are removed, the greater the chance the client will have lymphedema, an accumulation of lymph in soft tissue. An elastic sleeve may be worn for compression, and range-of-motion (ROM) exercises may reduce edema. A sodium-restricted diet may be ordered.

Reconstructive surgery after a mastectomy may be determined by the amount of breast tissue and muscle remaining after the initial procedure, the position of the mastectomy scar, and the probability of recurrent breast cancer. Breast reconstruction can help the client deal with the disfigurement that results from the mastectomy.

The client's desire for reconstruction and her psychological status play an important role in determining the personal value of additional surgery. In the United States particularly, the breast is associated with childbearing and female sexuality. It may be difficult for the client to express her concerns to her partner regarding her sexuality and desirability after the mastectomy. She may have difficulty facing the physical alteration immediately after surgery and for some time after. The nurse with good interpersonal communication skills can help the client identify and verbalize her feelings of loss, thus promoting the psychological healing process and acceptance of altered body image.

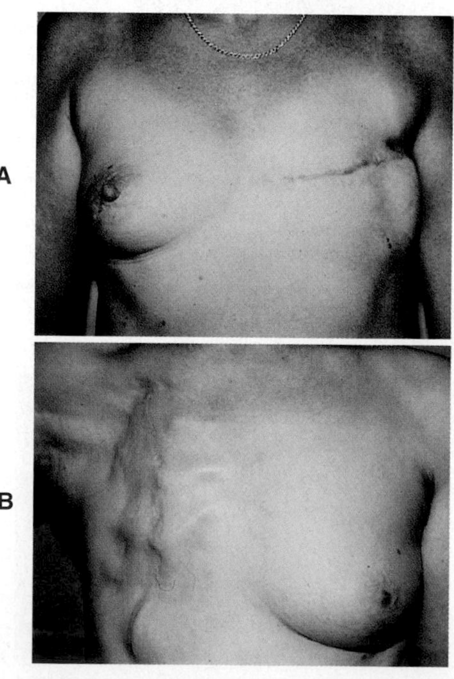

FIGURE 13-16 Mastectomy Clients; *A*, Modified Radical; *B*, Radical (*Courtesy of Steven M. Lynch, MD.*)

SAMPLE NURSING CARE PLAN (Continued)

NURSING DIAGNOSIS 3 *Acute **Pain***, related to surgical manipulation of tissues and excision of tissue as evidenced by client statement that she was glad she had the PCA pump to take care of the pain

Nursing Outcomes Classification (NOC)	Nursing Interventions Classification (NIC)
Symptom Severity	*Pain Management*
Pain Level	*Patient-Controlled Analgesia (PCA) Assistance*

PLANNING/OUTCOMES	NURSING INTERVENTIONS	RATIONALE
C.W. will verbalize that pain is controlled.	Assess C.W.'s pain level and response to analgesia every 2 hours.	Alerts the nurse to increasing pain and C.W.'s tolerance of the pain medication.
	Instruct C.W. how to use the PCA pump.	Allows C.W. control over analgesia and provides consistent pain relief.
	Evaluate the effectiveness of analgesia every 2 hours.	Allows the nurse to identify any untoward effects and effectiveness of the medication.
	Reposition C.W. every 2 hours.	Helps improve vascular flow and relieves pressure on bony prominences.
	Elevate the right arm on pillows.	Decreases edema and discomfort due to pressure on nerves in the area.

EVALUATION

C.W. reports pain is controlled at less than 2 on a 1 to 10 scale.

CERVICAL CANCER

An abnormal condition of the cervix known as dysplasia may be an early sign of developing cervical cancer. Dysplasia is a change in the size and shape of the cervical cells, and it is classified as mild, moderate, or severe. An abnormal Papanicolaou (Pap) smear may be the first indication of a problem.

Cervical cancer is the most preventable gynecological cancer. Sexual habits constitute a major factor in the development of cancer of the cervix. Sexually transmitted infection, particularly the human papillomavirus (HPV), is a particularly significant factor (ACS, 2009c). Other factors associated with cervical cancer include smoking, long-term use of oral contraceptives, immunosuppression, multiple pregnancies, family history, diet low in fruits and vegetables, obesity, a history of multiple sexual partners and maternal use of diethylstilbestrol (DES) during pregnancy. The most common sign of cervical cancer is abnormal bleeding, which progresses from a thin, watery, blood-tinged discharge to frank bleeding. Contact bleeding may also occur after intercourse. Advanced disease is indicated by odor, pain in the lower back and groin, difficulty in voiding, hematuria, and rectal bleeding. The Pap smear is the key to early detection. Promotion of regular pelvic exams and education regarding risk are essential.

Although cervical cancer can occur at any age, it occurs most frequently in women between 30 and 50 years of age. It is insidious because it is asymptomatic. Cervical cancer has a high cure rate in the early stages, and it is easily detected by the routine annual Pap smear. The overall 5-year survival rate is 74% (ACS, 2009c). The two main types of cervical cancer are squamous-cell carcinoma (80% to 90%) and adenocarcinoma (10% to 20%) (ACS, 2009c).

The nurse should immediately bring any abnormal Pap smear results to the attention of the physician or nurse practitioner so the client can be notified and the appropriate follow-up treatment initiated. A repeat Pap smear may be indicated after treatment with a vaginal antibiotic cream, or a colposcopy may be performed.

Staging of the cancer progresses from I to IV (Figure 13-19). Carcinoma *in situ* (CIS) means that the cancerous cells remain within the cervix and have not yet spread to adjacent areas. The greater the number on the staging table, the more the cancer has metastasized to other structures.

MEDICAL–SURGICAL MANAGEMENT

Surgical

Treatment modalities may include conization, a surgical excision of a cone-shaped section of the abnormal cervical tissues.

STAGING SYSTEM FOR CANCER OF THE CERVIX	
Stage	Characteristics
I	• Carcinoma is strictly confined to cervix (extension to corpus should be disregarded)
IA	• Preclinical carcinoma
IA1	• Minimal microscopically evident stromal invasion
IA2	• Microscopic lesions no more than 5 mm depth measured from base of epithelium surface or glandular from which it originates, and horizontal spread not to exceed 7 mm
IB	• All other cases of stage I; occult cancer should be marked "occ"
II	• Carcinoma extends beyond cervix but has not extended to pelvic wall; it involves vagina, but not as far as lower third
IIA	• No obvious parametrical involvement
IIB	• Obvious parametrical involvement
III	• Carcinoma has extended to pelvic wall; on rectal examination, there is no cancer-free space between tumor and pelvic wall; tumor involves lower third of vagina; all cases with hydronephrosis or nonfunctioning kidney should be included, unless they are known to be due to another cause
IIIA	• No extension to pelvic wall, but involvement of lower third of vagina
IIIB	• Extension to pelvic wall, or hydronephrosis or nonfunctioning kidney due to tumor
IV	• Carcinoma has extended beyond true pelvis or has clinically involved mucosa of bladder or rectum
IVA	• Spread of growth to adjacent pelvic organs
IVB	• Spread to distant organs (lungs, liver)

FIGURE 13-19 Cervical Cancer Screening

This procedure is desirable if the client is of childbearing age and wants children in the future.

Laser surgery, cryosurgery (freezing of the cells with liquid nitrogen), or cauterization (burning) may be performed as alternative methods of treatment if the cervical lesions are easily visible for the procedure. A total hysterectomy or radical pelvic surgery may be required to eradicate the cancer. If the spread of the disease has become too extensive, treatment will be directed toward palliative measures.

Other Therapies

The physician may recommend the use of radium implants or radiation therapy before the surgical excision of the cervix. The nurse must be cautious in providing nursing care for the client with radium implants. Pregnant nurses or female nurses of childbearing age should not care for this client or spend extended periods at the bedside. Direct client care should be organized to optimize time spent at the bedside. A sign should be hung on the door to indicate that radiation is being used in the room and provide a warning for visitors to limit their visit time. With the implants in place, the client will remain on complete bed rest.

In addition, chemotherapy may be utilized as an adjunct therapy to help shrink the tumor or slow its growth.

Nursing Management

Provide therapeutic emotional support to the client to help her cope with the diagnosis. After surgery, monitor vital signs and I&O. Encourage client to ambulate as ordered and to turn, cough, deep breathe, and use a spirometer. Assist with active and passive ROM exercises. Provide careful catheter care.

NURSING PROCESS

Assessment

Subjective Data

The client may describe postcoital bleeding (bleeding after intercourse) or spotting between menstrual periods or after menopause and, occasionally, a foul-smelling vaginal discharge. As the disease progresses, she may describe increased or bloody discharge, weight loss, and pain that radiates down the lower back and legs.

Objective Data

Objective data may include the presence and appearance of a vaginal discharge. The cervix may appear eroded or raw and may bleed easily when touched with a cotton-tipped applicator or Pap scraper. Necrotic tissue may be present and cause a foul odor. Pap smear results can indicate dyplasia. Tissue samples obtained through colposcopic examination may show cellular changes. In advanced disease, weight loss and anemia may be present. Laparotomy may be performed to stage the disease and along with other laboratory and diagnostic testing to identify metastases, which are most likely to occur in the rectum, vagina, bladder, and pelvis.

Nursing diagnoses for a client with cervical cancer include the following:

NURSING DIAGNOSES	PLANNING/OUTCOMES	NURSING INTERVENTIONS
Anxiety related to unknown outcome and possible treatments	The client will verbalize having less anxiety about treatment and possible outcome.	Be aware of the client's emotional state throughout the course of care and use effective interpersonal communication to facilitate the client's acceptance of her condition and the treatments. Explain diagnostic tests and procedures to client to decrease her anxiety. Provide therapeutic emotional support to client to help her cope with feelings.
Sexual Dysfunction related to vaginal bleeding, discomfort, and procedures	The client will return to normal sexual function after recovery from treatment for cervical cancer.	Inform client that she may experience dyspareunia related to vaginal dryness after radiation therapy. Instruct client to use a water-soluble lubricant during intercourse or to use lubricated condoms to decrease irritation. Listen to client's concerns.
Impaired Urinary Elimination related to sensory motor impairment from radiation effects	The client will regain normal urinary elimination.	Assess the function of the Foley catheter to ensure patency and drainage. Provide careful catheter care. Promote urination when catheter is removed. Record I&O, including color of urine. Encourage the client to drink fluids to flush the kidneys and decrease risk of UTI.

Evaluation: Evaluate each outcome to determine how it has been met by the client.

ENDOMETRIAL CANCER

Postmenopausal women are at the greatest risk for endometrial cancer, especially if they have taken estrogen replacement therapy for several years (usually more than 5 years). Research has shown that unopposed estrogen stimulation of the endometrial lining has a strong relationship with the development of endometrial cancer. During the normal menstrual cycle, estrogen and progesterone rise and fall. These hormonal fluctuations affect the stimulation of the endometrial tissue to grow and be sloughed off. Without the progesterone effects, the endometrial tissue is not sloughed off at regular intervals and may undergo cellular changes, leading to a high risk for endometrial dysplasia or cancer. For this reason, many physicians and nurse practitioners have recommended estrogen-progesterone therapy for clients who experience menopausal symptoms.

In summer 2002, the data and safety monitoring board for the Women's Health Initiative study of estrogen/progestin recommended stopping the trial because of an increased risk of invasive breast cancer (Fletcher & Colditz, 2002). It is recommended that long-term use of this combination be stopped.

Other risk factors associated with endometrial cancer may include never having borne a child, being Caucasian, being middle class, never having had sexual intercourse, use of oral contraceptives, total number of menstrual cycles, use of tamoxifen, obesity, diabetes, and family history.

Cancer of the endometrium usually does not produce symptoms until it becomes relatively advanced. Routine Pap smear and pelvic examinations are inadequate for early diagnosis. An endometrial biopsy, which examines the tissue from the uterine lining under a microscope, is the best diagnostic tool to identify cellular changes. This may be done on an annual basis when the client has a routine examination. The medical follow-up treatment plan depends on the biopsy results. D&C has a potential for spreading the cancer cells to adjacent tissues because the malignant cells may escape into the bloodstream at the time of the procedure. This is not usually a problem with the biopsy because the amount of tissue removed is so small and blood loss is minimal. A D&C is also more expensive, higher risk, and requires some type of anesthesia.

MEDICAL–SURGICAL MANAGEMENT

Treatments for endometrial cancer may range from radiation, radium implants, chemotherapy, or surgery to a combination of any of the above. The choices of treatment are related to the staging of the cancer.

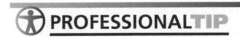

Radiation Exposure Risk

Because of the risk of radiation exposure to the caregiver from the radiation implant device, keep procedures that require exposure to the client's perineal area at a minimum.

Medical

Intravenous fluid administration will be implemented to replace fluids lost by the excessive bleeding. A blood transfusion may be ordered for a low hemoglobin. A hemoglobin above 10 gm/dL is preferred before surgical intervention. The physician may order whole blood or packed red blood cells to increase the hemoglobin rapidly.

Surgical

Surgery for endometrial or cervical cancer includes hysterectomy. A total hysterectomy is removal of the cervix and the uterus. In a subtotal hysterectomy, only the uterus is removed and the cervix remains. A radical or pan hysterectomy includes removal of the ovaries, cervix, uterus, fallopian tubes, pelvic lymph nodes, and part of the vagina. Vaginal hysterectomy procedures have been refined with the laparoscopic approach so that many clients are released from the hospital within 24 to 36 hours postoperatively. If the cancer has spread beyond the uterus into the pelvic region, an abdominal hysterectomy may be the best approach for visualization during surgery. The physician may recommend a course of radiation therapy after surgery.

Pharmacological

Drug therapy includes the use of the chemotherapy agents doxorubicin (Adriamycin), cisplatin, carboplatin, and paclitaxel (Taxol). Two or more drugs may be combined for treatment such as cisplatin and doxorubicin. Side effects of chemotherapy depend on the drug taken, the amount, and the length of time the client has been taking the drug.

Other Therapies

There is a tendency for endometrial cancer to confine itself to the uterus, which increases the client's 5-year survival prognosis. Endometrial cancer also usually responds well to the therapies available at this time, including radiation. Radiation may be delivered to the pelvic region via external sources, or it may be delivered via intracavitary devices or implants with radium or cesium. There is a potential danger for injury to adjacent pelvic structures during radiation therapy. The nurse should be alert for signs of complications, such as bleeding from the rectum, moderate to severe abdominal pain, constipation, or diarrhea.

Nursing Management

One of the earliest symptoms reported by many clients is vaginal bleeding. For the postmenopausal client, it is imperative that all bleeding be investigated immediately unless it is from hormonally induced periods. Late in the progression of the cancer, the client may experience symptoms similar to those discussed with cervical cancer. Pain is often associated with the spread of cancer to adjacent organs and is considered a late sign.

Objective data may be collected from the client's physical exam findings, biopsy reports, and a history of hormone replacement therapy with or without the estrogen-progesterone combination.

OVARIAN CANCER

Ovarian cancer most often originates in the epithelial tissue of the ovary, and, like cervical and endometrial cancer, does not produce symptoms until it is in an advanced, inoperable stage. It is sometimes called "the silent killer." Its symptoms are vague and may be ignored for a long time before the client seeks medical attention. According to Lehman (2007), the first national consensus statement on ovarian cancer symptoms was issued and recognizes that the symptoms of bloating, abdominal or pelvic pain, difficult eating, feeling full quickly, and urinary urgency or frequency are more likely to occur in woman with ovarian cancer than women in the general population (Lehman, 2007).

Ovarian cancer causes more deaths than does any other gynecological cancer, an estimated 14,600 in 2009 (ACS, 2009d; Lehman, 2007). The incidence is greatest in women between 45 and 65 years of age. Nulliparity (never having borne a child), smoking, alcohol use, infertility, and a high-fat diet are factors that place the client at higher risk for developing ovarian cancer. Metastasis occurs in more than 75% of cases before diagnosis, and often the cancer has spread beyond the pelvis. The colon is the most frequent site of ovarian cancer metastasis, then the stomach, and diaphragm.

Unfortunately, medical research has not yet developed an early diagnostic or screening tool to detect ovarian cancer. It is believed, however, that there is an increased risk of ovarian cancer for clients with breast cancer and vice versa. A family history of two or more female relatives with breast or ovarian cancer provides a sound rationale for more frequent breast and pelvic examinations. Often, the physician or NP palpates an ovarian mass on a routine bimanual examination. This finding is cause for further investigation by pelvic ultrasound or CT scan to determine the size, character, and consistency (solid or fluid-filled) of the mass and whether other pelvic structures are involved. Some experts believe that there is a link between the occurrence of ovarian cysts and the development of ovarian cancers in certain women.

General diagnostic studies, such as a lower GI series, chest x-ray, intravenous pyelogram (IVP), transvaginal ultrasound, and laparoscopy may be useful in determining the extent of the primary and secondary lesions. A blood test, CA-125 assay, measures a tumor marker CA-125 that is often higher than normal in women with ovarian cancer (Lehman, 2007). If the client develops peritoneal fluid or ascites as the cancer progresses, it may be removed by paracentesis for cytologic examination.

Recurrent disease is common and may occur in 2 years or less. Continued medical surveillance is recommended every 2 months for a period of 2 years for the earliest possible detection of new lesions. The 5-year survival rate is 45% (ACS, 2009d).

Medical–Surgical Management

Surgical

Surgical excision of the ovary is rarely successful because of the extensiveness of the disease. A total abdominal hysterectomy with a bilateral salpingo-oophorectomy or omentectomy is performed for most stages of the disease. Most often, a combination of radiation, chemotherapy, immunotherapy, and surgery produces the best results, even if they are only palliative for the client. The client must be actively involved and informed of her treatment options as well as her prognosis to enable her to make sound choices in the treatments chosen.

Pharmacological

Chemotherapy drugs that are used with ovarian cancer treatment include cyclophosphamide (Cytoxan), doxorubicin hydrochloride (Adriamycin), mitomycin (Mutamycin), cisplatin (Platinol), paclitaxel (Taxol) and carboplatin. For intravenous chemotherapy, carboplatin is preferred over cisplatin due to being as effective and having less side effects (ACS, 2009d). In 2006, the National Cancer Institute encouraged physicians to use a combined approach of intraperitoneal (IP) chemotherapy in addition to intravenous chemotherapy (Lehman, 2007). Intraperitoneal chemotherapy administers paclitaxel (Taxol) or cisplatin (Platinol) directly into the client's abdominal cavity. This technique can add a year to the lives of women with advanced stages of ovarian cancer. Combination chemotherapy is the standard approach for treatment of ovarian cancer. These may be administered by regional or intraarterial perfusion techniques. These percutaneous modes direct the drugs to the lesion's vascular supply. If the cancer has not metastasized, a regimen of chemotherapy using a single drug, such as Cytoxan, may be administered over the course of 5 days and repeated again at regular intervals over the course of a year. A combination of the chemotherapy agents, used in a rotating series, is often more effective for reproductive cancers in advanced stages. For example, the client would receive one drug over the course of 5 days, then switch to another drug for 5 days, and then a third drug for 5 days. This series may be repeated over the year in a similar pattern to that used with a single agent.

Sometimes two or three different medications are necessary to achieve pain control. Intravenous medications are often given by a PCA pump with continuous low-dose narcotics. This method seems more effective for the client than IV bolus doses every 4 hours. Medications may also be given slow IV push (an RN procedure), orally in tablets or liquids, intramuscularly, or by transdermal patches (Duragesic). A liquid mixture of syrup, cocaine, morphine, alcohol, flavoring, and water called "Brompton's mixture, elixir, or cocktail" may be ordered. The client may drink up to 20 mL every 3 to 4 hours for pain relief. Most of these methods of narcotic administration are equally effective and may be used in the home care or hospice setting. Other types of medication that may be given include tranquilizers, antiemetics, and laxatives.

NURSING MANAGEMENT

Accurately measure the client's legs to ensure the proper fit of antiembolic stockings. Provide comfort measures of back rub and position change. Teach client about skin care if receiving radiation. Assess bowel sounds and for abdominal distention. Maintain an accurate I&O record.

NURSING PROCESS

ASSESSMENT

Subjective Data

The client may describe fatigue, malaise, diarrhea or constipation, pelvic pressure, frequency of urination, loss of appetite, nausea, weight gain or loss, vaginal bleeding or spotting with intercourse, a foul-smelling vaginal discharge, and pain in the lower back. The list of symptoms is very vague and could be related to many reproductive and nonreproductive disorders.

Objective Data

Objective data pertinent to all cancers of the pelvic reproductive organs may include information from the client's previous health history, reproductive history (onset of menses, pregnancies, contraceptive methods, infections, hormonal replacement therapy, and surgeries), the discovery of a palpable mass during a bimanual examination, an abnormal appearance of the cervix or adjacent tissues, abnormal Pap smear results greater than Class II dysplasia, abnormal cervical or endometrial biopsies, increased abdominal girth, or the presence of ascites and pleural effusion.

Diagnostic tests and laboratory studies may include all or some of the following: Pap smear, pelvic ultrasound, chest x-ray, IVP, kidney/ureters/bladder x-ray (KUB), CBC with differential, blood chemistry studies, bleeding and clotting time, endometrial biopsy, cervical biopsy, D&C tissue specimens, Schiller's test and colposcopy, laparoscopy, barium enema, and bone scan.

Nursing diagnoses for a client with endometrial or ovarian cancer include the following:

NURSING DIAGNOSES	PLANNING/OUTCOMES	NURSING INTERVENTIONS
Preoperative:		
Fear related to tentative diagnoses, pending surgical procedures, cancer treatment and its side effects, incapacitating or extended illness with resulting dependence, and possible death	The client will verbalize fears and have behaviors consistent with reduced fear before and after surgery.	Facilitate client's expression of fear by encouraging the client's open discussion of her concerns. Be alert for nonverbal cues as well. Arrange a consultation with a social worker or chaplain, if appropriate.
Chronic ***Pain*** related to the spread of cancer throughout the pelvis and adjacent structures	The client will have pain controlled at a level that allows continual functioning in her activities of daily living as long as possible.	Administer analgesics as ordered. Provide comfort measures, such as position changes and back rub.

(*Continues*)

Nursing diagnoses for a client with endometrial or ovarian cancer include the following: (Continued)

NURSING DIAGNOSES	PLANNING/OUTCOMES	NURSING INTERVENTIONS
Postoperative:		
*Impaired **S**kin Integrity* related to surgical interventions, radiation, and chemotherapy side effects	The client's skin integrity will be maintained.	Provide client with proper skin-care instructions during and after radiation therapy that may include avoiding soaps, creams, powder, deodorants, and other substances around the incision that may irritate the skin; not washing off the radiation markings; and avoiding tight clothing around the area. Teach client to look for signs of reactions to radiation therapy, such as tenderness, flushed color (like a sunburn), delayed wound healing, and itching. Perform daily cleansing of the incisional area with water only. If client is on complete bed rest due to radium implant therapy, provide a complete bedbath as well as morning and bedtime skin care. Organize time near the client's bedside to brief periods to avoid overexposure to radiation. Wear rubber gloves when disposing of soiled materials. Put soiled dressings in a biohazard waste container.
*Impaired **U**rinary Elimination, **B**owel Incontinence, or **C**onstipation* related to the proximity of surgical site to bowel and bladder, spread of cancer to adjacent structures, manipulation of organs during surgery, administration of narcotic analgesics, lack of activity, and changes in dietary intake	The client will have adequate bowel and bladder function during the postoperative period.	Explain dietary modifications designed to reduce residue. The diet should be limited in dairy products, raw fruits, grains, and vegetables. Meats must be well cooked and possibly ground. If client is not receiving radium implant therapy, weigh her daily on the same scale at the same time of the day. Review client's normal elimination patterns from the baseline assessment data to help identify early changes in bowel or bladder elimination. Forewarn client of radiation enteritis and cystitis, and common tissue responses to radiation therapy. Instruct her to report symptoms, such as diarrhea, cramping, frequency, urgency, and dysuria. Assess bowel sounds and abdominal distention at least every 4 to 8 hours. Carefully monitor the client's urinary pattern and maintain an accurate intake and output record. Observe urine and stool for color, consistency, amount, and the presence of blood. Monitor client for other gastrointestinal problems, such as nausea, vomiting, and **tenesmus** (spasmodic contraction of the anal or bladder sphincter, causing pain and a persistent urge to empty the bowel or bladder).
*Impaired Physical **M**obility* related to intracavity radiation	The client will not develop deep vein thrombosis.	Accurately measure client's legs to ensure the proper fit of the hose. Apply thigh-high antiembolic stockings (TEDS) as ordered. Assist client to ambulate when allowed.

Evaluation: Evaluate each outcome to determine how it has been met by the client.

PROSTATE CANCER

Prostate cancer is the second leading cause of cancer deaths in men. According to 2009 estimates by the ACS, 192,280 new cases were diagnosed. Survival rate for all cases is nearly 100%. Incidence increases with age, as 70% of all prostate cancers are diagnosed in men older than age 65. Improved detection methods have greatly increased the number of individuals having positive outcomes. Diagnostic tests that may be performed are measurement of serum prostate-specific antigen (PSA), transrectal ultrasonic examination, DRE, and prostatic biopsy. Studies indicate that the PSA alone for routine screening is not especially useful. The American Cancer Society (2009f) recommends a yearly PSA level and digital rectal examination to screen for prostate cancer in men age 50 and older with a life expectancy of more than 10 years.

Most prostatic cancers are adenocarcinomas, slow-growing tumors that spread through the lymphatics. Early symptoms include dysuria, a weak urinary stream, and increased urinary frequency. Later symptoms are related to complete urethral obstruction or hematuria. Blood in the urine (**hematuria**), which can lead to anemia, occurs because of the rupture of blood vessels that have been overstretched.

MEDICAL–SURGICAL MANAGEMENT

Treatment depends on the extent of the disease and the age of the client.

Medical

Radiation is the traditional alternative to surgical removal of the malignant prostate gland; however, radiation may fail to eradicate the tumor or may lead to diarrhea, bowel obstruction, lymphocele formation, edema of the extremities, pulmonary embolism, wound infections, infection, impotence, incontinence, or radiation cystitis. An alternate successful radiation treatment option for early-stage prostate cancer is transrectal assisted radioactive seed implant. With the use of ultrasound, the physician is able to precisely position the rice-sized radioactive seeds inside the malignant prostate gland.

Surgical

Surgical treatment of prostatic cancer involves removal of the entire prostate gland, including the capsule and adjacent tissue. The urethra is then anastomosed to the bladder neck. Sometimes the perineal approach is used, but the usual approach is retropubic prostatectomy. Since 2003, a newer approach is the robotic-assisted laparoscopic radical prostatectomy using a robotic interface called the "da Vinci" system. The surgeon sits at a panel controlling the robotic arms to perform the operation through small incisions in the client's abdomen. This method has shown less blood loss and shorter recovery time than the standard radical prostatectomy.

Because of the proximity of the bladder sphincters to the prostate gland, urinary incontinence may be a complication. Other complications include sexual dysfunction and the universal surgical risks of hemorrhage, infection, thrombosis, and strictures. Removal of the testes (**orchiectomy**) may also be done as a palliative measure to help eliminate the androgenic effect that promotes tumor growth.

Cryosurgery (freezing) was used in the 1960s but abandoned because of tissue sloughing and fistula development. With the advent of the transrectal ultrasound and the transurethral warming device, cryosurgery is again a viable alternative.

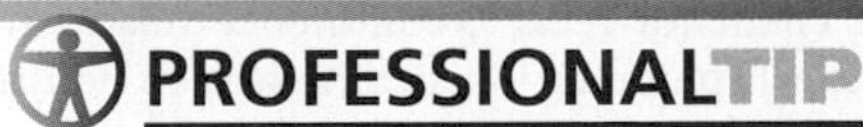

Risk Factors for Prostate Cancer

- Advancing age (more than 55 years)
- First-degree relative with prostate cancer
- African American heritage
- High level of serum testosterone (Estes, 2010)

The ultrasound allows the surgeon to selectively freeze prostate gland tissue while the temperature of the prostatic urethra is kept at 44°C by irrigation with heated water. This approach is an option for those who cannot tolerate more extensive surgery, have a localized tumor, or do not have successful radiation treatment. It can be performed more than once, involves a shorter hospital stay, and produces fewer side effects.

Pharmacological

Hormonal agents such as diethylstilbestrol (DES), luteinizing hormone releasing hormone agonist (LHRH) leuprolide acetate (Lupron), and nonsteroidal antiandrogens flutamide (Eulexin) may be used in the management of advanced prostate cancer. Chemotherapy drugs used to treat prostate cancer include paclitaxel (Taxol), carboplatin (Paraplatin), mitoxantrone (Novantrone), and vinblastine (Velban). A combination of prednisone and docetaxel (Taxotere) is used in clients with advanced prostate cancer.

NURSING MANAGEMENT

Encourage all male clients older than age 40 to have an annual rectal examination of the prostate and a PSA serum level. Monitor vital signs (*no rectal temperature*), urinary output, and fluid intake. Assess urine for signs of bleeding. Objectively assess for pain and administer analgesics as ordered. Keep perineal area clean and dry.

NURSING PROCESS

ASSESSMENT

Subjective Data

The client may seek care for BPH, which often accompanies cancer of the prostate. He may describe back pain or sciatica, frequency, dysuria, or nocturia.

Objective Data

Complete a physical assessment, including palpation of the abdomen and skin assessment. Palpate the abdomen to determine if there is any bladder distention. Skin assessment is important because the client is at risk for skin breakdown. There may or may not be hematuria present. Vital signs, the incisional site, and intake and output must all be assessed. Report hyperthermia, hypotension, tachycardia, or increased incisional drainage to the physician immediately.

A catheter is used postoperatively to maintain urinary drainage and as a splint for the urethral anastomosis rather than for hemostasis, so there are minimal bladder spasms. Monitor catheter patency by assessing the drainage for color, amount, and presence of clots. If the tubing is not draining freely, reposition or milk it. Call the physician if these measures fail to restore patency. During the first week of the postoperative period, monitor the client for fecal incontinence related to relaxation of the perineal sphincter. This complication occurs when the perineal surgical approach is used because the incision is made between the scrotum and the rectum.

Nursing diagnoses for a client (postoperative) with prostate cancer include the following:

NURSING DIAGNOSES	PLANNING/OUTCOMES	NURSING INTERVENTIONS
Urinary Retention related to urethral obstruction, secondary to urethral anastomosis.	The client will not experience urinary retention.	Monitor the client's urinary output, noting the amount, color, and presence of clots. The urine should not appear bright red for more than a few hours postoperatively, after which time it should be dark red. Reposition or milk the catheter tubing if not patent. If these interventions fail, notify the physician. Monitor the client's intake, encouraging a fluid intake of 2,500 to 3,000 mL/day.
Bowel Incontinence related to loss of rectal sphincter control becauseof perineal incision	The client will achieve rectal sphincter control.	Teach the client that temporary fecal incontinence frequently occurs after a perineal incision. Teach the client perineal exercises that will help him regain bowel control. Avoid the use of rectal thermometers, rectal examinations, and enemas.
Risk for Impaired Skin Integrity related to incontinence	The client will not experience skin breakdown.	Keep the client clean and dry, especially if he is experiencing fecal or urinary incontinence and reposition every 2 hours.

Evaluation: Evaluate each outcome to determine how it has been met by the client.

TESTICULAR CANCER

Although testicular cancer accounts for only 1% of all cancer in men, it is the most common cancer in young men between the ages of 15 and 35. According to the ACS (2009g), advances in treatment have made the 5-year survival rate 96%. The etiology is unknown, but the incidence is highest in men with undescended testicles and those whose mothers had taken hormones during pregnancy. A small, hard, painless lump is usually the first symptom noted.

Because early diagnosis of testicular cancer is so essential for a positive surgical outcome, men need to be taught how to perform a testicular self-examination (TSE) and be encouraged to routinely perform that examination (Figure 13-20).

TSE is performed as follows:

- Perform TSE after a bath or shower when scrotum is warm and most relaxed.
- Grasp testis with both hands and palpate gently between thumbs and forefingers.
- The testis should feel smooth, egg-shaped, and firm to the touch.
- The epididymis, located behind the testis, should feel like a soft tube.
- Any abnormal lumps or changes in the testes should be reported to a physician.

Medical–Surgical Management

Medical

Testicular ultrasound is used to study the testes for enlargement or lesions. In addition to a testicular ultrasound, the client may have a blood test for alpha-fetoprotein (AFP) and human chorionic gonadotropin (hCG). These proteins are called tumor markers, and when elevated levels are present in the blood it suggests testicular cancer.

Surgical

Biopsy of the testis is contraindicated because of the increased potential for metastases. Surgical removal of the testis, spermatic cord, and inguinal canal contents, with examination of the nodes, is indicated for testicular cancers. If unilateral removal of a testis is indicated, the remaining healthy testis will continue to maintain sperm and androgen production.

Pharmacological

Although chemotherapy and radiation are used as adjuvant treatments, radical inguinal orchiectomy remains the primary intervention. Combination chemotherapy with cisplatin (Platinol), vinblastine sulfate (Velban), and bleomycin sulfate (Blenoxane) is effective.

CRITICAL THINKING

Testicular Self-Examination

How would you teach a client to do a testicular self-examination? Make a teaching plan.

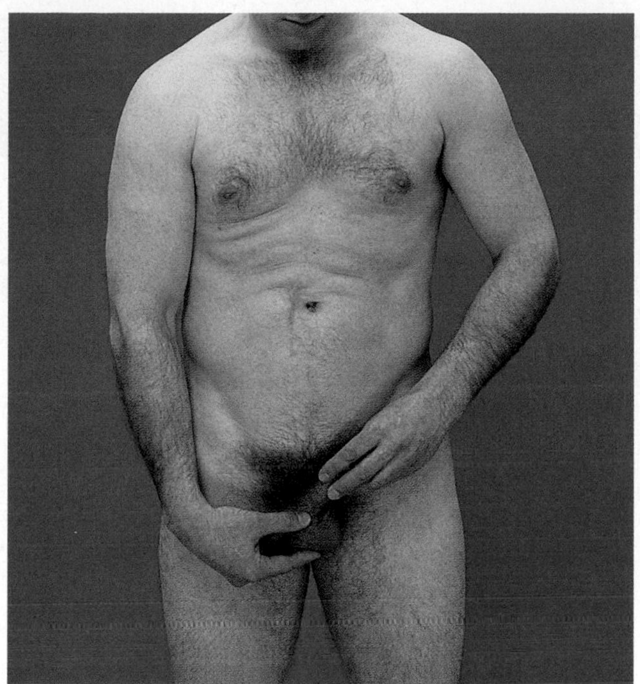

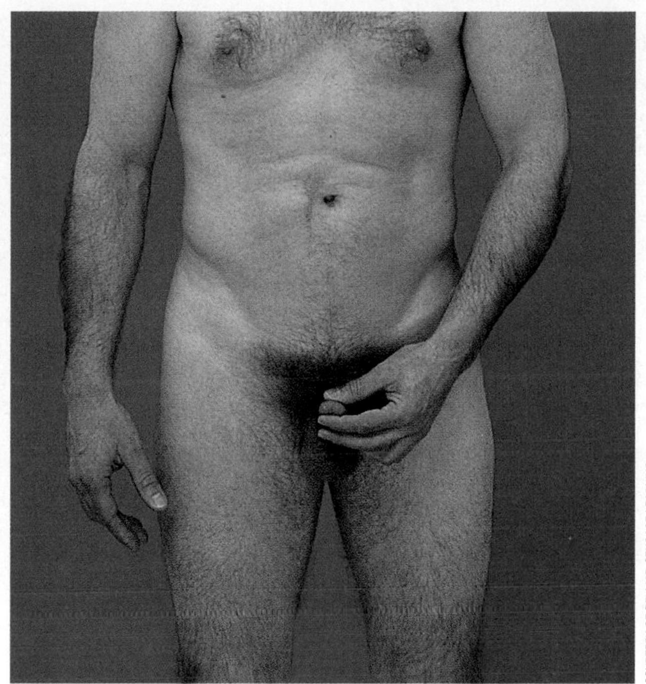

FIGURE 13-20 Performing a Testicular Self-Examination

NURSING MANAGEMENT

Encourage all male clients older than age 15 to perform testicular self-examination monthly. Cancer is suspected in a testicle that is hard. Postoperatively, monitor vital signs and incisional drainage. Maintain strict asepsis when changing dressings. Provide opportunities for the client to voice fears and concerns.

NURSING PROCESS

ASSESSMENT

Subjective Data

The client may describe a feeling of heaviness in the scrotum and may mention weight loss. During the postoperative phase, the client needs to be assessed for pain, using a pain scale to objectify data. Assess his emotional and educational needs. Monitor his behaviors and statements for signs of anxiety or depression.

Objective Data

A physical examination should include palpation of the abdomen and assessment of the scrotum. Positive findings in the scrotum include a firm, painless mass in the testis and an enlarged scrotum. Because gynecomastia (breast enlargement) is another symptom of testicular cancer, the client's breast tissue should be assessed for enlargement.

Nursing diagnoses for the client with testicular cancer include the following:

NURSING DIAGNOSES	PLANNING/OUTCOMES	NURSING INTERVENTIONS
*Risk for **Injury*** due to infection and hemorrhage related to surgery	The client will experience minimal bleeding and avoid infection.	Monitor the client's vital signs and incisional drainage. Report hyperthermia, tachycardia, hypotension, increased incisional drainage, and swelling or redness around the incision to the physician immediately. Maintain strict asepsis when handling wound dressings.
*Disturbed **Body** Image* related to surgery	The client will maintain or regain a positive body image.	Provide client with opportunities to voice concerns and ask questions. Monitor the client for statements and behaviors that indicate concern about loss of masculinity. Educate client that unilateral removal of a testis will not cause him to be sterile or demasculinized. Suggest sexual counseling if he does not appear to be resolving these issues. Sperm may be frozen before treatment.

(*Continues*)

Nursing diagnoses for the client with testicular cancer include the following: (Continued)

NURSING DIAGNOSES	PLANNING/OUTCOMES	NURSING INTERVENTIONS
*Deficient **K**nowledge* related to surgery and post operative care	The client will demonstrate understanding of postoperative activity restrictions and medical follow-up.	Teach the client that he needs to be on bed rest for 12 to 24 hours postoperatively. Instruct the client to wear tight-fitting underwear or an athletic supporter when ambulating and to avoid heavy lifting for 4 to 6 weeks.

Evaluation: Evaluate each outcome to determine how it has been met by the client.

PENILE CANCER

Penile cancer is rare and has a high correlation with poor hygiene and delayed or no circumcision. The bacteria harbored in the foreskin of the uncircumcised male are irritants to the glans penis and the prepuce. The chronic nature of this irritation is thought to be carcinogenic. Males with a history of sexually transmitted infections (STIs) are also predisposed to developing penile cancer. Symptoms of penile cancer include a painless, nodular growth on the foreskin, fatigue, and weight loss. Metastases are common in the inguinal nodes and adjacent organs.

MEDICAL–SURGICAL MANAGEMENT

Medical

The primary penile cancer treatment is surgery. Treatment with radiation alone is ineffective, and chemotherapy alone is used only for palliative treatment of penile cancer with deep, distant metastases; however, the client may receive adjuvant therapy with either radiation or chemotherapy.

Surgical

If the tumor is not extensive and no metastases are involved, the remaining penis should be long enough for the client to void standing and avoid soiling himself. If a penectomy is necessary, a perineal urethrostomy may be created.

NURSING MANAGEMENT

Provide emotional support if penectomy is required. Monitor vital signs and I&O. Elevate the scrotum to prevent edema. Objectively assess pain and administer analgesics as ordered.

NURSING PROCESS

ASSESSMENT

Subjective Data

Although the tumor is painless, ask the client if he is experiencing any pain, to rule out other possible diagnoses. Also ask about fatigue or weight loss. Preoperatively, assess the client for emotional and educational needs. Ask questions that can determine his understanding of the surgical procedure and the need for counseling. Postoperative assessment includes monitoring for pain and using a pain scale to objectify data.

Objective Data

The client's physical assessment should include inspection of the penis for the presence of painless, nodular growths. During the postoperative phase, monitor vital signs, incisional site, and intake and output. Hypotension, tachycardia, excessive incisional drainage, redness or swelling around the incision, or bright red or low urinary output could be signs of complications.

Nursing diagnoses for a client with penile cancer include the following:

NURSING DIAGNOSES	PLANNING/OUTCOMES	NURSING INTERVENTIONS
*Risk for **I**njury* due to infection and hemorrhage related to surgery	The client will experience minimal bleeding and avoid infection.	Monitor client's vital signs and incisional drainage. Report hyperthermia, tachycardia, hypotension, increased incisional drainage, and swelling or redness around the incision to the physician immediately. Maintain strict asepsis when handling wound dressings.
***A**nxiety* related to surgery	The client will discuss anxieties.	Provide client with information about the operative procedure, postoperative and discharge care. When available, a video may be used to present this information, with the nurse being available to answer the client's questions.

Nursing diagnoses for a client with penile cancer include the following: (Continued)

NURSING DIAGNOSES	PLANNING/OUTCOMES	NURSING INTERVENTIONS
Ineffective Sexuality Patterns related to the altered body function or structure	The client will maintain satisfactory sexuality patterns postoperatively.	Recommend the client to seek sexual counseling for both himself and his partner if he is unable to maintain normal sexuality patterns.

Evaluation: Evaluate each outcome to determine how it has been met by the client.

MENSTRUAL DISORDERS

Abnormalities of menstruation may be associated with an increase or decrease in secretion from any of the following glands: hypothalamus, pituitary, ovaries, adrenals, and thyroid. The normal menstrual pattern is controlled by a series of hormonal negative feedback mechanisms. The average menstrual cycle occurs every 28 to 30 days when the endometrial lining of the uterus sloughs off in the absence of a fertilized ovum.

DYSMENORRHEA

Painful menstruation, dysmenorrhea, also called "menstrual cramps," is more common in nulliparous women and in women who are not having intercourse. The exact pathophysiology is unknown, but it may be related to endocrine secretions such as prostaglandin F, which causes uterine cramping, irritation, and contractions. Other causes may include uterine anatomical anomalies, chronic illness, or psychological factors.

The primary symptom is pelvic pain before or at the onset of menses that may be caused by spasms of the uterus, cervical stenosis, uterine fibroids, emotional factors, endometriosis, pelvic inflammatory disease, or the presence of an intrauterine contraceptive device (IUD). The client may also state that the pain radiates across the lower back and downward into the legs.

The condition is diagnosed on the basis of the client's complaints and description of the timing of the onset of symptoms. Obtain information pertaining to the menstrual history and general health status of the client. A thorough physical exam is performed by the physician, including a bimanual exam to rule out other possible causes. A pelvic ultrasound may be ordered.

One effective preventive intervention may begin before the young woman begins menstruation. A positive parental attitude toward the onset of menstruation can aid the young girl in adjusting to the physiologic and psychological changes that occur with puberty.

Some medications are effective in the treatment of dysmenorrhea. Analgesics such as acetaminophen (Tylenol) and ibuprofen (Motrin) are useful in relieving pain. Oral contraceptives have been used for some clients to inhibit ovulation, which appears to be an associated cause. Prostaglandin inhibitors such as naproxen sodium (Aleve) and mefenamic acid (Ponstel) are useful if taken at the earliest sign of discomfort.

AMENORRHEA

Amenorrhea, the absence of menstruation, may be primary or secondary. Primary amenorrhea is defined as the absence of menstruation by the age of 16. Possible causes are related to anatomical or genetic abnormalities (Turner's syndrome). The treatment depends on the cause. Secondary amenorrhea is defined as the absence of menstruation after 6 months of regular periods or after 12 months of irregular periods. Several etiologies are possible for secondary amenorrhea, including anatomic abnormalities, nutritional deficits (anorexia nervosa), excessive exercise with significant decreases in body fat, endocrine dysfunction, emotional disturbances, side effects of medications, pregnancy, and lactation.

Diagnosis is based on the length of menstruation absence. A complete physical examination is performed, including a pelvic examination to rule out many other factors. A pregnancy test will be one of the first tests ordered, to rule out pregnancy. A progestin challenge test may be administered in an attempt to force the body to respond hormonally. Medroxyprogesterone acetate (Depo-Provera) is taken orally for 5 to 10 days as ordered by the physician. When the medication is finished, the client should have a menstrual period within 3 or 4 days. A menstrual flow after taking the medication may be an indicator that the client has not been ovulating. If no bleeding occurs, further investigation may be necessary to uncover other causes. Hormonal imbalances, microscopic pituitary tumors, and nutritional deficits are common etiologies of secondary amenorrhea. A microscopic pituitary tumor will cause an elevation in the prolactin level and result in anovulation and amenorrhea. A serum prolactin level should be ordered, especially if the client has noticed any breast discharge. Normal prolactin level should not exceed 15 ng/dL. With pituitary tumors, the prolactin level may exceed 400 ng/dL. In these cases, the drug of choice is bromocriptine mesylate (Parlodel), which had been used in the past to suppress lactation in mothers who did not breastfeed their newborns. A careful examination of the client is needed before administration of Parlodel because of an increased potential for cardiovascular problems associated with this medication. Because of this risk, the medication is no longer used for the postpartum client to suppress milk production. Other medical or surgical interventions depend on the cause of the amenorrhea.

OTHER DISORDERS

Other menstrual disorders include menorrhagia and metrorrhagia. Both types of abnormal bleeding can be problematic for the client and require further investigation. **Polymenorrhea** is a term used to describe short menstrual cycles of less than 21 days in length. The causes are similar to those of the other menstrual disorders. **Oligomenorrhea**, is a diminished menstrual flow, but it is not classified as amenorrhea. It may be associated with low-dose oral contraceptives that inhibit the growth of the endometrium and result in minimal tissue sloughing at the end of the cycle. Other causes may be metabolic or hormonal. Again, treatment is specific to the etiology.

For conditions associated with heavy bleeding or bleeding between periods, a dilation and curettage (D&C) may be performed. In this case, the procedure may be diagnostic and therapeutic. Tissue removed from the uterus is examined microscopically and histologically to evaluate its stage in the menstrual cycle. A hysterectomy may be indicated if abnormalities are discovered or if the bleeding is so excessive that the client is significantly compromised. The client may require a blood transfusion to correct low hemoglobin and hematocrit levels before any other procedures are performed. Supplemental iron generally is prescribed by the physician to also help correct the deficiency.

NURSING PROCESS

ASSESSMENT

Subjective Data

Ask the client about the onset of the bleeding and its relationship to the timing of her normal menstruation, the color of the bleeding, amount, number of pads saturated, presence of clots, and presence of pain with the bleeding. A history of current medications, contraception, and the possibility of pregnancy are additional data needed. Explore any preexisting health problems that could affect bleeding and clotting times, as well as life stressors.

Objective Data

Assessment of vital signs may indicate hypertension and tachycardia. Monitor laboratory test results.

NURSING MANAGEMENT

Acknowledge the client's feelings about the problem. Explain diagnostic tests and procedures. Encourage good nutrition, good posture, and exercise. Emphasize the importance of follow-up care.

Possible nursing diagnoses for a client with any of the menstrual disorders discussed in this section may include:

- *Acute **Pain*** related to uterine cramping or heavy bleeding
- *Decreased **C**ardiac Output* related to excessive blood loss
- ***Fatigue*** related to decreased hemoglobin and hematocrit levels
- *Disturbed **B**ody Image* related to the absence of menstruation

PREMENSTRUAL SYNDROME

One-third to one-half of women between 20 and 50 years of age experience some of the symptoms known as premenstrual syndrome (PMS). Once, this condition was thought by many physicians to be a psychological problem of women; however, recent research has supported data that many physiologic as well as psychological factors are involved. PMS often occurs during the secretory phase of the menstrual cycle, after ovulation. Risk factors associated with the development of PMS include age (older than 30), multiple life stressors, inappropriate nutritional status, a previous reaction to or side effects from oral contraceptive use, a sedentary lifestyle, marital status, a history of preeclampsia in pregnancy, and multiparity.

More than 150 symptoms have been reported that have been related to PMS. These include weight gain, bloating, irritability, edema, headache, mood swings, inability to concentrate, food cravings, acne, and numerous others. For many women, the PMS symptoms are merely a monthly nuisance, but for others, the symptoms are so incapacitating that they cannot function in their normal roles or responsibilities. The onset of symptoms is usually 7 to 10 days before the menstrual period starts; symptoms end after the menstrual flow begins.

Research has correlated hormonal imbalances of estrogen, progesterone, ACTH, and androgens with the symptoms of PMS. The presence of prostaglandin F in the tissue may also be a cause of some of the symptoms. Prostaglandins are associated with many inflammatory responses in the tissues.

The first step in identifying PMS is a physical examination to rule out other possible disorders of the reproductive system. The client may be asked to keep a monthly calendar of symptoms to see if there are patterns in severity, type, or onset. Blood tests may be ordered to assess estrogen and progesterone levels, as well as checking the glucose level. Low blood glucose level has been associated with irritability that sometimes accompanies PMS symptoms. The client should receive counseling, if needed, to facilitate coping with life stressors that may be complicating the complexity of the PMS symptoms.

MEDICAL–SURGICAL MANAGEMENT

Pharmacological

Some physicians and NPs recommend medication such as acetaminophen (Tylenol), naproxen (Naprosyn), mefenamic acid (Ponstel), and ibuprofen (Advil) for the relief of minor discomforts of PMS. Several PMS symptoms are thought to be related to a low progesterone level. For some clients, the use of progesterone suppositories or oral progesterone to supplement their own production during the secretory phase of the menstrual cycle has been useful. Selective serotonin reuptake inhibitors used to treat and relieve PMS symptoms include citalopram hydrobromide (Celexa), fluvoxamine maleate (Luvox), fluoxetine hydrochloride (Prozac), sertraline hydrochloride (Zoloft), escitalopram oxalate (Lexapro), and paroxetine hydrochloride (Paxil) (Daniels, Nosek, & Nicoll, 2007).

Diet

A thorough diet history should be included in the assessment data collected. Certain nutritional deficits or cravings have been linked to the worsening of PMS. Items such as sugar, salt, caffeine, and chocolate are in this category. Many studies have shown that limiting intake of these substances may be helpful. Caffeinated beverages may increase anxiety, irritability, and deplete vitamin B stores in the body. Dairy products interfere with the absorption of magnesium, which helps stabilize the mood. Chocolates have been related to increased sugar cravings, mood swings, fluid retention, and increased vitamin B demands. Oranges and other fruits or vegetables that are highly acidic may worsen PMS. Foods that are recommended are whole grains, nuts, pasta, legumes, root vegetables, fruits such as apples and pears, poultry, and seafood. A good vitamin supplement rich in vitamin B-complex, calcium, magnesium, and zinc should be taken daily, especially during the PMS period. Herbal tea formulas have shown some promise as alternative methods of relieving PMS.

Activity

A regular exercise routine, coupled with the use of stress-management techniques such as deep breathing and relaxation exercises, help the client cope with the increased sense of anxiety or irritability that may accompany PMS. Meditation, positive affirmation, visualization, and imagery may be helpful, as well as acupressure, neurolymphatic or neurovascular massage, and yoga.

Nursing Management

Encourage client to keep a monthly PMS calendar of events. Recommend that the client limit sodium, sugar, alcohol, caffeine, nicotine, and refined carbohydrate intake, and increase calcium intake to reduce PMS symptoms (Daniels, Nosek, & Nicoll, 2007).

NURSING PROCESS

Assessment

Subjective Data

Ask the client to describe her symptoms and the impact on her lifestyle. Many times, clients will seek medical attention for their PMS symptoms when the emotional impact has caused friction in the home, marriage, work, or family environment. Symptoms described may include weight gain, bloating, irritability, headache, mood swings, inability to concentrate, or food cravings. Ask the client to relate symptoms to time of menstrual cycle.

Objective Data

Assess the client for weight gain and edema. Review laboratory test results.

Nursing diagnoses for a client with premenstrual syndrome include the following:

NURSING DIAGNOSES	PLANNING/OUTCOMES	NURSING INTERVENTIONS
*Excess **Fluid** Volume* related to hormonal imbalance and increased sodium or sugar intake	The client's intake and output will be balanced, and edema will be decreased.	Educate client that a certain amount of fluid retention is normal before the onset of the menstrual period and cannot be avoided, but by limiting sodium and sugar intake, she may be able to influence the amount of fluid retained.
***Health**-Seeking Behaviors*, related to finding methods to cope with symptoms of PMS	The client will develop effective health-promotion skills to increase coping with PMS symptoms or to decrease symptom severity or frequency.	Teach client how to keep a monthly PMS calendar of events. Discuss prescribed medications with the client, including the dosage, expected effects, and side effects. Discuss relationship of foods to PMS.

Evaluation: Evaluate each outcome to determine how it has been met by the client.

MENOPAUSE

Menopause, or climacteric, is the cessation of menstruation. It may occur as a natural hormonal decline or it may be surgically induced by removal of the uterus and ovaries. Many people think of menopause as the "change of life" and accept it as part of aging. Most women will begin to experience signs and symptoms of approaching menopause around 50 years of age; however, the range of onset is from 45 to 60 years old. During this perimenopause transition, menstrual cycles become further apart and the flow decreases. The onset is usually gradual, and it may take more than a year before the woman has completely ceased menstruation. Reproductive capability is also lost with menopause. For some women this is a sad time perceived as the loss of womanhood; for others it is a welcome relief. Postmenopause is considered the time period one year after the last menstrual cycle and lasts the rest of a woman's lifetime.

The decreasing level of ovarian hormone production affects women in a variety of ways, more than just the end of menstruation. There may be a relaxation of the pelvic support structures, loss of skin turgor and elasticity, and thinning of the hair on the head, axilla, and pubic regions. Other signs of decreasing hormones (estrogen and progesterone) are vaginal dryness, thinning of the vaginal mucosa, weight gain, dry skin, and stress incontinence. The estrogen level plays an important protective role in maintaining an adequate calcium balance in the bones and preventing coronary artery disease. Without calcium, bones become brittle, and there is an increased risk of fractures and osteoporosis. A baseline bone density study may be recommended before menopause.

Some women experience psychological responses to menopause, such as mild to moderate depression, nervousness, and insomnia. Consultation with a psychologist, minister, or counselor may be useful in facilitating the transition through this period for some women.

Women may also experience mild to moderate periods of profuse perspiration called "hot flashes." These usually move from the waist upward. They are caused by the decreased estrogen level and its effect on the hypothalamus. The sensation may last from 30 seconds to 10 minutes. It appears that many different things can trigger a hot flash—drinking hot beverages, eating spicy foods, smoking, and consuming caffeine and alcohol.

Medical–Surgical Management

Pharmacological

For some women, estrogen replacement therapy is recommended, especially if they are experiencing moderately uncomfortable symptoms. Estrogen replacement therapy (ERT) may help decrease some symptoms, such as insomnia, hot flashes, mood swings, and lack of concentration. Estrogen elevates the high-density lipoproteins (healthy ones) and lowers the low-density lipoproteins (unhealthy) in the circulation. Estrogen may be administered orally, as a transdermal patch, or as a vaginal cream. Conjugated estrogen (Premarin), estradiol (Estrace), and synthetic conjugated estrogens Cenestin and Enjuvia are examples of oral estrogens available. Estrogen creams or water-soluble gels such as Lubrifax or K-Y may be used to combat the vaginal dryness and resulting dyspareunia (The North American Menopause Society, 2009).

Diet

Provide the client with instructions regarding the importance of an adequate daily intake of calcium-rich products, such as dairy products. Many low-fat, high-calcium products are available if the client has a concern about weight gain. Calcium supplements may also be taken in a tablet form. The woman should consult her health care provider before adding a calcium supplement because too much calcium increases the risk for other health problems. Herbal teas, vitamin E, magnesium, and primrose oil have been used as alternative methods to alleviate or decrease hot flashes and promote relaxation for some women.

Activity

One important way that the client can decrease the potential for calcium loss from weight-bearing bones is to exercise. A planned 30-minute program performed at least 3 times per week is adequate to maintain bone density. Exercises such as walking or swimming are excellent. Swimming provides good non–weight-bearing activity and promotes active movement of all extremities. Biking is a good exercise to maintain joint mobility in the lower extremities, but it does not require the use of the same muscle groups as walking.

Nursing Management

Encourage the client to exercise regularly, especially walking. Explain nutritional requirements for vitamins and calcium. Advise the client to try water-soluble gels for vaginal dryness and body lotion to prevent dry skin.

NURSING PROCESS

Assessment

Subjective Data

The client may describe decreasing regularity of menstruation or hot flashes. Obtain information from the client about gynecological and obstetrical history, including menstruation. It is helpful to know when the client began experiencing symptoms in predicting the length of time they may continue.

Objective Data

These include a physical examination and Pap smear. The results of the Pap smear can indicate if there is less estrogen present in the cervical tissue than normal.

Nursing diagnoses for a client experiencing menopausal symptoms include the following:

NURSING DIAGNOSES	PLANNING/OUTCOMES	NURSING INTERVENTIONS
Health-Seeking Behaviors related to perceived physiological and psychologic impact of decreased estrogen	The client will develop effective health promotion skills to increase coping with menopausal symptoms or to decrease symptom severity or frequency.	Encourage client to continue to see her health care provider for annual Pap smears and breast examinations. Explain nutritional requirements for vitamins and calcium that increase with menopause. Encourage client to begin a regular exercise program that includes weight-bearing activities such as walking to prevent loss of calcium from the bones.
Impaired Tissue Integrity related to vaginal dryness and dry skin	The client will maintain skin integrity, and vagina will not be dry.	Recommend that the client try estrogen creams or water-soluble gels such as Lubrifax or K-Y to combat the vaginal dryness and resulting dyspareunia. Encourage client to use body lotion to prevent dry skin.
Decisional Conflict related to taking supplemental estrogen therapy	The client will make informed decisions about taking supplemental estrogen.	Discuss the advantages and disadvantages of estrogen replacement therapy with the client. Remind client that if she has a uterus and takes hormonal replacements, she will continue to have monthly menstrual cycles.

Evaluation: Evaluate each outcome to determine how it has been met by the client.

STRUCTURAL DISORDERS

Structural anomalies are separated into female and male disorders.

CYSTOCELE, URETHROCELE, RECTOCELE, PROLAPSED UTERUS

Cystocele, urethrocele, rectocele, and prolapsed uterus are often associated with relaxation of the pelvic muscles that support the uterus, bladder, and rectum. A **cystocele** is a downward displacement of the bladder into the anterior vaginal wall. A **urethrocele** is a downward displacement of the urethra into the vagina, and a **rectocele** is an anterior displacement of the rectum into the posterior vaginal wall. **Prolapsed uterus** is a downward displacement of the uterus into the vagina (Figure 13-21). Possible causes for the four conditions are multiple pregnancies, third- or fourth-degree perineal lacerations with childbirth, and age-related weakening of the pelvic muscles.

A prolapsed uterus is often accompanied by a cystocele and/or rectocele. With a first-degree prolapse, the cervix is visible at the vaginal introitus, or opening, without straining. With a second-degree prolapse, the cervix extends beyond the vaginal opening to the perineum. With a third-degree prolapse, the uterus protrudes outside of the vagina. This severe condition is called *procidentia uteri*.

MEDICAL–SURGICAL MANAGEMENT

Medical and surgical interventions for the treatment of each of these conditions are focused on relief of discomfort and restoration of the structure and function of the pelvic organs.

Medical

The pessary is a small molded plastic or rubber apparatus that fits into the vagina behind the pubic bone and in front of the rectum. Its function is to provide an artificial or mechanical support for the uterus. Pessaries are not uncomfortable and should not be felt by the client if properly fitted and in the correct position. The client should be taught how to insert and remove the pessary so it can be cleaned. The pessary may be washed in warm, soapy water once every 1 to 2 weeks. Prolonged use of a mechanical device such as a pessary may result in vaginal necrosis and ulceration. Periodic examination by a health care professional is recommended.

Surgical

Surgery for a prolapsed uterus may require a hysterectomy. If the prolapse is accompanied by a cystocele or rectocele, an A&P repair may also be performed. An A&P repair (anterior/posterior colporrhaphy) may be performed vaginally to replace the bladder, urethra, or rectum in the correct anatomic position. Another procedure, the Marshall-Marchette-Krantz, may be performed to attach the bladder to the inferior surface of the pubic bone. Postoperatively, the client may be sent home with an indwelling Foley catheter because of the potential inability to void. This is a common postoperative situation that usually resolves itself spontaneously within 1 or 2 weeks after discharge.

Activity

The Kegel exercise is performed by tightening and releasing the perineal muscles. An important muscle group, called the "levators," helps lift and support the organs inside the pelvis.

CLIENT TEACHING

Kegel Exercises

- Suggest that the client practice when she has a full bladder. If she can successfully start and stop the flow of urine from the bladder, she is identifying and using the correct muscle groups.
- The muscles should be tightened and held for 5 to 10 seconds and then released slowly.
- Repeat the exercises at least 10 times.
- Kegel exercise can be practiced anytime and anyplace.
- A secondary benefit of increasing the strength and contractility of the pelvic and perineal muscles is seen in an improvement in pelvic sensations for both partners during intercourse.

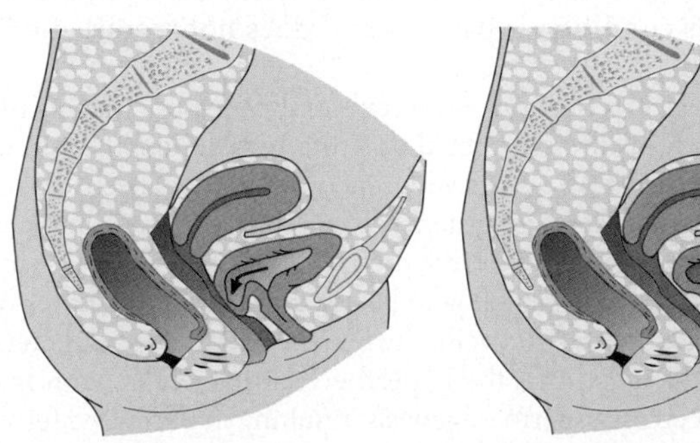

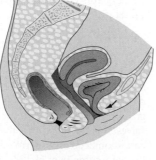

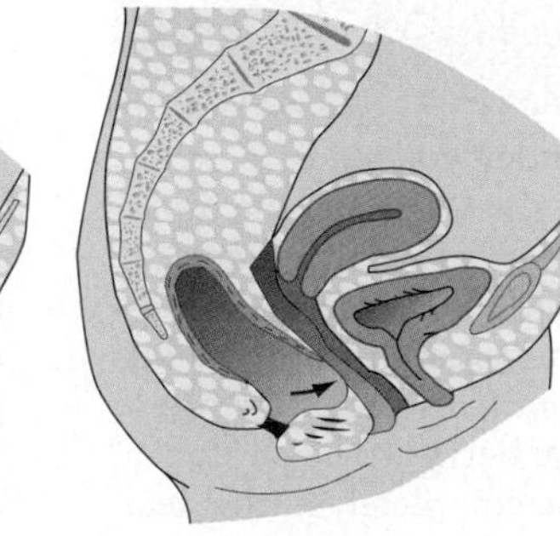

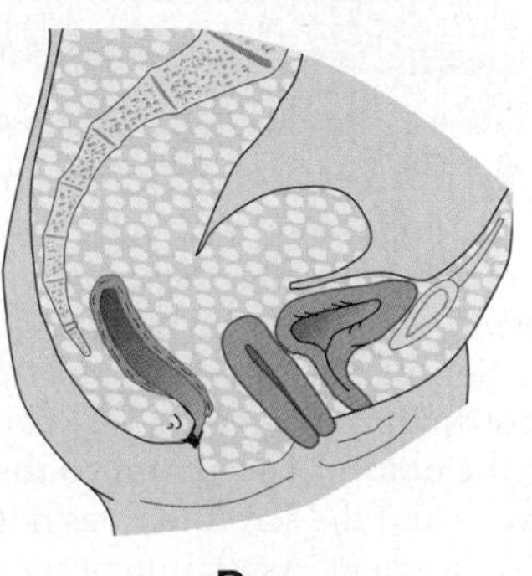

FIGURE 13-21 *A,* Cystocele; *B,* Urethrocele; *C,* Rectocele; *D,* Uterine Prolapse

NURSING MANAGEMENT

Teach client Kegel exercise and encourage daily practice. Describe to the client how a high-fiber diet and drinking plenty of fluids will help prevent constipation. Postoperatively, monitor vital signs and I&O. Cleanse perineal area following surgical asepsis. Encourage early ambulation.

NURSING PROCESS

ASSESSMENT

Subjective Data

The client often describes stress incontinence, a loss of urine when she coughs, sneezes, laughs, or jumps. She may describe it as "a leaky bladder." She may notice that her panties are damp or that she dribbles urine. Many women complain of frequent urination in small quantities with a feeling of urgency without burning or dysuria. The client may notice constipation or a sense of bearing-down pressure in the pelvis with a rectocele. Many of these symptoms will decrease or subside completely when lying down. Ask about the client's childbearing history, onset of current symptoms, and any other pertinent gynecological data.

Objective Data

These include the visualization of a bulging of the bladder, urethra, or rectum into the vagina. The bulging increases when the client is asked to bear down. Urinalysis results should be evaluated.

Nursing diagnoses for a female client with a structural disorder of the reproductive system include the following:

NURSING DIAGNOSES	PLANNING/OUTCOMES	NURSING INTERVENTIONS
Stress Urinary Incontinence related to relaxation of the pelvic muscles	The client will have less stress incontinence.	Teach the client Kegel exercise and encourage daily practice. Encourage client to empty bladder frequently.
Constipation related to relaxation of the anterior rectal wall into the vagina and decreased function	The client will not have constipation.	Encourage client to defecate at same time each day. Encourage client to eat high-fiber foods, drink plenty of fluids, and exercise regularly.
Risk for Infection related to exposure of internal tissues to external environmental factors	The client will be free of signs and symptoms of infection.	Monitor client's vital signs. Encourage client to practice proper personal hygiene and wear clean undergarments daily.
Sexual Dysfunction related to discomforts with intercourse	The client will have a fulfilling sexual relationship without discomfort.	Be sensitive to client cues related to her sexual concerns. Help the client set realistic goals during her recovery period to facilitate a new outlook on her relationship. Encourage client to openly discuss her feelings with her partner.

Evaluation: Evaluate each outcome to determine how it has been met by the client.

HYDROCELE, SPERMATOCELE, VARICOCELE, TORSION OF THE SPERMATIC CORD

A hydrocele is a benign, nontender collection of clear, amber fluid within the space of the testes and the tunica vaginalis or along the spermatic cord. Scrotal swelling may result, which can be painful if it develops suddenly. Inflammation of the epididymis or testis or a lymphatic or venous obstruction may cause this condition. Congenital hydrocele in the newborn occurs when the canal between the peritoneal cavity and the scrotum does not close completely during fetal development. Aspiration of the fluid is only a temporary measure and can lead to secondary infection. Therefore, treatment for the condition is surgery.

A spermatocele is a benign nontender cyst of either the epididymis or the rete testis. It contains milky fluid and sperm. Usually, this condition is painless and does not require medical treatment.

A varicocele is dilation of the veins of the scrotum that occurs when the venous system that drains the testicle lengthens and enlarges. This dilation occurs when incompetent or absent valves in the spermatic venous system permit blood to accumulate, resulting in increased hydrostatic pressure. This condition is most commonly found on the left side because of the increased retrograde pressure of the renal vein, the length, and fewer competent valves. It is theorized that the hyperthermia that occurs with this condition decreases spermatogenesis, resulting in decreased fertility. Symptoms may include a bluish discoloration of the scrotal skin or palpation of a wormlike mass when the male bears down. This condition seldom requires treatment.

Torsion of the spermatic cord occurs when the vascular pedicle of the testis twists, resulting in partial or complete venous occlusion. The three forms of this disorder are (1) rotation of the spermatic cord, (2) torsion of a testicular appendage, or (3) torsion of the spermatic cord and epididymis. Testicular torsion may be related to recent trauma, and the onset of symptoms often occurs suddenly. Symptoms of testicular torsion may include abdominal and scrotal pain, scrotal edema, nausea and vomiting, and, possibly, a slight fever. The pain caused by testicular torsion is not relieved by bed rest or scrotal support.

Medical–Surgical Management

Medical/surgical management of male structural disorders is specific to the condition. In some newborns, a hydrocele may resolve without medical intervention. Clients of all ages may have aspiration performed to reduce the swelling caused by fluid or a hematoma; however, this solution is usually only temporary, and surgical removal of the sac provides the only permanent solution to the problem. Although a spermatocele usually does not require treatment, sometimes surgical aspiration or excision is necessary.

Because a common complication of a varicocele is male infertility, ligation of the spermatic vein may be performed if infertility is a concern. Sometimes this does not resolve infertility problems because varicoceles may recur after surgery. When fertility is not a concern, the varicocele may be treated simply with scrotal support.

Torsion of the spermatic cord is one disorder that does require immediate surgery to perform surgical detorsion (untwisting) and suturing of the testicle to the scrotum.

Nursing Management

Maintain the client on bed rest with scrotal support and ice to the area. Objectively assess the client's pain and administer analgesics as ordered. Monitor vital signs, incisional drainage, and dressing. Use strict asepsis when changing dressings.

NURSING PROCESS

Assessment

Subjective Data

Ask the client about the type and location of his pain and related symptoms such as alteration in urinary patterns, warmth, fatigue, nausea, or vomiting. Assess the client's knowledge of his condition, treatment, follow-up care, and the implications of sterility and impotence to the client's life.

Objective Data

Inspect and palpate the genitals to detect the presence of swelling, testicular enlargement, scrotal immobility, redness, and warmth of the scrotum. Large varicoceles may be visible through the scrotal skin as a bluish discoloration.

Nursing diagnoses for a male client with a structural disorder of the reproductive system may include the following:

NURSING DIAGNOSES	PLANNING/OUTCOMES	NURSING INTERVENTIONS
*Risk for **Injury*** related to inflammation and hemorrhage	The client will experience minimal bleeding and avoid infection.	Monitor client's vital signs and incisional drainage. Maintain strict asepsis when handling wound dressings. Report hyperthermia, tachycardia, hypotension, increased incisional drainage, and swelling or redness around the incision to the physician immediately.
*Deficient **Knowledge*** related to the condition and possible complications	The client will demonstrate understanding of the possible complications of his condition.	Monitor statements made by the client to determine if there is any misunderstanding about how the surgery will affect his masculinity and fertility. Provide client with opportunities to voice his feelings and ask questions.

Evaluation: Evaluate each outcome to determine how it has been met by the client.

FUNCTIONAL DISORDERS AND CONCERNS

Included in this category are impotence, infertility, and contraception.

IMPOTENCE

Impotence is defined as the inability of an adult male to have an erection firm enough or to maintain it long enough to complete sexual intercourse. There are three types of impotence: functional, atonic, and anatomic. Psychological factors that lead to concerns about sexual performance may contribute to functional impotence. These factors include aging and difficulty with communication or relationships.

Atonic impotence may be the result of medications such as antihypertensives, sedatives, antidepressants, or tranquilizers. For example, antihypertensives lower blood pressure in all arteries of the body, and reduction of the blood pressure to penile arteries may lead to failure of the penis to fill sufficiently to achieve erection. The use of alcohol, cocaine, and nicotine can also decrease potency. Disease processes leading to atonic

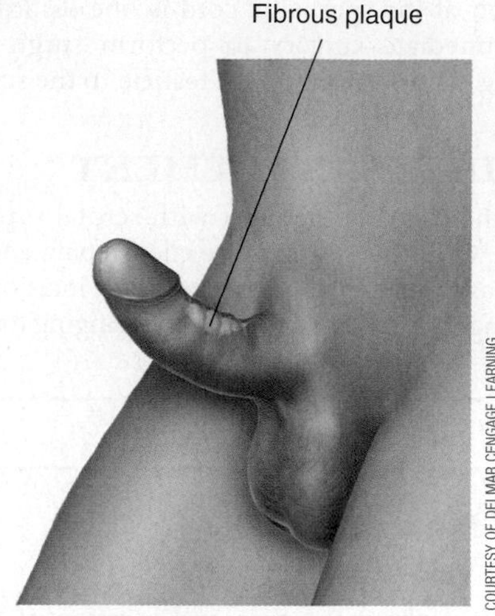

FIGURE 13-22 Dorsal Curvature of the Penis in Peyronie's Disease Caused by Fibrous Plaque

impotence include diabetes and vascular and neurological disorders. Diabetic clients are at increased risk for impotence because of their tendency to develop atherosclerosis and autonomic neuropathy. Vascular and neurological disorders include atherosclerosis, hypertension, spinal cord injuries, and multiple sclerosis. End-stage renal disease and chronic obstructive pulmonary disorders can also decrease potency.

Peyronie's disease is the development of nonelastic, fibrous tissue just beneath the penile skin, leading to anatomic impotence. The resulting loss of elasticity leads to a decreased ability of the penis to fill with and store blood during an erection. Peyronie's disease often causes the penis to bend upward, possibly leading to pain and an inability to penetrate the vagina (Figure 13-22).

Medical–Surgical Management

Medical

The first step in treating impotence is to determine whether the client's lifestyle is a factor. Further assessment may include nocturnal penile tumescence monitoring or dynamic infusion cavernosometry and cavernosography (DICC). Treatment will be based on the assessment findings and test results. Treatment may include changes in lifestyle to reduce the need for medications, manage stress, lose weight, and exercise. These changes often help improve the client's physical health, self-image, and attitude about his ability to function sexually.

External devices can be used to promote an erection. A vacuum constriction device (VCD) may be used to increase the blood supply to the penis, causing engorgement and rigidity. The client inserts his penis into a plastic cylinder and squeezes a pump to withdraw the air from the cylinder, creating a vacuum that draws blood into the penis. Once an erection has been achieved in this manner, a rubber ring is moved from the bottom of the cylinder to the base of the penis. This permits the blood to be safely trapped in the penis for up to one-half hour. Advantages of the VCD over surgical intervention are less expense and fewer complications.

Surgical

Surgical interventions for impotency include revascularization and penile implants. For clients with impotence related to blocked arteries, revascularization is done to bypass blocked arteries and remove veins that are causing excessive drainage. For clients who are not candidates for revascularization, penile prostheses are another option. One type is a semirigid implant, which is a silicone cylinder that may be flexible or inflexible. Another type is a hydraulic implant that has a cylinder that can be inflated by squeezing a pump located in the scrotum or at the end of the penis. Because of its ability to fill and empty, the hydraulic implant, unlike the silicone implant, which is always semirigid, most closely mimics flaccidity and erection. The disadvantages of surgical interventions are expense and postoperative complications, the most serious being postoperative infection.

Pharmacological

Medications that promote erections are sildenafil citrate (Viagra), vardenafil hydrochloride (Levitra), and tadalafil (Cialis), which belong to a class of drugs called phosphodiesterase (PDE) inhibitors. These drugs should not be used by men for whom sexual activity is not advisable because of underlying cardiovascular problems (Spratto & Woods, 2009). One side effect of drug therapy is prolonged erection that does not occur in response to sexual stimulation (**priapism**). Oral neurotransmitters have been used with variable success, and sublingual apomorphine shows some promise as an erectogenic agent. When administered sublingually rather than subcutaneously, as was done in the past, there are fewer side effects. Self-injections of vasodilators or other drugs may result in serious complications.

NURSING PROCESS

Assessment

Subjective Data

The client may describe a history of illicit and prescribed drug use, and alcohol consumption. Previous diagnoses, lifestyle, sexual functioning, and family disorders must be explored. Assess the client's emotional and educational needs to determine whether anxiety about sexual performance or lack of knowledge are contributing factors to impotence.

Objective Data

If the client has surgery, the nurse needs to monitor vital signs, incisional site, and I&O.

Nursing Management

Teach client how to take prescribed medications. If an implant has been inserted, teach client the signs of infection such as tenderness, fever, and dysuria.

Nursing diagnoses for a client who is impotent may include the following:

- *Sexual Dysfunction* related to altered body function or structure
- *Ineffective **S**exuality Patterns* related to altered body function or structure
- *Disturbed **B**ody Image* related to impotence
- *Deficient **K**nowledge* related to impotence

INFERTILITY

Approximately one in every eight couples experiences infertility, the inability to produce offspring. Infertility may be primary or secondary. In primary infertility, the couple have never achieved a pregnancy or have never carried a pregnancy to viability. Secondary infertility involves problems that arise after the couple has had a successful pregnancy. Many factors may be investigated as causes of infertility in both female and male clients. Forty percent of infertility factors are female-related, 40% are male-related, and 20% are a combination of multiple factors that involve both partners. The more factors that are involved, the more difficult the infertility resolution.

The etiology of infertility may be related to anatomic or endocrine problems. The female anatomic or structural abnormalities may include blocked passages through the cervix or fallopian tubes caused by failed development or by past infections, such as PID, or STIs. Uterine and cervical abnormalities may also occur. The cervix may be too narrow or closed, and sperm are unable to navigate through the passage. The uterus may have a partial or complete septum inside that limits the internal cavity space. Immune problems involve the development of antibodies by the woman's system to the male's sperm. These antibodies may be present in the cervical mucus and kill the sperm on contact. Hyposecretion or hypersecretion of FSH, LH, estrogen, or progesterone have been associated with infertility.

The causes of infertility in males include varicoceles, cryptorchidism, impaired sperm, insufficient number of sperm, and hormonal imbalance. The use of hot tubs, saunas, tight underwear, and laptop computers may decrease the sperm count.

The first step in treating an infertile couple is to obtain a history of sexual practices. In addition, detailed health histories need to be obtained and physical examinations performed.

A basic infertility workup may be initiated when the client has been unable to conceive after 6 to 12 months of unprotected intercourse. One simple, noninvasive procedure is the use of a basal body temperature chart. The chart is kept for a minimum of 3 months and then reviewed for normal ovulatory fluctuations in the basal temperature. During the first half of the menstrual cycle, the body temperature may remain below 98°F. At ovulation, there is often a slight decrease in the temperature for a 24-hour period. This is the optimal period of fertility. After ovulation, the woman's basal body temperature should go above 98°F and remain in that range for a period of 14 days. The length of the luteal phase (secretory phase) of the cycle following ovulation is a critical factor in some infertility disorders. Variations in the temperature chart may indicate that the client has had an anovulatory cycle or has a shortened luteal phase. Because the fertilized ovum does not implant in the endometrium until 6 to 8 days after conception, the luteal phase is critical to maintain the blood-rich lining long enough for implantation to occur. A low progesterone level during the luteal phase may result in spontaneous **abortion** (ending a pregnancy before the age of viability) of the fertilized ovum before implantation. Diagnostic tests that may be ordered include the following:

- Endometrial biopsy to detect tissue responses during both phases of the enstrual cycle
- Semen analysis, including sperm count, motility, and morphology
- Testicular biopsy (done when sperm are absent from the semen) to ascertain the presence of sperm
- Endocrine imbalance testing, which measures pituitary, gonadotropin, testosterone, estrogen, and progesterone levels
- Male–female interaction studies (Huhner test) to determine motility and number of sperm 2 to 4 hours after intercourse
- Laparoscopy to discover conditions such as endometriosis, adhesions, or scar tissue that potentially immobilize the fimbriae or polycystic ovarian disease (Stein-Leventhal syndrome)

MEDICAL–SURGICAL MANAGEMENT

There is no one treatment for infertility problems. The goal of treatment is successful achievement of a pregnancy that is carried to full term and produces a healthy offspring.

Medical

Infertility treatment may include artificial insemination with either the partner's sperm or donor sperm. This method is particularly useful if the male partner has a low sperm count, abnormal sperm, or no sperm production. With the procedure, the semen is placed directly into the cervix or uterus with a small flexible catheter and a syringe.

Surgical

Assisted reproductive technology (ART) has revolutionized infertility treatment. It is fertility treatment in which the eggs are surgically removed and combined with sperm in the laboratory and then returned to the woman's body. One method is *in vitro* fertilization. This may be by GIFT (gamete-intra-fallopian transfer) or ZIFT (zygote-intra-fallopian transfer). With the GIFT technique, the female partner receives monthly cyclic hormone injections that cause ova to ripen. The hormones may cause more than one ovum to ripen during each cycle, which enhances the possibility that more than one ovum will be fertilized and implanted in the uterus. A semen specimen is collected from the male partner 1 to 2 hours before the GIFT procedure and the sperm placed into a special catheter. The ripened ovum is obtained from the female via laparoscopy or ultrasound aspiration and is loaded into the catheter in a sequential manner with the sperm and then injected through the fimbrial end of the fallopian tube, also by laparoscopy. This procedure takes approximately 1 hour to complete. Pregnancy is confirmed within 7 to 10 days with a blood hormonal test (Beta hCG) or an ultrasound, or both.

The ZIFT procedure is similar to GIFT; however, several ova are obtained just before ovulation and are placed in a special fluid for several hours while the sperm are prepared. The ova and sperm are then carefully mixed and closely observed for 2 to 3 days. The fertilized ova (now zygotes) are transferred into the fallopian tube or into the uterine cavity. Another name for the ZIFT procedure is IVF-ER (in vitro fertilization and embryo replacement), which more clearly defines what actually occurs.

Both GIFT and ZIFT are relatively expensive procedures and may or may not be covered by health insurance. For many couples, these are final efforts to conceive.

Pharmacological

Several medications are used in the treatment of infertility disorders, and most are focused on hormone imbalances or deficiencies. Clomiphene citrate (Clomid) stimulates release of follicle-stimulating hormone (FSH) and luteinizing hormone (LH), and is used to induce ovulation. Clomid is administered orally beginning on the fifth day of the menstrual cycle. If ovulation does not occur, the dosage will be increased for 5 days in the next cycle. If ovulation does not occur by the time the dose has been increased 4 or 5 times, it may be considered a Clomid failure. There is some chance of multiple gestation while the client is taking Clomid, and she should be so informed. Most often it is a twin pregnancy, but occasionally triplets may be conceived.

Menotropins (Pergonal) mimics FSH and LH, causing follicular growth and maturation. It is administered by intramuscular injection. Although Pergonal is an expensive drug, it has been shown to increase the possibility for ovulation in clients who have not responded to other medications.

Human chorionic gonadotropin (Pregnyl) may also be administered with the Clomid or Pergonal therapy to help maintain the endometrial lining for implantation. It stimulates the production of progesterone from the ovary until the fertilized ovum implants and the placenta begins to function. Progesterone suppositories may be used vaginally two times per day to help correct a luteal phase defect by lengthening the time from ovulation until the onset of the menses or through implantation and pregnancy. Some clients continue with the progesterone suppositories throughout the first few weeks of the pregnancy to ensure that the endometrium remains intact. If the sperm count or motility is low, testosterone or thyroid extracts may be prescribed.

Health Promotion

Seeking prompt medical treatment for infections that involve the reproductive system is an essential means of preventing infertility problems, especially with STIs and PID. PID causes scarring of the outside of the fallopian tubes, and gonorrhea can result in scarring or strictures of the internal fallopian tube. Either cause can result in an ectopic pregnancy when the fertilized ovum cannot pass through the tube.

Other considerations may include wise choices in contraceptive methods. The use of oral contraceptives has been associated with primary and secondary infertility caused by decreased pituitary function. This condition may resolve spontaneously, or medications may be required to stimulate ovulation in order to conceive.

Multiple sexual partners have also been associated with an increased risk of sexually transmitted disease, infections, and cervical cancer.

CONTRACEPTION

Contraception, or prevention of pregnancy, has been accomplished by many methods over the centuries. In weighing the options, safety, ease of use, effectiveness, and cost should be considered. Both partners' wishes should be considered in this decision-making process.

Contraception may be accomplished by natural means or medical interventions. This section of the chapter discusses a basic overview of the types of contraceptive methods currently available, the advantages and disadvantages, the effectiveness of each kind, the mechanisms by which they work, and the client education that should accompany the methods (Table 13-2).

NATURAL METHOD

Natural methods of contraception may include what is called the "rhythm method." During the woman's fertile period of the month, usually lasting 7 days (3 days before ovulation to 3 days after), the couple should abstain from intercourse. The determination of the fertile period is based on the time of ovulation. Sperm can live up to 72 hours after ejaculation, and it is possible for sperm to still be in the cervix or uterus if the couple had intercourse 3 days before ovulation. The couple may also decide to maintain a basal body temperature chart to more accurately

TABLE 13-2 Contraception Methods: Effectiveness and Concerns

METHOD	EFFECTIVENESS RATE	RISKS	POSSIBLE SIDE EFFECTS	OTHER ADVANTAGES
Abstinence	100%	None known	Psychological reactions	Prevents infections including HIV
Hormonal				
Oral contraceptives	97%	Cardiovascular complications such as stroke, blood clots, high blood pressure, and heart attacks with the higher-dose combined oral contraceptive	Possible nausea, headaches, dizziness, spotting, weight gain, breast tenderness, chloasma, cramping	Protects against PID, decreases risk of ovarian and endometrial cancer, decreases menstrual blood loss and dysmenorrhea (cramps), decreases benign breast disease, regulates irregular menses, protects bone density, decreases risk of atherosclerosis, lessens the risk of rheumatoid arthritis, decreases uterine fibroids, and decreases ovarian cysts
Depo-Provera	98%	Pulmonary embolism	Headache, depression, hypertension, edema, nausea	Effective to treat obstructive sleep apnea
Lunelle	99%	None known	Breast tenderness, weight gain	None known

TABLE 13-2 Contraception Methods: Effectiveness and Concerns (Continued)

METHOD	EFFECTIVENESS RATE	RISKS	POSSIBLE SIDE EFFECTS	OTHER ADVANTAGES
Mirena	99.8%	None known	Headache, acne, breast tenderness first few months	Decreases menstrual blood loss, may protect against endometrial cancer
Transdermal patch	99%	None known	Skin reaction at application site	None known
Vaginal ring	97%	None known	Vaginal infections or irritation, headache, weight gain, nausea	None known
Nonhormonal				
IUD	94%	Pelvic inflammatory disease, uterine perforation, anemia	Menstrual cramping, spotting, increased bleeding	None known
Barriers				
Diaphragm Cervical cap Spermicide	84% 73–92% 79%	Mechanical irritation, vaginal infections, toxic shock syndrome	Pelvic pressure, cervical erosion, vaginal discharges if left in too long	Protects to some degree against sexually transmitted infections
Condoms	86%	None known	Decreased sensation, allergy to latex, less spontaneity in lovemaking	Protects against sexually transmitted infections, including AIDS; delays premature ejaculation
Sterilization				
Female Male	99.6% 99.8%	Infection	Pain at surgical site, psychological reaction with subsequent regret	None known

pinpoint ovulation each month. Another method to determine the approaching ovulation is to monitor the stretchiness of the cervical mucus. This is called "spinnbarkeit." As the woman nears ovulation, estrogen causes the cervical mucus to become clear, thin, and stretchy. This type of mucus provides a favorable environment for the sperm and helps their motility toward the ova. Immediately after ovulation, the cervical mucus becomes hostile to sperm. It becomes thick, cloudy, and more acidic. It also loses its stretchiness. Kits are available for purchase from the local drug store or pharmacy that react to chemicals in the cervical mucus and predict the time of ovulation. The kits are inexpensive and simple to use, much like home pregnancy tests.

HORMONAL METHODS

The many forms of hormonal contraceptives are discussed following.

ORAL CONTRACEPTIVES

The "pill" has been available as a contraceptive method for many years. Since its earliest form, it has been refined and the level of hormones reduced. Oral contraceptives work by suppressing ovulation. In a sense, the body thinks it is pregnant when the pill is used. Some oral contraceptives contain estrogen and progesterone; others contain only progestins.

In response to the pseudopregnancy state, the client may experience mild side effects and discomforts often associated with pregnancy such as nausea, headache, breast tenderness, or weight gain. Major side effects from oral contraceptives may include cardiovascular accidents or thrombophlebitis.

There is approximately a 1 in 200 chance of becoming pregnant while taking the oral contraceptive. If the woman thinks that she might be pregnant, she should stop the pill immediately and contact her physician. When the woman and her partner decide that it is time for a pregnancy, she should discontinue the oral contraceptive for at least 2 to 3 cycles before having unprotected intercourse. This "rest period" will lessen the possibility that pill effects will remain in her system and will allow her body to return to its own natural rhythm. Some women find that they experience primary or secondary infertility problems after being on the pill for several years because of pituitary suppression. The remedy is often fertility drugs such as clomiphene citrate (Clomid). Women who have never established a regular pattern of menstruation may not be good candidates for oral contraceptives, except as being used to regulate the cycle by artificial means. Other clients who should not take oral contraceptives include women with a history of hypertension, diabetes, cardiovascular disease, or thrombophlebitis. Some physicians may consider oral contraceptives in the newer low-dose combinations for clients who were previously in this high-risk group.

Depo-Provera

The medroxyprogesterone acetate (Depo-Provera) injection is administered intramuscularly (IM) every 12 weeks. It works like oral contraceptives to suppress ovulation. The client may experience breakthrough bleeding after the first injection, but this is not an indication that the hormone is not working. It usually requires about 3 weeks after the first injection before the contraceptive is effective, so the client should be advised to use a barrier contraceptive method during that period. The client must receive the injections at regular intervals to ensure effectiveness. Depo-Provera is a good option for the client who is approaching her forties or who smokes because it contains only progestins, which decreases the risk of cardiovascular problems.

Lunelle

The combination of estradiol cypionate and medroxyprogesterone acetate (Lunelle) is administered by IM injection every 28 to 30 days. It suppresses ovulation, thickens cervical mucus, and thins the endometrial lining. Monthly clinic visits are necessary, or the client must learn self-injection (Akert, 2003).

Mirena

Mirena, a levonorgestrol-releasing intrauterine system device, is placed in the uterus, providing contraception for 5 years. The small, soft T-shaped polyethylene frame has a hormone reservoir on the vertical stem that slowly releases the hormone. Cervical mucus thickens, sperm migration is inhibited, and endometrial growth is reduced. Mirena must be placed and removed by a health care provider (Akert, 2003).

Transdermal Patch

This first contraceptive patch, called OrthoEvra, contains norelgestromin and ethinyl estradiol. A new patch is applied every 7 days for 3 weeks. No patch is worn for the fourth week. Skin reactions are possible at the application site. The patch adheres during exercise, swimming, and hot tub/whirlpool use. It may not be as effective if the client weighs more than 198 pounds (Akert, 2003).

Vaginal Ring

The NuvaRing contains etonogestrel and ethinyl estradiol in a nonbiodegradable, flexible, transparent ring and provides constant delivery of hormones. It is inserted into the vagina and left for 3 weeks and then removed for 1 week. Precise ring position is not critical (Akert, 2003).

NONHORMONAL METHODS

Intrauterine Device

The intrauterine device (IUD) has been used for many years and has undergone several changes. The IUD is a T-shaped device wrapped with copper wire, which acts like a spermicide. The intrauterine device is recommended for women who have had children because the cervix has been dilated. This allows for easier insertion of the device. The IUD is inserted or removed by a clinician while the client is having her period because there is slight dilation of the cervix at that time. A string attached to the distal end of the device hangs out of the cervix into the vagina. The client is instructed to check the string each month after the menstrual period to make sure the device has not been expelled. Some women with an IUD experience more dysmenorrhea and a heavier menstrual flow. The IUD lasts 10 years. Fertility returns immediately upon removal.

Barriers

Methods of barrier contraception include male and female condoms, the diaphragm, and the cervical cap. Barrier devices work by blocking the pathway of the sperm through the cervix into the uterus. This type of contraceptive requires some preplanning on the part of one or both of the partners and may reduce the spontaneity of the sex act.

Spermicides

Spermicides contain a chemical, nonoxynol-9, that kills sperm on contact. If used alone, spermicidal agents have a lower efficacy rate than if used with a condom. The nurse should advise the couple to use a spermicidal gel, foam suppository, or film in addition to another barrier method for the greatest effectiveness. Foam should not be used with the diaphragm because it can result in deterioration of the latex. These agents must be placed in the vagina at least 15 minutes before intercourse to promote the spermicidal reaction. This method is safe and inexpensive but requires a high level of compliance each time or the effectiveness of the method drops significantly.

STERILIZATION METHOD

Sterilization is considered a permanent and very effective method of contraception. In a rare incident, a woman will become pregnant after a tubal ligation or after her partner has had a vasectomy. The female procedure interrupts the pathway through the fallopian tube. Sterilization may be performed on an outpatient basis in a surgical clinic or the outpatient department at the hospital. The tubal ligation is done under a general or epidural anesthetic with laparoscopy. The procedure takes about 30 to 60 minutes. The abdomen is distended with a gas to permit better visualization of the pelvic structures during the procedure.

The male sterilization, **vasectomy** (surgical resection of the vas deferens), is usually performed with local anesthesia on an outpatient basis. Rest, with ice to the scrotum, for 4 hours should follow. The client should not engage in strenuous activity or exercise for 1 week.

It may take up to 6 weeks for the semen to be clear of sperm. The client is instructed to return to the clinic for a sperm count after 20 ejaculations. If he is sexually active, during those ejaculations he should use a condom or some other form of contraception. At 6 months, a sperm count should be repeated and then monitored annually thereafter.

The female sterilization is more expensive and, because it requires more anesthesia, carries a slightly higher risk than the male procedure.

Refined microsurgical techniques have made it possible to reverse sterilization procedures. The reversals are not always successful, and the couple need to consider the odds of success before venturing into the expense of this type of surgery.

CASE STUDY

M.A. is a 70-year-old Caucasian man with a diagnosis of benign prostatic hyperplasia. Before his hospital admission for a TURP, he had been in good health. He returned from surgery 3 hours ago with a three-way Foley catheter and continuous bladder irrigation. His vital signs 1 hour ago were as follows: temperature 98.9°F, apical pulse 68, blood pressure 130/84, and respirations 18. When the nurse enters his room to take another set of vitals, M.A. is restless and moaning and has cool, moist skin; his catheter is not draining properly. His pulse is now 120 and blood pressure is 88/50. The nurse calls the physician to report the change in M.A.'s condition. The physician orders a STAT hematocrit and a bleeding and clotting time. An increase in the IV fluid drip rate is also ordered. The doctor is planning to arrive at the hospital within the next hour.

The following questions will guide your development of a nursing care plan for the case study.

1. List symptoms and clinical manifestations, other than M.A.'s, that a client may experience after a TURP.
2. List reasons why the doctor has ordered the STAT blood work and the IV changes.
3. List other diagnostic tests that may have been ordered for M.A.
4. Mentally do a head-to-toe or functional assessment on M.A. List subjective and objective data a nurse would want to obtain.
5. Write three individualized nursing diagnoses and goals for M.A.
6. Upon assessing M.A., the doctor decides to inject additional fluid into the balloon that anchors the indwelling catheter and apply increased traction to the catheter. List pertinent nursing actions a nurse would do following these medical interventions.
   - Medications
   - Comfort/rest
   - Cardiac output
   - Intake and output
   - Activity
   - Teaching
7. List resources within the medical center and the local area that could assist M.A. with his postoperative recovery.
8. List teaching that M.A. will need before his discharge.
9. List at least three successful outcomes for M.A.

SUMMARY

- Potential complications from PID may include sterility or infertility from scarring of fallopian tubes.
- Toxic shock syndrome occurs during the menses, and a strong correlation exists between the onset and use of super-absorbent tampons.
- Common male reproductive system inflammatory disorders include epididymitis, orchitis, and prostatitis. Bilateral epididymitis and orchitis can lead to sterility. Treatment includes antibiotic therapy.
- A BSE is an important method for detecting breast changes and should be practiced each month. Breast cancer is the most common female cancer in the United States.
- Benign prostatic hyperplasia is a common disorder in males older than age 50. Early symptoms include hesitancy, decreased force of stream, urinary frequency, and nocturia.
- Cervical cancer is most common in women with multiple sexual partners.
- Endometrial cancer often produces symptoms only after it is widespread. Any unusual vaginal bleeding should be investigated, especially if it occurs after menopause.
- Male cancers related to the reproductive system involve the prostate, testes, breast, and penis. Emphasis should be placed on testicular self-examination and regular physical examinations in order to facilitate early diagnosis and treatment.
- Menstrual disorders are often associated with hormonal imbalances, increased or decreased function of the endocrine glands, or neoplasms.
- Menopause is a normal, gradual decline in the ovarian production of female hormones that occurs around age 50.
- Infertility affects at least 1 in every 8 couples in the United States and is caused by hormonal imbalances and structural or physiologic abnormalities in both male and female clients.
- Women who smoke and are older than age 40 are at greater risk for major complications while using oral contraceptives. Major health risks include cardiovascular accidents and deep vein thrombosis.
- Impotence may be caused by emotional or physical factors. Treatment includes counseling, medications, circulatory aids, and surgery.

REVIEW QUESTIONS

1. A postoperative prostatectomy client has a three-way indwelling catheter for continuous bladder irrigation. During second shift, 2,700 mL of irrigation solution was instilled. At the end of the shift, 3,250 mL of fluid was drained from the catheter collection bag. The total urine output for the shift is:
   1. 6,250 mL
   2. 3,250 mL
   3. 2,700 mL
   4. 550 mL
2. A client complains of pain and discomfort in the lower abdominal area after a suprapubic prostatectomy. The initial nursing action should be to:
   1. administer the intravenous antibiotic as ordered.
   2. inspect the drainage tube for occlusion.
   3. increase the intravenous rate.
   4. administer oxygen at 2 liter per minute per nasal cannula.
3. The nurse is teaching a female client about fibrocystic breast changes. Which of the following should be included in the teaching plan?
   1. Breast self-examination should not be performed because it will aggravate fibrocystic breasts.
   2. Caffeine and sodium intake should be limited.
   3. Wearing a bra will increase breast discomfort.
   4. Take hot showers to promote comfort.
4. The nurse is teaching a 20-year-old man how to perform a testicular self-examination. Which of the following is an abnormal finding?
   1. The right testes is larger than the left testes.
   2. The testes are slightly sensitive to compression.
   3. The testes are oval shape and movable.
   4. The left testes hangs lower than the right testes.
5. A client has been informed that her sister has been diagnosed with ovarian cancer. The client asks the nurse if she is at risk of developing this type of cancer. The nurse informs the client that risk factors associated with ovarian cancer include: (Select all that apply.)
   1. nulliparity.
   2. infertility.
   3. low-fat diet.
   4. smoking.
   5. family history.
   6. multiparity.
6. The nurse is teaching a female client about breast self-examination (BSE). Which of the following statements indicates that the client correctly understands when she should perform a BSE?
   1. "I should perform a BSE a few days before my menstrual period begins."
   2. "During the time I am ovulating is when I should do a BSE."
   3. "I should do a BSE right after my menstrual period."
   4. "I can perform a BSE anytime of the month."
7. Which nursing intervention must be included in a care plan for a 12-day post radical mastectomy client?
   1. Maintain NPO status for 24 hours.
   2. Place client on complete bed rest for 24 hours.
   3. Place commode at bedside.
   4. Elevate operative arm for 24 hours.
8. A 21-year-old female client makes an appointment with her physician to ask about beginning oral contraceptives. Which of the following questions asked by the nurse would determine if oral contraceptives are an appropriate method of contraception for this client?
   1. "Have you ever had a blood clot or deep vein thrombosis?"
   2. "Do you exercise every day?"
   3. "Are you married?"
   4. "Have you been pregnant before?"
9. What information should be included in a teaching plan for a women's health program to raise awareness of toxic shock syndrome? (Select all that apply.)
   1. Most often caused by Streptococcus group A.
   2. Hypothermia occurs due to inflammatory process.
   3. There is a strong relationship with the use of tampons.
   4. A macular erythematous rash may develop.
   5. Bed rest is usually prescribed.
   6. Hypertensive crisis is a common complication.
10. A 45-year-old male client asks the nurse why he is experiencing impotence since he started taking antihypertensive medication. The best response from the nurse is:
    1. "Antihypertensive medication lowers blood pressure to penile arteries leading to failure of the penis to fill sufficiently to achieve erection."
    2. "You should not be experiencing impotence and need to notify your physician immediately."
    3. "Impotence is only a temporary side effect and will go away within 3 weeks of taking the medication."
    4. "Antihypertensive medication only causes impotence in diabetic men that smoke."

REFERENCES/SUGGESTED READINGS

Akert, J. (2003). A new generation of contraceptives. *RN, 66*(2), 54–61.

American Cancer Society (ACS). (2003). Cancer facts & figures—2003. Retrieved from http://www.cancer.org/downloads/ STT/CFF2003DUSSecured.pdf

American Cancer Society. (2008). Breast cancer. Retrieved August 9, 2009 from http://www.cancer.org/downloads/PRO/BreastCancer.pdf

American Cancer Society. (2009a). Cancer statistics 2009 a presentation from the American Cancer Society. Retrieved August 9, 2009 from http://www.cancer.org/docroot/PRO/content/PRO_1_1_Cancer_Statistics_2009_Presentation.asp

American Cancer Society. (2009b). Detailed guide: Breast cancer—how is breast cancer staged? Retrieved August 9, 2009 from http://www.cancer.org/docroot/CRI/content/CRI_2_4_3X_How_is_breast_cancer_staged_5.asp?sitearea=

American Cancer Society. (2009c). Detailed guide: Cervical cancer—what is cervical cancer? Retrieved August 9, 2009 from http://www.cancer.org/docroot/CRI/content/CRI_2_4_1X_What_is_cervical_cancer_8.asp?sitearea=

American Cancer Society. (2009d). Detailed guide: Ovarian cancer—chemotherapy. Retrieved August 9, 2009 from http://www.cancer.org/docroot/CRI/content/CRI_2_4_4X_Chemotherapy_33.asp?rnav=cri

American Cancer Society. (2009e). Detailed guide: Prostate cancer—chemotherapy. Retrieved August 9, 2009 from http://www.cancer.org/docroot/CRI/content/CRI_2_4_4X_Chemotherapy_36.asp?rnav=cri

American Cancer Society. (2009f). Detailed guide: Prostate cancer—what are the key statistics about prostate cancer? Retrieved August 9, 2009 from http://www.cancer.org/docroot/CRI/content/CRI_2_4_1X_What_are_the_key_statistics_for_prostate_cancer_36.asp?rnav=cri

American Cancer Society. (2009g). Detailed guide: Testicular cancer—what are the key statistics about testicular cancer? Retrieved August 9, 2009 from http://www.cancer.org/docroot/CRI/content/CRI_2_4_1X_What_are_the_key_statistics_for_testicular_cancer_41.asp?sitearea=

Arbique, D., Carter, S., & Van Sell, S. (2008). Endometriosis can evade diagnosis. *RN, 71*(9), 28–32.

Aschenbrenner, D. (2006). Over-the-counter access to emergency contraception. *American Journal of Nursing, 106*(11), 34–36.

Baird, S., Donehower, M., Stalsbroten, V., & Ades, T. (Eds.). (1997). *A cancer source book for nurses* (7th ed.). Atlanta: American Cancer Society.

Carroll, C. (2006). Sorting out breast biopsy options. *Nursing2006, 36*(3), 70–71.

Centers for Disease Control and Prevention. (2008). Pelvic inflammatory disease—CDC fact sheet. Retrieved August 8, 2009 from http://www.cdc.gov/std/PID/STDFact-PID.htm#What

Choma, K. (2003). ASC-US HPV testing. *AJN, 103*(2), 42–50.

Conversations with Colleagues. (2003). Endometriosis sufferers risk other diseases. *AWHONN Lifelines, 6*(6), 502–504.

Crandall, L. (1997). Menopause made easier. *RN, 60*(7), 46–50.

D'Arcy, Y. (2002). What is postmastectomy pain syndrome? *Nursing2002, 32*(11), 17.

Daniels, R. (2010). *Delmar's guide to laboratory and diagnostic tests* (2nd ed.). Clifton Park, NY: Delmar Cengage Learning.

Daniels, R., Nosek, L. & Nicoll, L. (2007). *Contemporary medical-surgical nursing*. Clifton Park, NY: Delmar Cengage Learning.

Dell, D. (2001). Regaining range of motion after breast surgery. *Nursing2001, 31*(10), 50–52.

Estes, M. (2010). *Health assessment & physical examination*. (4th ed.). Clifton Park, NY: Delmar Cengage Learning.

Ficorelli, C., & Weeks, B. (2006). Facing up to prostate cancer. *Nursing2006, 36*(5), 66–68.

Fink, J. (2003). Beyond the shock of an abnormal Pap. *RN, 66*(6), 56–61.

Fletcher, S., & Colditz, G. (2003). Editorial: Failure of estrogen plus progestin therapy for prevention. *Journal of the American Medical Association, 288*(3). Available from http://jama.ama-assn.org/issues/v288n3/ffull/jed20042.html

Fu, M., Ridner, S., & Armor, J. (2009). Post-breast cancer lymphedema. *American Journal of Nursing, 109*(7), 48–54.

Gordon, S., Brenden, J., Wyble, J., & Ivey, C. (1997). When the Dx is penile cancer. *RN, 60*(3), 41–44.

Harris, L. (2002). Ovarian cancer: Screening for early detection. *AJN, 102*(10), 46–52.

Held-Warmkessel, J. (2002). Prostate cancer. *Nursing2002, 32*(12), 36–42.

Hurley, M. (2007). More evidence that race affects breast cancer survival. *RN*, 70(4).

Hutti, M. (2003). New & emerging contraceptive methods. *AWHONN Lifelines, 7*(1), 32–39.

Katz, A. (2007a). 'Not tonight, dear': The elusive female libido. *American Journal of Nursing*, 107(12), 32–34.

Katz, A. (2007b). When sex hurts: Menopause-related dyspareunia. *American Journal of Nursing*, 107(7), 34–39.

Katz, A. (2009). Fertility preservation in young cancer patients. *American Journal of Nursing*, 109(4), 44–47.

Kessenich, C. (1999). Myths & facts about menopause. *Nursing99, 29*(4), 67.

Kring, D. (2003). Benign prostatic hyperplasia. *Nursing2003, 33*(5), 44–45.

Lehman, M. (2007). Ovarian cancer it whispers so listen. *RN*, 70(10), 28–32.

Machia, J. (2002). Breast cancer: Risk, prevention, & tamoxifen. *AJN, 101*(4), 26–34.

Marchbanks, P., McDonald, J., Wilson, H., et al. (2002). Oral contraceptives and the risk of breast cancer. *New England Journal of Medicine, 346*(26), 2025.

Marieb, E. (2003). *Human anatomy and physiology* (6th ed.). Redwood City, CA: Benjamin/Cummings.

Martini, F. (2002). *Fundamentals of anatomy & physiology* (6th ed.). Englewood Cliffs, NJ: Prentice Hall.

Mayo Clinic. (2008a). Endometriosis treatments and drugs. Retrieved August 8, 2009 from http://www.mayoclinic.com/health/endometriosis/DS00289/DSECTION=treatments-and-drugs

Mayo Clinic. (2008b). Fibrocystic breasts lifestyle and home remedies. Retrieved August 8, 2009 from http://www.mayoclinic.com/health/fibrocystic-breasts/DS01070/DSECTION=lifestyle-and-home-remedies

McDaniel, C. (2007). Uterine fibroid embolism: the less invasive alternative. *Nursing2007, 37*(7), 26–27.

Miller, K. (1999). Testicular torsion. *AJN 99*(6), 33.

Moorhead, S., Johnson, M., Maas, M., & Swanson, E. (2007). *Nursing Outcomes Classification (NOC)* (4th ed.). St. Louis, MO: Mosby.

National Cancer Institute (NCI). (2002a). What you need to know about breast cancer (NIH Publication No. 00-1556). Retrieved from http://www.nci.nihl.gov/cancerinfo/wyntk/ breast

National Cancer Institute (NCI). (2002b). What you need to know about cancer of the cervix (NIH Publication No. 95-2047). Retrieved from http://www.nci.nih.gov/cancerinfo/wyntk/cervix

National Cancer Institute (NCI). (2002c). What you need to know about cancer of the uterus (NIH Publication No. 01-1562). Retrieved from http://www.nci.nih.gov/cancerinfo/ wyntk/uterus

National Cancer Institute (NCI). (2002d). What you need to know about ovarian cancer (NIH Publication No. 00-1561). Retrieved from http://www.nci.nih.gov/cancerinfo/wyntk/ovary

National Institute of Diabetes, and Digestive and Kidney Disease (NIDDK). (2002). Prostate enlargement: Benign prostatic hyperplasia. Retrieved from http://www.niddk.nih.gov/ health/urolog/pubs/prostate/index.htm

National Institutes of Health. (2006). Prostate enlargement: benign prostatic hyperplasia. Retrieved August 8, 2009 from http://kidney.niddk.nih.gov/kudiseases/pubs/prostateenlargement/index.htm

Neighbors, M., & Tannehill-Jones, R. (2006). *Human disease* (2nd ed). Clifton Park, NY: Delmar Cengage Learning.

North American Nursing Diagnosis Association International. (2010). *NANDA-I nursing diagnoses: Definitions and classification* 2009–2011. Ames, IA: Wiley-Blackwell.

Otto, S. (2001). *Oncology nursing* (4th ed.). St. Louis, MO: Mosby–Year Book.

Pasacreta, J., Jacobs, L., & Cataldo, J. (2002). Genetic testing for breast and ovarian cancer risk: The psychosocial issues. *AJN, 102*(12), 40–47.

Pickar, G., & Abernethy Pickar, A. (2008). *Dosage calculations* (8th ed.). Clifton Park, NY: Delmar Cengage Learning.

Resnick, B., & Belcher, A. (2002). Breast reconstruction. *AJN, 102*(4), 26–33.

Rizzo, D. (2010). *Fundamentals of anatomy & physiology* (3rd ed). Clifton Park, NY: Delmar Cengage Learning.

Sarvis, C. (2003). When lymphedema takes hold. *RN, 66*(9), 32–36.

Spratto, G., & Woods, A. (2009). *2009 PDR nurse's drug handbook.* Clifton Park, NY: Delmar Cengage Learning.

The North American Menopause Society. (2009). Hormone products for postmenopausal use in the United States and Canada. Retrieved August 9, 2009 from http://www.menopause.org/htcharts.pdf

U. S. Food and Drug Administration (FDA). (2002). Update on advisory for Norplant contraception kits. Retrieved from http//:www.fda.gov/medwatch/safety/2002/norplant.htm

Wallace, M. (2008). Assessment of sexual health in older adults using the PLISSIT model to talk about sex. *American Journal of Nursing, 108*(7), 52–60.

Walter, L., Bertenthal, D., et al. (2006). PSA screening among elderly men with limited life expectancies. *Journal of American Medical Association, 296*(19), 2336.

Workman, L. (2002). Breast cancer. *Nursing2002, 32*(10), 58–63.

Wynd, C. (2002). Testicular self-examination in young adult men. *Journal of Nursing Scholarship, 34*(3), 251–255.

Zaccognini, M. (1999). Prostate cancer, *AJN, 99*(4), 34–35.

Zuckerman, D. (2002). The breast cancer information gap. *RN, 65*(2), 39–41.

RESOURCES

American Association of Sex Educators, Counselors, and Therapists, http://www.aasect.org

American Cancer Society, Inc., http://www.cancer.org

American College of Obstetricians and Gynecologists (ACOG), http://www.acog.org

American Society of Reproductive Medicine, http://www.asrm.org

Association of Women's Health, Obstetric, and Neonatal Nurses (AWHONN), http://www.awhonn.org

Breast Cancer Network of Strength, http://www.networkofstrength.org

National Cancer Institute (NCI), http://www.cancer.gov

National Ovarian Cancer Coalition, http://www.ovarian.org

North American Menopause Society (NAMS), http://www.menopause.org

Older Women's League, http://www.owl-national.org

Ovarian Cancer National Alliance, http://www.ovariancancer.org

RESOLVE: The National Infertility Association, http://www.resolve.org

CHAPTER 14
Sexually Transmitted Infections

MAKING THE CONNECTION

Refer to the following chapters to increase your understanding of sexually transmitted infections:

Adult Health Nursing

- ***Reproductive System***
- ***Immune System***

LEARNING OBJECTIVES

Upon completion of this chapter, you should be able to:

- Define key terms.
- List the most prevalent STIs, including causative agents.
- Describe currently used methods of prevention of STIs.
- Describe signs and symptoms, diagnostic aids, and treatment of the common STIs.
- Utilize the nursing process to plan the care of a client with an STI.
- Demonstrate the ability to teach self-care and reinfection prevention measures to the client with an STI.

KEY TERMS

abstinence
asymptomatic
chancre
exposure
incidence
incubation period

INTRODUCTION

Sexually transmitted infections (STIs) are transmitted or passed from one person to another primarily through sexual contact. The STIs covered in this chapter are chlamydia, gonorrhea, syphilis, genital herpes, cytomegalovirus, genital warts, trichomoniasis, and hepatitis B. Acquired immunodeficiency syndrome (AIDS) is not solely an STI, although sexual activity is one of the primary modes of transmission. AIDS is discussed in detail in Chapter 16 and will be briefly discussed here.

The **incidence** (frequency of disease occurrence) of STIs has been increasing worldwide, with chlamydia and gonorrhea being the most widespread STIs today. Syphilis has been described as an STI for centuries. An estimated 19 million Americans are diagnosed annually with an STI (CDC, 2007). Almost half of the newly diagnosed infections are among young people who are 15 to 24 years of age. Chlamydia remains to be the most commonly reported STI with approximately 2.8 million new cases infecting Americans every year. Gonorrhea is the second most commonly reported STI in the United States, infecting an estimated 700,000 people (Mayo Clinic, 2009a). Syphilis, although less common than either chlamydia or gonorrhea, has seen a 17.5% increase from 2006 to 2007 in the United States (CDC, 2007a).

The development of antibiotic treatment for STIs in the 1940s caused a dramatic decrease in the prevalence of STIs, and for awhile, it was predicted that STIs would be eradicated completely. However, a variety of factors have contributed to the dramatic increase of STIs, such as casual sex, asymptomatic carriers of the disease, the use of nonbarrier methods of birth control, and lack of knowledge of methods of preventing STIs.

Another factor that has contributed to the vast increase in STIs in recent years is the increased consumption of alcohol and the use of illegal drugs. The sharing of needles among intravenous (IV) drug abusers is a factor in the increased incidence of STIs, as is the lessening of inhibitions that occurs with drug and alcohol abuse. The trading of sex for drugs is also a factor in the spread of STIs.

Inadequate reporting of STIs may also cause statistics to be inaccurate. There is no uniformity in reporting requirements for STIs. Regulations differ from state to state and from disease to disease. Health-care providers are required to report new cases of chlamydia, gonorrhea, syphilis, and hepatitis to state health departments and the CDC (Freedom Network, 2009). The Centers for Disease Control and Prevention (CDC) keeps statistics on reportable diseases.

Public education regarding the causes, methods of transmission, and methods of prevention of STIs is the most important weapon in the battle against STIs. Although many STIs caused by bacterial infection are curable with modern antibiotics, the viruses are not. The CDC (2007a) estimates that STIs cost the U.S. health-care system $15.3 billion annually.

Because sexual activity is beginning at earlier ages today, sex education, including information about STIs, is being presented in elementary schools. Many schools have comprehensive education programs already in place to teach about STIs and recommendations to prevent the spread of STIs. Television, especially educational programs, has been helpful in informing the public of the dangers of having sex without protection against STIs.

Many messages have been disseminated to the general public regarding the best methods of prevention of STIs. The only 100% effective method of prevention of STIs is **abstinence** (refraining from sexual intercourse or mucous membrane–to–mucous membrane contact altogether). Couples who are mutually monogamous are also not at risk, unless one of them was previously infected. The popularity of the birth control pill has decreased consistent condom use. Most current methods of birth control are not effective in preventing the transmission of STIs. Only a barrier method, such as the latex condom, has been effective in preventing the spread of STIs, although even this method provides only safer sex, not completely safe sex.

Once the diagnosis of an STI is made, identification of all sexual contacts is important. Many people are reluctant to be candid regarding sexual activity and sexual contacts because this is an area of life considered to be extremely private. One of the most difficult aspects in dealing with STIs is that many of the diseases are asymptomatic, especially in women. These asymptomatic partners can both transmit the disease to new partners and/or reinfect a treated partner, if they are not identified and treated.

An overview of the STIs covered in this chapter is presented in Table 14-1.

ANATOMY AND PHYSIOLOGY REVIEW

The major system affected by STIs is the reproductive system. Males are generally more symptomatic than females and will seek health care more readily because the signs of disease on the external genitalia are more visible. In females, the sex organs are internal; females, therefore, are more likely to have complications and increased severity of symptoms by the time the disease is identified.

In addition to the reproductive system, any area of sexual contact, such as oral and rectal areas, may also exhibit signs and symptoms of the disease process.

COMMON DIAGNOSTIC TESTS

Commonly used diagnostic tests for clients with symptoms of STIs are listed in Table 14-2.

CHLAMYDIA

Chlamydia is caused by a spherical bacterial organism known as *Chlamydia trachomatis*. Outside the body, the organism has difficulty surviving, but inside the body, chlamydia reproduces rapidly. The mode of transmission in chlamydia must be through intimate body contact because the organism is so fragile that it cannot survive long when outside of the body.

Because nearly 50% of chlamydia infections are **asymptomatic**, having no symptoms at all, it is known as the "silent STI" and usually goes untreated (Freedom Network, 2009). If left untreated, chlamydial infections cause tissue inflammation, ulceration, and scar tissue formation in both women and men. Salpingitis (inflammation of the fallopian tubes) or pelvic inflammatory disease (PID) can lead to scarring of the delicate fallopian tubes, ectopic pregnancy, or even infertility.

TABLE 14-1 Sexually Transmitted Infections: An Overview

DISEASE	CHARACTERISTICS	NURSING IMPLICATIONS
Chlamydia	Asymptomatic or may experience purulent discharge Painful urination Urethral discharge *Note:* If untreated, pelvic inflammatory disease (PID) can develop	Instruct client to notify sexual partner(s) of past 2 months of their need for treatment. Instruct client to avoid sexual activity or to use condoms until both client and partner(s) are symptom free. Provide instruction regarding medications prescribed.
Cytomegalovirus (CMV) (Human herpesvirus type 5 [HHV-5])	Often asymptomatic, occasionally fever, fatigue, and weakness Generally acquired during childhood or adolescence 50% to 80% of adults have antibodies to CMV by age 40	Implicated in some spontaneous abortions or mental retardation. Congenital infection produces cytomegalic inclusion disease. May be life threatening in a client with a poorly functioning immune system.
Genital Herpes: Herpes Simplex Virus 2 (HSV-2) (Human herpes-virus type 2 [HHV-2])	Vesicles on penis, vagina, labia, perineum, or anus Can progress to painful ulceration Lesions may last up to 6 weeks Recurrence common *Note:* May be asymptomatic	Refer sexual partner(s) for examination. Teach that virus can be transmitted even when the person experiences no symptoms. Instruct in use of condoms. Teach females of the need for annual Pap smears. Provide instruction regarding medications prescribed.
Gonorrhea	*Male:* Urethritis (inflammation of the urethra) Purulent discharge Urinary frequency Epididymitis (inflammation of the epididymis) *Female:* Often asymptomatic May lead to PID or salpingitis (inflammation of the fallopian tube) Can occlude the fallopian tubes, resulting in sterility	Instruct client to return if symptoms persist. Sexual partner(s) of past 60 days must be assessed. Instruct client to avoid sexual activity until symptoms subside in both client and partner(s). Provide instruction regarding medications prescribed.
Hepatitis B Virus (HBV)	Varies greatly from asymptomatic state, to severe hepatitis, to cancer	Partner(s) should receive medical prophylaxis within 14 days after exposure. For client and partner(s), recommend three-dose immunization series when this episode has abated.
Genital Warts (Human Papillomavirus) (HPV)	Fleshy, cauliflower-like growth on genitalia	Inform and treat sexual partner(s). Provide instruction regarding medications prescribed.

(*Continues*)

Table 14-1 Sexually Transmitted Infections: An Overview (Continued)

DISEASE	CHARACTERISTICS	NURSING IMPLICATIONS
Syphilis	Disease consists of four stages with distinct manifestations as follows:	Interview client to identify sexual contacts.
	Primary:	
	A painless papule on penis, vagina, or cervix (chancre)	All those exposed to the disease should be given penicillin or other antibiotic if allergic to penicillin.
	Usually negative serologic blood test	
	Highly infectious during this stage	
	Secondary:	
	Rash, especially prevalent on palms and soles	Educate client and sexual contacts about the disease.
	Low-grade fever	Provide instruction regarding medications prescribed.
	Sore throat	
	Headache	
	Early latency:	
	Possible infectious lesions, otherwise asymptomatic	Counsel and educate client.
	Reactive serologic tests	
	Late latency:	
	Possible lesions in central nervous and cardiovascular systems	Counsel and educate client.
	Noninfectious except to fetus of pregnant woman	
Trichomoniasis	Petechial lesions	Treat sexual partners simultaneously with metronidazole (Flagyl).
	Profuse urethral or vaginal discharge that is foul smelling, yellow, and foamy	Provide instruction regarding medication prescribed.

When symptoms of chlamydia appear in men, they include dysuria; watery white, cloudy discharge from the urethra; and testicular pain and swelling. Women may have grayish white mucopurulent vaginal drainage, bleeding between periods, dysuria, low abdominal pain, and bleeding or pain during or after sexual intercourse.

Medical–Surgical Management

Pharmacological

The treatment of choice is doxycycline (Vibramycin). If compliance with an extended period of drug therapy is thought to be a problem, azithromycin (Zithromax) can be given orally in a single dose. Pregnant women may be treated with erythromycin estolate (Ilosone) or amoxicillin (Amoxil), but they should be cultured again after treatment is completed to confirm the absence of chlamydial infection. Retesting is not required after treatment with doxycycline or azithromycin. It is important that all sexual partners are tested and treated for chlamydia because reinfection is probable if only one partner is treated.

Health Promotion

Persons who have more than one sexual partner, especially women less than 25 years old, should regularly be tested for chlamydial infection even when there are no symptoms. The current use of male latex condoms during sexual intercourse may help reduce transmission.

GONORRHEA

Gonorrheal infections are often seen in combination with chlamydia. Gonorrhea is a serious bacterial infection, caused by the gram-negative bacterial organism *Neisseria gonorrhea*. In 2007, more than 350,000 cases occurred in the United States (CDC, 2007a). The organism multiplies

Table 14-2 Common Diagnostic Tests for STIs

Blood Tests
- Enzyme immunoassay (EIA) (rapid test)
- Western Blot
- Venereal Disease Research Laboratories (VDRL)
- Rapid plasma reagin (RPR)
- Fluorescent treponemal antibody-absorption test (FTA-ABS)
- Reiter test
- Antigen test for HSV

Culture
- Tissue: Male urethra, female endocervix
- Discharge—swab test
- Tzanck
- Nucleic Acid Amplification Test (NAAT)

Urine
- Urine specimen
- NAAT

Other
- Dark field examination of wart screenings
- Microscopic examination
- OSOM Trichomonas rapid test
- Immunofloresence testing

COURTESY OF DELMAR CENGAGE LEARNING

quickly in warm, moist areas of the body, including the oral cavity, reproductive tract, and rectum. Mouth-to-mouth kissing does not transmit gonorrhea. It is spread during sexual intercourse—vaginal, oral, and anal. The cervix is the usual site of infection in women. The disease progresses in much the same manner as chlamydia and can cause many of the same complications, such as infertility from salpingitis and PID.

Symptoms of infection may occur within 2 to 10 days after **exposure** (contact with an infected person or agent). Men are more likely to exhibit symptoms such as white, yellow, or green thick discharge from the tip of the penis (Figure 14-1), swelling of the testicles and prostate gland, dysuria, and anal irritation and discharge. Many women are asymptomatic, but the remainder may have pain or burning on urination and/or a yellow or bloody vaginal discharge.

If a woman is infected with gonorrhea when she gives birth, the infection may be transmitted to the newborn's eyes as the baby travels through the birth canal. In the United States, all infants are treated with an antibiotic ophthalmic

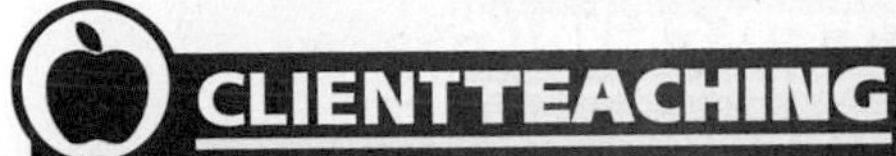

CLIENT TEACHING

Proper Use of Condoms

No method of barrier birth control works perfectly to protect against STIs. Therefore, the client should be educated regarding the proper use of both male and female condoms.

- Aside from abstinence, condoms provide the most protection against STIs by preventing mucous membrane contact.
- Clients should be advised to use condoms for every sexual encounter.
- Latex sheaths are available to prevent oral-genital mucous membrane contact.
- The client should be instructed to store condoms in a cool, dry place, away from sunlight.
- A new condom must be used for each sexual encounter; condoms cannot be reused.
- Proper condom disposal includes holding the condom at the base of the penile shaft after ejaculation so that the condom does not slip out of place.

CRITICAL THINKING

Chlamydia Treatment

1. Your client has been prescribed doxycycline for treatment of chlamydia. What precautions will the nurse include with the prescription?
2. The client asks you if she needs to continue taking the medication even though she no longer has any STI symptoms. What will the nurse tell her?
3. The client asks if she can continue to engage in sexual activity with her boyfriend while she is taking the antibiotic. What will the nurse recommend?

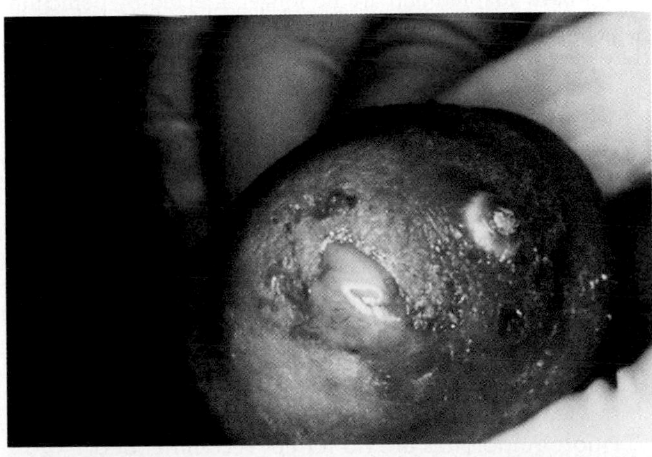

Figure 14-1 Male clients with gonorrhea exhibit purulent discharge from the penis. (*Courtesy of Centers for Disease Control and Prevention.*)

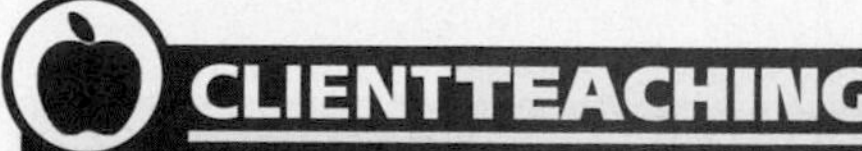

Reducing Your Risk

- Practice abstinence or mutual monogamy.
- The best method is to use latex condoms at the beginning of vaginal and/or anal sex until there is no longer skin contact.
- Water-based spermicides are not recommended for the prevention of gonorrhea.
- Recent studies have shown that nonoxynol-9 is not effective in preventing gonorrhea (American Social Health Association [ASHA], 2009).
- Do not share sex toys.
- You cannot catch gonorrhea from sharing toilet seats or sharing towels.
- Several barrier methods can be used to reduce the risk of transmission of gonorrhea during oral sex.
  - A nonlubricated condom can be used for mouth-to-penis contact.
  - A dental dam or food plastic wrap can be used during mouth-to vulva/vaginal or oral-anal (rimming) contact.

(ASHA, 2009; Freedom Network, 2009)

ointment at birth to prevent the gonorrheal-induced eye infection known as ophthalmia neonatorum.

Medical–Surgical Management

Once the presence of gonorrhea has been confirmed, both partners should be treated with a course of antibiotic therapy. Penicillin used to be the drug of choice when treating gonorrhea, but because penicillin has been so widely used against many types of infection, some strains of *Neisseria gonorrhea* have adapted and are no longer affected by penicillin. The current practice is to treat all cases of gonorrhea as though they were resistant to the traditional drug therapies.

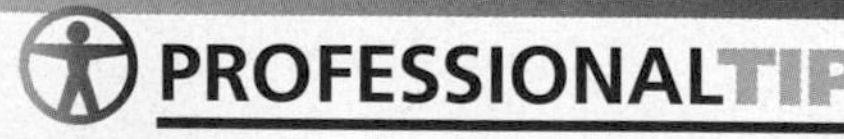

Antibiotic Resistance

In 2007, the CDC revised its gonorrhea treatment guidelines based on data indicating widespread drug resistance to fluoroquinolones, which were the leading antibiotic class to treat gonorrhea. Fluoroquinolones are no longer recommended to treat gonorrhea. Cephalosporins are now the antibiotic choice for treatment.

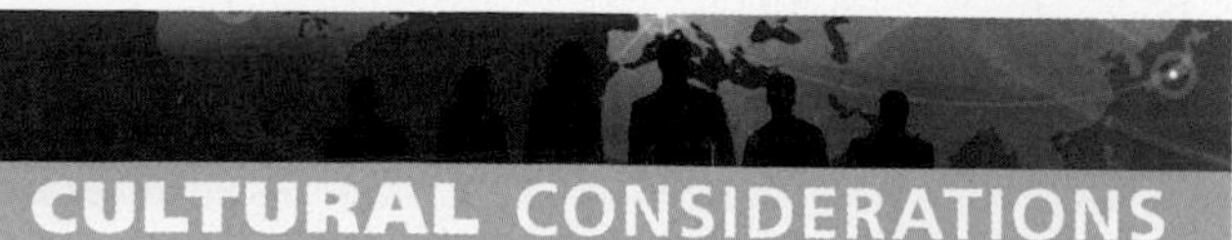

CULTURAL CONSIDERATIONS

Gonorrhea

Traditionally, ethnic minorities in the United States have had greater rates of reported gonorrhea and other STIs—in part, a reflection of limited access to quality health care. African-American subjects are most widely affected by gonorrhea, with a rate of infection approximately 19 times greater than that of Caucasian subjects. American Indians/Alaska Natives had the second highest gonorrhea rate in 2007, followed by Hispanics. Asians/Pacific Islanders had the lowest rates of gonorrhea (CDC, 2007b).

Pharmacological

A variety of antibiotics are effective against gonorrhea. One of the most effective therapies includes a single dose of ciprofloxacin (Cipro), followed by a 7-day course of oral doxycycline (Vibramycin). Because almost half of all clients with gonorrhea also have chlamydia, doxycycline (Vibramycin) is an appropriate choice of drug therapy because it combats both infections effectively. For pregnant clients, or those younger than 16 years of age, an injection of ceftriaxone sodium (Rocephlin), followed by oral erythromycin estolate (Ilosone), is recommended. Follow-up cultures to determine the success of the course of treatment are recommended when the treatment has been completed.

SYPHILIS

Syphilis, an STI that was almost eradicated after the discovery of antibiotic therapy in the 1940s, is on the upswing again, with 11,466 cases reported in 2007, a 15.2 % increase from 2006 (CDC, 2007a). The causative organism of syphilis is a spirochete, a spiral-shaped bacterium known as *Treponema pallidum,* which was first identified in 1905. Transmission of syphilis is either through sexual contact or congenitally (mother to child). Syphilis is often seen with human immunodeficiency virus (HIV) infection, just as chlamydia is often seen with gonorrhea.

Syphilis has four stages. In primary stage syphilis, the **incubation period**, time between exposure to an infectious disease and the first appearance of symptoms, can be 10 to 90 days with the development of a chancre usually occurring within 2 to 6 weeks. A **chancre** is a clean, painless ulcer that usually is present at the site of body contact (Figure 14-2). There is usually just one chancre present, but multiple chancres have been known to occur. Chancres may occur on the internal genitalia of women (e.g., the cervix) and thus not be noticed. The chancre will heal within a few weeks, even without treatment, and either leave a thin scar or none at all. If not identified and treated, about one-third will progress to secondary syphilis.

In secondary syphilis, the client has a skin rash of penny-sized brown sores that appear approximately 3 to 6 weeks after the chancre. The rash may be on all or any part of the body but almost always involves the palms of the hands and the soles of

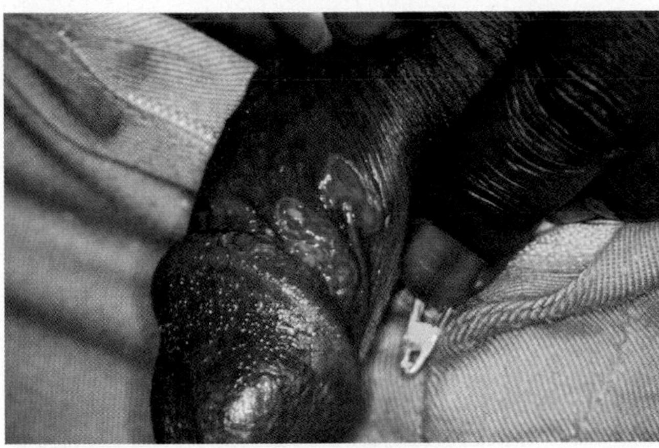

FIGURE 14-2 The primary stage of syphilis is usually marked by the appearance of a single sore called a chancre. (*Courtesy of Centers for Disease Control and Prevention.*)

the feet. Active bacteria are in the sores, so any contact, sexual or nonsexual, with the broken skin of the infected person may spread the infection. The rash heals within several months. Other symptoms, such as low-grade fever, fatigue, headache, sore throat, and generalized lymph node swelling, may occur. Occasionally, a wart-like growth known as condyloma latum may be present in the genital area of both men and women. Because this growth is so close in appearance to the condylomata acuminata of human papillomavirus infection, it may be confused with genital warts. Symptoms of secondary syphilis may come and go for 1 or 2 years. Because many of these symptoms are also common to many other diseases, syphilis has often been called "the great imitator."

When not treated, syphilis enters into a latent period when no symptoms are present and the disease is no longer contagious. Only approximately one-third of those clients with secondary syphilis will develop the symptoms of tertiary syphilis, that is, when the bacteria damages the heart, eyes, brain, nervous system, bones, joints, or any other part of the body. Tertiary syphilis can last for years or decades and may result in heart disease, blindness, neurologic problems, and death.

Medical–Surgical Management

Pharmacological

Since the time that syphilis was first treated with antibiotic therapy, penicillin has remained the drug of choice because

> **MEMORYTRICK**
> **RASH**
>
> A useful memory trick to use when assessing a client for signs and symptoms of syphilis is **RASH**:
>
> **R** = Rash (on palms and soles)
> **A** = A painless papule (on penis, vagina, or cervix)
> **S** = Sore throat
> **H** = Headache

> **CLIENTTEACHING**
> **Testing for Syphilis**
>
> - According to the CDC (2007a), regular screening of men who have sex with men (MSM), is an important step toward preventing the spread of syphilis.
> - Pregnant women being screened at their first prenatal visit is critical in protecting infants from congenital syphilis complications such as blindness.

no cases of penicillin-resistant syphilis have been identified. All types of penicillin are effective, but penicillin G benzathine (Bicillin L-A) is often preferred. Antimicrobial therapy will destroy Treponema pallidum at any stage, but any damage done to body organs is irreversible. If the client has a demonstrated allergy to penicillin, alternative medications may be administered, such as doxycycline (Vibramycin), tetracycline HCl (Achromycin V), or erythromycin estolate (Ilosone). For pregnant women who are allergic to penicillin, erythromycin is recommended as the best alternative therapy.

Clients being treated for syphilis must have periodic blood tests to ensure that the infecting agent has been completely destroyed.

GENITAL HERPES

Genital herpes affects an estimated 45 million persons in the United States. (1 out of 5 adolescents and adults) (CDC, 2009). It is caused by the human herpesvirus type 2, commonly called the herpes simplex virus (HSV-2). HSV-1 commonly causes sores on the lips (fever blisters, cold sores). HSV-2 causes genital sores. Either can infect the other area following oral-genital sex. Genital herpes is usually acquired through sexual contact with an infected person. That person may or may not be aware of having genital herpes.

When symptoms occur in the first episode, they usually appear in 2 to 10 days after infection and last an average of 2 to 3 weeks. Itching or burning sensations; pain in the genital area, legs, or buttocks; vaginal discharge; or abdominal pressure are the early symptoms. Within a few days, lesions (sores) appear at the infection site (perianal area), in the vagina or on the cervix of women, or in the urethra of women and men.

Small red bumps appear first, change into blisters (Figure 14-3), and then become open sores that crust over in a few days. Other symptoms with the first episode may include fever, muscle aches, headache, dysuria, vaginal discharge, and swollen glands in the groin.

With the first episode, the virus travels through the sensory nerves and remains inactive in nerve cells until the virus travels back to the skin, causing a recurrence. The frequency of recurrences vary greatly (some only 1 or 2 a year), but new sores may or may not be apparent. Symptoms are usually milder than the first episode and last approximately 1 week.

The most accurate method of diagnosis is a viral culture, which takes several days. A blood test detecting HSV antibodies only indicates that the person has been infected at some time.

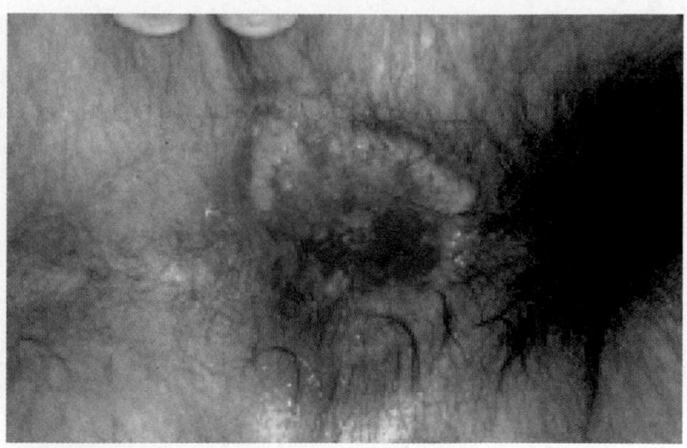

FIGURE 14-3 Chronic Mucocutaneous Perianal Herpes Infection (*Courtesy of Centers for Disease Control and Prevention.*)

MEDICAL–SURGICAL MANAGEMENT

Pharmacological

There is no known cure for the herpes simplex virus at this time. Treatment has been geared toward alleviating symptoms of the disease. Acyclovir (Zovirax) has been used in the treatment of herpes. A topical form may be applied to the lesions; the drug may also be taken orally to shorten the duration of the lesions in a primary outbreak. When taken daily, it prevents most recurrences. Famciclovir (Famivir) and valacyclovir (Valtrex) treat later episodes and prevent recurrences.

Cleansing the area of the lesions with mild soap and water, hydrogen peroxide, or Burow's solution often helps reduce the discomfort of the lesions and decrease the chance of secondary infections. The area should be blown dry with a hairdryer, and then the dry skin may be dusted with a cornstarch powder, which aids in decreasing client discomfort.

CYTOMEGALOVIRUS

Another virus in the herpes virus family is cytomegalovirus (CMV). Unlike the more commonly recognized herpes viruses, CMV rarely produces noticeable clinical symptoms.

CMV is primarily transmitted from person to person through contact with body fluids such as saliva, breast milk, urine, and blood. The virus has been identified in semen, vaginal fluids, and cervical mucus, so it can be spread by sexual contact. CMV is incurable; people are infected for life. The inactive virus may reactivate from time to time.

Most people acquire CMV during childhood or adolescence through contact with saliva and respiratory secretions and will not notice any symptoms. Occasionally, a client will present with fever, fatigue, and weakness. These symptoms may persist for several weeks and may lead to a tentative diagnosis of infectious mononucleosis, although the sore throat and swollen lymph nodes of "mono" are not present with CMV.

CMV has been implicated in some complications of pregnancy, such as spontaneous abortion or mental retardation of the neonate. Congenital infection of an infant produces cytomegalic inclusion disease that ranges from an asymptomatic condition to a severely debilitating condition that may even result in death. The central nervous system damage to the infant may be profound, although it rarely occurs. An estimated 8,000 children each year will suffer permanent disabilities caused by CMV such as mental retardation, blindness, deafness, or epilepsy (CDC, 2008a). CMV can also become a life-threatening illness in a client who has a poorly functioning immune system, such as a client with AIDS.

There is no antiviral agent specifically utilized for this disorder because most of the population will not have any symptoms.

> **PROFESSIONALTIP**
>
> **Client Support**
>
> The client may need emotional support, since the diagnosis of herpes means lifelong management. The disease will not be cured after a course of antiviral medication, and the client must thoroughly understand this fact. The client may be referred to a counselor or to a support group such as HELP at the Herpes Resource Center (ASHA, 2009a).

HUMAN PAPILLOMAVIRUS/ GENITAL WARTS

Another virus that is sexually transmitted is the human papillomavirus (HPV), which causes genital warts, also called condylomata acuminata. Genital warts may occur in the urogenital, perineal, or anal areas and may be either external or internal. The population at risk seems to be teenage girls or young women in their twenties. In the United States, it is estimated that there are approximately 25,000 new cases of HPV identified every year, and at least 20 million people are already infected (National Institutes of Health, 2008). The incubation period for genital warts appears to be approximately 1 to 2 months but may be up to 6 months. Unlike genital herpes, genital warts are usually painless, soft fleshy growths appearing most commonly in the genital area. Sometimes many warts may grow together to form a large cauliflower-shaped growth (Figure 14-4).

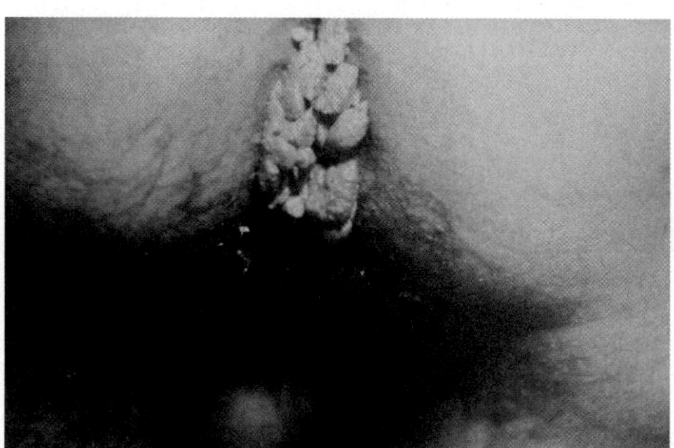

FIGURE 14-4 Genital warts (*Condylomata acuminate*) are caused by human papillomavirus (HPV), which presents as bumps or warts on the genitalia and within the perineal region. (*Courtesy of Centers for Disease Control and Prevention.*)

The greatest health threat that HPV poses to a female client is the potential development of cervical cancer. Although there are more than 100 different types of HPV, only 30 types are spread through sexual contact, and some of these can cause cervical cancer. Cigarette smoking has been linked to the development of cancerous cervical changes in women with HPV. Women who have HPV should be advised not to smoke. HPV appears to play a role in the development of cervical cancer, along with many other factors. An abnormal Pap test may be the first indication of HPV.

Genital warts are less common in men. If seen, they are usually on the tip of the penis or anal area.

Medical–Surgical Management

Because genital warts are caused by a virus, there is no cure for the disease. The focus is on preventing the spread of the disease to sexual partners and reducing the possibility of cancer. Use of a condom during sexual intercourse may provide some protection. Once the genital warts disappear, the disease may lie dormant for many years until there is a recurrence of the outbreak.

Surgical

The warts may be removed under local anesthesia. This is especially recommended if the warts have formed a large, fleshy cauliflower-like growth. Freezing the warts off with cryosurgery, surgical use of extreme cold, is the treatment of choice for small warts. The warts may also be removed with laser surgery or cauterized. Whatever treatment is recommended, it must be remembered that the treatment will not cure HPV, but only provide a palliative effect. The warts may recur after any treatment.

Pharmacological

A topical solution of podophyllum resin (Poddoen) may be applied to the genital warts. It is only recommended for treatment of one or two lesions at a time because it can be toxic if applied to too large an area at one time. Most people report experiencing a good deal of pain from the treatment. After the solution has been in contact with the genital warts for a period of 4 to 6 hours, it is then washed off with soap and water. If not thoroughly washed off, podophyllum may cause chemical burns that heal very slowly and are very painful. This therapy must not be used on a diabetic client, a client with poor circulation, or a pregnant client.

A cream, imiquimod (Aldara), is applied before bedtime and washed off in the morning. It can be used 3 times a week for 16 weeks or less.

Health Promotion

There is currently a vaccine (Gardasil) available that can protect females from the four types of HPV that cause the majority of cervical cancers and genital warts. The vaccine is recommended for females 11 to 26 years of age. The immunization schedule for the vaccine includes a series of three intramuscular injections. There are no vaccines available at this time for males. Studies are currently being conducted to find out if the vaccine is safe for females and effective in males.

AIDS

AIDS, or acquired immunodeficiency syndrome, is not truly an STI, but it needs to be discussed briefly here because sexual contact is one of the primary modes of its transmission. AIDS is the end stage of the disease process caused by the human immunodeficiency virus (HIV) (Chapter 16). Similar to the viruses previously discussed in this chapter, AIDS is not curable. Unlike the other viruses, herpes genitalis and genital warts, AIDS is ultimately fatal. AIDS results in a severe disorder of the body's immune system, leading to an inability of the body to fight off disease.

Persons at risk are those who have multiple sexual partners, IV drug users who share needles, and persons with hemophilia. There are three basic modes of transmission: sexual, bloodborne, and from mother to baby either prenatally, during the birth process, or when breastfeeding. When first identified in 1981, HIV infection was primarily found among homosexual men, but by 1990, the disease was moving into heterosexual populations with great rapidity. By the mid-1990s, cases of AIDS were occurring more frequently among women than among men. The greatest growth in AIDS rates among women occurred in African-American and Hispanic women. Teenagers also have one of the fastest growing rates of HIV infection.

The CDC's HIV/AIDS surveillance system is the nation's source for current information and statistics, tracking the epidemic, and collecting, analyzing, interpreting, and evaluating data regarding HIV/AIDS. The CDC also conducts research studies to find new treatment options and potential vaccines (Figure 14-5). It is estimated that 1.1 million

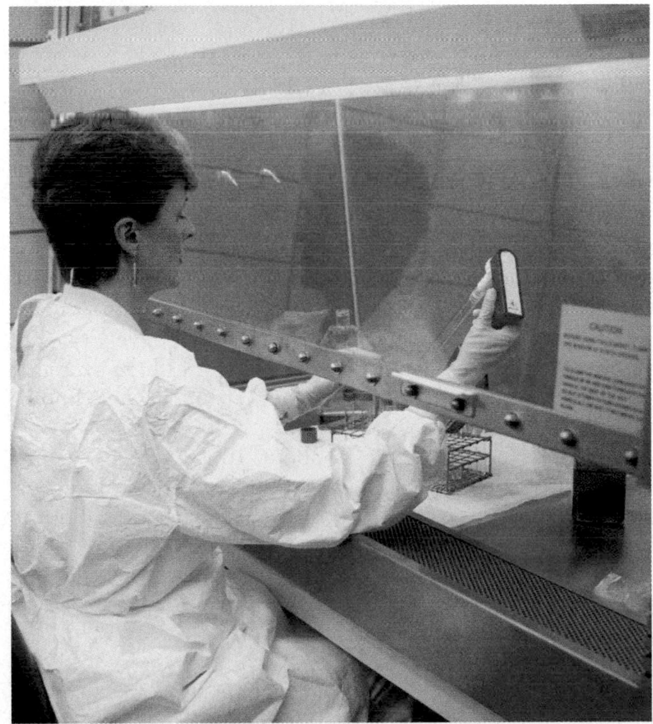

FIGURE 14-5 **Since the beginning of the AIDS epidemic, the CDC has been at the forefront of HIV investigation and lab research.** (*Courtesy of Centers for Disease Control and Prevention.*)

Americans are living with HIV and 33.2 million persons worldwide. Two-thirds of HIV infections are in sub-Saharan Africa (CDC, 2008c; WHO, 2009).

TRICHOMONIASIS

Trichomoniasis is caused by a parasitic protozoan called *Trichomonas vaginalis*. Trichomoniasis is a very common STI with an incidence of approximately 8 million new cases a year (CDC, 2008b). It is seen frequently in combination with gonorrhea. The most common method of transmission is sexual, although the protozoa can survive for a period of time in water, so other modes of transmission are possible.

The incubation period after initial exposure to trichomoniasis ranges from approximately 4 to 20 days. About 25% of women infected with trichomoniasis will have no symptoms, and men almost never have symptoms. In these clients, the *Trichomonas* organisms may remain dormant for years without becoming an active infection. Precipitating factors that may encourage the growth of *Trichomonas* include pregnancy, sexual intercourse, menstruation, or illness. Vulval and vaginal pruritus are the most common symptoms, with a vaginal discharge of a frothy, copious yellow-green mucus. Only 10% of women will present with the classic symptoms of a *Trichomonas* infection: severe itching of the vulva, redness, swelling of the vulva, pain on intercourse and urination, urinary frequency, a grayish, malodorous discharge, and the appearance of a "strawberry cervix" caused by hemorrhages with accompanying papules and vesicles. Men most often have a watery, whitish discharge and difficult or painful urination, but they may also have urethritis and an accompanying inflammation. In men, *Trichomonas* in the dormant state are usually harbored in the prostate or urethra.

MEDICAL–SURGICAL MANAGEMENT

Pharmacological

Both partners should be treated with metronidazole (Flagyl or Protostat) given either orally in a single dose or for a period of approximately 1 week. Metronidazole is effective against both protozoal and bacterial infections. If given vaginally, metronidazole (Flagyl) is not as effective. Pregnant women are usually treated after the first trimester to avoid the possibility of birth defects, because metronidazole is known to cross the placenta.

Adverse effects occur in about 10% of clients taking metronidazole (Flagyl) and usually affect the gastrointestinal system in the form of nausea, vomiting, diarrhea, and abdominal cramping. CNS effects such as headache or dizziness may also be seen.

> **CLIENT TEACHING**
>
> **Metronidazole (Flagyl or Protostat)**
>
> No alcohol should be consumed when taking this drug because it causes severe nausea and vomiting, flushing, palpitations, abdominal cramps, and headache (Cleveland Clinic, 2009).

HEPATITIS B

Hepatitis B, caused by the hepatitis B virus, is now recognized as an STI. Today, it is primarily transmitted through direct contact with blood, vaginal secretions, and semen. In 2006, approximately 46,000 people were newly infected with HBV. An estimated 800,000 to 1.4 million Americans have chronic HBV infection (CDC, 2008e).

Clients with hepatitis B experience inflammation of the liver, anorexia, vague abdominal discomfort, nausea, vomiting, fatigue, and jaundice. Fever may be mild or absent. Symptoms may progress to chronic liver disease, hepatic cancer, hepatic failure, and death.

MEDICAL–SURGICAL MANAGEMENT

Medical

There is no specific treatment for acute HBV infection. Treatment is based on relieving symptoms. Several antiviral medications are available to treat chronic HBV infection including adefovir dipivoxil (Hepsera), peginterferon (Pegasys), lamivudine (Epivir), and entecavir (Baraclude). Interferon, another antiviral agent, helps to stop the replication of HBV.

Health Promotion

Hepatitis B has two single-antigen vaccines and three combination vaccines currently available for administration in the United States. The immunization schedule most commonly followed consists of a series of three intramuscular injections. Recommendations for immunization include all newborns, health-care workers, and high-risk groups of all ages (CDC, 2008e).

NURSING MANAGEMENT

Follow proper hand hygiene technique. Teach the client hand hygiene to be followed after using the bathroom and every time the penis, vagina, or perineal areas are touched. Provide nonjudgmental support to all clients. Encourage clients to notify past and present sexual partners of the diagnosis and the need to seek medical care. Advise client to wear loose-fitting clothes and cotton underwear for comfort.

NURSING PROCESS

The following is a general nursing process for the client with an STI.

ASSESSMENT

Subjective Data

Data to be gathered from a client who presents with a suspected STI are very similar, regardless of the actual STI. A thorough history must be obtained. A relaxed, nonjudgmental attitude will help to elicit accurate information from the client. Confidentiality and privacy are extremely important

CRITICAL THINKING

Multiple Sexual Partners

What should a client who has multiple sexual partners be taught about STIs? Make a teaching plan while keeping in mind the sensitivity of the information to be shared and the client's receptivity.

when dealing with both the history and physical examination for STIs. Gather pertinent information regarding the client's sexual orientation (homosexual, heterosexual, bisexual), any prior treatment for an STI, and the number of sexual partners that the client has had in the last 6 months.

Ask women about symptoms such as vulval or vaginal itching, vaginal discharge, pain or discomfort, skin rashes or pruritus, and any changes in the menstrual periods or other abnormal bleeding. Question men regarding the presence of symptoms such as pain or burning on urination, abnormal penile discharges, skin rashes or itching, or lesions on external genitalia. Ask both men and women about urinary frequency or discomfort and systemic symptoms such as fatigue, malaise, or sore throat. Ask homosexual men about rectal symptoms such as abnormal discharge, itching, lesions, or pain on defecation (Table 14-3).

Objective Data

Carefully assess the reproductive, gastrointestinal, and integumentary systems. Determine the presence or absence of skin rashes or lesions and abnormal discharges. Females need a speculum examination of the vagina and cervix to closely observe internal organs for changes consistent with STIs. Examine the rectal area to look for any abnormal discharge, lesions, or tenderness. Palpate inguinal lymph nodes to look for signs of infection.

LIFE SPAN CONSIDERATIONS

Sexual Activity in Older Adults

Many young nurses find it difficult to think of older adults as sexual beings. As the "baby boomers" age, however, they are becoming very assertive about living life to the fullest, which includes continuing to enjoy an active sex life. An older adult who is single may still be sexually active and engage in high-risk sexual activities. A tactful, respectful approach will allow the nurse to obtain an accurate sexual history if symptoms seem to indicate the likelihood of an STI.

TABLE 14-3 Health History Questions: STIs

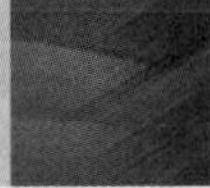

Questions for Women and Men

- Can you share with me your sexual orientation (homosexual, heterosexual, bisexual)?
- Have you been diagnosed with an STI in the past?
- If so, which STI(s) have you been diagnosed with?
- Have you been diagnosed with more than one STI? If so, which disease(s)?
- How many sexual partners have you had in the past 6 months?
- How many sexual partners have you had since you became sexually active?
- Do you have any skin rashes or itching? If so, where on your body?
- Does it burn or hurt when you urinate?
- Are you urinating more frequently than usual?
- Have you been more tired than usual?
- Do you have a sore throat?
- Have you had any sores or lesions on your lips, tongue, or in your mouth?
- Have you noticed any anal discharge or tenderness?

Questions for Women

- Have you experienced vaginal itching? Vaginal pain or discomfort?
- Are you experiencing any changes in your menstrual cycle?
- Do you have any abnormal vaginal bleeding or discharge?

Questions for Men

- Do you have any sores or lesions in your pubic area?
- Do you have any sores or lesions on your penis?
- Are you experiencing any discharge from the tip of your penis?
- Are your testicles swollen or tender?

Nursing diagnoses for the client with an STI include the following:

NURSING DIAGNOSES	PLANNING/OUTCOMES	NURSING INTERVENTIONS
Anxiety related to unknown procedures, embarrassment, or other factors (relates to nearly every client who presents with an STI)	The client will verbalize a lack of knowledge and embarrassment.	Provide a relaxed, nonjudgmental attitude which will aid in reducing client anxiety. Listen actively to both the spoken and unspoken concerns of the client. The nurse must examine own attitudes toward STIs and the clients who suffer from them.
*Deficient **Knowledge*** related to mode of transmission of the STI, prevention methods, and risk for spread of the STI	The client will accurately discuss the mode of transmission of an STI and list appropriate measures to avoid reinfection or future infection.	Teach mode of transmission, prevention of further infection, and risk for spread. Take time to make sure the client has a thorough understanding of all necessary aspects of the disease.
*Risk for **Infection*** related to incomplete treatment or lack of precautions with untreated, infected partners	The client will state the need for having all sexual partners notified and treated. The client will state understanding of the treatment regimen and of the importance of completing treatment. The client will explain appropriate use of latex condoms, including how and when to apply and remove the device.	Discuss the need for all sexual partners to be notified and treated. Discuss the importance of completing treatment regimen. Teach the importance of abstaining from sexual intercourse until the infection is resolved, or of using appropriate measures, such as latex condoms, to prevent reinfection.

Evaluation: Evaluate each outcome to determine how it has been met by the client.

SAMPLE NURSING CARE PLAN

The Client with Genital Herpes

J.B. is a single woman in her middle twenties who has been coming to the clinic for annual Pap smears and birth control for several years. She is a well-nourished, healthy-appearing young woman of medium height. She rescheduled her annual Pap smear to come into the clinic early because she noticed a cluster of small blisters on the inside of her left thigh that also involves the labia majora. She also reports that she has just gotten the flu as evidenced by headache, fever, and general achiness.

J.B. has used birth control pills in the past and reports satisfaction with this method of birth control. She reports that she and her new boyfriend became intimate about 2 weeks ago, so she wants to renew her birth control pill prescription. She also states that intercourse has been uncomfortable since the appearance of the lesions and that she does not feel comfortable with sexual activity while the lesions are present because they make her feel "ugly."

The assessment determines the presence of a cluster of small blisters as well as swollen, tender inguinal lymph nodes. A Tzanck smear test is obtained. J.B.'s test results come back positive for genital herpes.

NURSING DIAGNOSIS 1 *Ineffective **S**exuality Pattern* related to lesions as evidenced by her comment that intercourse has been uncomfortable since the appearance of the lesions

Nursing Outcomes Classification (NOC)
Psychosocial Adjustment: Life Change

Nursing Interventions Classification (NIC)
Sexual Counseling

SAMPLE NURSING CARE PLAN (Continued)

PLANNING/OUTCOMES	NURSING INTERVENTIONS	RATIONALE
J.B. will express her feelings about potential changes in her sexual behavior before leaving the clinic.	Provide a nonjudgmental atmosphere to encourage J.B. to express her feelings about this perceived change in her sexual identity.	Demonstrates the caregiver's positive feelings toward J.B. and concerns she may have regarding her future sexuality.
	Provide privacy and an uninterrupted amount of time to talk with J.B.	Shows respect and conveys reassurance in discussing sexuality issues and concerns with her.
	Provide accurate information to J.B. about genital herpes and include literature or videos for her to share with her boyfriend.	Helps J.B. focus on specific, necessary information and encourages her to ask questions.
	Offer the names of local support groups such as HELP (Herpetics Engaged in Living Productively) or other support persons who can provide information and group support to J.B.	Provides J.B. with resources for support once she has returned home and the reality of her diagnosis has set in.

EVALUATION

J.B. states that she is still in shock but thinks that she will be able to deal with her diagnosis. She also states that she will call back to the clinic in a few days with more questions after she has assimilated some of the information.

NURSING DIAGNOSIS 2 *Anxiety* related to threatened sexual identity, as evidenced by her comment that she is not comfortable with sexual activity while the lesions are present because they make her feel "ugly"

Nursing Outcomes Classification (NOC)
Acceptance: Health Status

Nursing Interventions Classification (NIC)
Teaching: Individual

PLANNING/OUTCOMES	NURSING INTERVENTIONS	RATIONALE
J.B. will be able to express feelings of anxiety and identify support systems to help her cope with these feelings before leaving the clinic.	Explain any procedures clearly and concisely before performing them.	Helps alleviate anxiety.
	Listen attentively to concerns or expressions of anxiety from J.B.	Helps identify anxious behaviors and source of her anxiety.
	Include J.B. in as many decisions related to her care and follow-up as is possible.	May reduce her feelings of anxiety and gives her some control.

EVALUATION

J.B. expresses feelings of anxiety about the diagnosis. States she has a cousin with herpes whom she will use as a resource person. Also states that she has a secure relationship with her boyfriend and will talk to him about herpes. Agrees to call the clinic for any further support or information that she may need.

(Continues)

SAMPLE NURSING CARE PLAN (Continued)

NURSING DIAGNOSIS 3 *Risk for Infection* related to break in skin integrity as evidenced by the presence of blisters

Nursing Outcomes Classification (NOC)
Risk Control: Sexually Transmitted Infections (STI)

Nursing Interventions Classification (NIC)
Teaching: Disease Process
Teaching: Sexuality

PLANNING/OUTCOMES	NURSING INTERVENTIONS	RATIONALE
J.B.'s herpes blisters will heal without secondary infection within 10 days.	Wear gloves when examining perineal area and when handling exudate from herpes lesions.	Prevents secondary infection in herpes blisters from caregiver's hands and protects caregiver when dealing with wound exudate.
	Teach J.B. how to wash hands very thoroughly after using the toilet or handling the area around the herpes lesions.	Prevents spread of herpes infection from genital area to other areas of J.B.'s body or to another person.
	Instruct J.B. in the importance of keeping the herpes lesions clean and dry until they heal.	Helps prevent the occurrence of a secondary infection that may delay healing for up to 6 weeks.
	Instruct J.B. to wear cotton underwear and loose-fitting clothing during herpes outbreaks.	Provides air circulation to promote healing and reduce further local irritation.

EVALUATION

J.B. has been taught to keep blisters clean and dry and states that she will contact the clinic if the lesions develop any signs of a secondary infection. She makes an appointment to return to the clinic in 10 days for a follow-up evaluation.

CASE STUDY

N.L., a 17-year-old student, has come to your clinic seeking treatment. N.L. is complaining of pain and burning on urination, as well as pain during intercourse. She states that she is infrequently sexually active with her 17-year-old boyfriend and is also seeking a form of birth control. She has not used any form of birth control in the past and neither has her boyfriend. She also complains of a yellowish vaginal discharge and has been wearing a panty liner to deal with this. Upon examination, N.L. complains of some abdominal tenderness but denies that she has had any tenderness before this time. N.L. is screened for chlamydia and gonorrhea. She denies having had sex with any other partners but does admit that she and her boyfriend had a fight and broke up temporarily about a month ago. They went back together about a week later. She does not know if he had any other sexual contacts during their period of separation. N.L. is concerned that she has contracted an STI and states, "I'll die of embarrassment!"

The following questions will guide your development of a nursing care plan for the case study.

1. What other information should be elicited from N.L.?
2. What other STIs will N.L. most likely be tested for in addition to chlamydia and gonorrhea?
3. Write three nursing diagnoses and goals for N.L.
4. List the medications that N.L. will be most likely to receive to treat a chlamydial infection.
5. List some complications that N.L. may experience if she does not receive treatment for an active chlamydial or gonorrheal infection.
6. What information will you include when you counsel N.L. regarding sexual activity and forms of birth control? (See the chapter on Reproductive Systems for additional information.)

SUMMARY

- STIs are among the most common infections occurring in the United States today.
- Despite massive education efforts, the number of new STI cases identified each year continues to grow.
- Early, intensive education regarding STIs is being used to help combat the high incidence of STIs, which virtually are an epidemic among young, urban-dwelling populations.
- Many STIs, such as gonorrhea, syphilis, and chlamydia, are treatable with antibiotics, but many others are caused by viruses and are not curable.
- Identification of groups at risk for STIs and appropriate prevention teaching are the most effective weapons in the ongoing battle against STIs.

REVIEW QUESTIONS

1. A female client comes to the health clinic because her boyfriend was recently diagnosed with chlamydia. She asks the nurse what would have happened to her if she had not found out and had gone without treatment. The nurse explains to her that lack of treatment could result in:
   1. development of a chancre.
   2. heart disease and blindness.
   3. scar tissue formation.
   4. nervous system damage.
2. A nursing diagnosis for a client with an STI is *Risk for Infection related to incomplete treatment and lack of precautions with an infected partner*. Which of the following are desired outcomes for the client? (Select all that apply.)
   1. The client will state the need for having all sexual partners notified and treated.
   2. The client will maintain adequate tissue perfusion as manifested by stable vital signs.
   3. The client will maintain adequate fluid balance.
   4. The client will state understanding of the treatment regimen and of the importance of completing treatment.
   5. The client will explain appropriate use of condoms, including how and when to apply and remove the device.
   6. The client will maintain skin integrity and vagina will not be dry.
3. A male client informs the nurse that his girlfriend is being treated for cytomegalovirus (CMV). What common symptoms of cytomegalovirus (CMV) will the nurse assess for in a male client?
   1. Urethritis, purulent drainage, and epididymitis.
   2. Often asymptomatic, occasionally fever, fatigue, and weakness.
   3. Fleshy cauliflower like growth on genitalia.
   4. Rash on palms and soles.
4. A 29-year-old male client is diagnosed with gonorrhea. Which of the following treatments are included in his plan of care? (Select all that apply.)
   1. A single dose of ciprofloxacin (Cipro) followed by a 7-day course of oral doxycycline (Vibramycin).
   2. Follow-up cultures to determine the success of the course of treatment.
   3. An injection of ceftriaxone sodium (Rocephin) followed by oral erythromycin estolate (Ilosone).
   4. Abstain from mouth-to-mouth kissing.
   5. An antibiotic ophthalmic ointment is administered in both eyes.
   6. Administer mild analgesics as ordered to minimize dysuria.
5. A 22-year-old male has recently been diagnosed with syphilis and presents with a skin rash, sore throat, headache, and small papules on the tip of his penis. The nursing assessment data indicates that the client is in which stage of syphilis?
   1. Primary.
   2. Secondary.
   3. Tertiary.
   4. Latent.
6. The nurse is teaching a classroom of college students the proper use of condoms to protect against STIs. Which of the following statements made by a student indicates that further teaching is needed?
   1. "I always wear a condom and use a water based lubricant when having sex with my girlfriend."
   2. "I never reuse a condom."
   3. "I keep extra condoms in the glove compartment of my car so I am always prepared."
   4. "I prefer lambskin condoms because they fit the best."
7. The nurse knows that which of the following is the best method for reducing the risk of acquiring an STI?
   1. Always wear a condom during sexual intercourse.
   2. Do not share sex toys.
   3. Use a barrier method when engaging in oral sex.
   4. Abstinence.
8. The client has been diagnosed with trichomonas and is prescribed the medication Flagyl for treatment. Which of the following is the most important information for the nurse to teach the client regarding the administration of Flagyl?
   1. Do not drink alcoholic beverages while taking this medication.
   2. Take with food.
   3. Do not drink grapefruit juice while taking this medication.
   4. Do not take use an antacid one hour before or after taking the medication.

9. When conducting a health history, which of the following questions is inappropriate to ask a client suspected of having an STI?
   1. Have you been diagnosed with a STI in the past?
   2. How many sexual partners have you had in the past 6 months?
   3. Have you noticed any anal discharge or tenderness?
   4. Why didn't you use a condom when having sex with your partner?
10. A 45-year-old male client has been recently diagnosed with chlamydia. His wife is in the room and asks the nurse why she has to be tested and treated as well, since she does not have any symptoms. The best explanation by the nurse is:
   1. "It is important that all sexual partners be tested and treated, because reinfection can occur if only one partner is treated."
   2. "The doctor requires that spouses be tested and treated even if they do not have any symptoms."
   3. "Because chlamydia is a silent disease with no symptoms."
   4. "It is something that all doctors require."

REFERENCES/SUGGESTED READINGS

American Social Health Association (ASHA). (2009). Gonorrhea: questions & answers. Retrieved January 17, 2009 from http://www.ashastd.org/learn/learn_gonorrhea.cfm

American Social Health Association (ASHA). (2009a). Herpes resource center: overview. Retrieved January 17, 2009 from http://www.ashastd.org/herpes/herpes_aboutcenter.cfm

Apoola, A. & Radcliffe, K. (2004). Antiviral treatment of genital herpes. *International Journal of STD & AIDS, 15*(7), 429–433.

Ballard, R. & Morse, S. (2003). Chancroid. In: *Atlas of sexually transmitted diseases and AIDS* (3rd ed.). Edinburgh: Mosby.

Baseman, J. & Koutsky, L. (2005). The epidemiology of human papillomavirus infections. *Journal of Clinical Virology, 32*(Suppl. 1), S16–S24.

Bulechek, G., Butcher, H., McCloskey, J., & Dochterman, J., eds. (2008). *Nursing Interventions Classification* (*NIC*) (5th ed.). St. Louis, MO: Mosby/Elsevier.

Centers for Disease Control and Prevention. (2007a). Trends in reportable sexually transmitted disease in the United States, 2007: national surveillance data for chlamydia, gonorrhea, and syphilis. Retrieved January 17, 2009 from http://www.cdc.gov/std/stats07/trends.htm

Centers for Disease Control and Prevention. (2007b). Sexually transmitted disease surveillance, 2007: gonorrhea. Retrieved January 17, 2009 from http://www.cdc.gov/std/stats07/gonorrhea.htm

Centers for Disease Control and Prevention. (2008a). About CMV: general information. Retrieved July 8, 2009 from http://www.cdc.gov/cmv/facts.htm

Centers for Disease Control and Prevention. (2008b). Division of parasitic diseases: trichomonas infection fact sheet. Retrieved January 18, 2009 from http://www.cdc.gov/ncidod/dpd/parasites/trichomonas/factsht_trichomonas.htm

Centers for Disease Control and Prevention. (2008c). HIV transmission rates in the United States. Retrieved January 18, 2009 from http://www.cdc.gov/hiv/topics/surveillance/resources/factsheets/transmission.htm

Centers for Disease Control and Prevention. (2008d). Vaccines and Preventable Diseases: HPV vaccination. Retrieved January 17, 2009 from http://www.cdc.gov/vaccines/vpd-vac/hpv/default.htm

Centers for Disease Control and Prevention. (2008e). Viral hepatitis: FAQs for health professionals. Retrieved January 17, 2009 from http://www.cdc.gov/hepatitis/HBV/HBVfaq.htm#overview

Centers for Disease Control and Prevention. (2009). Genital herpes—CDC fact sheet. Retrieved January 17, 2009 from http://www.cdc.gov/std/Herpes/STDFact-Herpes.htm

Cleveland Clinic. (2009). Sexually transmitted diseases: an overview. Retrieved January 18, 2009 from my.clevelandclinic.org/disorders/Sexually_Transmitted_Disease_STD/hic_Sexually_Transmitted_Diseases_An_Overview.aspx

Daniels, R. (2010). *Delmar's guide to laboratory and diagnostic tests* (2nd ed.). Clifton Park, NY: Delmar Cengage Learning.

Ehreth, J. (2005). The economics of vaccination from a global perspective: present and future. 2-3 December, 2004, Vaccines: all things considered. *Expert Rev. Vaccines, 4*, 19–21.

Estes, M. (2010). *Health assessment & physical examination* (4th ed.). Clifton Park, NY: Delmar Cengage Learning.

Freedom Network. (2009). Facts about STD. Retrieved January 17, 2009 from http://std-gov.org/

Keck, J. (2005). Ulcerative lesions. *Clinical Family Practice, 7*(1), 13–30.

Mayo Clinic. (2009a). Gonorrhea: definition. Retrieved January 16, 2009 from http://www.mayoclinic.com/print/gonorrhea/DS00180/DSECTION=all&method=print

Mayo Clinic. (2009b). HIV/AIDS. Retrieved January 18, 2009 from http://www.who.int/features/qa/71/en/index.html

Moorhead, S., Johnson, M., Maas, M., & Swanson, E. (2007). *Nursing Outcomes Classification (NOC)* (4th ed.). St. Louis, MO: Mosby.

National Institutes of Health. (2008). U.S. reported 25,000 cases of HPV-related cancers annually. Retrieved January 18, 2009 from http://www.nlm.nih.gov/medlineplus/news/fullstory_71187.html

National Institutes of Health. (2009). Sexually transmitted diseases. Retrieved January 18, 2009 from http://www.nlm.nih.gov/medlineplus/sexuallytransmitteddiseases.html

North American Nursing Diagnosis Association International. (2010). *NANDA-I nursing diagnoses: Definitions and classification 2009–2011*. Ames, IA: Wiley-Blackwell.

Ohio Department of Health. (2007). Genital warts. Retrieved January 18, 2009 from http://www.odh.ohio.gov/pdf/idcm/genwart.pdf

Roden, R., Ling, M., & Wu, T. (2004). Vaccination to prevent and treat cervical cancer. *Human Pathology, 35*, 971–982.

Rural Center for AIDS/STD Prevention. (2006). Rural methamphetamine use and HIV/STD risk. Fact sheet No. 18. Retrieved January 15, 2009 from http://www.indiana.edu/~aids/factsheets18.pdf

Spratto, G., & Woods, A. (2009). *2009 edition Delmar nurse's drug handbook*. Clifton Park, NY: Delmar Cengage Learning.

World Health Organization (WHO). (2009). HIV surveillance, estimates, monitoring and evaluation. Retrieved July 8, 2009 from http://www.who.int/hiv/topics/me/en/index.html

RESOURCES

American College of Obstetricians and Gynecologists (ACOG), http://www.acog.org

American Public Health Association (APHA), http://www.apha.org

American Social Health Association (ASHA), http://www.ashastd.org

Centers for Disease Control and Prevention (CDC), http://www.cdc.gov

National Foundation for Infectious Diseases, http://www.nfid.org

National Institute of Allergy and Infectious Diseases, http://www.niaid. nih.gov

Planned Parenthood Federation of America, Inc., http://www.plannedparenthood.org

U.S. Department of Health and Human Services (USDHHS), http://www.hhs.gov

World Health Organization (WHO), http://www.who.int

UNIT 6 Nursing Care of the Client: Body Defenses

CHAPTER 15
Integumentary System

MAKING THE CONNECTION

Refer to the following chapters to increase your understanding of the integumentary system:

Adult Health Nursing

- ***Oncology***
- ***Immune System***
- ***The Older Adult***

LEARNING OBJECTIVES

Upon completion of this chapter, you should be able to:

- Define key terms.
- Describe common disorders of the integumentary system.
- Relate the pathophysiology of each skin disorder.
- Discuss the common diagnostic tests used to differentiate skin disorders.
- State the usual treatment for each skin disorder.
- Assess the nursing care needs of a client with a disorder of the integument.
- Plan and implement effective nursing care.

KEY TERMS

alopecia
angiogenesis
angioma
blanching
cyanosis
debride
ecchymosis
erythema
eschar
exudate
friction
granulation tissue
hemorrhagic exudate
hemostasis
hyperthermia
hypothermia
inflammation
ischemia
jaundice
keloid
keratin
lipoma
melanin
nevi
pallor
petechiae
purulent exudate
sanguineous exudate
sebaceous cyst
sebum
serosanguineous exudate
serous exudate
shearing
telangiectasia
vitiligo
wound

INTRODUCTION

As an old adage asserts, the health of the skin mirrors the health of the body. Many systemic diseases have skin manifestations. Psychological stress can affect the condition of the skin, and skin rashes can be a complication of drug therapy. As the largest and the most visible system in the body, the integumentary system (skin, hair, scalp, nails, and mucous membranes) is vulnerable to injury and susceptible to several primary diseases. Although the outward appearance of the skin is important for psychological well-being, the healthy, intact status of the skin is also essential for physiologic well-being. Maintaining this status of the integumentary system is, therefore, an important independent nursing function. The focus of this chapter is to describe common skin disorders, identify the usual treatment modalities for these disorders, and discuss measures that nurses can implement to provide effective nursing care for clients with disorders of the integument.

ANATOMY AND PHYSIOLOGY REVIEW

As the external covering of the body, the skin performs the vital function of protecting internal body structures from harmful microorganisms and substances. The skin is continuous with mucous membranes at external body openings of the respiratory tract, the digestive system, and the urogenital tract. As appendages of the skin, the hair and nails also have protective functions. In addition to its vital protective role, the skin also plays other roles in the normal functioning of the human organism. These roles include participating in the regulation of body temperature, functioning as a sensory organ, helping to maintain fluid and electrolyte balance, producing vitamin D, and excreting certain waste products from the body.

STRUCTURE OF THE SKIN

The skin is composed of three layers: the epidermis, the dermis, and the subcutaneous fatty tissue (Figure 15-1).

Epidermis

The epidermis is a layer of squamous epithelial cells. Most of the cells are keratinocytes that produce a tough, fibrous protein called **keratin**. As new cells are produced in the deep layers of the epidermis, old cells are pushed to the surface of the skin. As these cells move from the deeper epidermal layers to the surface, they undergo a process of keratinization in which they become filled with keratin, thus hardening the outer layer of epidermal cells. The keratin creates a barrier that repels bacteria and foreign matter and is impermeable to most substances. The epidermal cells on the palms of the hands and soles of the feet, areas of the body subjected to increased friction and pressure, contain larger amounts of keratin, resulting in thickened skin and callouses.

The epidermis also contains specialized cells called melanocytes. These cells produce **melanin**, the pigment that gives the skin its color. The more melanin present, the darker the skin color. Exposure to ultraviolet light (sun) causes an increase in the production of melanin, which darkens (tans) the skin and provides some protection against the harmful effects of suntanning. Moles and birthmarks (**nevi**), pigmented areas in the skin, are aggregations of melanocytes. In **vitiligo**, melanocytes are destroyed, causing milk-white patches of depigmented skin surrounded by normal skin.

Dermis

The dermis is dense, irregular connective tissue composed of collagen and elastic fibers, blood and lymph vessels, nerves, sweat and sebaceous glands, and hair roots. The sebaceous glands secrete an oily substance called **sebum** that lubricates the skin, helping to keep it soft and pliable. Sweat (eccrine) glands are found in the skin over most of the body surface. Another type of sweat gland, apocrine glands, is concentrated in the axillae, anal region, scrotum, and labia majora. These glands secrete an organic substance that is odorless at first but is quickly metabolized by skin bacteria, causing the characteristic odor commonly referred to as body odor (Tate, 2008). Intradermal injections, such as the TB skin test, are given in the dermis.

Subcutaneous Tissue

The subcutaneous tissue is primarily connective and adipose (fatty) tissue. Here the skin is anchored to muscles and bones. An individual's nutritional status and genetic makeup dictate the amount of subcutaneous tissue present. Emaciated persons have very little subcutaneous tissue, whereas obese persons may have several inches of subcutaneous tissue. The amount of subcutaneous tissue is an important factor in body temperature regulation.

FUNCTIONS OF THE SKIN

Understanding the functions of the skin and contiguous mucous membranes guides the nurse in planning and implementing appropriate nursing care. Because intact, healthy skin and mucous membranes serve as the first line of defense against harmful agents, *maintaining skin integrity is one of the most important independent functions of the nurse.* Nursing interventions such as providing daily hygiene care and regularly turning and repositioning dependent clients are aimed at preventing skin breakdown.

Protection

The first and most important function of the skin is protection. As long as the skin is intact and healthy, it is a barrier against microorganisms and numerous substances that could be harmful to the individual. Not only is the skin a barrier to keep harmful substances out, it is also a barrier to keep essential

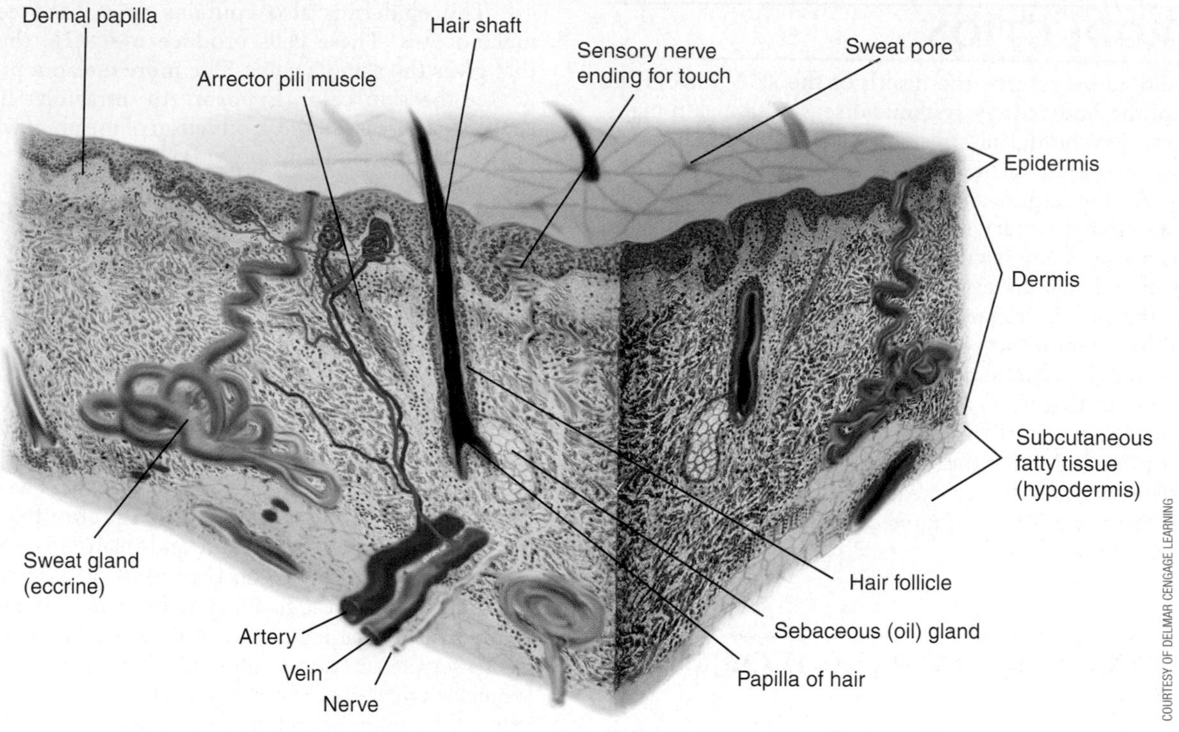

FIGURE 15-1 Cross Section of the Skin

substances such as water and electrolytes inside the body. It also cushions internal organs.

Temperature Regulation

The body produces heat as a result of metabolism of food. Exercise, fever, or a hot environment can raise body temperature. Through several mechanisms, the skin can either release or conserve body heat to maintain normal body temperature. Radiation is the primary means of heat loss. As body heat increases, arterioles in the dermis dilate, bringing body heat to the skin surface. By the process of radiation, waves of heat from uncovered body surfaces are released to the environment. Layering clothes in winter, for example, helps prevent excess loss of body heat by radiation. Heat is also lost by conduction. In conduction, heat is transferred from warmer surfaces to cooler ones. Placing a cool washcloth on a client's forehead is an example of using the principle of conduction. The washcloth becomes warmer, the forehead cooler. Evaporation is another way in which excess body heat is lost. As moisture on the skin—either from perspiration or from a tepid sponge bath—dries, the body is cooled. To conserve (prevent excess loss) body heat, arterioles in the dermis contract to decrease the flow of blood to the skin surface, thus decreasing heat lost by radiation. The phenomenon of "goose flesh" is another method of conserving body heat. Tiny hairs standing on end create a layer of air insulation decreasing loss of body heat to the environment.

Sensory Perception

The skin contains receptors for pain, touch, pressure, and temperature. The sensory receptors pick up information to help protect the body from environmental dangers as well as provide sensations of comfort and pleasure. The brain then processes the information and causes a response.

Fluid and Electrolyte Balance

The skin helps maintain the stability of the internal environment by preventing loss of body fluids and electrolytes and by preventing subcutaneous tissues from drying out. Skin damage, such as that occurring with severe burns, results in rapid loss of large quantities of fluid and electrolytes. This can lead to shock, circulatory collapse, and death.

Structure and Function of Hair

Hair is composed of dead epidermal cells that begin to grow and divide in the base of the hair follicle. As the cells are pushed toward the skin surface, they become keratinized and die. Hair color is genetically determined.

Scalp hair grows for 2 to 5 years, then the follicle becomes inactive. When the growth cycle begins again, a new hair is produced and the old hair is pushed out. Approximately 50 hairs are lost each day. Sustained hair loss of more than 100 hairs each day usually indicates that something is wrong.

There are 5 million hairs covering the entire human body except for the lips, palmar and plantar surfaces, nipples, and the glans penis. The amount and texture of hair vary with age, sex, race, and body part.

Hair on the head protects the scalp from the ultraviolet rays from the sun and cushions blows to the head. Eyelashes help prevent foreign particles from entering the eyes just as the hairs in the nostrils and external ear canals help keep particles from entering the nose and ears.

STRUCTURE AND FUNCTION OF NAILS

Nail production occurs in the nail root, an epithelial fold that cannot be seen from the surface (Figure 15-2). The nail plate covers the nail bed. The blood vessels under the nail bed give the nails their pink color.

The nails protect the ends of the fingers and toes.

STRUCTURE AND FUNCTION OF MUCOUS MEMBRANES

Mucous membranes have epithelium overlying a layer of loose connective tissue. Specialized cells within the mucous membrane secrete mucus.

The cavities and tubes that open to the outside of the body are lined with mucous membranes. These include the oral and nasal cavities and the tubes of the respiratory, gastrointestinal, urinary, and reproductive systems. Mucous membranes perform absorptive or secretory functions depending on their placement.

EFFECTS OF AGING

With advancing years, the blood flow to the skin is reduced. The skin becomes thinner and is more easily injured. Older skin breaks down easily from prolonged pressure. The long-accepted rule of thumb is to turn clients every 2 hours, but for the ill older client, every 2 hours may not be often enough. *Significant skin damage can occur in just 1 hour of unrelieved pressure.* Preventing skin breakdown in the elderly client depends on an accurate assessment of both the client's skin condition and mobility status.

Loss of subcutaneous tissue causes skin sagging and wrinkling. The activity of sebaceous and sweat glands diminishes, resulting in dry skin and a decreased ability to adapt to changes in environmental temperature. Extremes in temperature pose hazards for older adults. In very hot weather, they are susceptible to **hyperthermia**, a condition in which the core body temperature reaches 106°F (41.1°C). In hyperthermia, the hypothalamus no longer functions appropriately. Sweating stops, the skin becomes dry and flushed, and the person becomes confused and eventually comatose. Each summer many elderly persons die from the effects of hyperthermia. Winter puts older adults at risk for **hypothermia**, a condition in which the core body temperature drops below 95°F (35°C). The hypothermic client may become confused and disoriented. As the core body temperature continues to drop, the person becomes comatose. Each winter some older adults die from severe hypothermia (Tate, 2008).

On the hands and face, melanocytes increase in number, causing the age spots commonly seen in older adults. Gray hair occurs from a lack of melanin production. Skin exposed to sunlight ages faster.

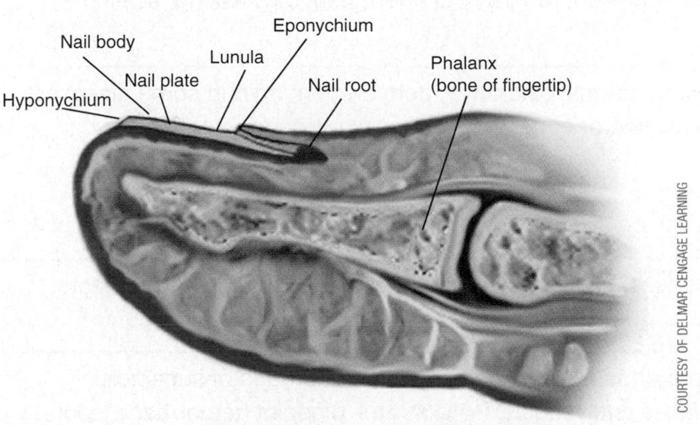

FIGURE 15-2 Structures of the Fingernail

LIFE SPAN CONSIDERATIONS

Effects of Aging on the Skin

- Skin vascularity and the number of sweat and sebaceous glands decrease, affecting thermoregulation.
- Inflammatory response and pain perception diminish, increasing the risk of adverse effects from noxious stimuli.
- A thinning epidermis and prolonged wound healing make the elderly more prone to injury and skin infections.
- Skin cancer is more common among the elderly.
- Use of skin lotions containing alcohol can cause drying of the skin, increasing the risk of injury. Moisture-enhancing products should be used instead.

ASSESSMENT

Assessing clients with disorders of the integument includes obtaining a health history and performing a physical assessment of the skin, hair, nails, and mucous membranes. The nurse's assessment skills, along with an understanding of the anatomy and physiology of the integumentary system, ensure a complete, factual database from which to plan and implement appropriate nursing care. Box 15-1 contains a list of questions to ask and observations to make in obtaining a health history.

ASSESSMENT OF SKIN

Seven parameters should be examined when performing a physical assessment of the skin. They are integrity, color, temperature and moisture, texture, turgor and mobility, sensation, and vascularity. Table 15-1 outlines these parameters with the normal and abnormal findings. Inspection and palpation are the two assessment techniques used when examining the skin. Good lighting is essential for accurate assessment.

Any skin lesions should be identified according to type and described regarding color, size, and location. Describe the amount, color, odor, and appearance of any drainage that might be present. Document assessment findings clearly, concisely,

BOX 15-1: QUESTIONS TO ASK AND OBSERVATIONS TO MAKE WHEN COLLECTING DATA

Subjective Data

- When did you first notice this problem?
- Where did the first symptom appear?
- What did the rash/lesion look like when it first appeared?
- Describe what happened in the days/weeks after the first symptom appeared.
- Are the symptoms worse at any particular time? Season?
- Have you experienced any itching or burning sensations?
- Are the lesions painful?
- What do you think might have caused this problem?
- Have you ever had a skin problem like this before?
- Has anyone in your family ever had a problem like this?
- What have you been doing to treat this problem?
- What kind of skin care products do you normally use?
- Have you changed any of your usual products/habits/routines?
- Is there anything else you would like to tell me about this problem?

Objective Data

- Check vital signs.
- Inspect color and integrity of skin.
- Observe skin for rashes, lesions, moles, calluses, tattoos, scars, and piercings.
- Inspect skin folds and creases.
- Inspect skin for edema.
- Observe for signs of bleeding and ecchymosis.
- Observe hair distribution, quality, and texture.
- Inspect scalp for dryness and lesions.
- Inspect nail curvature, color, thickness.
- Palpate skin for temperature, moisture, and texture.
- Assess skin turgor.
- Palpate the skin for pitting edema.
- Note any skin odor.
- Report diagnostic test results.

TABLE 15-1 Skin Assessment Parameters

PARAMETER	NORMAL	ABNORMAL
Integrity	Skin intact; no diseased or injured tissue	Broken skin; open areas such as fissures, ulcers, excoriations. Rash or lesions such as papules, nodules, vesicles, pustules, wheals, scales (Figures 15-3 and 15-4).
Color	Varies with skin type and race: pink, tanned, olive, brown	**Pallor**—pale skin, especially in face, conjunctiva, nail beds, and oral mucous membranes. **Cyanosis**—bluish discoloration noticed in lips, earlobes, and nail beds. **Jaundice**—a yellowing of the skin, mucous membranes, and sclera. **Erythema**—reddish hue to the skin as in sunburn and inflammation or increased blood flow.
Temperature and moisture	Usually warm and dry, depending on environmental temperature	Cool, cold, moist, clammy, or warmer than normal
Texture	Smooth, soft. Thickness varies in different areas.	Loose, wrinkled, rough, thickened, thin, oily, flaking, scaling
Turgor and mobility	An assessment of skin hydration. Normally skin moves freely. A pinched fold of skin returns immediately to normal position (Figure 15-5).	Taut with edema; slack with dehydration; rigid in some diseases such as scleroderma
Sensation	Distinguishes hot and cold, sharp and dull	Numbness, tingling, insensitive to pressure and sharp objects
Vascularity	Clear; no discoloration	**Telangiectasia**—permanent dilation of groups of superficial capillaries and venules. **Petechiae**—pinpoint hemorrhagic spots. **Ecchymosis**—large, irregular, hemorrhagic areas (Figure 15-6).

NONPALPABLE

A

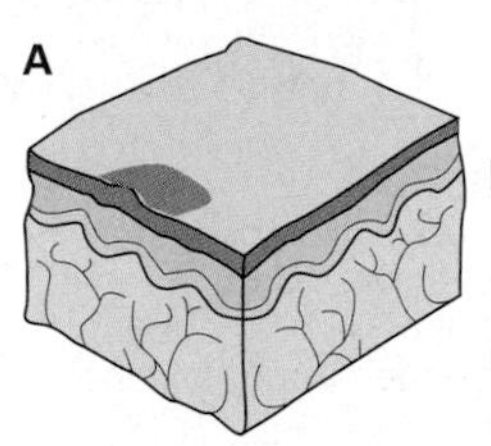

Macule:
Localized changes in skin color of less than 1 cm in diameter
Example:
Freckle

B

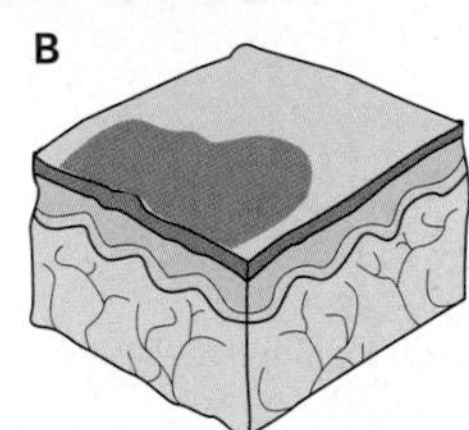

Patch:
Localized changes in skin color of greater than 1 cm in diameter
Example:
Vitiligo, stage 1 of pressure ulcer

PALPABLE

C

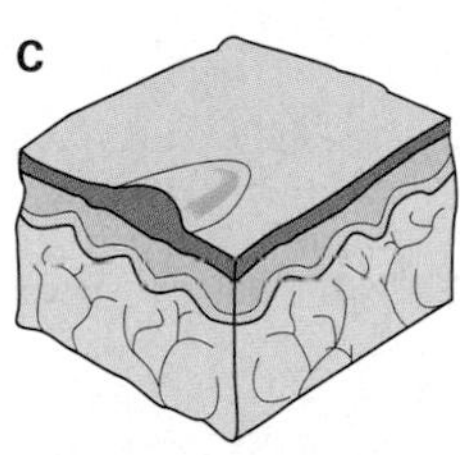

Papule:
Solid, elevated lesion less than 0.5 cm in diameter
Example:
Warts, elevated nevi, seborrheic keratosis

D

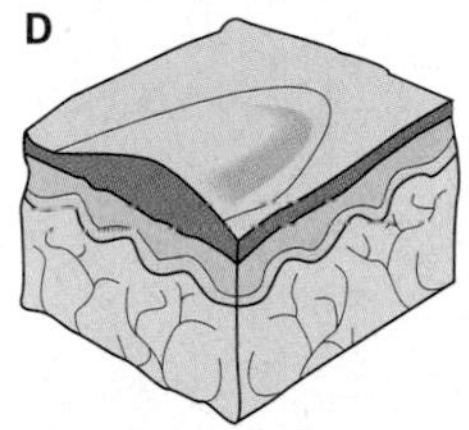

Plaque:
Solid, elevated lesion greater than 0.5 cm in diameter
Example:
Psoriasis, eczema

E

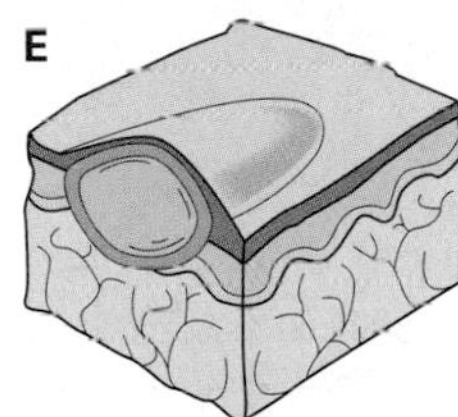

Nodules:
Solid and elevated; however, they extend deeper than papules into the dermis or subcutaneous tissues, 0.5–2 cm
Example:
Lipoma, erythema nodosum, cyst, melamoma, hemangioma

F

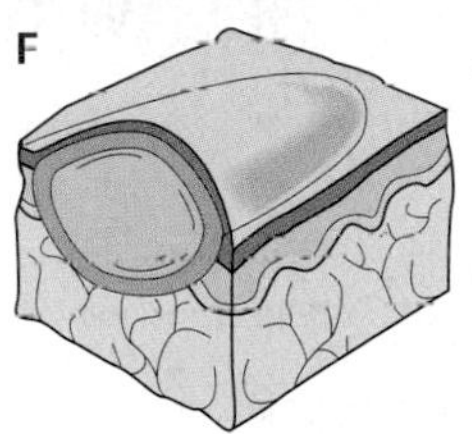

Tumor:
The same as a nodule only greater than 2 cm
Example:
Carcinoma (such as advanced breast carcinoma); **not** basal cell or squamous cell of the skin

G

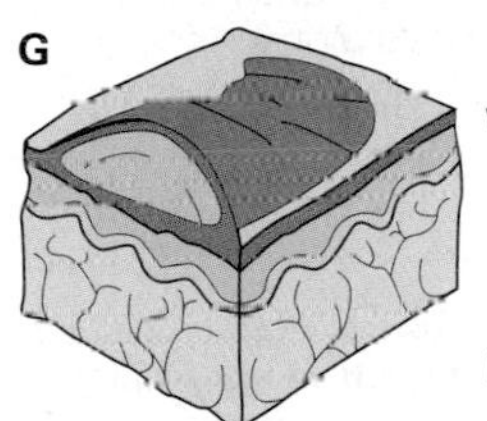

Wheal:
Localized edema in the epidermis causing irregular elevation that may be red or pale
Example:
Insect bite, hive, angioedema

FLUID-FILLED CAVITIES WITHIN THE SKIN

H

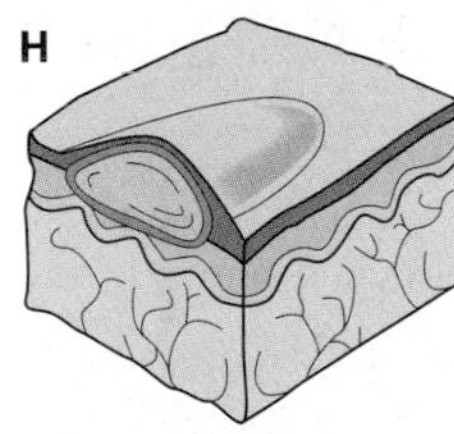

Vesicle:
Accumulation of fluid between the upper layers of the skin; elevated mass containing serous fluid; less than 0.5 cm
Example:
Herpes simplex, herpes zoster, chickenpox, scabies

I

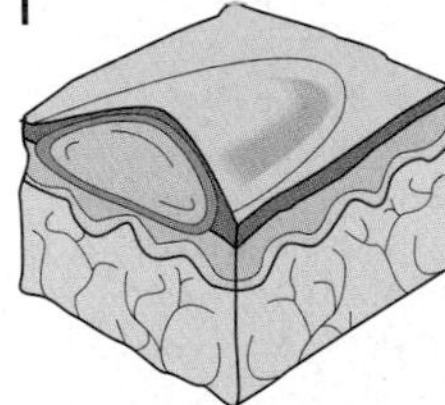

Bullae:
Same as a vesicle only greater than 0.5 cm
Example:
Contact dermatitis, large second-degree burns, bullous impetigo, pemphigus

J

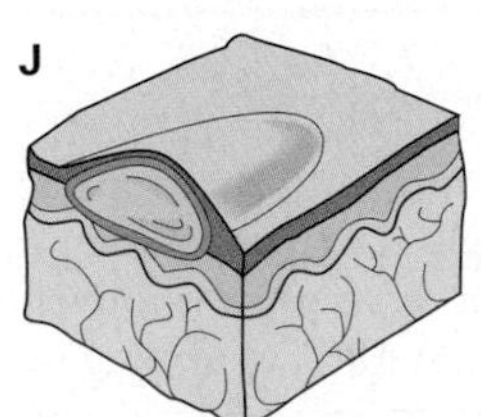

Pustule:
Vesicle or bullae that becomes filled with pus, usually described as less than 0.5 cm in diameter
Example:
Acne, impetigo, furuncles, carbuncles, folliculitis

K

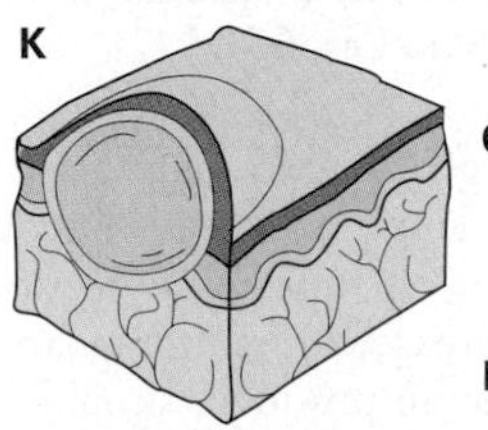

Cyst:
Encapsulated fluid-filled or semi-solid mass in the subcutaneous tissue or dermis
Example:
Sebaceous cyst, epidermoid cyst

FIGURE 15-3 Types of Primary Skin Lesions

ABOVE THE SKIN SURFACE

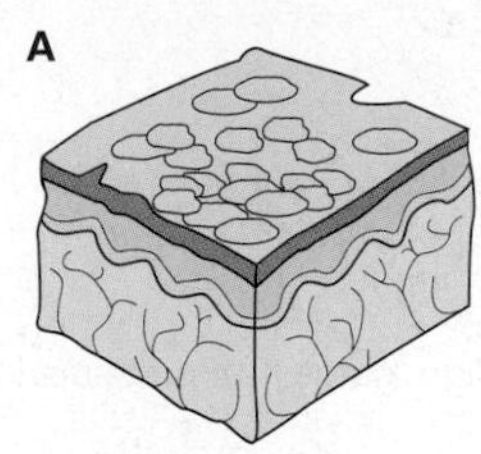

A
Scales:
Flaking of the skin's surface
Example:
Dandruff, psoriasis, xerosis

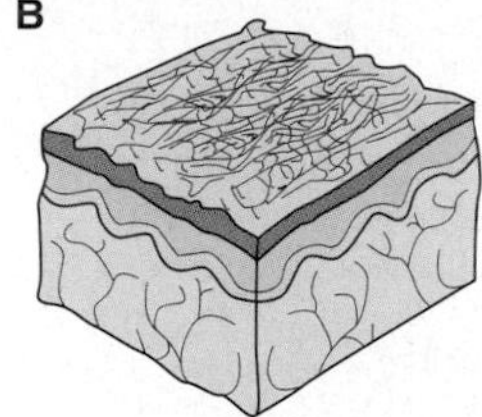

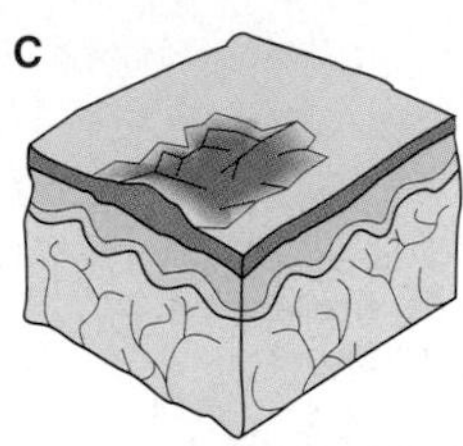

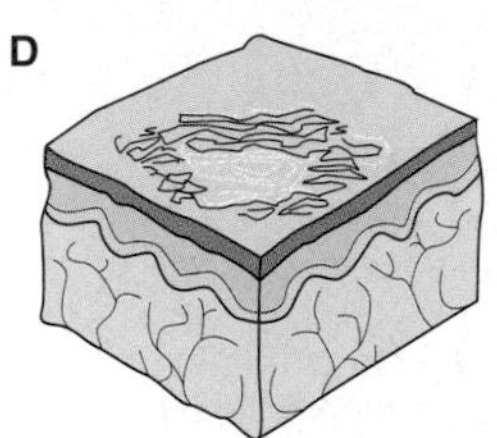

D
Atrophy:
Thinning of the skin surface and loss of markings
Example:
Striae, aged skin

BELOW THE SKIN SURFACE

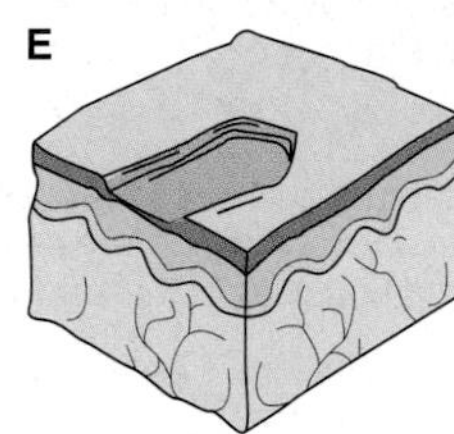

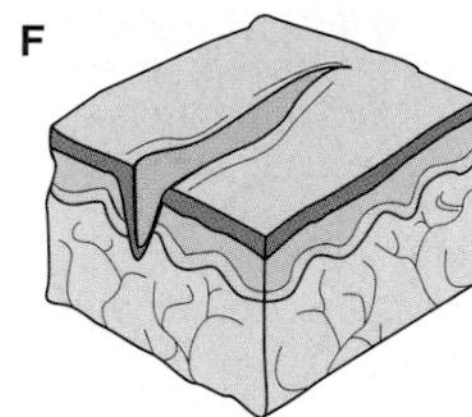

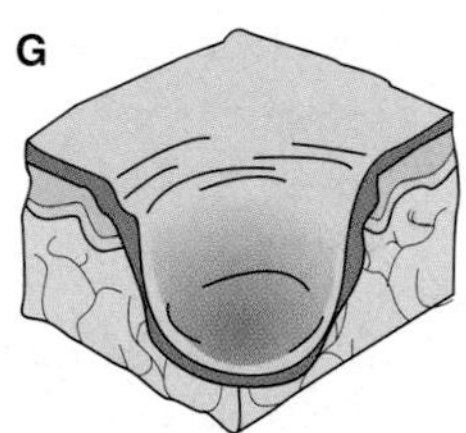

G
Ulcer:
A depressed lesion of the epidermis and upper papillary layer of the dermis
Example:
Stage 2 pressure ulcer

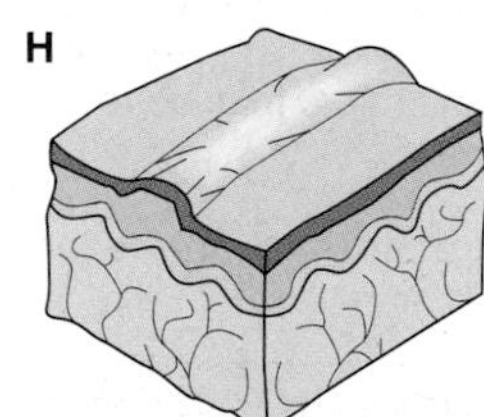

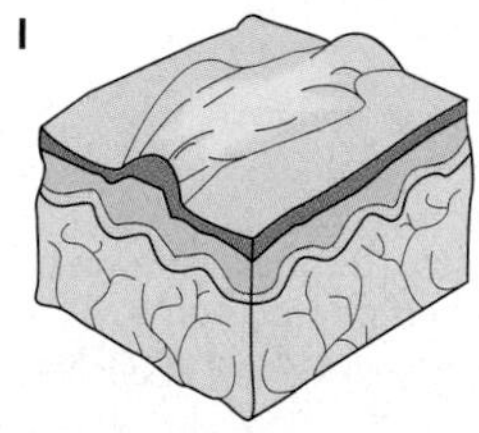

I
Keloid:
Enlarging of a scar past wound edges due to excess collagen formation (more prevalent in dark skinned persons)
Example:
Burn scar

J

Excoriation:
Loss of epidermal layers exposing the dermis
Example:
Abrasion

FIGURE 15-4 **Types of Secondary Skin Lesions**

and completely. The intent of nursing care is to maintain the integrity of intact skin and to restore damaged skin or mucous membranes to an intact state. Aging changes skin texture, moisture, and mobility, requiring increased nursing vigilance to maintain skin integrity. Daily hygiene products should be selected to meet the client's individual skin care needs.

ASSESSMENT OF HAIR, NAILS, AND MUCOUS MEMBRANES

Hair should be smooth, shiny, and resilient. Excess hair loss can result from drugs, radiation, dietary or hormonal factors, stress, and high fever.

Nails should be pink, smooth, and shiny and feel firm yet flexible when palpated. An angle of approximately 160° should be present between the nail body and the eponychium. Early clubbing is a nail angle of at least 180°. Clubbing occurs when long-standing hypoxia is present, particularly with cyanotic heart disease and advanced chronic obstructed pulmonary disease. Koilonychia, also known as "spoon nails," is a sign of iron deficiency anemia, malnutrition, or trauma of the nail bed. The nails are thin and concave. Beau's lines are white lines across the nail seen with acute severe illness, malnutrition, or trauma. Paronychia is an infection of the nail caused by bacteria or *Candida albicans* (Figure 15-7).

Mucous membranes normally appear pink and moist.

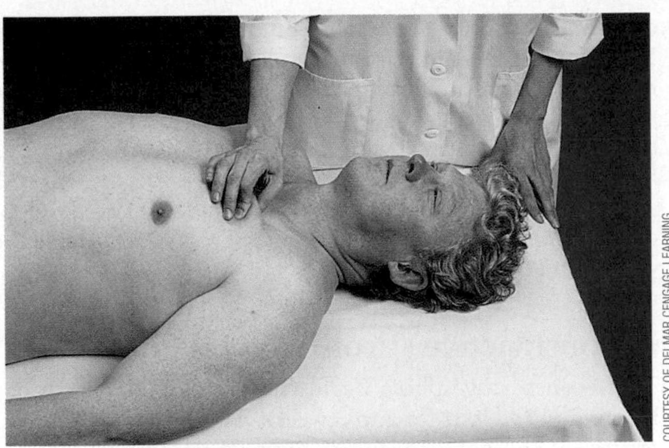

FIGURE 15-5 Assessment of Skin Turgor

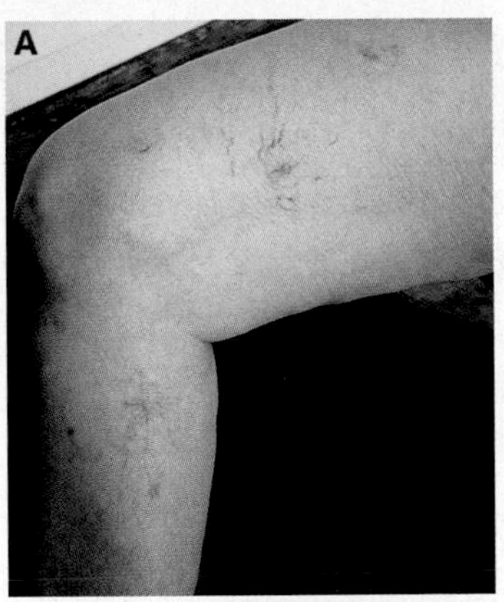

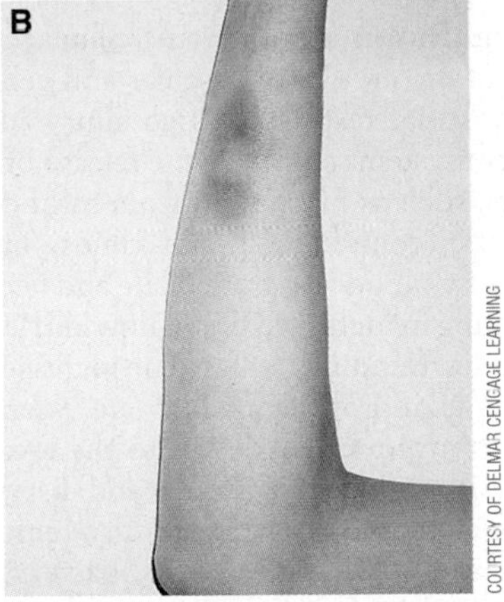

FIGURE 15-6 *A*, Telangiectasis (Spider Veins); *B*, Ecchymosis (Bruise)

COMMON DIAGNOSTIC TESTS

Commonly used diagnostic tests for clients with integumentary disorders are listed in Table 15-2.

WOUNDS

A disruption in the integrity of body tissue is called a **wound**.

Physiology of Wound Healing

When an injury is sustained, a complex set of responses is set into motion, and the body begins a three-phase process of wound healing. Understanding these physiological responses will assist the nurse in caring for clients with impaired skin integrity and promoting optimal wound healing.

Defensive (Inflammatory) Phase

The defensive phase occurs immediately after injury and lasts about 3 to 4 days. The major events that occur in this phase are hemostasis and inflammation. **Hemostasis**, or cessation of bleeding, occurs by vasoconstriction of large blood vessels in the affected area. Platelets, activated by the injury, aggregate to form a platelet plug and stop the bleeding. Activation of the clotting cascade results in the eventual formation of fibrin and a fibrinous meshwork, which further entraps platelets and other cells. The result is fibrin clot formation, which provides initial wound closure, prevents excessive loss of blood and body fluids, and inhibits contamination of the wound by microorganisms.

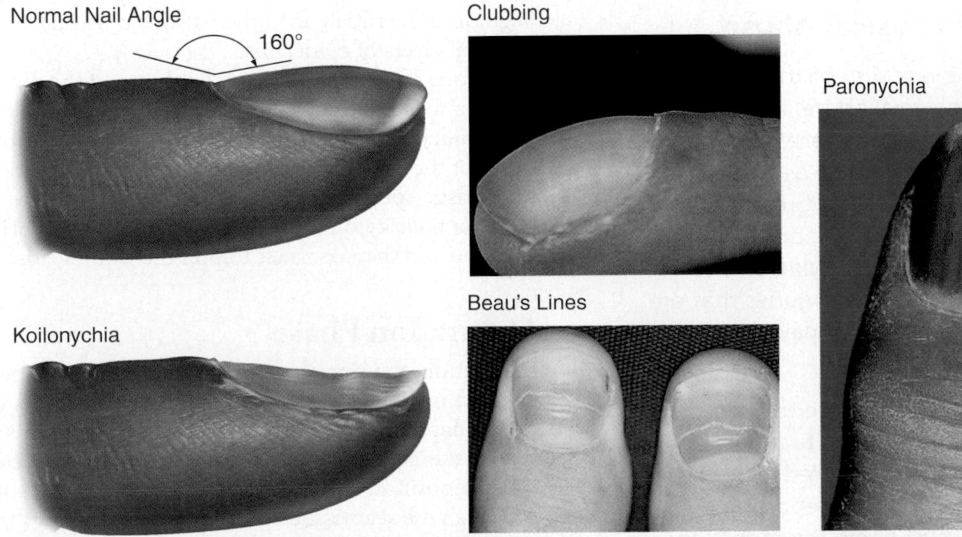

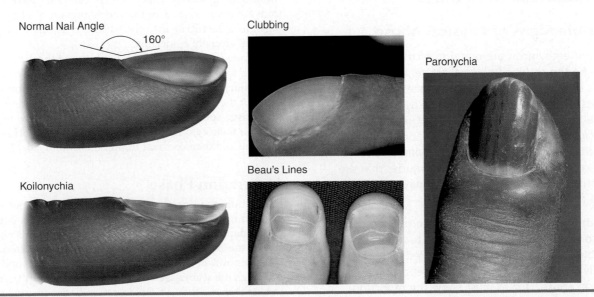

FIGURE 15-7 Nail Variations (*Photos of clubbing and Beau's line courtesy of Robert A. Silverman, MD, Clinical Associate Professor, Department of Pediatrics, Georgetown University; all other images courtesy of Delmar Cengage Learning.*)

TABLE 15-2 Common Diagnostic Tests for Integumentary Disorders

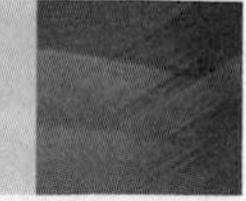

Biopsy (punch, incisional, excisional, shave)
Patch testing
Tzanck smear
Immunofluorescence (IF testing)
Wood's light examination
Skin scrapings
Culture and sensitivity

Inflammation is a nonspecific cellular response to tissue injury and involves both vascular and cellular responses. During the vascular response, tissue injury and activation of plasma protein systems stimulate the release of various chemical mediators, such as histamine (from mast cells), serotonin (from platelets), complement, and kinins. These vasoactive substances cause blood vessels to dilate and become more permeable, resulting in increased blood flow and leakage of serous fluid into the surrounding tissues. The increased blood supply carries nutrients and oxygen, which are essential for wound healing, and transports leukocytes to the area to participate in phagocytosis, or the envelopment and disposal of microorganisms. The increased blood supply also removes the "debris of battle," which includes dead cells, bacteria, and **exudate** (material, fluid, and cells slowly discharged from cells or blood vessels). The area is red, edematous, and warm to touch, and it has varying amounts of exudate.

During the cellular response, leukocytes move out of the blood vessel into the interstitial space. Neutrophils are the first cells to arrive at the injured site and begin phagocytosis. They subsequently die and are replaced by macrophages, which arise from blood monocytes. Macrophages perform the same function as neutrophils but remain for a longer time. In addition to being the primary phagocyte of debridement, macrophages are important cells in wound healing because they secrete several factors, including fibroblast activating factor (FAF) and angiogenesis factor (AGF). FAF attracts fibroblasts, which form collagen or collagen precursors. AGF stimulates the formation of new blood vessels. The development of this new microcirculation supports and sustains the wound and the healing process.

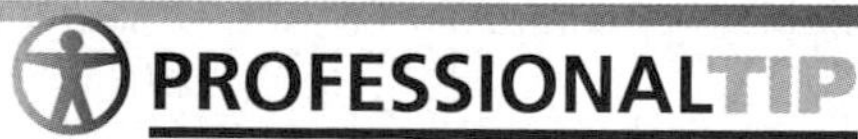

PROFESSIONALTIP

Possible Signs of Physical Abuse

Areas of ecchymosis are one sign of trauma that could be the result of physical abuse. Injuries noted at the base of the skull or on the face, buttocks, breasts, abdomen, or any area such as the top of the back that the client could not reach, are suspicious for abuse. Unusual marks on the skin such as cigarette burns and belt buckle or bite marks may also be signs of abuse. Injuries that are inconsistent with the client's story may also be the result of abuse.

Institutional policies generally relate to reporting and to whom to report when the situation of possible physical abuse is encountered. This is usually based on state laws about reporting physical abuse. Nurses must know the reporting laws of the state in which they are employed.

Reconstructive (Proliferative) Phase

The reconstructive phase begins on the third or fourth day after injury and lasts for 2 to 3 weeks. This phase contains the process of collagen deposition, angiogenesis, granulation tissue development, and wound contraction.

Fibroblasts, normally found in connective tissue, migrate into the wound because of various cellular mediators. They are the most important cells in this phase because they synthesize and secrete collagen. Collagen is the most abundant protein in the body and is the material of tissue repair. Initially, collagen is gel-like, but within several months it cross-links to form collagen fibrils and adds tensile strength to the wound. As the wound gains strength, the risk of wound separation or rupture is less likely. The wound can resist normal stress such as tension or twisting after 15 to 20 days. During this time, a raised "healing ridge" may be visible under the injury or suture line.

Angiogenesis (formation of new blood vessels) begins within hours after the injury. The endothelial cells in preexisting vessels begin to produce enzymes that break down the basement membrane. The membrane opens, and new endothelial cells build a new vessel. These capillaries grow across the wound, increasing blood flow, which increases the supply of nutrients and oxygen needed for wound healing.

Repair begins as granulation tissue, or new tissue, grows inward from surrounding healthy connective tissue. Granulation tissue is filled with new capillaries that are fragile and bleed easily, thus giving the healing area a red, translucent, granular appearance. As granulation tissue is formed, epithelialization, or growth of epithelial tissue, begins. Epithelial cells migrate into the wound from the wound margins. Eventually, the migrating cells contact similar cells that have migrated from the outer edges. Contact stops migration. The cells then begin to differentiate into the various cells that comprise the different layers of epidermis.

Wound contraction is the final step of the reconstructive phase of wound healing. Contraction is noticeable 6 to 12 days after injury and is necessary for closure of all wounds. The edges of the wound are drawn together by the action of myofibroblasts, specialized cells that contain bundles of parallel fibers in their cytoplasm. These myofibroblasts bridge across a wound and then contract to pull the wound closed.

Maturation Phase

Maturation, the final stage of healing, begins about the 21st day and may continue for up to 2 years or more, depending on the depth and extent of the wound. During this phase, the scar tissue is remodeled (reshaped or reconstructed by collagen deposition and lysis and debridement of wound edges). Although the scar tissue continues to gain strength, it remains weaker than the tissue it replaces. Capillaries eventually disappear, leaving an avascular scar (a scar that is white because it lacks a blood supply).

Types of Healing

Tissue may heal by one of three methods, which are characterized by the degree of tissue loss. *Primary intention* healing occurs in wounds that have minimal tissue loss and edges that are well-approximated (closed). If there are no complications, such as infection, necrosis, or abnormal scar formation, wound healing occurs with minimal granulation tissue and scarring.

Secondary intention healing is seen in wounds with extensive tissue loss and wounds in which the edges cannot be approximated. The wound is left open, and granulation tissue gradually fills in the deficit. Repair time is longer, tissue replacement and scarring are greater, and the susceptibility to infection is increased because of the lack of an epidermal barrier to microorganisms.

Tertiary intention healing, also known as delayed or secondary closure, is indicated when primary closure of a wound is undesirable. Conditions in which healing by tertiary intention may occur include poor circulation or infection. Suturing of the wound is delayed until the problems resolve and more favorable conditions exist for wound healing.

Kinds of Wound Drainage

Chemical mediators released during the inflammatory response cause vascular changes and exudation of fluid and cells from blood vessels into tissues. Exudates may vary in composition, but all have similar functions. These functions include the following:

- Dilution of toxins produced by bacteria and dying cells
- Transport of leukocytes and plasma proteins, including antibodies, to the site
- Transport of bacterial toxins, dead cells, debris, and other products of inflammation away from the site

The nature and amount of exudate vary depending on the tissue involved, the intensity and duration of the inflammation, and the presence and type of microorganisms.

Serous exudate is composed primarily of serum (the clear portion of blood), is watery in appearance, and has a low protein level. This type of exudate is seen with mild inflammation, resulting in minimal capillary permeability changes and minimal protein molecule escape (e.g., seen in blister formation after a burn).

Purulent exudate is also called pus. It generally occurs with severe inflammation accompanied by infection. Purulent exudate is thicker than serous exudate because of the presence of leukocytes (particularly neutrophils), liquefied dead tissue debris, and dead and living bacteria. The process of pus formation is called suppuration, and bacteria that produce pus are referred to as pyogenic bacteria. Purulent exudates may vary in color (e.g., yellow, green, brown) depending on the causative organism.

Hemorrhagic exudate or **sanguineous exudate** has a large component of red blood cells (RBCs) because of capillary damage, which allows RBCs to escape. This type of exudate is usually present with severe inflammation. The color of the exudate (bright red versus dark red) reflects whether the bleeding is fresh or old.

Mixed types of exudates may also be seen, depending on the type of wound. For example, a **serosanguineous exudate** is clear with some blood tinge and is seen with surgical incisions.

Factors Affecting Wound Healing

Wound healing depends on multiple influences, both intrinsic and extrinsic. Wounds may fail to heal or may require a longer healing period when unfavorable conditions exist. Factors that may negatively influence healing include age, oxygenation, smoking, drug therapy, and diseases such as diabetes. Such factors reduce local blood supply and impair wound healing. Nutrition and diet can also affect the healing process.

Hemorrhage

Some bleeding from a wound is normal during and immediately after initial trauma and surgery, but hemostasis usually occurs within a few minutes. Hemorrhage is abnormal and may indicate a slipped surgical suture, a dislodged clot, or erosion of a blood vessel. Swelling in the area around the wound or affected body part and the presence of sanguineous, bloody, drainage from the surgical drain may indicate internal bleeding. Other evidence of bleeding may include the signs and symptoms seen in hypovolemic shock (decreased blood pressure, rapid thready pulse, increased respiratory rate, diaphoresis, restlessness, and cool clammy skin). A hematoma (localized collection of blood underneath the tissues) may also be seen and appears as a reddish-blue swelling or mass. External hemorrhaging is detected when the surgical dressing becomes saturated with sanguineous drainage. It is also important to assess the linen under the client's wound site because it is possible for the blood to seep out from under the sides of the dressing and pool under the client. The risk for hemorrhage is greatest during the first 24 to 48 hours after surgery.

Infection

Bacterial wound contamination is one of the most common causes of altered wound healing. A wound can become infected with microorganisms preoperatively, intraoperatively, or postoperatively. During the preoperative period, the wound may become exposed to pathogens because of the manner in which the wound was inflicted, such as in traumatic injuries. Nicks or abrasions created during preoperative shaving may also be a source of pathogens. The risk for intraoperative exposure to pathogens increases when the respiratory, gastrointestinal, genitourinary, and oropharyngeal tracts are opened.

If the amount of bacteria in the wound is sufficient or the client's immune defenses are compromised, clinical infection may result and become apparent 2 to 11 days postoperatively. Infection slows healing by prolonging the inflammatory phase of healing, competing for nutrients, and producing chemicals and enzymes that are damaging to the tissues.

Wound Classification

Many different classification systems are used to describe wounds. These systems describe either how the wound was acquired, how clean it is, or which tissue layers are involved. A classification system will assist the nurse in planning wound care management. The following are commonly used classification systems.

Cause of Wound

Intentional wounds occur during treatment or therapy. These wounds are usually made under aseptic conditions. Examples include surgical incisions and venipunctures.

Unintentional wounds are unanticipated and are often the result of trauma or an accident. These wounds are created in an unsterile environment and therefore pose a greater risk of infection.

Cleanliness of Wound

This classification system ranks the wound according to its contamination by bacteria and risk for infection (Brunicardi, Anderson, Billiar, & Dunn, 2005).

- *Clean wounds* are intentional wounds that were created under conditions in which no inflammation was encountered and the respiratory, alimentary, genitourinary, and oropharyngeal tracts were not entered.
- *Clean-contaminated wounds* are intentional wounds that were created by entry into the alimentary, respiratory, genitourinary, or oropharyngeal tract under controlled conditions.
- *Contaminated wounds* are open, traumatic wounds or intentional wounds in which there was a major break in aseptic technique, spillage from the gastrointestinal tract, or incision into infected urinary or biliary tracts. These wounds have acute nonpurulent inflammation present.
- *Dirty and infected wounds* are traumatic wounds with retained dead tissue or foreign material or intentional wounds created in situations where purulent drainage was present.

Depth of Wound

The third classification system is based on the depth of the wound, taking into account the skin layers involved.

- *Superficial wounds* are confined to the epidermis layer, which comprises the four outermost layers of skin.
- *Partial-thickness wounds* involve the epidermis and part of the dermis, which is the layer of skin beneath the epidermis.
- *Full-thickness wounds* involve the entire epidermis and dermis. Deeper structures such as fascia, muscle, and bone may be involved.

Assessment

Nurses are confronted with wounds that are extremely diverse. The wound may have occurred traumatically just before the client presents to the emergency room, or the wound may be a slow-healing chronic ulcer. Approach wound assessment systematically, evaluating the wound's stage in the healing process. Show sensitivity to the client's pain and tolerance levels during assessment and always follow Standard Precautions to prevent transfer of pathogens. Following are some basic criteria for wound assessment.

Location

Assessment begins with a description of the anatomical location of the wound (e.g., "5-inch suture line on the right lower quadrant of the abdomen"). This task often becomes difficult if the client has multiple wounds close to each other, as is common in burn or multiple-trauma victims. Use of a skin documentation form that incorporates drawings of the body allows the nurse to number the location of the various wounds and then describe them.

Size

The length (head to toe), width (side to side), and depth of a wound are measured in centimeters. Single-use measurement guides (tape measures) often come with dressing supplies. To determine the depth of a wound, a sterile cotton swab, moistened with 0.9% saline solution, is inserted into the deepest point of the wound and marked at the skin surface level. Then the swab can be measured and the wound depth in centimeters documented. Tunneling, also called undermining, can be measured by using a cotton swab to gently probe the wound margins. If tunneling is noted, the location and depth are documented. For clarity in describing the location of the tunneling, the hands of the clock can be used as a guide, with 12 o'clock pointing at the client's head. Example: "Tunneling occurs at 1 o'clock and its depth is 2 cm."

General Appearance and Drainage

A general description of the color of the wound and surrounding area helps determine the wound's present phase of healing. Gently palpate the edges of the wound for swelling, and document the amount, color, location, odor, and consistency of any drainage.

Pain

Document and notify the physician of any pain or tenderness at the wound site. Pain may indicate infection or bleeding. It is normal to experience pain in a surgical incision wound for approximately 3 days. Report any sudden increase in pain accompanied by changes in the appearance of the wound to the physician immediately.

Laboratory Data

Cultures of wound drainage are used to determine the presence of infection and the identity of the causative organism. The sensitivity results list the antibiotics that will effectively treat the infection. An elevated WBC count indicates an infectious process. A decreased leukocyte count may indicate that the client is at increased risk for developing an infection related to decreased defense mechanisms. Albumin is a measure of the client's protein reserves; if the albumin is decreased, the client will have decreased resources of protein for wound healing.

Nursing Diagnoses

Nursing diagnoses for clients with wounds focus on prevention of complications and promotion of the healing process through proper wound care and client teaching. Following are NANDA-approved nursing diagnoses with a partial list of related factors:

- *Impaired **T**issue Integrity* related to surgical incision, pressure, shearing forces, decreased blood flow, immobility, mechanical irritants
- *Risk for **I**nfection* related to malnutrition, decreased defense mechanisms
- *Acute **P**ain* related to inflammation, infection
- *Disturbed **B**ody Image* related to changes in body appearance secondary to scars, drains, removal of body parts
- *Deficient **K**nowledge (Wound Care)* related to lack of exposure to information, misinterpretation, lack of interest in learning

Planning/Outcome Identification

After identifying the nursing diagnoses, establish targeted outcomes for wound healing based on the client's identified needs and individualized to the client's condition. Changes in the health care delivery system have brought about early discharge from the hospital, so clients are often sent home with wounds that need continued care; the goals for clients with wounds generally focus on promoting wound healing, preventing infection, and educating the client.

Implementation

Nursing interventions to promote wound healing and prevent infection include emergency measures to maintain homeostasis (state of internal constancy of the body), and cleansing and dressing of the wound.

Emergency Measures

Assess the type and extent of injury that the client has sustained. If hemorrhage is detected, apply sterile dressings and pressure to stop the bleeding, and notify the physician immediately. Always implement Standard Precautions. Monitor the client's vital signs frequently.

When dehiscence or evisceration occurs, instruct the client to remain quiet and avoid coughing or straining. Position the client to prevent further stress on the wound. Use sterile dressings, such as ABD pads soaked with sterile normal saline, to cover the wound and internal contents. This reduces the risk of bacterial contamination and drying of the viscera. Notify the surgeon immediately and prepare the client for surgical repair of the area.

Cleansing the Wound

The goal of cleansing the wound is to remove debris and bacteria from the wound bed with as little trauma to the healthy granulation tissue as possible. Choice of cleansing agent depends on the physician's prescription as well as agency protocol. It is recommended that isotonic solutions such as normal saline or lactated Ringer's be used to preserve healthy tissue.

PROFESSIONALTIP

Wound Cleansing

Following are the major principles to keep in mind when cleansing a wound:

- Use Standard Precautions at all times.
- When using a swab or gauze to cleanse a wound, work from the clean area out toward the dirtier area. For example, when cleaning a surgical incision, start over the incision line, and swab downward from top to bottom. Change the swab and proceed again on either side of the incision, using a new swab each time.
- When irrigating a wound, warm the solution to room temperature, preferably to body temperature, to prevent lowering of the tissue temperature. Be sure to allow the irrigant to flow from the cleanest area to the contaminated area to avoid spreading pathogens.

Dressing the Wound

A dressing serves several purposes:

1. To protect the wound from bacterial contamination
2. To promote homeostasis
3. To provide a moist environment to enhance epithelialization
4. To support healing by absorbing drainage
5. To enhance debridement of the wound
6. To provide thermal insulation of the wound
7. To provide splinting or support of the wound site
8. To shield the client from seeing the wound when perceived as unpleasant

Keeping these purposes in mind, determine an appropriate dressing for the client's wound. There are thousands of different wound care products on the market. The physician may prescribe a specific dressing, or follow agency policy. Remember that dressing plans must be modified as the wound changes.

Monitoring Drainage of Wounds

During the inflammatory response, exudates develop within a wound. When excessive drainage accumulates in the wound bed, tissue healing is delayed. If the outer surface is allowed to heal while the drainage remains entrapped within the wound, infection and abscess may form. To facilitate drainage of any excess fluid, the physician may insert a tube or drain.

Other Therapies

Negative-pressure wound therapy, also called vacuum-assisted closure (VAC), increases healing rates. It supports the wound-healing efforts of the body by increasing cellular proliferation, reducing edema around the wound, and providing a moist, protected wound bed.

Biodebridement or maggot debridement therapy (MDT) is mainly used for chronic wounds. Maggots ingest and digest bacteria and dead tissue, thus they debride and disinfect the wound. This decreases wound odor. Maggots excrete a variety of substances, such as calcium carbonate and urea that promotes granulation tissue formation. The Food and Drug Administration regulates MDT since only certain types of maggots are therapeutic. The first intentional use occurred during the Civil War (Hunter, Langemo, Thompson, Hanson, & Anderson, 2009). Unintentional use can occur if flies are allowed to land on open wounds.

Electrical stimulation helps speed healing by increasing capillary density and perfusion, improving wound oxygenation, and encouraging fibroblast activity and granulation. Placement of the electrodes varies with the stage of healing. A physical therapist determines electrode placement and polarity (Ramadan & Zyada, 2008).

Evaluation

Evaluate the client's achievement of the goals established during the planning phase to achieve or maintain skin integrity. Goals for clients with wounds generally focus on wound healing, prevention of infection, and client education. If the goals are not achieved, examine the nursing interventions and strategies that were employed and revise the nursing care plan accordingly. Review techniques and procedures, especially those performed by the client or other caregivers in the client's support system.

BURNS

Burns are among the most devastating injuries an individual can suffer. Burns can be painful and disfiguring, requiring long hospitalizations. Many are fatal. Most burns occur in the home and are preventable. Often, the burn injury is the result of the individual's own action. Feelings of anger and guilt can complicate recovery. Often, the individual suffers self-image disturbances, and family relationships can be strained.

MAJOR CAUSES

There are many different causes for burns to the skin. A major source of burn injury for all ages is overexposure to the sun. Most burn injuries to adults are associated with cigarette smoking and cooking. The elderly are more likely to spill hot liquid on themselves or catch their clothes on fire as they cook or smoke. Young children are especially prone to burn injuries from spilling scalding liquids on themselves and playing with matches or cigarette lighters. Industrial accidents account for a significant number of burn injuries in young adults.

SEVERITY

Burns are classified according to the depth of the burn and the extent of skin surface involved. First- and second-degree burns are partial-thickness (within the epidermis/dermis) burns. First-degree burns involve only the epidermis. The skin is hot, red, and painful. Sunburn is an example of a first-degree burn. First-degree burns heal in about a week without scarring. Second-degree burns damage the dermis and the epidermis. The skin is red, hot, and painful; blisters form and tissue around the burn is edematous. An example of a second-degree burn is spilling boiling water on the skin. Usually, second-degree burns heal in about 2 weeks without scarring; however, if deep layers of the dermis are involved, healing might take months and scarring can occur. Second-degree burns involving deep layers of the dermis may appear white, tan, or red in color.

When the dermis and epidermis are completely destroyed and deeper tissues are involved, burns are classified as full-thickness burns. Third-degree and fourth-degree burns are full-thickness burns. In third-degree burns all dermal structures are destroyed and cannot be regenerated. Subcutaneous tissue is also damaged. Full-thickness burns can be white, tan, brown, black, charred, or bright red in color. Fourth-degree burns, which extend to the underlying muscles and bones, appear white to black or charred with dark networks of thrombosed capillaries visible inside the wound. Fourth-degree burns result from fires, explosions, and nuclear radiation. Figure 15-8 depicts the various layers of skin involved in burn injuries.

Severely burned individuals generally have both partial-thickness and full-thickness burns. Whereas first- and second-degree burns are painful, third- and fourth-degree burns are not painful because sensory nerve endings are destroyed. The client, however, will still be in severe pain. Body movement causes pain in areas of first- and second-degree burns that often surround the full-thickness burns. Skin can regenerate

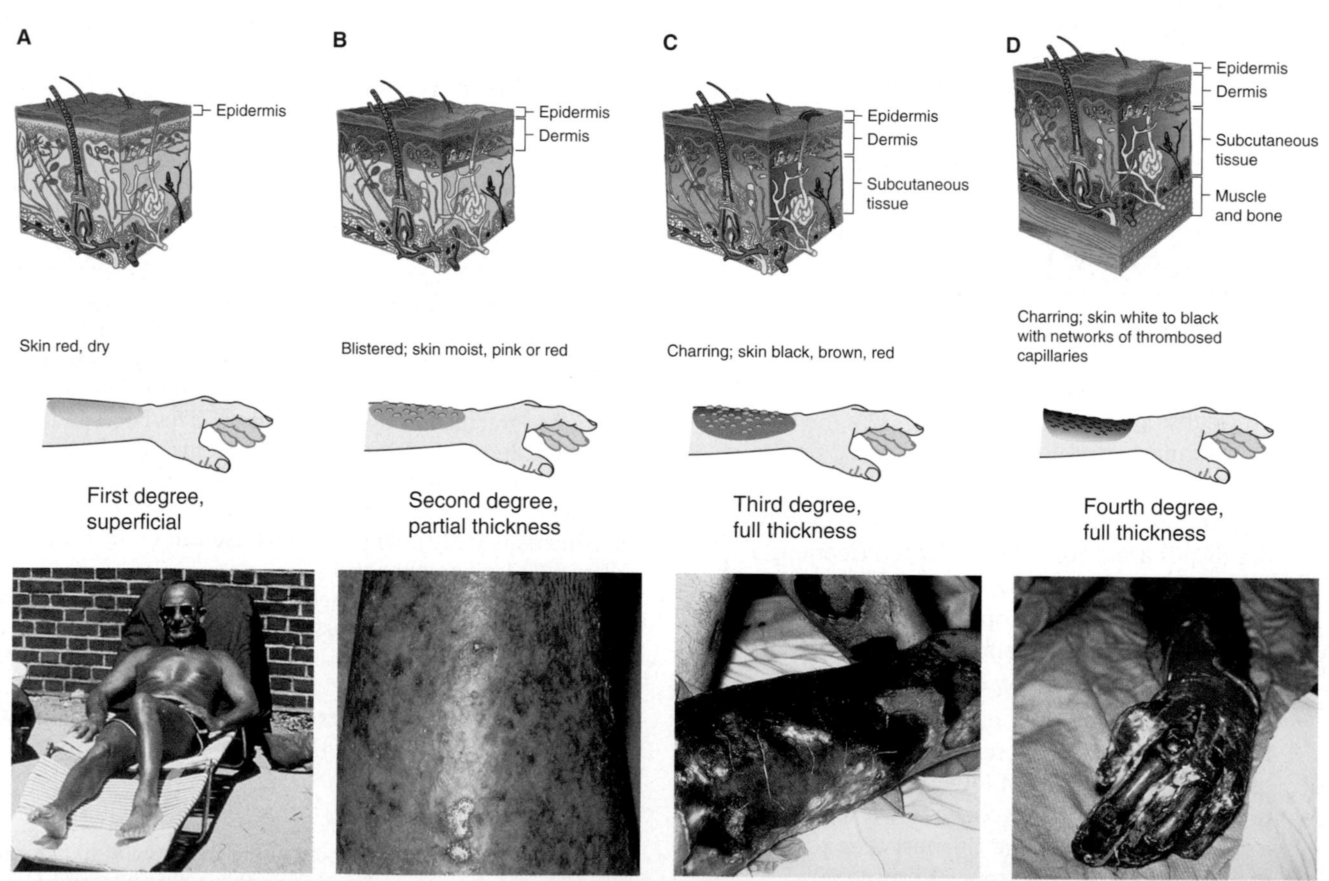

FIGURE 15-8 Skin Layers Involved in Burn Injuries; *A*, First-Degree Burn; *B*, Second-Degree Burn; *C*, Third-Degree Burn; *D*, Fourth-Degree Burn (*Photos courtesy of the Phoenix Society of Burn Survivors, Inc.*)

only from the edges of full-thickness burns. Scarring is inevitable. Skin grafting is necessary to promote healing because the section of skin destroyed by the burn cannot regenerate itself.

Prognosis in burn cases depends on the severity of the burn, the surface area of the body burned, and the preinjury health status of the individual. Local tissue injury response from burns becomes systemic when more than 20 percent of the body is involved. These clients have an increased susceptibility to multiple organ failure and sepsis. The most frequent burn related problem is inhalation injury, and it has the most significant effect on survival (Grunwald & Warren, 2008). Elderly burn victims whose physiologic reserves are already reduced as an effect of aging will have an extended recovery period and a greater risk of complications.

For years, documenting the extent of burn injuries was done by using the Rule-of-Nines method to estimate the body surface area burned for adults. The body is divided into areas that are about 9% (or multiples of 9%). The head comprises 9% (4.5% anterior and 4.5% posterior). Each arm is 9% (4.5% anterior and 4.5% posterior). The anterior trunk and posterior trunk are each 18%. Each leg is 18% (9% anterior and 9% posterior). The genitalia comprise the remaining 1%.

More recently, Milner (2001), inventor of the "Burn Wheel" (Figure 15-9), incorporated a chart similar to the Rule-of-Nines. His chart has a specific percentage for the upper and lower parts of the arms and legs and for the hands and feet, making a more accurate assessment. One side is for infants and children; the other side is for adults.

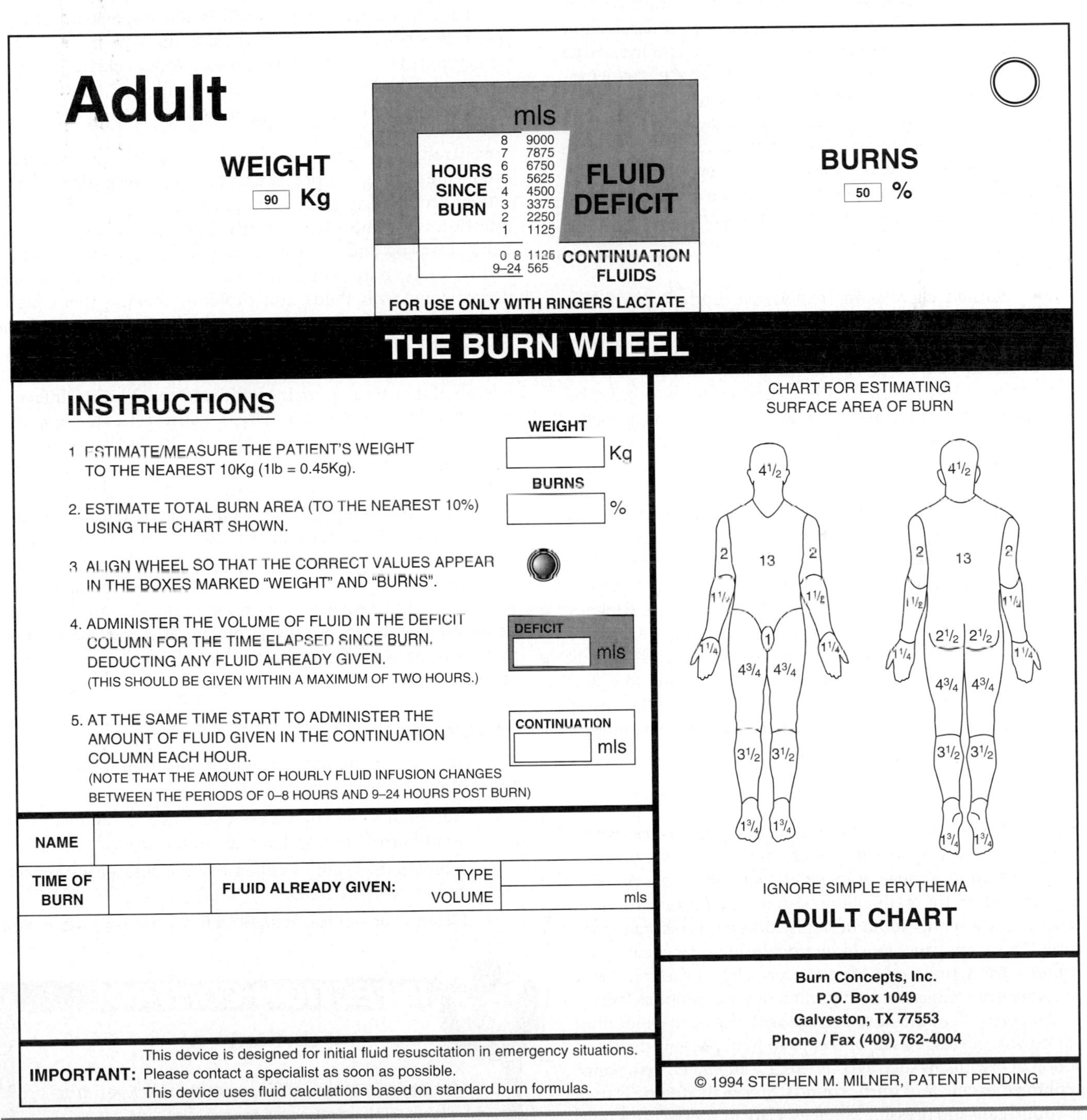

FIGURE 15-9 Burn Wheel (*Invented by Stephen M. Milner.*)

COMPLICATIONS

Destruction of the skin renders it unable to fulfill its functions. Vast amounts of internal fluids and electrolytes are lost. The ability to maintain body temperature is altered, and the individual is susceptible to serious infections. Initially, the complications that are the most life threatening are respiratory failure and massive loss of body fluids.

Smoke Inhalation and Carbon Monoxide Poisoning

Heat and smoke can cause serious damage to the respiratory tract. Signs and symptoms of potential respiratory tract damage include facial burns, singed nasal hairs, changes in voice, difficulty breathing, wheezing, coughing, and carbon-tinged sputum (National Institutes of Health, 2008a). Inhaling heat and smoke in a closed-space fire causes airway inflammation and edema of the respiratory mucosa. The carbon-monoxide that is inhaled along with the heat and smoke attaches to hemoglobin, forming the compound carboxyhemoglobin. A high level of carboxyhemoglobin in the blood means that oxygen is not being delivered to vital body tissues. The client may be stuporous because of cerebral anoxia. Keeping an open airway and administering 100% humidified oxygen are essential for treating these two conditions. Intubation is often necessary.

Shock

Severely burned clients may experience both hypovolemic shock (a life-threatening condition caused by massive loss of blood and circulating fluids) and neurogenic shock (a form of shock that occurs when peripheral vascular dilation occurs causing hypotension). Fluids and electrolytes must be replaced as fast as they are being lost. Tremendous amounts of fluids are lost through the burn wounds themselves as well as into surrounding tissues in the form of edema. The fluid loss shock that results can lead to circulatory collapse and renal shutdown. The Burn Wheel was developed for use in hospitals and emergency departments (EDs) because the first 24 hours after a burn injury are crucial (Milner, 2001). The Burn Wheel uses the client's weight (in Kg) along with the percentage of area burned to identify the amount of Ringer's lactate solution to be given IV within 2 hours and the amount to be continued for 24 hours. Use of the wheel takes seconds to determine fluid replacement, whereas remembering and figuring formulae may take much longer and mistakes can be easily made. At least two large-bore venous catheters are used to give large volumes of fluid rapidly.

Infection

Once the client has been stabilized, infection poses a serious risk. *Staphylococcus aureus*, an ever-present organism in the environment, is a common cause of infections. Of grave concern is an infection caused by methicillin-resistant *Staphylococcus aureus* (MRSA) because this strain of staphylococcus is resistant to all antibiotics except vancomycin hydrochloride (Vancocin). This antibiotic has serious side effects, especially to the otic nerve and to the liver, and is used only when other antibiotics fail.

All persons coming into contact with the burn client must wear gowns, gloves, masks, and caps to help prevent the introduction of organisms such as *S. aureus, Pseudomonas aeruginosa*, or coliform bacilli, into burn wounds. Sterile technique is used for wound care and dressing changes. Care in special burn units reduces the chance of infection because of stringent infection control precautions and a carefully controlled environment.

MEDICAL–SURGICAL MANAGEMENT

Medical

Immediate Care Initially, medical management of the client involves keeping an open airway, maintaining an adequate level of oxygenation, replacing body fluids and electrolytes, monitoring kidney function, controlling pain, and protecting the burns with sterile dressings to minimize the loss of body temperature and the risk of infection. In cases of severe burns, the client usually requires endotracheal intubation and administration of 100% humidified oxygen. A multiport central venous catheter or two large-bore peripheral venous catheters are needed for fluid and electrolyte replacement. A Foley catheter is inserted and urine output measured hourly to help monitor kidney function.

Pain is controlled with small intravenous doses of morphine. Emotional and psychological trauma can intensify pain perception. The client will be anxious about survival, physical appearance, and the effect this injury will have on the family. Prophylactically, the client is given tetanus toxoid.

Stabilized Care Once the client's condition has been stabilized, care focuses on promoting healing, preventing complications, controlling pain, and restoring function. Preventing infection is an important priority. Burn wounds may require daily cleansing and dressing changes. Because of the nature of the injury, burn wounds contain a large amount of dead tissue along with fluids and proteins, making them highly susceptible to infection even with the best of care. Antibiotics and strict aseptic technique are essential. The dead tissue of full-thickness burns forms a dry, dark leathery **eschar** (a scab of denatured protein) within 48 to 72 hours. Infection can often begin under the eschar, causing tissue sloughing. Loose eschar must be **debrided** before skin grafting can occur. Debriding, removing dead and damaged tissue or foreign material within the burn wound, can sometimes be done mechanically by hydrotherapy. Burn wounds may require surgical debridement. The base of the wound must be free of infection and necrotic tissue before it can be covered with skin grafts.

Use of specialty beds, such as fluidized or alternating air-filled mattresses, minimizes pressure on skin surfaces, thus promoting comfort. Limiting movement and maintaining normal body alignment with the use of splints can also help alleviate client discomfort.

Surgical

Skin grafts cover the burn wound to promote healing. Four types of skin grafts might be used:

1. Autograft—the client's own skin that is removed from an unburned area and applied to the wound
2. Homograft—skin obtained from a cadaver within 6 to 24 hours after death
3. Heterograft—skin obtained from an animal, such as a pig

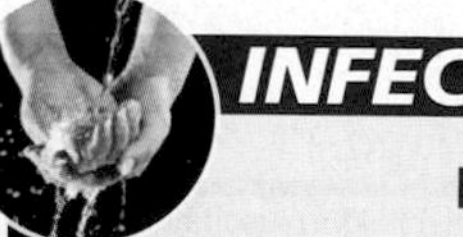

INFECTION CONTROL

Debridement

Strict aseptic techniques must be followed during burn debridement procedures.

4. Synthetic skin substitute—a manmade product that has properties similar to skin (Fritsch & Yurko, 2003)

Homografts, heterografts, and synthetic skin substitutes are temporary grafts that facilitate healing. These grafts prevent water, electrolyte, and protein loss. They decrease pain and allow more freedom of movement for the client. When the client's condition is stable and the wound beds have healthy **granulation tissue** (delicate connective tissue consisting of fibroblasts, collagen, and capillaries), permanent closure of the burn wounds is done with autographs. Granulation tissue is red and provides a base for healing (Tate, 2008).

Autografts are taken from areas of healthy skin. They may be either split-thickness grafts or full-thickness grafts. Split-thickness grafts include the epidermis and part of the dermis. They are not so deep as to prevent regeneration of skin at the donor site.

The application of pressure dressings during the rehabilitative phase reduces the development of hypertrophic scarring, a condition in which the scar becomes elevated and has a "Swiss cheese" appearance. Pressure dressings, which may be elastic wraps, stockinettes, or custom-made pressure garments, must be worn constantly and are to be removed only for daily hygiene care. Full maturation of the burn scar may take 1 to 2 years. As the physical wounds heal, so do the emotional and psychological wounds. The client's ability to cope with daily stresses and resume social and work activities typically coincides with the physical healing process.

Pharmacological

Dressing changes, wound debridement, as well as any movement or manipulation, are extremely painful for clients. Many clients become extremely anxious, fearing pain as well as permanent disfiguration and loss of function. Intravenous narcotics, usually morphine, may be administered 10 to 15 minutes before procedures. By decreasing anxiety and fear, daily doses of psychotropic drugs can enhance the effectiveness of pain medications and help the client cope with the prospect of long-term rehabilitation.

Treatment of the burn wound with topical agents can decrease infection and promote healing. Common topical agents used are mafenide acetate (Sulfamylon); silver sulfadiazine (Silvadene); povidone-iodine (Betadine); nitrofurazone (Furacin); and antibiotic agents such as neomycin sulfate (Myciguent), bacitracin (Baciguent), and gentamicin sulfate (Garamycin). Mafenide acetate (Sulfamylon) can penetrate thick eschar and is effective against gram-negative and gram-positive organisms, including *P. aeruginosa*. Silver sulfadiazine (Silvadene) is effective against many gram-positive and gram-negative organisms as well as *Candida* organisms. It is painless and somewhat soothing but may cause a skin rash. Povidone-iodine (Betadine) has broad-spectrum microbial action against a wide variety of bacteria, fungi, yeasts, viruses, and protozoa. Application of povidone-iodine (Betadine) to large open areas could lead to elevated serum iodine levels. Nitrofurazone (Furacin) has broad-spectrum activity and is effective against *S. aureus*. It is not absorbed systemically and has a low incidence of sensitivity.

Antibiotic ointments are used to decrease infection. Neomycin sulfate (Myciguent) and gentamicin sulfate (Garamycin) can be absorbed systemically and have serious side effects of ototoxicity and nephrotoxicity. Bacitracin (Baciguent) has minimal antimicrobial activity, but it is especially useful to prevent drying of the wound. Topical agents must be applied in a thin layer with a sterile glove. The wound may be left open to air or covered with a gauze dressing, depending on the properties of the medication and the physician's orders. Application of these medications can be painful because of manipulation of the burned tissue. Administration of pain medication may be necessary before providing wound care. The surrounding skin should be assessed for any allergic rashes.

INFECTION CONTROL

Skin Grafts

Follow strict aseptic care of both the donor sites and the newly grafted burn wounds to prevent infection.

Diet

After experiencing a moderate to severe burn, the client's need for calories and protein increases. Actual protein loss occurs with the burn injury itself, and some protein is metabolized to meet the increased energy requirements brought on by stress. For tissue repair and healing, daily protein needs of the client increase significantly. Twice the normal caloric requirement may be needed to meet the body's energy needs. Supplemental vitamins and minerals are given.

Initially, the client's daily nutritional needs may be met with total parenteral nutrition (TPN) because of a paralytic ileus and gastric dilation. Following a severe burn, decreased enteric circulation leads to slowed or stopped peristalsis. Food and fluids cannot be given orally or by tube feeding until peristalsis is restored. Hearing active bowel sounds is one indication of peristaltic activity in the bowel. Immobility, stress, and the negative nitrogen balance brought on by protein catabolism depress appetite. Curling's ulcer may develop. Meeting the client's nutritional needs can be a challenge. Six to eight small feedings daily and high-protein milkshakes or protein supplements can help meet daily nutritional needs. Involving the family in bringing in favorite foods can also stimulate the client's appetite.

Activity

Contractures, among the most serious complications of severe burns, can be prevented with a program of positioning,

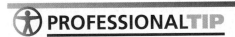

Serving Meals

Serve foods attractively and put an occasional small "surprise" on the tray (e.g., a flower, a small, brightly colored seasonal decoration, a funny card) so that the client will look forward to meals.

CRITICAL THINKING

Burns and Self-Image

How might a person's self-image be affected when the person has burns on the face, arms, or legs?

LIFE SPAN CONSIDERATIONS

Burn Injuries in the Elderly

- Normal physiologic changes that occur with aging delay recovery and put the older adult at greater risk for complications following a burn injury.
- As a person ages, the physiologic reserves of organ systems decrease.
- While the older person may have adequate pulmonary and cardiac functions at rest, the stress of a severe burn can leave the body unable to cope with demands for increased oxygen and increased cardiac output.
- Renal changes that occur with aging, such as decreased renal blood flow, fewer nephrons, and a decreased glomerular filtration rate, put the older adult at higher risk for kidney failure after a severe burn.
- With loss of subcutaneous tissue and decreased secretion of sebum, the older person's skin is normally more fragile.
- Circulation, especially in the lower extremities, may already be compromised, so healing will be delayed.
- Skin-grafting procedures may not be successful because of impaired circulation and impaired tissue nutrition.

splinting, exercising, and ambulating. When repositioning, the client's body must be kept in correct alignment. Use pillows to keep limbs in alignment and splints on limbs to prevent contractures or to immobilize joints following skin grafting. Range-of-motion exercises maintain joint mobility. Whenever possible, encourage active rather than passive range-of-motion exercises. Active exercise increases circulation, maintains joint flexibility, and improves muscle tone. As the client recovers, activities of daily living can be increased and ambulation can be initiated.

Nursing Management

Immediate care includes establishing an airway and administering oxygen. (The physician often inserts an endotracheal tube). Initiate IV fluid therapy with Ringer's lactate solution. Insert a Foley catheter and monitor output, which should be 30 to 50 mL per hour. Administer analgesic IV as ordered. Monitor vital signs, noting respiratory pattern, effort, and breath sounds. Assess pulse oximetry, client's color, and level of consciousness. Accurately record I&O. Monitor client's laboratory results, especially electrolytes.

When the client is stabilized, continue monitoring vital signs, I&O, respiratory pattern, daily weight, and for pain. Strictly follow Standard Precautions. Monitor wounds for signs of infection. Assess mental status. If client is on TPN or enteral tube feedings, monitor client's reaction to feedings. Assess abdomen for bowel sounds. Use pillows and splints, if ordered, to keep client's body in good alignment and turn and reposition every 2 hours. Perform passive ROM exercises when able. Explain the healing process to the client and family. Provide opportunities for the client to express feelings. Listen actively. Encourage the client to look at the wounds to see evidence of healing. Maintain an open, honest approach with the client and family. Assist client and family to prepare for discharge.

NURSING PROCESS

Assessment

Subjective Data

Observe for emotional reactions such as anger, self-consciousness, embarrassment, or isolation. Clients with burns are likely to be frightened and anxious. Feelings of guilt, anger, and depression are also common following burns. Ask the client to describe the pain according to location, intensity, and duration, and also to rate the pain on a scale of 0 to 10. Hypoxia or fluid and electrolyte imbalances can cause confusion, disorientation, and decreased level of consciousness. The client may be nauseated.

Objective Data

Assess vital signs, level of consciousness, and breath sounds. If the client has a productive cough, the amount, consistency, and color of sputum should be noted. Black/gray sputum indicates smoke inhalation. Clients with smoke inhalation may also have crackles, wheezing, or diminished breath sounds. Observe burn wounds for signs of infection such as redness, swelling, purulent drainage, and a foul odor. Measure urine output hourly. Monitor intake and output and daily weight. Routinely check for bowel sounds. As rehabilitation progresses, continue to assess wounds for signs of healing, such as a moist, clean, red wound base and decrease in the size of the wound. Note the client's mobility status and degree of involvement in care. Assess daily dietary intake. Monitor laboratory test results for the following:

- Red blood cell count and hemoglobin level give information about the body's ability to meet oxygen demands of body tissues and organs.
- Creatinine and blood urea nitrogen as well as urine specific gravity give information about kidney function.
- Total protein and albumin levels yield information about the ability to maintain the volume of circulating fluid as well as information about nutritional status.
- White blood cell count indicates the presence of infection and the body's ability to fight it.
- Wound culture and sensitivity data indicate the specific organisms causing infection and the specific antibiotics effective against these organisms.
- Electrolytes yield information about the homeostasis of body fluids. Alterations in pH and electrolyte levels affect cell function in every body tissue, particularly vital body organs such as the heart and cerebrum.

Nursing diagnoses for a client with a burn injury include the following. Initially, the greatest dangers to the client will be:

NURSING DIAGNOSES	PLANNING/OUTCOMES	NURSING INTERVENTIONS
*Impaired **G**as Exchange* related to edema and inflammation of the respiratory tract	The client will achieve a regular respiratory pattern and oxygen saturation level >90%.	Monitor the client's vital signs every 4 hours if stable; otherwise, every 1 to 2 hours. Listen to breath sounds, especially noting respiratory pattern and effort. If the client is on continuous oximetry, note the oxygen saturation reading each time vital signs are assessed. Assess the client's color and level of consciousness. Document assessments and keep the physician informed about the client's condition. Elevate the head of the bed 30 degrees to facilitate full chest expansion with each breath.
*Deficient **F**luid Volume* related to increased capillary permeability with loss of large amounts of fluid through open burn wounds	The client will maintain electrolytes within normal limits and an hourly urine output >30 mL per hour.	Administer intravenous fluids at the ordered rate. Monitor for signs and symptoms of fluid overload such as shortness of breath, crackles auscultated in lung bases, changes in heart rate and/or heart sounds, changes in blood pressure, increased anxiety, or changes in mental status. Measure urine output hourly, report outputs below 30 mL to the physician. Record intake and output. Involve the client and family in keeping a bedside record of fluid intake. Weigh client daily, preferably before breakfast, and in the same type of clothing each day. When the client can tolerate oral fluids, set a fluid intake goal for each shift (e.g., 1,200 mL during the day; 800 mL during the evening; 500 mL during the night). Explain to the client and family the reasons for a high fluid intake. Involve family members in helping the client achieve the fluid maintenance goal. Keep fluids available at the bedside, including, within dietary restrictions, the client's favorite fluids. Monitor for signs and symptoms of electrolyte imbalances such as increased muscle weakness, muscle cramps, cardiac arrhythmias, fatigue, nausea, dizziness. Monitor the client's laboratory results.

Evaluation: Evaluate each outcome to determine how it has been met by the client.

During the stabilization and recovery period after a burn, the nursing diagnoses include the following:

NURSING DIAGNOSES	PLANNING/OUTCOMES	NURSING INTERVENTIONS
*Risk for **I**nfection* related to risk factors of tissue destruction and inadequate primary defenses	The client's burn wounds will exhibit signs of healing without serious or life-threatening infections.	Wash hands with an antibacterial skin cleanser before and after gloving. Wear clean gloves when giving client care. Wear an isolation gown over your uniform when giving client care. Whenever the client's wounds are exposed, wear gown, cap, mask, and sterile gloves. Use sterile technique for wound care and dressing changes. Monitor wound daily for signs of infection: redness, swelling, purulent drainage, pain. Assess for signs of systemic infections. Observe for increased pulse and respirations, decreased blood pressure, fever, and any changes in mentation such as disorientation and delirium.

(Continues)

During the stabilization and recovery period after a burn, the nursing diagnoses include the following: (Continued)

NURSING DIAGNOSES	PLANNING/OUTCOMES	NURSING INTERVENTIONS
		Note urinary output and assess for hypoactive bowel sounds. Monitor the client's white blood cell count. Assist client with personal hygiene, and keep noninjured areas of the body clean.
*Acute **Pain*** related to physical injury	The client will verbalize that pain is controlled at a tolerable level.	Assess for pain every 2 to 4 hours by asking client to rate pain level on a scale of 0 to 10. Observe for nonverbal signs of pain such as grimacing or crying. Administer pain medications as ordered, especially prior to wound care or exercise and mobilization activities. Monitor and document response to medications. Implement comfort and diversional measures: a. Reposition client; use pillows or foam supports to keep all body parts in good alignment. b. Teach client to use progressive relaxation exercises or to use guided imagery. c. Encourage the client to use diversionary activities of his choice such as television or music, or place him so that he can see into the hallway.
*Imbalanced **Nutrition**: Less than Body Requirements*, related to increased caloric requirements and difficulty ingesting sufficient quantities of food	The client will ingest sufficient calories daily to meet increased metabolic needs.	If the client is currently on TPN or enteral tube feedings, administer the ordered nutrients at the correct rate and closely monitor the client's reaction. When oral intake is tolerated, encourage the client to eat 90% to 100% of daily diet. Provide oral hygiene before meals to stimulate salivation and eliminate any bad taste in the client's mouth. Give 6 to 8 small feedings daily of the client's favorite foods within dietary restrictions and encourage family members to bring in home-prepared foods and to eat with the client. When permitted, encourage the client to sit up in a chair for each meal. Plan care so that painful procedures are not done immediately before meals. A rest period of 20 to 30 minutes before meals helps the client feel more like eating. Determine the time of day when the client feels most like eating and does indeed eat most of the meal, and serve the highest calorie/protein nutrients at that time.
*Impaired Physical **Mobility*** related to pain and decreased muscle strength	The client will participate in daily activity to maintain joint mobility and prevent contractures.	Perform passive ROM exercises 4 times a day by supporting the limb above and below the joint and performing exercises slowly and smoothly. As the client is able, have him perform active ROM exercises every 3 to 4 hours. Turn and reposition the client every 2 hours. Use small pillows and foam supports to keep the client's body in good alignment. Use splints as ordered by the physician to keep hands, wrists, feet, and ankles in natural alignment and explain the reason for these activities to the client. As healing and rehabilitation progress, encourage progressive ambulation and self-care activities.

During the stabilization and recovery period after a burn, the nursing diagnoses include the following: (Continued)

NURSING DIAGNOSES	PLANNING/OUTCOMES	NURSING INTERVENTIONS
		Gradually guide and assist the client to resume activities of daily living (ADLs). Encourage family members to participate in ADLs and provide positive reinforcement as the client becomes involved in his care.
*Disturbed **B**ody Image* related to change in physical appearance with loss of body tissues or body parts	The client will state realistic expectations for recovery and participate in rehabilitation.	Provide time for the client to express feelings (fear, anger, frustration, regret, and depression are commonly expressed by clients with burns) and practice active listening. Explain the healing process to the client. Give the client daily updates on the degree of wound healing and on his progress in rehabilitation. Encourage the client to look at the wounds to see evidence of healing. Stress that wound healing following serious burn injuries proceeds slowly and that complete healing with improved skin appearance may take a year or more.
*Interrupted **F**amily Processes* related to the shift in health status of a family member	The client and family members will verbalize feelings to nurses and each other and will participate in client care.	Involve family members in the client's care and encourage daily visits. Encourage family members to express their fears and concerns, especially any feelings of anger, blame, or guilt. Guide family members in recognizing and reflecting to the client small, step-by-step progress that is made. Maintain an honest, open approach with the client and family but do not give false reassurance. Collaborate with counselor, social worker, and chaplain to help the client and family cope with the condition. Assist the family to appraise the situation and plan for discharge. What is at stake? What is realistic for the future? What can they expect during the rehabilitation phase? What are their choices? Where can they get help?

Evaluation: Evaluate each outcome to determine how it has been met by the client.

NEOPLASMS: MALIGNANT

Skin cancer is one of the most common malignant neoplasms in the United States and is the most preventable cancer. In 2009, the American Cancer Society estimates more than one million new diagnoses of basal cell carcinoma (approximately 800,000–900,000) and squamous cell carcinoma (approximately 200,000–300,000) in the United States (American Cancer Society [ACS], 2008a). Approximately 68,720 new diagnoses of melanomas are expected to occur in 2009 (ACS, 2008b). These are the three most common skin cancers.

Skin lymphoma is another type of malignancy. Exposure to the sun is the leading cause of skin cancer. Skin damage from sun exposure is cumulative. The ability of skin to tan is not fully developed until the teenage years, meaning that most of the long-term skin damage from sun exposure occurs during childhood. By age 20, most adults have already experienced significant skin damage; however, it takes 10 to 20 years before unprotected sunbathing results in skin cancer.

BASAL CELL CARCINOMA

Basal cell carcinoma, the most frequent type of skin cancer, arises from the basal cell layer of the epidermis. Prolonged sun exposure, poor tanning ability, and previous therapy with x-rays for facial acne are risk factors for basal cell carcinoma (Figure 15-10). Metastasis is rare.

It is generally found on the face and upper torso, and is scaly in appearance. As the disease develops, it extends into the dermis and may form an open ulcer. Surgical removal cures this type of cancer.

SQUAMOUS CELL CARCINOMA

Squamous cell carcinoma appears as a nodular lesion in the epidermis. It is much less common than basal cell carcinoma. Risk factors include prolonged sun exposure and exposure to gamma radiation and x-rays. The sun-exposed lower lip is a common site for squamous cell carcinoma. Without treatment, it can extend into the dermis and ultimately metastasize

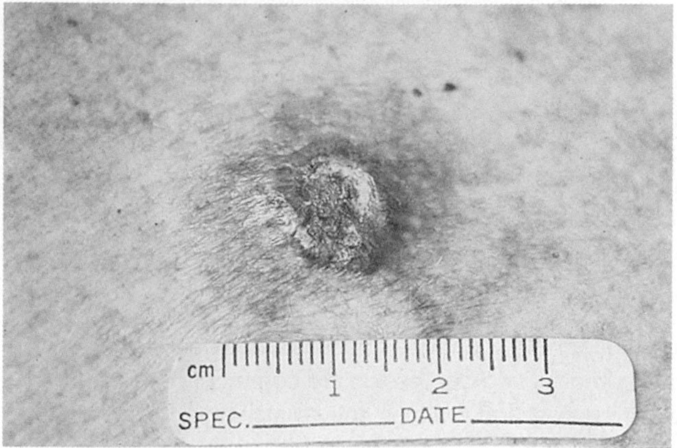

FIGURE 15-10 Basal Cell Carcinoma (*Courtesy of Robert A. Silverman, MD, Clinical Associate Professor, Department of Pediatrics, Georgetown University.*)

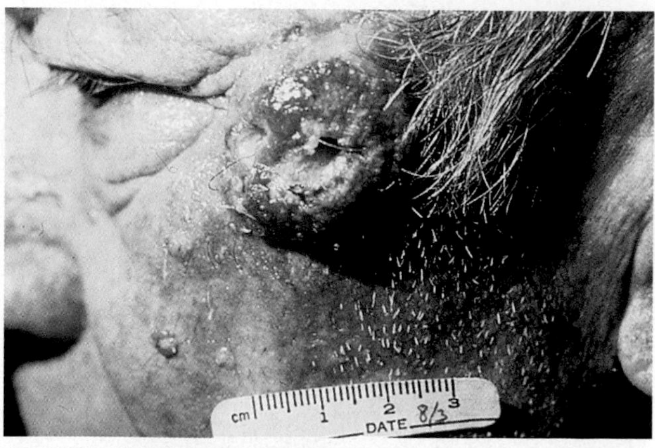

FIGURE 15-11 Squamous Cell Carcinoma (*Courtesy of Robert A. Silverman, MD, Clinical Associate Professor, Department of Pediatrics, Georgetown University.*)

to other body tissues, causing death (Figure 15-11). Treatment, for squamous cell carcinoma may be by excision of lesion, electrodesiccation (cautery) and curettage (scraping of lesion), cryosurgery (freezing with liquid nitrogen), Mohs surgery (a microscopic surgical procedure of removing layers of cancerous tissue with very high rates of success), radiation therapy, lymph node dissection, and/or chemotherapy (ACS, 2008c).

MALIGNANT MELANOMA

In malignant melanoma, atypical melanocytes are present in both the dermis and epidermis. Malignant melanoma is the most serious of the three types of skin cancers and may begin in a preexisting mole (nevus). These moles have an irregular shape. Contrasted to normal moles, they are larger than 6 mm in diameter and do not have a uniform color (see ABCD rule). Malignant melanoma can metastasize to every organ in the body through the bloodstream and lymphatic system.

Melanoma is more common in fair-skinned individuals and occurs most often on the trunk of males and the lower legs on females, but can occur on any area of the body and in all skin tones. Malignant melanomas can arise from a mole that has been present for a client's entire life as well as from skin independent of mole existence. Any mole that looks significantly different from other moles present on the body whether or not it has always been present should be examined carefully, photographed, followed, and/or biopsied.

MEMORY**TRICK**

ABCD rule: Usual warning signs for melanoma

- **A** = ASYMMETRICAL – Both halves of the mole or birthmark do not match.
- **B** = BORDER – Borders are irregular, blurred, or. notched.
- **C** = COLOR – Color is uneven, in different shades of black, brown, or red, white or blue.
- **D** = DIAMETER – Diameter is greater than 6 mm (¼ inch).

The most significant warning sign is a mole or birthmark that is changing in size, shape, or color over time (ACS, 2009e).

The incidence of malignant melanoma is increasing in the United States as a result of increased sun exposure and use of artificial ultraviolet light (tanning lights/beds). Clearly, the best hope of preventing skin cancer lies in education. Limiting sun exposure (and artificial ultraviolet light) and using sunscreen at least SPF 15 on exposed skin markedly reduce damage from ultraviolet rays and ultimately decrease the risk of skin cancer. Figure 15-12 shows lentigo malignant melanoma.

CUTANEOUS T-CELL LYMPHOMA

Cutaneous T-cell lymphoma is also known as mycosis fungoides and skin lymphoma. It is a malignant disease involving T-helper cells that has both skin manifestations and multiple organ system manifestations. In the early stages, it resembles psoriasis or seborrheic dermatitis. Later, fissures and skin ulcers develop. Pruritus can be severe. Even if the

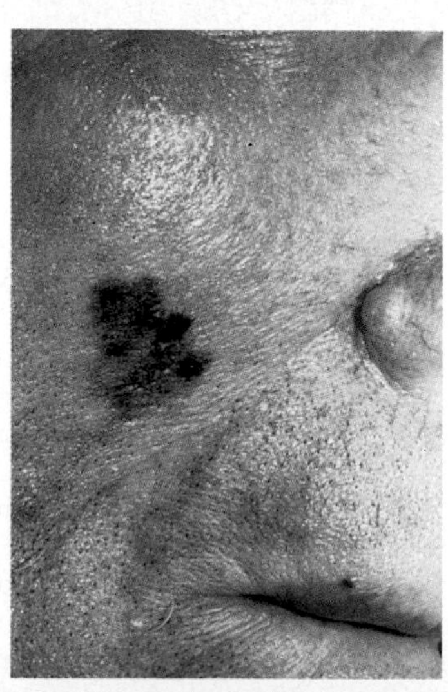

FIGURE 15-12 Lentigo Malignant Melanoma (*Courtesy of Robert A. Silverman, MD, Clinical Associate Professor, Department of Pediatrics, Georgetown University.*)

skin condition can be improved with topical steroids and chemotherapeutic agents, the disease is ultimately fatal because of the involvement of vital organ systems. Clients with AIDS can develop cutaneous T-cell lymphoma.

Medical–Surgical Management

Surgical

Treatment is determined by the size of the lesion, the type of neoplasm, and the stage of the disease. The primary treatment is surgery: a simple excision or a wide excision (removing skin in a large area around the lesion), amputation if on fingers or toes, and/or lymph node dissection if lymph nodes are enlarged or a sentinel node biopsy confirms the presence of malignant cells. If indicated, chemotherapy may be used either systemically or directly into the affected extremity. By injecting chemo into an artery of the affected limb, high doses are targeted to the tumor area without affecting the entire body. Radiation therapy may also be used (ACS, 2009d). With early detection, melanoma can be successfully treated, but presently there is no cure with advanced melanoma. Melanomas have a rapid rate of metastasis.

Nursing Management

Careful assessment of the client's skin can reveal suspicious skin lesions. Clients with blue eyes, fair complexion, blonde or red hair, and freckles have the greatest risk. Clients who have had one skin cancer are likely to have more. Early referral and prompt care can ensure a good prognosis. Because most skin cancers are treated by excision, client teaching and follow-up care focus on proper wound care to promote healing and prevent infection. Many clients will experience body image disturbance; the nurse can help the client cope with this. All other nursing care should be focused on prevention.

NEOPLASMS: NONMALIGNANT

Benign tumors of the skin include a variety of lesions such as skin tags, lipomas, keloids, sebaceous cysts, nevi (moles), and angiomas. In general, they do not require medical or nursing intervention except for cosmetic reasons or unless they are subject to continual irritation that might predispose to a break in skin integrity and infection. **Lipomas** (benign, fatty tumors) or **sebaceous cysts** (distended sebaceous glands filled with sebum) might cause pressure on surrounding nerves or interfere with normal body function. In these instances they would be surgically removed. A **keloid** is abnormal growth of scar tissue that is elevated, rounded, and firm with irregular, clawlike margins. Surgical removal is not always successful; healing following surgery can again result in a keloid. Steroids or radiation have been helpful in some conditions. **Angiomas**, commonly known as birthmarks, are vascular tumors involving skin and subcutaneous tissue. They can be raised, bright red nodular lesions (strawberry birthmarks) or dark red/purple patches (port-wine angiomas). Cosmetics can be used to camouflage them. Laser treatments are being used on some angiomas with some success.

INFECTIOUS DISORDERS OF THE SKIN

Given an accessible portal of entry and decreased host resistance, virulent organisms can invade the skin, causing inflammation, infection, itching, and pain. Bacteria, viruses, fungi, or parasites can cause infectious disorders of the skin (Figure 15-13). Treating the client's disease is only one aspect of the treatment plan; preventing the spread of infection is the other. Table 15-3 outlines several disease conditions and

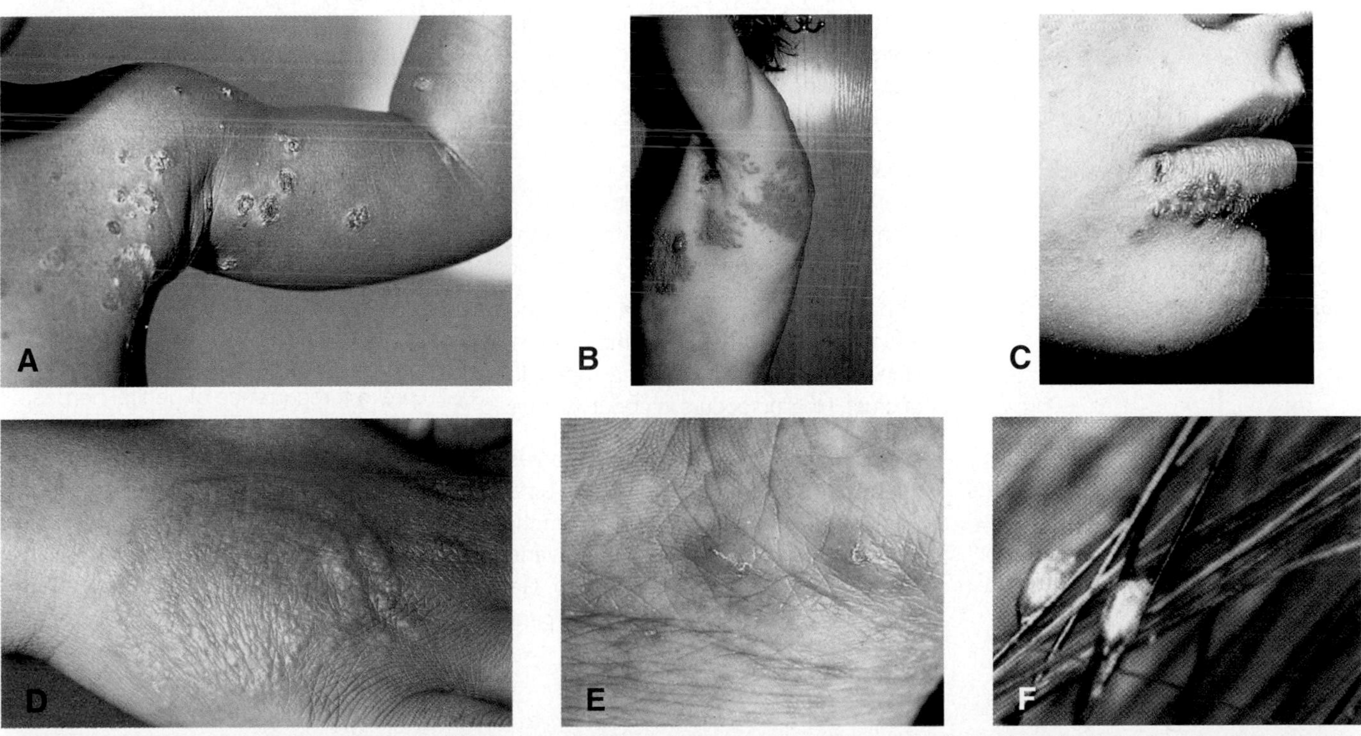

Figure 15-13 Infectious Disorders of the Skin; *A*, Impetigo Contagiosa; *B*, Herpes Zoster (Shingles); *C*, Herpes Simplex Type 1; *D*, Tinea Corporis (Ringworm); *E*, Scabies; *F*, Pediculosis (Head Lice) (*Images A, B, C, D and E courtesy of Robert A. Silverman, MD, Clinical Associate Professor, Department of Pediatrics, Georgetown University; image F courtesy of Hogil Pharmaceutical Corporation.*)

TABLE 15-3 Infectious Disorders of the Skin

DISEASE	ORGANISM	CLINICAL MANIFESTATIONS	MANAGEMENT
Bacterial Infections			
Impetigo contagiosa	*Staphylococcus aureus*	Begins as a small vesicle; becomes weeping lesion; forms a light brown crust. Usually on the face and upper trunk (Figure 15-13A). More common in children. More common in spring and fall. Poor hygiene coupled with warm weather facilitates the spread of the disease.	Cleanse the affected area at least 3 times a day. Apply an antibiotic ointment. Occasionally, systemic antibiotics are needed.
Carbuncle	*Staphylococcus aureus*	Begins as infected hair follicles in the dermis. Symptoms are redness, swelling, pain. Yellow cores of pus develop. Carbuncles usually occur on the nape of the neck and upper back. Obese or malnourished persons with poor hygiene as well as diabetics are most susceptible to carbuncles.	Warm, moist soaks may help "bring the boil to a head." Once the carbuncle ruptures or is incised and drained, pain subsides. Carbuncles tend to recur. The *Staphylococcus* organism may be resistant to topical antibiotics. Systemic antibiotics may be needed.
Viral Infections			
Herpes zoster (shingles)	V-Z (varicella-zoster)	Clusters of small vesicles over the course of a peripheral sensory nerve. Two-thirds of clients have lesions just in the thoracic region. Lesions can occur over the trigeminal nerve, affecting the face, scalp, and eyes (Figure 15-13B). Crusts develop in several days. Symptoms are mild to severe pain, itching, fever, malaise. In older adults, pain can last for months or years. Persons who have not had chickenpox risk contracting the disease if they care for herpes zoster clients with open lesions. Persons who previously had chickenpox, but developed only partial immunity to it, may still be susceptible to herpes zoster.	Acyclovir (Zovirax), valacyclovir (Valtrex), or famciclovir (Famvir) may be given to clients in severe pain or to immunosuppressed clients. Analgesics help control the pain. Narcotic analgesics are prescribed for severe pain. Antipruritic topical medications decrease the itching. Shingles (herpes zoster) vaccine is recommended for adults 60 and older even if they have had shingles in the past (Harvard Health Letter, 2008).
Herpes simplex, Type 1 (fever blisters, cold sores) Type 2 (genital)	*Herpes simplex virus*	Type 1—a cluster of vesicles on an erythematous base occurring most commonly at the corners of the mouth (Figure 15-13C) or at the edge of the nostrils. Type 2—lesions in the vagina or cervix of a woman or on the penis of a man. The lesions itch, burn, and frequently break open, forming a crust. Healing occurs in about 10 days.	Topical use of antiviral agents such as acyclovir decreases discomfort. Even with treatment, cold sores and fever blisters tend to recur, especially with fever, upper respiratory infections, and stress. Oral administration of acyclovir helps prevent recurrence of genital herpes.
Warts	Human papillomavirus	Seen as small, painless round papules on hands, face, and neck. On the bottom of the feet, warts grow inward from the pressure and are painful (plantar warts). Warts in the anogenital region itch. Genital warts increase the risk of cervical cancer.	No treatment is indicated for painless warts; they tend to disappear eventually. Plantar warts may be removed by cryosurgery or with locally applied chemicals such as nitric acid. Warts are not highly contagious from person to person but may be spread on the person's own body by rubbing or scratching. Genital warts are spread by sexual intercourse.

(Continues)

TABLE 15-3 Infectious Disorders of the Skin (Continued)

DISEASE	ORGANISM	CLINICAL MANIFESTATIONS	MANAGEMENT
Fungal Infections			
Tinea (ringworm) Tinea capitis (ringworm of the scalp) Tinea corporis (ringworm of the body) Tinea cruris (jock itch) Tinea pedis (athlete's foot)	*Microsporum audouini*	Tinea is a superficial infection of the skin called ringworm because of its circumscribed appearance, typically round, and reddened with slight scaling (Figure 15-13D). Lesions of tinea corporis have a pale center. Itching is common with tinea cruris. Itching and burning occur with tinea pedis. Tinea is spread easily. Jock itch and athlete's foot are more common among men than women.	Treat mild infections with a topical antifungal drug such as miconazole nitrate (Micatin) or tolnaftate (Aftate). Severe infections are treated with oral administration of griseofulvin microsize (Grisactin).
Parasitic Infections			
Scabies	*Sarcoptes scabiei* (female itch mite)	The itch mite burrows under the skin, lays eggs, and deposits fecal material. Short, dark-red wavy lines may be seen on hands, wrists, elbows, axillary folds, nipples, waistline, and gluteal folds (Figure 15-13E). Pruritis is severe and can persist for up to 3 months after treatment. Scratching leads to secondary infection. Scabies is spread by prolonged contact and is frequently seen in several members of a family.	Apply the scabicide, lindane (Kwell), topically to the entire body at bedtime so that the medication remains on the skin 8 to 12 hours. Treat all family members even if they do not have symptoms. Wash all underclothing and bed and bath linens in hot water and dry in dryer. Change linens daily. Items that cannot be washed should be dry cleaned.
Pediculosis (lice)	*Pediculus capitis* (head lice) *Pediculus corporis* (body lice) *Phthirus Pubis* (pubic lice)	Eggs, or nits, of pediculosis capitis attach themselves firmly to a hair shaft on the head or in a beard (Figure 15-13F). Nits have a gray, pearly appearance. The pubic louse resembles a tiny crab that attaches itself to pubic hair. Body lice live in the seams of clothing. The bite of the louse causes severe pruritis. Scratching leads to secondary infection.	Lindane (Kwell) is applied topically to the hair as a shampoo or to the body as a cream or lotion. Repeat the treatment again in 8 to 10 days. Wash or dry clean clothing and linens. Disinfect combs and brushes. Vacuum carpets and furniture; then spray with a pediculicide. All nits must be removed to prevent reinfection.

identifies the organism responsible, clinical manifestations, and the management for each disorder.

NURSING MANAGEMENT

Teach the client and family about preventing the spread of infection. Follow Standard Precautions. Stress the importance of not scratching lesions. Provide emotional support to client and family. Encourage expression of feelings.

CRITICAL THINKING

Preventing Spread of Skin Infections

How can the spread of skin infections be prevented? Prepare a teaching plan for a client with a skin infection.

NURSING PROCESS

ASSESSMENT

Subjective Data

Ask the client how long the problem has existed, if there is any itching or pain, and what treatment has been used. Clients with infectious disorders of the skin may feel shame or embarrassment because of stigmas attached to some of these conditions, so also note the client's mood.

Objective Data

A complete skin assessment is performed, describing the size, appearance, and distribution of all lesions, as well as any drainage, itching, odor, or pain present.

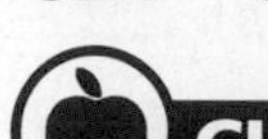

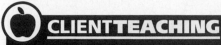

CLIENTTEACHING

Herpes Zoster

- Take the full course of prescribed medications.
- Use topical measures along with NSAIDs for pain management.
- Avoid persons who have not had chickenpox, especially pregnant women, so they do not get chickenpox.
- When dark crusts form over pustules, the client is no longer contagious.
- In older adults, pain may last for months or years.

Nursing diagnoses for a client with an infectious disorder of the skin include the following:

NURSING DIAGNOSES	PLANNING/OUTCOMES	NURSING INTERVENTIONS
*Impaired **S**kin Integrity* related to invasion of skin structures by pathogenic organisms	The client will regain skin integrity.	Wear gloves when caring for the client with skin lesions. Cleanse the skin thoroughly, but gently. In the case of bacterial infections or lesions with secondary infections, use an antibacterial soap. Gently remove crusts, scales, and traces of old medication before applying fresh creams or lotions. Administer prescribed medications; apply creams and lotions; then monitor their effectiveness. Explain what you are doing and why.
*Acute **P**ain*, related to itching, burning, and infection	The client will report less pain.	Instruct client to keep the environmental temperature cool because warmth increases itching; also cleanse skin lesions with tepid water, not hot. Stress the importance of not scratching the lesions.
*Disturbed **B**ody Image* related to unsightly skin lesions and embarrassment	The client will verbalize a positive body image.	Encourage client to ask questions and to talk about feelings. Provide positive reinforcement as the client learns to care for the skin lesions. When possible, suggest ways to camouflage the lesions or minimize their appearance. When there is no danger of spreading the infection, encourage client to participate in social and work activities.

Evaluation: Evaluate each outcome to determine how it has been met by the client.

SAMPLE NURSING CARE PLAN

The Client with Scabies

E.E., 68, has had a skin rash for the past 2 weeks. The dark red lesions occur mainly on her hands, wrists, and elbows, around her nipples, at her waistline, and in her gluteal folds. The itching has become increasingly intense. She states that she has been scratching the lesions, sometimes until they are open and bleeding. Upon examination, some of the lesions are open with small amounts of serosanguineous drainage. Other lesions are scabbed. She lives with her daughter and two teenaged granddaughters. Because the lesions were getting steadily worse, her daughter finally convinced her to seek medical attention. She was horrified when the doctor told her that she had scabies. She had always associated "the itch" with "dirty people who didn't take care of themselves."

NURSING DIAGNOSIS 1 *Impaired **S**kin Integrity* related to scratching scabies lesions as evidenced by open lesions draining serosanguineous fluid, scabbed lesions, and client statements of scratching the lesions until they bleed

(Continues)

SAMPLE NURSING CARE PLAN (Continued)

Nursing Outcomes Classification (NOC)
Tissue Integrity: Skin & Mucous Membranes
Self-Care: Hygiene

Nursing Interventions Classification (NIC)
Skin Care: Topical Treatments
Skin Surveillance

PLANNING/OUTCOMES	NURSING INTERVENTIONS	RATIONALE
E.E. will follow the prescribed treatment protocol to promote healing of skin lesions and regain skin integrity.	Instruct E.E. to cleanse lesions carefully using an antibacterial soap and tepid water. The lesions can be cleaned 1 to 3 times daily.	Reduces the number of microorganisms present and decreases the risk of infection. Tepid water does not intensify itching as hot water does.
	Teach E.E. to apply antipruritic lotions as prescribed by the doctor after cleansing the skin.	Lotions applied just after bathing help to retain skin moisture.
	Instruct E.E. to keep fingernails short with smooth edges.	Less likely to break the skin if the client scratches.
	Teach E.E. to press itching lesions, and not to scratch them.	Stimulates nerve endings and reduces the sensation of itching. Prevents breaks in the skin, which would be portals of entry for microorganisms.
	Explain that itching can persist up to 3 months following treatment with the scabicide but persistent itching does not mean that treatment was ineffective.	Skin reaction to the toxins and secretions of the itch mite can persist for up to 3 months after the itch mites are killed by the scabicide.
	Keep room temperature between 68° and 72°F and humidity constant at 30% to 35%.	Itching is intensified in hot, humid environments.

EVALUATION

E.E.'s lesions are still red, but none are open and draining. Some lesions are still scabbed. No new open lesions have developed. E.E. states that the recommended measures "help," but that the itching is still "pretty bad." Goal of promoting healing of skin lesions is being met. Encourage E.E. to continue outlined protocols. Reassure her that itching will gradually subside as healing progresses.

NURSING DIAGNOSIS 2 *Deficient Knowledge (infection control measures),* related to lack of familiarity with treatment and prevention protocols as evidenced by client's inability to recognize the skin lesions as infectious and by statements about scabies happening only to people with poor hygiene

Nursing Outcomes Classification (NOC)
Knowledge: Infection Control

Nursing Interventions Classification (NIC)
Teaching: Disease Process
Teaching: Prescribed Medication

PLANNING/OUTCOMES	NURSING INTERVENTIONS	RATIONALE
E.E. will apply the scabicide correctly and state ways to avoid spreading infection to others.	Assess E.E's knowledge of scabies, its treatment regimen and infection control measures. Ask specific questions.	Provides a frame of reference for the client, helping her relate new information and integrate it into her behavior.

(Continues)

SAMPLE NURSING CARE PLAN (Continued)

PLANNING/OUTCOMES	NURSING INTERVENTIONS	RATIONALE
	Explain that scabies is transmitted by skin-to-skin contact or by contact with articles freshly contaminated by infected persons, and affects persons of all social, economic, and age levels.	Teaching that does not "talk down" to the client communicates respect.
	Stress the importance of following treatment protocol exactly. Review salient points such as (1) shower before applying the scabicide; (2) apply the scabicide to the entire body surface, including skin without scabies lesions; and (3) apply the scabicide at bedtime so that the medication remains on the skin 8 to 12 hours.	Failure to apply the scabicide as directed and/or failure to leave the lotion on the skin for the prescribed length of time will not kill the itch mite.
	Give E.E. step-by-step written instructions.	Enhances compliance with the treatment regimen.
	Instruct E.E. to wash hands under warm running water with plenty of soap (preferably an antibacterial soap) for at least 10 seconds after touching lesions and clean carefully under fingernails while washing hands.	Thorough handwashing is the single most effective means of preventing the spread of infection. Large numbers of bacteria reside under the fingernails.
	Advise E.E. not to share washcloths, towels, clothing, pillows, or bed linens with other family members.	Disease-causing microorganisms can be spread to well individuals indirectly when their skin comes into contact with contaminated items.
	Instruct E.E. to wash underclothing and bed and bath linens in detergent and hot water and dry outside in sunlight or in a dryer on the hot setting.	Soap reduces surface tension. When fat or protein substances that shield organisms are broken down, the organisms are exposed to the killing effects of heat. Prolonged exposure to heat or ultraviolet rays from direct sunlight kills microorganisms.
	Advise E.E. to shower daily, use an antibacterial soap, rinse thoroughly, and dry carefully, especially in skin folds and between toes, using a towel and washcloth only once before laundering it.	Reduces the number of microorganisms on the skin. Moisture encourages the growth of microorganisms. Laundering the towel and washcloth after only one use prevents the indirect transfer of the itch mite.

SAMPLE NURSING CARE PLAN (Continued)

PLANNING/OUTCOMES	NURSING INTERVENTIONS	RATIONALE
	Assess lesions daily for signs of healing. Report any signs and symptoms of infection in secondary lesions such as redness, swelling, pain, drainage (describe characteristics of the drainage) to the physician or clinic.	Increases the probability of effective treatment with fewer complications.
	Teach E.E. and family members the early signs and symptoms of scabies infection, such as any reddened papules with wavy, threadlike lines visible on the skin around the papules and severe itching, especially at night.	Early recognition and treatment of scabies can minimize the severity of the infection.
	Instruct them to assess their skin daily.	A daily examination allows treatment to begin as soon as the problem is identified.

EVALUATION

E.E. and her family did apply the scabicide as prescribed. The client can describe how scabies are transmitted but continues to express fear that she will give "this awful thing to somebody." Goal of correctly applying scabicide met. Although E.E. can state how scabies are transmitted, she still has doubts; hence, the goal of stating ways to avoid spreading the infection to others has only been partially met. Reinforce that even though red skin lesions are still visible, the itch mites were killed by treatment and cannot be transmitted to others even if the client does shake hands, hug, or touch someone else.

NURSING DIAGNOSIS 3 *Disturbed Body Image* related to unsightly lesions and embarrassment as evidenced by distribution of lesions on exposed skin areas and client statements of being horrified about the diagnosis and associating scabies with "dirty people"

Nursing Outcomes Classification (NOC)
Body Image

Nursing Interventions Classification (NIC)
Anxiety Reduction
Mutual Goal Setting

PLANNING/OUTCOMES	NURSING INTERVENTIONS	RATIONALE
E.E. will assume self-care of lesions.	Explain that by using the scabicide, lindane (Kwell), as directed and by following measures to prevent secondary infection of the scabies lesions, she can expect complete healing of the lesions without any visible scars within a few weeks.	Reassurance that scabies can be cured enhances the client's self-image.
E.E. will maintain relationships with family and friends.	Encourage E.E. to express her feelings about herself and her opinions about scabies.	Brings feelings and opinions out into the open where they can be dealt with appropriately.

(Continues)

SAMPLE NURSING CARE PLAN (Continued)

PLANNING/OUTCOMES	NURSING INTERVENTIONS	RATIONALE
	Provide information to correct any misconceptions she might have.	Accurate information dispels misconceptions.
	Encourage E.E. to verbalize the perceptions she has about her family's and friends' feelings about persons with scabies.	A person perceiving derogatory opinions of her is likely to socially isolate herself from them.
	Be alert to verbal and nonverbal messages.	Nonverbal messages give insight into the client's real feelings. Identifying and discussing feelings can lead to behavioral changes.
	Reassure her that she will not infect friends and family members by sitting beside them or being in the same room with them for prolonged periods.	The client will be unlikely to avoid friends or make disparaging remarks about herself when she realizes that she is not a danger to them.
	Share with E.E. that wearing long-sleeved cotton blouses or dresses will hide most of the visible lesions.	Makes the client less self-conscious and embarrassed. Cotton fabric allows good air circulation. Cool skin itches less.

EVALUATION

The client has assumed self-care responsibilities. She does interact with her family but emphasizes that she "doesn't want to get too close to them until these things are completely gone." She has refused to go to church, social gatherings, or activities outside of the house.

Goal has been partially met in that the client does follow proper procedures when caring for her skin lesions, but goal has not been met in so far as maintaining relationships is concerned. Encourage the client to talk about her feelings, particularly feelings of embarrassment. Point out to her the evidence that her lesions are healing. Emphasize that symptoms of intense itching, worsening of present skin lesions, and signs of more skin lesions would be present if the itch mites were alive and still spreading. Encourage her to go on at least one outing with her family during the coming week. Reevaluate in 1 week.

INFLAMMATORY DISORDERS OF THE SKIN

Included in this category are dermatitis and psoriasis.

DERMATITIS

By definition, dermatitis is an inflammatory condition of the skin. In current usage, eczema has almost become synonymous with dermatitis, although eczema tends to be used most often to refer to chronic forms of dermatitis. Most clients with dermatitis are treated as outpatients. Patch testing may identify a specific allergen that is causing the dermatitis. Avoiding the allergenic substance may prevent future dermatitis. In some cases, application of a topical corticosteroid is all that is needed. Other types of this inflammatory disorder include contact dermatitis and exfoliative dermatitis.

ECZEMA

Eczema is an atopic dermatitis often associated with allergic rhinitis and asthma. It is a chronic superficial inflammation that evolves into pruritic, red, weeping, crusted lesions (Estes, 2010). See Figure 15-14. Mostly infants get eczema, but older children and adults may have it. The common allergens are chocolate, orange juice, wheat, and eggs. Heredity is a major factor. Elimination of dietary substances is used to identify the client's allergen(s). Tiny cracks in the skin allow body fluid to escape, so skin hydration is the major treatment.

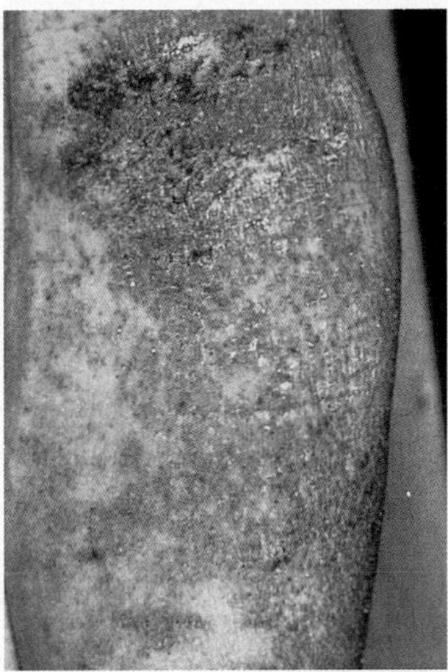

FIGURE 15-14 Eczema (***Courtesy of Centers for Disease Control and Prevention.***)

NURSING MANAGEMENT

Nursing management is directed toward promoting healing, providing comfort, preventing infection, and fostering a positive attitude to help the client cope with an altered body image. Nursing diagnoses may include *Impaired **S**kin Integrity; Risk for **I**nfection; Acute **P**ain*; and *Disturbed **B**ody Image*.

Affected areas are soaked in warm water for 15 to 20 minutes and then an occlusive ointment is applied, as directed, to retain the water. Following a bath or shower, pat the skin dry and immediately apply the occlusive ointment. Wet dressings may be ordered to maximize skin hydration. Moisturizing lotions such as Curel or Lubriderm may be used as the lesions heal. Client teaching is focused on identifying and avoiding substances that cause dermatitis, care for the lesions, how to prevent infection, and how to cope with the conditions.

CONTACT DERMATITIS

In contact dermatitis the skin reacts to external irritants such as (1) allergens like cosmetics, (2) harsh chemical substances like detergents or insecticides, (3) metals such as nickel, (4) mechanical irritation from wool or glass fibers, and (5) body substances like urine or feces. Symptoms include pruritus, burning, and erythema. Often, a maculopapular rash or a combination of papules and vesicles develops. Scratching the lesions may spread the dermatitis as well as lead to secondary infections of the skin (Figure 15-15).

Treatment of symptoms may include a corticosteroid ointment and an oral antihistamine such as diphenhydramine hydrochloride (Benadryl).

> **LIFE SPAN CONSIDERATIONS**
>
> **Skin Integrity in the Older Adult**
>
> The thinning and drying of the skin due to aging makes older adults more susceptible to irritants that cause dermatitis. Restoring skin integrity in older adults takes longer and requires persistent nursing effort.

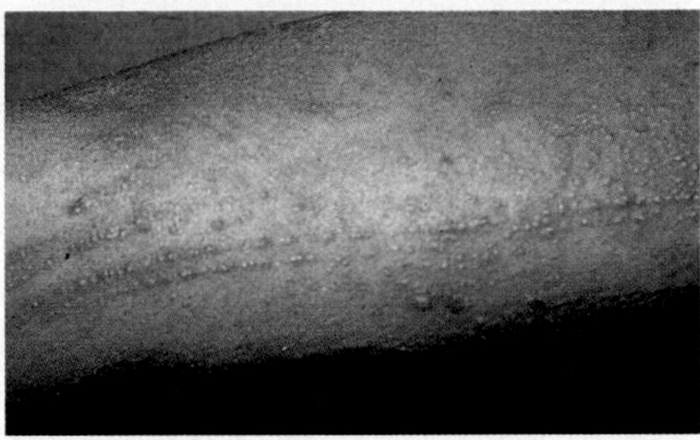

FIGURE 15-15 Allergic Contact Dermatitis from Poison Oak: Note Linear Pattern to Lesions (***Courtesy of Centers for Disease Control and Prevention.***)

NURSING MANAGEMENT

Assist the client in identifying the causative allergen. Use aseptic technique when caring for open lesions. Apply dressings wet with Burow's solution as ordered. Advise the client that a cool, moist environment reduces pruritis.

DERMATITIS VENENATA AND MEDICAMENTOSA

Dermatitis venenata is a specific type of contact dermatitis when the allergen is from a plant (e.g., poison ivy, poison oak). The first exposure sensitizes the client's body to form antigens against the allergen. Later exposures lead to inflammation, pruritis, edema, and vesicle formation.

Dermatitis medicamentosa is a skin reaction to a medication (e.g., penicillin, codeine). Symptoms range from mild to severe erythema and vesicle formation. Respiratory distress may occur.

NURSING MANAGEMENT

For dermatitis venenata, wash the affected area immediately. Calamine lotion relieves the pruritis. Corticosteroids may be needed for more severe cases to decrease inflammation and itching.

For dermatitis medicamentosa, notify the physician immediately so the medication can be discontinued and treatment of symptoms initiated. Advise the client to wear a Medic Alert bracelet or necklace and to notify all health care members of the allergy.

EXFOLIATIVE DERMATITIS

In exfoliative dermatitis, inflammation of the skin gradually worsens. Localized symptoms include erythema, severe pruritus, extensive scaling, and skin sloughing. Exfoliative dermatitis affects the entire body, not just the skin. Systemic symptoms include chills, fever, and malaise. With the loss of

LIFE SPAN CONSIDERATIONS

Exfoliative Dermatitis

Older adults have a greater risk of fatal complications from exfoliative dermatitis. As body systems age, they are less able to respond quickly and effectively to the stress of illness.

large areas of skin surface, the individual has difficulty maintaining body temperature, loses body fluids and electrolytes, and is susceptible to infection.

In most cases, the cause of exfoliative dermatitis is unknown. Severe reactions to drugs such as penicillin may sometimes cause exfoliative dermatitis. It may also be associated with other types of dermatitis or lymphoma. Exfoliative dermatitis can be fatal, primarily because of overwhelming systemic infections and/or massive loss of body fluids and electrolytes.

Nursing Management

When clients are hospitalized with exfoliative dermatitis, management is directed toward maintaining fluid balance, preventing infection, decreasing inflammation, and promoting comfort. The client requires intravenous fluids to maintain the volume of circulating fluid, corticosteroids to decrease inflammation, and antibiotics to treat infection. Medicated baths, topical steroids, and mild analgesics may be prescribed to ease the pruritus.

PSORIASIS

Psoriasis, a chronic, inflammatory, noninfectious autoimmune disease of the skin, affects about 7.5 million Americans, especially young adults. Psoriasis is more prevalent in Caucasians. The parts of the body most commonly affected are the scalp, elbows, palms, knees, lower back, and soles of the feet (National Psoriasis Foundation, 2009) (Figure 15-16). The exact cause of psoriasis is unknown, although a genetic component may be involved. Emotional stress, infections, trauma, and seasonal and hormonal changes trigger exacerbations of psoriasis. It may improve for a while only to recur. This process of subsiding and recurring continues throughout the client's life. Psoriasis is not curable. In psoriasis, the process of keratinization has gone awry. Instead of producing cells that provide a natural barrier against harmful substances and microorganisms, abnormal keratinization causes large, red patches covered with thick silvery scales in the outermost layer of the epidermis (Tate, 2008). If these scales are scraped away, bleeding occurs. When fingernails are affected, pitting and yellow discoloration is seen.

Medical–Surgical Management

Medical

Treatment is directed toward slowing down the rate of cell formation in the epidermis or toward altering the abnormal process of keratinization. Treatment regimens can be effective in reducing the scaling and itching. The client must recognize that psoriasis can only be controlled, not cured. Furthermore, the client must be committed to lifetime therapy.

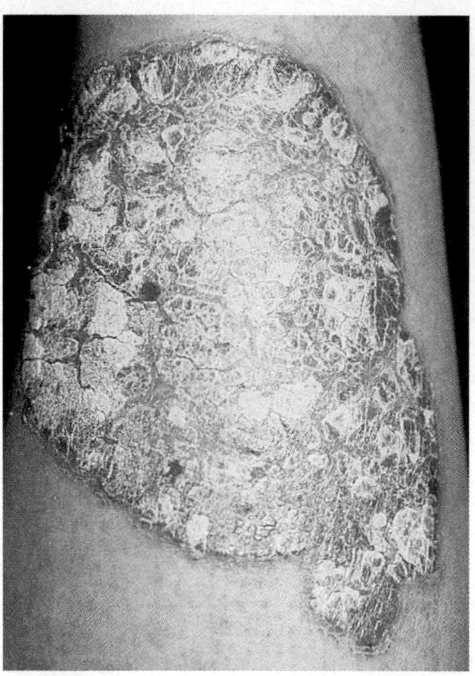

Figure 15-16 Psoriasis (*Courtesy of Robert A. Silverman, MD, Clinical Associate Professor, Department of Pediatrics, Georgetown University.*)

Pharmacological

Keratolytic agents such as salicylic acid preparations and coal tar preparations are applied topically to the lesions. Corticosteroids may also be used to reduce inflammation. Ultraviolet light and methotrexate (Mexate) inhibit DNA synthesis in the epidermal cells, thus slowing the rate of cell division and the process of abnormal keratinization. Because of its toxicity to the liver, methotrexate is used only in severe cases of psoriasis that do not respond to any other form of treatment. The Goeckerman regimen, which combines the use of coal tar and ultraviolet light, is one of the oldest effective treatments available but is not offered in many centers in the United States (American Academy of Dermatology [AAD], 2007).

Photochemotherapy is used for severe psoriasis. Photochemotherapy (psorafen and ultraviolet A-range, or PUVA) combines the use of psorafen with ultraviolet A light waves. Psorafen is a photosensitizing agent that reacts with ultraviolet A light waves to markedly reduce DNA synthesis, thereby slowing cell division in psoriasis lesions and relieving symptoms. PUVA is effective in approximately 85% of cases, but approximately 25 treatments occur over several months before clearing of psoriasis occurs. Continued treatments are needed to maintain control over this disease (AAD, 2007).

Etretinate (Tegison), a compound related to retinoic acid vitamin A, is used in severe psoriasis not amenable to other therapies. It may be used alone or in combination with ultraviolet A light waves. Etretinate has numerous adverse effects, including liver damage and severe birth defects. The client must be monitored closely. Women of childbearing age must use effective contraception during treatment and for at least 1 month after treatment.

Alternative therapies, such as aloe vera, may decrease itching, scaling, redness and inflammation. Capsaicin cream may lessen itching, and Omega 3 fatty acids (fish oil) may reduce inflammation. These treatments are considered safe to use (Mayo Clinic, 2009).

Nursing Management

Assist the client to understand and comply with the treatment. Teach the client proper hand hygiene. Listen to the client's feelings and frustrations.

NURSING PROCESS

Assessment

Subjective Data

Psoriasis lesions are generally very visible and likely to make the client feel self-conscious and uncomfortable. Many clients tend to suffer self-esteem and body image disturbances, and sometimes depression, because psoriasis requires lifelong treatment. The treatment can be time-consuming, bothersome, and, from the client's point of view, not completely effective. Encourage the client to verbalize feelings. Ask about itching, burning, and discomfort, as well as the client's mood.

Objective Data

Check the skin carefully, noting the distribution, size, and appearance of lesions. Note signs of infection such as redness, swelling, pain, or drainage.

Nursing diagnoses for a client with psoriasis include the following:

NURSING DIAGNOSES	PLANNING/OUTCOMES	NURSING INTERVENTIONS
*Deficient **K**nowledge* related to psoriasis and its treatment	The client will discuss condition and adhere to treatment.	Help client gain an understanding of psoriasis and comply with the treatment regimen. Support and encourage the client. Explain the purpose of each medication.
*Risk for **I**nfection* related to open lesions	The client will not get an infection.	Teach client how to prevent infections by proper hand hygiene and not scratching the lesions.
*Disturbed **B**ody Image* related to scaly lesions	The client will identify positive attributes about self.	Listen actively and encourage client to express feelings and frustrations. Reinforce positive behavior.
*Situational Low **S**elf-Esteem* related to appearance	The client will demonstrate behaviors that promote self-esteem.	Guide client in identifying effective coping techniques. Help client focus on personal attributes that contribute to effective functioning and a positive self-image. Encourage work and social interactions.

Evaluation: Evaluate each outcome to determine how it has been met by the client.

ULCERS

The two most common types of ulcers of the skin are venous ulcers and pressure ulcers.

VENOUS ULCERS

Poor venous circulation, especially in lower extremities, can lead to a condition known as stasis dermatitis (Figure 15-17). The skin changes in texture, turgor, and color. The skin develops a brownish discoloration and a brawny induration—that is, skin in the affected area becomes dry and looks rough; subcutaneous tissue atrophies; and it loses its usual resiliency and feels hard to the touch. Body hair is lost in this area. Pruritus is common. Scratching or small injuries can lead to ulcer formation because of the poor circulation.

Venous ulcers begin as small, tender, inflamed areas above the ankle. Any slight trauma to the area causes an open area that develops into an ulcer. Some edema surrounds the ulcer, which can easily become infected, most often with *Staphylococcus* or *Streptococcus*. Healing is very slow. In an effort to decrease venous congestion and improve circulation, varicose veins, if present, may be removed. Ulcers that do not heal may require surgery. If diagnostic testing reveals adequate circulation, skin grafting will result in the healing of large venous ulcers. In cases that do not respond to treatment, the affected leg has to be amputated.

Medical–Surgical Management

Medical

Vacuum-assisted closure (VAC) therapy may be used for chronic open wounds such as venous ulcers. Applying negative pressure to the wound is painless for the client. The negative pressure stretches or distorts the cells, causing the epithelial cells to multiply rapidly and form granulation tissue. As the vacuum pulls fluid from the surrounding tissues, reducing edema that compressed blood vessels, blood flow to the wound is improved.

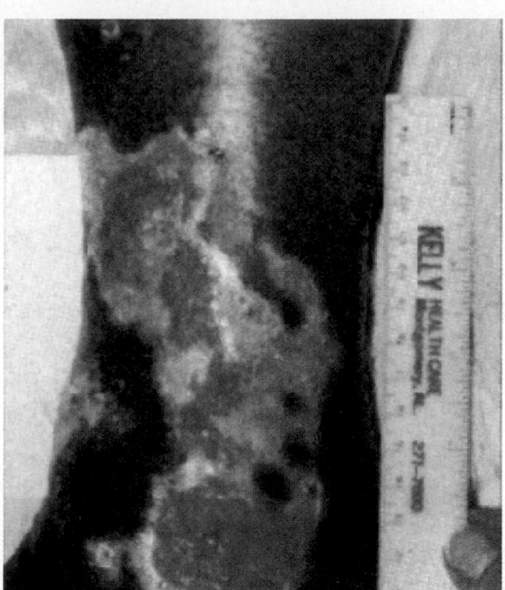

FIGURE 15-17 Venous Stasis Ulcer (*Courtesy of Carrington Laboratories, Inc., Irving, TX.*)

Elevation and compression are the keys to reducing edema of the leg and improving blood return to the heart. This reduces venous hypertension and helps the venous ulcer heal. The legs should be elevated 7 inches above the heart at night and for several hours during the day. Many types of compression therapy products are available, including Unna's boot, elastic wraps, intermittent pneumatic or sequential compression stockings, compression pumps, and sustained graduated compression using an elastic, multilayered bandage system.

Pharmacological

For healing to occur, the ulcer must have adequate circulation and be free of infection and necrotic tissue. Usually, antibiotics are prescribed. Enzyme preparations such as fibrinolysin and desoxyribonuclease (ELASE) or wet-to-dry dressings may be used to debride the ulcer. Normal saline is the solution most often used in wet-to-dry dressings because it is not irritating to healthy tissue.

Diet

A diet high in protein and vitamin C is needed for tissue regeneration. If the client is anemic, lean meats, whole grains, and green, leafy vegetables should be encouraged.

Nursing Management

Maintain peripheral tissue perfusion by encouraging the client to elevate legs when sitting, wear support hose, and not cross legs. Promote comfort by encouraging the client to keep legs elevated, cleansing the venous ulcer as prescribed, and keeping the area covered as ordered. Promote wound healing by reviewing the client's diet and encouraging foods high in iron, protein, and vitamin C.

NURSING PROCESS

Assessment

Subjective Data

Ask the client to describe any pain and rate its severity on a scale of 0 to 10. Note whether the pain is worse with the leg in a dependent position or when the client is standing. Document measures used to relieve the pain. Note if the skin around the ulcer itches, the length of time the client had the ulcer before seeking care, and any palliative measures tried.

Objective Data

Describe the size and location of the ulcer, as well as the appearance of the ulcer and surrounding skin. Observe for necrotic tissue inside the ulcer. It may be yellow and look like thin strands of fibers. The base of the ulcer may have a dark red, "beefy" appearance. Document the color and appearance of the extremity in both a dependent and an elevated position as well as any drainage, including its odor and characteristics. Edema may be present, and the lower extremity may appear swollen. Hardened and indurated tissue may surround the ulcer. Tissue farther away from the ulcer may "pit" with firm pressure. Assess peripheral pulses.

Nursing diagnoses for a client with a venous ulcer include the following:

NURSING DIAGNOSES	PLANNING/OUTCOMES	NURSING INTERVENTIONS
Ineffective Tissue Perfusion (Peripheral) related to edema and pooling of venous blood	Client will follow prescribed measures to improve peripheral circulation.	Assess for edema. Encourage client to elevate legs while sitting or when in bed and to avoid standing for more than a few minutes at a time. Advise client to wear elastic stockings when walking and that new stockings should be purchased every few months because continual wear and laundering tend to decrease the elasticity of the stockings. Instruct not to sit with legs crossed. Note the client's hemoglobin level because anemic clients will have difficulty meeting tissue demands for oxygen.

Nursing diagnoses for a client with a venous ulcer include the following: (Continued)

NURSING DIAGNOSES	PLANNING/OUTCOMES	NURSING INTERVENTIONS
*Chronic **Pain*** related to exposed sensory nerve endings and edema	Client will report decreased pain after implementing recommended measures.	Assess for pain. Encourage client to elevate legs. Cleanse ulcer with prescribed solutions. Keep ulcer covered with prescribed medications and dressings.
*Risk for **Infection*** related to poorly nourished tissue in and around the ulcer and to nonintact skin	Client will describe and implement measures to minimize the risk of infection.	Assess the ulcer daily for signs of healing. Assess the client's ability to care for the ulcer physically and financially. Review diet with the client and instruct in food choices as needed. Encourage foods high in iron such as fortified cereal, lean meats, whole grains, and leafy green vegetables.

Evaluation: Evaluate each outcome to determine how it has been met by the client.

PRESSURE ULCERS

Pressure ulcers, also known as bedsores or decubitus ulcers, are localized areas of tissue necrosis that tend to develop when soft tissue is compressed between a bony prominence and an external surface such as a mattress or chair seat for a prolonged period. Pressure ulcers are caused by **ischemia**, a local and temporary decrease in blood supply, and commonly occur in areas subject to high pressure from body weight on bony prominences.

Physiology of Pressure Ulcers

A pressure ulcer occurs when pressure on the skin is sufficient to cause collapse of blood vessels in the area. Ischemia and redness can occur at the site within 1 hour; when pressure continues for more than 2 hours, necrosis (tissue death) may occur in the involved area. Bony prominences such as the occipital skull, pinna of ears, sacrum, ischial tuberosities, trochanter area of hips, ankles, and heels are the areas most likely to develop a pressure ulcer.

Other forces acting in conjunction with pressure contribute to pressure ulcer formation. **Shearing** is the force exerted against the skin by movement or repositioning. The skin and subcutaneous tissue tend to adhere to the bed surface and remain stationary while deeper underlying tissues pull away and slide in the direction of movement. This action results in stretching and tearing of blood vessels, reduced blood flow, and necrosis.

Friction is the force of two surfaces moving across one another. When a client moves or is pulled up in bed, rubbing of the skin against the sheets creates friction. Friction can remove the superficial layers of the skin, making it more prone to breakdown.

The reduction of blood flow causes **blanching** (white color) of the skin when pressure is applied. When pressure is relieved, the skin takes on a brighter color (reactive hyperemia) because of vasodilation, the body's normal compensatory response to the absence of blood flow. If this area blanches with fingertip pressure or if the redness disappears within an hour, no tissue damage is anticipated. If, however, the redness persists and no blanching occurs, then tissue damage is present.

Pressure ulcers are staged to classify the degree of tissue damage (Figure 15-18). The National Pressure Ulcer Advisory Panel (NPUAP, 2008) recommends the following staging system:

- *Suspected Deep Tissue Injury*: Discolored intact skin, either maroon or purple, caused by shear or pressure resulting in soft tissue damage to underlying tissue. This localized area may be warmer or cooler, firmer or boggy in comparison to surrounding tissue.
- *Stage I*: Nonblanchable erythema of intact skin; the heralding lesion of skin ulceration. No blanching may be noticeable in darkly pigmented skin. A change in color usually occurs in comparison to surrounding tissue.
- *Stage II*: Partial-thickness skin loss involving epidermis, dermis, or both. The ulcer is superficial and presents clinically as an abrasion, blister, or shallow crater.
- *Stage III*: Full-thickness skin loss involving damage or necrosis of subcutaneous tissue that may extend down to, but not through, underlying fascia. The ulcer presents clinically as a deep crater with or without undermining and tunneling.
- *Stage IV*: Full-thickness skin loss with extensive destruction, tissue necrosis, or damage to muscle, bone, or supporting structures. Undermining and tunneling may also be associated with stage IV pressure ulcers.
- *Unstageable*: A full-thickness tissue loss where slough (yellow, gray or tan) or eschar (black or brown) covers the base of the wound bed. This ulcer is unstageable until debridement of the slough and/or eschar occurs.

The NPUAP (1999) has developed an assessment tool, Pressure Ulcer Scale for Healing (PUSH Tool). It uses three parameters: the surface area of the wound, amount of exudate, and type of tissue present in the wound. The scores for each parameter are added together and plotted to show wound healing or worsening. This PUSH Tool is available on the Internet (www.npuap.org/push3-0.htm).

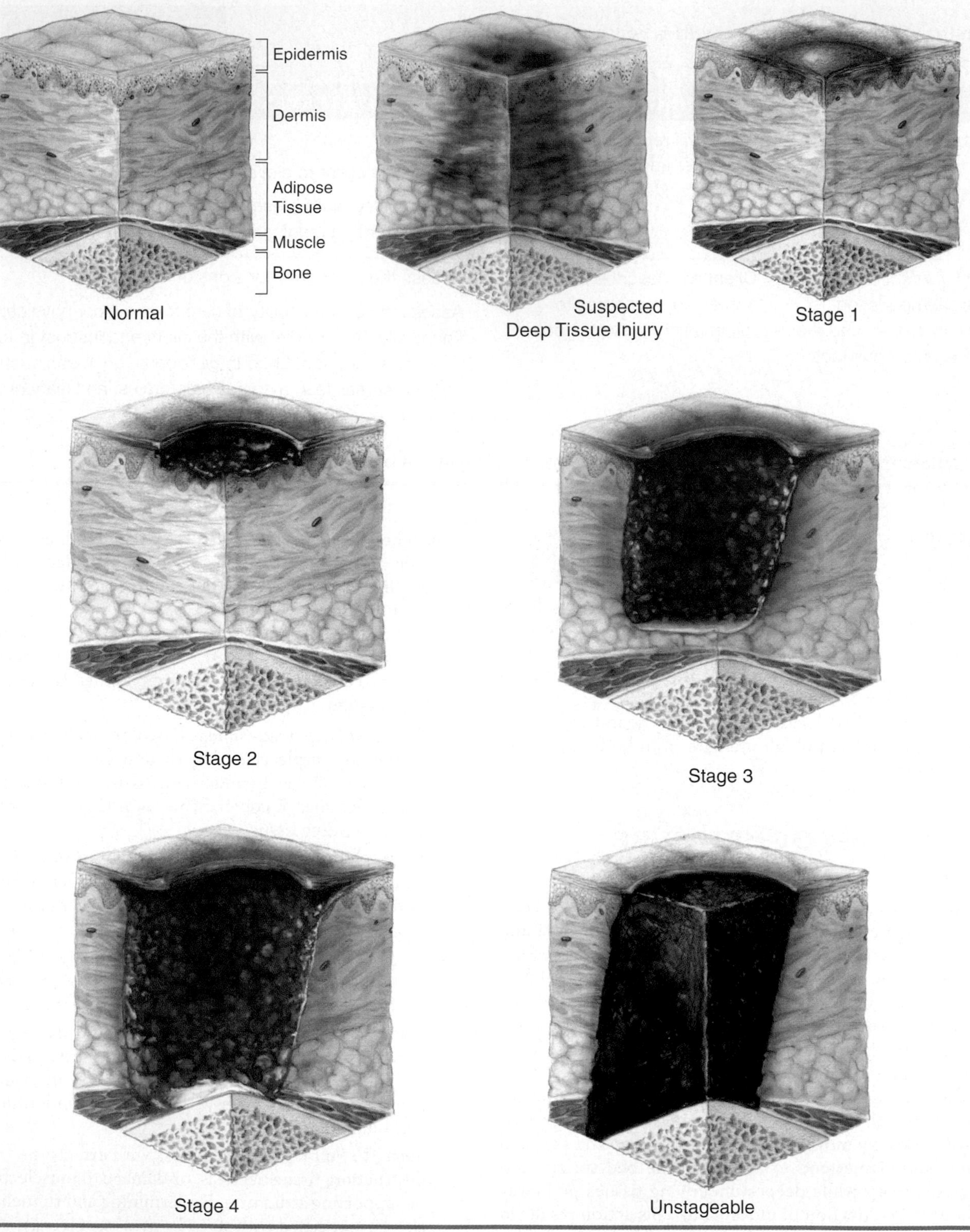

FIGURE 15-18 Pressure Ulcers (*Courtesy of the NPUAP. Reproduction of the National Pressure Ulcer Advisory Panel [NPUAP] materials in this document does not imply endorsement by the NPUAP of any products, organizatons, companies, or any statements made by any organization or company.*)

The Braden Scale for Predicting Pressure Sore Risk (Table 15-4) is a research-based tool that estimates risk level for pressure ulcers and predicts those clients who are most likely to develop pressure ulcers.

Risk Factors for Pressure Ulcers

Pressure ulcers can be prevented if at-risk individuals are identified and the specific factors placing them at risk are reduced or eliminated. More than 2.5 million clients each year have pressure ulcers, and most of these clients are in their 70s and 80s (Institute for Healthcare Improvement, 2008). Both intrinsic and extrinsic factors may influence tissue response to pressure. Intrinsic factors include impaired immobility, incontinence, nutritional status, and altered level of consciousness. Extrinsic factors include pressure, shearing, friction, and moisture. Any condition that decreases tissue perfusion, such

TABLE 15-4 Braden Scale for Predicting Pressure Sore Risk

Patient's Name ________		Evaluator's Name ________		Date of Assessment				
SENSORY PERCEPTION ability to respond meaningfully to pressure-related discomfort	**1. Completely Limited** Unresponsive (does not moan, flinch, or grasp) to painful stimuli, due to diminished level of consciousness or sedation OR has limited ability to feel pain over most of body.	**2. Very Limited** Responds only to painful stimuli. Cannot communicate discomfort except by moaning or restlessness OR has a sensory impairment which limits the ability to feel pain or discomfort over ½ of body.	**3. Slightly Limited** Responds to verbal commands, but cannot always communicate discomfort or the need to be turned OR has some sensory impairment which limits ability to feel pain or discomfort in 1 or 2 extremities.	**4. No Impairment** Responds to verbal commands. Has no sensory deficit which would limit ability to feel or voice pain or discomfort.				
MOISTURE degree to which skin is exposed to moisture	**1. Constantly Moist** Skin is kept moist almost constantly by perspiration, urine, etc. Dampness is detected every time patient is moved or turned.	**2. Very Moist** Skin is often, but not always moist. Linen must be changed at least once a shift.	**3. Occasionally Moist** Skin is occasionally moist, requiring an extra linen change approximately once a day.	**4. Rarely Moist** Skin is usually dry, linen only requires changing at routine intervals.				
ACTIVITY degree of physical activity	**1. Bedfast** Confined to bed.	**2. Chairfast** Ability to walk severely limited or non-existent. Cannot bear own weight and/or must be assisted into chair or wheelchair.	**3. Walks Occasionally** Walks occasionally during day, but for very short distances, with or without assistance. Spends majority of each shift in bed or chair.	**4. Walks Frequently** Walks outside room at least twice a day and inside room at least once every two hours during waking hours.				
MOBILITY ability to change and control body position	**1. Completely Immobile** Does not make even slight changes in body or extremity position without assistance.	**2. Very Limited** Makes occasional slight changes in body or extremity position but unable to make frequent or significant changes independently.	**3. Slightly Limited** Makes frequent though slight changes in body or extremity position independently.	**4. No Limitation** Makes major and frequent changes in position without assistance.				

(Continues)

TABLE 15-4 Braden Scale for Predicting Pressure Sore Risk (Continued)

NUTRITION usual food intake pattern	**1. Very Poor** Never eats a complete meal. Rarely eats more than ⅓ of any food offered. Eats 2 servings or less of protein (meat or dairy products) per day. Takes fluids poorly. Does not take a liquid dietary supplement OR is NPO and/or maintained on clear liquids or IVs for more than 5 days.	**2. Probably Inadequate** Rarely eats a complete meal and generally eats only about ½ of any food offered. Protein intake includes only 3 servings of meat or dairy products per day. Occasionally will take a dietary supplement OR receives less than optimum amount of liquid diet or tube feeding.	**3. Adequate** Eats over ½ of most meals. Eats a total of 4 servings of protein (meat, dairy products) per day. Occasionally will refuse a meal, but will usually take a supplement when offered OR is on a tube feeding or TPN regimen which probably meets most nutritional needs.	**4. Excellent** Eats most of every meal. Never refuses a meal. Usually eats a total of 4 or more servings of meat and dairy products. Occasionally eats between meals. Does not require supplementation.				
FRICTION & SHEAR	**1. Problem** Requires moderate to maximum assistance in moving. Complete lifting without sliding against sheets is impossible. Frequently slides down in bed or chair, requiring frequent repositioning with maximum assistance. Spasticity, contractures or agitation leads to almost constant friction.	**2. Potential Problem** Moves feebly or requires minimum assistance. During a move, skin probably slides to some extent against sheets, chair, restraints, or other devices. Maintains relatively good position in chair or bed most of the time but occasionally slides down.	**3. No Apparent Problem** Moves in bed and in chair independently and has sufficient muscle strength to lift up completely during move. Maintains good position in bed or chair.					
				Total Score				

as edema, anemia, or atherosclerosis, also increases the risk. Other factors are decreased mental status, diminished sensation, and age-related changes.

Individuals should be assessed for pressure ulcer risk on admission to acute care hospitals and at least every 48 hours, long-term care facilities at least daily, and home health care at every RN visit.

Medical–Surgical Management

Medical

Follow sterile technique in the care of all pressure ulcers to prevent secondary infection. Cleanse the wound with normal saline or a noncytotoxic wound cleaner at each dressing change. Such agents as povodine-iodine, iodophor, sodium hypochlorite, hydrogen peroxide, or acetic acid should not be used because they can damage the cells. A 35-mL syringe with a 19-gauge needle or angiocatheter provides enough pressure to cleanse the wound and enhance wound healing without causing trauma to the tissue.

Debridement must be done as needed. Topical enzyme agents may be applied or a mechanical method of wet-to-dry dressings, or hydrotherapy, may be used. Refer to the discussion of VAC therapy in the section on venous ulcers; this therapy can also be used for pressure ulcers.

There are many commercial products available for treatment and dressing of pressure ulcers. Whichever products the physician prescribes, everyone should be taught how to use them and have a commitment to use them properly.

Support Surfaces and Beds A variety of support surfaces and beds are available to support the entire body and evenly distribute pressure. These devices help reduce pressure, but they are no substitute for frequent positioning.

In addition to pressure reduction or relief, many support surfaces reduce shear and friction and control moisture. Pressure-reducing support surfaces include overlays filled with foam, gel, or water.

- *Egg-crate mattress*: The egg-crate mattress is composed of thick foam with a unique, egg-crate design. The purposes of the egg-crate mattress include minimizing pressure and shearing force. The open design of the mattress surface allows air to circulate to dissipate heat and moisture. Egg-crate foam is also used as wheelchair cushions, heel-ankle protectors, wrist restraint cushioning pads, and ulnar protectors.
- *Air-filled mattresses*: The air-filled mattress is placed over the mattress of the hospital bed for weight redistribution. Varieties of air-filled mattresses include some with a pump and alternating bands of inflation and deflation and some that are inflated continuously with air. Mattresses are covered with a sheet for client comfort. These types of mattresses are frequently used in long-term care situations.
- *Clinitron® bed*: A Clinitron® bed (Figure 15-19) is a specialized bed that has a mattress filled with small glass sand particles. Moisture from urine, stool, or drainage flows through the mattress, preventing moisture exposure to the skin. Because warm air is circulating through the mattress, the accumulation of moisture next to the skin is inhibited. The mattress aids in positioning the client because it is constructed to mold against the client's body.
- *Kin Air bed*: A Kin Air bed, another type of specialized bed, has a mattress of air-inflated pillows divided in sections for the head, back, seat, legs, and feet. The pressure can be adjusted in each of the sections for the client's specific needs. Air flows from the mattress to eliminate moisture. The bed frame can be adjusted for various positions such as Fowler's, Trendelenburg, prone, or supine. A trapeze can be connected to the bed frame (Figure 15-20).

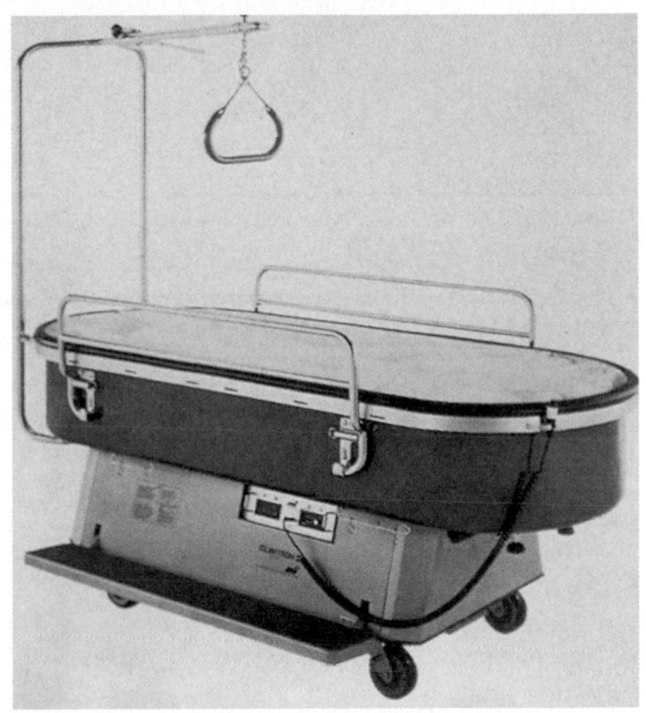

Figure 15-19 Clinitron® Air-Fluidized Therapy Unit Model C11 (*Courtesy of Hill-Rom, Batesville, IN.*)

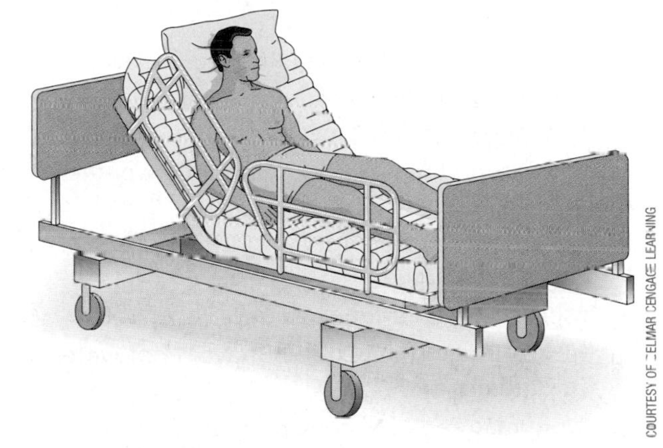

Figure 15-20 Kin Air Bed

- *Roto Kinetic bed*: A Roto Kinetic bed is a specialized bed that rocks slowly from side to side, thus relieving pressure areas and countering the effects of immobility. The client is placed on the mattress, with dividers between the legs and dividers between the trunk and arms. Clients can be maintained in traction while on this bed.

Regardless of the type of surface or bed on which the client is lying, the 30-degree side-lying position prevents pressure on the sacrum and trochanters. This position is illustrated in Figure 15-21.

Surgical

Occasionally, surgical debridement may be necessary.

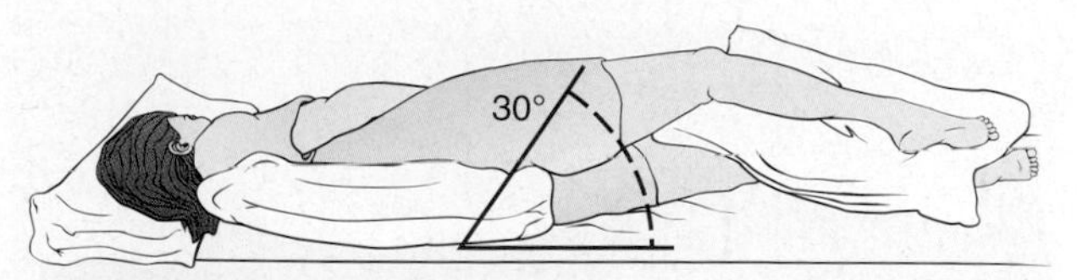

COURTESY OF DELMAR CENGAGE LEARNING

FIGURE 15-21 Avoiding Pressure Points with the 30-Degree Lateral Position

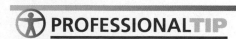

> **PROFESSIONALTIP**
>
> **Preventing Pressure Ulcers**
>
> - Establish written repositioning/turning schedule for clients, including those on pressure-reducing support surfaces.
> - Use 30-degree position when side-lying position is used.
> - Prevent direct contact between bony prominences by using pillows and foam wedges.
> - Use a lifting sheet.
> - Encourage clients in wheelchairs to shift their weight every 15 minutes.
> - Raise heels off the bed with pillow lengthwise to support legs.
> - Use knee gatch when head of bed is elevated.
> - Keep head of bed elevated to less than 30 degrees except at mealtimes.
> - Limit sitting time to 1 hour at a time whether in bed, chair, or wheelchair.
> - Use proper positioning, transferring, and turning techniques.
> - Inspect skin at least once a day.
> - Use mild cleansing agent, but avoid hot water for bathing.
> - Avoid massage over bony prominences.
> - Use moisturizer on skin.
> - Use protective barrier on skin if client is incontinent.
> - Cleanse skin at time of soiling and at routine intervals.

Pharmacological

Vitamin and mineral supplements may be ordered. Antibiotics may also be ordered.

Diet

Eating a well-balanced diet should be encouraged, including 2 half-cup servings of orange juice or other juice high in vitamin C and 6 ounces of a high-protein drink. Adequate calories, protein, vitamins, and minerals, especially vitamin C and zinc, improve wound healing and prevents tissue breakdown. Offering small, frequent feedings enhances nutritional needs.

Activity

Active ROM exercises should be performed, if possible. If not, passive ROM exercises should be performed with the client several times a day.

NURSING MANAGEMENT

Assess skin several times a day. Keep linens clean, dry, and free from wrinkles. Provide daily bath and skin care when the client is incontinent of bowel or bladder. Encourage adequate fluid intake, a well-balanced diet, and active or passive ROM exercises. Turn client at least every 2 hours. Use the 30-degree lateral position to avoid pressure on the sacrum and trochanters. Position client on unaffected areas and protect skin as ordered. Monitor vital signs, especially temperature.

NURSING PROCESS

ASSESSMENT

Subjective Data

Statements such as, "I'm tired of lying on my side"; "I wish I could move more"; or "my hips (back, heels, and so on) are sore" may be expressed.

Objective Data

Symptoms may include any of the risk factors already mentioned; shiny, erythematous area; small blisters or erosions or ulcerations. Check for reddened areas and blanching of those areas.

Nursing diagnoses for a client at risk for pressure ulcers or who has a pressure ulcer include the following:

NURSING DIAGNOSES	PLANNING/OUTCOMES	NURSING INTERVENTIONS
Risk for Impaired Skin Integrity related to immobility	The client will maintain skin integrity.	Assess skin 3 times a day for pressure areas. Provide daily bath and skin care as needed for incontinence of urine or stool. Use mild cleansing agents with warm water, use moisturizing lotion, and minimize exposure to cold and low humidity.

(*Continues*)

Nursing diagnoses for a client at risk for pressure ulcers or who has a pressure ulcer include the following: (Continued)

NURSING DIAGNOSES	PLANNING/OUTCOMES	NURSING INTERVENTIONS
		Avoid massage over bony prominences. Keep bed linen clean, dry, and free from wrinkles. Encourage adequate fluid intake and a well-balanced diet, including 2 half-cup servings of orange juice or other juice high in vitamin C, and 6 ounces of a high-protein drink. Encourage active ROM exercises or provide passive ROM exercises. Turn and reposition client at least every 2 hours. If reddened area does not blanch when you press it, turn the client more often. Use the 30-degree lateral position to avoid pressure on the sacrum and trochanters. Use pressure-reducing surfaces. Do not use donut-shaped cushions; they put pressure around the pressure ulcer.
*Impaired **S**kin Integrity* related to pressure ulcer formation	The client will show healing of pressure ulcer.	Assess skin daily, identifying the stage of pressure ulcer development (size, color, odor, and exudate). Continue all preventive nursing interventions. Position client on unaffected areas. Protect skin surface and affected area as per facility protocol or as ordered. Monitor temperature. Administer antibiotics as ordered.
*Disturbed **B**ody Image* related to trauma or injury (pressure ulcer)	The client will make a positive statement about body image.	Encourage client to discuss meaning of pressure ulcer to the client. Provide information as requested by client.
Anxiety related to threat to or change in health status (pressure ulcer)	The client will discuss concerns about pressure ulcer with caregivers.	Schedule time to be with client, other than care times. Encourage client to discuss fears and concerns. Provide information as requested by client.

Evaluation: Evaluate each outcome to determine how it has been met by the client.

ALOPECIA

Alopecia, which is partial or complete baldness or loss of hair, can be caused by illness, malnutrition, effects of certain drugs such as those used in cancer therapy, hormonal imbalances, heredity, or diseases that affect the scalp.

There are many types of alopecia, ranging from head or beard hair loss to loss of all hair over the entire body. Treatment depends on the cause. Hair transplants may be performed on the head, but this is very expensive. In some clients, minoxidil (Rogaine) can promote hair growth, but hair growth stops when the drug is stopped. This is also very expensive.

CASE STUDY

M.M., age 68, noticed that the skin on the outside of her left lower leg just above the ankle was changing in color and texture. The skin felt rigid and did not move as easily as skin on the upper part of her leg did. Itching was becoming a problem. Inadvertently, she would scratch the area, sometimes causing small excoriations. One day she bumped her leg against the rough edge of the outside steps as she was going into the house. The cut was only an inch long and was not very deep. Over the next few weeks, she noticed that instead of healing, it was getting bigger and was becoming quite painful. The skin around the wound was red and swollen. The yellow drainage coming from the wound had a bad smell. She had never had this kind of problem before. She did have varicose veins in that leg, and while she knew that she was uncomfortable if she was standing for long periods, she did not think the problem was serious. When she went to the doctor, he diagnosed a venous stasis ulcer and cultured the drainage. He ordered the following treatment:

1. Cefaclor (Ceclor) 500 mg p.o. every 8 hours for 2 weeks (culture of the wound identified *Staphylococcus aureus*)
2. Wet-to-dry dressings with normal saline solution. Change every 8 hours.
3. Bed rest with left leg elevated. May have bathroom privileges and be up for meals.

The doctor explained that he would be ordering an Unna's boot after the wound was debrided and the infection controlled so that she could be ambulatory, but that even after the Unna's boot was applied, he would want her to have rest periods during the day with her leg elevated. M.M. thought she could learn to change the dressings, but she expressed doubt that she could stay in bed most of the time. She was used to being up and active and getting her work done each day.

The following questions will guide your development of a nursing care plan for the case study.

1. List the clinical manifestations of a venous stasis ulcer.
2. What is the usual medical treatment?
3. List the subjective and objective assessment data that the nurse should obtain from M.M.
4. Write two to four individualized nursing diagnoses to address these problems.
5. What will be the goals (expected outcomes) of nursing treatment?
6. List appropriate nursing actions for each diagnosis. Include basic nursing care measures. Be specific about client education needs. Address nutrition and pharmacologic implications. Give a rationale for each action.
7. Describe how to evaluate goal achievement for M.M.

SUMMARY

- Maintaining intact skin and mucous membranes to protect internal body structures from harmful substances and from invasion by microorganisms is an important independent nursing responsibility.
- Burns are devastating, traumatic injuries that can often be prevented.
- In general, skin cancers can be prevented by avoiding excessive sun exposure.
- Treatment of benign skin tumors such as nevi, lipomas, keloids, sebaceous cysts, and angiomas depends on the kind of tumor and its location.
- Psoriasis is a chronic skin condition that can be treated but not cured.
- Skin infections caused by bacteria, viruses, fungi, or parasites are effectively treated with medications and supportive nursing care.
- Dermatitis, an inflammation of the skin, can have many causes.
- Eczema is a term that is often used for chronic forms of dermatitis.
- Venous ulcers are more common in older persons, heal slowly, and often recur following a slight injury.
- Alopecia, or baldness, can be caused by illness, drugs, hormonal imbalances, or heredity.

REVIEW QUESTIONS

1. A client is brought into the emergency room with facial burns, singed nasal hairs, and change in voice. The client states he is having pain of a 7 on a 0–10 pain scale in the facial area and he appears anxious. Based on these clinical findings, what is the most important initial nursing intervention?
   1. Attempt to calm client.
   2. Maintain an adequate level of oxygenation.
   3. Protect burns with a sterile dressing.
   4. Administer pain medication.
2. The nurse charted that the client's skin was loose, wrinkled, and thin with mild scaling. The nurse was describing:
   1. integrity.
   2. texture.
   3. turgor and mobility.
   4. vascularity.
3. An effective nursing intervention related to the care of open burn wounds that require daily dressing changes would be:
   1. keep the head of the bed elevated 30 degrees with all four side rails up.
   2. set a fluid intake goal of 2,500 mL/24 hours (1,200 mL during the day; 950 mL during the evening; 350 mL during the night).
   3. wear a cap, gown, mask, and sterile gloves when providing wound care.
   4. weigh daily, preferably before breakfast, and in the same type of clothing each day.

4. The client has lesions on his scalp and on his arms near his elbows. The lesions appear as red patches covered with thick silvery scales. The most likely cause of these lesions is:
   1. herpes zoster (shingles).
   2. pemphigus vulgaris.
   3. psoriasis.
   4. tinea (ringworm).
5. A nursing care plan for a client with an infectious disorder of the skin would include interventions to teach the client:
   1. how to avoid spreading the infection to others.
   2. how to do range-of-motion exercises to maintain joint flexibility.
   3. ways to conserve energy.
   4. which foods are most likely to cause allergic reactions.
6. The nursing care plan of a client at risk for impaired skin integrity is likely to include:
   1. turning and repositioning client every 4 hours.
   2. massaging bony prominences.
   3. using a donut shaped cushion around the pressure ulcer.
   4. using the 30-degree lateral positioning when turning client.
7. The nurse is assessing a client's dressing after an abdominal surgery. The nurse notices clear with some blood-tinged drainage on the dressing. The nurse would document the drainage to be:
   1. purulent exudates.
   2. serosanguineous exudates.
   3. serous exudates.
   4. sanguineous exudates.
8. When admitting a new client, the nurse performs a physical assessment of the client's skin. What parameters will the nurse assess? (Select all that apply.)
   1. Integrity and color.
   2. Temperature and moisture.
   3. Texture and vascularity.
   4. Culture and sensitivity.
   5. Turgor and mobility.
   6. Sensation.
9. A 75-year-old man comes to the outpatient clinic. He has long-standing severe chronic obstructive pulmonary disease. He is short of breath at rest with oxygen at 3 yes L per minute via nasal cannula. When inspecting his nail beds, you would expect his nail angle to be:
   1. greater than 160 degrees.
   2. less than 140 degrees.
   3. less than 90 degrees.
   4. greater than 90 degrees.
10. The nurse is teaching a client's wife about preventing pressure ulcers. Which statement best demonstrates that the wife correctly understands the risk factors for pressure ulcers?
    1. "I need to assess the skin once a week for redness or open areas."
    2. "If my husband is wearing Depends®, they will absorb his urine incontinence, so I will need to change his Depends only when saturated."
    3. "He has his favorite foods, so as long as he is eating, I will not need to worry."
    4. "I will try to encourage him to change positions frequently during the day."

REFERENCES/SUGGESTED READINGS

American Academy of Dermatology (AAD). (2007). Psoriasis & psoriatic arthritis. Retrieved May 20, 2009 from http://www.aad.org/public/publications/pamphlets/common_psoriasis.html

American Cancer Society (ACS). (2008a). What are the key statistics about squamous and basal cell skin cancer? Retrieved May 22, 2009 from www.cancer.org/docroot/CRI/content/CRI_2_4_1X_What_are_the_key_statistics_for_skin_cancer_51.asp?sitearea=cri

American Cancer Society (ACS). (2008b). What are the risk factors of melanoma? Retrieved May 22, 2009 from www.cancer.org/docroot/CRI/content/CRI_2_4_2X_What_are_the_risk_factors_for_melanoma_50.asp?rnav=cri

American Cancer Society (ACS). (2008c). What are the key statistics about melanomas? Retrieved May 20, 2009 from www.cancer.org/docroot/CRI/content/CRI_2_4_1X_What_are_the_key_statistics_for_melanoma_50.asp?sitearea=

American Cancer Society (ACS). (2008d). Treating squamous cell carcinoma. Retrieved May 25, 2009 from www.cancer.org/docroot/CRI_2_4_4X_Treatment_of_Squamous_Cell_Carcinoma_51.asp?sitearea=

American Cancer Society (ACS). (2008e). Skin (pressure) sores. Retrieved May 20, 2009 from http://www.cancer.org/docroot/MBC?content/MBC_2_3X_Skin_Pressure_Sores.asp

American Cancer Society (ACS). (2009a). How is melanoma skin cancer treated? Retrieved May 25, 2009 from www.cancer.org/docroot/CRI/content/CRI_2_2_4X_How_Is_Melanoma_Skin_Cancer_Treated_50.asp?rnav=cri

American Cancer Society (ACS). (2009b). The ABCD rule for early detection of melanoma. Retrieved May 25, 2009 from www.cancer.org/docroot/SPC/content/SPC_1_ABCD_Mole_Check_Tips.asp

Bolton, L. (2008). Compression in venous ulcer management. *Journal of Wound, Ostomy & Continence Nursing*, 35(1), 40–49.

Brunicardi, F., Anderson, D., Billiar, T., & Dunn, D. (2005). *Schwartz's principles of surgery* (8th ed.). New York: McGraw-Hill.

Bulechek, G., Butcher, H., McCloskey, J., & Dochterman, J., eds. (2008). *Nursing Interventions Classification (NIC)* (5th ed.). St. Louis, MO: Mosby/Elsevier.

Daniels, R. (2010). *Delmar's guide to laboratory and diagnostic tests* (2nd ed.). Clifton Park, NY: Delmar Cengage Learning.

Davidson, M. (2002). Sharpen your wound assessment skills. *Nursing2002, 32*(10), 32hn1–32hn4.

Drisdelle, R. (2003). Maggot debridement therapy: A living cure. *Nursing2003, 33*(6), 17.

Estes, M. (2010). *Health assessment & physical examination* (4th ed). Clifton Park, NY: Delmar Cengage Learning.

Goldsmith, J. (2003). Nit-Picking. *AJN, 103*(9), 22–23.

Grunwald, T., & Garner, W. (2008). Acute burns. *Plastic and Reconstructive Surgery: Journal of the American Society of Plastic Surgeons, 121*(5), 311e–319e.

Harvard Health Letter. (2008). Should you get the shingles vaccine? 33(12), 6–7.

Hayes, J. (2003). Are you assessing for melanoma? *RN, 66*(2), 36–40.

Hess, C. (2003a). Managing a patient with a venous ulcer. *Nursing2003, 33*(4), 73–74.

Hess, C. (2003b). Treating a fungal rash. *Nursing2003, 33*(9), 20–22.

Hill, M. (1998). Nursing management of adults with skin disorders. In P. G. Beare & J. L. Myers (Eds.), *Principles and practice of adult health nursing* (3rd ed., pp. 2089–2115). St. Louis, MO: Mosby.

Hilton, G. (2001). Thermal burns. *AJN, 101*(11), 32–34.

Hunter, S., Langemo, D., Thompson, P., Hanson, D., & Anderson, J. (2009). Maggot therapy for wound management. *Advances in Skin & Wound Care, 22*(1), 25–27.

Institute for Healthcare Improvement. (2008). The 5 million lives campaign. getting started kit: prevent pressure ulcers how-to-guide. Retrieved May 31, 2009 from www.ihi.org/IHI/Programs/Campaign

Kloth, L. (2002). How to use electrical stimulation for wound healing. *Nursing2002, 32*(12), 17.

Leukemia-Lymphoma Society. (2006). Skin lymphoma. Retrieved May 20, 2009 from www.leukemia-lymphoma.org/all_mat_toc.adp?item_id=9846

Magnan, M. & Maklebust. J. (2009). The nursing process and pressure ulcer prevention: Making the connection. *Advances in Skin & Wound Care, 22*(2), 83–92.

Martin, S. (2001). There's what in the wound? *RN, 64*(2), 44–47.

Martini, F., & Bartholomew. E. (2008). *Essentials of anatomy and physiology* (4th ed.). Englewood Cliffs, NJ: Prentice-Hall.

Mayo Clinic. (2009). Psoriasis. Retrieved May 27, 2009 from www.mayoclinic.com/health/psoriasis/DS00193?DSECTION=treatments-and-drugs

McCain, D., & Sutherland, S. (1998). Skin grafts for patients with burns. *AJN, 98*(7), 34–39.

Mendez-Eastman, S. (1998). When wounds won't heal. *RN, 61*(1), 20–23.

Mendez-Eastman, S. (2002). New treatment for an old problem: Negative-pressure wound therapy. *Nursing2002, 32*(5), 58–63.

Milner, S., Mottar, R., & Smith, C. (2001). The burn wheel. *AJN, 101*(11), 35–37.

Moorhead, S., Johnson, M., Maas, M., & Swanson, E. (2007). *Nursing Outcomes Classification (NOC)* (4th ed.). St. Louis, MO: Mosby.

Moses, M. (2003). A simple matter of grooming. *AJN, 103*(9), 11.

National Institutes of Health (NIH). (2008). Burns. Retrieved May 25, 2009 from http://www.nlm.nih.gov/medlineplus/ency/imagepages/1078.htm

National Institutes of Health (NIH). (2009). Psoriasis. Retrieved May 20, 2009 from www.nlm.nih.gov/medlineplus/psoriasis.html

National Pressure Ulcer Advisary Panal (NPUAP). (1998). PUSH Tool Version 3.0. Retrieved May 20, 2009 from http://www.npuap.org/push3-0.htm

National Psoriasis Foundation. (2009). About psoriasis. Retrieved May 27, 2009 from http://www.psoriasis.org/netcommunity/learn_statistics

North American Nursing Diagnosis Association International. (2010). *NANDA-I nursing diagnoses: Definitions and classification 2009–2011.* Ames, IA: Wiley-Blackwell.

Ramadan, A., & Zyada, R. (2008). Effect of low-intensity direct current on the healing of chronic wounds: A literature review. *Journal of Wound Care, 17*(7), 292–296.

Regojo, P. (2003). Burn care basics. *Nursing2003, 33*(3), 50–53.

Roy, D., & Stotts, N. (2002). Targeting cellulitis. *Nursing2002, 32*(12), 46–47.

Sarvis, C. (2007). Calling on NERDS for critically colonized wounds. *Nursing2007, 37*(5), 26–27.

Schweon, S., & Novatnack, E. (2002). What's causing that itch? *RN, 65*(8), 43–46.

Smeltzer, S., Bare, B., Hinkle, J., & Cheever, K. (2008). *Brunner & Suddarth's textbook of medicalsurgical nursing* (11th ed.). Philadelphia, PA: Lippincott Williams & Wilkins.

Spratto, G., & Woods, A. (2008). *2009 Edition Delmar nurse's drug handbook*. Clifton Park, NJ: Delmar Cengage Learning.

Tate, P. (2008). *Seelay's principles of anatomy & physiology*. New York McGraw-Hill.

Thompson, J. (2003). Maximizing your pressure ulcer care. *Travel Nursing Today, a supplement to RN,* (April 2003), 16–24.

Wiebelhaus, P., & Hansen, S. (2001a). Another choice for burn victims. *RN, 64*(9), 34–37.

Wiebelhaus, P., & Hansen, S. (2001b). What you should know about burn emergencies. *Nursing2001, 31*(1), 36–41.

Zulkowski, K., & Ratliff, C. (2006). Perineal dermatitis or pressure ulcer: How can you tell? *Nursing2006, 36*(12), 22–23.

RESOURCES

American Burn Association, http://www.ameriburn.org

American Hair Loss Council, http://www.ahlc.org

Dermatology Foundation, http://www.dermfnd.org

National Burn Victim Foundation, http://www.nbvf.org

National Decubitus Foundation, http://www.decubitus.org

National Pressure Ulcer Advisory Panel (NPUAP), http://www.npuap.org

National Psoriasis Foundation, http://www.psoriasis.org

Skin Cancer Foundation, http://www.skincancer.org

Wound Healing Society, http://www.woundheal.org

Wound, Ostomy and Continence Nurses Society, http://www.wocn.org

TABLE 16-4 Common Diagnostic Tests for Immune System Disorders

- Antinuclear antibodies (ANA)
- Complement assay (Total complement, C3 and C4)
- C-reactive protein test (CRP)
- CD4 T-cells
- Enzyme-linked immunosorbent assay (ELISA)
- Erythrocyte sedimentation rate (ESR or Sed Rate Test)
- Human leukocyte antigen DW4 (HLA-DW4)
- Lupus erythematosus test (LE Prep)
- Polymerase chain reaction (PCR)
- Red blood cell count (RBC count)
- Rheumatoid factor (RF)
- Total white blood cell count
  - Differential count
  - Neutrophils
    - —Segs (mature neutrophils)
    - —Bands (immature neutrophils)
  - Eosinophils
  - Basophils
  - Lymphocytes
  - Monocytes
- Western blot

COMMON DIAGNOSTIC TESTS

Commonly used diagnostic tests for clients with symptoms of immune system disorders are listed in Table 16-4.

HYPERSENSITIVE IMMUNE RESPONSE

Hypersensitive immune responses include allergies, anaphylaxis, transfusion reactions, transplant rejection, and latex allergy.

ALLERGIES

Allergic disorders are the result of **hypersensitivity** (excessive reaction to a stimulus) of the immune system to **allergens** (a type of antigen commonly found in the environment). Allergens may be inhaled, injected, ingested, or contacted. There are four types of hypersensitivity reactions based on how tissue is injured.

Type I reactions occur immediately upon exposure to a specific antigen. Upon first exposure to an allergen, IgE antibodies are produced. They adhere to mast cells. When a subsequent exposure occurs, these cells attach to the antigen and activate the release of chemical mediators, such as histamine, bradykinin, and serotonin. These chemicals cause vasodilation, enhanced capillary permeability, and bronchoconstriction (Figure 16-3).

The most common Type I reactions include allergic rhinitis, urticaria, and angioedema. Anaphylaxis is the most severe and is covered separately.

Allergic rhinitis, also known as *hay fever* or *pollinosis,* is a common allergy in our society caused by airborne allergens such as pollen, mold, animal dander, dust, and ragweed. Symptoms include nasal congestion; thin, clear, watery discharge; sneezing; itching; swelling; and redness of the eyes. Headaches and ear infections may also develop. Approximately 12.2 million office visits to health care providers each year are for allergic rhinitis (Centers for Disease Control and Prevention, 2008e).

Urticaria (hives) are raised pruritic, red, nontender wheals on the skin. They are usually on the trunk and on the areas of the extremities closest to the trunk.

Angioedema, edema of subcutaneous layers and mucous membranes, is painless and only slightly pruritic.

Drug and food allergies are also Type I hypersensitivity. Any drug potentially may cause a drug reaction, but common ones include penicillin, cephalosporins, codeine, pain medications, vaccines, and local anesthetics. Reactions vary from mild to severe. Usually, symptoms do not occur until the client has taken several doses of the medication, although they can occur at first exposure. The most common reaction is the sudden development of a bright red, itchy rash, often appearing initially on the trunk or arms. Occasionally, a client may develop an anaphylactic reaction.

Although individuals may be allergic to any edible substance, certain foods, such as milk, shellfish, eggs, wheat, and nuts, are common allergens. According to the CDC (2008a), 1 of every 100 children in the United States have a food allergy. Diarrhea is a result of immunological reaction in the intestinal

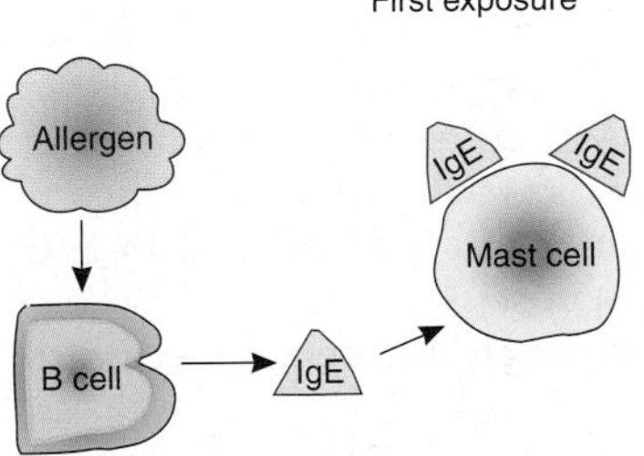

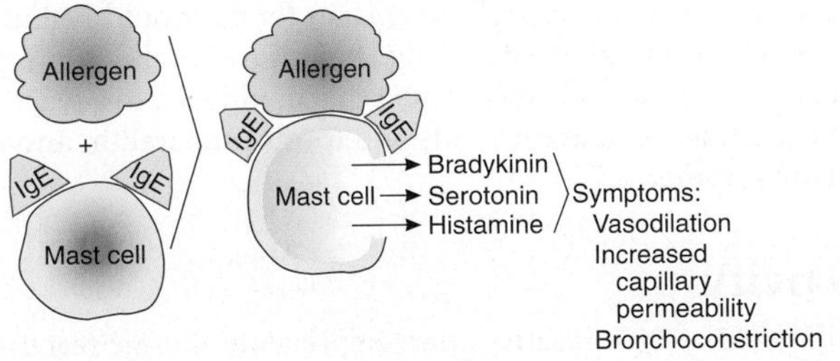

FIGURE 16-3 Allergic Response

mucosa. Headache, nausea, vomiting, rash, itching, and wheezing may also develop.

Type II reactions are the destruction of cells or substances with antigens attached that either immunoglobulin G (IgG) or immunoglobulin M (IgM) senses as being foreign. Antibodies cause either lysis of the cells or accelerated phagocytosis. Hemolytic transfusion reactions are this type of reaction. Transfusion reactions are discussed in detail later.

Type III reaction involves IgG immune antigen-antibody complexes. It is a local reaction evident after several hours that may change from red skin to hemorrhage and tissue necrosis. Occasionally, this is noted after penicillin or sulfonamide use.

Type IV is a delayed reaction involving sensitized T-lymphocytes coming in contact with the allergen. Contact dermatitis and transplant rejection are examples of this type of reaction. Poison ivy and poison oak are the most common causes of contact dermatitis. Latex rubber is a more recently discovered cause of contact dermatitis or occasionally a Type I (anaphylactic) reaction. Transplant rejection and latex allergy are covered separately.

LIFE SPAN CONSIDERATIONS

Allergy to Foods

- Food allergies have increased among children in the United States during the past 10 years by 18%.
- Boys and girls have similar rates of food allergies.
- Children younger than the age of 5 have a greater rate of reported food allergies than children between the ages of 5 to 17 years.
- Children with food allergies are two to four times more likely to have other related conditions such as asthma, compares with children without food allergies.

(CDC, 2008a)

MEDICAL–SURGICAL MANAGEMENT

Medical

Medical management of clients experiencing an allergic response (reaction to allergen) includes drug therapy to treat symptoms and identification of precipitating agents. Allergen **immunotherapy** (treatment to suppress or enhance immunological functioning) involves repeated injections of the diluted allergen. Decreased levels of histamine are released upon subsequent exposure to the allergen. Venom can be used to treat allergies to bees, wasps, yellowjackets, and hornets.

Pharmacological

Several medications are employed to treat the symptoms of an allergic response. Antihistamines counteract the effects of histamine. They may be taken orally, topically, or intravenously, depending on the type of allergic response and urgency for treatment. Nasal decongestants help relieve respiratory symptoms. Topical corticosteroids effectively relieve inflammation associated with contact dermatitis and dermatitis medicamentosa. Oral or injectable forms of corticosteroids may be used either alone or in combination with antihistamines and nasal decongestants.

Skin testing by a physician can determine the specific causative allergen.

Diet

Individuals who are allergic to certain foods should be taught to check food labels carefully, be aware of how food is prepared, and not eat any product that could lead to a reaction. This includes restaurant foods and foods prepared in another person's home.

Activity

Avoidance of the causative allergen prevents allergic reactions. Activities should be centered around this, if at all possible. For instance, individuals who are allergic to pollen may need to stay in air-conditioned environments on those days when the pollen count is extremely high.

NURSING MANAGEMENT

Teach the client that with allergic rhinitis to stay indoors when airborne allergens are present in great numbers. Ask about pets in the house. Encourage the client to read labels if there are food allergies and to inform all health care personnel if there are drug allergies. Assist the client to plan lifestyle changes to avoid exposure to allergens. Emphasize the importance of following the medication regimen prescribed. Figure 16-4 outlines the differences between a cold and an airborne allergy.

NURSING PROCESS

ASSESSMENT

Subjective Data

Take detailed, comprehensive client history, including information about previous allergic reactions, foods eaten or medications taken recently, and contact with environmental pollutants or anything not normally encountered. The client may describe having nausea, pruritus, and being uneasy.

Objective Data

Assess gastrointestinal and respiratory functioning, cardiovascular and neurological status, and the presence of urticaria, angioedema, sneezing, excessive nasal secretions, diarrhea, wheezes, cough, or hypotension.

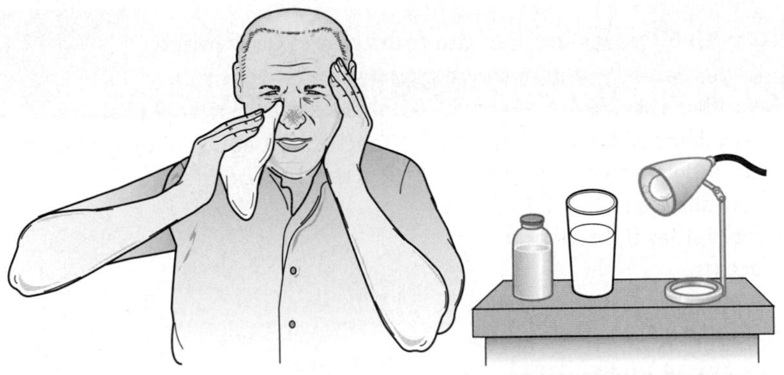

Is It a Cold or an Allergy?

Symptoms	Cold	Airborne Allergy
Cough	Common	Sometimes
General Aches, Pains	Slight	Never
Fatique, Weakness	Sometimes	Sometimes
Itchy Eyes	Rare or Never	Common
Sneezing	Usual	Usual
Sore Throat	Common	Sometimes
Runny Nose	Common	Common
Stuffy Nose	Common	Common
Fever	Rare	Never
Duration	3 to 14 days	Weeks (for example, 6 weeks for ragweed or grass pollen seasons)

Treatment	Antihistamines Decongestants Nonsteroidal anti-inflammatory medicines	Antihistamines Nasal steroids Decongestants
Prevention	Wash your hands often with soap and water Avoid close contact with anyone with a cold	Avoid those things that you are allergic to such as pollen, house dust mites, mold, pet dander, cockroaches
Complications	Sinus infection Middle ear infection Asthma	Sinus infection Asthma

FIGURE 16-4 Differences Between a Cold and an Airborne Allergy (*National Institute of Allergy and Infectious Diseases. (2008). http://www3.naid.nih.gov/topics/allergicDiseases/PDF/ColdAllergy.pdf.*)

Nursing diagnoses for clients with allergies include the following:

NURSING DIAGNOSES	PLANNING/OUTCOMES	NURSING INTERVENTIONS
Risk for Injury, related to an allergic reaction	The client will identify factors that increase the potential of a reaction.	Assist client in identifying those factors that increase the potential for a reaction.
Health-Seeking Behaviors related to causative allergen, therapeutic modalities, and/or preventive measures	The client will relate methods to avoid exposure to allergens.	Assist client in planning lifestyle changes that will help in avoiding exposure to allergens.

(*Continues*)

Nursing diagnoses for clients with allergies include the following: (Continued)

NURSING DIAGNOSES	PLANNING/OUTCOMES	NURSING INTERVENTIONS
Deficient Knowledge related to lack of information about allergens, treatment, or preventive measures	The client will demonstrate an understanding of and compliance with therapeutic modalities if a reaction occurs. The client will demonstrate an understanding of and compliance with preventive measures to avoid subsequent allergic reactions.	Teach client about allergy treatments and what to do if a reaction occurs.

Evaluation: Evaluate each outcome to determine how it has been met by the client.

ANAPHYLACTIC REACTION

Anaphylaxis is a type I systemic reaction to allergens and is the most serious type of allergic reaction. It occurs in individuals who are extremely sensitive to an allergen. Symptoms develop suddenly and can progress to severe levels within minutes. Usually, the faster the reaction, the worse it is. Foods, drugs, hormones, insect bites, blood, and vaccines all are associated with anaphylactic reactions. Shellfish, eggs, nuts, berries, and chocolates are the most common foods involved. According to the National Institute of Allergy and Infectious Diseases (2008a), peanut and tree nut allergies are the leading causes of anaphylaxis in the United States. Any medication has the potential of causing a reaction, but antibiotics (especially penicillin), insulin, muscle relaxants, and x-ray dyes are the most frequent precipitating agents. Bee, wasp, hornet, and snake bites may also cause anaphylactic reactions. According to Golden (2007), anaphylaxis to insect bites occurs in 3% of adults and can be fatal on the first reaction.

Anaphylactic reactions may be life-threatening. Symptoms involve the skin, GI tract, and cardiovascular and respiratory systems. Clients experience peripheral tingling, flushing, fullness in the mouth, throat/nasal congestion, tearing and swelling around the eyes, itching, cough, laryngeal edema, bronchospasms, severe dyspnea, vasodilation, and cyanosis. If untreated, these catastrophic effects lead to respiratory failure, severe hypotension, anaphylactic shock, and death. Therefore, it is crucial that symptoms be identified early and treatment initiated immediately because death can occur in minutes.

CLIENT TEACHING

Severe Allergies

- Advise clients with severe allergies to wear a Medic Alert tag.
- Encourage clients who are allergic to insect stings to carry an emergency anaphylactic kit containing epinephrine at all times.

CASE STUDY

Allergic Reaction

A client is stung by a bee and experiences an allergic reaction with severe shortness of breath. The client is transported to the local emergency department.

Answer the following questions and state the rationale for your answer.

1. Briefly describe the role of B-cells and T-helper lymphocytes in immune physiology.
2. What role does the antigen play in an immune response?
3. What is the difference between an "allergen" and an "antigen"?

MEDICAL–SURGICAL MANAGEMENT

Medical

Medical management centers around establishing an intravenous line, administering fluids and emergency drugs, and maintaining an airway. Provide oxygen via a nonrebreather oxygen mask. In severe cases, endotracheal intubation or a tracheotomy may be required.

Pharmacological

Epinephrine is administered subcutaneously as soon as symptoms develop to dilate bronchioles, increase heart contractions, and constrict blood vessels. Antihistamines, such as diphenhydramine hydrochloride (Benadryl), block the effects of histamine in bronchioles, blood vessels, and the GI tract. Corticosteroids are given for their anti-inflammatory effect. Vasopressors, such as norepinephrine bitartrate (Levophed) or dopamine hydrochloride (Intropin), may be needed to increase blood pressure. If bronchoconstriction and spasms are severe, albuterol (Proventil), metaproterenol sulfate (Alupent), and/or aminophylline (Aminophyllin) may be administered.

Diet

Clients will be NPO until normal respiratory and circulatory function have been restored.

Activity

Clients will remain on bed rest until vital signs are stable and normal breathing patterns have been restored. Those experiencing severe anaphylactic responses are generally transferred to intensive care units for continued treatment and observation.

Nursing Management

Monitor vital signs frequently as well as I&O. Administer IV fluids and medications as ordered. Teach client and family the importance of providing the name of the causative agent and a description of the reaction when asked about allergies.

NURSING PROCESS

Assessment

Subjective Data

Client history may reveal a previous anaphylaxis reaction. The client may describe feelings of uneasiness, anxiety, weakness, itching, dizziness, nausea, peripheral tingling, and a generalized warm sensation throughout the body.

Objective Data

Because anaphylaxis is a sudden, unexpected event, be aware that variations in a client's cardiovascular and respiratory status may be signs of an impending anaphylactic reaction. The first symptoms are sweating, sneezing, tachycardia, hypotension, dysrhythmias, cyanosis, edema of tongue and larynx, wheezing, bronchospasms, vascular collapse, and cardiac arrest. Regularly assessing client's vital signs and cardiovascular, respiratory, and neurological status will detect changes before the severe signs of respiratory distress and impending shock develop.

Nursing diagnoses for clients with anaphylaxis include the following:

NURSING DIAGNOSES	PLANNING/OUTCOMES	NURSING INTERVENTIONS
Ineffective Tissue Perfusion, related to increased capillary permeability and vasodilation	The client will have adequate tissue perfusion.	Monitor vital signs frequently. Place client in Trendelenburg position for hypotension. Monitor I&O. Administer IV fluids and medications as ordered.
Ineffective Breathing Pattern related to bronchoconstriction, laryngeal edema, and increased secretions	The client will have effective breathing patterns.	Monitor vital signs. Maintain patent airway. Suction secretions as needed. Administer oxygen and medications as ordered.
Deficient Knowledge related to causative allergen, therapeutic modalities, and/or preventive measures	The client will relate causative allergen, therapeutic modalities, and preventive measures.	Teach client and family importance of avoiding allergen and symptoms of anaphylactic reactions. Teach client to provide the name of the causative agent and a description of reaction experienced when asked about allergies. Document allergy on all medical records.

Evaluation: Evaluate each outcome to determine how it has been met by the client.

TRANSFUSION REACTIONS

Blood components, such as whole blood, packed or frozen red blood cells (RBCs), leukocytes, platelets, and plasma, may be administered to clients when their own bodies are incapable of manufacturing them at a rate required to maintain vascular homeostasis. Any client receiving blood products that are **allogeneic**, or from a donor of the same species, may develop a transfusion reaction. For this reason, some clients are arranging to have their own blood collected, saved, and available for infusion, if needed, during or following elective surgeries. This is known as an **autologous** blood transfusion. Immunological reactions do not develop with this type of blood transfusion.

There are five types of transfusion reactions: febrile nonhemolytic, allergic urticarial, delayed hemolytic, acute hemolytic, and anaphylactic. Febrile nonhemolytic reactions are the most common and occur in clients who have had previous blood transfusions as a result of an antibody-antigen reaction to WBCs. Symptoms may develop soon after the infusion has started or up to 5 to 6 hours after completion. Fever is the classic symptom and may be accompanied by chills, nausea, headache, hypotension, and respiratory problems. Clients who have allergic urticarial reactions develop a skin rash during or within 1 hour following the transfusion. A delayed hemolytic reaction may occur days to weeks following the transfusion. The client's hemoglobin level falls because of incompatibility of RBC antigens. This type of reaction is often misdiagnosed

CRITICAL THINKING

Donor Blood Transfusion

What are the pros and cons of receiving a blood transfusion from a donor?

and thought to be related to the condition that created the need for blood replacement rather than a transfusion reaction. An acute hemolytic reaction is potentially a life-threatening situation. Symptoms, resulting from the incompatibility of ABO groups, usually occur during the first 15 minutes of administration, but can develop anytime during the transfusion. Clients complain of chills, nausea, and back pain. Fever, drop in blood pressure (hypotension), vomiting, hematuria, or oliguria may be observed. As the condition progresses, chest pain, dyspnea, anuria, and shock develop. Anaphylactic reactions, although rare, are also life-threatening. Symptoms of acute gastrointestinal malfunctioning and cardiovascular and respiratory collapse develop moments after the transfusion has started.

Medical–Surgical Management

Medical

Medical management of clients experiencing a blood transfusion reaction depends on the type of reaction. Treatment of a febrile nonhemolytic reaction includes stopping the blood, infusing normal saline, and treating the symptoms. For clients experiencing an allergic urticarial reaction, the transfusion should be slowed and an antihistamine administered. Delayed hemolytic reactions often go undetected and untreated. Both acute hemolytic reactions and anaphylactic reactions are medical emergencies. The transfusion must be stopped immediately. Normal saline and emergency drugs are given intravenously.

Pharmacological

If a febrile nonhemolytic or allergic urticarial reaction occurs, diphenhydramine hydrochloride (Benadryl) and a corticosteroid (hydrocortisone or prednisone) are administered to counteract the immunological response. Antipyretics are ordered to control fever. For life-threatening conditions, emergency medications are employed. (Refer back to Anaphylactic Reaction.)

Diet

Clients should not be fed if a reaction is occurring, especially if respiratory symptoms have developed, because aspiration could occur.

Activity

Clients should remain in bed until symptoms of the reaction have subsided.

Nursing Management

Follow agency protocol for use and administration of blood products. Assess vital signs before administration of blood products and at 15-minute intervals four times. Stay with the client for at least the first 15 minutes of administration. When reaction occurs, stop transfusion, but keep saline going for IV access if needed. Notify physician immediately.

NURSING PROCESS

Assessment

Subjective Data

Occasionally, clients verbalize the feeling of something "not being right" or "something strange is going on in my body" before actual symptoms become apparent. They may have itching, headache, or low-back pain.

Objective Data

Assess for any signs of a transfusion reaction, such as fever, chills, or respiratory problems.

A nursing diagnosis for clients with transfusion reactions is:

NURSING DIAGNOSES	PLANNING/OUTCOMES	NURSING INTERVENTIONS
Risk for Injury related to infusion of allogeneic blood components	The client will not have injury from infusion of allogeneic blood products.	Follow protocol for blood products and administration. Check client's identification and blood product with another nurse. If a reaction occurs, stop transfusion immediately, then call the physician. Administer medications as ordered. Send blood tubing and a urine specimen to the lab for analysis. Monitor and document client's condition. Teach client who has a blood transfusion reaction to inform health care providers whenever questioned about allergies.

Evaluation: Evaluate each outcome to determine how it has been met by the client.

TRANSPLANT REJECTION

In 2005, more than 163,000 organ transplants were performed in the United States (Department of Health and Human Services, 2007). The success of these procedures is directly related to matching antibodies and antigens of the donor and recipient and to the effectiveness of immunosuppressive medications in preventing rejection. Immunosuppressive medications make the client prone to the development of infections and cancers. Clients must have a regular medical checkup, including cancer screening tests.

Medical–Surgical Management

Medical

Although blood components are the most common type of tissue transplants, today it is possible to transplant bone marrow, corneal tissue, skin, kidneys, pancreas, hearts, livers, and lungs. Bone marrow and blood components often employ autologous donations. Allogeneic donations may be from living related donors or living nonrelated donors. Cadaveric donations are harvested from individuals after they are pronounced clinically dead. It is important to match ABO blood groups and **human leukocyte antigen** (antigens present in human blood) to prevent rejection when allogeneic and cadaveric donors are used.

Pharmacological

A combination of immunosuppressive medications is used to hinder rejection. Steroids such as prednisone (Deltasone) and methylprednisolone sodium succinate (Solu-Medrol) decrease the inflammatory response. Cyclosporine (Sandimmune), antithymocyte globulin (equine), ATG (Atgam), and tacrolimus (Prograf) inhibit T-cells. Azathioprine (Imuran) inhibits purine synthesis. Muromonab-CD3 (Orthoclone, OKT 3) prevents acute rejection in kidney transplant clients. Clients taking immunosuppressive medications are especially prone to developing infections. Antibiotics may be prescribed prophylactically.

Steroids cause fluid and sodium retention, low potassium level, elevated blood pressure, moon face, muscle wasting, elevated glucose level, impaired wound healing, mood swings, and masculinization in women. Cyclosporine may be toxic to the kidneys and liver. Imuran may cause hair loss and lower platelet level. OKT 3 also causes fluid retention.

Activity

Activity depends on the type of transplant. Clients who receive a major organ, such as a heart, lung, pancreas, or liver, are placed in reverse isolation in the hospital setting for at least 2 weeks. They are carefully observed for signs of rejection. Exposure to others is limited. Before discharge, they are taught to avoid contact with anyone who may have an infection and to wear a mask whenever out in public.

Nursing Management

Monitor vital signs, fluid balance, nutritional status, mental status, and cardiovascular and respiratory functioning. Prevent contact with anyone who may have an infection. Teach client and family proper hand hygiene. Emphasize the importance of taking all medications as prescribed.

NURSING PROCESS

Assessment

Subjective Data

Client history may reveal fear of possible transplant rejection. The client generally describes tenderness at the transplant site.

Objective Data

After transplantation, carefully monitor clients' vital signs, nutritional status, fluid balance, urinary output, mental status, and respiratory and cardiovascular functioning. Weigh client daily. Check wound sites frequently. Signs of rejection include fever, weight gain, and swelling or tenderness at the transplant site.

Nursing diagnoses for clients with organ transplants include the following:

NURSING DIAGNOSES	PLANNING/OUTCOMES	NURSING INTERVENTIONS
Fear related to possible transplant rejection.	The client will relate less fear regarding rejection.	Allow client to verbalize concerns and develop realistic expectations. Set aside time to sit down and talk to client.
Deficient Knowledge related to home care following transplantation	The client will discuss signs and symptoms of rejection.	Teach client and family about signs of rejection and infection.
	The client will demonstrate an understanding of the side effects of immunosuppressive drugs and lifestyle changes to adapt to their effects.	Teach client and family ramifications of taking immunosuppressive medications. Teach client to watch for side effects and report them to physician.

(Continues)

Nursing diagnoses for clients with organ transplants include the following: (Continued)

NURSING DIAGNOSES	PLANNING/OUTCOMES	NURSING INTERVENTIONS
Risk for Infection related to immunosuppressive medications	The client will demonstrate appropriate wound care. The client will be free of infection.	Teach client and family appropriate wound care and proper hand hygiene. Teach client importance of taking antibiotics as ordered, wearing a mask whenever out in public, and regular checkups, including cancer screening tests.

Evaluation: Evaluate each outcome to determine how it has been met by the client.

LATEX ALLERGY

Since 1987, when universal precautions (now called Standard Precautions) were mandated, exposure to latex by health care workers has dramatically increased. Today, between 8% and 17% of health care workers and less than 1% of the general population are sensitized to natural rubber latex (American Latex Allergy Association, 2009).

The latex proteins can enter the body through the skin and mucous membranes, intravascularly, and by inhalation. The cornstarch powder on gloves absorbs the latex proteins and becomes airborne when the gloves are put on or taken off. From the air, the latex proteins may be inhaled or may be in contact with the skin and mucous membranes. Anyone, client or health care worker, who after exposure to latex develops red, watery, itchy eyes; sinus or nasal irritation; hives; shortness of breath; dry cough; wheezing; chest tightness; or flushing, tachycardia, and hypotension should be suspected of latex allergy.

Latex allergy has the potential to induce a life-threatening anaphylactic reaction with repeated exposure; avoidance of latex products is of utmost importance. Synthetic versions of products are often available. An individual product may be "latex free," but an environment is "latex safe" only when all items of latex that might come in contact with the allergic individual are removed.

CLIENT TEACHING

Latex Safety

- Clients with latex allergy are at risk for cross-reactivity to banana, avocado, chestnuts, kiwi, and passion fruit (NIAID, 2003).
- Clients with spina bifida, or who need multiple surgeries, have a risk of nearly 50% of developing allergies to latex (American Academy of Allergy Asthma & Immunology, 2007). These clients need to avoid exposure to latex products such as gloves, band-aids, rubber bands, condoms, and latex birthday balloons.
- Health care workers and others whose job requires wearing latex gloves have nearly a 10% risk of developing a latex allergy (American Academy of Allergy Asthma & Immunology, 2007).
- Clients with latex allergy are instructed to avoid all latex products, including the powder/dust from inside latex gloves.

SAFETY

Latex Allergy

A Medic Alert tag stating "latex allergy" should be worn by any individual with a latex allergy.

AUTOIMMUNE DISEASES

Disorders in this category include rheumatoid arthritis, systemic lupus erythematosus, and myasthenia gravis.

RHEUMATOID ARTHRITIS

Rheumatoid arthritis (RA) is a chronic, systemic autoimmune disease characterized by joint stiffness. It affects 1.3 million people in the United States, and occurs in women two to three times more often than men (Arthritis Foundation, 2009e). Rheumatoid arthritis can affect anyone, including children, and onset usually occurs between 30 to 50 years of age. Clients with the genetic marker HLA-DR4 may have an increased risk of developing rheumatoid arthritis (Arthritis Foundation, 2009f).

The cause of RA is unknown, but there seems to be a genetic predisposition (susceptibility) in many, but not all, persons affected. It is believed that something must trigger the disease process such as a virus, bacterium, hormonal factors, or stress. The person's immune system attacks the cells inside the joint(s), producing substances that act as antigens. Immune complexes are formed within the joint, causing inflammation, swelling, and increased synovial fluid. As this chronic, systemic condition progresses, surrounding cartilage, tendons, and ligaments become involved. Thickening of synovial tissue eventually leads to calcification of the joint, joint pain, limited mobility, and deformity.

It is believed that the damage to the bones begins within the first two years of the onset of RA. Early diagnosis and aggressive treatment are important to control the disease. Usually, the joints of the hand and wrist are affected initially. As the disease progresses, shoulder, elbow, hip, knee, ankle, and cervical spine joints become affected. The pattern of joint involvement is symmetrical (i.e., if a joint is affected on the right side of the body, the same joint will also be affected on the left side) (Arthritis Foundation, 2009). Other areas of the body where connective tissue is present may also be involved, such as blood vessels, lining of the lungs, and pericordial sac.

Clients experience periods of **remission**, a decrease or absence of symptoms, and **exacerbations**, an increase in symptoms. Both physical and emotional stressors lead to increased symptomatology. This means that simple tasks such as answering the telephone or buttoning clothes may become very challenging.

Medical–Surgical Management

Medical

Medical management centers around reducing inflammation, relieving pain, slowing down or a stopping joint damage, and promoting general health. Therapeutic regimen includes medications, exercise, rest, hot and cold applications, and stress management. Currently researchers are working on developing and testing a vaccine for the prevention of rheumatoid arthritis (Arthritis Foundation, 2009a).

Surgical

Hip, knee, and finger joints may be surgically replaced. Refer to the Musculoskeletal System chapter for a discussion of joint replacement.

Pharmacological

Nonsteroidal anti-inflammatory drugs (NSAIDs) and salicylates have the potential to relieve symptoms such as joint pain, stiffness, and swelling but do not control the disease. Disease-modifying antirheumatic drugs (DMARDs) have the potential to modify the disease and should be given early in the disease to control progression. The commonly used DMARDs include prednisone (Deltasone), gold salts, and sulfasalazine (Azulfidine EN-Tabs) (Table 16-5). Aggressive treatment includes disease-modifying

Table 16-5 Medications Used to Treat Rheumatoid Arthritis

DRUG	USE/ACTIONS	SIDE EFFECTS	NURSING CONSIDERATIONS
Salicylates			
• aspirin	Inhibit prostaglandin synthesis resulting in decreased pain. (Analgesia) antipyretic and anti-inflammatory effects.	GI upset, tinnitus, easy bruising, nausea, prolonged bleeding time.	Instruct client to take with food or take enteric coated aspirin and to report ringing in ears. Do not give to clients on oral anticoagulants. Assess for bleeding/bruising.
Nonsteroidal Anti-inflammatory Drugs (NSAIDs)			
• ibuprofen (Motrin, Rufen) • naproxen (Naprosyn) • phenylbutazone (Butazolidin) • nabumetone (Relafen)	Inhibit prostaglandin synthesis. Reduce joint swelling stiffness. Analgesic and antipyretic properties.	GI irritation, nausea, vomiting, heartburn. GI bleeding and ulceration, dizziness, headache, liver toxicity.	Administer with food. May prolong bleeding time, may require frequent blood count.
Indole Analogues			
• indomethacin (Indocin) • sulindac (Clinoril)	Analgesic anti-inflammatory effect.	Gastric bleeding, headaches, dizziness, psychiatric disturbances.	Administer with food. Instruct client to report any bleeding (tarry stools, hematemesis). Avoid giving aspirin.
Corticosteroids			
• prednisone (Deltasone)	Decreases inflammation.	GI irritation, muscle weakness, fluid retention, moon face, muscle wasting, impaired wound healing.	Administer with food. Weigh daily. Monitor BP, sleep pattern, and serum potassium.
Antimalarials			
• hydroxychloroquine sulfate (Plaquenil Sulfate)	Not a drug of choice.	Visual disturbances, nightmares, skin lesions, nausea, diarrhea, low blood count.	Monitor CBC and liver function tests. Discontinue after 6 months if no beneficial effects noted.

(*Continues*)

TABLE 16-5 Medications Used to Treat Rheumatoid Arthritis (Continued)

DRUG	USE/ACTIONS	SIDE EFFECTS	NURSING CONSIDERATIONS
Gold Salts			
• auranofin (Ridaura)	Anti-inflammatory effect.	Diarrhea, nausea, vomiting, jaundice.	Remind client to keep all physician appointments. Beneficial effects may take 3 months to appear.
Chelating Agent			
• penicillamine (Depen)	Palliative when other medications have failed.	Bone marrow depression, fever, rashes, blood dyscrasias, liver toxicity.	Give on empty stomach. Have epinephrine 1;1,000 handy for anaphylaxis. Fluids to 3,000 mL/day to prevent renal failure.
Sulfonamide			
• sulfasalazine (Azulfidine EN-TABS)	For clients who do not respond well to NSAIDs.	Anorexia, headache, nausea, vomiting, gastric distress, reversible oligospermia.	Give with food. May discolor urine or skin yellow-orange. Take at least 2–3 L/day of water. May increase sensitivity to sun.
Immunomodulator			
• adalimumab (Humira)	Decreases inflammation and inhibits progression of structural damage.	Increased risk for infections, redness and pain, itching, swelling and/or bruising at the injection site.	Drug must be refrigerated but not frozen. Comes in pre-filled syringes and is injected into the abdomen, upper arm, or thigh.
• etanercept (Enbrel)	Delays structural damage and improves physical function.	Redness and pain, itching, swelling and/or bruising at the injection site.	Comes in pre-filled syringe or pen device. The needle cover contains latex; do not handle if sensitive to latex. Drug must be refrigerated and allowed to come to room temperature before administration.
Immunosuppressant			
• azathioprine (Imuran)	For clients that are nonresponsive to conventional therapy.	Bone marrow depression, loss of appetite, liver problems, low blood counts, unusual tiredness or weakness.	Take with food. Improvement may take 6 to 12 weeks.
Antibiotic			
• minocycline (Minocin)	Increasingly being used for clients that do not respond to conventional therapy.	Cramps or burning of the stomach, diarrhea, darkening of the skin, dizziness, light-headed or unsteadiness, liver problems, and sun sensitivity.	Take on an empty stomach.
Antimetabolite			
• methotrexate (Rheumatrex, Trexall)	For clients that do not respond well to NSAIDS.	Bone marrow depression, increased sun sensitivity, hair loss, liver problems, low blood counts, mouth sores, yeast infections.	Take tablets at bedtime with an antacid to minimize GI upset. Monitor CBC and liver function tests.

antirheumatic drugs such as methotrexate, hydroxychloroquine (Plaquenil), sulfasalazine (Azulfidine), a biologic agent such as etanercept (Enbrel), or adalimumab (Humira), or a combination of both a biologic and a DMARD (Arthritis Foundation, 2009b). Because of the large doses required to control inflammation and the long-term use because of the chronicity of this condition, side effects often develop. In severe cases, azathioprine (Imuran), hydroxychloroquine sulfate (Plaquenil Sulfate), D-penicillamine (Depen), or methotrexate sodium (Rheumatrex) may be used. These medications also have serious side effects. Minocycline, an antibiotic, is increasingly being used to treat rheumatoid arthritis. Researchers have been investigating the use of the antimalarial drug, hydrochloroquine in protecting clients with RA from developing diabetes (Arthritis Foundation, 2009b).

Diet

Clients should eat a nutritious, well-balanced diet. Poorly nourished individuals are prone to infections. For clients with RA, an infection results in exacerbation of symptoms. Foods high in iron are encouraged when RBCs are low.

Activity

Because joint mobility is a major problem, occupational and physical therapists are part of the therapeutic team. Range-of-motion exercises, resting splints, and assistive devices such as canes and hand rails are often employed to promote mobility.

Nursing Management

Encourage the client to practice relaxation techniques and take a warm shower to relieve joint stiffness and pain. Emphasize the importance of doing ROM exercises several times a day and to have planned rest periods. Teach the client to use assistive devices such as handrails, tools to pick up objects, raised toilet seat, walker, or cane.

NURSING PROCESS

Assessment

Subjective Data

Client history frequently reveals a gradual development of symptoms, beginning initially with early-morning stiffness and pain in finger joints. Eventually, other joints become involved. Fatigue, weight loss, temperature elevation, and anemia develop, along with malaise, loss of appetite, fatigue, and muscle weakness. Obtain information about periods of remissions and exacerbations as well as the client's understanding of and compliance with the treatment regimen.

Objective Data

Assessment of the hands may reveal the classic deformities associated with RA: boutonniere deformity (fixed flexion of the proximal interphalangeal joint and hyperextension of the distal interphalangeal joint), ulnar drift (deviation of the fingers to the ulnar side of the hand), and swan-neck deformity (fixed flexion of the distal interphalangeal joint and hyperextension of the proximal interphalangeal joint). Figure 16-5 illustrates these changes in the hands.

Skin may show the presence of ulcers, caused by vasculitis, and moveable, subcutaneous skin nodes, known as *rheumatoid nodules*. Eye tissue may be inflamed. Reduction in tear and saliva production can occur, causing dryness of the eyes, mouth, and mucous membranes. This is known as Sjögren's syndrome. The client may have weight loss and an elevated temperature.

X-rays demonstrate the amount and degree of deformity. No specific laboratory test confirms a diagnosis of RA, although alterations in the following may occur: RBCs decrease (anemia) as the disease progresses, elevation of WBCs, erythrocyte sedimentation rate (ESR), antinuclear antibodies (ANAs), C-reactive proteins, and platelet count. The rheumatoid factor (RF) is present in about 75% of adult clients with RA (Daniels, 2010).

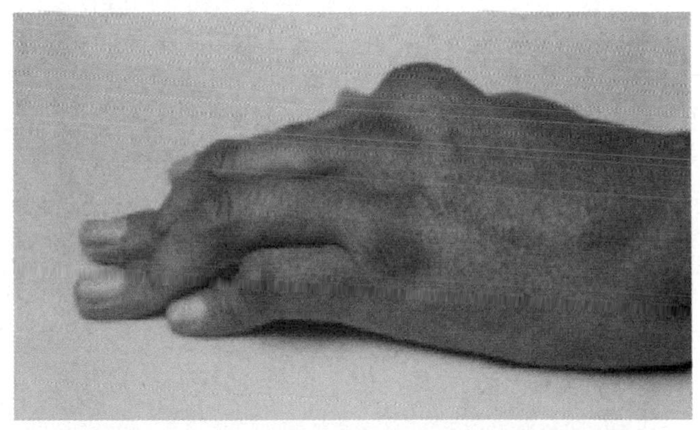

FIGURE 16-5 Arthritic Hands (*Courtesy of the Arthritis Foundation.*)

Nursing diagnoses for clients with rheumatoid arthritis include the following:

NURSING DIAGNOSES	PLANNING/OUTCOMES	NURSING INTERVENTIONS
Chronic Pain related to swollen, inflamed joints	The client will relate appropriate use of anti-inflammatory medications. The client will relate methods to decrease pain.	Teach client about prescribed analgesics and anti-inflammatory medications. Encourage client to practice relaxation techniques and take warm shower to relieve early morning joint stiffness and pain. Use hot and cold packs to decrease muscle spasms. Teach client proper body alignment and to avoid using pillows under the knees, which leads to pooling of blood in the feet.

(*Continues*)

Nursing diagnoses for clients with rheumatoid arthritis include the following: (Continued)

NURSING DIAGNOSES	PLANNING/OUTCOMES	NURSING INTERVENTIONS
Impaired Physical Mobility related to edema, and joint immobility	The client will demonstrate measures to maintain joint mobility.	Teach hospitalized clients to use the overhead trapeze when moving in bed and to change position frequently.
	The client will demonstrate use of adaptive devices.	Assist with ROM exercises and maintain planned rest periods.
		Teach client use of assistive devices, such as handrests, tools to pick up objects, or three-legged canes, as needed.
		Check with occupational and physical therapists for available equipment. Assist client to use handrails in tub, shower, and toilet; raised toilet seat; and rubber-tipped walker or cane.
Bathing/Dressing/Grooming Self-care Deficit related to joint inflammation or deformity	The client will bathe, dress, and groom to abilities.	Encourage client to stop and rest when tired.
		Teach self-care using assistive devices, as required. Recommend shoes with Velcro® closures.
		Assist with routine plan for ADLs.
Fatigue related to chronic inflammatory process	The client will state less fatigue.	Explain that fatigue is a common symptom of autoimmune disorders. Plan rest periods between activities.
	The client will establish priorities for daily activities.	Allow the client to express feelings about altered lifestyle.
		Inform client of community services such as Meals on Wheels.
	The client will balance daily activities with periods of rest.	Help identify activities client should perform and what can be delegated. Instruct client to record level of fatigue and activities performed on an hourly basis for 24 hours. One method uses 0 to 10 scale (0 = not tired, peppy; 10 = totally exhausted).
		Help plan important tasks during high-energy periods and distribute difficult ones throughout the week.

Evaluation: Evaluate each outcome to determine how it has been met by the client.

SYSTEMIC LUPUS ERYTHEMATOSUS

Systemic lupus erythematosus (SLE) is a chronic, progressive, incurable autoimmune disease affecting multiple body organs. It is characterized by periods of exacerbation (flares) and remission. SLE occurs most commonly in women during their childbearing years and is 2 to 3 times more common in African-American women (Lupus Foundation of America, 2009). In clients with SLE, abnormal B-lymphocyte cells produce autoantibodies that destroy body cells. Immune complexes are formed and circulate in serum, causing inflammation and tissue damage in the skin, brain, kidney, lung, heart, or joints. Production of these autoantibodies is influenced by genetic predisposition, medications, infections, stress, and sunlight (ultraviolet light rays).

No single test is conclusive for a diagnosis. The American College of Rheumatology has established criteria for SLE. These criteria include a malar rash (over cheeks); discoid rash; photosensitivity; oral ulcers; arthritis; serositis (pleuritis or pericarditis); excessive protein or cellular casts in the urine; seizures or psychosis; hemolytic anemia, or leukopenia, or lymphopenia, or thrombocytopenia; and positive for LE cells, or anti-DNA antibody, or anti-Sm, or a false-positive syphilis test. If four or more of these criteria are present, a client is diagnosed with SLE.

MEDICAL–SURGICAL MANAGEMENT

Medical

Medical treatment is aimed at decreasing tissue inflammation and destruction. A knowledgeable client can assist in controlling the disease process through stress management, rest, exercise, taking medications as prescribed, and immediately reporting symptoms to the health care provider. During acute exacerbations, plasmapheresis may be used. This treatment modality involves removal

CLIENT TEACHING

Systemic Lupus Erythematosus

- Get adequate rest.
- Use stress-reduction techniques such as visualization, guided imagery, meditation, or yoga.
- Avoid exposure to sunlight; use sunscreen.
- Involve family and friends in care.
- Report fever, chills, anorexia, or symptom worsening to health care provider immediately.
- Never just stop taking medications.
- Contact the Lupus Foundation of America, Inc., for information and support (see Resources at the end of chapter).

of the client's plasma, processing it through a special machine to eliminate various cellular elements, and reinfusing the cleansed plasma. In SLE, autoantibodies are removed.

Because clients with SLE are prone to a variety of complications, they are carefully monitored for renal, cardiac, pulmonary, hematological, and neurological damage. A large percentage of SLE clients eventually develop renal failure, requiring dialysis to maintain life.

Pharmacological

NSAIDs are used for muscle and joint pain. The lowest possible dose of corticosteroid is used to suppress immune system activity. During periods of exacerbations, higher doses may be required. Prolonged use of these medications leads to multiple side effects. Hydroxychloroquine sulfate (Plaquenil sulfate), an antimalarial agent, is used. Although the exact mechanism involved is unknown, it does work effectively in decreasing joint and skin problems. It can lead to the development of retinal toxicity; therefore, clients should have yearly eye exams. Cyclophosphamide (Cytoxan) or azathioprine (Imuran) may be used for severe SLE.

Diet

Clients on corticosteroids are prone to developing hypernatremia, hyperglycemia, hypokalemia, and fluid retention. Diet should be low in sodium and glucose and high in potassium. Excessive fluid intake should be discouraged.

Activity

Clients should be encouraged to sleep at least 8 hours a night and rest periodically during the day. Regular exercise helps prevent muscle weakness and fatigue.

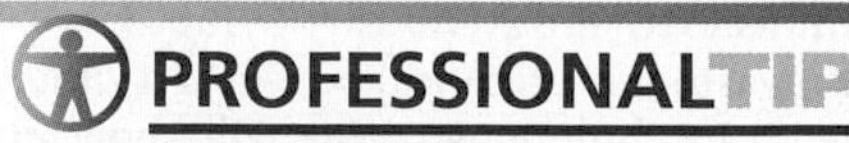

PROFESSIONAL TIP

RA and SLE

Clients with RA and SLE have common nursing diagnoses of fatigue and impaired mobility. Clients with SLE have an additional risk for infection if WBC count is low.

CRITICAL THINKING

Lifestyle Implications

What are the lifestyle implications of being diagnosed with a chronic disease such as rheumatoid arthritis or systemic lupus erythematosus?

Nursing Management

Teach the client the importance of avoiding direct sunlight and the use of protective clothing and sunscreen (SPF 15 or higher). Encourage the client to balance rest and activity and to eat a balanced diet with reduced sodium. Emphasize the signs of exacerbation (rash, fever, cough, or increased joint and muscle pain) and early signs of infection. Provide emotional, psychosocial, and spiritual support.

NURSING PROCESS

ASSESSMENT

Subjective Data

Ask when the disease began, what symptoms have developed, and how they have been treated. Note information about medications the client is taking and side effects, activity level, and degree of fatigue. Determine client's understanding of the disease process, how lifestyle has changed, and how effectively client is coping. The client may describe having malaise, photosensitivity, pain in joints, irregular menses, irritability, confusion, or hallucinations.

Objective Data

Most common findings include joint swelling and pain, fever, swollen glands, nausea, vomiting, anorexia, hypertension, respiratory and cardiac infections, renal involvement, enlarged liver and spleen, and skin lesions, especially the classic "butterfly" rash. Figure 16-6 shows an individual with a "butterfly" rash. If exposed to the cold, Raynaud's phenomenon (intermittent attacks of diminished blood supply to fingers, toes, ears, and nose) may develop.

Laboratory tests frequently reveal serum antinuclear antibodies (ANA) and anti-DNA antibodies. Lupus erythematosus cells (LE cells) are present in most clients. Anemia, leukopenia, and thrombocytopenia are evident.

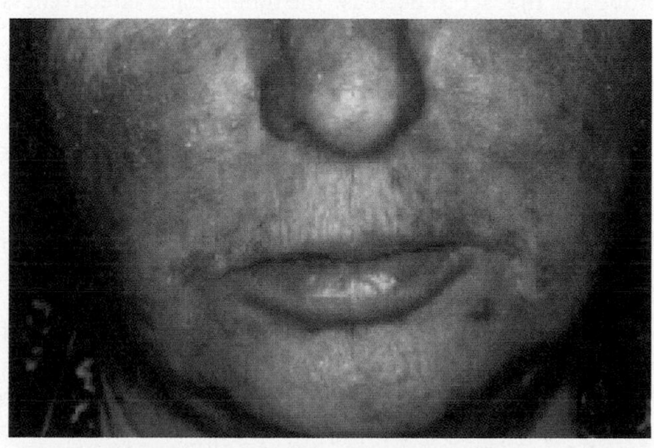

FIGURE 16-6 Butterfly Rash (*Courtesy of the American Academy of Dermatology.*)

Nursing diagnoses for a client with SLE include the following:

NURSING DIAGNOSES	PLANNING/OUTCOMES	NURSING INTERVENTIONS
Impaired Skin Integrity related to presence of butterfly rash, skin lesions, Raynaud's phenomenon, and/or oral ulcers	The client will participate in a plan to promote wound healing.	Teach client to clean and dry area prior to application of topical corticosteroids. Warn client that sunlight and ultraviolet rays increase symptoms and tanning sessions are contraindicated. Encourage client to wear protective clothing, sunscreen of at least SPF 15, and sunglasses. In cold weather, client should wear a hat and gloves. Encourage client in regular oral care to promote healing of mouth sores.
Deficient Knowledge related to adapting lifestyle with treatment and prevention of complications	The client will describe disease process, factors contributing to symptoms, and regimen for control.	Teach client effects of disease and methods to control complications. Teach stress management techniques. Allow client to vent feelings. Help client plan methods to adapt lifestyle. Encourage client to visit the physician on a regular basis to monitor for early symptoms of major organ involvement. Advise client to have regular eye exam if taking Plaquenil Sulfate. Inform client of community support groups available through the Lupus Foundation of America, Inc. (see Resources).

Evaluation: Evaluate each outcome to determine how it has been met by the client.

MYASTHENIA GRAVIS

Myasthenia gravis (MG) is an autoimmune disease characterized by extreme muscle weakness and fatigue caused by the body's inability to transmit nerve impulses to voluntary muscles. It is thought that clients with MG develop antibodies that act to decrease the number and effectiveness of acetylcholine receptor sites at neuromuscular junctions. Voluntary muscles are most commonly involved, especially those innervated by cranial nerves. Muscle weakness increases during periods of activity and improves after a period of rest.

Severity of symptoms varies. In mild conditions known as Group I ocular myasthenia, only the eye muscles are involved. As severity increases, symptoms of Group II generalized myasthenia develop: Facial, neck, skeletal, and respiratory muscles become affected. The thymus gland is enlarged in most clients. Anti-ACh receptor antibodies are produced in this organ. MG affects men more frequently than women, with the onset of symptoms after age 50. Periods of remission and exacerbation occur, usually during the first few years.

There are three possible complications: respiratory distress, myasthenic crisis, and cholinergic crisis. Clients need to be carefully monitored for early signs of respiratory distress, such as dyspnea, tachypnea, tachycardia, and diaphoresis.

Myasthenia crisis is an acute emergency characterized by increased muscle weakness; difficulty swallowing, chewing, or talking; and respiratory distress. It occurs in newly diagnosed clients who are not responding to anticholinesterase medications following infections, surgery, or delivery of a child.

Cholinergic crisis is the result of an overdose of anticholinesterase medications. Physical symptoms of both myasthenia crisis and cholinergic crisis are the same. An edrophonium chloride (Tensilon) test is used to differentiate between the two. Tensilon is administered intravenously; symptoms of clients experiencing a myasthenia crisis will be relieved within seconds, whereas clients in cholinergic crisis will show no response. Atropine is administered to counteract the effects of excessive amounts of anticholinesterase drugs. The treatment goal for both is restoration of normal respiratory functioning and alleviation of symptoms.

Medical–Surgical Management

Medical

Medical management involves the use of anticholinesterase medications and plasmapheresis, which removes anti-ACh receptor antibodies. Because it affords only temporary relief of symptoms, it is used primarily for clients in acute crisis who are not responding to drug therapy or before a thymectomy. A client's relief of symptoms is a good indicator of how successful surgery might be.

Surgical

Surgical removal of the thymus gland has shown the best results in young people early in the course of the disease. In some people, the weakness may completely disappear, but it varies with each client.

Pharmacological

Anticholinesterase medications, such as pyridostigmine bromide (Mestinon), neostigmine bromide (Prostigmin), and ambenonium chloride (Mytelase), are prescribed early in the course of the disease and act to increase acetylcholine at the neuromuscular junction. Dosages need to be individually determined. Early side effects of overdosage include nausea, abdominal cramping, vomiting, diarrhea, increased saliva, diaphoresis, and low pulse rate. Variation may occur in muscle group responses for the same client. Steroids may slow down the immunological response.

Diet

Clients need to be encouraged to eat a snack before taking anticholinesterase medications to avoid GI irritation. If the client's ability to chew and swallow is affected, food should be chopped, mashed, or pureed. A commercial thickener can be added to liquids to reduce the risk of aspiration. Sit upright when eating and do not talk.

Activity

Symptoms of MG increase with exercise. Clients should avoid excessive muscular activity and should rest periodically throughout the day. ROM exercises, braces, splints, and walkers assist in keeping the client independent.

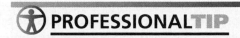

Myasthenia Gravis

Clients with myasthenia gravis experience problems similar to those with RA and SLE (e.g., fatigue and impaired physical mobility). Although the cause, in this case, is weakness of voluntary muscles, client goals and nursing interventions are the same.

Nursing Management

Teach the client airway protective techniques (e.g., double swallowing, chin tuck). Encourage the client to change daily activity pattern for minimal energy expenditure, and to do ROM exercises to help maintain muscle function. Emphasize the need to see the physician at the first sign of an upper respiratory infection. Advise client to avoid crowds during cold and flu season and anyone known to have either.

NURSING PROCESS

Assessment

Subjective Data

Client describes muscle weakness, fatigue, and possibly difficulty chewing or swallowing.

Objective Data

Assess muscle groups affecting the eyes, face, neck, and chest, looking for **diplopia** (double vision), **ptosis** (drooping upper eyelids), and facial symmetry. Note chewing or swallowing problems and weakness in arm and legs muscles as well as muscles used for breathing. Assess vocal tones and breath sounds.

ACh receptor antibody and LE cell tests are often positive. X-rays and CT scans of the thymus gland are used to detect enlargement. Electromyogram (EMG) determines the extent of muscle damage.

Nursing diagnoses for a client with MG include the following:

NURSING DIAGNOSES	PLANNING/OUTCOMES	NURSING INTERVENTIONS
Ineffective Breathing Pattern related to muscle weakness	The client will have normal respiratory rate and rhythm and normal breath sounds bilaterally.	Monitor client's respiratory rate and rhythm and breath sounds frequently. Administer oxygen as ordered. Notify physician immediately if respiratory problem develops. Elevate head of client's bed.

(*Continues*)

Nursing diagnoses for a client with MG include the following: (Continued)

NURSING DIAGNOSES	PLANNING/OUTCOMES	NURSING INTERVENTIONS
Risk for Aspiration related to impaired swallowing	The client will not experience aspiration.	Have client eat in a sitting position or with head of the bed elevated. Teach client to chew food well and swallow only small bites. Request a special diet of thickened, soft foods. Suction oral secretions as required. Teach client to suction secretions as needed.
Deficient Knowledge related to disease process and understanding of methods to control disease and prevent complications	The client will describe disease process, factors contributing to symptoms, and regimen for control. The client will practice health behaviors needed to manage the effects of MG and methods to prevent complications.	Teach client stress management techniques and methods to avoid infections. Teach clients to take medications at regularly scheduled times to maintain appropriate level. Encourage client to wear a Medic Alert bracelet indicating the name and dosage of medications being taken. Refer to the Myasthenia Gravis Foundation for information and support groups (see Resources).

Evaluation: Evaluate each outcome to determine how it has been met by the client.

SAMPLE NURSING CARE PLAN

The Client with Myasthenia Gravis

M.H., a 29-year-old mother of two preschool children, was diagnosed with myasthenia gravis 2 years ago. Initially, she had double vision and drooping eyelids, but after beginning a course of pyridostigmine bromide (Mestinon), she went into remission. Recently, she has been experiencing facial, neck, and chest muscle weakness and is now admitted to the hospital for evaluation. Occasionally, she has difficulty swallowing and breathing. Her thymus gland is enlarged. She has asked the nurse to teach her some strategies for managing this chronic illness.

NURSING DIAGNOSIS 1 *Ineffective Breathing Pattern* related to respiratory muscle fatigue as evidenced by facial, neck, and chest weakness

Nursing Outcomes Classification (NOC)
Respiratory Status: Ventilation

Nursing Interventions Classification (NIC)
Airway Management
Energy Management
Neurologic Monitoring

PLANNING/OUTCOMES	NURSING INTERVENTIONS	RATIONALE
M.H.'s respiratory rate and rhythm and breath sounds will remain within normal limits.	Assess M.H.'s breathing patterns q2h.	Detects early signs of respiratory distress.
	Ask M.H. to notify the nurse immediately if she has any breathing difficulties.	May be reluctant to call the nurse and needs to be encouraged to do so.
	Notify physician immediately if respiratory problems develop.	Physician must determine the cause and if a tracheostomy is needed.

SAMPLE NURSING CARE PLAN (Continued)

EVALUATION

M.H.'s respiratory rate and rhythm have remained within normal limits.

NURSING DIAGNOSIS 2 *Risk for Aspiration* related to impaired swallowing as evidenced by difficulty swallowing

Nursing Outcomes Classification (NOC)
Neurological Status
Respiratory Status: Ventilation

Nursing Interventions Classification (NIC)
Aspiration Precautions
Neurologic Monitoring

PLANNING/OUTCOMES	NURSING INTERVENTIONS	RATIONALE
M.H. will not experience aspiration.	Position M.H. to eat in a sitting position.	Promotes passage of food into the stomach.
	Teach M.H. the importance of thoroughly chewing food, and swallowing only small bites.	Can cause aspiration.
	Have oral suctioning equipment at the bedside.	Readily available if required.

EVALUATION

M.H. has not aspirated. She makes a point of always sitting up when eating.

NURSING DIAGNOSIS 3 *Deficient Knowledge*, related to disease process and understanding of methods to control effects of myasthenia gravis and prevent complications as evidenced by verbalization of need for future teaching

Nursing Outcomes Classification (NOC)
Knowledge: Disease Process
Knowledge: Energy Conservation

Nursing Interventions Classification (NIC)
Teaching: Disease Process
Teaching: Individual

PLANNING/OUTCOMES	NURSING INTERVENTIONS	RATIONALE
M.H. will practice health behaviors needed to manage the effects of MG and prevent complications.	Assess M.H.'s prior knowledge of MG and methods of controlling the effects of prescribed medications and preventing complications.	Provides a basis for planning teaching.
	Include M.H.'s family members in teaching sessions.	Fosters implementation of regimen at home.
	Teach M.H. and family members basic information about MG, the actions of anticholinesterase medication, the need to take it on a regular basis with a snack, side effects of overdose, and the importance of notifying the physician of any signs of respiratory problems or infection.	Information about one's disease, medications, and when to notify the physician is essential knowledge the client and family members need to effectively manage this chronic illness.

(Continues)

SAMPLE NURSING CARE PLAN (Continued)

PLANNING/OUTCOMES	NURSING INTERVENTIONS	RATIONALE
	Encourage M.H. to wear a Medic Alert bracelet, which lists here name, diagnoses, and dosage of prescribed medications.	Provides accurate information to medical personnel in case of an emergency.
	Provide M.H. with the address and telephone number of the Myasthenia Gravis Foundation and encourage her to contact them for additional information and support.	Facilitates future attainment of knowledge and possible involvement with a support group.

EVALUATION

M.H. and her husband related information about MG, action and side effects of Mestinon, signs and symptoms to watch for, and when to notify the physician. She has obtained a Medic Alert bracelet and has contacted the MG Foundation. She plans to attend the next local chapter meeting.

INADEQUATE IMMUNOLOGICAL RESPONSE

This category includes HIV/AIDS; pulmonary, gastrointestinal, oral, gynecological, and central nervous system opportunistic infections; and opportunistic malignancies.

HIV/AIDS

Although allergies are hypersensitive immune responses, and autoimmune diseases literally have the body attacking itself, acquired immunodeficiency syndrome (AIDS) is a disease that causes an inadequate immunological response by the body. The human immunodeficiency virus (HIV) may be acquired anytime after conception.

The **human immunodeficiency virus (HIV)**, a retrovirus that causes **acquired immunodeficiency syndrome (AIDS)**, was first reported in the United States in 1981. AIDS is a progressively fatal disease that destroys the immune system and the body's ability to fight infection. By the end of 2007, it was estimated that 33 million people in the world were living with HIV/AIDS (World Health Organization [WHO], 2008a). In the United States, 1,051,875 cases of AIDS had been reported by the end of 2007, and as many as 1,106,400 may be infected with HIV (CDC, 2008d).

Following exposure to HIV and an incubation period of 2 to 4 weeks, some individuals, but not all, will experience flulike symptoms such as fever, sweats, headache, myalgia, neuralgia, sore throat, GI distress, and photophobia (Figure 16-7). Many persons, if tested at this time, will test negative because antibodies may not yet be present in the blood. In 2 or 3 weeks, these symptoms disappear. Infected individuals are very infectious during this period, with large quantities of HIV present in genital secretions.

Most individuals will remain symptom free for years (10 or more), but some may begin to have symptoms in a few months. During this "asymptomatic" period, HIV is multiplying, infecting, and killing the CD4 T-cells of the immune system.

A variety of symptoms become evident as the CD4 T-cells disappear. Lymph nodes enlarged for more than 3 months are one of the first symptoms. Others may include weight loss, lack of energy, fevers and sweats, persistent skin

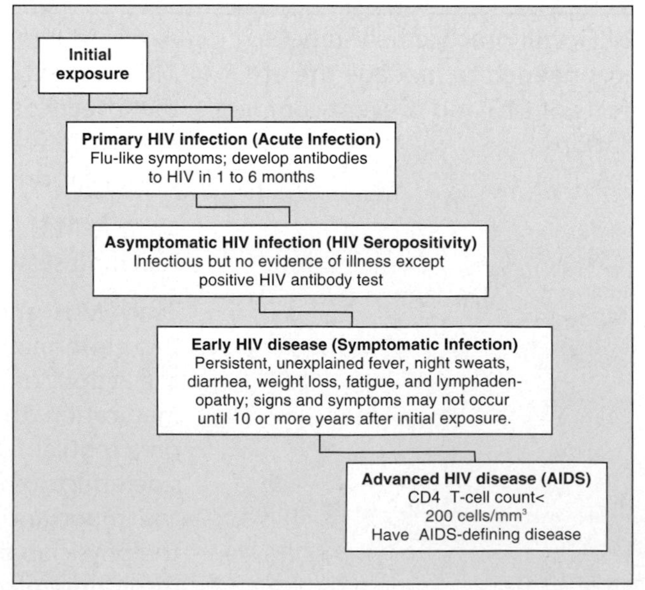

FIGURE 16-7 Continuum of HIV Disease

PROFESSIONAL TIP

Prevention for Health Care Workers

Health care workers are at risk for contracting HIV because of being near blood, semen, vaginal fluids, and placentas. The health care worker needs to follow standard precautions and wear gloves at all times when in contact with these fluids. The health care worker should wear goggles and a gown if there is potential of HIV contaminated fluids spraying or splashing into their eyes or on their clothes.

rashes or flaky skin, persistent or frequent oral or vaginal yeast infections, PID that does not respond to treatment, and short-term memory loss. Oral, genital, or anal herpes infection or shingles may also develop.

When the CD4 T-cell count is less than 200 cells/mm^3 (healthy persons have 1,000 or more CD4 cells/mm^3) and the individual has 1 or more of the 26 clinical conditions that affect persons with advanced HIV disease, the individual is considered to have AIDS. Most of the AIDS-defining conditions are **opportunistic infections** (infections in persons with a defective immune system that rarely cause harm in healthy individuals). Tuberculosis is the most common life-threatening opportunistic infection affecting people living with HIV/AIDS (WHO, 2008b). It kills nearly 250,000 people living with HIV each year, and is the leading cause of death among HIV-infected people living in Africa (WHO, 2008b).

The **enzyme-linked immunosorbent assay (ELISA)** is the basic screening test to detect antibodies to HIV. A positive test result is always retested to rule out false-positive results and/or technician error. A confirmatory test, the **Western blot** test, is always employed when the ELISA test is positive. Results of both the ELISA and Western blot taken together have an extremely high accuracy rate.

Obtaining a signed informed consent for testing is often a nursing responsibility. Most states mandate a consent form solely for HIV testing. Some states allow verbal consent and a statement of the client's consent signed by the health care provider.

The FDA has approved the OraQuick Rapid HIV-1 Antibody Test, which provides results with over 99.3% accuracy in 20 minutes (FDA, 2004).

Demographics of AIDS in the United States

Demographics are viewed in terms of clients' age, gender, and race.

Age

AIDS mainly affects people during the most productive years of their life. As of 2007, the age group with the highest number of new HIV diagnoses (219, 601 cases) was persons between the ages of 35-39 (CDC, 2009).The estimated number of new cases of AIDS among individuals younger than 13 in the United States fell from 954 in 1992 to 28 in 2007 (CDC, 2009).

Gender

Trends in HIV-related mortality reflect changes in the demographic patterns of the HIV epidemic. Although more men than women are infected with HIV, the number of AIDS cases in women in the United States has increased from 7% in 1985 to 25% in 2001. By the end of 2005, the proportion had decreased to 23% (CDC, 2008c).

Race Of the new AIDS cases reported in the United States in 2005:

- African Americans accounted for 71.3/100,000 population.
- Hispanic Americans accounted for 27.8/100,000 population.
- Caucasians accounted for 8.8/100,000 population.
- American Indian/Alaska Natives accounted for 10.4/100,000 population.
- Asian American/Pacific Islanders accounted for 7.4/100,000 population (CDC, 2008)

The HIV/AIDS epidemic is growing most rapidly among some minority populations (see Figure 16-8) and is a leading cause of death of African-American men ages 25 to 44 (CDC, 2009b).

Modes of Transmission

There are many way to become infected with HIV. The virus may be found in blood, semen, vaginal secretions, and breast milk of infected individuals. There is no evidence that HIV is spread through sweat, tears, urine, or feces. The saliva of infected individuals has the virus, but there is no evidence that it is spread to others through kissing. The risk of infection from "deep kissing" and oral sex is unknown. Tissue transplantation (including artificial insemination), blood transfusion, and needlesticks are high-risk situations but are relatively rare methods of transmission in the United States today. Having another sexually transmitted infection such as chlamydia, genital herpes, syphilis, or gonorrhea seems to make an individual more susceptible to becoming infected with HIV during sexual intercourse with an infected partner. Theoretically, HIV is present in sufficient quantities in amniotic fluid,

LIFE SPAN CONSIDERATIONS

Life Span Considerations

Mark Cichocki (2007) wrote in an article for amazon.com titled *HIV and the Older Adult—A Growing Population*, that there is a myth regarding the population aged 50 years and older not having sex. This age group is sexually active, contracting HIV, and needs to be assessed closely and asked the same questions as the other population age groups as to their sexual behaviors. The 50 years of age and older population also need to be educated about HIV, and how it is contracted to help reduce the risk of transmission.

Percentages of AIDS Cases by Race/Ethnicity, Reported in 2007—50 States and DC

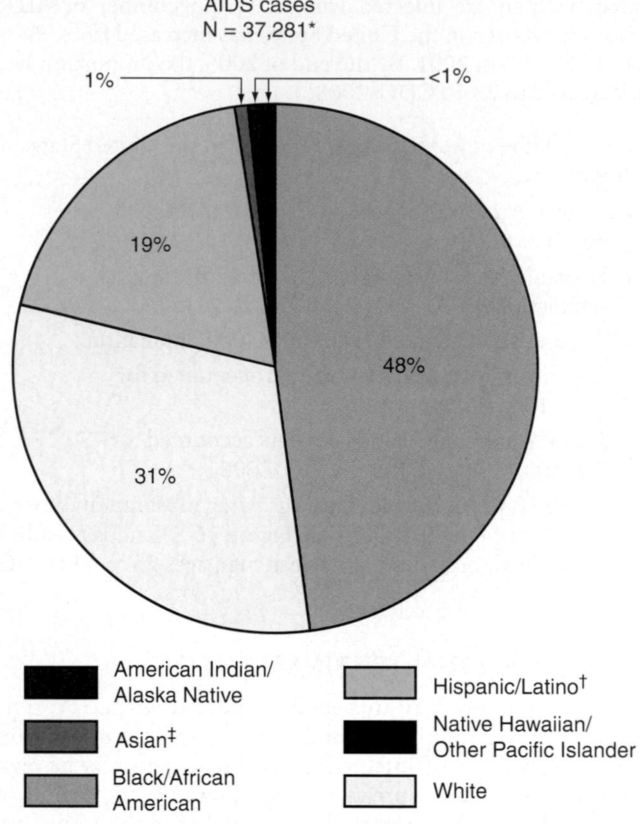

*Includes 411 persons of unknown race or multiple races.
†Hispanics/Latinos can be of any race.
‡Includes Asian and Pacific Islander legacy cases.

Taken from: HIV/AIDS surveillance by race/ethnicity (through 2007). Retrieved 4-27-09 from www.cdc.gov/hiv/topics/surveillance/resources/slides/race-ethnicity/index.htm

FIGURE 16-8 Percentages of AIDS Cases by Race/Ethnicity in 2007 (*Centers for Dieseas Control and Prevention, 2009b, Atlanta, GA.*)

cerebrospinal fluid, pleural fluid, peritoneal fluid, and pericardial fluid whereby infection could occur with exchange of these body fluids, particularly in health care settings where contact with these fluids may occur. Behaviors associated with increased risk of sexual transmission of HIV by infected persons include unprotected sexual intercourse, multiple sex partners, failure to disclose HIV status, and trading sex for money or drugs. Transmission of HIV can also take place by having contact with infected blood or sharing needles or syringes; it may also transmit from mother to fetus during pregnancy or birth.

Sexual intercourse (anal, oral, vaginal) without using a condom is the most frequently reported risk behavior for infection with HIV. Injection-drug use is the second most frequently reported risk behavior for infection with HIV. When HIV seropositive women take zidovudine (AZT) during pregnancy and labor and zidovudine is given to the newborn, perinatal transmission is significantly reduced.

MEDICAL–SURGICAL MANAGEMENT

Medical

The goal of care is to keep the disease from progressing for as long as possible. The client's chance of disease progression can now be monitored by a viral load test that measures copies of HIV RNA. The approved **viral load test** is the Amplicor HIV-1 Monitor test, better known as the *polymerase chain reaction (PCR) test*. It can be used to see if individuals with HIV are at risk for getting sick, for checking the effects of drugs taken by individuals with HIV to see if they are working against the virus, and to distinguish the difference between actual HIV infection in a newborn and maternally acquired antibodies. The "ultra-sensitive" PCR test can measure as few as 50 copies/mL of HIV RNA. There is no "safe" level of viral load. The risk is less, but HIV can be passed to another person if the viral load is undetectable.

Pharmacological

The goal of anti-HIV treatment is to keep the viral load as low as possible for as long as possible, ideally below what the viral load test can detect. Currently available antiretroviral drugs do not cure HIV/AIDS. Treatment is usually begun at the time of **seroconversion** (evidence of antibody formation in response to disease or vaccine). In high-risk occupational exposures, treatment may be started immediately.

One group of drugs, called *nucleoside analog reverse transcriptase inhibitors* (NRTIs), interrupt HIV's life cycle at an early stage. The spread of HIV in the body may be slowed and the onset of opportunistic infections may be delayed by NRTIs, but these drugs do not prevent HIV transmission to other individuals. This group includes zidovudine (Retrovir), formerly known as AZT, zalcitabine (Hivid), didanosine (Videx), stavudine (Zerit), lamivudine (Epivir), and abacavir (Ziagen). A combination of zidovudine and lamivudine (Combivir) is available. Zidovudine (Retrovir) may cause depletion of red or white blood cells. If this depletion is severe, the drug must be discontinued. Painful nerve damage and pancreatitis may be caused by didanosine (Videx).

Non-nucleoside reverse transcriptase inhibitors (NNRTIs) are available to be used only in combination with

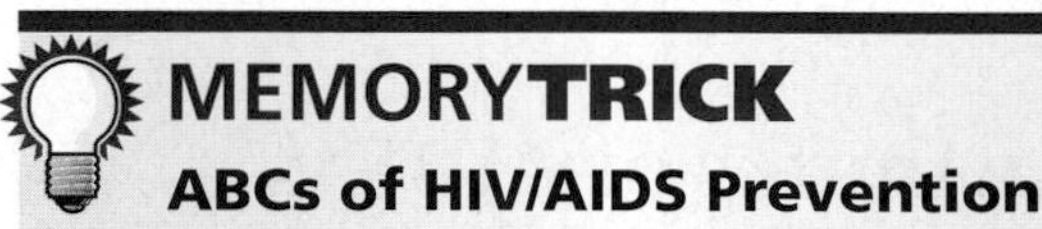

To protect oneself from acquiring HIV/AIDS, remember these **ABC**s:

A = Abstinence

B = Be Faithful

C = Condoms

(CDC, 2008)

Nursing diagnoses for the HIV-positive client with gastrointestinal disorders include the following: (Continued)

NURSING DIAGNOSES	PLANNING/OUTCOMES	NURSING INTERVENTIONS
		Offer commercially prepared nutritional supplements between meals. Weigh client daily. Administer supplemental vitamins and minerals as prescribed. Administer antiemetics and antidiarrheals as ordered. Teach client to keep a food diary and a log of exacerbation and remission of signs and symptoms.
Risk for Impaired Skin Integrity related to diarrhea, malnutrition, decreased mobility	The client will maintain skin integrity.	Monitor stool for presence of blood, fat, undigested food and stool cultures for evidence of new infections. Protect the perirectal area by keeping it clean and using compounds such as Aloe Vesta cream. Avoid prolonged pressure on bony prominences by a scheduled turning plan. If nonambulatory, provide client with a pressure relief mattress. Use soft sheets on the bed and avoid wrinkles. Teach client to use nondrying soaps and to pat skin dry.

Evaluation: Evaluate each outcome to determine how it has been met by the client.

ORAL OPPORTUNISTIC INFECTIONS

Candidiasis and leukoplakia are discussed following.

ORAL AND ESOPHAGEAL CANDIDIASIS

Oral candidiasis (thrush) is a fungal infection caused by *Candida albicans* (Figure 16-9), and usually only appears if CD4 levels fall below 300 (Mayo Clinic, 2007). Many clients complain of an unpleasant taste or mouth dryness. Other clinical signs and symptoms include creamy, white oral plaques and mucosal tenderness. When the white oral plaques are wiped off, they leave an erythematous or even bleeding mucosal lesions. Esophageal candidiasis, an AIDS-defining disease, causes dysphagia and painful swallowing.

These symptoms may interfere with the client's eating, nutrition, and weight. Diagnosis is established by the presence of the characteristic lesions in the oral cavity. Microscopic examination of oral or esophageal lesions reveals budding yeast cells.

Treatment for esophageal candidiasis is oral fluconazole (Diflucan). Oral candidiasis is treated with nystatin suspension (Mycostatin) and clotrimazole (Mycelex Troches). Another medication used to treat candidiasis is ketoconazole (Nizoral). Amphotericin B (Amphotericin B) is used to treat disseminated candida infection. The antiulcer drug sucralfate (Carafate) may be used as a slurry to relieve mouth pain before eating.

ORAL HAIRY LEUKOPLAKIA

Oral hairy leukoplakia (OHL) usually appears as a white patch on the lateral borders of the tongue as shown in Figure 16-10. It is caused by the Epstein-Barr virus. The lesions are rarely in other areas of the mouth and are different in appearance from candidiasis. The irregular surface of the lesion appears as projections that resemble hairs and cannot be scraped off. Diagnosis is made by visual inspection of the lesion. OHL is

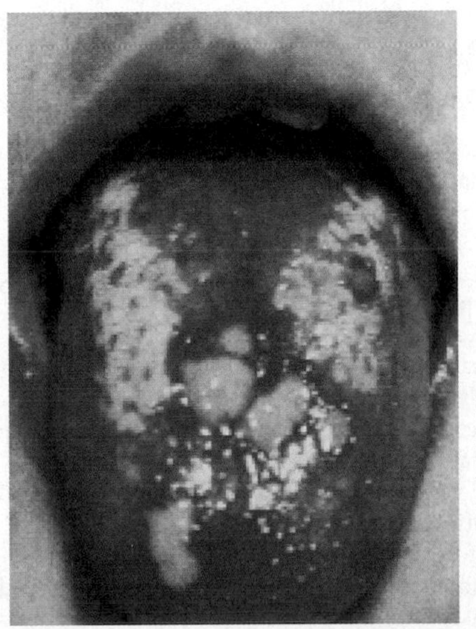

FIGURE 16-9 Oral Candidiasis (Thrush)

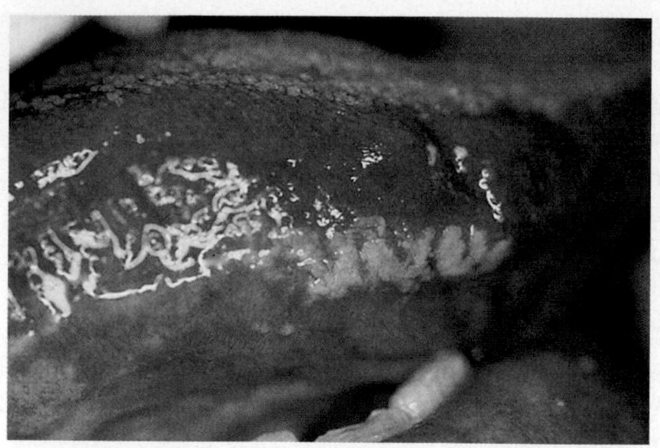

FIGURE 16-10 **Oral Hairy Leukoplakia** (*Courtesy of Dr. Joseph Konzelman, School of Dentistry, Medical College of Georgia.*)

not usually bothersome to the client and may regress spontaneously. No treatment is necessary for most cases of OHL; however, oral acyclovir (Zovirax) may be given to selected clients.

NURSING MANAGEMENT

Assess oral cavity frequently. Assist with oral hygiene before and after meals. Administer prescribed medications. Teach client to avoid mouthwashes containing alcohol or glycerine because they are very drying.

NURSING PROCESS

ASSESSMENT

Subjective Data

Assess the client's symptoms and oral hygiene habits. Ask about recent nutritional intake, use of alcohol and tobacco, and current medications.

Objective Data

Assess the client's lips, tongue, and buccal mucosal surfaces for lesions, white cheesy patches, and bleeding. Note any difficulty swallowing.

A nursing diagnosis for an HIV-positive client with oral manifestations is:

NURSING DIAGNOSES	PLANNING/OUTCOMES	NURSING INTERVENTIONS
*Impaired **O**ral Mucous Membrane* related to oral lesions	The client will be free from oral lesions.	Administer prescribed medications. Frequently assess the oral cavity. Provide oral hygiene with a small soft toothbrush before and after meals. Instruct client to avoid commercial mouthwashes containing alcohol or glycerine.

Evaluation: Evaluate each outcome to determine how it has been met by the client.

GYNECOLOGICAL OPPORTUNISTIC INFECTIONS

Gynecological infections discussed include vaginal candidiasis and cervical intraepithelial neoplasia.

VAGINAL CANDIDIASIS

Vaginal candidiasis is a fungal infection caused by *Candida albicans.* It is the most common initial infection occurring in HIV-infected women. Clinical manifestations include a white, clumped-appearing vaginal discharge, vaginal wall inflammation, and vaginal itching. Diagnosis is made by microscopic identification of yeast.

Most cases of vaginal candidiasis are treated with topical antifungal agents such as clotrimazole (Gyne-Lotrimin). For clients who do not respond to treatment with clotrimazole, ketoconazole (Nizoral) or fluconazole (Diflucan) is recommended.

CERVICAL INTRAEPITHELIAL NEOPLASIA

Women infected with HIV have a much higher incidence of cervical intraepithelial neoplasia (CIN) than women who are not infected. CIN and cancer of the cervix are considered to be on a continuum of abnormal cervical cells, ranging from mild abnormality (Grade I) to severe abnormality and cancer Grade III). CIN in HIV-infected women progresses more rapidly and is less responsive to standard treatments than in noninfected women. Factors related to increased risk of CIN in HIV-positive women include a decreased number of CD4 T-cells and infection with human papilloma virus (HPV). It is thought that HIV activates HPV, causing cellular abnormalities.

The early stages of CIN have no symptoms. Clinical manifestations of cervical cancer include painless postcoital bleeding and blood-tinged vaginal discharge. As CIN progresses, back pain, abdominal or pelvic pain, weight loss, anorexia, and leg edema caused by obstruction of lymph nodes may occur. Initial diagnosis is made by Pap smear to determine the presence of abnormal cells. Clients with abnormal Pap smears are referred for cervical biopsy and colposcopy.

Treatment for CIN includes laser therapy, conization, and hysterectomy. Treatment for invasive cervical cancer depends on the stage of the disease and may include chemotherapy, surgery, and radiation.

NURSING MANAGEMENT

Encourage the client to have a Pap test every 6 months, to keep vaginal area clean and dry, and to wear loose-fitting cotton underwear. Inquire about bleeding following sexual intercourse, pelvic and abdominal pain, and vaginal itching or discharge.

NURSING PROCESS

ASSESSMENT

Subjective Data

Assess the client's history of symptoms, and ask the client about bleeding after intercourse, abdominal and pelvic pain, and vaginal itching or discharge.

Objective Data

Assess vaginal discharge for white or blood-tinged secretions. Note weight loss and edema.

Nursing diagnoses for a female HIV-positive client with gynecological manifestations include the following:

NURSING DIAGNOSES	PLANNING/OUTCOMES	NURSING INTERVENTIONS
Impaired Tissue Integrity related to vaginal mucosal lesions	The client will be free of vaginal infections.	Teach the client to have Pap smears every 6 months. Assess the frequency and consistency of vaginal discharge. Teach client to keep the vaginal area clean and dry and to wear loose-fitting cotton underwear to prevent irritation.
Disturbed Body Image related to chronic vaginal infections or surgery, radiation, or removal of cervix	The client will verbalize feelings and concerns about body image.	Encourage client to verbalize feelings and concerns about body image. Refer client to a support group for women with HIV.

Evaluation: Evaluate each outcome to determine how it has been met by the client.

CENTRAL NERVOUS SYSTEM OPPORTUNISTIC INFECTIONS

Disorders covered include AIDS dementia complex, toxoplasmosis, and cryptococcosis.

AIDS DEMENTIA COMPLEX

The most common central nervous system complication in persons with AIDS is AIDS dementia complex (ADC). This disorder is chronic and progressive, with cognitive, motor, and behavioral dysfunction. ADC is caused by infection of glial cells in the brain with HIV. Signs and symptoms are sometimes vague during the initial stages of ADC. Early signs include poor concentration, forgetfulness, loss of balance, leg weakness, apathy, and social withdrawal. Clients with advanced ADC may exhibit psychotic behaviors and delirium and progress to a catatonic-like state with minimal responsiveness to the environment.

Diagnosis is made by neurological testing of cognitive, motor, and behavioral functioning. Other diagnostic tests include brain imaging to look for cerebral atrophy. Cerebrospinal fluid analysis can show elevated proteins and will exclude other pathogens. Clients treated with zidovudine (Retrovir) have shown a delay in disease progression in asymptomatic HIV-infected clients (FDA, 2003).

TOXOPLASMOSIS

Toxoplasmosis is caused by the protozoan *Toxoplasma gondii.* Cats and other animals serve as a reservoir for this organism. It is spread to humans by ingestion of oocytes found in contaminated water, soil, or food, especially raw or undercooked meat. After entering the body, *Toxoplasma gondii* reproduces and spreads via the blood or lymph system. A person with an intact immune system may have no symptoms or mild symptoms, and the organism may remain dormant for years. In the immunocompromised person, the infection may be reactivated (secondary) or occur with the ingestion of oocytes from contaminated sources. Clinical signs and symptoms may be vague and nonspecific, or range from a mild headache, fever, and lethargy to poor coordination, seizures, and coma. Diagnosis is made by identification of a lesion through brain imaging (computerized tomography or magnetic resonance imaging), presence of serum antibodies to *Toxoplasma gondii*, and recent onset of a neurologic abnormality.

The treatment of choice is oral pyrimethamine (Daraprim) and sulfadiazine (Microsulfon). Lifelong suppressive therapy of pyrimethamine plus sulfadiazine and leukovorin calcium (Wellcovorin) is needed.

CRYPTOCOCCOSIS

Cryptococcosis is a fungal infection caused by *Cryptococcus neoformans*. Cryptococcosis is one of the most life-threatening fungal infections in clients with AIDS (National Institutes of Health, 2008). The organism is acquired in the environment, usually from bird droppings. In the noncompromised host, the fungus is inhaled and contained in the lungs. In the immunocompromised host with AIDS, *Cryptococcus neoformans* can be disseminated, remain in the lungs, or infect the brain and meninges. Clinical manifestations include fever, headache, nausea and vomiting, dizziness, photophobia, mental status changes, seizures, and a stiff neck. Detection of cryptococcal antigen in cerebrospinal fluid, urine, or blood can be used for diagnosis. If untreated, this condition is fatal.

Treatment for acute cryptococcal infections includes intravenous amphotericin B (Fungizone Intravenous) to be given for at least 2 weeks, followed by fluconazole (Diflucan) for 10 to 12 weeks. Once treatment for acute infection is complete, lifelong suppressive therapy with oral fluconazole daily is recommended.

NURSING MANAGEMENT

Monitor client for forgetfulness, poor concentration, loss of balance, leg weakness, social withdrawal, apathy, stiff neck, seizures, nausea, and headache. Assess vital signs. Provide cues for orientation (e.g., calendar, clock) and a structured environment and activities for social interaction.

NURSING PROCESS

ASSESSMENT

Subjective Data

Ask the client about forgetfulness, missing appointments, ability to complete activities of daily living, and if there have been any recent falls or accidents. Ask the client's family and significant others about behavior changes such as social withdrawal or unusual behavior.

Objective Data

Assess the client for subtle mental status changes such as poor concentration and inability to remember instructions or previous conversations. Assess the client for motor impairment such as dropping things, poor coordination, or changes in writing ability. Assess the client's ability to remember usual medication schedule. Observe the environment for safety.

Nursing diagnoses for an HIV-positive client with central nervous system manifestations include the following:

NURSING DIAGNOSES	PLANNING/OUTCOMES	NURSING INTERVENTIONS
Disturbed Thought Processes related to mental status changes	The client will maintain cognitive functioning.	Assess client's mental and neurologic status and emotional, cognitive, and motor skills. Provide cues for orientation (clock, calendar). Monitor client for adherence to medical regimen.
Social Isolation related to alteration in mental status	The client will have contact and interact with significant others.	Encourage family and significant others to visit client. Provide structured activities and environment for social interaction. Encourage client to verbalize feelings and concerns.

Evaluation: Evaluate each outcome to determine how it has been met by the client.

OPPORTUNISTIC MALIGNANCIES

Kaposi's sarcoma and non-Hodgkin's lymphoma are discussed.

KAPOSI'S SARCOMA

Kaposi's sarcoma (KS) is a vascular malignancy that can occur any place in the body, including internal organs. The first lesions often appear subtly on the face or in the oral cavity. The more immunosuppressed the person is, the more aggressive the spread of KS. Clinical manifestations of KS are red to purple lesions, which are painless, nonblanching, and palpable (Figure 16-11). These lesions are sometimes mistaken for bruises. Edema in the face, penis, scrotum, and legs can occur as a result of blockages in the lymphatic system. KS can also be found in the GI tract and lungs. Diagnosis is made by tissue biopsy.

Treatment involves a variety of options depending on whether the lesions are local or systemic. Radiation therapy, intralesional therapy with interferon alpha 2a or 2b (Roferon A, Intron A) or vinblastine sulfate (Velban), laser therapy, and cryotherapy are used on single or isolated

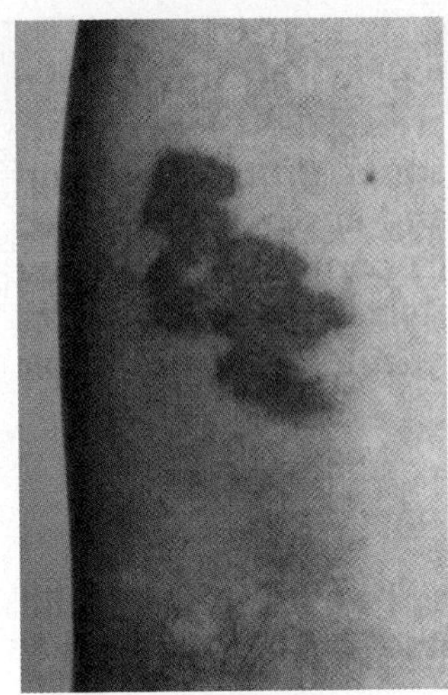

FIGURE 16-11 Kaposi's Sarcoma (*Courtesy of Daniel J. Barbaro, MD, Fort Worth, TX.*)

KS lesions. For clients with advanced widespread symptomatic disease, single or combination chemotherapeutic regimens include vinblastine sulfate (Velban), vincristine sulfate (Oncovin), etoposide (VePesid), bleomycin sulfate (Blenoxane), doxorubicin Hcl (Rubex), and mitoxantrone Hcl (Novantrone).

NON-HODGKIN'S LYMPHOMA

Lymphomas are malignant tumors of the immune system. B-cells are the origin of malignancy for most clients with AIDS-related non-Hodgkin's lymphoma (NHL). Clinical manifestations are nonspecific and may include fever, night sweats, and weight loss. Confusion, lethargy, and memory loss may be present in persons with CNS involvement.

Diagnosis of NHL is complicated because of the nonspecific symptoms. Examination of tissue is the recommended diagnostic procedure. There is no standard treatment of NHL. Individualized treatment may include a combination of chemotherapy, antiretroviral agents, prophylaxis against opportunistic infections, and colony-stimulating factors to enhance bone marrow production of blood cells; however, in many clients with advanced HIV disease, treatment of NHL is withheld because it is not tolerated well and may even lead to earlier death.

NURSING MANAGEMENT

Assess client for fever, night sweats, weight loss, confusion, lethargy, memory loss, and ability to perform ADLs. Emphasize no scratching of skin lesions, not using drying soaps, and making sure clothing and linens are thoroughly rinsed of detergent. Encourage significant others to participate in the client's care. Provide access to clergy, social worker, or HIV counselor.

NURSING PROCESS

ASSESSMENT

Subjective Data

Ask the client about frequency, onset, and persistence of current symptoms. Note the effect of current symptoms on ability to perform activities of daily living and relationships with others, as well as the effect of treatment plan on quality of life.

Objective Data

Assess skin lesions. Document increased frequency, intensity, or recurrence of nonspecific symptoms, including fever, night sweats, and weight loss.

Nursing diagnoses for an HIV-positive client with a malignancy include the following:

NURSING DIAGNOSES	PLANNING/OUTCOMES	NURSING INTERVENTIONS
Risk for Impaired Skin Integrity related to lesions or treatment	The client will maintain skin integrity.	Teach client to avoid scratching skin lesions, to avoid drying soaps, and to make sure clothing and linen have been thoroughly rinsed of detergent.
Social Isolation related to change in appearance	The client will maintain usual social interactions and identify factors that enhance quality of life.	Facilitate the client's interaction with others. Keep client and significant others aware of treatment plan. Encourage significant others to participate in the care of the client. Encourage physical closeness between the client and significant others. Provide client with access to clergy, social worker, or HIV counselor. Encourage the client to join a support group or obtain peer support. Assist client in identifying positive coping strategies.

Evaluation: Evaluate each outcome to determine how it has been met by the client.

CASE STUDY

J.H., a 37-year-old man, suspects that he is HIV positive. He enters the medical unit with chronic symptoms such as fever, night sweats, diarrhea, weight loss, shortness of breath, and a nonproductive cough. On the initial assessment, he is alert and oriented, color is pale, temperature 100.6°F, pulse 92, respirations 36, and blood pressure 140/70. He has generalized lymphadenopathy. His height is 5'11", and his weight is 125 pounds. J.H. states that he is not currently taking any medications, although he is "familiar" with the drug zidovudine (Retrovir).

The following questions will guide your development of a nursing care plan for the case study.

1. List symptoms/clinical manifestations, other than J.H., that a client may experience when HIV-positive.
2. List two reasons zidovudine (Retrovir) may be initiated for J.H.
3. List two diagnostic tests that will confirm the diagnosis of HIV.
4. List subjective and objective data the nurse would want to obtain about J.H.
5. Write three individual nursing diagnoses and goals for J.H.
6. List pertinent nursing actions the nurse would perform in caring for J.H. related to:
   - hydration
   - fatigue
   - nutrition
   - oxygenation
   - medications
7. List resources that could assist J.H. with his diagnosis.
8. List teaching J.H. will need before leaving the medical unit.

SUMMARY

- The immune system identifies substances as self or nonself and protects the body by neutralizing or destroying foreign organisms.
- Immunity to a disease is either natural or acquired.
- Age, sex, nutritional status, medications, and stress influence the immune response.
- Clients receiving blood transfusions must be carefully monitored, especially during the first half-hour, for signs of a reaction.
- Anaphylactic reactions, which may occur as a result of exposure to foods, medications, blood, or insect bites, can potentially be life-threatening.
- Organ transplant clients must understand the implications of taking immunosuppressive medications.
- Clients with rheumatoid arthritis must be taught methods of adapting to the effects of synovial joint inflammation, immobility, and deformity.
- Systemic lupus erythematosus affects multiple body systems.
- Clients with myasthenia gravis experience extreme muscle weakness and fatigue and must be carefully monitored for signs of respiratory distress, and myasthenic or cholinergic crisis.
- Diagnosis of HIV/AIDS is made by the ELISA and Western blot test. These tests determine the presence of antibodies to HIV, not the virus itself.
- *Pneumocystis carinii* pneumonia is the most common opportunistic infection associated with HIV.
- Oral candidiasis can be painful and interfere with the client's nutritional status.
- AIDS dementia complex is a progressive disorder with cognitive, motor, and behavioral dysfunction.

REVIEW QUESTIONS

1. A client has just been diagnosed with syphilis and has an order for 1,000,000 units of penicillin IM. She has no history of allergies to medications. She has never had penicillin. When giving her the injection in the right upper outer quadrant of her buttocks, you note a tattoo. Several minutes after receiving the injection, she tells you she feels anxious and weak. You note she is diaphoretic, scratching her forearm, and is breathing faster than normal. Based upon this assessment data, you would conclude:
   1. she is embarrassed because you saw her tattoo.
   2. she is probably anxious since you know she has a sexually transmitted disease.

3. her syphilis is getting worse.
4. these are early signs of an anaphylactic reaction.

2. Which of the following statements shows that the client understands a diagnosis of HIV positive?
   1. "Being HIV positive means that I have AIDs."
   2. "Since I am only HIV positive, I cannot infect others."
   3. "Because I am HIV positive, I have the virus that causes AIDS."
   4. "I became infected by donating blood."
3. The nurse is caring for a client who is experiencing diarrhea and weight loss. Which of the following nursing interventions is appropriate for him?
   1. Encourage fluids with meals.
   2. Substitute a milk shake for lunch.
   3. Offer small, frequent meals.
   4. Suggest he eat more sweets.
4. The nurse is caring for a client who asks when zidovudine (Retrovir) is normally started. Which of the following would be the nurse's correct response?
   1. When the client becomes symptomatic.
   2. When CD4 level reaches 500/mm3.
   3. After the client's first opportunistic infection.
   4. As soon as the client is diagnosed as HIV positive.
5. The nurse is discussing transmission of HIV with a client. Which of the following statements indicates that the client needs more education?
   1. "I should not share needles with anyone."
   2. "I can spread the virus through sexual contact."
   3. "I can no longer donate blood."
   4. "I should not hug or kiss anyone."
6. The nurse enters the room of an HIV client who cannot remember where he is. What is the first priority for the nurse to implement?
   1. Call the physician.
   2. Perform a neurological assessment on the client.
   3. Tell the client where he is.
   4. Give the client his medication that is due at this time.
7. The client tells the nurse, "I am going to quit taking my HIV medication because I have no symptoms and the medication makes me very nauseated" What would be the best response from the nurse?
   1. "I agree with you and I will not give you your medication."
   2. "Let me ask the physician first to see what he thinks."
   3. "Taking the medication with food will help with the nausea."
   4. "I am going to continue to give you your medications, it is up to you if you decide to take the medications or not."
8. A client diagnosed with AIDS spends most of his day sitting at a window. The nurse wants the client to implement a physical activity plan. The nurse knows that the purpose of this plan is to:
   1. Help the client discuss the problems creating his depression.
   2. Help reduce the client's risk for obesity.
   3. Encourage socialization.
   4. Increase the client's appetite.
9. A client is admitted to the hospital with a diagnosis of AIDS and is being treated for Kaposi's sarcoma. Which client would be an appropriate roommate for this client?
   1. A client who just had abdominal surgery.
   2. A client that has pneumonia.
   3. A client that has lymphoma.
   4. A client that has Kaposi's sarcoma.
10. Which client is at highest risk for developing an infection?
   1. A 16-year-old student who plays football on the high school team.
   2. A 34-year-old pregnant school teacher.
   3. A 45-year-old homemaker who smokes two packages of cigarettes daily.
   4. A 73-year-old retired banker who lives in an assisted living facility.

REFERENCES/SUGGESTED READINGS

American Academy of Allergy Asthma & Immunology (AAAAI). (2007). Tips to remember: latex allergy. [Online] Retrieved April 26, 2009, from www.aaaai.org/patients/publicedmat/tips/latexallergy.stm

American Latex Allergy Association. (2009). Latex allergy statistics. [Online] Retrieved April 26, 2009, from www.latexallergyresources.org/topics/LatexAllergyStatistics.cfm

Arthritis Foundation. (2009a). Arthritis today: a vaccine for rheumatoid arthritis. [Online] Retrieved April 26, 2009, from www.arthritistoday.org/conditions/rheumatoid-arthritis/news-and-research/rheumatoid-arthritis-vaccine.php

Arthritis Foundation. (2009b). Arthritis today: antimalarial drug may help rheumatoid arthritis and diabetes. [Online] Retrieved April 26, 2009, from www.arthritistoday.org/conditions/rheumatoid-arthritis/news-and-research/antimalarial-drug.php

Arthritis Foundation. (2009c). Arthritis today: how rheumatoid arthritis is diagnosed. [Online] Retrieved April 26, 2009, from www.arthritistoday.org/conditions/rheumatoid-arthritis/all-about-ra/diagnosing-ra.php

Arthritis Foundation. (2009d). Arthritis today: how to treat rheumatoid arthritis. [Online] Retrieved April 26, 2009, from www.arthritistoday.org/conditions/rheumatoid-arthritis/ra-treatment/how-to-treat-ra.php

Arthritis Foundation. (2009e). Rheumatoid arthritis what is it? [Online] Retrieved April 27, 2009, from www.arthritis.org/disease-center.php?disease_id=31

Arthritis Foundation. (2009f). Rheumatoid arthritis: who is at risk? [Online] Retrieved April 27, 2009, from www.arthritis.org/disease-center.php?disease_id=31&df=whos_at_risk

Arnold, L. (2001). Living with AIDS. *Nursing2001*, 31(10), 53.

Barroso, J. (2002). HIV-related fatigue. *AJN*, 102(5), 83–86.

Bradley-Springer, L. (2001). HIV prevention: what works? *AJN*, 101(6), 45–50.

Bulechek, G., Butcher, H., McCloskey, J., & Dochterman, J., eds. (2008). *Nursing Interventions Classification (NIC)* (5th ed.). St. Louis, MO: Mosby/Elsevier.

Bursaw, M., Keenan, K., & Ehrhart, M. (2001). HIV update. *Nursing2001*, 31(2), 62–63.

Carroll, P. (2001). Anaphylaxis. *RN*, 64(12), 45–49.

Centers for Disease Control and Prevention. (2006). Revised recommendations for HIV testing of adults, adolescents, and pregnant women in health-care settings. *Morbidity and Mortality Weekly Report*, 55(RR14), 1–17.

Centers for Disease Control and Prevention. (2008). Basic information. [Online] Retrieved May 3, 2009, from www.cdc.gov/hiv/topics/basic/index.htm

Centers for Disease Control and Prevention. (2008a). Food allergy among U.S. children: trends in prevalence and hospitalizations. [Online] Retrieved April 26, 2009, from www.cdc.gov/nchs/data/databriefs/db10.htm

Centers for Disease Control and Prevention. (2008b). HIV/AIDS among American Indians and Alaska Natives. [Online] Retrieved April 29, 2009, from www.cdc.gov/hiv/resources/factsheets/aian.htm

Centers for Disease Control and Prevention. (2008c). HIV/AIDS among women. [Online] Retrieved April 29, 2009, from www.cdc.gov/hiv/topics/women/resources/factsheets/women.htm

Centers for Disease Control and Prevention. (2008d). HIV prevalence estimates-United States, 2006. *Morbidity and Mortality Weekly Report*, 57(39), 1073–1076.

Centers for Disease Control and Prevention. (2008e). National ambulatory medical care survey: 2006 summary. [Online] Retrieved April 26, 2009, from www.cdc.gov/nchs/data/nhsr/nhsr003.pdf

Centers for Disease Control and Prevention. (2009). Basic statistics. [Online] Retrieved May 3, 2009, from www.cdc.gov/hiv/topics/surveillance/basic.htm#aidsage

Centers for Disease Control and Prevention. (2009a). Guidelines for prevention and treatment of opportunistic infections in HIV-infected adults and adolescents. *Morbidity and Mortality Weekly Report*, 58(RR-4), 1–207.

Centers for Disease Control and Prevention. (2009b). HIV/AIDS surveillance by race/ethnicity (through 2007). [Online] Retrieved April 27, 2009, from www.cdc.gov/hiv/topics/surveillance/resources/slides/race-ethnicity/index.htm

Cichocki, M. (2007). HIV and the older adult—a growing population. [Online] Retrieved May 17, 2008 from http://aids.about.com/cs/aidsfactsheets/a/seniors.htm

Cohen, S. (2001). Myths & facts ... about latex allergy. *Nursing2001*, 31(2), 76.

Coyne, P., Lyne, M., & Watson, A. (2002). Symptom management in people with AIDS. *AJN*, 102(9), 48–55.

Daniels, R., Nosek, L., & Nicoll, L. (2007). Contemporary medical-surgical nursing. Clifton Park, NY: Delmar Cengage Learning.

Daniels, R. (2010). *Delmar's guide to laboratory and diagnostic tests* (2nd ed.). Clifton Park, NY: Delmar Cengage Learning.

D'Arcy, Y. (2002). How to treat arthritis pain. *Nursing 2002*, 32(7), 30–31.

Daughtry, L., Bankston, J., & Deshotels, J. (2002). HIV meds: keeping trouble at bay. *RN*, 65(2), 31–35.

Department of Health and Human Services. (2007). OPTN/SRTR annual report: transplant data 1997-2006, chapter 1, trends in organ donation and transplantation in the United States, 1997-2006. [Online] Retrieved April 26, 2009, from www.ustransplant.org/annual_reports/current/chapter_i_AR_cd.htm?cp=2

Estes, M. (2010). *Health assessment & physical examination* (4nd ed.). Clifton Park, NY: Delmar Cengage Learning.

Food and Drug Administration (FDA). (2003). Retrovir. [Online] Retrieved May 3, 2009, from www.fda.gov/medwatch/SAFETY/2003/03Oct_PI/Retrovir_PI.pdf

Food and Drug Administration (FDA). (2004). OraQuick ADVANCE Rapid HIV-1/2 antibody test. [Online] Retrieved May 3, 2009, from www.fda.gov/cber/pma/p01004716.htm

Golden, D. (2007). Insect sting anaphylaxis. [Online] Retrieved April 26, 2009, from www.pubmedcentral.nih.gov/articlerender.fcgi?artid=1961691.

Goldrick, B. (2005). Emerging infections: infection in the older adult. *American Journal of Nursing*, *105*(6), 31–34.

Halzemer, W. (2002). HIV and AIDS: the symptom experience. *AJN*, 102(4), 48–52.

Jones, S. (2001). Taking HAART: How to support patients with HIV/AIDS. *Nursing2001*, 31(2), 36–41.

Jurewicz, M. (2000). Anaphylaxis: When the body overreacts. *Nursing2000*, 30(7), 58.

Lenehan, G. (2002). Latex allergy: Separating fact from fiction. *Nursing2002*, *32*(3), 58–63.

Lenehan, G. (2003). Latex allergy. *Nursing2003*, 33(6), 54–55.

Litton, K. (2003). Defenses gone awry: lupus. *RN*, 66(3), 53–59.

Lupus Foundation of America (LFA). (2009a). How lupus affects the body. [Online] Retrieved April 27, 2009, from www.lupus.org/webmodules/webarticlesnet/templates/new_learnaffects.aspx?articleid=2268&zoneid=526

Lupus Foundation of America (LFA). (2009b). Living with lupus. [Online] Retrieved April 27, 2009, from www.lupus.org/webmodules/webarticlesnet/templates/new_learnliving.aspx?articleid=2252&zoneid=527

Lupus Foundation of America (LFA). (2009c). Medications to treat lupus symptoms. [Online] Retrieved April 27, 2009, from www.lupus.org/webmodules/webarticlesnet/templates/new_learntreating.aspx?articleid=2246&zoneid=525

Lupus Foundation of America (LFA). (2009d). What is lupus. [Online] Retrieved April 27, 2009, from www.lupus.org/webmodules/webarticlesnet/templates/new_learnunderstanding.aspx?articleid=2232&zoneid=523

Mayo Clinic. (2007). Oral thrush. [Online] Retrieved May 3, 2009, from www.mayoclinic.com/print/oral-thrush/DS00408/DSECTION=all&METHOD=print

Moorhead, S., Johnson, M., Maas, M., & Swanson, E. (2007). *Nursing Outcomes Classification (NOC)* (4th ed.). St. Louis, MO: Mosby.

National Institute for Occupational Safety and Health (2009). Latex allergy a prevention guide. [Online] Retrieved April 26, 2009, from www.cdc.gov/niosh/98-113.html

National Institute of Allergy and Infectious Diseases (NIAID). (2003). Current trends in allergic reactions: a multidisciplinary approach to patient management. [Online] Retrieved April 26, 2009, from www3.niaid.nih.gov/about/organization/dait/PDF/Allergic_Reactions.pdf

National Institute of Allergy and Infectious Diseases (NIAID). (2008a). Food allergy: living with food allergies. [Online] Retrieved April 26, 2009, from www3.niaid.nih.gov/topics/foodAllergy/living.htm

National Institute of Allergy and Infectious Diseases (NIAID). (2008b). Is it a cold or an allergy? [Online] Retrieved April 26, 2009, from www3.niaid.nih.gov/topics/allergicDiseases/PDF/ColdAllergy.pdf

National Institutes of Health. (2008). Cryptococcosis. [Online] Retrieved May 3, 2009, from www.nlm.nih.gov/medlineplus/ency/article/001328.htm

Putnam, J., & May, K. (2001). Relief for patients with severe allergies. *RN*, 64(6), 26–30.

Spratto, G., & Woods, A. (2009). *2009 PDR nurses' drug handbook.* Clifton Park, NY: Delmar Cengage Learning.

Trzcianowska, H., & Mortensen, E. (2001). HIV and AIDS: Separating fact from fiction. AJN, 101(6), 53–59.

Veronesi, J. (2003). Rheumatoid arthritis. *RN, 66*(8), 46–52.

World Health Organization (2008a). Global summary of the AIDS epidemic, December 2007. [Online] Retrieved April 27, 2009, from www.who.int/hiv/data/2008_global_summary_AIDS_ep.png

World Health Organization (2008b). HIV/AIDS. [Online] Retrieved April 27, 2009, from www.who.int/features/qa/71/en/index.html

World Health Organization (2009). TB/HIV facts 2009. [Online] Retrieved April 27, 2009, from www.who.int/tb/challenges/hiv/factsheet_hivtb_2009.pdf

Yee, C. (2002). Getting a grip on myasthenia gravis. *Nursing2002,* 32(1), 32hn1–32hn4.

RESOURCES

The American Academy of Allergy, Asthma, and Immunology, http:// www.aaaai.org

American Association of Blood Banks, http:// www.aabb.org

American College of Rheumatology, http:// www.rheumatology.org

American Latex Allergy Association, http:// www.latexallergyresources.org

Arthritis Foundation, http:// www.arthritis.org

Association of Nurses in AIDS Care, http:// www.anacnet.org

Asthma and Allergy Foundation of America, http:// www.aafa.org

CDC National STD & AIDS Hotlines, 800-232-4636

Lupus Foundation of America, Inc., http:// www.lupus.org

Myasthenia Gravis Foundation of America, http:// www.myasthenia.org

National Institute of Arthritis and Musculoskeletal and Skin Diseases (NIAMS), http:// www.niams.nih.gov

United Network for Organ Sharing, http:// www.unos.org

UNIT 7 Nursing Care of the Client: Physical and Mental Integrity

CHAPTER 17
Mental Illness

MAKING THE CONNECTION

Refer to the following chapters to increase your understanding of mental illness:

Adult Health Nursing

- ***Immune System***
- ***Substance Abuse***
- ***The Older Adult***

LEARNING OBJECTIVES

Upon completion of this chapter, you should be able to:

- Define key terms.
- Identify and describe the components of a therapeutic nurse–client relationship.
- Cite nursing interventions for working with clients who are angry, aggressive, homicidal, and/or suicidal.
- Detail nursing interventions for working with clients who are experiencing anxiety.
- Identify and explain the potential side effects associated with antianxiety medications.
- Recount nursing interventions for working with clients who are depressed.
- Identify and explain the potential side effects associated with antidepressant medications.
- Detail nursing interventions for working with clients who have schizophrenia.
- Identify and explain the potential side effects associated with antipsychotic medications.
- Detail nursing interventions for working with clients who have bipolar disorder.
- Identify and explain the potential side effects associated with mood stabilizers.
- Cite nursing interventions for working with clients who have attention-deficit/hyperactivity disorder.
- Recount nursing interventions for working with clients who have been neglected or abused or who have been exposed to domestic violence.
- Discuss nursing interventions for working with clients who have an eating disorder.

KEY TERMS

abuse
actively suicidal
affect
anger-control assistance
anxiety
anxiolytic
auditory hallucination
brief dynamic therapy
cognitive-behavior therapy
command hallucination
crisis
cycling
delusion
depression
domestic violence
electroconvulsive therapy (ECT)
empathy
euphoric
flashback
genuineness
hallucination
hypervigilant
hypomania
mania
mental disorder
mental illness
mood
neglect
paradoxical reaction
physically aggressive
pressured speech
psychoanalysis
psychosis
psychotherapy
rapport
respect
seclusion
serum lithium level
startle response
suicidal ideation
tolerance
trust
verbally aggressive
visual hallucination
word salad

INTRODUCTION

Because they will encounter clients who are emotionally disturbed and/or mentally ill, it is imperative that nurses understand and feel comfortable working with such individuals—not just on psychiatric units, but in all types of circumstances and settings. This chapter is designed to give LP/VNs a beginning knowledge base regarding mental health and illness and to better prepare them for working with individuals who are in a state of crisis or who have emotional needs and/or psychiatric problems.

As the nurse becomes more knowledgeable about mental illness, opportunities arise to increase self-awareness and to examine any personal experiences, preconceived ideas, or prejudices that might negatively affect the nurse's ability to work effectively with clients. For example, the nurse who has unresolved issues regarding sexuality or becomes embarrassed when discussing sexuality will probably be uncomfortable talking about the potential problems in sexual functioning secondary to antidepressant therapy. Examining personal ideas and prejudices before working with clients will facilitate a positive nurse–client relationship.

MENTAL HEALTH AND ILLNESS

In general, people are considered mentally healthy when they possess knowledge of themselves; meet their basic needs; assume responsibility for their behavior; have learned to integrate thoughts, feelings, and actions; can successfully resolve conflicts; maintain relationships; communicate directly with others; respect others; and adapt to change. **Mental illness** occurs when an individual is not able to view self clearly or has a distorted view of self; is unable to maintain satisfying personal relationships; and is unable to adapt to the environment (Frisch & Frisch, 2010). The American Psychiatric Association defines **mental disorder** as "clinically significant behavior or psychological syndrome or pattern that occurs in an individual and is associated with present distress (i.e., negative response to stimuli that are perceived as threatening) or disability (i.e., impairment in one or more important areas of functioning) or with a significantly increased risk of suffering, death, pain, disability, or an important loss of freedom."

One of the ways to conceptualize psychiatric disorders is to think of a continuum, with mental health being situated at one end and mental illness at the other (Figure 17-1). Between these two extremes lie a variety of psychiatric disorders ranging in nature from mild to severe. The fourth edition of the *Diagnostic and Statistical Manual of Mental Disorders* (better known as the DSM-IV) (American Psychiatric Association [APA], 2000) is the reference tool used to identify and establish psychiatric diagnoses. The psychiatrist is the individual most often involved in this process, although other mental health care practitioners may give input and make recommendations for diagnoses.

One of the primary roles of the nurse in working with clients who have mental illness is that of teaching. The nurse is responsible not only for teaching clients about their illnesses, including the probable courses of their given disorders, but also for adequately preparing and educating the client's family. The nurse is usually the first individual to have contact with the family and is most often the one with whom family members maintain consistent contact. Because of the highly personal and sensitive nature of mental disorders, the concept of confidentiality, the nondisclosure of the identity of or personal information about an individual, is vitally important in psychiatric nursing.

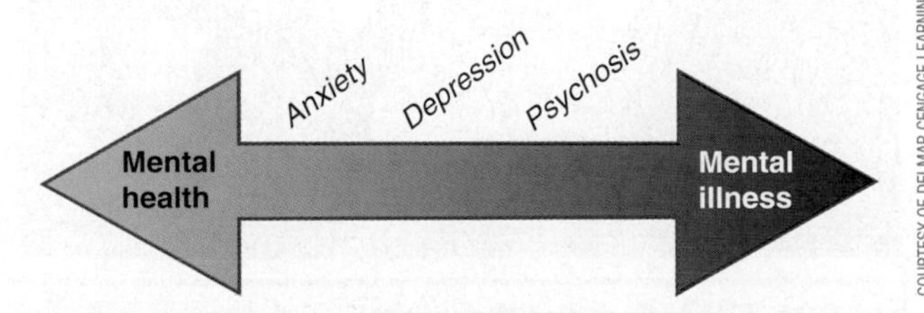

FIGURE 17-1 Mental Health Continuum

RELATIONSHIP DEVELOPMENT

Psychiatric nursing differs from some of the other fields of nursing in that the primary skill the nurse employs is what is referred to as "the therapeutic use of self." Many theorists such as Rogers and Peplau have been instrumental in identifying and exploring the factors that significantly influence the development of therapeutic relationships. Townsend (2008) identifies five components necessary to the development of a therapeutic working relationship and of particular importance in the therapeutic nurse–client relationship. These five components are trust, rapport, respect, genuineness, and empathy.

TRUST

Trust is the ability to rely on an individual's character and ability. Trust must be present for help to be given and received. A therapeutic relationship is firmly rooted in trust. Three major activities facilitate the development of trust: consistency, respect, and honesty. Consistency includes following through on plans, adhering to the schedule, being straightforward with no hidden motives, and seeking extra time for client interaction. Respect includes addressing clients the way they wish to be addressed (e.g., Mr., Mrs., Ms., first name), listening to the clients, and providing clear explanations. Honesty includes keeping promises and maintaining confidentiality. Being consistently trustworthy is an expression of the nurse's personal integrity and builds the foundation for nursing effectiveness (Figure 17-2).

Many clients with emotional and/or psychiatric problems have great difficulty trusting and having confidence that others will be good to their word. They may have been lied to or hurt in the past, and this makes it difficult for them to trust again, even with health care professionals who are trying to help them. It is very important, therefore, that the nurse fulfill any promise made to the client.

RAPPORT

Rapport is a bond or connection between two people that is based on mutual trust. Such a bond does not just happen spontaneously; it is planned by the nurse, who purposefully implements behaviors that promote trust. The nurse sets the tone of the relationship by creating an atmosphere wherein the client feels free to express feelings. When seeking to develop trust, the nurse acts in a manner that indicates recognition of the client as a unique individual and reinforces that individuality. Such actions, which serve to humanize the client, are therapeutic. To establish rapport, the nurse must show that the client is important. Actions are implemented to boost the level of the client's self-esteem. Nonverbal interventions are of utmost importance in helping establish rapport. Interacting with family and significant others is also helpful in establishing rapport with the client. Recognizing the importance of the family and its influence on the healing process allows the nurse to bond with those who will encourage and support the client during recovery.

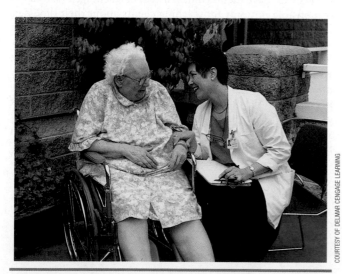

COURTESY OF DELMAR CENGAGE LEARNING

FIGURE 17-2 Spending time with the client one-to-one helps promote a trusting relationship.

RESPECT

Respect is the acceptance of an individual as is, in a nonjudgmental manner. The concept of respect is an integral component of the nurse–client relationship. Respect means caring for clients whose vvalue system may differ greatly from that of the nurse. To show respect, the nurse must not react with shock, surprise, or disapproval toward a client's lifestyle, dress, or behaviors. The nurse respects the client's choices and actions yet sets limits on unhealthy or undesirable behavior.

GENUINENESS

Genuineness (sincerity) is an attribute easily perceived by the client and can be the most significant aspect of the nurse–client relationship. Nurses are often concerned about whether they will say the right thing to a client; though saying the right thing is important, more important is that the nurse be honest and genuine in communications with the client.

EMPATHY

Empathy (the ability to perceive and relate to another's personal experience) is an important quality necessary to successful nurse–client interactions. The empathic nurse understands that the client's perception of the situation is real to him. By perceiving the client's understanding of her own needs, the nurse is better able to assist the client in determining what will work best. Empathy enables the nurse to assist the client to become a fully participating partner in treatment, rather than a passive recipient of care. Through empathy, the nurse validates the experiences of the client (Figure 17-3).

THE CLIENT EXPERIENCING A CRISIS

In psychological terms, a **crisis** is a stressor that forces an individual to respond and/or adapt in some way. Emotions may intensify during a crisis situation or serious illness, and any situation or illness can potentially become a crisis if the stressors are severe enough. The understanding of crisis is particularly important in psychiatric and mental health nursing. A crisis taxes the individual's coping resources, and each person responds differently to seemingly identical situations. Crisis requires that an individual call on all of her personal skills as well as on the outside social and familial supports that she has built through her life (Frisch & Frisch, 2010). Each individual has personality strengths, interpersonal networks, and socioeconomic resources that offer some protection against the threat of crisis. When any (or all) of these protections are weak, however, a person's

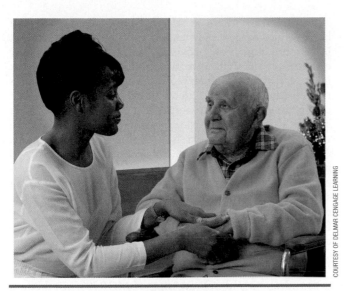

FIGURE 17-3 Through empathic listening, the nurse can reach an understanding of the client's experience and help the client see the positive aspects of the experience.

response to crisis may be dysfunctional, and the result may be one or more symptoms of mental illness. Although theories differ in their definitions of crisis and stress, it is generally accepted that most psychiatric problems result from or are strongly influenced by the interaction of stress and overwhelmed coping mechanisms (Frisch & Frisch, 2010). The client experiencing crisis may be anxious, angry, aggressive, homicidal, suicidal, psychotic, or any combination of these.

ANXIETY

Anxiety is a state wherein a person feels a strong sense of dread frequently accompanied by physical symptoms of increased heart and respiratory rates and elevated blood pressure in the absence of a specific source or reason for these emotions or responses. Nurses frequently encounter clients and family members who are anxious because of alterations in or threats to health and physical well-being. Peplau (1963) identifies four escalating stages of anxiety beginning with mild anxiety, moving to moderate anxiety, followed by severe anxiety, and, finally, to the stage of panic, if not effectively treated. Intervention can occur at any point along the continuum, preferably before the stages of severe anxiety or panic are reached.

MILD ANXIETY

The mildly anxious client is beginning to experience some of the signs and symptoms of anxiety, such as irritability and restlessness; however, the person is still able to concentrate and focus on the task at hand. In fact, *mild* anxiety can actually benefit an individual as far as enhancing performance ability (Townsend, 2008).

MODERATE ANXIETY

The individual with moderate anxiety experiences additional physiologic and cognitive symptoms. Blood pressure, pulse, and respirations increase, and the client becomes diaphoretic. The moderately anxious individual begins to have difficulty concentrating or learning new material. This is important to recognize before teaching a client about a medication or test, or performing a procedure. Before teaching can be effective, the client must be assisted in lowering the level of anxiety (Townsend, 2008).

SEVERE ANXIETY

Severely anxious clients are significantly impaired in several areas. Their ability to cognitively process material may drastically diminish, they may experience tunnel vision, their focus may become very limited, and the physiologic symptoms of anxiety become much more pronounced. Clients at this high level of anxiety are often very fearful and may be irrational in their thought processes (Townsend, 2008).

PANIC

The individual experiencing panic may begin to manifest symptoms of **psychosis** (losing touch with reality), such as **delusions** (false beliefs that misrepresent reality) and/or **hallucinations** (perceptions that something is present when it is not, e.g., hearing voices that are not really there). The individual with this level of anxiety requires constant reassurance and continuous assessment for suicide risk and maladaptive coping behaviors (Antai-Otong, 2008).

ANXIETY DISORDERS

Some of the most common psychiatric diagnoses related to anxiety are Generalized Anxiety Disorder, Panic Disorder, Obsessive-Compulsive Disorder, and Post-Traumatic Stress Disorder. It is estimated that 40 million adult Americans have an anxiety disorder (Anxiety Disorders Association of America [ADAA], 2009a).

GENERALIZED ANXIETY DISORDER

The client with Generalized Anxiety Disorder (GAD) exhibits symptoms of excessive anxiety, chronic worry, or dread. Clients usually realize that their symptoms are out of proportion to any real threat. The symptoms include three or more of the following: restlessness, easy fatigue, difficulty concentrating, irritability, trembling, muscle tension, abdominal upsets, and sleep disturbance. For anxiety to be termed excessive, clients must experience symptoms frequently over a period of 6 months or more (ADAA, 2009b).

PANIC DISORDER

Panic Disorder is diagnosed when the client experiences at least two panic attacks followed by at least 1 month's concern about having another panic attack (ADAA, 2009d). These attacks begin abruptly and peak within 10 minutes and are characterized by a set of any four of the following symptoms: palpitations or rapid heart rate, sweating, trembling, shortness of breath, sensation of choking, chest pain, nausea, dizziness, fear of losing control, fear of dying, numbness or tingling, chills or hot flushes, and some sense of altered reality. The client has a strong desire to run away or escape from the situation that triggered the attack. In some individuals, the attack is brought about by specific stimuli or a particular setting, for example the dentist's office. In others, the attacks come on "out of the blue."

OBSESSIVE-COMPULSIVE DISORDER

In Obsessive-Compulsive Disorder (OCD), the individual has persistent, recurring thoughts or impulses (obsessions) that are intrusive or inappropriate, causing anxiety or fears leading the individual to perform repetitive behaviors or rituals (compulsions) to neutralize the anxiety caused by the obsession. The obsessions and/or compulsions may take up at least several hours a day and interfere with the individual's normal routine, occupation, social activities, or relationships (ADAA, 2009c).

POST-TRAUMATIC STRESS DISORDER

Clients suffering from Post-Traumatic Stress Disorder (PTSD) have experienced a serious trauma. Being severely beaten or emotionally, physically, or sexually abused or living through or witnessing a catastrophic event or natural disaster such as a flood, earthquake, hurricane, war, or plane crash might lead to PTSD. The response to the trauma must have been one of fear or helplessness, and the event is persistently reexperienced through recurrent recollections, dreams, or hallucinatory-like flashbacks. Individuals with this disorder have symptoms for more than 1 month and exhibit impairment of social functioning, anxiety symptoms, avoidance of stimuli associated with the trauma, and a general numbness. More than 7.7 million Americans are diagnosed with PTSD (ADAA, 2009e).

MEDICAL–SURGICAL MANAGEMENT

Medical

Psychotherapy (the treatment of mental and emotional disorders through psychological rather than physical methods) continues to be widely used in the treatment of anxiety disorders. Psychotherapy can be viewed as falling into two general categories: those therapies based on helping individuals achieve insight into *why* they feel anxiety and those that emphasize behavioral means of controlling the anxiety.

Psychotherapy based on insight into symptoms may sometimes be valuable, especially for highly motivated individuals whose symptoms are not disabling. **Psychoanalysis** (therapy focused on uncovering unconscious memories and processes) is among the best known of the insight therapies and has been widely employed to assist persons with anxiety.

In contrast, there is strong empirical evidence that behaviorally based treatments are effective in treating at least some anxiety disorders. Cognitive-behavior therapy often results in significant benefit for persons experiencing panic attacks. **Cognitive-behavior therapy** assumes that clients can learn to identify the common stimuli that create their anxiety, develop plans to respond to those stimuli with nonanxious responses, and problem solve when unanticipated anxiety-provoking situations arise. Although insight is very much involved in this process, it is not insight into deep psychological causes, as in psychoanalysis, but rather, practical, commonsense problem solving. Treatment appears both to be effective during the relatively brief course of therapy and to remain effective for some months after therapy finishes. Sometimes medical and psychological follow-up are important to ensure satisfactory improvement.

A new treatment method for PTSD is eye-movement desensitization and reprocessing (EMDR). This method involves asking a client to imagine a traumatic event or anxiety provoking occurrence and processing the traumatic event in a non-threatening manner. Special training is necessary to perform EMDR (Antai-Otong, 2008).

Pharmacological

The drugs of choice for treating clients with anxiety are usually the **anxiolytics** or antianxiety agents (Table 17-1). Some of the antianxiety medications such as alprazolam (Xanax) and lorazepam (Ativan) may also be helpful in alleviating the symptoms of anxiety, nervousness, and sleeplessness frequently associated with panic disorder and PTSD.

Most of these medications can be used on either a routine or as-needed (PRN) basis and belong to the family of benzodiazepines. Onset of action for the benzodiazepines usually occurs within 30 minutes after oral administration, and most individuals respond favorably to these medications; that is, a reduction or cessation of the symptoms of anxiety is experienced.

Clients should be warned about the potential risk of addiction associated with antianxiety medications. These particular medications should be used with extreme caution because long-term use can lead to an increased **tolerance**, acquired resistance to the effects of the drug. Tolerance results in the need to increase the frequency and amount of medication in order to achieve the same benefit. Over time, this may cause a dependency on the medication, actually creating another serious problem for the client. Therefore, the antianxiety agents are usually indicated for short-term management of anxiety rather than for long-term use. The benefits of a particular medication for the client must always be weighed against the possible risk of addiction, particularly if long-term use is or may be indicated. The *one exception* is buspirone hydrochloride (BuSpar), a nonbenzodiazepine antianxiety medication, which does not appear to have any addictive potential; however, the therapeutic effectiveness of BuSpar is not reached for approximately 7 to 10 days; thus, although it can be given as a regularly scheduled antianxiety agent, BuSpar has absolutely no value as a PRN medication. When initiating therapy with BuSpar, another antianxiety medication such as alprazolam (Xanax) or lorazepam (Ativan) may be given concurrently until the therapeutic level is reached; then the other medication can be gradually decreased.

TABLE 17-1 Antianxiety Medications

GENERIC NAME	TRADE NAME	TYPE	POTENTIAL SIDE EFFECTS
aprazolam	Xanax	Benzodiazepine	Dizziness, drowsiness, lethargy, physical and psychological dependence, tolerance
buspirone hydrochloride	BuSpar	Nonbenzodiazepine	Blurred vision, chest pain, clamminess, dizziness, drowsiness, excitement, fatigue, headache, insomnia, nasal congestion, numbness, myalgia, nausea, nervousness, palpitations, paresthesia, skin rashes, sore throat, syncope, tachycardia, tinnitus, incoordination, weakness
clonazepam	Klonopin	Benzodiazepine	Ataxia, behavioral changes, drowsiness, physical and psychological dependence, tolerance
diazepam	Valium	Benzodiazepine	Dizziness, drowsiness, fatigue, hypotension, hypertension, CV collapse, dependence, tolerance
lorazepam	Ativan	Benzodiazepine	Agranulocytosis, CV collapse, dizziness, drowsiness, lethargy

Data from *Delmar Nurses's Drug Handbook 2010 Edition*, by G. Spratto and A. Woods, 2010, Clifton Park, NY: Delmar Cengage Learning.

Activity

The anxious client's activity level may be negatively affected by both the anxiety disorder and the side effects of the prescribed medication. The side effects of sedation and drowsiness can pose safety hazards for certain activities and must be emphasized to the client.

NURSING MANAGEMENT

Remain with the client while fear level and/or anxiety level is high and speak in a calm, soothing voice. Reassure the client that she is in a safe place. Explore with the client what things are relaxing and calming. Teach the client relaxation exercises. Encourage participation in recreation or sports activities.

Do not touch the client with PTSD without permission. If the client is confused or disoriented, orient the client to reality.

MEMORYTRICK

CALM

A memory trick to remember nursing management methods for anxiety is **CALM**:

C = Cognitive-behavior therapy

A = Anxiolytic medication management

L = Learn methods to reduce/control anxiety

M = Maintain a safe, calm environment

NURSING PROCESS

ASSESSMENT

Subjective Data

Clients experiencing anxiety report problems concentrating, and fear that something dreadful is about to happen. They may verbalize an overwhelming feeling of impending doom. They may also report that the anxiety is very frightening to them and that they are afraid of losing control. Table 17-2 lists questions that may help in identifying a client's anxiety.

Clients with PTSD may describe unwanted memories of an event, express suicidal ideation, or express fantasies of retaliation toward the identified source of trauma. The client with PTSD may describe feeling extremely fearful and "on guard" at all times and may report having **flashbacks** (reliving of the original trauma as if currently experiencing it) along with recurrent dreams and/or nightmares.

Objective Data

Changes in vital signs, such as an increase in blood pressure, pulse, and respirations, as well as restlessness, irritability, pacing, and agitation may become more pronounced as anxiety level increases.

Clients with PTSD may exhibit an exaggerated **startle response** (overreaction to minor sounds or noises), or they may be **hypervigilant** (constantly scanning the environment for potentially dangerous situations). Clients with PTSD may react with survival responses appropriate for the trauma they survived. For example, abused children may seek to placate adults and female incest victims may become flirtatious or seductive with men.

TABLE 17-2 Asking Clients about Symptoms of Anxiety Disorders

Following are questions that have proven useful in eliciting information from clients about symptoms of anxiety disorders. You may find that you prefer to word these questions somewhat differently, but the important thing is to ask them. Many clients experience anxiety symptoms for years before a doctor, nurse, or psychologist takes the time to ask about these symptoms.

Generalized Anxiety Disorder	Do you find yourself worrying frequently about a number of different things, such as the way things are going for you at home, work, or school? Do you find yourself feeling anxious or tense much of the time without any obvious reason?
Panic Disorder	Have you ever experienced sudden, intense fear for no reason? Have you found yourself experiencing intense physical symptoms of chest pain, shortness of breath, dizziness, or sweating, along with a sense that something terrible or life threatening was happening to you?
Post-Traumatic Stress Disorder	Have you ever had a particularly traumatic experience such as witnessing or experiencing violence or a catastrophic event (such as a flood or fire)? Have you ever found yourself reexperiencing a violent or catastrophic event through dreams or waking "flashbacks"?

From *Psychiatric Mental Health Nursing*, by N. Frisch and L. Frisch (4th ed.). 2010, Clifton Park, NY: Delmar Cengage Learning.

Nursing diagnoses for the client with anxiety include the following:

NURSING DIAGNOSES	PLANNING/OUTCOMES	NURSING INTERVENTIONS
Anxiety related to a subjective sense of uneasiness and tension	The client will learn how to demonstrate and utilize new and more effective methods of managing anxiety.	Teach the client relaxation exercises. Explore with the client those things that are calming and relaxing. Encourage physical movement or participation in some type of recreational or sporting activity to release excess energy.
Fear related to a specific object (e.g., hospitals)	The client will report feeling less fearful.	Remain with the client while level of fear is high. Talk to the client in a calm, soothing voice. Reassure the client that he is in a safe place.
Post-Trauma Syndrome related to anxiety felt following a significant life-threatening event	The client will experience a decrease in frequency and intensity of symptoms.	Orient the client to reality, if the client is confused, disoriented, or experiencing flashbacks. Do not touch the client without permission. Teach the client, family, and significant others about the symptoms of PTSD, including flashbacks, amnesia, memory loss, and nightmares.

Evaluation: Evaluate each outcome to determine how it has been met by the client.

DEPRESSION

Depression is the state wherein an individual experiences feelings of extreme sadness, hopelessness, and helplessness. Several symptoms may be seen with depression, which can range anywhere from mild to severe and be manifested in many different ways.

It involves an imbalance of neurotransmitters and is treatable. The direct cause of depression is unclear; however, changes in body chemistry caused by experiencing a traumatic event, hormonal changes, altered health habits, presence of another illness, or substance abuse can bring on depression (Depression and Bipolar Support Alliance [DBSA], 2007).

Symptoms of depression include prolonged sadness; significant changes in appetite and sleep patterns; irritability, agitation, anxiety, worry; pessimism; loss of energy; feelings of guilt, worthlessness; inability to concentrate; inability to take pleasure in former interests; unexplained aches and pains; and recurring thoughts of death or suicide. Adult Americans of all ages, races, ethnic groups, and social class experience depression every day. According to the

PROFESSIONALTIP

Achieving a State of Relaxation

Clients who are anxious and feeling overwhelmed will often require assistance in achieving a state of relaxation. Help the client identify activities that are relaxing, such as listening to favorite music, watching television, reading a book, playing a game, drawing a picture, working a puzzle, or whatever is calming to the client. Teach the client a variety of stress-management techniques such as deep-breathing exercises, progressive deep-muscle relaxation, and guided imagery. All of these can assist the client in reaching a greater state of relaxation. Explore with the client the possibility of enrolling in a course such as Tai Chi. In addition to providing physical activity, it assists the client in achieving a state of balance and an increasing ability to focus.

CRITICAL THINKING

Anxiety

A client shares with you that she is feeling anxious and cannot stop worrying about who will take care of her cat, how she will afford her health care, and she is anxiously waiting for her lab results.

1. Which client concern do you think should be addressed first?
2. How will you handle this situation?

Substance Abuse and Mental Health Services Administration (SAMHSA) (2008), 16.5 million adult Americans had at least one major depressive episode (MDE) between the years 2006-2007. Clients can experience mild, moderate, or severe depression with varying degrees of symptomatology.

MILD DEPRESSION

Individuals with mild depression may notice a difference in the way they are feeling and their ability to function in certain situations, but they may not be able to identify the problem at this point in time. Although they are still able to function and carry on their daily routines, doing so may put quite a strain on them both physically and mentally.

MODERATE DEPRESSION

Moderate depression interferes with the individual's life in a variety of ways. A decrease in the ability to perform on the job may be noticed. Relationships are affected as the individual becomes increasingly withdrawn and isolated and disinterested in things that previously were pleasurable, such as hobbies and leisure-time activities. Interventions performed at this stage are most effective in arresting the depression before the individual's mental health deteriorates any further.

PROFESSIONALTIP

Flashbacks

The client experiencing a flashback is usually not aware of current surroundings and often does not recognize familiar individuals. For the duration of the flashback, the client is actually reexperiencing and reliving the original trauma once again. For this reason, it is extremely important to never touch a client during a flashback, as the client may perceive you as dangerous and react to you as if you are trying to inflict harm. Talk to the client in a soft, calm voice and gently let the client know who you are, where the client is, and what is happening.

SEVERE DEPRESSION

When depression progresses to a severe state, the individual becomes seriously impaired. The individual with severe depression may experience psychosis, or a loss of contact with reality, in addition to the symptoms of depression.

DEPRESSION DISORDERS

Some of the psychiatric diagnoses associated with depression include Major Depressive Disorder and Dysthymic Disorder.

MAJOR DEPRESSIVE DISORDER

To qualify for the diagnosis of Major Depressive Disorder, *DSM-IV* requires the presence of at least one major depressive episode that (1) lasts at least 2 weeks, (2) represents a change from previous functioning, and (3) causes some impairment in a person's social or occupational functioning. Five or more symptoms of depression must also be present. One of these symptoms *must* be either depressed mood or loss of interest in previously enjoyable activities. The other four symptoms may include changes in appetite or weight; sleep disturbance (usually trouble staying asleep); fatigue or loss of energy; feelings of worthlessness or guilt; difficulty concentrating, thinking, or making decisions; or recurrent thoughts of death or suicide.

Some individuals, particularly adolescents, exhibit irritability or crankiness rather than sadness. Family members or close friends will notice a change in the individual, most commonly a social withdrawal and a neglect of activities that previously brought the person pleasure.

Major depressive episodes frequently develop over a few days or weeks, and without treatment commonly last longer than 6 months (Frisch & Frisch, 2010).

DYSTHYMIC DISORDER

Whereas the essence of Major Depressive Disorder is discrete episodes of depression, persons with Dysthymic Disorder feel depressed nearly all of the time. The *DSM-IV* criteria for Dysthymic Disorder include "depressed mood for most of the day, for more days than not . . . for at least 2 years." A person with Dysthymic Disorder must also have at least two of the following symptoms: appetite disturbance, sleep disturbance, fatigue, low self-esteem, poor concentration or difficulty making decisions, and feelings of hopelessness. As with Major Depressive Disorder, the symptoms must cause clinically significant distress or impairment in social or occupational functioning. Dysthymic Disorder is somewhat rarer than Major Depressive Disorder, occurring during a lifetime in approximately 6% of persons (Frisch & Frisch, 2010).

MEDICAL–SURGICAL MANAGEMENT

Medical

Psychotherapy refers to any of more than 250 types of largely verbal techniques designed to help individuals surmount psychological stresses including depression. Psychotherapy based on psychoanalytic interventions emphasizes helping clients gain insight into the causes of their depression. This approach is long term and requires much motivation on the part of the client to invest considerable time, effort, and money (Frisch & Frisch, 2010).

Brief dynamic therapy focuses on core conflicts from personality and living situations. The goal is to resolve depressive symptoms by improving these conflicts and resolving stresses. The therapist in this approach takes an active role to direct sessions toward resolution of conflicts. Techniques of confrontation and interpretation of behaviors and events are frequently used. Conflicts, their meanings, and individuals' choices are emphasized. This type of therapy can be done either with individuals or in a group format.

Cognitive therapy focuses on removing symptoms by identifying and correcting perceptual biases in clients' thinking and correcting unrecognized assumptions. The therapy concentrates on changing negative thoughts and behaviors into alternatives that do not sustain depression.

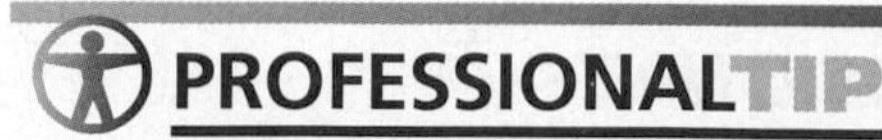

Journaling

Suggest to depressed clients that they keep personal journals in which they write down their thoughts and feelings. Putting thoughts and emotions down on paper may help clarify issues relating to depression and is an excellent way of venting or releasing pent-up feelings.

Electroconvulsive therapy (ECT) is used for clients with severe depression who have not responded to medications. The client under anesthesia is treated with pulses of electrical energy sufficient to cause a brief convulsion or seizure. Muscle-depolarizing agents are also given so that no actual convulsive movements occur; the primary effect of ECT is on the brain. Studies show that clients do not find the actual ECT treatment frightening, painful, or unpleasant. Although deaths have occurred from ECT, particularly in elderly clients or those with heart disease, the risk is quite low. Side effects depend on the specific technique used but are mostly limited to memory deficits (Frisch & Frisch, 2010).

Pharmacological

The main classification of medications usually prescribed for treatment of depression is the antidepressants. Within this classification are several groups, including the tetracyclic and atypical antidepressants (Table 17-3), the selective serotonin reuptake inhibitors (SSRIs) (Table 17-4), the tricyclic antidepressants (Table 17-5), and the monoamine oxidase inhibitors (MAOIs) (Table 17-6). These antidepressant families have unique properties, as do the individual medications within each. Many of these medications must be taken at bedtime. It is a nursing responsibility to adequately educate the client and family about the prescribed medications.

Diet

The client experiencing depression often has a disturbance in eating patterns. Some individuals will not be hungry and will

TABLE 17-3 Tetracyclic and Atypical Antidepressants

GENERIC NAME	TRADE NAME	TYPE	POTENTIAL SIDE EFFECTS
mirtazapine	Remeron	Tetracyclic	Agranulocytosis, drowsiness, dry mouth, nausea, suicidal ideation
nefazodone hydrochloride	Serzone	Antidepressant	Constipation, dizziness, dry mouth, insomnia, nausea, weight loss
venlafaxine hydrochloride	Effexor	Antidepressant	Abnormal dreams, altered taste, anorexia, constipation, diarrhea, dizziness, dry mouth, dyspepsia, headache, nausea, nervousness, paresthesia, rectal hemorrhage, rhinitis, seizures, sexual dysfunction, visual disturbances, vaginal/uterine hemorrhage, weakness, weight loss

Data from *Delmar Nurses's Drug Handbook 2010 Edition*, by G. Spratto and A. Woods, 2010, Clifton Park, NY: Delmar Cengage Learning.

eat very little or sometimes not at all, whereas others will overeat. A nutritional assessment should be done as part of the health history obtained by the nurse, and if any significant problem areas are identified, a dietary consult may be indicated.

When a client is started on antidepressant therapy, the client and family must be educated regarding any special dietary needs, depending on the type of medication prescribed. The client receiving SSRI therapy may experience an initial loss of appetite during the first part of therapy, because of the gastrointestinal (GI) side effects frequently associated with these medications (Table 17-4). Anorectic clients or those at risk for weight loss must be closely monitored. The client receiving MAOI therapy must be especially alert to the dietary restrictions associated with this particular type of medication (Table 17-6).

Table 17-4 Selective Serotonin Reuptake Inhibitors (SSRIs)

GENERIC NAME	TRADE NAME	POTENTIAL SIDE EFFECTS
fluoxetine hydrochloride	Prozac	Headache, abnormal dreams, anxiety, diarrhea, drowsiness, excessive sweating, insomnia, nervousness, palpitations, pruritus, seizures, tremors, visual disturbances, weight loss
fluvoxamine maleate	Luvox	Constipation, convulsions, impotence, dry mouth, drowsiness, dyspepsia, headache, heart failure, insomnia, MI, nausea, nervousness, weakness
paroxetine hydrochloride	Paxil	Anxiety, constipation, diarrhea, dizziness, drowsiness, dry mouth, ejaculatory disturbance, headache, insomnia, nausea, seizures, sweating, weakness, tremors
sertraline hydrochloride	Zoloft	Diarrhea, dizziness, drowsiness, dry mouth, fatigue, headache, increased sweating, insomnia, nausea, palpitations, sexual dysfunction, tremors, vomiting when given with pimozide (Orap) raises pimozide concentration by about 40% (FDA, 2002)

Data from *Delmar Nurses's Drug Handbook 2010 Edition*, by G. Spratto and A. Woods, 2010, Clifton Park, NY: Delmar Cengage Learning.

Table 17-5 Tricyclic Antidepressants

GENERIC NAME	TRADE NAME	POTENTIAL SIDE EFFECTS
amitriptyline hydrochloride	Elavil	Arrhythmia, blurred vision, constipation, dry eyes, dry mouth, heart block, hypotension, lethargy, MI, sedation, stroke
imipramine hydrochloride	Tofranil	Arrhythmia, blurred vision, constipation, drowsiness, dry eyes, dry mouth, fatigue, hypotension, seizures, urinary retention

Data from *Delmar Nurses's Drug Handbook 2010 Edition*, by G. Spratto and A. Woods, 2010, Clifton Park, NY: Delmar Cengage Learning.

Table 17-6 Monoamine Oxidase Inhibitors (MAOIs)

GENERIC NAME	TRADE NAME	POTENTIAL SIDE EFFECTS
isocarboxazid	Marplan	Arrhythmia, blurred vision, diarrhea, dizziness, headache, orthostatic hypotension, insomnia, restlessness, seizures, weakness; these medications usually have the side-effect of lowering blood pressure. A potentially fatal hypertensive crisis can result when MAOIs are taken in combination with certain foods and drugs such as broad beans, certain cheeses (e.g., brie, cheddar), liver, caffeine, figs, dry sausage (pepperoni), tea, yogurt, amphetamine, cocaine, dopa, and many OTC cold products, hay fever medications, and nasal decongestants.
phenelzine sulfate	Nardil	
tranylcypromine sulfate	Parnate	

Data from *Delmar Nurses's Drug Handbook 2010 Edition*, by G. Spratto and A. Woods, 2010, Clifton Park, NY: Delmar Cengage Learning.

PROFESSIONALTIP

Antidepressant Therapy

Before initiating antidepressant therapy, a baseline electrocardiogram (EKG) is needed to determine whether any preexisting underlying cardiac problems are present. If the client develops cardiac difficulties during antidepressant therapy, another EKG is obtained and compared to the original to assist in ascertaining whether the antidepressant exacerbated the cardiac condition.

CLIENTTEACHING

Tricyclic Antidepressants

Be sure to instruct each client taking a tricyclic antidepressant medication in the following:

- Do not drink alcohol while on the medication.
- Do not take any other medications unless prescribed by your physician.
- Drowsiness and sedation may impair the ability to drive and operate heavy machinery.
- Some of the side effects may diminish in intensity once your body adjusts to the medication.
- Do not stop taking the medications without physician approval.
- Increase fluid intake to assist in combating dry mouth and constipation.
- Sugarless candy and gum can help decrease the side effect of dry mouth.
- Increase dietary fiber to decrease the side effect of constipation.
- Rise slowly from a lying position to prevent dizziness and a sudden drop in blood pressure.

CLIENTTEACHING

Potential Adverse Drug–Drug Reactions with MAOIs

A serious drug–drug reaction can occur when an MAOI is taken concurrently with certain other medications. The combination of an MAOI and some common prescription or OTC medications can result in a hypertensive crisis that is often fatal. Some of the most dangerous reactive medications include meperidine (Demerol), stimulants, decongestants, and weight-reduction aids.

CLIENTTEACHING

Tetracyclic and SSRI Antidepressants

Be sure to instruct each client taking a tetracyclic, atypical, or SSRI antidepressant medication in the following:

- Take the medication *only* as directed by your physician.
- Do not take the medication unless prescribed by your physician.
- Do not take fluoxetine (Prozac), paroxetine (Paxil), or sertraline (Zoloft) on an empty stomach.
- Mirtazapine (Remeron) does not need to be taken with food.
- Ability to drive and/or operate heavy machinery may be impaired while taking the medication.
- Do not drink alcohol while taking the medication.
- If female, advise your physician if you are breastfeeding, suspect you are pregnant, or are planning a pregnancy while taking the medication.
- Wear sunscreen and protective clothing while outdoors, as fluoxetine (Prozac), paroxetine (Paxil), and sertraline (Zoloft) increase susceptibility to sunburn.
- The medications may cause drowsiness.
- If taking fluoxetine (Prozac), mirtazapine (Remeron), or nefazodone (Serzone), rise slowly from a lying position to prevent dizziness and a sudden drop in blood pressure.
- Utilize good oral hygiene in conjunction with sugarless candy or gum to minimize the discomforting side effect of dry mouth associated with fluoxetine (Prozac), mirtazapine (Remeron), nefazodone (Serzone), paroxetine (Paxil), and sertraline (Zoloft).
- Monitor weight, as mirtazapine (Remeron) may cause an increase in appetite.
- Do not take any over-the-counter (OTC) cold medications with mirtazapine (Remeron).
- If taking mirtazapine (Remeron), inform your physician of the medication regimen prior to surgery.
- If taking venlafaxine (Effexor), fluvoxamine (Luvox), or nefazodone (Serzone), inform your physician if signs of allergic reaction occur.

CLIENTTEACHING

MAOIs

Be sure to instruct each client taking an MAOI antidepressant medication in the following:

- *Do not take any other medications, including OTC medications,* unless prescribed by your physician.
- Take the medication exactly as prescribed.
- Do not drink alcohol while on the medication.
- Rise slowly from a lying position to prevent dizziness and a sudden drop in blood pressure.
- *Avoid all foods containing tyramine,* including alcoholic beverages, especially beer and wine; aged cheeses; avocados; bananas; caffeine; chocolate; and smoked or pickled meats (such as salami, pepperoni, smoked fish, and summer sausage).

CRITICAL THINKING

Coworker Depression

What actions would you take if you felt a coworker was suffering from depression?

Activity

Clients experiencing depression often experience a significant decrease in level of activity and report feeling tired and lethargic. Clients experiencing depression will often require encouragement to engage in any type of physical activity.

Nursing Management

Spend time with the client one-on-one to build rapport and develop a therapeutic relationship. Encourage the client to initiate conversation and interact with others. Guide the client to bathe, groom, and wear clean clothes. Praise the client verbally for conversing and interacting with others and for taking care of hygiene and grooming.

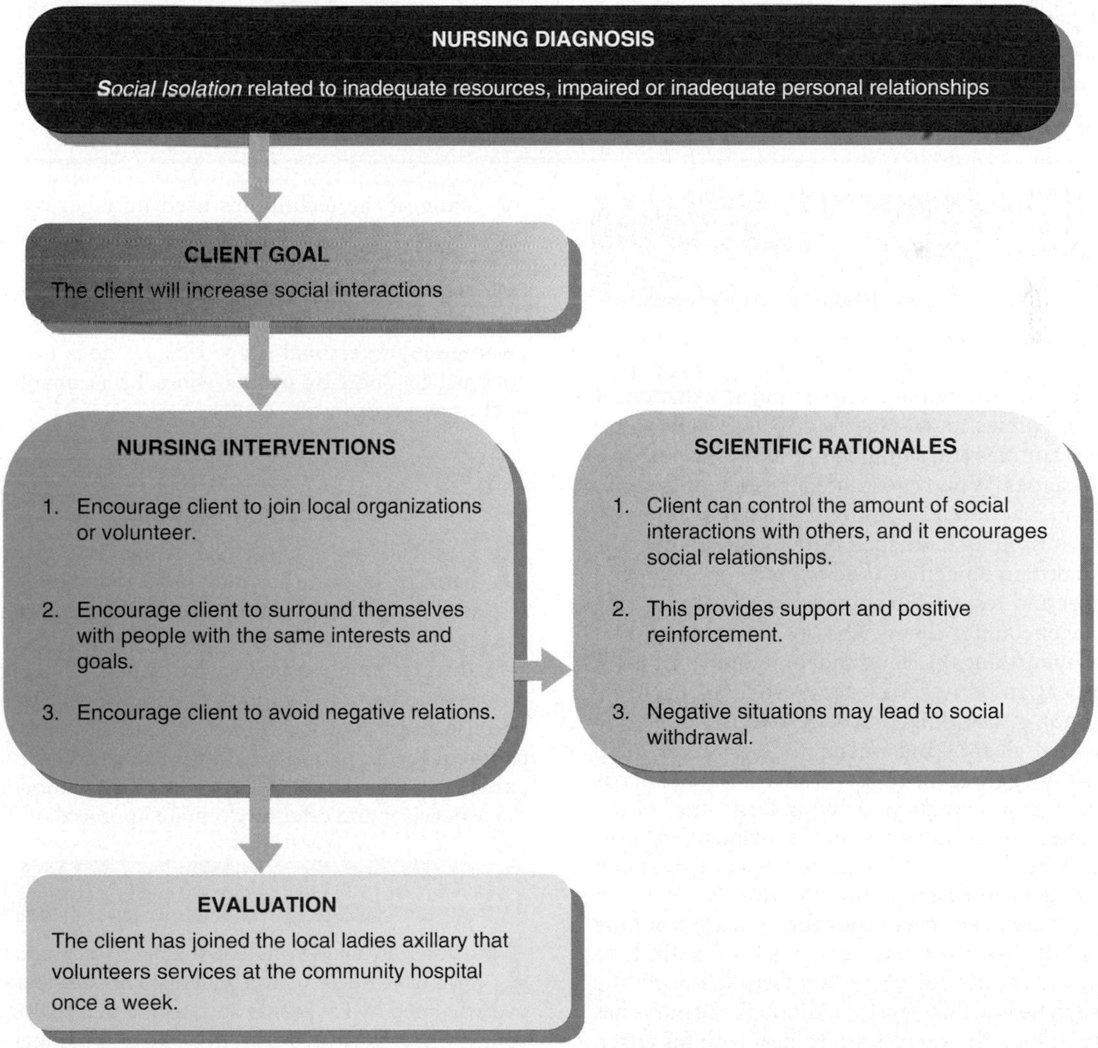

NURSING DIAGNOSIS

Social Isolation related to inadequate resources, impaired or inadequate personal relationships

CLIENT GOAL

The client will increase social interactions

NURSING INTERVENTIONS	SCIENTIFIC RATIONALES
1. Encourage client to join local organizations or volunteer.	1. Client can control the amount of social interactions with others, and it encourages social relationships.
2. Encourage client to surround themselves with people with the same interests and goals.	2. This provides support and positive reinforcement.
3. Encourage client to avoid negative relations.	3. Negative situations may lead to social withdrawal.

EVALUATION

The client has joined the local ladies axillary that volunteers services at the community hospital once a week.

Concept Care Map 17-1

NURSING PROCESS

ASSESSMENT

Subjective Data

The client may verbalize overwhelming feelings of sadness, thoughts of suicide, a loss of interest and pleasure in activities that were previously enjoyable, and problems with memory, recall, and concentration. In addition, a decreased libido, extreme lethargy, and having insufficient energy to complete activities of daily living (ADLs) and needed tasks may be reported. The depressed client who has become increasingly withdrawn and socially isolated may experience problems in intimate, personal, and social relationships.

Objective Data

The client may manifest a noticeable decline in personal hygiene and grooming, possibly because of a lack of energy and an inability to perform even the simplest of tasks. Weight loss resulting from the client's failure to eat may also be noted.

Nursing diagnoses for the client with depression include the following:

NURSING DIAGNOSES	PLANNING/OUTCOMES	NURSING INTERVENTIONS
Social Isolation related to inability to engage in satisfying personal relationships	The client will increase the number of interactions with other individuals.	Build rapport and develop therapeutic relationship with client. Spend time with client individually. Encourage client to initiate conversation and interact with others. Verbally praise client for increasing interactions and initiating conversation.
Bathing/Dressing and Feeding Self-care Deficit related to lack of concern or regard toward self	The client will attend to own basic health care needs.	Encourage client to bathe and wear clean clothes. Teach client the importance of balanced nutrition. Praise client for each activity done on own.

Evaluation: Evaluate each outcome to determine how it has been met by the client.

THE CLIENT WHO IS POTENTIALLY VIOLENT

In today's society, violence has become increasingly common and widespread. The media routinely and graphically reports the numerous violent crimes and acts that occur on a daily basis. Nurses may come face to face with angry clients and their families and significant others and, perhaps, even angry colleagues. When confronted by someone who is angry, the natural reaction is to respond in a like manner or, perhaps, to feel intimidated. In such difficult situations, it is important to maintain objectivity and not get "hooked" into the client's anger and respond in an inappropriate manner.

Nurses may encounter clients who are **verbally aggressive** (prone to saying things in a loud and/or intimidating manner), **physically aggressive** (prone to threatening or actually harming someone), or a combination of the two. Mind-altering substances such as alcohol and phencyclidine (PCP) often increase the risk of aggression. **Anger-control assistance** is defined as a nursing intervention aimed at facilitation of the expression of anger in an adaptive and nonviolent manner. Anger control includes establishing a basic level of trust and rapport with the client and using a calm and reassuring manner. The nurse should use every means possible to learn from the client (or his family/friends) those situations that are likely to bring on anger, and should encourage the client to inform the nursing staff when he is feeling tension. Although the nurse has a responsibility to help the client learn to deal with his anger, she also has a clear duty to assess for inappropriate aggression and to intervene before such aggression is expressed.

Some of the techniques used in anger control include limiting access to frustrating situations, providing physical outlets for expression of anger or tension (such as punching bags, large motor activities [sports], and anger journals), and ensuring that a client for whom anger is a problem is given enough personal space that he does not have to feel encroached upon by others when he is unable to tolerate environmental stimuli.

HOMICIDAL INTENT

The client who is homicidal is planning or threatening to harm or kill another individual or individuals. It is the responsibility of health care personnel to attempt to ascertain the seriousness of the intent; that is, whether the individual is actually threatening someone else or just "blowing off steam." Once aware of an individual's threat or intent to harm someone else, the nurse must inform the individual(s) at risk of the potential for harm and/or notify the proper authorities and enlist their help. The first step in such a situation is to contact the supervisor and offer an accurate appraisal of the situation.

SUICIDAL INTENT

Purposefully taking one's own life, or suicide, is the ultimate form of self-destruction. Clients who are suicidal often feel overwhelmed by life events and decide that the only relief will come from ending their own lives. Intense feelings of fear, loss, anger, or despair can drive individuals to commit suicide, and the effects of an attempted or completed suicide can be devastating

PROFESSIONALTIP

Assessing for Risk of Violence

- Be aware of those clients with past history of violence and poor impulse control.
- Observe the client's body language: Notice changes in behavior, words, or dress.
- Assess for aggressive behaviors, increasing tension, clenched fists, loud or angry tone of voice, narrowed eyes, and pacing.
- Remember that hostility tends to be contagious. Do not reciprocate with anger and hostility!

and long lasting. Nurses must learn to recognize the danger signs of clients at risk for suicide and know the appropriate interventions to help clients preserve their health and dignity.

Suicide is the eleventh leading cause of death in the United States, claiming more than 32,000 lives each year (CDC, 2008a). The populations at greatest risk are individuals with diagnosed mood disorders such as Major Depressive Disorder, elders, and those with serious or life-threatening medical illnesses such as cancer or human immunodeficiency virus.

SUICIDAL IDEATIONS

The client experiencing **suicidal ideations** has thoughts of hurting or killing himself but may or may not be planning to act on these thoughts. It is important to understand the difference between thoughts and actions; that is, having a thought does not necessarily mean that the behavior will follow. When confronted with a client's verbalization of possible suicide, however, it is always wise to take the client's expression of intent seriously. Because suicide is a leading cause of death in the United States, nurses must know how to evaluate a client for the likelihood of a completed suicide. It is critical to thoroughly assess the client and attempt to accurately ascertain the degree of danger the client is experiencing. Once this is done, take the precautions necessary to maintain the client's safety (Table 17-7).

ACTIVELY SUICIDAL

The **actively suicidal** client is intent on hurting or killing himself and is in imminent danger of doing so. This situation requires immediate and appropriate action to protect the client from potentially fatal self-destructive behavior. If the client is in a supervised setting, it is the nurse's responsibility to maintain the safety of the client and to inform other staff members of the client's suicidal intentions. The client at risk for self-inflicted injury must be monitored closely (per institutional policy and the frequency as ordered by the physician).

The frequency of client observation is determined by the degree of suicide risk and is written as a specific order from the physician. Observations of the client are documented. Some clients must be checked a minimum of once every 15 minutes. Other clients may require more frequent observation and monitoring. If the client is *actively* suicidal and/or homicidal and is indicating an imminent intent to harm self or others, a specific staff member will be assigned to that client at all times on a one-to-one basis.

All pertinent observations such as verbalizations and behaviors that indicate self-harm potential should be documented in the client's record. Any changes in the client's condition should be reported immediately to the physician. The conversation

Table 17-7 Assessment of Risk for Suicide

The following areas are to be assessed in all potentially suicidal clients:

1. Does the client have a *plan* to commit suicide?	
Example: Client plans to "end it all" after wife leaves for work on a Monday.	***Rationale:*** Some clients may be experiencing thoughts of wishing they were dead or killing themselves, but may not have a plan for doing so. *The client who has a plan for committing suicide is at increased risk.*
2. How *specific* is the plan to commit suicide?	
Example: Client states he plans to overdose on sleeping pills.	***Rationale:*** *A specific plan increases the risk of completing a suicide.*
3. Does the client have access to the *means* to commit suicide?	
Example: Client states he will use his spouse's sleeping pills to overdose.	***Rationale:*** *Easy availability of the means to kill oneself increases the risk of suicide.*
4. How *lethal* is the intended means to commit suicide?	
Example: Client states he will "blow his brains out" with a gun.	***Rationale:*** Some means of suicide are more likely to result in a completed suicide. *Gunshots are the most common cause of completed suicide.* The lethality of guns makes the potential for a successful intervention very slim. Intervention in light of means that are less lethal may yield a more favorable outcome (e.g., overdose, cutting of wrists).

with the doctor, as well as any new orders or changes in orders, must also be documented in the client's record.

Medical–Surgical Management

Medical

The client who is severely agitated, aggressive, actively suicidal, and/or homicidal and who is exhibiting or threatening violent acts may need to be restrained or placed in seclusion in order to be safely contained. The physical holding of someone or use of mechanical restraints severely restricts movement and can constitute a violation of the client's rights unless sufficient clinical justification exists. Thus, all of the client's comments and behaviors plus any nursing interventions must be documented in the client record per agency policy. This documentation provides the necessary justification for the use of restraints or seclusion. In addition, the physician must write a specific, time-limited order that spells out the reason restraints or seclusion was indicated for use with the client.

Physical Restraints Physical restraints, usually leather straps, are used to immobilize a person who is clearly dangerous to self or others and who poses sufficient risk of harm. Physical restraints may be applied only under the direction and supervision of a registered nurse (RN) and must comply with state laws regarding their use. In almost all cases, there must be a physician's order to apply the restraints, and there must be clearly documented evidence that the restraints were needed. Some of the observable behaviors indicating that restraints are necessary include increased motor activity, verbal and/or physical threats, overresponsiveness to stimuli, and actual physical assault (Frisch & Frisch, 2010).

Seclusion Seclusion is the process of confining a client to a single room. The room may be locked or unlocked, and it may or may not have furnishings. The purpose of seclusion is to provide security, to remove the client from a situation of escalating anger and violence, or to remove the client who is hypersensitive to environmental stimuli from the stimulation of a hospital unit. Seclusion, like the use of physical restraints, can be used only when all other avenues for control have been exhausted. The client must be told what is happening and why. He must not be left alone; a staff member should be assigned to observe the client, usually from the doorway. Seclusion is an enforced "time-out," where the client is removed from the situation only long enough to allow him to calm down, regain a sense of control, and then reenter the unit.

Therapy Psychotherapy is often indicated and initially may focus on personal and social conditions that bring about and/or perpetuate suicidal thoughts. Cognitive-behavioral therapy may be particularly useful, as may techniques to deal with frustration and anger. Substance use and abuse are often involved and may require separate outpatient or inpatient interventions.

Pharmacological

The severely agitated, aggressive, suicidal, and/or homicidal client who is violent or threatening violence may require a medication with strong anxiolytic (antianxiety) and/or sedative properties, such as one of the antianxiety agents or a sedative-hypnotic (Table 17-1). Additionally, the suicidal client who is depressed may be evaluated for treatment with one of the many available antidepressants such as fluoxetine hydrochloride (Prozac), sertraline hydrochloride (Zoloft), paroxetine hydrochloride (Paxil), fluvoxamine maleate (Luvox), mirtazapine (Remeron), or one of the many others (Tables 17-3, 17-4, 17-5, and 17-6).

Diet

Foods are not restricted because a client is severely agitated, aggressive, actively suicidal, and/or homicidal, but may be restricted depending on the medications being taken. The food tray should be inspected for any potentially dangerous objects such as glassware or silverware. Even plasticware can be broken in such a way as to yield a very dangerous weapon for hurting self or others.

Activity

The activity level of the client who is severely agitated, aggressive, actively suicidal, and/or homicidal may need to be restricted for a period of time in order to maintain the client's safety and the safety of others.

> **PROFESSIONALTIP**
>
> **Providing a Safe Environment**
>
> When a client verbalizes an intention to inflict self-harm, measures must be taken to ensure the client's safety. One way is to provide and maintain a safe, secure environment for the client. This may require a change in items allowed in the client's surroundings and living space. For example, a pencil or pen could be used as a dangerous weapon; an empty soda can could be used to deeply cut the wrists or to seriously injure someone else; and the broken glass from a bottle of make-up could cause great harm. These and all other potentially dangerous items must be removed from the client's immediate area.

Nursing Management

Assess the client for suicidal thoughts. If the client has a specific plan, evaluate the degree of risk for the client and contact the physician. Assess the environment for potentially dangerous items. Increase the level of client observation.

NURSING PROCESS

Assessment

Subjective Data

The client may argue, yell, curse, and make numerous verbal threats in a loud voice. The suicidal client may indicate intentions verbally, nonverbally, or a combination of the two. The client contemplating suicide may verbalize his thoughts either directly or indirectly. A direct statement may be something as straightforward as "I am planning to kill myself." An indirect

PROFESSIONALTIP

No-Suicide Contract

Obtaining a "No-Suicide Contract" from the client is one way to help reduce the risk of suicide attempts. There are several guidelines to follow in working through this process:

- Ask the client whether he is able to make a promise *to himself* that he will not do anything to harm himself. ***Rationale:*** It is important for the client to make the contract with himself, because if the contract is made with someone else, such as a nurse, and the client later becomes angry or upset with that person, he may then harm himself in order to "get back" at that person.
- If the client is unable to commit to the No-Suicide Contract for the rest of his life, work with him on establishing a time frame to which he can commit, for example, 1 week, 24 hours, 8 hours, or some other time frame. Always meet with the client at the end of the allotted time frame and review/renew the contract at that time. ***Rationale:*** The suicidal individual may feel overwhelmed at the thought of promising *never* to harm himself, but may be able to sincerely commit for a shorter length of time.
- Ask the client whether he is able to maintain the No-Suicide Contract *no matter what happens.* ***Rationale:*** Some clients will leave a way out of the contract. For example, the suicidal client may outwardly make a promise to not commit suicide but inwardly think "unless something really bad happens, like if my wife leaves me." If the wife then files for a divorce, the client may feel that he has "permission" to kill himself. Adding the *no matter what happens* clause blocks off this avenue of escape from the contract.
- Ask the client whether he can make a promise to himself that if thoughts of suicide return, he will talk to someone before taking any action. ***Rationale:*** If the client talks to someone regarding his thoughts of suicide *before* he attempts suicide, a successful intervention and suicide prevention are more likely.
- Assist the client in developing a detailed plan of action regarding those persons he will contact in the event that he again experiences suicidal thoughts. Include names and phone numbers of all significant and supportive individuals. ***Rationale:*** During a crisis, the suicidal individual is not able to think rationally and will behave and act in an impulsive manner. Having a well-developed plan of action increases the likelihood that the suicidal individual can follow these guidelines.
- At the bottom of the list, put the name and phone number of the local suicide crisis hotline and/or local emergency number (911). ***Rationale:*** Including these numbers ensures that there will always be someone available for the suicidal client to talk to 24 hours a day, 7 days a week, 365 days a year.
- Assist the client in putting the No-Suicide Contract in writing and in his own words. Give the client the original and put a copy in the client's chart ***Rationale:*** When the contract is in writing and the client has a copy, he will be more likely to follow through with his promise to not commit suicide.

statement might be "I'm not going to be around here anymore" or "Everyone will be better off without me."

Objective Data

The client may exhibit restlessness, pacing, and "poor impulse control"; may be physically intimidating; and may use or try to use items in the environment, such as books, furniture, or a coffee pot, as weapons. A nonverbal signal of possible intentions of suicide may be seen in the client who begins making arrangements for people and pets to be taken care of, putting personal affairs in order, and giving away personal possessions, especially treasured items.

Nursing diagnoses for the client who is severely agitated, aggressive, actively suicidal, and/or homicidal include the following:

NURSING DIAGNOSES	PLANNING/OUTCOMES	NURSING INTERVENTIONS
Risk for Self-Directed Violence related to risk factors such as mental health, emotional status, or suicidal plan	The client will not harm self.	Assess for the presence of suicidal thoughts and whether a specific plan is present. Evaluate the degree of risk associated with the client's verbalization of suicide intent. Contact the attending physician or psychiatrist and inform of the client's intentions and current condition.

(*Continues*)

Nursing diagnoses for the client who is severely agitated, aggressive, actively suicidal, and/or homicidal include the following: (Continued)

NURSING DIAGNOSES	PLANNING/OUTCOMES	NURSING INTERVENTIONS
		Assess and evaluate the client's surroundings and environment for any potentially dangerous items or objects that could be used for self-harm. Remove or secure any potentially harmful items. Increase the level of observation so that the client is frequently monitored. Assist the client in developing a No-suicide Contract.
Risk for Other-Directed Violence related to risk factors such as history of violence against others, suicidal behavior, impulsivity	The client will not harm anyone.	Assess for the presence of homicidal ideations. If the client is verbalizing a plan to harm someone, immediately notify the proper authorities so they can alert this individual.

Evaluation: Evaluate each outcome to determine how it has been met by the client.

SAMPLE NURSING CARE PLAN

The Suicidal Client with Major Depression

A.J. is a 27-year-old woman who was brought to the emergency department of a county hospital by ambulance after a serious suicide attempt via ingesting a bottle of insecticide. After being treated in the emergency room, she spent 2 days in the intensive care unit (ICU) and then was transferred to a locked adult inpatient psychiatric unit for evaluation and treatment. A.J. reports she became suicidal following the recent ending of a 4-year relationship with her boyfriend and decided to take her life because she felt "completely hopeless," that "there was nothing left to live for," that "no one would miss her" if she were dead, that she "would never be loved," and that she "could never be happy again." Before the suicide attempt, A.J. reports that she had not been eating, had only been sleeping 1 to 2 hours per night, and had been crying almost continuously throughout the day. Since admission to the psychiatric unit, A.J. has been started on sertraline (Zoloft).

NURSING DIAGNOSIS 1 *Risk for Self-Directed Violence* related to recent loss, feelings of abandonment, and impulsive behavior as evidenced by suicide attempt of drinking bottle of insecticide, verbalizations that "there was nothing left to live for" and that "no one would miss her" if she were dead

Nursing Outcomes Classification (NOC)
Depression Level
Suicide Self-Restraint

Nursing Interventions Classification (NIC)
Self-Esteem Enhancement
Coping Enhancement

PLANNING/OUTCOMES	NURSING INTERVENTIONS	RATIONALE
A.J. will verbalize that she is no longer at risk of harming herself.	Assist A.J. in developing a No-Suicide Contract. Obtain in writing if possible, make a copy for her chart, and give her the original.	May help deter self-destructive behavior in the future.
	Explore with A.J. factors that contributed to her becoming suicidal.	Can be the first step in preventing another attempt.

(Continues)

SAMPLE NURSING CARE PLAN (Continued)

PLANNING/OUTCOMES	NURSING INTERVENTIONS	RATIONALE
	Encourage A.J. to verbalize her feelings related to the recent break-up and to explore any unresolved past issues that this loss might have triggered.	Current feelings of loss and abandonment are often magnified and intensified by unresolved past situations and circumstances that were never effectively handled.
	Explore with A.J. her usual methods of coping with stressful situations and whether these have been effective for her.	Can lead to a better understanding of those behaviors that must be changed.
	Assist A.J. in identifying and then developing stress-management methods as alternatives to attempting suicide.	Assists the client in recognizing alternate methods of managing stressful situations.
	Assist A.J. in developing a suicide-prevention plan and in identifying supportive individuals and resources that she can turn to in the event that she begins to again have suicidal thoughts.	Plans to prevent suicide must be developed ahead of time, because individuals contemplating suicide are impulsive and unable to problem solve or think clearly. They may, however, be able to follow through with a previously defined plan of action.
	Teach A.J. about possible side effects associated with sertraline (Zoloft), such as nausea and GI upset, and encourage her to have something to eat prior to taking this medication.	Medication education is an integral part of treatment.
	Emphasize the importance of taking this medication as prescribed and not stopping the medication on her own, even if she starts to feel better and thinks that she no longer needs it.	If medications are discontinued prematurely, symptoms usually reappear and are often much more serious.
	Encourage A.J. to keep a journal to reflect on her thoughts and feelings.	Writing in a journal can be a safe and effective method of identifying, expressing, and releasing feelings and emotions.
	Encourage A.J. to keep follow-up appointments for medication to monitor progress.	Recommended to evaluate effectiveness and to monitor for any side effects.
	Assist A.J. in setting up an appointment for outpatient counseling/therapy upon discharge per recommendation from the treatment team. Encourage A.J. to keep counseling appointments.	Recommended after a suicide attempt in order to address the underlying issues and to prevent future attempts.

(Continues)

SAMPLE NURSING CARE PLAN (Continued)

EVALUATION

At the time of discharge from the adult inpatient psychiatric unit, A.J. was no longer actively suicidal or intent upon harming herself. She still had occasional suicidal ideations; however, she did not feel compelled to act on them. She had made a promise to herself that she would never try to kill herself again no matter what happened, and that if those thoughts returned, she would find someone to talk to before she did anything. She also had developed a written list of friends and relatives she could call if she again experienced thoughts of suicide.

NURSING DIAGNOSIS 2 *Hopelessness* related to feelings of loss about her life and future as evidenced by verbalizations of feeling: "completely hopeless," that she "would never be loved," and that she "could never be happy again"

Nursing Outcomes Classification (NOC)
Depression Control
Mood Equilibrium

Nursing Interventions Classification (NIC)
Suicide Prevention
Patient Contracting

PLANNING/OUTCOMES	NURSING INTERVENTIONS	RATIONALE
A.J. will be less hopeless as indicated by verbalizations of plans for her future	Develop a therapeutic nurse–client relationship with A.J. using the components of trust, rapport, respect, genuineness, and empathy.	Fosters the development of a therapeutic nurse–client relationship.
	Encourage A.J. to become involved in activities on the unit, for example, interacting with staff and other clients and attending and participating in therapy groups and recreational activities.	Helps distract the mind from a preoccupation with losses, overwhelming feelings of depression, and suicidal ideations.
	Provide things for A.J. to do when she is feeling down, for example, go for a walk with the staff, read a newspaper or book, or play a game.	Provides time to allow for something to shift for her, to see the situation as not so utterly and permanently hopeless or for her to begin to feel better and think differently once she has started responding to medication.
	Assist A.J. in identifying the irrational beliefs or thoughts that she is having, for example, when she says no one will ever love or want her again.	Changing the way a person thinks by replacing irrational thoughts with rational or healthier ones, will change the way the person feels.

EVALUATION

A.J. continued to have fleeting thoughts of hopelessness as far as ever having another significant relationship or being in love again; however, she now was beginning to catch herself and could identify these thoughts as being irrational and negative in nature and not helpful to her in any way.

THE CLIENT WHO IS PSYCHOTIC

Psychosis is a state wherein an individual loses the ability to recognize reality. A psychotic person may experience hallucinations, wherein he hears voices or sees images of persons or things that others cannot see or hear. A psychotic person is frequently unable to care for basic needs of safety, security, nutrition, and so on. Such an individual is hospitalized for his own safety and to initiate treatment (usually involving some form of medication) to bring the symptoms under control. A psychotic person may slip into and out of reality.

Psychosis can be a component of several illnesses, including Schizophrenia and Bipolar Disorder.

SCHIZOPHRENIA

The client with schizophrenia can be very difficult to understand and treat because the symptoms of schizophrenia can be confusing and frightening to caregivers. Clients with schizophrenia frequently have belief systems that have become distorted, so that they hold firmly to false ideas or delusions, even when presented with evidence to the contrary. When confronted with an opposing belief system, they may become even more entrenched in their mistaken views and begin to believe others are "against them," when, in fact, they are not. This makes them even more paranoid and suspicious, adding to their already distorted views of reality. As a result, these individuals are often struggling to determine the difference between that which is real and that which is unreal or delusional.

Hallucinations can occur in relation to any of the five senses (hearing, sight, touch, taste, and smell), but the most common types of hallucinations are auditory and visual. Individuals experiencing **auditory hallucinations** hear someone talking to them, when, in reality, no one is. The voice may be that of someone the individual recognizes, or the voice may be unknown to the person. If the voice or voices are comforting, the individual will be very resistant to "giving them up." Most of the time, however, the voices are derogatory in nature, telling the person that there is something wrong with him.

The individual experiencing a **visual hallucination** perceives or sees someone or something that is not actually there. Depending on the nature of the hallucination and whether the individual perceives it as threatening, the situation can be very frightening.

The most serious type of hallucination is referred to as the **command hallucination**, which occurs when the voice or voices tell the individual to harm himself or someone else. For example, the voices may tell the individual to jump off a bridge or building, step in front of a moving motor vehicle, or take an overdose of medication. These hallucinations are extremely dangerous because the demands are so strong that the individual is very likely to act on them.

MEDICAL–SURGICAL MANAGEMENT

Medical

At this time, there is no cure for schizophrenia; however, it is possible for some clients with schizophrenia to lead functional lives with minimally debilitating symptoms through psychosocial treatments.

The goals of psychosocial treatment can be divided into three categories: clinical and family support services, rehabilitative services, and humanitarian aid/public safety. Clinical support involves outpatient management and family/community services. Rehabilitation involves increasing clients' capacities, both for social interactions and for productive activity (including gainful employment, when feasible). Humanitarian interventions are those efforts that maximize an individual's independence and quality of life within the bounds of the mental disability. Public safety involves balancing personal liberty with the recognition that some social control may be needed to prevent harm, both to the individual and to society.

Pharmacological

The most commonly prescribed classification of medications for the client experiencing schizophrenia is the antipsychotics (Tables 17-8 and 17-9). This group of medications is given to reduce the signs and symptoms of psychosis, with a long-term goal of the client eventually being symptom free. If this is not possible, the goal is to reduce symptoms to a manageable level.

Because several side effects are associated with the antipsychotics, client teaching is an important part of the nurse's role. In addition to common side effects, some antipsychotic medications also have the potential for causing adverse reactions such as extrapyramidal symptoms (EPS), tardive dyskinesia (TD), and neuroleptic malignant syndrome (NMS).

One of the most important factors in symptom management for schizophrenia is medication compliance. In most cases, individuals who are schizophrenic must take some type of antipsychotic medication for the remainder of their lives. Clients suffering from schizophrenia are often extremely resistant to taking their medications as prescribed and usually require multiple repeat hospitalizations for stabilization. Multiple reasons exist for noncompliance, one being the client's denial of the diagnosis or the illness or of the seriousness of the illness. As a result of denial, the individual with schizophrenia resists taking medication, because to the client, taking medication equates to acceptance of having a serious mental disorder. Clients may

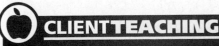

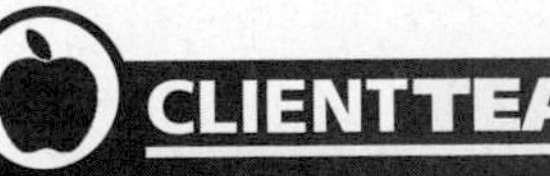

Schizophrenia

Family involvement is important for all clients, but it is especially critical for the client with schizophrenia. Because the client may be too ill or confused to be trusted to take medications reliably, it becomes the responsibility of family members to help ensure medication compliance. Most hospital readmissions for the client with schizophrenia are a result of noncompliance with the prescribed medication regimen. If the family understands the important role psychotropic medications can play in preventing decompensation (a return of the psychiatric symptoms) and subsequent hospital readmission, the client has a much better chance of remaining stabilized.

Table 17-8 Atypical Antipsychotics

GENERIC NAME	TRADE NAME	POTENTIAL SIDE EFFECTS
clozapine	Clozaril	Agranulocytosis, angina, constipation, dizziness, orthostatic hypotension, increased salivation, leukopenia, NMS, drowsiness, seizures, tachycardia, weight gain
olanzapine	Zyprexa	Agitation, acute renal failure, amblyopia, constipation, CVA, dizziness, dry mouth, headache, NMS, orthostatic hypotension, restlessness, rhinitis, sedation, seizures, tachycardia, TD, tremors, weakness, weight gain
quetiapine fumarate	Seroquel	Dizziness, headache, NMS, seizures, TD, weight gain
risperidone	Risperdal	Acute renal failure, constipation, cough, decreased libido, diarrhea, dizziness, dry mouth, dysmenorrhea/menorrhagia, headache, increased dreams, increased sleep duration, insomnia, itching/skin rash, MI, nausea, NMS, pharyngitis, rhinitis, sedation, visual disturbances

Data from *Delmar Nurse's Drug Handbook 2010 Edition*, by G. Spratto and A. Woods, 2010, Clifton Park, NY: Delmar Cengage Learning.

Table 17-9 Phenothiazines (Antipsychotics)

GENERIC NAME	TRADE NAME	POTENTIAL SIDE EFFECTS
chlorpromazine, hydrochloride	Thorazine	Agranulocytosis, blurred vision, constipation, dry eyes, dry mouth, hypotension, laryngeal edema, NMS, photosensitivity, sedation, TD
fluphenazine hydrochloride	Prolixin	Agranulocytosis, EPS, photosensitivity, TD
thioridazine hydrochloride	Mellaril	Agranulocytosis, blurred vision, constipation, dry eyes, dry mouth, hypotension, NMS, photosensitivity, sedation, TD

Data from *Delmar Nurse's Drug Handbook 2010 Edition*, by G. Spratto and A. Woods, 2010, Clifton Park, NY: Delmar Cengage Learning.

CLIENTTEACHING

Adverse Reactions to Antipsychotic Medications

- *Extrapyramidal side effects:* a common adverse reaction of some antipsychotic medications (especially the older ones) involving muscle rigidity and involuntary muscle movements; reversible if the dose is lowered or an anti-Parkinson agent is administered
- *Tardive dyskinesia:* irreversible reaction to antipsychotics (usually associated with high doses over a long period) consisting of involuntary muscle and body movements
- *Neuroleptic malignant syndrome:* a rare and potentially fatal reaction to antipsychotic medications characterized by a very high fever, severe muscle stiffness, and changes in sensorium progressing to coma

also become noncompliant after a period of time on medication; once they start to feel better, they think the medication is no longer needed and stop taking it. After a short time of being off the prescribed medication, however, most individuals with schizophrenia will experience a return or significant worsening of their previous symptoms.

Probably the most common reason for medication noncompliance, however, is the number of troublesome side effects and potentially dangerous adverse reactions historically associated with antipsychotic medications. Fortunately, newer antipsychotic medications are now available that have fewer side effects and are much better tolerated. Even with the advent of these newer and more effective medications, however, many individuals are unable to benefit from them because of the high cost and the difficulties sometimes associated with accessing these medications.

Diet

Some of the antipsychotics such as clozapine (Clozaril), olanzapine (Zyprexa), quetiapine fumerate (Seroquel), and risperidone (Risperdal) can cause weight gain over time. For the individual who has schizophrenia and its multiple

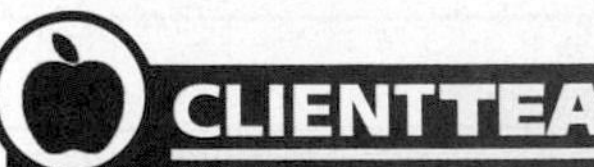

Phenothiazines

Be sure to instruct each client taking a phenothiazine medication in the following:

- Do not drink alcohol while on the medication.
- Do not take any other medications unless prescribed by your physician.
- Do not stop taking the medication abruptly.
- The ability to drive and/or operate heavy machinery may be impaired while taking the medication.
- Be aware of possible side effects of the medication.
- Increase fluid intake to minimize the side effects of dry mouth and constipation.
- Increase dietary fiber to minimize the side effect of constipation.
- Rise slowly from a lying position to prevent dizziness and a sudden drop in blood pressure.
- These medications are contraindicated during pregnancy and lactation. Female clients should advise their physicians immediately if they are either pregnant or planning to become pregnant.
- Wear sunscreen and protective clothing while outdoors, as the medication increases susceptibility to sunburn.
- Some of the side effects may diminish in intensity after an initial period of adjustment.
- The medication may increase your risk of developing EPS, TD, and NMS.

associated problems, weight gain can constitute yet one more stressor. Teaching for the client who is at risk for gaining weight must therefore emphasize the importance of being cognizant of and conservative with regard to caloric and fat intake, avoiding a sedentary lifestyle, and increasing physical activity.

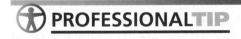

Refrain from Making Judgments

Changing the words we use may help the client and family feel less defensive and may open the door for more effective communication. One example of an often-used term that carries negative connotations is *noncompliance*. Ward-Collins (1998) encourages nurses to consider using another term such as *nonadherence*, which does not carry the same degree of negative connotations.

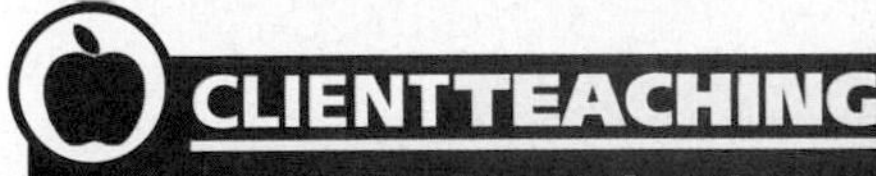

Atypical Antipsychotics

Be sure to instruct each client taking an atypical antipsychotic medication in the following:

- Do not drink alcohol while taking the medication.
- Do not take any other medications, prescription or OTC, unless prescribed by your physician.
- Do not stop taking the medication without authorization from your physician.
- Do not stop taking the medication abruptly.
- The ability to drive and/or operate heavy machinery may be impaired while taking the medication.
- Rise slowly from a lying position to prevent dizziness and a sudden drop in blood pressure.
- The medication is contraindicated during pregnancy and lactation. Reliable contraception should be utilized while taking the medication. Female clients should advise their physicians immediately if they suspect they are either pregnant or planning to become pregnant.
- Be aware of the potential side effects of the medications.
- Notify your physician immediately of unexplained fever, sore throat, bleeding, bruising, or petechiae.
- Wear sunscreen and protective clothing while outdoors, as olanzapine (Zyprexa) and risperidone (Risperdal) increase susceptibility to sunburn.
- Avoid temperature extremes if taking olanzapine (Zyprexa), quetiapine fumerate (Seroquel), or risperidone (Risperdal), as the body's ability to regulate internal temperature is affected by these medications.
- Utilize good oral hygiene in conjunction with sugarless candy or gum to minimize the discomforting side effect of dry mouth associated most frequently with clozapine (Clozaril) and olanzapine (Zyprexa).
- Beware of associated risks including EPS, NMS, and a high risk of agranulocytosis and seizures with clozapine (Clozaril); EPS, TD, and NMS with olanzapine (Zyprexa), quetiapine (Seroquel), and risperidone (Risperdal); and seizures with olanzapine (Zyprexa) and quetiapine fumerate (Seroquel).
- Treatment with clozapine (Clozaril) requires weekly white blood cell (WBC) monitoring to assess for onset of agranulocytosis. Medication is dispensed in 7-day increments to maintain policy compliance and prevent this potentially life-threatening occurrence.

Activity

Clients with schizophrenia tend to be tired and lethargic, probably because of multiple factors including the disease process and, possibly, the sedative properties associated with some of the antipsychotics, especially some of the older ones such as chlorpromazine (Thorazine) and thioridazine (Mellaril).

Nursing Management

Carefully observe the client's behavior. Listen to the client but neither agree nor disagree with what the client is saying. Accurately document what is seen and heard. Include the family in client care. Encourage the client to perform ADLs.

NURSING PROCESS

Assessment

Subjective Data

The client may be very frightened, confused, and have disorganized thought processes, using a nonsensical combination of words that is meaningless to others (**word salad**), talk out loud even when no one is present, or respond to internal stimulation or hallucinations.

Objective Data

The client may be isolated, withdrawn, experience great difficulty in any type of social interaction or situation, and stay in bed and sleep. Thus, the client may require a great deal of assistance and encouragement to perform ADLs and complete basic hygiene needs.

Nursing diagnoses for the client with schizophrenia include the following:

NURSING DIAGNOSES	PLANNING/OUTCOMES	NURSING INTERVENTIONS
*Disturbed **S**ensory Perception (Visual, Auditory)* related to altered sensory perception	The client will experience a decrease in the intensity and frequency of symptoms.	Assess for the presence of hallucinations. Assist the client in beginning to exert some control over the hallucinations. Educate the client about ways to decrease the intensity and power of the hallucinations.
*Deficient **K**nowledge* related to medication therapy	The client will verbalize an understanding of the disorder and the ongoing need for medications.	Educate the client and family about the disorder of Schizophrenia, the need for antipsychotic medications, and the importance of continuing the prescribed medication regimen.

Evaluation: Evaluate each outcome to determine how it has been met by the client.

BIPOLAR DISORDER

Bipolar Disorder (previously known as manic–depressive disorder) is characterized by wide fluctuations in **mood** (the way an individual reports feeling, e.g., depressed, elated, happy, sad) and **affect** (the objective or outward manifestation of the way an individual is feeling). Nearly 6 million Americans have bipolar disorder (DBSA, 2009). Bipolar disorders are a personal and public health concern with as many as 19 % of bipolar individuals dying from suicide, and bipolar disorder ranking sixth as a leading cause of disability in the United States (Antai-Otong, 2008). In addition to having a wide range of both affect and mood, the individual with bipolar disorder may experience fluctuations between depression and **mania** (extremely elevated mood with accompanying agitated behavior). The client with bipolar disorder may experience these fluctuations in mood and affect in varying degrees and over varying time frames. For example, an individual may experience changes in mood and affect every few years, at certain times of the year, every few months, every few weeks, or even every few days. The alterations in mood between depression and mania are often referred to as cycling. Individuals who suffer what is known as rapid cycling may experience multiple swings between depression and mania in the same day. There are also several degrees of both depression and mania that the individual can experience. As is the case with depression, an individual can experience mild, moderate, or severe mania. The degrees of mania range on a continuum from **hypomania** (a mild form of mania without significant impairment) to severe or delirious mania (DBSA, 2006).

An individual in the depressed phase of bipolar disorder will manifest the same signs and symptoms as an individual with depression. The client in the manic phase of bipolar disorder may be very irritable and agitated and can be intimidating toward others, both verbally and physically. The client exhibiting manic behavior is often hyperactive, unable to sit down or remain still, and may display a **euphoric** (being elated out of context to the situation) affect and mood. Once in the manic phase of illness, clients will often exhibit behaviors incongruent with their usual personalities. For example, the manic client may dress in a flamboyant and provocative manner; spend money and buy things in a very lavish fashion; and become sexually promiscuous and engage in risky behaviors that would otherwise be out of character. After a while, the client may experience a great deal of conflict in social, familial, and personal relationships. It often becomes the responsibility of a significant other or family member to seek professional assistance for the individual. This already difficult situation is compounded by the fact that the client

Table 17-10 Mood Stabilizer: Antimanic

GENERIC NAME	TRADE NAME	POTENTIAL SIDE EFFECTS	SIGNS AND SYMPTOMS OF TOXICITY
lithium carbonate	Eskalith, Lithonate	Abdominal pain, acneiform eruption, anorexia, arrhythmia, bloating, diarrhea, dizziness, drowsiness, EKG changes, fatigue, folliculitis, GI upset, headache, hypothyroidism, impaired memory, irritability, leukocytosis, muscle weakness, nausea, polyuria, seizures, tinnitus, tremors	Ataxia, change in level of orientation, confusion, diarrhea, drowsiness, excessive urination, lack of coordination, muscle weakness, tremors, vomiting

Data from *Delmar Nurse's Drug Handbook 2010 Edition,* by G. Spratto and A. Woods, 2010, Clifton Park, NY: Delmar Cengage Learning.

in the manic phase of bipolar disorder is frequently in denial about the illness, does not perceive the erratic behavior as problematic, and enjoys the "high" created by the disorder. As a result, the individual often refuses any type of help, and the family may be required to seek involuntary hospitalization in order to obtain the much-needed treatment.

Medical–Surgical Management

Medical

The severely agitated client in the manic phase of bipolar disorder may need to be secluded and/or restrained in order to protect against self-inflicted injury and/or the risk of injury to others.

Psychotherapy may be helpful to the client experiencing bipolar disorder, but it is not recommended as the only intervention. These clients typically require some type of medication management for the remainder of their lives in order to function adequately.

Pharmacological

The drug of choice for treatment of bipolar disorder is lithium carbonate (Lithonate) (Table 17-10). Lithium is a naturally occurring salt that has proven highly effective for many individuals in managing the severe mood swings associated with bipolar disorder. Lithium is referred to as a "mood stabilizer," meaning that it helps level or even out the wide mood swings associated with the disorder; however, some individuals either cannot tolerate lithium therapy or become resistant to its therapeutic effectiveness after a period of time. Fortunately, some other medications are often prescribed for clients who cannot take lithium. These include the anticonvulsants valproic acid (Depakene) and carbamazepine (Tegretol) (Table 17-11) and the anxiolytic/anticonvulsant clonazepam (Klonopin).

Lithium has a very narrow range of therapeutic effectiveness. The amount of lithium the individual has available and whether this level is appropriate is measured by a blood test called serum lithium level. The acceptable therapeutic range for the **serum lithium level** is 0.4 to 1.0 mEq/L; however, the value may vary slightly depending on the laboratory that is performing the test (Spratto & Woods, 2008). A lithium level that is too low will not produce any benefit, and one that is too high may be toxic, or poisonous. It is therefore critical that the serum lithium level be obtained every 5 days until the client is stabilized on the medication. Blood should then be drawn monthly for as long as the client is taking the medication (Spratto & Woods, 2008). Before initiating lithium therapy, a 24-hour urine creatinine clearance test is done to evaluate the functioning of the kidneys and their ability to adequately excrete the lithium.

Diet

Because lithium is a salt that is chemically similar to sodium chloride (table salt), lithium and sodium compete for

Table 17-11 Mood Stabilizers: Anticonvulsants

GENERIC NAME	TRADE NAME	POTENTIAL SIDE EFFECTS
carbamazepine	Tegretol	Agranulocytosis, aplastic anemia, ataxia, drowsiness, drug induced hepatitis, thrombocytopenia
valproic acid	Depakene	Depression, dizziness, indigestion, hepatotoxicity, leukopenia, nausea, thrombocytopenia, vomiting, weight gain

Data from *Delmar Nurse's Drug Handbook 2010 Edition*, by G. Spratto and A. Woods, 2010, Clifton Park, NY: Delmar Cengage Learning.

LIFE SPAN CONSIDERATIONS

Lithium Use in Older Adults

Because older adults have a reduced creatinine clearance, they are at greater risk for developing toxicity while taking lithium. Use caution in the older adult because lithium is more toxic to the central nervous system. The older adult may also develop a lithium-induced goiter and hypothyroidism (Spratto & Woods, 2010).

CLIENT TEACHING

Lithium

Be sure to instruct each client taking lithium in the following:

- Do not drink alcohol while taking this medication.
- Do not take any other medications, prescribed or OTC, unless authorized by your physician.
- Do not stop taking this medication without authorization from your physician.
- Female clients should utilize a reliable form of contraception while taking this medication. Immediately inform your physician if pregnancy is suspected.
- Drink 2,000 to 3,000 mL of fluid (10–12 glasses) per day.
- Maintain a consistent level of salt in the diet.
- The ability to drive or operate heavy machinery may be impaired while on this medication.
- Serum lithium level must be checked at scheduled intervals throughout therapy.
- Be aware of signs and symptoms of lithium toxicity.

absorption at receptor sites. This relationship is inversely proportional; thus, any changes in the body's sodium level will directly affect lithium level. Adequate fluid intake is very important for the client on lithium therapy. It is recommended that the client taking lithium consume a minimum of 2,000 to 3,000 mL of water per day. Because of the stimulating effects of caffeine, clients taking lithium should avoid any beverages containing caffeine.

Activity

The balance of sodium chloride to lithium can also be affected by the client's level of activity. An increase in activity, especially in hot and/or humid conditions when excessive perspiration is likely, can deplete the client's sodium level, thereby causing a drastic increase in lithium level and, potentially, lithium toxicity. A sudden increase in a client's activity level requires close monitoring and replacement of both fluid and electrolytes in order to prevent a sudden increase in the lithium level.

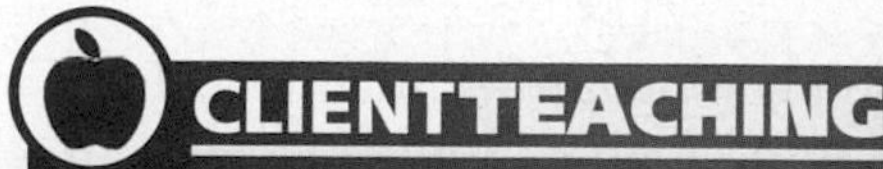

Anticonvulsants

Be sure to instruct each client taking an anticonvulsant medication in the following:

- Do not drink alcohol while taking the medication.
- Do not take any other medications, prescribed or OTC, unless authorized by your physician.
- Take the medication exactly as prescribed.
- Do not stop taking the medication without authorization from your physician.
- Do not stop taking the medication abruptly.
- The medications are contraindicated during pregnancy and lactation. Female clients should advise their physicians immediately if they are either pregnant or planning to become pregnant.
- Carbamazepine (Tegretol) can impair the effectiveness of hormonal forms of contraception. Female clients should practice an alternate form of birth control while on this medication.
- The ability to drive or operate heavy machinery may be impaired while on the medication.
- Laboratory tests monitoring complete blood count (CBC), platelet count, bleeding time, and hepatic functioning must be performed periodically throughout therapy.
- Notify your physician immediately of unexplained fever, sore throat, bleeding, bruising, or petechiae.
- Serum level must be checked at scheduled intervals throughout therapy.

NURSING MANAGEMENT

Include the family in client education about the disease process, illness progression, medications, and importance

CASE STUDY

Bipolar Disorder

A 28-year-old male client is admitted to the psychiatric unit with a diagnosis of Bipolar Disorder. He is unable to sleep, in constant motion, very talkative, exaggerating and glamorizing life events, and inappropriately talking about sexual promiscuity to other clients.

1. The client is exhibiting which phase of bipolar disorder?
2. The drug of choice for treatment of bipolar disorder is?
3. List two types of treatment for bipolar disorder.

of taking the medications as prescribed (even if the client's condition improves dramatically). Emphasize the need to keep follow-up appointments and to have lab work done for lithium level. Encourage the family to help the client maintain a regular eating and sleeping schedule.

NURSING PROCESS

ASSESSMENT

Subjective Data

The client may deny having a problem or may view the problem as residing in other people. The client may also be quite loud, flamboyant, and grandiose in verbalizations and manifest very quick and **pressured speech** (rapid, intense speech).

Objective Data

The client may be sleeping very little or not at all and may not be eating or drinking, if in the manic phase. The client may at times be very irritable, agitated, quick to anger, and, possibly, violent. Clients with bipolar disorder often have extreme difficulty in interpersonal and social relationships because they have no personal boundaries. They may also be invasive and intrusive in their interactions with others, both verbally and physically.

Nursing diagnoses for the client with bipolar disorder include the following:

NURSING DIAGNOSES	PLANNING/OUTCOMES	NURSING INTERVENTIONS
*Disturbed **Sleep** Pattern* related to sensory alterations	The client will sleep 6 hours per night.	Provide a quiet, peaceful environment. Decrease external stimulation and environmental distractions. Teach client relaxation exercises.
***N**oncompliance (medication and treatment regimen)* related to health beliefs	The client will demonstrate increased compliance with medication and treatment.	Educate the client and family about the disease process and the progression of the illness over time, prescribed medication, indications for use, dosage, times, and any possible side effects or untoward reactions, and the importance of taking the medication as prescribed. Teach the client to continue taking medication and to not miss doses *even if the condition improves dramatically.*

Evaluation: Evaluate each outcome to determine how it has been met by the client.

THE CLIENT REQUIRING SPECIAL CONSIDERATION

Several disorders require special attention and consideration on the part of the nurse. These include disorders commonly associated with childhood and adolescence and with individuals who have been violated in some manner, such as via neglect and/or abuse.

ATTENTION-DEFICIT/ HYPERACTIVITY DISORDER

The *DSM-IV* identifies 18 diagnostic criteria for Attention-Deficit/Hyperactivity Disorder (ADHD) that fall under the categories of *inattention, hyperactivity,* and *impulsivity* (APA, 2000). There are three varieties of Attention-Deficit/Hyperactivity Disorder listed in the DSM-IV: Attention-Deficit/Hyperactivity Disorder, Predominantly Hyperactive-Impulsive Type; Attention-Deficit/Hyperactivity Disorder, Predominantly Inattentive Type; and Attention-Deficit/Hyperactivity Disorder, Combined Type. The child with ADHD may exhibit one or more of these behaviors in any combination (inattention, hyperactivity, and impulsivity). The problematic behaviors associated with these disorders vary in severity for each individual. Once thought to be a disorder only of childhood, it is now known that ADHD may continue well into adulthood. Individuals with ADHD are extremely sensitive to their environments and surroundings and respond immediately to any type of stimuli or distraction that most individuals would not even notice.

PROFESSIONALTIP

Token-Economy System

A token-economy system is a form of behavior modification used to shape a client's behavior over time. The client receives a "token" (poker chips work well) each time an appropriate or desired behavior is exhibited. In the classroom, the desired behavior might be working 15 minutes on a math assignment; at home, it might be picking up dirty clothes from the floor. Receiving the token is a form of positive reinforcement for the client and provides immediate gratification. At the end of a designated period, the client may "cash in" earned tokens for a prize (game, puzzle) or a special privilege (going to get an ice cream). The cashing in of tokens emphasizes the concept of delayed gratification, which in turn teaches patience.

PREDOMINANTLY HYPERACTIVE-IMPULSIVE TYPE

Hyperactivity is the hallmark feature of Predominantly Hyperactive-Impulsive Type ADHD, which is usually diagnosed in childhood when the symptoms first manifest. The pediatric client with ADHD may be referred for evaluation and treatment by parents or teachers because of impulsive and disruptive behavior in the classroom and/or at home. In many cases, there seems to be a familial or possible genetic link, as seen in health histories, which often reveal a parent or immediate family member as having had a similar problem as a child.

PREDOMINANTLY INATTENTIVE TYPE

In some children with ADHD predominantly inattentive type, the symptom of hyperactivity is not always present. The children have problems primarily with attention span. The inattentive child cannot maintain attention on one task, does not appear to listen when spoken to, and is easily distracted and forgetful.

COMBINED TYPE

Children with ADHD of the combined type exhibit symptoms of hyperactivity, impulsivity, and inattention. The characteristics must typically be exhibited for a period of at least 6 months in order to qualify for the diagnosis.

MEDICAL–SURGICAL MANAGEMENT

Medical

Counseling and therapy are often recommended to the client and family to assist in managing the child. The parents will require assistance in developing an effective behavior-modification program, such as a token-economy system that rewards desired behaviors, to help manage some of the child's problematic behaviors.

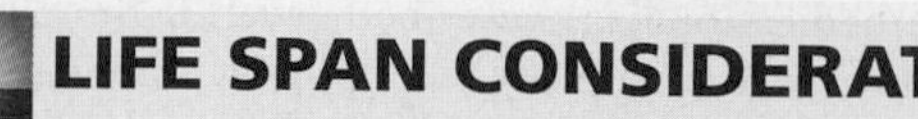

LIFE SPAN CONSIDERATIONS

ADHD

In the past, it was believed that most children would outgrow ADHD. Today, it is known that symptoms of ADHD can continue into adulthood (Antai-Otong, 2008).

Pharmacological

The central nervous system (CNS) stimulants, which include methylphenidate hydrochloride (Ritalin), pemoline (Cylert), dextroamphetamine sulfate (Dexedrine), and amphetamine sulfate (Adderall), are usually prescribed to treat ADHD (Table 17-12). When one of the CNS stimulants is given to someone with ADHD, however, it has the opposite effect, or **paradoxical reaction**. Thus, instead of making someone with ADHD more hyperactive, it actually helps calm him. Because most of the symptoms of the child with ADHD, such as hyperactivity and the inability to concentrate and remain on task, are manifested in the classroom, any improvement will likely first be noted in this setting. When a child begins a new medication, it is vitally important that the family communicate openly with the child's teacher to ensure close monitoring of the child's response to medication. The child with ADHD who has been hyperactive, unable to stay on task, or complete assignments before receiving medication may now be less disruptive in the classroom and better able to remain on task and complete assignments. In addition, the medication can be a useful adjunct to facilitate the child's ability to develop and strengthen internal mechanisms for improving behavior.

Table 17-12 Central Nervous System Stimulants

GENERIC NAME	TRADE NAME	POTENTIAL SIDE EFFECTS
dextroamphetamine sulfate	Dexedrine	Anorexia, headache, hyperactivity, hypertension, insomnia, palpitations, physical and psychological dependence, restlessness, tachycardia, tolerance, tremors, urticaria, weight loss
amphetamine sulfate	Adderall	Anorexia, hyperactivity, insomnia, palpitations, physical and psychological dependence, restlessness, tachycardia, tremors
methylphenidate hydrochloride	Ritalin	Anemia, anorexia, hyperactivity, hypertension, insomnia, leukopenia, physical and psychological dependence, restlessness, skin rash, suppression of weight gain, tolerance, tremors
pemoline	Cylert	Insomnia, anorexia, aplastic anemia, decreased growth, drug-induced hepatitis, nausea, physical or psychological dependence, seizures, stomachache, tolerance, weight loss
atomoxetine hydrochloride	Strattera	Fatigue, decreased appetite, aggression, nausea, vomiting, postural hypotension

Data from *Delmar Nurse's Drug Handbook 2010 Edition*, by G. Spratto and A. Woods, 2010, Clifton Park, NY: Delmar Cengage Learning.

Teaching the client and family about the prescribed medication is very important, as there are some common side effects associated with the CNS stimulants, such as insomnia. To help decrease the risk of insomnia, these medications are usually given in the morning at breakfast, and if more is needed, another dose is given again at lunchtime. In some cases, a late-afternoon dose may be needed after school; however, this decision must be made very cautiously, because the later in the day that the dose is given, the greater the risk of insomnia that night for the child.

The client on CNS stimulants must be monitored for any vocal or motor tics, which might indicate the development of Tourette's syndrome. The CNS stimulant should be discontinued immediately if these symptoms are noted.

Diet

One potential problem associated with the CNS stimulants is that of decreased appetite, which can become serious if the child begins losing weight as a side effect of the medication. If this occurs, the medication may be given immediately after a meal to decrease the chance of appetite suppression. The family can adjust the timing and amount of food intake, such as eating larger meals later in the day, when the effects of the medication have worn off, or having a larger snack in the evening before bedtime.

The role and importance of diet in the management of ADHD continues to be highly controversial; however, some data supports the restriction of certain foods as an effective method of managing this disorder. Foods that contain sugar and caffeine are sometimes recommended to be excluded from the diet of the child with ADHD. The theory behind this recommendation is that sugar and caffeine tend to energize and increase any child's activity level, and in the case of some children with ADHD, this effect seems to be even more accentuated. Another controversial issue surrounding the significance of diet is that of food sensitivities and allergies. Food allergies sometimes manifest in symptoms such as irritability and hyperactivity, which may then be confused or misdiagnosed as ADHD.

Activity

The child with ADHD will usually respond best to a highly structured environment, which includes clear expectations and firm, consistent limits as well as appropriate consequences for unruly and disruptive behaviors. For example, a "time-out" may be used when the child must be temporarily removed from a setting or the environment.

Nursing Management

Monitor growth (height and weight) and development. Explain to the client what comprise acceptable behaviors. Provide positive reinforcement for appropriate behavior. Teach the client and family about prescribed medications.

NURSING PROCESS

Assessment

Subjective Data

The child or adolescent frequently verbalizes feeling "bad" about being unable to control hyperactive and disruptive behaviors and feeling like a failure, especially in the classroom. After only a single dose of medication, however, the child sometimes states a noticeable difference in the ability to remain centered and focused.

Objective Data

Although usually described as being hyperactive, unable to concentrate, unable to focus, and unable to remain on task, children with ADHD may sometimes be able to concentrate and remain quite attentive and focused. This usually happens in situations that the child enjoys and sometimes in situations that are new to the child. It can be quite frustrating for parents to bring in their child for an evaluation or screening, only to have the child not exhibit any of the usual problematic behaviors. The knowledgeable practitioner or evaluator will be aware of what is happening and will obtain the necessary information from the parental report of the child's health history.

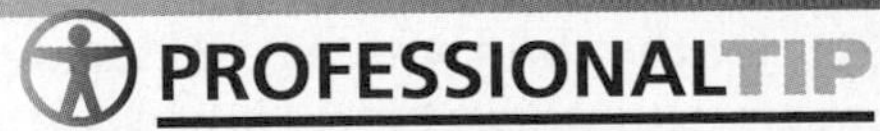

CNS-Stimulant Abuse

Another consideration often overlooked in terms of the CNS stimulants is the risk for abuse because of the strong addictive potential of these medications. Not only is the client with ADHD at risk for abusing these medications, but sometimes the client "shares" prescribed medication with schoolmates and friends interested in drug experimentation. Another problem that may be encountered is abuse of the prescribed medication by a family member with a substance-abuse problem.

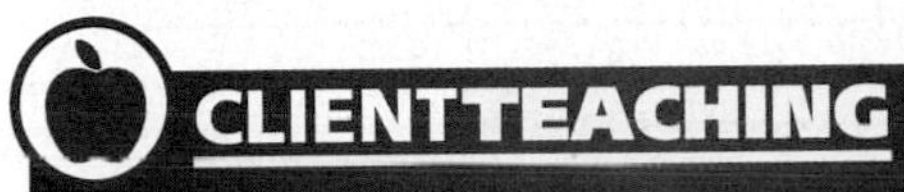

CNS Stimulants

For each client taking a CNS-stimulant medication, instruct the client or, if the client is too young to understand or reliably carry out the instructions, the client's caregivers in the following:

- Take the medication only as prescribed.
- Do not take any other medications without physician approval.
- Be alert for decreased appetite and adjust meals and mealtimes accordingly.
- Do not take any doses after 5 p.m. because doing so will increase the risk of insomnia.
- Obtain periodic liver function tests if taking pemoline (Cylert).
- Obtain periodic CBC, platelet count, and differential if taking methylphenidate (Ritalin).
- Limit caffeine intake.

Nursing diagnoses for the child with ADHD include the following:

NURSING DIAGNOSES	PLANNING/OUTCOMES	NURSING INTERVENTIONS
Deficient Knowledge (medications and disease process) related to new diagnosis of disorder and treatment regimen	The child and parents will verbalize an increased understanding of the disorder. The child and parents will verbalize an understanding about the role medications can play in treatment.	Educate the child and family about the disorder, including signs and symptoms, about the medication, including indications for use, dosages, when to take the medication, possible side effects, and the benefits that can be expected with the particular medication. Emphasize the importance of taking the medication as prescribed.
Impaired Social Interaction related to unaccepted social behaviors	The child will demonstrate an increase in appropriate peer interactions.	Explain to the child those behaviors that are acceptable. Observe the child in social situations with peers. Provide positive reinforcement for demonstration of appropriate behaviors. Immediately intervene when unacceptable behaviors are observed.

Evaluation: Evaluate each outcome to determine how it has been met by the client.

NEGLECT AND/OR ABUSE

There are many types of **neglect** (a situation wherein a basic need of the client is not being provided) and **abuse** (an incident involving some type of violation to the client). Neglect can be quite evident, such as a lack of adequate food, clothing, or shelter, or less tangible, such as emotional neglect or an absence of nurturing. Abuse can be physical, emotional, psychological, financial, or sexual in nature, or any combination of these. Abuse can also take the form of **domestic violence**, which is aggression and violence involving family members. Neglect and abuse often go hand in hand.

A client experiencing neglect or abuse is usually dependent on another individual for the meeting of basic care and needs. In many neglectful or abusive situations, the clients are vulnerable individuals such as children, adolescents, or elders. Others who are neglected or abused include individuals with some type of illness or incapacitation. Neglect and abuse can take many shapes and forms, ranging anywhere from mild cases to situations so severe that death is the end result.

ELDER ABUSE AND NEGLECT

Elder abuse became nationally recognized in 1981 after the House Select Committee on Aging issued its landmark report *Elder Abuse: An Examination of a Hidden Problem.* The committee found that elder abuse was simply "alien to the American ideal." Because it is such a difficult concept to come to grips with, even abused elders are reluctant to admit that their loved ones have abused them.

The committee defined the following types of elder abuse: physical, passive physical, financial, psychological, sexual, and violation of rights. There is no federal legislation to protect elders from abuse, neglect, or exploitation. All 50 states, including the District of Columbia, have some form of elder abuse prevention laws (AoA, 2003). Adult abuse and protection laws are based on the legal premise that society (represented by the state) has the authority to act in a parental capacity for persons who are unable to care for and protect themselves and thus prevent them from suffering from abuse, neglect, or exploitation by those responsible for their care or from self-abuse (Frisch & Frisch, 2010). The purposes of adult protection service laws are to facilitate the identification of functionally impaired elders who are being abused, neglected, or exploited by others; to encourage expeditious reporting; and to extend protective services while protecting the rights of the abused. In most states, the adult protective services (APS) agency is the principal agency designated to receive and investigate allegations of elder abuse and neglect. In most jurisdictions, the county departments of social services maintain the APS unit.

The National Elder Abuse Incidence Study of 1996 found that almost 450,000 persons age 60 and older experienced abuse and/or neglect in domestic settings. Only 16% were reported to APS; that is, less than 1 of 5 cases were reported. Persons age 80 and older were abused and neglected two to three times their proportion of the elderly population.

LIFE SPAN CONSIDERATIONS

Teen Dating Violence

Teen dating violence is a serious public health concern in the United States. Three common types of dating violence are physical, emotional, and sexual. Approximately 10% of students report being physically hurt by a boyfriend or girlfriend in the past 12 months (CDC, 2008b).

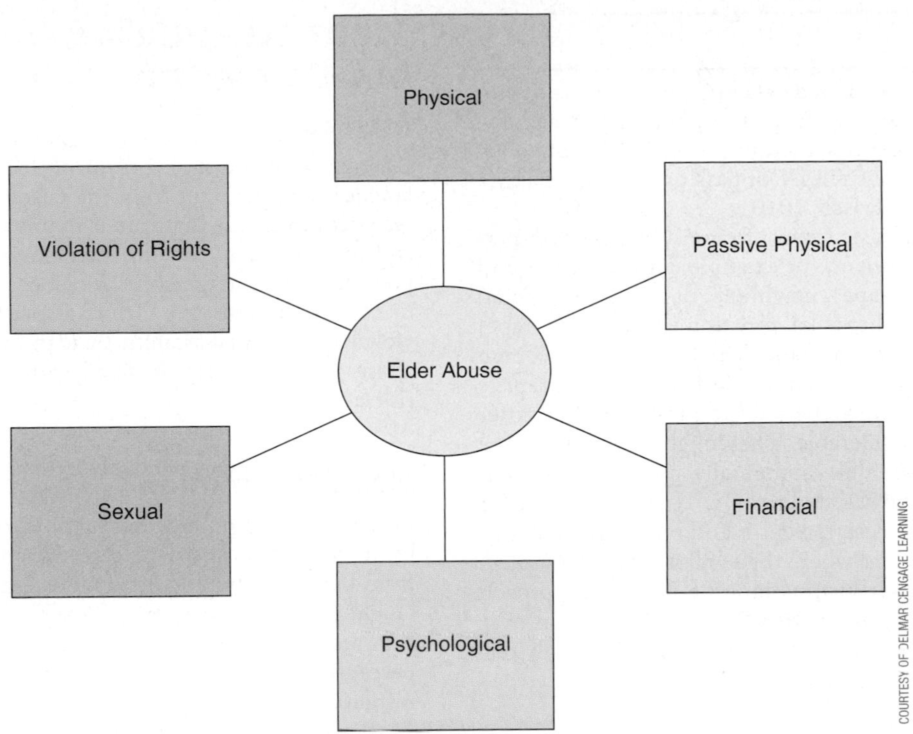

FIGURE 17-4 Types of Elder Abuse

DOMESTIC VIOLENCE

Domestic violence is a pattern of controlling behavior and assaults, including physical, sexual, and psychological attacks and economic control, that adolescents and adults use against their intimate partners. It is common and lethal, affecting people of all ages, cultures, religions, sexual orientations, educational backgrounds, and income levels.

Domestic violence occurs in relationships where conflict is the continuous result of power inequality between partners. One of the partners is afraid of and harmed by the other. In all cultures, the perpetrators are most often men and the victims are most often women (National Coalition Against Domestic Violence [NCADV], 2005).

In all states, domestic violence is a crime, but the laws in each state are a little different. The nurse is responsible for knowing the laws, especially mandatory reporting, about domestic violence in the state of employment. Each state has a coalition against domestic violence, which are valuable resources. The National Domestic Violence Hotline is 800-799-7233 (SAFE).

CRITICAL THINKING

Domestic Violence

What are your feelings about domestic violence? How would you react to a client who was a victim of domestic violence? Would you be able to respond appropriately? What if the client refuses your attempt to assist her to leave the abusive situation?

PROFESSIONALTIP

Caring for the Abused Client

When questioning clients about the possibility of interpersonal violence or sexual assault, the nurse must quickly develop a rapport and create an environment indicating that personal experiences are acceptable topics to discuss. This allows them the opportunity to express their fears and concerns. This can be done by:

- Treating them with dignity and concern.
- Giving priority to them over nonemergency clients.
- Placing them in quiet and private areas.
- Not leaving them alone.
- Speaking quietly and in a nonjudgmental manner.
- Using active and empathic listening skills.
- Not acting shocked or surprised at the details of their experiences.
- Reassuring them that the abuse was not their fault.
- Explaining any delays in treatment.
- Asking permission to call family members, friends, or in the case of rape, rape crisis advocates.
- Providing information about community resources.

RAPE

Rape is a legal term, not a medical entity. It is a crime of violence. Rapists use sexual violence to dominate and degrade their victims and to express their own anger. It is not an act of lust or an overzealous release of passion done to satisfy a sexual urge (Frisch & Frisch, 2010).

There are three basic types of rape: (1) rape by a person known to the survivor, for example, father, former and current friends (date rape), neighbors, partner or separated partner, dissatisfied clients of prostitutes; (2) gang rape; and (3) stranger-to-stranger rape. The latter, which women fear the most, follows an identifiable pattern. Such rapists look for women who are vulnerable, even though they differ on defining who is vulnerable. They might attempt to rape elders, people who are developmentally, physically, or mentally challenged, or intoxicated people. They might look for environments that are easy to enter and relatively safe (e.g., women's bedrooms) and where they will not be interrupted. They often select their victims long before they approach them and repeat the same pattern of victim selection over and over again. All types of rape can be an emotionally terrorizing experience for the survivors.

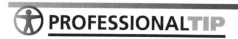

PROFESSIONALTIP

Interviewing the Survivor of Abuse or Violence

The type of questions will depend on the type of violence and whether survivors have told you they have been abused. If they have told you they have been abused, you must ask specific questions about the abuse. If they have not, you must ask more open-ended questions to allow them to disclose sensitive information. Generally speaking:

- Inform the client that it is necessary to ask some very personal questions.
- Use language appropriate for the age and developmental level of the survivor.
- Use conversational language or street language.
- Keep questions simple, nonthreatening, and direct.
- Pose questions in a manner that permits brief answers.
- Indicate sensitivity to and acceptance of the client's state of confusion.
- Avoid using leading statements that can distort the client's report.
- Do not criticize the client's family.
- Do not promise not to report the abuse; indicate that you are required by law to report the abuse.

MEDICAL–SURGICAL MANAGEMENT

Medical

Planning care for survivors of neglect and abuse and their families requires input from the clients and a survey of their resources to ensure that care is in line with their expectations and commitments. Nursing interventions directed at primary prevention of interpersonal violence are those that reduce or control the causative factors associated with interpersonal violence and sexual assaults. By identifying families at risk for abuse, nurses can help the family plan efforts to modify those risk factors.

Health Promotion

Primary prevention includes empowering survivors of abuse by helping them learn to care for and protect themselves from the imposition by others. For example, children can be taught in health care settings or schools those things to do if they are being abused. It also includes changing the family's perceptions of violence as an acceptable mode of conflict resolution.

Provide anticipatory guidance. For example, by anticipating the challenges of toddlerhood, acknowledge that this can be a difficult period for parents and provide practical advice about constructive discipline. Teach college freshmen about date rape and to avoid vulnerable situations. Encourage families with dependent elderly members to use respite care services and day care programs. Such support and anticipatory guidance can enhance the family's and client's competence and diminish the likelihood of violence or abuse.

NURSING MANAGEMENT

Know the mandatory reporting laws in your state of employment. When assessing clients, ask about bruises, scars, and burns when seen. Provide anticipatory guidance for challenging events in a client's family life that will enhance the family's competence and diminish the probability of abuse or violence.

NURSING PROCESS

ASSESSMENT

Subjective Data

There is no comprehensive assessment tool that offers conclusive evidence that neglect, abuse, or violence has occurred. Act like detectives when assessing clients, given that clients or their abusers will rarely admit to abuse or violence. Make direct observations of the client and family members (e.g., Does the child seem afraid of the caregiver? Does the caregiver hit the child?). These observations are clues that more probing is necessary.

To properly assess survivors of abuse, the symptoms that are commonly seen in interpersonal violence and sexual assaults and the common characteristics of the abusers must be known. Many of the symptoms are subjective, so the health care team must piece together the evidence to ascertain whether interpersonal violence has occurred or clients are at risk for violence. Psychological abuse is a particularly difficult area to assess because emotional relationships are very culture bound, and words and emotions that may be harmful in one family are not necessarily so in another family.

Objective Data

A more extensive examination is warranted when the history or behavioral symptoms indicate interpersonal abuse. Clients need to have physical examinations to assess the extent of their injuries and to collect forensic evidence to prove who assaulted them. A traumagram, or body map (a drawing of the front and back of a nude human figure), is generally used to mark the location of all visible injuries. Each state has legally mandated procedures for collecting evidentiary material, and it is a nursing responsibility to be sure that the legal "chain of evidence" pertaining to collection of forensic samples is unbroken. The medical record should document the injuries and nursing and medical treatment that may serve as legal evidence of the client's condition.

Nursing diagnoses for the client experiencing neglect or abuse include the following:

NURSING DIAGNOSES	PLANNING/OUTCOMES	NURSING INTERVENTIONS
*Interrupted **Family** Processes* related to neglect	The client will not experience any further Neglect.	Provide support for the client. Document the evidence of neglect with which the client presents via written observations, laboratory reports, and/or pictures, if indicated. Report the case of neglect to the proper authorities: police, child protective services (CPS), APS, and any others that might be indicated.
Fear related to abuse	The client will verbalize being less fearful.	Reassure the client that the client is in a safe place and that you are there to help in any way that you can. Provide emotional support to the client in a nonjudgmental manner.
*Risk for **Injury*** related to abusive home life	The client will not experience any further injury or abuse.	Address the client's safety needs and attempt to assess whether abuse is occurring. If you suspect that abuse is occurring notify your supervisor so the proper authorities can be notified (Ladebauche, 1997).

Evaluation: Evaluate each outcome to determine how it has been met by the client.

EATING DISORDERS

Eating disorders include anorexia nervosa and bulimia nervosa. Anorexia nervosa is characterized by self-imposed starvation by restricting caloric intake and compulsive exercising. Bulimia nervosa is characterized by periods of binge eating of up to 10,000 calories at one time followed by self-induced vomiting and other forms of purging such as laxative and diuretic abuse. In bulimia nervosa, the client's weight is normal or above normal. In anorexia nervosa, body weight is low and keeps getting lower. Most clients with these disorders are female and younger than age 30.

Complications can be serious and include cardiac abnormalities such as bradycardia, hypotension, arrhythmias, CHF, and cardiovascular collapse; oral and esophageal erosions and dental caries from vomiting; renal abnormalities that affect the kidney's ability to filter urine; skin rashes from malnutrition; and bruising from vomiting.

Clients with anorexia nervosa tend to be high achievers, perfectionists, have a distorted body image in that they see themselves as fat, and are rigid and ritualistic.

Bulimia nervosa occurs more frequently than anorexia nervosa, with clients experiencing a fear of not being able to stop eating. Clients often experience guilt and depression after a binge.

MEDICAL–SURGICAL MANAGEMENT

Diet

During severe cases, clients may be admitted for enforced feeding, including the placement of a feeding tube or TPN, IV fluid rehydration, and electrolyte replacement. Clients need to be monitored for refeeding complications such as pancreatitis and gastric dilation. Small quantities are given at first, and very gradually the amount is increased.

Other Therapies

Treatment is primarily psychiatric, involving the client and family, and is typically done on an outpatient basis.

NURSING MANAGEMENT

Monitor weight, calorie intake, I&O, and exercise program. Assess behavior around mealtime. Administer IV fluid and electrolyte replacement. Check vital signs and laboratory test results.

NURSING PROCESS

ASSESSMENT

Subjective Data

Clients with either anorexia nervosa or bulimia nervosa may verbalize feelings of helplessness and being out of control, and may exhibit low self-esteem. They may also have overprotective parents. Clients with anorexia nervosa may also describe bad dreams and cold intolerance.

Objective Data

Clients with anorexia nervosa are underweight, usually lost over a short period of time, reluctant to eat with others, move food around the plate without eating it, hypotensive, have heart irregularities, and altered thinking patterns.

Clients with bulimia nervosa have normal weight, tooth erosions and dental caries, puffy face, callused knuckles, broken blood vessels in the eyes and face, reluctance to eat with others, and going to the bathroom immediately after eating.

Laboratory analysis will include a CBC, which may show low Hgb, Hct, and platelets; electrolytes, which may show low sodium, potassium, and chloride; an SMA-22 that shows low protein, phosphate, and magnesium; and elevated BUN.

Nursing diagnoses for a hospitalized client with anorexia nervosa or bulimia nervosa include the following:

NURSING DIAGNOSES	PLANNING/OUTCOMES	NURSING INTERVENTIONS
*Imbalanced **N**utrition: Less than Body Requirements* related to psychological restriction of food intake, excessive activity	The client will demonstrate increased consumption of nutrients as evidenced by weight gain daily and improved laboratory values.	Weigh daily. Monitor calorie intake. Monitor I&O every shift. Administer IV rehydration, electrolyte replacement, and TPN or tube feedings as ordered. Monitor behavior at and around meal time, such as going to the bathroom right after eating. Monitor exercise patterns.
*Risk for Deficient **F**luid Volume* related to inadequate intake of liquids, self-induced vomiting, laxative and diuretic use	The client's intake and output will be approximately equal by the fourth hospital day. The client's electrolytes will be within normal limits, by the third hospital day. The client's fluid intake will be at least 2,000 mL per day.	Monitor I&O every shift and bowel movements for diarrhea (a sign of continued laxative abuse). Monitor laboratory reports for electrolyte levels as ordered. Administer IV fluid and electrolyte replacement as ordered.
*Ineffective **C**oping (Individual)* related tomaturational crisis andattempting to control environment	The client will verbalize feelings regarding disease process and hospitalization, by discharge. The client will identify current coping strategies, by discharge. The client will identify personal strengths, by discharge.	Provide opportunities for the client to express feelings regarding hospitalization. Encourage client to identify coping mechanisms and strengths. Give positive feedback regarding identified personal strengths.

Evaluation: Evaluate each outcome to determine how it has been met by the client.

SUMMARY

- The components of a therapeutic nurse–client relationship include trust, rapport, respect, genuineness, and empathy.
- An individual's anxiety level may range anywhere from mild to panic level.
- The nurse often encounters clients and/or family members who are angry, aggressive, homicidal, and/or suicidal in the midst of a crisis situation.
- The depressed individual must be evaluated for risk of suicide.
- The individual with schizophrenia may be out of touch with reality and influenced by delusions and/or hallucinations.
- Individuals with bipolar disorder may experience wide mood swings ranging from depression to mania.
- Neglect and abuse can occur among any age group.
- Anorexia nervosa and bulimia nervosa are psychological disorders affecting mostly women. Severe nutritional imbalances can occur leading to serious effects on the cardiovascular system.

REVIEW QUESTIONS

1. The client who is experiencing severe or panic level anxiety should:
   1. be left alone to calm down.
   2. be taught new information.
   3. never be left alone.
   4. be given an antidepressant immediately.
2. A nurse who is aware of a client's plan to kill someone else should:
   1. do nothing; it is not her responsibility.
   2. contact the physician and alert the proper authorities.
   3. discourage the client from following through with the plan.
   4. continue preparing the client for discharge per orders in the chart.
3. Components of a therapeutic nurse–client relationship include: (Select all that apply.)
   1. genuineness.
   2. rapport.
   3. independence.
   4. trust.
   5. mild anxiety.
   6. respect.
4. A client experiencing panic level anxiety informs the nurse that she is hearing the voice of her deceased husband and wants it to stop. The most appropriate nursing action is to:
   1. provide constant reassurance, monitoring, and supervision.
   2. apply wrist restraints.
   3. place all four bed side rails up.
   4. medicate the client with a sedative and supervise for safety.
5. The nurse notices that a client on your unit is giving away prized personal possessions to his family and friends. This action is indicative of:
   1. a client that is schizophrenic.
   2. a client that is contemplating suicide.
   3. a client that is experiencing excessive anxiety.
   4. an anorexic client that is recovering.
6. A client has an order for Paxil 12.5 mg one tablet every morning. Which of the following client statements indicates that further teaching is needed?
   1. "I should take the medication on an empty stomach."
   2. "Paxil can cause drowsiness."
   3. "I cannot drink alcohol while taking Paxil."
   4. "I should put on sunscreen when outside because I will be more susceptible to sunburn."
7. The nurse is assessing a client admitted to the psychiatric unit with a diagnosis of Bipolar Disorder The nurse can expect the client to exhibit all but which of the following behaviors?
   1. Conflict in relationships.
   2. Sexual promiscuousness.
   3. Euphoria.
   4. Drug seeking behavior.
8. Before the administration of MAOI antidepressant medication to a client with depression symptoms, it is imperative for the nurse to teach the client which of the following?
   1. It is safe to drink alcohol while taking this medication.
   2. Over the counter medications can be taken with MAOIs.
   3. Avoid all foods containing tyramine.
   4. MAOIs do not affect blood pressure.
9. A 45-year-old female client is diagnosed with depression. An appropriate nursing intervention for working with this client is:
   1. to allow plenty of alone time to think through issues.
   2. to provide at least 14 hours of sleep time each day.
   3. to encourage her to engage in any type of physical activity.
   4. to do her activities of daily living for her since she cannot.
10. The nurse is assessing a client admitted with schizophrenia. The nurse can expect to observe which of the following signs and symptoms?
    1. Able to care for basic needs.
    2. Alert and oriented.
    3. Speech clear and appropriate.
    4. Delusional.

REFERENCES/SUGGESTED READINGS

American Psychiatric Association. (APA). (2000). *Diagnostic and statistical manual of mental disorders (4th ed.)*. (DSM-IV-TR [text-revision]) Washington, DC: Author.

Antai-Otong, D. (2008). *Psychiatric nursing, biological & behavioral concepts.* Clifton Park, NY: Delmar Cengage Learning.

Anxiety Disorders Association of America (ADAA). (2009a). Brief overview of anxiety disorders. [Online] Retrieved May 18, 2009, from www.adaa.org/GettingHelp/Briefoverview.asp

Anxiety Disorders Association of America (ADAA). (2009b). Generalized anxiety disorder *(GAD).* [Online] Retrieved May 18, 2009, from www.adaa.org/GettingHelp/AnxietyDisorders/GAD.asp

Anxiety Disorders Association of America (ADAA). (2009c). Obsessive-compulsive disorder (OCD). [Online] Retrieved May 18, 2009, from www.adaa.org/GettingHelp/AnxietyDisorders/OCD.asp

Anxiety Disorders Association of America (ADAA). (2009d). Panic disorder (panic attack). [Online] Retrieved May 18, 2009, from www.adaa.org/GettingHelp/AnxietyDisorders/Panicattack.asp

Anxiety Disorders Association of America (ADAA). (2009e). Posttraumatic stress disorder (PTSD). [Online] Retrieved May 18, 2009, from www.adaa.org/GettingHelp/AnxietyDisorders/PTSD.asp

Berlinger, J. (2002). Domestic violence: How you can make a difference. *Nursing2001, 31*(8), 58–63.

Bulechek, G., Butcher, H., McCloskey, J., & Dochterman, J., eds. (2008). *Nursing Interventions Classification (NIC)* (5th ed.). St. Louis, MO: Mosby/Elsevier.

Centers for Disease Prevention and Control (CDC). (2008a). Suicide-datasheet. [Online] Retrieved May 19, 2009, from http://www.cdc.gov/ViolencePrevention/pdf/Suicide-DataSheet-a.pdf

Centers for Disease Prevention and Control (CDC). (2008b). Youth risk behavioral surveillance – United States, 2007. *Morbidity and Mortality Weekly Report, 57*(No. SS #4).

Daniels, R. (2010). *Delmar's guide to laboratory and diagnostic tests* (2nd ed.). Clifton Park, NY: Delmar Cengage Learning.

Depression and Bipolar Support Alliance (DBSA). (2006). *Types of bipolar disorder.* [Online] Retrieved May 19, 2009, from www.dbsalliance.org/site/PageServer?pagename=about_bipolar_types

Depression and Bipolar Support Alliance (DBSA). (2007). Depression and other illnesses. [Online] Retrieved May 18, 2009, from www.dbsalliance.org/site/PageServer?pagename=about_depression_otherillnesses

Depression and Bipolar Support Alliance (DBSA). (2009). Bipolar disorder. [Online] Retrieved May 19, 2009, from www.dbsalliance.org/site/PageServer?pagename=about_bipolar_overview

Ferri, R., Sofer, D., & Zolot, J. (2003). Depression in America, *AJN, 103*(9), 17.

Frisch, N., & Frisch, L. (2010). *Psychiatric mental health nursing.* (4th ed.). Clifton Park, NY: Delmar Cengage Learning.

Gale, G. (2002). A useful screening tool. *RN, 65*(9), 41–43.

Koschel, M. (2003). Is it child abuse? *AJN, 103*(4), 45–46.

McGlotten, S. (2003). Attempted suicide. *Nursing*2003, 33(4), 96.

Moorhead, S., Johnson, M., Maas, M., & Swanson, E. (2007). *Nursing Outcomes Classification (NOC)* (4th ed.). St. Louis, MO: Mosby.

Morris, R. (1998). Elder abuse: What the law requires. *RN, 61*(8), 52–53.

National Coalition against Domestic Violence (NCADV). (2005). The Problem. [Online]. Retrieved from www.ncadv.org/problem/what.htm

North American Nursing Diagnosis Association International. (2010). *NANDA-I nursing diagnoses: Definitions and classification 2009-2011.* Ames, IA: Wiley-Blackwell.

Orbanic, S. (2002). Understanding bulimia. *AJN, 101*(3), 35–41.

Peplau, H. (1962). Interpersonal techniques: The crux of psychiatric nursing. *AJN, 62*(6), 50–54.

Peplau, H. (1963). A working definition of anxiety. In S. Burd & M. Marshall (Eds.), *Some clinical approaches to psychiatric nursing.* New York: Macmillan.

Peplau, H. (1991). *Interpersonal relations in nursing.* New York: Springer.

Richardson, B. (2007). *Clinical decision making, case studies in psychiatric nursing.* Clifton Park, NY: Delmar Cengage Learning.

Rother, L. (2003). Electroconvulsive therapy sheds its shocking image. *Nursing2003, 33*(3), 48–49.

Ryan, B. (2003). Do you suspect child abuse? *RN, 66*(9), 73–77.

Spratto, G., & Woods, A. (2010). *Delmar nurse's drug handbook 2010 edition.* Clifton Park, NY: Delmar Cengage Learning.

Substance Abuse and Mental Health Services Administration (SAMHSA). (2008). Results from the 2007 national survey on drug use and health: national findings. [Online] Retrieved May 19, 2009, from www.oas.samhsa.gov/NSDUH/2k7nsduh/2k7results.cfm#8.1

Townsend, M. (2008). *Psychiatric mental health nursing: Concepts of care in evidence-based practice* (6th ed.). Philadelphia: F. A. Davis.

Townsend, M. (2009). *Nursing diagnoses in psychiatric nursing: Care plans and psychotropic medications* (7th ed.). Philadelphia: F. A. Davis.

U. S. Food and Drug Administration. MedWatch. (2002). Zoloft (sertraline hydrochloride). [Online]. Retrieved from www.fda.gov/medwatch/SAFETY/2002/safety02.htm#zoloft

U. S. House of Representatives, Select Committee on Aging (1981, April 3). *Elder Abuse (an examination of a hidden problem)* (Comm. Pub. No. 97–277). Washington, DC: U. S. Government Printing Office.

U. S. Preventive Services Task Force (2002). Screening for depression: Recommendations and rationale. *Annals of Internal Medicine,* 136(10), 760.

United States Code Annotated, Title 42, The Public Health and Welfare, Chapter 67, Child Abuse Prevention and Treatment and Adoption Reform; Subchapter 1, Child Abuse Prevention and Treatment; Definitions; Title II, Victims of Child Abuse Act of 1990; Subtitle D, Federal Victims' Protection and Rights; Section 226, Child Abuse Reporting. St. Paul, MN: West.

Vernarec, E. (2002). The hidden threat to our nation's kids. *RN,* 65(9), 36–40.

Woods, A. (2003). Depression. *Nursing2003,* 33(3), 54–55.

RESOURCES

Administration on Aging (AoA), http://www.aoa.gov

American Anorexia/Bulimia Association, http://www.aabainc.org

American Psychiatric Association, http://www.psych.org

American Psychiatric Nurses Association, http://www.apna.org

Anxiety Disorders Association of America, http://www.adaa.org

Depression and Bipolar Support Alliance, http://www.dbsalliance.org

Family Violence Prevention Fund (FVPF), http://www.endabuse.org

National Alliance for Research on Schizophrenia and Depression (NARSAD), http://www.narsad.org

National Alliance for the Mentally Ill (NAMI), http://www.nami.org

National Association of Anorexia Nervosa and Associated Disorders, http://www.anad.org

National Center on Elder Abuse, http://www.ncea.aoa.gov

National Coalition against Domestic Violence (NCADV), http://www.ncadv.org

National Domestic Violence Hotline, http://www.ndvh.org

National Eating Disorders Association, http://www.nationaleatingdisorders.org

National Institute of Mental Health, http://www.nimh.nih.gov

Parents Anonymous, The National Organization, http://www.parentsanonymous.org

Recovery, Inc.: The Association of Nervous and Former Mental Patients, http://www.recovery-inc.com

Victims of Incest Can Emerge Survivors (VOICES), http://www.healthywomen.org

CHAPTER 18
Substance Abuse

MAKING THE CONNECTION

Refer to the following chapters to increase your understanding of substance abuse:

Adult Health Nursing

- ***Respiratory System***
- ***Gastrointestinal System***
- ***Sexually Transmitted Infections***
- ***The Older Adult***

LEARNING OBJECTIVES

Upon completion of this chapter, you should be able to:

- Define key terms.
- Differentiate among dependence, abuse, and intoxication.
- Describe issues related to drug testing.
- Discuss substances frequently abused.
- Use assessment skills to identify possible substance abuse.
- Describe nursing interventions in working with substance abusers.
- Describe stages of alcoholism and the impact on the individual, family, and society.
- Discuss medications frequently used in the treatment of substance abuse.
- Describe an impaired nurse.
- Identify goals of programs for impaired nurses.

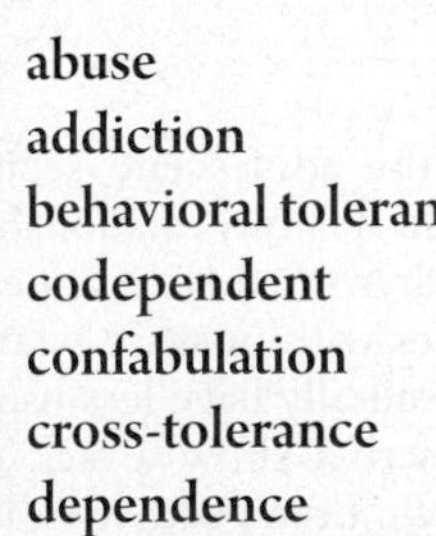

KEY TERMS

abuse
addiction
behavioral tolerance
codependent
confabulation
cross-tolerance
dependence
detoxification
hallucination
intoxication
Johnsonian intervention
misuse
opisthotonos
relapse
reverse tolerance
substance
synesthesia
teratogenic
tolerance
withdrawal

INTRODUCTION

Substance use has taken place for many centuries. It is not a new problem for society. A **substance** is a drug, legal or illegal, that may cause physical or mental impairment. With the great increase in world population, there are more people involved in substance abuse. Today's speed of travel and communication has facilitated the broad distribution of substances.

Many street drugs are "cut" (mixed) with substances that should not be consumed, such as talcum powder, rodent exterminating powder, or even strychnine. The purity (strength) of the drug is then not known and overdose easily occurs. Fatalities can occur from the substance with which the drug is cut.

In the United States, substance disorders affect males and females, all ethnic groups, and persons of all levels of education and income. From the newborn to the elderly, all ages can be affected.

Substance disorders may be classified as intoxication, abuse, or dependence (addiction); definitions are based on the criteria presented in the *American Psychiatric Association's Diagnostic and Statistical Manual of Mental Disorders*, fourth edition (DSM-IV). The reversible effect on the central nervous system (CNS) soon after the use of a substance is termed **intoxication**. **Abuse** is the misuse, excessive, or improper use of a substance, the abstinence of which does not cause withdrawal symptoms. **Dependence (addiction)** is reliance on a substance to such a degree that abstinence causes functional impairment, physical withdrawal symptoms, and/or a psychological craving for the substance.

According to the National Institute on Drug Abuse (NIDA, 2008h), substances interfere with normal brain function, inducing powerful feelings of pleasure and having long-term effects on brain metabolism and activity. At some point, changes in the brain turn substance abuse into addiction, a chronic, relapsing illness. Table 18-1 shows diagnostic criteria for abuse and dependence.

HISTORICAL PERSPECTIVES

Nearly 6,500 years ago, ancient Egyptians used opium for pain relief. Later they used it for recreation when they discovered it provided anxiety relief, a pleasurable experience, and an escape from reality. Drug problems began in the United States with the Civil War in 1861. Wounded soldiers were given their own supply of morphine. Its use was uncontrolled. Dependence-producing drugs such as cocaine, heroin, and morphine were given freely to clients by doctors. Patent medicines, many containing alcohol, cocaine, and heroin, were said to cure almost any ailment a person might have.

The Pure Food and Drug Act of 1906, requiring accurate labeling of drugs, was the first measure designed to control drugs in the United States. In 1914, The Harrison Act made the use of certain narcotics illegal. Physicians then became unwilling to give individuals these drugs, and drug use actually increased as those persons already using drugs turned to illegal markets for a supply. In 1919, Congress passed the 19th Amendment to the Constitution declaring the making and selling of alcohol illegal. Prohibition lasted until 1933, when the 19th Amendment was finally repealed because it had not controlled drunkenness or alcoholism as it was intended.

Many medical, law enforcement, and legislative efforts in the 1930s slowed narcotic abuse and addiction. Then marijuana flooded the market. The Marijuana Tax Act of 1937 was intended to raise revenue, identify the persons involved in its use, and discourage the recreational use of marijuana. Marijuana was removed in 1941 from the official list of drugs U.S. physicians could prescribe. World War II disrupted supply routes of drugs from Asia and Europe, and large-scale drug use disappeared in the United States.

The 1960s, saw drug use move into the mainstream of life in the United States. Drugs were used as a form of relaxation. The Comprehensive Drug Abuse Prevention and Control Act was passed in 1970; it is commonly referred to as the Controlled Substance Act. This act regulates the manufacture, distribution, and dispensing of controlled substances. To enforce the provisions of this act, the Drug Enforcement Administration (DEA) was organized.

There are five classifications or schedules of controlled substances. The categories are based on the drugs' potential to cause psychological and/or physical dependence, and also on their potential for abuse. Table 18-2 identifies and explains the five schedules.

In the 1980s, marijuana and other drug use declined, especially among high school students. Cocaine and its derivative, crack, were the new drugs of choice. The increased supply hooked many people into heavy drug use. The early 1990s saw an increase in the use of all substances. Adolescent illicit drug use is decreasing for almost all of the specific types of drugs. Combined data for 8th, 10th, and 12th graders show an overall decline in illicit drug use by 24% between 2001 and 2007 (NIDA, 2008g).

FACTORS RELATED TO SUBSTANCE ABUSE

Many factors interact to influence a person's substance abuse. Many people who have stopped substance abuse **relapse** (return to a previous behavior or condition) because of these same factors. These factors may be categorized as individual, family, lifestyle, environmental, and developmental.

INDIVIDUAL FACTORS

Genetic factors are being researched as a possible reason for a person's susceptibility to substance abuse. Research suggests that variations in the intensity of the flow of neurotransmitters may cause certain individuals to be more susceptible to addiction. The personality traits of sensation seeking and being impulsive may make it easier for the person to experiment with substances.

FAMILY PATTERNS

Substance abuse, especially in the adolescent, seems to be related to family relationships. Close family relationships, with the parents involved in their children's activities, appear to discourage substance abuse. Families with positive relationships between parents and children generally have less use of illicit drugs. Parent–child interactions that show a lack of closeness, lack of involvement in the children's activities, lack of or inconsistent discipline, and low aspirations for the children's education contribute to the prediction of substance abuse by the children.

Families of adolescent substance abusers generally have negative communication patterns. That is, there is a lack

TABLE 18-1 Diagnostic Criteria for Substance Dependence and Abuse

SUBSTANCE DEPENDENCE

A maladaptive pattern of substance use, leading to clinically significant impairment or distress, as manifested by three (or more) of the following, occurring at any time in the same 12-month period:

(1) tolerance, as defined by either of the following:
  (a) a need for markedly increased amounts of the substance to achieve intoxication or desired effect
  (b) markedly diminished effect with continued use of the same amount of the substance
(2) withdrawal, as manifested by either of the following:
  (a) the characteristic withdrawal syndrome for the substance (refer to Criteria A and B of the criteria sets for Withdrawal from the specific substances)
  (b) the same (or a closely related) substance is taken to relieve or avoid withdrawal symptoms
(3) the substance is often taken in larger amounts or over a longer period than was intended
(4) there is a persistent desire or unsuccessful efforts to cut down or control substance use
(5) a great deal of time is spent in activities necessary to obtain the substance (e.g., visiting multiple doctors or driving long distances), use the substance (e.g., chain-smoking), or recover from its effects
(6) important social, occupational, or recreational activities are given up or reduced because of substance use
(7) the substance use is continued despite knowledge of having a persistent or recurrent physical or psychological problem that is likely to have been caused or exacerbated by the substance (e.g., current cocaine use despite recognition of cocaine-induced depression, or continued drinking despite recognition that an ulcer was made worse by alcohol consumption)

SUBSTANCE ABUSE

A. A maladaptive pattern of substance use leading to clinically significant impairment or distress, as manifested by one (or more) of the following, occurring within a 12-month period:
  (1) recurrent substance use resulting in a failure to fulfill major role obligations at work, school, or home (e.g., repeated absences or poor work performance related to substance use; substance-related absences, suspensions, or expulsions from school; neglect of children or household)
  (2) recurrent substance use in situations in which it is physically hazardous (e.g., driving an automobile or operating a machine when impaired by substance use)
  (3) recurrent substance-related legal problems (e.g., arrests for substance-related disorderly conduct)
  (4) continued substance use despite having persistent or recurrent social or interpersonal problems caused, or exacerbated by the effects of the substance (e.g., arguments with spouse about consequences of intoxication, physical fights)

B. The symptoms have never met the criteria for Substance Dependence for this class of substance.

TABLE 18-2 Schedules of Controlled Substances

Schedule I (C-I)	High abuse and dependence potential. No accepted medical use in the United States. Includes heroin, mescaline, LSD, marijuana, and other hallucinogens and certain opiates. Can be obtained legally for limited research programs.
Schedule II (C-II)	High abuse and dependence potential. Have currently accepted medical use. Includes narcotics, barbiturates, and amphetamines. Obtained only with physician's prescription, nonrefillable.
Schedule III (C-III)	Less abuse potential, moderate dependence likely. Includes nonbarbiturate sedatives and some narcotics in limited doses. Prescription refills good for 6 months. Fewer controls than for Schedule II.
Schedule IV (C-IV)	Even less abuse potential, limited dependence likely. Includes some sedatives and antianxiety agents and nonnarcotic analgesics.
Schedule V (C-V)	Limited abuse potential. Includes cough medicines containing codeine and antidiarrheals. May be sold over-the-counter in pharmacies to persons over 18 years old. A record is kept of the buyer's name.

of praise and a great deal of blaming and criticism. Often there are unreal expectations of the children by the parents, inconsistent or unclear behavioral limits, and a pattern of self-medication by family members.

Lifestyle

All dimensions of a person's life that influence how that person lives are termed *lifestyle*. First is the physical dimension, which includes food, clothing, shelter, and health care. The second is the social dimension, which includes friends, organizations, and activities with others. Third is the intellectual/emotional dimension, including education, parental support of education, self-esteem, and how the individual is treated by others. The fourth dimension is spiritual and includes a belief in a "higher being," caring and compassion for others, and being in touch with the inner self. Substance use, abuse, or dependence may be the coping mechanism used by an individual who has problems in any dimension of lifestyle.

Environmental Factors

Many environmental factors may encourage or predispose an individual to substance abuse. The social environment in which persons find themselves, the groups, clubs, gangs, sororities, fraternities, and other organizations influence the acceptance or rejection of substance abuse. Stresses in a person's life, including accidents, disabilities, illnesses, stressful family relations, frequent job changes, divorce, death, or precarious financial conditions may be too much for that person to handle. The maladaptive coping of substance abuse offers temporary relief. Because the symptoms of the stressors are reduced, substance abuse is reinforced.

Social traditions, especially in the use of alcohol, may open the door for abuse in certain individuals. Examples of these social traditions are having wine with meals, making toasts at weddings and other celebrations, serving "holiday cheer," and going to "happy hour." For some individuals, these situations may predispose them to alcohol abuse or dependence.

Peer activities, especially during adolescence, may result in substance abuse. Even adults often feel they must go along with certain activities, such as drinks after work or cocktail hour, to get ahead in their careers.

Some occupations, like health care, seem to be more associated with substance problems than others. Physicians and nurses, particularly, have access to many substances that can be abused.

Developmental Factors

Many individuals have not had good role models in their lives. They have not learned to identify with others and do not understand that their behavior affects others. Not learning the skills and attitudes of problem solving leaves individuals unable to apply personal resources to situations, and escape seems the only answer. Substances provide that escape.

Learning the intrapersonal skills of self-discipline, self-control, and self-assessment helps the individual cope with tension and stress. These skills also work to prevent dishonesty with self, inability to defer gratification, and low self-esteem. A lack of interpersonal skills results in dishonesty with others, resistance to feedback, and inability to share feelings and give or accept help. Not learning to take responsibility or adapt one's behavior to a situation results in irresponsibility, not accepting the consequences of behavior, and seeing oneself as a victim of circumstances. Individuals who do not view themselves as empowered may choose substance use as a means of gratification.

PREVENTION

Prevention of substance abuse must be a proactive process to empower people to constructively confront stressful situations in adaptive ways. There are three levels of prevention. *Primary prevention* focuses on preventing the initial use or preventing further uses that may lead to abuse or dependence. This is usually aimed at school-age children. Children need to hear the message that drugs are not good for them. Education about substances and their effects must also emphasize personal, social, and health risks. Children need role models to teach them how to cope with life without drugs, to resist social and peer pressure, and to make effective decisions.

Secondary prevention focuses on preventing ongoing use from becoming a situation of abuse or dependence. If abuse is already evident, the focus is to return the client to a state of abstinence or at least reduced use.

Tertiary prevention focuses on returning the client to a drug-free state. If this is not possible, the goal is then to prevent physical and psychosocial problems from getting worse.

DIAGNOSTIC TESTING

Clients who have a problem with substance abuse or dependence often have abnormal liver function tests and electrolyte levels. Diagnostic criteria for specific substance-related disorders can be found in DSM-IV.

Tests may be done with either a blood or urine specimen. A positive test indicates only that the person has been exposed to the substance. It does not indicate abuse, addiction, or intoxication (except alcohol). Positive screening tests should be confirmed by a more specific test using a different process. Drugs for which tests can be done include alcohol, benzodiazepines, barbiturates, cocaine, crack, amphetamines, opiates, synthetic narcotic analgesics, marijuana, and PCP.

Urine is usually the body fluid tested because it is easily obtained and tested. When obtaining a urine specimen for drug screening, the client should be observed to prevent adulteration of the specimen by the client, such as substituting another person's drug-free urine. A "chain of custody" is maintained by having each person who handles the specimen sign an attached paper until the specimen has been tested.

Detection of a substance depends on the amount used and the time since last used. Most substances are detectable for less than 7 days. Chronic marijuana use, however, may be detected for up to 30 days. Barbiturates, amphetamines, and opiates are detectable for less than 2 days and alcohol less than 1 day. A false negative may result if the client's drug level falls below the threshold of sensitivity for the test.

Positive results for reasons other than substance abuse can occur. This is called a false positive. Poppy seeds may give a positive result for opiates for up to 60 hours after ingestion. Using a Vicks® inhaler or over-the-counter diet aids may give a positive result for amphetamines. The client should be asked about the use of these items.

Breath specimens can be used to determine alcohol levels. Law enforcement officials do this with the breathalyzer tests.

If hair is not cut, hair analysis can detect cocaine and heroin use for up to a year or more after the person has used the drug. Testing meconium (first stools) from a newborn can detect illicit drug use by the mother during pregnancy.

TREATMENT/RECOVERY

Treatment depends on many factors, including the amount and frequency of substance use, age, health, diet, and overall lifestyle of the individual. Infection from the use of unsterile needles and/or tissue or organ damage caused by the substance used, such as lung damage from smoking crack or marijuana or using inhalants, will also require treatment.

Recovery requires abstinence along with intrapersonal and interpersonal changes. Most individuals need professional treatment and participation in a self-help program. There are four areas of recovery: physical recovery, psychological and behavioral recovery, social and family recovery, and spiritual recovery.

Physical recovery means eliminating the substance from the body. This is termed **detoxification**. If the client cannot stop using the substance or if withdrawal symptoms are present, admission to a detoxification unit is usually necessary. After detoxification, treatment must focus on restoring the client's physical health and dealing with the cravings for the substance now removed from the client's body. It helps if environmental cues such as drug paraphernalia and alcohol bottles or cans are removed.

Psychological and behavioral recovery becomes evident when the client no longer denies the problem and accepts the inability to consistently control the substance abuse. The client will have developed a desire for abstinence and accepted the need for long-term recovery and support. Emotional stability will be restored when the client learns to cope with uncomfortable emotional states without the use of the abused substance.

Social and family recovery occurs when the client no longer denies the impact on the family and makes amends to family members and significant others who have been negatively affected by the substance abuse. The client works to improve family relationships and develops a recovery support system. Also, the client learns to resist social pressures to use alcohol or other drugs and participates in healthy leisure-time activities. The client's family should also attend a program for recovery. If a client returns to a dysfunctional family, it may be difficult for the client to maintain recovery.

Spiritual recovery is attained when the client has resolved the feelings of guilt and shame and developed a meaning for life and a relationship with a higher power.

SUBSTANCE USE PATTERNS

Patterns of substance use have changed throughout the years. Coffee (caffeine) and cigarettes (nicotine) are legal in our society and widely used. Although many people still drink coffee, more are using decaffeinated coffee. Cigarette use has decreased in the older population as the addictive nature and negative effects of nicotine have become more evident; however, cigarette use has increased in the adolescent population.

The substance of choice is alcohol, which is legal and easily obtained. Many high school seniors have been drunk and some are already regular drinkers. There are still more alcoholic men than women, but the number of identified women alcoholics is increasing.

> **CRITICAL THINKING**
>
> **Attitude toward Substance Abusers**
>
> What is your attitude toward substance abusers? How would you respond to a client who is a substance abuser? Discuss with your classmates.

Elderly persons are more commonly addicted to prescription medications, especially minor tranquilizers and sleeping pills. Alcohol may be used by the elderly to soothe feelings of isolation and loneliness. Depression and paranoia may be misidentified as senility rather than a problem with alcohol.

Moderate consumption of alcohol may have been influenced by Mothers Against Drunk Driving (MADD) and Students Against Destructive Decisions (SADD) (founded as Students Against Driving Drunk). Laws that make bars and individuals liable if they let guests leave and drive while drunk, called social host laws, and famous people like Betty Ford and Liza Minelli sharing with the public their illness and recovery, are other influences.

The National Institute on Drug Abuse (2008h) report on the ongoing study of illicit drug use among 8th-, 10th-, and 12th-grade students shows a decrease in use.

CNS DEPRESSANTS

Central nervous system depressants usually decrease the heart and respiratory rates as well as voluntary muscle responses. Substances in this category include alcohol, benzodiazepines, and marijuana.

ALCOHOL

Low doses of alcohol depress areas of the brain that are inhibitory, causing diminished self-control and impaired judgment. Continued alcohol ingestion may cause unconsciousness and even death. According to the National Institute on Alcohol Abuse and Alcoholism (NIAAA) (2006), 39.5% of all traffic crash fatalities were alcohol related.

The active ingredient in alcoholic beverages is ethanol. Depending on the alcoholic beverage consumed, varying amounts of ethanol are ingested (Figure 18-1). It is metabolized at an average rate of 10 mL/hr. Table 18-3 shows the alcohol content in some beverages.

One ounce of alcohol provides 200 Kcal but no other nutrients. It is not converted to glycogen. The blood alcohol level depends on the size of the person, the amount ingested, and the time since ingestion. Most states have set the legal limit for blood alcohol while driving a motor vehicle at 0.08%, but driving skills are affected at a much lower level.

INCIDENCE

Several national surveys have found that approximately two-thirds of the population has more than an occasional drink. Men are likely to drink more frequently and in greater quantity than women. Some alcoholics drink little or nothing in public or with friends. They are "at home" or "hidden" alcoholics and

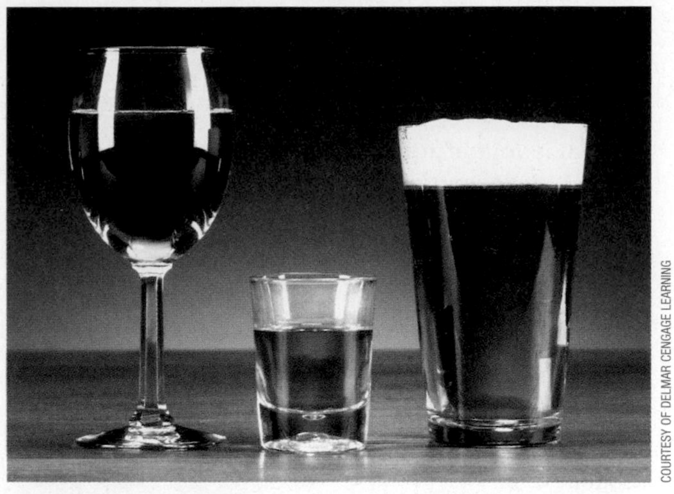

FIGURE 18-1 Each of these drinks contains approximately the same level of alcohol.

are more likely to be women. It often takes a family quite awhile to realize that one of its members has an alcohol problem.

The individual with an alcohol problem often learns **behavioral tolerance**, a compensatory adjustment made by an individual under the influence of a particular substance. The person under the influence of alcohol learns how to compensate for the deterioration of motor performance and speech.

SIGNS AND SYMPTOMS

The ingestion of alcohol causes a feeling of euphoria, relaxation of skeletal muscles, changes in mental activity such as altered judgment, and reduced self-control. It has a diuretic effect that, in heavy drinkers, may cause increased loss of electrolytes, especially potassium, magnesium, and zinc. An increased level of alcohol depresses the cardiovascular and respiratory systems and produces a toxic effect on the intestinal mucosa, resulting in decreased absorption of thiamine, folic acid, and vitamin B_{12}. Excess long-term consumption of alcohol often results in a severe lack of nutrient intake.

Psychosocial aspects include memory blackouts, secretive drinking, rationalization of drinking behavior, trouble with family and employer, loss of outside interests, neglect of food intake, impaired thinking, and moral deterioration. **Confabulation**, making up information to fill in memory gaps, is used by individuals abusing or depending on alcohol. Alcohol may be detected in the blood for 6 to 10 hours after ingestion.

POTENTIAL FOR ADDICTION

The potential for addiction is high. Alcohol is not a scheduled or controlled drug.

TABLE 18-3 Alcohol Content in Selected Beverages

BEVERAGE	PERCENT ALCOHOL	EQUIVALENT AMOUNTS
Beer	4	12 ounces
Wine cooler	4	12 ounces
Wine	14	4 ounces
Hard liquor	40	1½ ounces

ASSOCIATED PROBLEMS/ DISORDERS

Excessive and prolonged alcohol intake can affect numerous body systems.

Liver Deterioration

Chronic alcohol abuse causes three distinct diseases of the liver: *fatty liver*, an accumulation of triglycerides in the liver caused by obesity, excessive alcohol consumption, and certain drugs; *alcoholic hepatitis*, an acute toxic liver injury from excess alcohol consumption; and *cirrhosis*, a chronic degenerative liver disease that can be caused by alcohol consumption. Fatty liver is reversible, but alcoholic hepatitis and cirrhosis are not. Liver cells will not function once the scar tissue of cirrhosis develops. In 2005, 45.9% of deaths from cirrhosis of the liver were related to alcohol consumption (NIAAA, 2008a). Esophageal varices are associated with cirrhosis and could cause death if they bleed.

Gastrointestinal Disturbances

Alcohol damages the lining of the stomach and esophagus by irritating the mucosa and causing inflammation or ulcer formation. Aspirin with alcohol can result in greater irritation and bleeding in the gastrointestinal (GI) tract. Gastric pain, vomiting, and diarrhea are common in alcohol abuse and are often what brings the individual to the health care system.

Pancreatitis

An alcoholic has a higher risk of developing pancreatitis than an abstainer. Severe pancreatitis can result in death.

Wernicke's Encephalopathy

This inflammatory hemorrhagic and degenerative condition of the brain is caused by a thiamine deficiency. It is characterized by delirium, memory loss, unsteady gait, a sense of apprehension, and an altered level of consciousness. Thiamine intake improves the situation.

Korsakoff's Psychosis

Disorientation, amnesia, insomnia, hallucinations, and peripheral neuropathologies characterize this psychosis. Both thiamine and B_{12} deficiencies contribute to the degeneration of the brain and peripheral nervous system. Frequently, there is bilateral foot drop and pain. Thiamine and B_{12} intake may improve the situation.

Cardiovascular Disturbances

Moderate amounts of alcohol cause cutaneous vasodilation (flushed skin). This causes rapid heat loss, and the core temperature may drop to a dangerous level. Blood pressure decreases with intoxicating doses of alcohol. There may be irregularities in cardiac rhythm. Hematologic alterations such as bone marrow depression, anemia, leukopenia, or thrombocytopenia may also occur.

Fetal Alcohol Syndrome

Fetal alcohol syndrome (FAS) is caused by the **teratogenic** (causing abnormal development of the embryo) effects of alcohol related to the amount of alcohol ingested and the stage of pregnancy when the alcohol is ingested. Even a small amount of alcohol can be detrimental and have lifelong consequences for the infant. For a diagnosis of FAS, the infant must meet these criteria:

- Prenatal and/or postnatal growth retardation (weight, length, or head circumference below the 10th percentile)
- CNS involvement (signs of neurologic abnormality, developmental delay, or intellectual impairment)
- Craniofacial anomalies, at least two of the following (microcephaly or head circumference below 3rd percentile, microophthalmia or short palpebral fissure, poorly developed philtrum, thin upper lip, or flattening of maxillary area)

If only some of the FAS criteria are met, it is called fetal alcohol effects (FAE). The only treatment for FAS or FAE is prevention. Women who are pregnant or are trying to get pregnant should abstain from alcohol consumption.

Withdrawal

Withdrawal refers to the symptoms produced when a substance on which an individual has dependence is no longer used by that individual. Alcohol withdrawal syndrome (AWS) appears when the blood alcohol concentration of the alcoholic decreases. The onset of symptoms usually occurs 6 to 12 hours after drinking stops and may last up to 8 days. Chronologically, how long the drinking has occurred and the amount of alcohol consistently consumed are factors in the severity of the withdrawal symptoms. Figure 18-2 shows alcohol withdrawal patterns.

Alcohol withdrawal has three stages:

- *Stage 1* (minor withdrawal) includes restlessness, anxiety, sleeping problems, agitation, and tremors; other signs include low-grade fever, tachycardia, diaphoresis, and hypertension.
- *Stage 2* (major withdrawal) includes stage 1 signs and symptoms plus visual and auditory hallucinations, whole-body tremors, pulse >100 beats/min, diastolic BP >100 mm Hg, pronounced diaphoresis, and possibly vomiting.
- *Stage 3* (delirium tremens) includes a temperature >37.8°C (100°F); disorientation to time, place, and person; global confusion; and inability to recognize familiar objects or persons. This is a medical emergency with a mortality rate of 1% to 5% (Kasser, Geller, Howell, & Wartenberg, 2004).

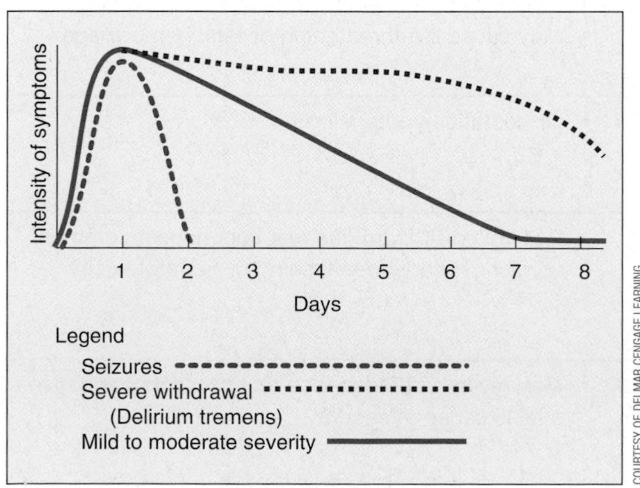

FIGURE 18-2 **Alcohol Withdrawal Patterns**

CRITICAL THINKING

Alcohol Withdrawal

A client, who is going through alcohol withdrawal and is on the appropriate medication protocol, is not clear mentally and is becoming very agitated. What would you investigate and how would you communicate your findings to the physician?

If alcohol abuse continues, symptoms of subsequent withdrawals are generally more severe. It is recommended that withdrawal be medically monitored to decrease the chance of fatality.

Treatment/Rehabilitation

Many treatment programs are based in hospital or residential treatment centers. These are generally called inpatient programs and last 30 days. Many insurance companies are encouraging clients to participate in lower-cost outpatient programs. Currently, there is no evidence that inpatient programs are more effective than outpatient programs.

Many outpatient programs have both day and evening sessions so clients can maintain their usual occupations. The programs usually consist of a 4-week intensive session with follow-up sessions for 6 to 24 months. The first part of either type of treatment program is detoxification.

Detoxification

The goal of detoxification (DETOX) is to halt or control the neuronal overactivity that occurs when the alcohol level is reduced or alcohol is no longer present in the client's body. This is done by substituting a pharmacologically similar drug and gradually reducing the dose given. The benzodiazepine drugs, chlordiazepoxide (Librium), diazepam (Valium), lorazepam (Ativan), and clorazepate dipotassium (Tranxene), are the most commonly used.

During DETOX, other problems such as malnutrition, vitamin deficiencies (B vitamins, especially thiamine), dehydration, and potassium and magnesium deficiencies must also be treated. A client with hypoglycemia should be given thiamine before administering dextrose to prevent Wernicke's encephalopathy. Ignoring these problems complicates the management of detoxification.

Psychological Intervention

The classic psychological intervention technique was originally described by Johnson in 1973 (Johnson, 1990 & 2001). Although several modifications have been published and used since then, the technique is still used and is known as **Johnsonian intervention**, which is a confrontational approach to a client with a substance problem that lessens the chance of denial and encourages treatment before the client "hits bottom." The client's significant others (spouse, teenage or older children, one or two close friends, possibly employer) meet with a professional addiction counselor. This group rehearses so that they may present a united front when confronting the client. They present specific examples of painful or embarrassing behaviors by the client while intoxicated that caused problems and concerns. It is difficult for the client to maintain denial in this situation. Then the group encourages the client to accept professional help. If the client refuses help, each individual of the group must plan to minimize codependent behavior in the future. This technique can also be used for substances other than alcohol. Examples of confrontations may be found in Johnson's books (1989, 1990, 2001). Codependency is discussed later in the chapter.

Education

The abuse of or dependence on alcohol is a maladaptive way to cope with life stressors. Learning basic life skills to improve personal competence and provide adaptive coping mechanisms helps the individual resist the use of alcohol.

One adaptive coping mechanism is exercise. Assist clients to become active in an exercise program and encourage them to participate. Exercise helps relieve feelings of stress and promotes feelings of well-being.

Teach clients about the Food Guide Pyramid for an adequate, balanced diet. Most alcoholics have, in the past, received most of their calories from alcohol. They must now learn how to maintain health by eating nutritious foods.

The interaction of alcohol with other drugs should also be taught. Some effects can be life-threatening. Table 18-4 shows the interaction of alcohol with some classifications of drugs.

Self-Help Groups

Alcoholics Anonymous (AA), begun in 1935, is the model for other self-help groups such as AL-ANON for adults, AL-ATEEN for teenage children, and AL-ATOT for younger children in the family of an alcoholic. The holistic approach of AA to the individual with alcohol problems is described in the Twelve Steps (Table 18-5).

Disulfiram

Disulfiram (Antabuse) may be given to some alcohol abusers as a deterrent to drinking. It inhibits the enzyme needed to metabolize alcohol (NIAAA, 2008b). Drinking alcohol with disulfiram in the body causes flushing of the neck and face, blurred vision, nausea, vertigo, anxiety, palpitations, tachycardia, and hypotension. Clients must be instructed not to use cologne, mouthwash, aftershave, over-the-counter cold preparations, cough syrups, vitamin-mineral tonics, as well as candies, sauces, and foods made with alcohol. These items will cause the same reaction as if the person took a drink of alcohol.

Therapy should not be started until at least 12 hours after the last drink of alcohol. The effects of disulfiram with alcohol can occur for 6 to 12 days after taking the disulfiram. As with any drug, there are side effects such as drowsiness, fatigue, and impotence. Garlic-like breath occurs frequently and is sometimes used as an indicator of compliance in taking

TABLE 18-4 Alcohol Interaction with Other Drugs

DRUG CLASSIFICATIONS WITH EXAMPLES	INTERACTION
Narcotic analgesics • meperidine hydrochloride (Demerol) • morphine sulfate (Morphine) • proproxyphene HCl (Darvon) • hydromorphone HCl (Dilaudid)	• Loss of effective breathing (respiratory arrest) • Can be fatal
Nonnarcotic analgesics • aspirin • acetaminophen (Tylenol)	• Stomach and intestinal bleeding • Liver damage
Anticoagulants • warfarin sodium (Coumadin, Panwarfin) • dicumarol	• Increases drugs' ability to stop blood clotting • May cause life-threatening or fatal hemorrhage
Antihypertensives • reserpine (Serpasil) • methyldopa (Aldomet)	• Orthostatic hypotension
Antimicrobials • metronidazole (Flagyl) • cefotetan disodium (Cefotan) • rifampin (Rifadin)	• Possible disulfiram-like reaction, nausea, cramps, vomiting, headache, flushing or hepatotoxicity
CNS stimulants • most diet pills • dextroamphetamine sulfate (Dexedrine) • caffeine (No Doz) • methylphenidate HCl (Ritalin)	• May reverse depressant effect of alcohol and give a false sense of security

TABLE 18-4 Alcohol Interaction with Other Drugs (Continued)

DRUG CLASSIFICATIONS WITH EXAMPLES	INTERACTION
Diuretics • chlorothiazide (Diuril) • furosemide (Lasix)	• May reduce blood pressure and cause dizziness
Antidepressants • imipramine HCl (Tofranil) • desipramine HCl (Pertofrane) • perphenazine and amitriptyline HCl (Triavil)	• Reduces CNS functioning • Chianti wine may cause hypertensive crisis
Antihistamines • Most cold remedies • pseudoephedrine HCl and triprolidine HCl (Actifed) • chlorpheniramine maleate and acetaminophen (Couricidin)	• Increased calming effect • Person becomes very drowsy • Driving is hazardous
Antipsychotics • thioridazine HCl (Mellaril) • chlorpromazine HCl (Thorazine)	• Added CNS depression and impairs voluntary movements • Causes respiratory depression • Can be fatal
Sedative-hypnotics • glutethimine (Doriden) • pentobarbital (Nembutal)	• Reduces CNS functioning • Sometimes causes coma and respiratory arrest • Can be fatal
Antianxiety agents • diazepam (Valium) • chlordiazepoxide (Librium)	• Reduces CNS functioning • Decreased alertness and judgment • Can lead to household and driving accidents

TABLE 18-5 Alcoholics Anonymous

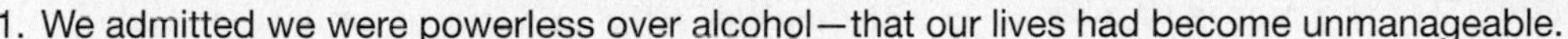

1. We admitted we were powerless over alcohol—that our lives had become unmanageable.
2. Came to believe that a Power greater than ourselves could restore us to sanity.
3. Made a decision to turn our will and our lives over to the care of God *as we understood Him*.
4. Made a searching and fearless moral inventory of ourselves.
5. Admitted to God, to ourselves and to another human being the exact nature of our wrongs.
6. Were entirely ready to have God remove all these defects of character.
7. Humbly asked Him to remove our shortcomings.
8. Made a list of all persons we had harmed, and became willing to make amends to them all.
9. Made direct amends to such people wherever possible, except when to do so would injure them or others.
10. Continued to take personal inventory and when we were wrong promptly admitted it.
11. Sought through prayer and meditation to improve our conscious contact with God, *as we understood Him*, praying only for knowledge of His will for us and the power to carry that out.
12. Having had a spiritual awakening as the result of these steps, we tried to carry this message to alcoholics, and to practice these principles in all our affairs.

the disulfiram. Disulfiram is contraindicated in clients with cardiovascular disease, hypothyroidism, suicide ideation, and in clients receiving antihypertensives or monoamine oxidase inhibitors (MAOI).

BENZODIAZEPINES AND OTHER SEDATIVE-HYPNOTICS

With the introduction in 1961 of chlordiazepoxide (Librium), the benzodiazepines have replaced most of the short-acting barbiturates and other nonbarbiturate sedative-hypnotics that were in use before that time. Examples of benzodiazepines include diazepam (Valium), secobarbital (Seconal), paraldehyde (Paral), and flunitrazepam (Rohypnol). Rohypnol when mixed with alcohol can incapacitate and prevent the person from resisting sexual assault or remembering what she experiences under the effects of the drug. It is known as the "date rape drug" (NIDA, 2008b). Street names include roofies, tranks, ludes, and barbs.

INCIDENCE

Benzodiazepines are not commonly used as recreational drugs but are widely prescribed and are thus available for abuse. Statistics are not available because some clinicians still deny that addiction to these drugs occurs. Withdrawal symptoms are subtle and delayed, and the symptoms are not always connected to the benzodiazepines.

Barbiturates and other sedative-hypnotics are more abused but less prescribed. These are available on the illegal market.

SIGNS AND SYMPTOMS

Benzodiazepines in low doses produce drowsiness or sedation. Larger doses produce sleep, but surgical anesthesia cannot be induced. Respirations are not depressed, and there is little effect on the cardiovascular system unless extremely large doses are taken. Then a decrease in systolic blood pressure and an increase in heart rate may result. Side effects may include motor incoordination, ataxia, increased hostility or rage, confusion, metallic-like aftertaste, headache, and blurred vision. **Tolerance** (a decreased sensitivity to subsequent doses of the same substance; an increased dose of a substance is needed to produce the same desired effect) to other benzodiazepines and **cross-tolerance** (a decreased sensitivity to other substances in the same category) to other CNS depressants occur with chronic use. In some clients, particularly pediatric, geriatric, or autistic, a paradoxical reaction can occur. They show excessive movement, increased talkativeness, agitation, violent behavior, and physical assault instead of the expected calming effect (Bramness, J., Skurtveit, S., & Morland, J., 2006, Mancuso, C.E., Tanzi, M.G., & Gabay, M., 2004).

Barbiturates depress all areas of the CNS, some selectively according to the dosage. They do not reduce pain. Respirations are depressed but not significantly when therapeutic doses are taken. When a barbiturate is given to a client in pain, excitement rather than sedation may occur. Side effects may include drowsiness, residual effects on motor skills, and especially in the elderly, excitement, irritability, or delirium. An overdose of barbiturates causes decreased respirations, rapid and weak pulse, cyanosis, coma, and sometimes respiratory paralysis. Tolerance results from chronic use or abuse. Benzodiazepines may be detected for 1 to 6 weeks.

POTENTIAL FOR ADDICTION

The potential for addiction is high for all of these substances. Benzodiazepines are schedule IV drugs; barbiturates may be either schedule II, III, or IV drugs; and methaqualone is a schedule I drug.

WITHDRAWAL

Symptoms of withdrawal for benzodiazepines, which may not manifest for a week or more, include cramping, sweating, disorientation, confusion, tremors, depression, hallucinations, and paranoia. Barbiturate withdrawal symptoms include anxiety, weakness, anorexia, insomnia, tremors, delirium, and seizures that occur within 72 hours of the last use. Withdrawal reactions related to other sedative-hypnotics include nausea, headache, cramping, toxic psychosis, insomnia, and convulsions.

The withdrawal pattern is the same as for alcohol.

TREATMENT/REHABILITATION

Ideally, treatment for benzodiazepine abuse is a gradual reduction in the amount taken until the client is no longer taking any. A cross-tolerant drug such as phenobarbital is sometimes given to control symptoms and then its dosage is reduced. Hospital treatment is likely to be needed. Treatment for barbiturate and other sedative-hypnotics overdose or withdrawal is symptomatic.

Rehabilitation that focuses on teaching clients alternative methods of coping with the anxiety and stressors in their lives is necessary. Supportive individual psychotherapy or a self-help recovery group is almost always advisable. The goal is to assist the client to identify the consequences of the behavior and to understand the risks of relapse.

MARIJUANA (CANNABIS)

Marijuana is the most common type of cannabis used. It is composed of dried leaves, stems, and flowers of the plant *Cannabis sativa* and can be smoked or added to food. Hash or hashish is a potent concentrate of the resin from the flowers. Hash oil is extremely concentrated, made by boiling hashish in a solvent and filtering out the solid matter. Street names include grass, pot, reefer, smoke, weed, and Mary Jane. "Blunts" are cigars emptied of tobacco and refilled with marijuana. It is the most commonly used illicit drug in the United States (NIDA, 2009d). Often, it is the "gateway" drug leading to the abuse of other drugs.

INCIDENCE

Use in the United States began in the early 1900s, peaked in the period 1978 to 1980, and has steadily decreased since. According to Johnston, O'Malley, and Buchman (1991, 1998, 2008a, and 2008b), the prevalence of marijuana use by high school seniors increased from 20% in the class of 1969 to 60.4% in the class of 1979 and decreased to 50.2% in the class of 1987 and decreased again to 40.7 percent in the class of 1990. Use increased between 1990 and 1997 but declined in 1998 to 49%. A National Institute on Drug Abuse study (NIDA, 2007) showed that 10.3% of 8th, 24.6% of 10th, and 31.7% of 12th graders had abused marijuana at least once in 2006. The 2007 National Survey of Drug Use and Health (Substance Abuse and Mental Health Services Administration (SAMHSA, 2008) showed that of the 2.7 million Americans aged 12 or older who used illicit drugs for the first time within the past 12 months, 56.2 % reported that their first drug was marijuana (Figure 18-3).

Signs and Symptoms

Short-term effects of marijuana use include memory and learning problems; distorted perception; difficulty in thinking and problem solving; loss of coordination; and increased heart rate, anxiety, and panic attacks. Long-term use produces changes in the brain that make a person more at risk of becoming addicted to alcohol and cocaine. Long-term effects of marijuana use may lead to lung cancer, impairment of the immune system, and a greater risk of getting lung infections (NIDA, 2009d). A **reverse tolerance** can develop whereby a smaller amount of marijuana will elicit the desired psychic effects. Marijuana may be detected in urine for up to 3 to 30 days depending on how much and how long it has been used.

Potential for Addiction

The potential for psychological addiction is moderate. More than 290,000 persons seek treatment each year for their primary marijuana addiction (NIDA, 2009d). Marijuana is a schedule I drug.

Associated Problems/Disorders

Critical skills related to attention, learning, and memory are impaired in heavy marijuana users even 24 hours after the last use. Also, persons who use marijuana tend to be more accepting of deviant behavior, have more aggression and delinquent behavior, act more rebellious, and have poorer relationships with parents.

Withdrawal

Nausea, myalgia, restlessness, irritability, nervousness, insomnia, and depression may appear after ceasing marijuana use. Symptoms may not appear for up to 1 week after the last use.

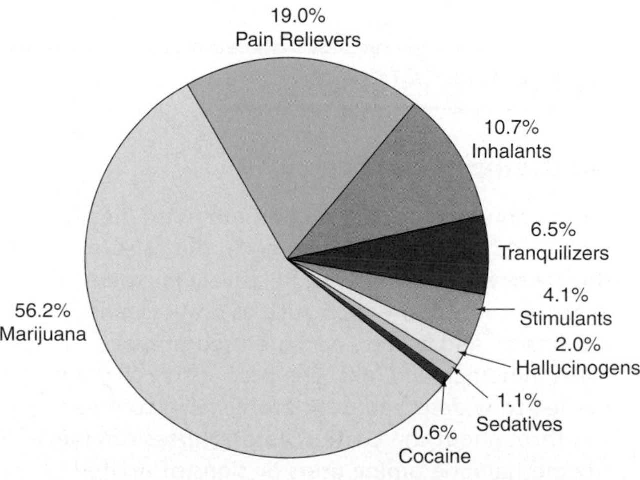

Figure 18-3 **Specific Drug Used When Initiating Illicit Drug Use among Persons Aged 12 or Older** (***Results from the 2007 National Survey on Drug Use and Health: National Findings, Department of Health and Human Services, Substance Abuse and Mental Health Services Administration [SAMHSA] [2008].***)

Treatment/Rehabilitation

Treatment focuses on relapse prevention and the development of new coping mechanisms, ways of living, and means of having fun without drugs. Weekly group therapy sessions to maintain a commitment to abstinence and enhance interpersonal skills are often used. Participation in a self-help group is encouraged.

CNS STIMULANTS

Drugs that stimulate the CNS include cocaine, amphetamines, caffeine, nicotine, and methylphenidate hydrochloride (Ritalin). They increase cortical alertness and electrical activity in the brain and spinal cord. There is tachycardia and an increase in blood pressure.

COCAINE

Cocaine is extracted from the leaves of the coca plant, *Erythroxylum coca*. It may be heated and the fumes inhaled. This is termed *free-basing*. As a white powder, cocaine is snorted by inhaling it through the nose or heated to a liquid state and injected intravenously. Crack is a crystallized form of cocaine that is melted in a water pipe and smoked. Street names include coke, crack, flake, rocks, snow, "C," and blow.

Incidence

Cocaine abuse and dependence was the major illicit drug problem for the United States in the 1980s. The introduction of crack dramatically increased cocaine abuse among the poor. Crack is low cost and gives an intense "high." It is estimated that 1.6 million Americans are dependent on or abuse cocaine (SAMHSA, 2008).

Signs and Symptoms

The immediate reaction, less than 10 seconds, is an intense euphoria that lasts 10 to 15 minutes. This short response time leads people to repeatedly use cocaine trying to maintain the euphoria.

The heart rate increases, blood pressure goes up, pupils dilate, peripheral blood vessels constrict, and temperature increases. Normal pleasures are magnified, anxiety decreases, self-confidence increases, social inhibitions are reduced, communication is facilitated, and sexual feelings are enhanced. Other psychological effects are inability to concentrate, insomnia, reduced sense of humor, antisocial behavior, hallucinations, and compulsive behavior.

An overdose may occur with the first use because there is little quality control of drug strength in the street drug culture. A client with an overdose may have arrhythmias, tremors, convulsions, respiratory failure, cardiovascular collapse, and death. Cocaine may be detected for up to 2 to 3 days in urine and for up to several months to years in hair.

Potential for Addiction

The potential for addiction is high. Cocaine is a schedule II drug.

Associated Problems/Disorders

Many types of heart disease are linked to cocaine use, especially ventricular fibrillation, heart attack, and hypertension. When cocaine is snorted regularly, respiratory problems occur, including loss of sense of smell, nosebleeds, hoarseness, and respiratory failure.

When cocaine is taken with alcohol, the two drugs are converted in the body to cocaethylene, which is more toxic than either drug alone (NIDA, 2008a).

Withdrawal

The crash, a period of exhaustion, occurs with symptoms of depression, anxiety, and a great need for sleep. The depression may be to the point of suicidal behavior. The client has no energy, shows little interest in the surroundings, and seems to have little ability to experience pleasure. These symptoms are the most intense during the first 3 days but continue for 1 to 4 months. An intense craving for cocaine is felt, including dreaming about cocaine. Then there is a period of less intense craving for cocaine called extinction, which may last months or even years. Withdrawal does not result in a medical emergency as seen with alcohol.

Treatment/Rehabilitation

Treatment is aimed at reducing the craving and managing the severe depression. Careful monitoring of the client is necessary to identify and prevent actions aimed at carrying out the idea of suicide. An individual with a history of cocaine usage has an intense craving for cocaine and a strong denial that cocaine is addicting. This creates a problem in engaging an individual in treatment. Inpatient programs are necessary for some clients with cocaine dependence, whereas other clients can be effectively treated in outpatient programs.

Medications

Bromocriptine mesylate (Parlodel) in small doses seems to reduce the withdrawal symptoms. Amantadine hydrochloride (Symmetrel) also has some success in treating cocaine withdrawal. Desipramine hydrochloride (Pertofrane) seems to reduce the craving for cocaine.

Education

Individual or group therapy should focus on helping the client feel pleasure again, improve energy level, and reduce cocaine craving. Peer support groups and self-help groups, such as Cocaine Anonymous, may be very effective. Random and regular urine testing is an external support to promote abstinence.

AMPHETAMINES

Amphetamines (also called uppers, speed, bennies) include dextroamphetamine sulfate (Dexedrine), amphetamine sulfate (Amphetamine), and methamphetamine hydrochloride (Desoxyn). Medically they are used to treat attention deficit hyperactivity disorder (ADHD), narcolepsy, and obesity.

Incidence

Amphetamines have been abused since the early 1930s. World War II greatly increased use and abuse when military personnel used amphetamines to decrease fatigue and increase alertness. Today, abuse ranges from truck drivers and college students who want to ward off sleep and increase alertness to the heavy abuser who injects or smokes homemade methamphetamine, known as meth, chalk, ice, crystal, crank, and glass. An estimated 10.4 million people in the United States have tried methamphetamine at some time (NIDA, 2005b).

Signs and Symptoms

Besides suppressing fatigue and increasing alertness, amphetamines enhance psychomotor performance, induce a temporary state of well-being, and give an instantaneous euphoria. Like cocaine, after several days the person becomes exhausted and lapses into a long period of sleep and depression (crash). The action of amphetamines lasts much longer than that of cocaine, and there is a greater potential for adverse reactions and severe toxicity (Figure 18-4).

High abuse doses may cause insomnia, tachycardia, headache, arrhythmias, hypertension followed by hypotension, nausea, vomiting, cramping, diarrhea, hyperreflexia, convulsions, and death. The psychological effect is termed *amphetamine psychosis* and closely resembles paranoid schizophrenia. Symptoms include paranoid ideation, confusion, compulsive behaviors, and visual and auditory hallucinations. Tolerance does develop. Amphetamines may be detected for up to 2 days.

Potential for Addiction

The potential for addiction is high. Amphetamines are schedule II drugs.

Associated Problems/Disorders

Cardiovascular problems occur, including irregular and rapid heartbeat; hypertension; and irreversible, stroke-producing

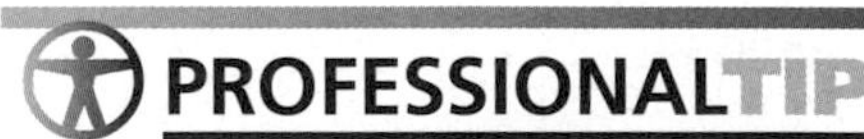

Methamphetamine

Methamphetamine, known as meth, is an illegal highly addictive drug belonging to the class of drugs known as stimulants. Relatively inexpensive over the counter products such as drain cleaner, antifreeze, and battery acid are used to make meth in homemade labs. The production of meth has led to widespread drug problems in communities throughout the United States. Nurses can identify methamphetamine users by signs of excited speech, agitation, decreased appetite, weight loss, nausea, vomiting, diarrhea, increased physical activity and energy level, dilated pupils, hypertension, angina, dyspnea, and hyperthermia.

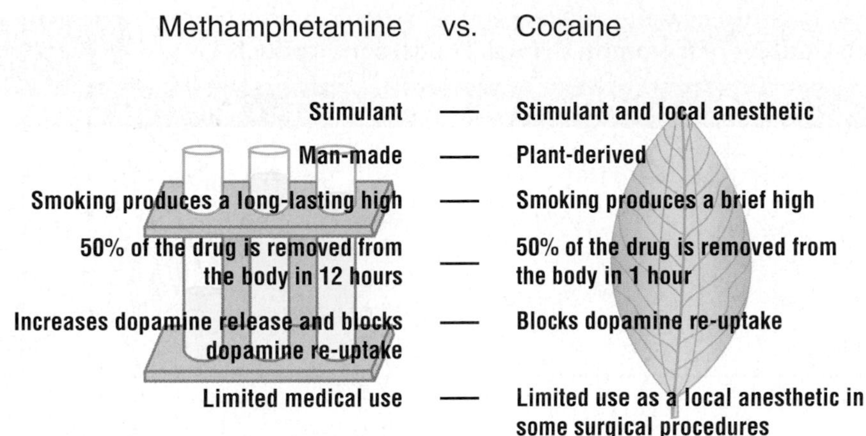

Methamphetamine vs. Cocaine
Stimulant — Stimulant and local anesthetic
Man-made — Plant-derived
Smoking produces a long-lasting high — Smoking produces a brief high
50% of the drug is removed from the body in 12 hours — 50% of the drug is removed from the body in 1 hour
Increases dopamine release and blocks dopamine re-uptake — Blocks dopamine re-uptake
Limited medical use — Limited use as a local anesthetic in some surgical procedures

FIGURE 18-4 **Basic Differences between Methamphetamine and Cocaine** (*Adapted from Research Report Series—Methamphetamine Abuse and Addiction, National Institute on Drug Abuse, 2008.*)

damage to small blood vessels in the brain (NIDA, 2008j). Injecting the drug may damage blood vessels and cause skin abscesses, and if injection equipment is shared, there is an increased risk of HIV/AIDS and hepatitis B and C transmission.

Withdrawal

Symptoms of withdrawal include apathy, fatigue, irritability, depression, disorientation, anxiety, paranoia, aggression, and an intense craving for the drug.

Treatment/Rehabilitation

Urinary acidifiers, such as ascorbic acid (vitamin C), increase the excretion of amphetamines. Diazepam (Valium) is given for sedation to ease the withdrawal crash. Bromocriptine mesylate (Parlodel) or levodopa (Dopar) may help decrease the craving. A quiet environment is also helpful.

Behavioral therapy is used to help the client recognize and accept the need to stop using amphetamines. Supportive individual or group therapy, and especially self-help groups, aids the client to stay abstinent and in treatment.

CAFFEINE

Caffeine is found in coffee, tea, cola beverages, energy drinks, cocoa, chocolate, and some nonprescription drugs (Table 18-6).

Incidence

Caffeine is probably the best known and most frequently used and abused CNS stimulant.

Signs and Symptoms

Caffeine causes relaxation of smooth muscles in blood vessels and bronchi, diuresis, an increased gastric acid secretion, suppression of appetite, increased feeling of energy, and constriction of cerebral blood vessels. An increased level of caffeine intake causes jitteriness, restlessness, nervousness, excitement, flushed face, palpitations, and nausea.

Potential for Addiction

The potential for addiction is moderate. Caffeine is not a scheduled drug.

Withdrawal

Withdrawal produces headache, irritability, and tremulousness.

Treatment/Rehabilitation

A gradual reduction of caffeine intake can reduce or eliminate the withdrawal symptoms. The client can then drink decaffeinated coffee and tea and caffeine-free soft drinks. The intake of cocoa and chocolate should be greatly reduced or eliminated. Caffeine can be avoided by reading labels and not using nonprescription products that contain caffeine.

NICOTINE

Nicotine is found in tobacco in a 1% to 2% concentration. There is no therapeutic use for nicotine. Smoking and other uses of tobacco have been in and out of favor several times during the past five centuries. This century has seen the greatest degree of abuse. Reasons for this increase are related to the mass production of tobacco products, mass advertising campaigns, and the psychological dependence produced by nicotine. Tobacco, even when used in moderation, will likely produce disease and death. Tobacco kills more than 430,000 U.S. citizens and 5 million persons worldwide each year (World Health Organization (WHO, 2008), Centers for Disease Control and Prevention (CDC, 2008c).

Incidence

In the United States 19.8% of the population, (43.4 million people) are current cigarette smokers (CDC, 2008a). Among high school students, 20% were current smokers in 2007 (CDC, 2008b).

Signs and Symptoms

Nicotine causes decreased skeletal muscle tone, decreased sensitivity of some receptor sites (pain, heat, taste buds),

TABLE 18-6 Caffeine Content of Common Drinks, Foods, and Products

SUBSTANCE	SERVING SIZE	CAFFEINE CONTENT (MILLIGRAMS)
Coffee		
Brewed, drip method	8 oz.	65–150
Instant	8 oz.	60–130
Decaffeinated	8 oz.	2–9
Espresso	1 oz.	30–64
Starbucks Cafe Latte	16 oz.	150
Starbucks Coffee Grande	16 oz.	330
Tea		
Brewed	8 oz.	20–110
Instant	8 oz.	10–35
Green tea, brewed	8 oz.	30–50
Canned or bottled	8–12 oz.	10–75
Lipton Brisk Iced Tea, lemon flavored	12 oz.	10
Nestea, sweetened or unsweetened	12 oz.	17
Snapple Iced Tea	16 oz.	18
Soft Drinks		
Mountain Dew (Regular & Diet)	12 oz.	54
Mello Yellow	12 oz.	53
Diet Coke	12 oz.	47
Sunkist Orange	12 oz.	41
Pepsi	12 oz.	38
Coca-Cola	12 oz.	35
Diet Pepsi	12 oz.	35
Sprite	12 oz.	0
Sports/Energy Drinks		
Spike Shooter	8.4 oz.	300
No Name (formerly known as Cocaine)	8.4 oz.	280
Monster Energy	16 oz.	160
Rockstar	16 oz.	160
Full Throttle	16 oz.	144
Red Bull	8.3 oz.	76
Vault	8 oz.	47
Foods & Products		
Milk chocolate candy bar	1–1.5 oz	2–10
Dark chocolate candy bar	1–1.5 oz.	5–35
Hot cocoa	8 oz.	2–10
Jolt Caffeinated Gum	1 stick	33
Foosh Energy Mints	1 mint	100
Coffee ice cream	8 oz.	8–85
NoDoz Maximum Strength	1 tablet	200
Vivarin	1 tablet	200
Excedrin Extra Strength	2 tablets	130

Data from Johns Hopkins University School of Medicine, Johns Hopkins Bayview Campus, Behavioral Biology Research Center, 2009, www.caffeinedependence.org/caffeine_dependence.html#sources; Mayo Clinic, 2007, *How much caffeine is in your daily habit?* Retrieved from http://www.mayoclinic.com/health/caffeine/AN01211/METHOD=print; Center for Science in the Public Interest, 2007, *Caffeine content of food and drugs.* Retrieved from http://www.cspinet.org/new/cafchart.htm

LIFE SPAN CONSIDERATIONS

Smoking

- Menopause generally occurs earlier in women who smoke.
- The older smoker is often less motivated to quit because of the feeling that "I've survived this long."

reduced appetite, vasoconstriction, decreased body temperature, and increased blood pressure. Tolerance develops so the daily intake must increase to continue the desired effect.

Potential for Addiction

The potential for addiction is high. Even first-time users can become dependent within weeks of their initial use. Nicotine is not a scheduled drug.

Associated Problems/ Disorders

Other ingredients in the smoke (tar, carbon monoxide, and incompletely burned waste products) are largely responsible for the negative health consequences.

Respiratory

Chronic obstructive pulmonary disease is caused by the many changes tobacco use makes in the respiratory system. Smokers are more prone to developing pneumonia, and asthma is exacerbated by smoking. Chronic exposure to smoke inhalation gives children higher rates of otitis media and respiratory illnesses.

Cardiovascular

Ischemic heart disease is twice as likely to develop in a smoker than in a nonsmoker. Cerebrovascular accidents and peripheral vascular disease are strongly associated with smoking. Cessation of smoking, about 10 years, reduces the risks for these three vascular diseases to the nonsmoker's level.

Cancer

Many cancers—oral, pharyngeal, laryngeal, esophageal, lung, pancreatic, kidney, and bladder—are strongly associated with tobacco. Secondhand smoke causes lung cancer in nonsmoking adults. Tobacco use is by far the most important risk factor in lung cancer development (American Cancer Society, 2007).

Withdrawal

Short-term effects of nicotine withdrawal include nausea, diarrhea, headache, drowsiness, insomnia, irritability, and poor concentration. Increased appetite along with an intense craving for tobacco may persist for 6 months or longer.

Treatment/Rehabilitation

Nicotine replacement therapy by patch, nasal spray, inhaler, or gum helps individuals break the habit. It is important that the client not smoke while using the patch. Serious adverse effects may be experienced with a high serum nicotine level. It can be toxic. Later, a gradual withdrawal of the nicotine patch can be accomplished. The first non-nicotine prescription drug to treat nicotine addiction, bupropion (Zyban), was approved by the Food and Drug Administration in 1996.

An exercise program will help with stress management and minimize possible weight gain. Relaxation techniques will also reduce stress. Support by family and significant others for the person quitting tobacco use may help the process. A lack of support may greatly increase the difficulty of quitting for the individual. The rate of relapse is highest in the first few weeks and diminishes considerably after 3 months.

METHYLPHENIDATE HYDROCHLORIDE (RITALIN)

Currently, there is an increase in the use (misuse and overuse) of Ritalin that is becoming a growing problem. Ritalin is an accepted treatment for children with attention deficit hyperactivity disorder (ADHD). Although Ritalin is a CNS stimulant, there is a paradoxical calming effect on children with ADHD. Many children are being given Ritalin without thorough testing to eliminate other causes of attention deficit. These children have the potential for dependence. Ritalin is also used for narcolepsy. It can be detected for 1 to 2 days and is a schedule II drug.

HALLUCINOGENS

Hallucinogens refers to a group of naturally occurring and synthetic agents that produce essentially the same mind-altering effects.

Psilocybin and psilocin are naturally occurring organic compounds found in some mushrooms that grow in the United States and Mexico. These mushrooms have been used for centuries in southern Mexico, primarily in religious ceremonies. Fresh or dried mushrooms, sometimes mixed with food, are ingested orally.

Dimethyltryptamine (DMT) and diethyltryptamine (DET) are found in tropical plant leaves and seeds. For centuries they have been dried and powdered and used as snuff. They are not orally active. Sometimes the powder is added to tobacco or marijuana.

There are several amphetamine-like hallucinogens. Probably the two best known are 2,5 dimethyl-4-ethylamphetamine (DOM) and methylene-dioxyamphetamine (MDMA, ecstasy), which are chemically manufactured compounds. These are usually taken orally but may be injected intravenously or inhaled.

LYSERGIC ACID DIETHYLAMIDE

Lysergic acid diethylamide (LSD), a manufactured chemical compound, is perhaps the most widely known and used hallucinogen. In the past, LSD has been used as a legitimate medication and in research. In the 1960s, when its abuse became so widespread, the manufacturer refused to supply it for research. It had already been discontinued as a useful medication. It is generally taken orally but can be injected intravenously.

Incidence

The use of hallucinogens declined throughout the 1980s. In the early 1990s, LSD made a comeback. The 1990 and 1991 annual survey of high school seniors found that for the first time since 1976, more seniors had used LSD than cocaine in the previous 12 months. The 1998 survey showed a slight downward movement in LSD use. The 2007 survey showed that in 2006 more than 23 million Americans aged 12 or older had used LSD in their lifetime (SAMHSA, 2008). Other names for LSD are acid, blotter, and microdot.

Signs and Symptoms

The functioning of both the peripheral nervous system and the central nervous system is altered by LSD. Physical effects include hypertension, increased temperature, sweating, loss of appetite, dilated pupils, and dry mouth. Time and distance are distorted, rational judgment is impaired, and visual **hallucinations** (perceiving things that are not really there) and delusions along with **synesthesia** (hearing colors and seeing sounds) occur. A state of either euphoria or depression is experienced. The depression with feelings of anxiety, panic, or suicidal tendencies is termed a "bad trip." Flashbacks occur suddenly days or years after LSD use. Their occurrence and frequency are unpredictable but seem to happen in times of high stress. LSD may be detected up to 8 hours after use.

Potential for Addiction

LSD is not considered an addictive drug, but it does produce tolerance. It is a schedule I drug.

Associated Problems/ Disorders

Personality changes occur with LSD use and may happen after a single LSD experience. Acceptable social behaviors seem to diminish with use.

Withdrawal

There is no withdrawal seen.

Treatment/Rehabilitation

A person on a "bad trip" should be carefully watched to prevent self-injury. Reassurance, support, and "talking down" should be done in a quiet, pleasant manner. The person should be encouraged to sit up or walk. Closing the eyes intensifies the "bad trip." The person should be reminded that the drug is causing the effects, which will soon go away.

After cessation of chronic LSD use, long-term psychotherapy is usually required to determine what needs were fulfilled by the use of this drug. A 12-step program and family assistance are usually necessary to reinforce the decision to remain abstinent. If the client is upset by flashbacks or the fear of flashbacks, an anxiolytic drug such as diazepam (Valium) may be ordered.

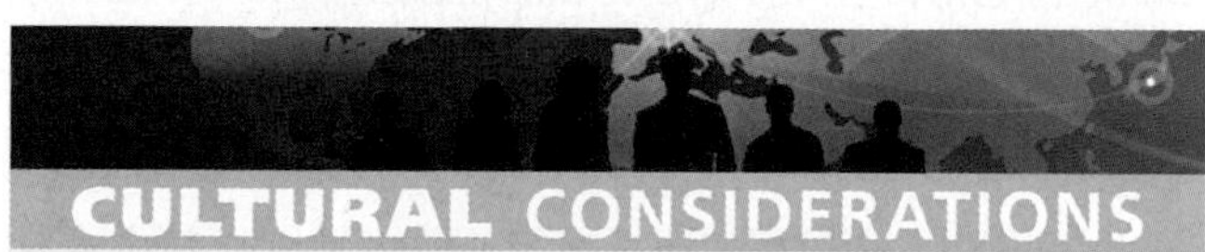

CULTURAL CONSIDERATIONS

Mescaline

Mescaline is the active ingredient in peyote cactus found growing in the southwestern United States and Mexico. It is the only legally used hallucinogen. Members of the Native American Church of the United States may use it for religious purposes. It is ingested orally. A cross-tolerance to LSD and psilocybin occurs.

PHENCYCLIDINE

Phencyclidine (PCP) was made for use as an anesthetic agent, but it produced such adverse reactions that it was withdrawn from clinical trials; however, it can easily be manufactured in an unsophisticated laboratory from simple materials. The degree of purity varies widely. It is often found as a contaminant in other street drugs. The anesthetic is used in veterinary medicine.

Incidence

PCP is primarily used by adolescents and young adults, with the first use between the ages of 13 and 15 years. Approximately 12.8% of those between the ages of 12 and 17 years had used PCP in 1979. The use decreased to 2.4% in 1992 and increased to 3.9% in 1997. In 2006, *The National Survey on Drug Use and Health* reported that 6.6 million persons aged 12 or older had used PCP in their lifetime (SAMHSA, 2008). The *Monitoring the Future Survey* showed that in 2007, 2.1% of high school seniors had tried PCP (NIDA, 2007). Other names for PCP are angel dust, ozone, wack, and rocket fuel. Marijuana combined with PCP is called killer joints or crystal super grass.

Signs and Symptoms

There are usually four phases, with the symptoms dose related. Acute toxicity is characterized by visual disturbances, auditory hallucinations, combativeness, catatonia, convulsions, and coma, and lasts about 3 days. The toxic psychosis phase has visual and auditory hallucinations, agitation, paranoid delusions, and disturbed judgment, and lasts about 7 days. The third phase has psychotic episodes, including thought disorders, paranoid ideation, and affect disorders much like schizophrenia and lasts a month or more. Depression is the fourth phase that may end in suicide. The use of other street drugs may alleviate the depression. Behavior is highly unpredictable. Death can occur from respiratory depression. For 2 to 8 days, PCP can be detected.

Potential for Addiction

Even chronic use does not produce physical dependence. Psychological dependence does develop as evidenced by a craving for PCP. It is a schedule I and II drug.

Associated Problems/ Disorders

Seizures are a common occurrence with PCP. Hypertension and hyperthermia must be treated before they become a crisis situation. **Opisthotonos**, a complete arching of the body with only the head and feet on the bed, usually is relieved as the blood level of PCP decreases. Cardiac arrhythmias may need interventions by a cardiologist. Acute renal failure may result from the use of PCP. Strokes also have been reported.

WITHDRAWAL

PCP is fat soluble and its effects are felt weeks after the last use as it is gradually released from the fatty tissue into the circulation.

TREATMENT/REHABILITATION

Treatment should begin in an inpatient setting because of the high risk of suicide. The goal is to keep the client from resuming drug use. Sedatives may be used, and urinary acidifiers such as ascorbic acid may be given to increase excretion of PCP. Minimal confrontation should be used in a nonthreatening, nonstimulating, supportive environment. No effort should be made to "talk down" or calm the individual. Diazepam (Valium) may be ordered.

Vocational counseling and training may enhance self-esteem. Body awareness, yoga, and progressive relaxation help the client focus and improve attention span and concentration. Participation in a self-help group such as Narcotics Anonymous (NA) should be encouraged, although initial involvement is usually minimal.

OPIOIDS

Opioids is a term used to refer to naturally occurring opiates, semisynthetic opiates, synthetic opiates, and agonist-antagonists. Table 18-7 provides examples of these opioids. Heroin is the most abused and the most rapid acting of the opioids (NIDA, 2008i).

INCIDENCE

Kleber (1999) described the 1990s as the decade of heroin. Cocaine addicts switched to heroin. Heroin was easily available, the purity was higher than in decades, and it could now be sniffed or smoked instead of injected (NIDA, 2008i). In 2006, 560,000 Americans age 12 and older had abused heroin at least once in the year before being surveyed (SAMHSA, 2008). Other names for heroin are horse, smack, "H," skag, and junk.

SIGNS AND SYMPTOMS

All of these drugs affect the CNS, causing mental changes, euphoria, drowsiness, analgesia, constricted pupils, and depressed respirations (Figure 18-5). These changes become more pronounced as the dose is increased.

Opioids increase stomach tone, decrease intestinal peristalsis, and increase the tone of the anal sphincter. This all adds up to constipation. Prolonged drug use may result in a fecal impaction.

Peripheral blood vessels are dilated by opioids, and orthostatic hypotension frequently occurs. The work of the heart is not changed by opioids, so they are frequently used to treat the severe pain of a myocardial infarction.

TABLE 18-7 Opioids

TYPE	EXAMPLE
Natural Opiates	morphine sulfate codeine sulfate
Semisynthetic Opiates	heroin hydromorphone hydrochloride (Dilaudid) oxymorphone hydrochloride (Numorphan) oxycodone (in Percodan) hydrocodone (in Hycodan)
Synthetic Opiates	meperidine hydrochloride (Demerol) methadone hydrochloride (Dolophine) propoxyphene (Darvon)
Agonist-Antagonists	pentazocine (Talwin) nalbuphine hydrochloride (Nubain) butorphanol tartrate (Stadol)

Tolerance may develop to one or more of the effects of opioids but not to others. For example, morphine addicts will always have pinpoint pupils even when the euphoric effects are not experienced. Tolerance to one opioid usually means tolerance to other opioids as well. Withdrawal symptoms from one opioid can be suppressed by using another opioid.

POTENTIAL FOR ADDICTION

The potential for addiction is high. Heroin is a schedule I drug; methadone, schedule II; morphine, schedule II or III; and codeine and opium are schedule II, III, or IV.

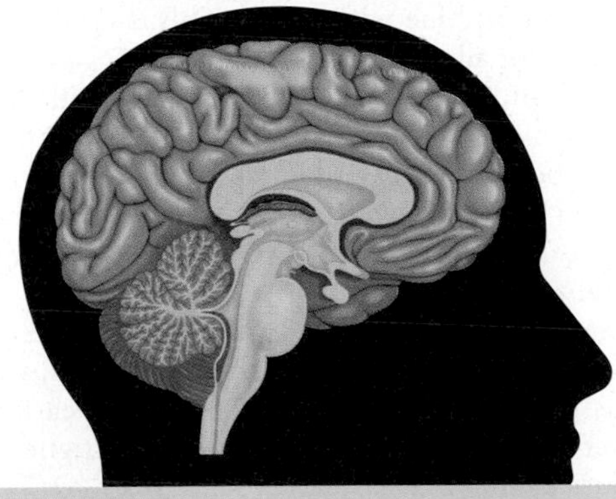

The Short-Term Effects of Opiates
• Opiates can depress breathing by changing neurochemical activity in the brain stem, where automatic body functions are controlled.
• Opiates can change the limbic system, which controls emotions, to increase feelings of pleasure.
• Opiates can block pain messages transmitted through the spinal cord from the body.

FIGURE 18-5 **Opiates act on many places in the brain and spinal cord.** (*From Research Report Series—Heroin Abuse and Addiction, National Institute on Drug Abuse, 2008.*)

CRITICAL THINKING

Narcotic Addiction

A client who has had a series of abdominal surgeries with recurrent infections told his wife that he is afraid that he is becoming addicted to narcotics, but he does not want anyone to know. The wife confides in you and asks for advice. How would you respond to the wife?

Associated Problems/Disorders

Chronic heroin injection may cause scarred and collapsed veins, bacterial infections of heart valves and blood vessels, abscesses, and liver or kidney disease. Pneumonia may result from the respiratory-depressing effect of heroin. Additives to street heroin may clog blood vessels or cause immune reactions, leading to arthritis or other rheumatologic conditions. Sharing injection equipment can lead to infections of hepatitis B and C, HIV, and other blood-borne viruses, which can be passed on to sexual partners and children.

Withdrawal

Withdrawal symptoms depend on drug purity, dose, and route of administration. Withdrawal is characterized by a rebound excitability of those functions that had been depressed. Symptoms include stomach cramps, nausea, vomiting, diarrhea, diaphoresis, hypertension, aching of bones and muscles, lacrimation, rhinorrhea, cold flashes with goose bumps, yawning, mydriasis, anxiety, irritability, restlessness, and sometimes paranoia, violence, fear, or depersonalization.

Morphine withdrawal symptoms begin within 8 to 12 hours after the last dose, and the acute phase is over in about 10 to 14 days. Figure 18-6 illustrates the signs and symptoms of morphine withdrawal. This is the basic pattern of withdrawal for all opioids.

Codeine withdrawal symptoms may be a little less severe than those of morphine withdrawal. Dilaudid and heroin withdrawal may begin slightly earlier than morphine withdrawal. Meperidine (Demerol) withdrawal begins within 3 hours and peaks in 8 to 12 hours. Propoxyphene (Darvon) withdrawal is considerably milder.

Methadone withdrawal is slower to develop and lasts longer. Symptoms may not occur for 1 to 2 days, with acute symptoms lasting 2 to 3 weeks but not disappearing until 6 weeks after abstinence begins. Symptoms of fatigue, sluggishness, and irritability may last up to 6 months.

Withdrawal from the agonist-antagonists begins in 6 to 8 hours and is usually over in 8 days. The symptoms are the same as for morphine only in a milder form.

Treatment/Rehabilitation

Initial treatment is symptomatic and supportive of vital functions until the acute phase is over.

Detoxification

Several methods currently used for opioid detoxification are methadone, LAAM, and naltrexone.

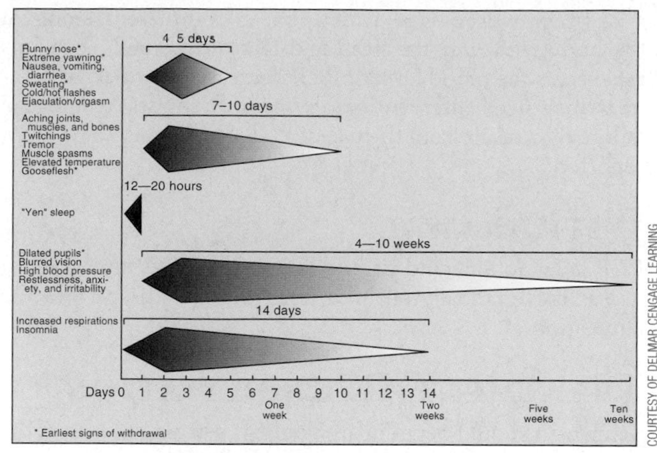

FIGURE 18-6 Duration of Morphine Withdrawal Signs and Symptoms (Basic Pattern for All Opioids)

Methadone Methadone is given and the dose adjusted to keep withdrawal symptoms under control. The daily dose is gradually reduced over a period of 3 to 6 months. Routine and random urine testing is usually done to ensure no other drug use.

Levo-alpha-acetyl-methadol Levo-alpha-acetyl-methadol (LAAM) is a synthetic opiate, like methadone, used to treat heroin addiction. It blocks the effects of heroin for up to 72 hours, so it need be taken only 3 times a week.

Naltrexone Naltrexone (ReVia) blocks the effects of morphine, heroin, and other opiates. Its effects last for 1 to 3 days, depending on the dose. The pleasurable effects of heroin are blocked, making it useful to treat highly motivated individuals. It is also used to prevent relapse in former opiate addicts.

Counseling/Self-Help Groups

Individual and/or group counseling must go hand in hand with the detoxification to help the client learn new methods of coping with life's stresses. Participation in Narcotics Anonymous (NA) helps the client maintain abstinence from drugs.

Behavioral Therapy

Contingency management therapy employs a voucher system. Clients earn "points" for having negative drug tests. These can be exchanged for items encouraging healthy living.

INHALANTS

Inhalants are inexpensive and easy to obtain. Examples are toluene (glues), gasoline, kerosene, isopropyl alcohol, lacquer thinner, acetone, benzene, naptha, carbon tetrachloride, fluorocarbons (aerosol propellants), correction fluid, and nitrous oxide. They are rapidly absorbed into the brain and stored in body fat. Common names for inhalants are whippets, poppers, and snappers.

Incidence

In 1997, 21% of 8th graders, 18.3% of 10th graders, and 16.1% of 12th graders reported using inhalants at least once. By 2002, 15.2% of 8th graders, 13.5% of 10th graders, and 11.7% of 13th graders reported using inhalants at least once. The Monitoring the Future Study (NIDA, 2005a) revealed that 17.3% of 8th graders have abused inhalants. Several National Surveys have reported that more than 22.9 million Americans have abused inhalants at least once in their lives (NIDA, 2005a). Inhalants are not scheduled drugs.

Signs and Symptoms

The desired effect of euphoria is followed by nausea, headache, and amnesia. Other effects of using inhalants include dizziness, unsteady gait, slurred speech, auditory and visual hallucinations, drowsiness, hypotension, heightened sexual response caused by profound vasodilation, stupor, unconsciousness, and coma. Heavy use can lead to hypoxia, multiple organ damage, and death. Airway freezing and/or laryngospasm can be caused by nitrous oxide.

Behaviors that may indicate inhalant abuse include decreased school performance; loss of interest in extracurricular, family, and social activities; and the onset of legal problems.

Potential for Addiction

The potential for addiction is high for psychological dependence only.

Associated Problems/Disorders

Chronic pulmonary irritation and/or chemical pneumonitis may be caused by the use of inhalants. Toluene may cause renal tubular acidosis, hearing loss, and brain damage. Fluorocarbons sensitize the myocardium to catacholemines and may cause arrhythmias.

Withdrawal

There are no withdrawal symptoms.

Treatment/Rehabilitation

Initial treatment is to provide oxygen and respiratory support. Participation in a traditional chemical dependency program is often needed. An adolescent 12-step group is very helpful. Individual and family counseling are essential.

ECSTASY

Ecstasy, also called MDMA (3,4-methylenedioxymethamphetamine), is a complex drug having similarities to methamphetamine, a stimulant, and mescaline, a hallucinogen (NIDA, 2008f). It produces stimulant effects and distorted time and perception rather than true hallucinations. Street names include "X", "E", "XTC", Adam, hug, beans, clarity, lover's speed, and love drug. Ecstasy tablets also often contain one or more of the following: caffeine, methamphetamine, dextromethorphan, ephedrine, or cocaine.

Incidence

Americans using ecstasy for the first time increased from 615,000 in 2005 to 860,000 in 2006. Most of these new users were 18 or older (SAMHSA, 2008).

Signs and Symptoms

Ecstasy provides an enhanced sense of pleasure and self-confidence; feelings of peacefulness, acceptance, and closeness with others; and increased energy. Research has shown that ecstasy can lead to disruptions in body temperature and cardiovascular regulation. It also damages the nerves in the brain's serotonin system and appears to produce long-term deficits in memory and cognition (NIDA, 2001b). It appears that the more ecstasy taken, the greater the deficit (NIDA, 2001a).

Potential for Addiction

The potential for addiction is currently being researched by clinical studies. For some people, studies have found that ecstasy can be addictive (NIDA, 2008f).

Associated Problems/Disorders

MDMA interferes with the metabolism of other drugs, including some that may be in the tablet with the ecstasy.

ANABOLIC STEROIDS

Anabolic steroids are synthetic derivatives of testosterone. They cause both androgenic (masculinizing) and anabolic (tissue building) effects. Most people use anabolic steroids for their anabolic effects. Medically, they are used in the treatment of some anemias and in some cancer therapies. The use of anabolic steroids is banned by the International Olympic Committee and the National Collegiate Athletic Association.

Incidence

Primary users are athletes seeking to improve their performance. Other people use anabolic steroids to improve their physical appearance. In 2000, 3% of 8th graders, 3.5% of 10th graders, and 2.5% of 12th graders had used anabolic steroids. The *2007 Monitoring the Future Study* (NIDA, 2009e) reported that 0.8% of 8th, 1.1% of 10th, and 1.4% of 12th graders had abused anabolic steroids at least once in the year prior to being surveyed.

PROFESSIONALTIP

Club Drugs

Club drugs are being used by young adults at all-night parties such as "raves" or "trances," dance clubs, and bars. MDMA (Ecstasy), GHB, Rohypnol, ketamine, methamphetamine, and LSD are some of the club or party drugs. These drugs can cause serious health problems. Used in combination with alcohol, the drugs are even more dangerous (NIDA, 2009b).

Signs and Symptoms

The commonly perceived effects of anabolic steroids are an increase in skeletal muscle mass, enhanced physical performance of the skeletal muscles, and improved athletic ability; however, there is no conclusive evidence that these perceived effects are medically accurate.

Potential for Addiction

The potential for addiction is moderate. Anabolic steroids are schedule III drugs.

Associated Problems/ Disorders

Other effects found when anabolic steroids are used include hepatocellular damage, cholestasis, hepatoadenoma, hepatocarcinoma, acne, hirsutism, male-pattern baldness, a deepening of the voice, increased cholesterol level, increased blood pressure, decreased glucose tolerance, mood swings, aggressiveness, depression, psychosis, and hepatitis or HIV infection if needles are shared. In males, there is also testicular atrophy, oligospermia, impotence, prostatic hypertrophy, prostatic carcinoma, and gynecomastia. In females, there is also amenorrhea, clitoromegaly, uterine atrophy, breast atrophy, facial hair growth, and teratogenicity.

These effects seem to be reversible when the anabolic steroids are no longer taken, except for the male-pattern baldness, liver tumors, and gynecomastia in males and clitoral enlargement, virilization, and male-pattern baldness in females. The increased aggressiveness and euphoria are probably beneficial during athletic competitions but otherwise may cause severe social problems.

Withdrawal

Symptoms of withdrawal include lethargy, abdominal muscle cramps, constipation, headache, and depression.

Treatment/Rehabilitation

Treatment of withdrawal focuses on providing symptom relief for the client and counseling to build self-esteem and self-confidence in abilities without the use of anabolic steroids.

NURSING PROCESS

Nursing care is an essential component of the multidisciplinary approach to substance abuse treatment.

Assessment

The subjective and objective data given are related to substance abuse and dependence in general.

Subjective Data

The client will often describe being very relaxed; feeling wonderful; or having a headache, fatigue, depression, sleep disturbance, suppression of appetite, dizziness, hallucinations, paranoia, anxiety, emotional lability, memory loss, heightened sexual desire (with early use), or loss of sexual desire (with continued use). Problems in various areas of life are common, such as frequent job changes; marital conflict, separation and/or divorce; work-related accidents, lateness, absenteeism; and legal problems, including arrest for driving while intoxicated. The client may describe having falls or fights and financial problems. Normal diet pattern and the presence of any disease conditions should be noted.

The client should be asked health history questions regarding substance abuse (Table 18-8). The information received from the client may not always be accurate. Validation with the family or significant other is helpful.

Objective Data

Neglect of health and personal care is often evident. The client may have dental caries, bad breath, gingivitis, unkempt appearance, and be undernourished or malnourished. If substances have been inhaled, there may be irritation and bleeding of the nasal mucosa, destruction of the nasal mucosa and cartilaginous structures, or depression of respirations. If substances have been injected intravenously, there will be scarring of veins (needle marks, track marks), possibly skin infections, enlarged lymph nodes, and hematomas.

Table 18-8 Obtaining a Client History of Substance Abuse Problems

How often do you use drugs/alcohol?

How much do you usually use?

Have you ever used drugs/alcohol more than you use them now? When?

Under what circumstances?

What substance did you last use?

Has anyone ever told you to cut back or quit using drugs/alcohol?

Have you tried?

Have you or are you having interpersonal, occupational, physical, psychological or legal problems due to drugs/alcohol?

MEMORY TRICK

Substance Abuse Client Assessment

An easy memory trick for general assessment findings for a client participating in substance abuse is **DRUGS**:

- **D** = Depression
- **R** = Reduced self-control
- **U** = Unkept appearance
- **G** = Gives excuses (for absenteeism, memory loss, etc.)
- **S** = Sleep disturbance

The client may appear older than the stated age and have a chronic cough producing brown to black sputum, dilated or pinpoint pupils, tremors, slurred speech, lack of coordination, frequent episodes of sexually transmitted diseases, jaundice, or vomiting. There may be tachycardia, hypertension, ascites, or petechiae.

Nursing Diagnoses

NANDA-International (2009) nursing diagnoses for a client with substance abuse or dependence may include the following:

- *Imbalanced* ***Nutrition****: Less than Body Requirements*
- ***Self-Care*** *Deficits*
- *Risk for* ***Injury***
- *Disturbed* ***Sleep*** *Pattern*
- ***Activity*** *Intolerance*
- *Impaired Physical* ***Mobility***
- *Disturbed* ***Sensory*** *Perception*
- *Impaired Verbal* ***Communication***
- *Risk for* ***Infection***
- *Excess or Deficient* ***Fluid*** *Volume*
- *Disturbed* ***Thought*** *Processes*
- *Ineffective* ***Coping***
- *Situational Low* ***Self-Esteem***
- *Risk for* ***Violence*** *(Other-Directed or Self-Directed)*
- ***Anxiety***
- *Impaired* ***Social*** *Interaction*
- ***Hopelessness***
- ***Powerlessness***
- *Compromised Family* ***Coping***
- *Defensive* ***Coping***
- *Self-****Neglect***

Planning/Outcome Identification

There are several overall goals for the care of a client with a substance abuse problem. The client will do the following:

1. Abstain from using psychoactive substances
2. Adhere to the treatment plan
3. Make lifestyle changes to maintain abstinence
4. Engage in behaviors that foster good health

Possible outcomes from Nursing Outcomes Classification (NOC) include:

- Distorted Thought Control
- Risk Control: Alcohol Use
- Risk Control: Drug Use

Nursing Interventions

Nursing interventions include active listening, providing care in a nonjudgmental manner, teaching health promotion, and referral to self-help groups or individual counseling. Other nursing interventions must be specific for the goals and nursing diagnoses identified for the individual client. Examples might include the following:

1. Provide a well-balanced diet. Monitor intake and results of lab tests. Assess for GI bleeding.
2. Assist with personal hygiene. Encourage self-care.
3. Administer medications as ordered to decrease or prevent symptoms of withdrawal. Keep call light in client's reach. Keep siderails up.
4. Provide warm milk at bedtime. Plan with client a time for bed. Encourage use of relaxation techniques. Reassure client that insomnia will improve.
5. Encourage client to do active ROM exercises.
6. Assist client to turn in bed. Assist client to ambulate as able. Answer call light promptly.
7. Do not argue with a client having hallucinations. Remind client of day, time, and place.
8. Monitor the client's nonverbal communication.
9. Encourage good personal hygiene. Inspect skin for integrity.
10. Administer antibiotics as ordered. Monitor vital signs, I&O, and results of diagnostic testing.
11. Administer vitamins as ordered. Provide cues as needed. Encourage adequate diet intake.
12. Assess coping patterns to identify strengths and weaknesses. Actively listen to client. Refer to appropriate community agencies.
13. Assist client to identify areas of low self-esteem. Encourage client participation in group therapy. Refer to individual counseling as needed.
14. Monitor client closely. Use restraints as ordered. Keep bed in low position and side rails up.
15. Introduce client to other recovering persons. Encourage client to participate in self-help group.
16. Provide spiritual support if asked.
17. Involve client in decision making when possible. Give positive reinforcement for abstinence.
18. Encourage family to participate in treatment program.

LIFE SPAN CONSIDERATIONS

Substance Misuse or Abuse

In the older adult:

- Misuse (using a legal drug for something other than intended or exceeding the recommended dose of a drug) is more common than abuse or dependence.
- Substances that decrease respirations can increase the frequency of mental confusion.
- Decreased coordination from alcohol or other substances is associated with falling more often and fracturing the wrist, back, and hips.
- Chronic medical conditions can be made worse from even minimal use of alcohol or other drugs because these substances can change the effect of prescribed medications.
- Unrealistic expectations of retirement may lead to use of mood-altering substances to relieve depression and boredom.

Possible interventions from Nursing Interventions Classification (NIC) include:

- Delusion Management
- Hallucination Management
- Anxiety Reduction
- Delirium Management
- Mood Management

EVALUATION

Each goal must be evaluated to determine how it has been met by the client and modified as necessary.

CODEPENDENCY

Codependency was first recognized by those working with families of alcoholics. It is a learned pattern of feeling and behaving, a problem with relationships. In healthy relationships, people share love, concern, and respect for each other. There is equal give-and-take. This is termed *interdependence*. In unhealthy relationships, people are often out of touch with their own needs and feelings. They may be unwilling or unable to take care of themselves and have little self-esteem. Only by fulfilling the expectations of others do they feel good about themselves. This is termed *codependence*. **Codependent** persons live based on what others think of them. They always try to meet the needs of others, demand love from others, and manipulate and control the lives of others.

Serious family problems like addictions, abuse, family secrets, or other major stresses cause confusion and put a family at risk. Codependent behavior thrives when fear, guilt, blame, and low self-esteem become evident. When family members do not relate to each other in positive ways or when their interactions do not provide a healthy environment, the family is called *dysfunctional*. Many children grow up in dysfunctional families and learn to be codependent.

Codependency tends to run in families. Parents cannot teach their children how to cope in healthy ways if they do not know how themselves. Without intervention or a conscious change by the individual, a pattern of codependent behavior will continue in other relationships.

CHARACTERISTICS

Persons who are codependent have specific characteristics or traits. They have low self-esteem, never feel they are good enough, and often feel shame. Emotions are denied. They are out of touch with their own feelings and deny their own needs. Their smile is phony much of the time. Problems with communication become evident as they have trouble expressing their needs and feelings. Often they say the opposite to hide their true feelings. They expect others to read their minds. Relationship problems occur because they are afraid of being hurt or that others might learn of their secret feelings and reject them. They cannot risk loving and losing. Relationships are desired, but walls are always put up.

Codependent persons live through others. They are people pleasers who would rather give than take. The approval of others means they are okay. They think they can fix others. The feeling of powerlessness occurs because they give power to others by looking to them for approval. They go to extremes. For a while they will try very hard for approval, and then they will not try at all or they will keep negative feelings inside with a smile on their face and then blow up over some little thing. Table 18-9 lists some characteristics of the codependent person.

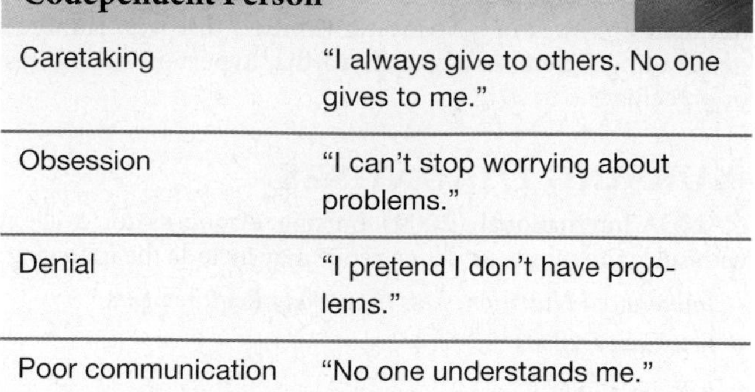

TABLE 18-9 Characteristics of the Codependent Person

Caretaking	"I always give to others. No one gives to me."
Obsession	"I can't stop worrying about problems."
Denial	"I pretend I don't have problems."
Poor communication	"No one understands me."
Lack of trust	"I don't trust myself."
Anger	"I resent feeling controlled and manipulated."

From *Mental Health Concepts* (5th ed.), by C. Waughfield, 2002, Clifton Park, NY: Delmar Cengage Learning. Copyright 2002 by Delmar Cengage Learning. Adapted with permission.

TREATMENT

Professional help is usually necessary to change codependent behavior. The goal of treatment is to help the codependent person feel happy and good about himself or herself. Therapy sessions focus on identifying and reconnecting with the true self, dealing with feelings, learning how to communicate feelings, learning to trust, setting boundaries for relationships, and taking charge of their own life.

THE IMPAIRED NURSE

Most states now have peer assistance programs to help nurses who are impaired by either alcohol or other substances. Substance abuse and dependence are greater problems among nurses than among the general public because nurses have access to many controlled substances. The impaired nurse often requests to give medications, makes medication errors, and "wastes" drugs frequently. This nurse may wear long sleeves and spend an extraordinary amount of time in the bathroom.

Peer assistance programs first appeared in 1980. They have been formed through the state nursing association or the state board of nursing, or through joint effort of both. The goals of the peer assistance programs are to assist the impaired nurse to receive treatment; protect the public from impaired nurses; help the recovering nurse reenter the nursing

RESOURCES

Al-Anon Family Group, http://www.al-anon.org
Alcoholics Anonymous (AA), http://www.aa.org
American Council for Drug Education, http:// www.acde.org
Codependents Anonymous (CODA), http://www.codependents.org
Drug Abuse Resistance Education (DARE), Local Police Department, http://www.dare-america.com
Drug Enforcement Administration (DEA), http://www.usdoj.gov/dea
Families Anonymous, (Families of Substance Abusers), http://www.familiesanonymous.org
Mothers Against Drunk Driving (MADD), http://www.madd.org
Narcotics Anonymous (NA), http://www.na.org
National Clearinghouse for Alcohol and Drug Information, http://www.health.org
National Council on Alcoholism and Drug Dependence, http://www.ncadd.org
Students Against Destructive Decisions (Founded as Students Against Driving Drunk), http://www.saddonline.com

UNIT 8 Nursing Care of the Client: Older Adult

CHAPTER 19
The Older Adult

MAKING THE CONNECTION

Refer to the following chapters to increase your understanding of the older adult:

Adult Health Nursing

- ***Surgery***
- ***Respiratory System***
- ***Cardiovascular System***
- ***Gastrointestinal System***
- ***Urinary System***
- ***Musculoskeletal System***
- ***Neurological System***
- ***Sensory System***
- ***Endocrine System***
- ***Reproductive Systems***
- ***Integumentary System***
- ***Mental Illness***
- ***Substance Abuse***

LEARNING OBJECTIVES

Upon completion of this chapter, you should be able to:

- Define key terms.
- Describe stereotypes associated with older adults.
- Discuss the biological and psychosocial theories of aging.
- Cite the normal physiologic changes that occur with aging.
- List the normal functional changes that occur with aging.
- Describe key factors of optimal health maintenance in the aging adult.
- Identify funding and policy changes that have influenced older-adult care.
- Identify common disorders related to aging.
- Detail nursing interventions for each disorder.
- Discuss areas wherein the nurse can advocate for older adults on the individual, community, state, and national levels.

KEY TERMS

activities of daily living
ageism
delirium
dementia
gerontological nursing
gerontologist
gerontology
polypharmacy

INTRODUCTION

Gerontology is the study of the effects of normal aging and age-related diseases on human beings. It is a general term used by all health care and social services disciplines. Aging (senescence) is a complex phenomenon that occurs on a continuum, beginning with birth and continuing throughout the life span.

The phrase *older adult* is very subjective and has historically meant persons who are 65 years of age and older. However, there is a great deal of debate among **gerontologists** (gerontological specialists in advanced-practice nursing, geriatric psychiatry, medicine, and social services) as to whether this specific age delineation should continue to be used. The practice of using 65 years of age as a dividing line for social welfare benefits began in the 1880s when Otto von Bismark randomly selected that age for benefits in Germany. It should be noted that there was no standardized clinical basis for establishing this age as the dividing line between young and old. Longer average life-expectancy rates (84 years for both sexes, 82.4 years for men, and 85.3 years for women) (AoA, 2009b) along with a decrease in the average number of children per family since the late 1960s have changed U.S. demographics. As a result, there is a great need to support and strengthen independence among older adults, and to value and use their life experiences in the areas of career, family, and community.

Retirement age is now less consistently determined by a mandatory age limit. Rather, retirement frequently is offered when the employee meets a formula of combined age and years of service. Since the 1990s, benefit penalties have been imposed on Social Security beneficiaries up to 70 years of age and who continue to earn incomes over a minimum amount. This was changed in April 2000 when the Senior Citizens' Freedom to Work Act of 2000 was signed into law by the president. This eliminates the Social Security retirement earnings test in and after the month in which a person is 65 years of age (the current full retirement age) (Social Security Administration [SSA], 2000).

Currently, the clinical delineation of an older adult is still someone who is 65 years of age or older; older-old adults are defined as those individuals 85 years of age or older. In 1900, there were a total of 3.1 million individuals older than age 65 in the United States; by 1996, there were 33.2 million, 3.8 million of whom were older than age 85 years (AARP, 1998). In 2001, there were 4.2 million people aged 85 and older in the United States (NCOA, 2002). It is projected that by the year 2030, the number of older individuals in the United States will reach 72.1 million (Figure 19-1)(AoA, 2009a). The most rapid increase is expected to occur in the years 2010–2030, when the "baby boomers" reach age 65.

The future will also place demands on those who were born from the late 1950s to the late 1960s. Many in this age group chose to focus first on career, delaying marriage and childrearing until in their thirties. They have thus been labeled "the sandwich generation" to denote the challenges they will face in meeting social and financial responsibilities later in life as they work to provide for children entering college and for aging parents and, sometimes, grandparents and, in a few instances, great-grandparents.

This chapter presents an overview of influences on the older adult, including the social impacts of aging. Also examined are theories of aging; myths and realities of aging; health promotion and aging; physiologic and functional changes that normally occur with aging; and some common disorders of aging along with nursing interventions to assist clients to achieve optimal outcomes related to those disorders.

As caregivers for older adults, nurses and other members of the health care team must understand the budgetary and policy decisions that can affect the care they will provide to their clients. Thus, this chapter concludes with a short discussion on health care financing for older adult care in the 21st century.

GERONTOLOGICAL NURSING

The acceptance of **gerontological nursing** as a separate nursing specialty that addresses and advocates for the special care needs of older adults has not been realized without a struggle. In 1961, gerontological nursing attained national recognition with the creation of its own division of nursing within the American Nurses Association (ANA). Nurses in the United States who were aware of the trends toward an aging population realized the importance of taking such a step. The charter members of the Division of Gerontological Nursing deserve a great deal of credit for their vision and commitment to developing gerontology education and recognizing the special nursing care needs of older adults. The major topics addressed in the expanding scope of practice for gerontological nursing included:

- The historical evolution of gerontological nursing practice based on population statistics
- The way that ageism in U.S. society has affected the profession of nursing, the health care delivery system, and the care of older adults
- Nursing education and care of older adults with a perspective derived from studies of the attitudes and interests of nursing personnel and nursing students
- The delineation of various aspects of nursing care of older adults, including clinical practice based on the ANA Standards of Nursing Practice; select theories of nursing applied to the care of older adults; and the expanding scope of gerontological nursing, in general, and the roles of clinical nurse specialists and geriatric nurse practitioners, in particular
- Trends in gerontological nursing and long-term care

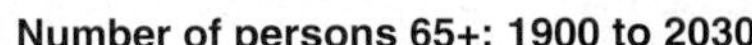

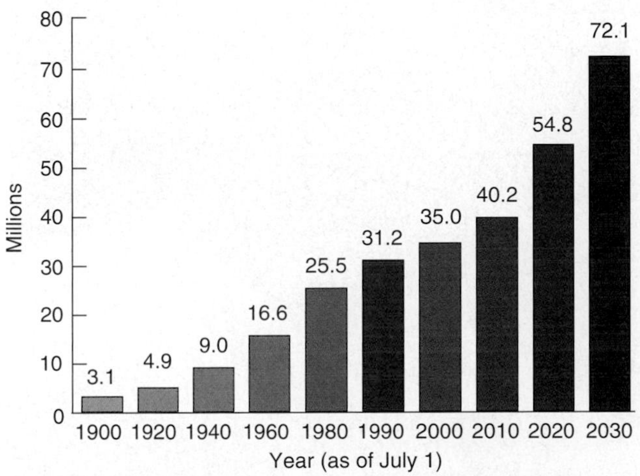

FIGURE 19-1 **Number of Persons Older Than Age 65: 1900–2030** (*Data from Administration on Aging [AOA], 2009a.*)

The battle continues against stereotyping older adults, both in the health professions and in the community at large. Health professionals, in particular, must be diligent in avoiding age prejudice. Stereotypes can influence interactions between older adults and caregivers. The caregiver may treat the older adult as a child in an old body. This approach is demeaning to older adults and strips them of their self-esteem and dignity. Clients with cognitive or expressive deficits cannot always process questions or comments quickly or follow through with responses. Nurses and caregivers must never make the mistake of believing that clients do not understand verbal and, especially, nonverbal messages. Older adults are a diverse group; they deserve respect and, through their memories and life examples, can teach a great deal to younger persons about life and survival and coping skills. Learning from clients and their families and assisting clients to find activities that enhance the quality of life (regardless of state of health) make caring for older adults a rewarding and satisfying experience.

Aging is universal, progressive, and irreversible, and eventually leads to death. The aging process itself, however, is very individualized and is independent of chronological age. The way an individual ages is influenced by genetics, lifestyle, availability and quality of health services, cultural beliefs, and socioeconomic status. Certain physiologic changes are expected with aging (Figure 19-2), although there exists considerable variation in the time of onset, rate, and degree of these changes. In order to render effective and compassionate care to older clients, nurses working in gerontology must be familiar with the normal processes as well as the common disorders of aging.

THEORIES OF AGING

At this time, no single theory of aging has been universally accepted by practitioners in gerontology. Aging is a complex issue that takes into account the psychosocial, cultural, and experiential aspects of living. Several biological theories of aging have been proposed to explain the physiologic and functional changes that are observed in older adults. Psychosocial theories of aging strive to explain the behaviors and social interactions of older adults. These theories are summarized in Table 19-1. Also, as more knowledge is garnered from scientific studies (e.g., the study of the impact on cells of auto-oxidization by free radicals and the study of dietary chemical exposure) and gene sequencing efforts (e.g., the human genome project), it is likely that the biological theories of aging will change as well.

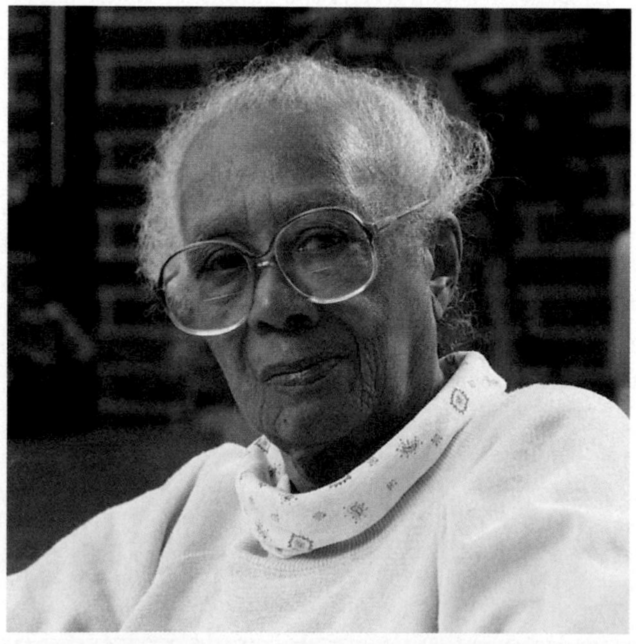

COURTESY OF DELMAR CENGAGE LEARNING

FIGURE 19-2 The aging process is a normal and natural part of growth and development.

MYTHS AND REALITIES OF AGING

Myths are fictitious ideas. Myths about the older adult are abundant and do not reflect the reality of the aging population. **Ageism** is the stereotyping of older adults based upon myths. Some common ageism myths based in part on data from the National Institute on Aging (2009), the U.S. Census Bureau, and *A Profile of Older Americans* developed by the American Association of Retired Persons (AARP) in 1998 are:

Myth: Senility is an expected result of aging.
Reality: Senility is an outdated term once used to refer to any form of dementia that occurred in older people. Dementia is a result of disease, can affect adults of all ages, and is not a natural consequence of aging. Although some slight declines are noted in short-term memory from the age of 40 on, most people adjust through the use of memory aids such as lists and calendars. Although long-term memory can remain somewhat intact long into a dementia disease process, there is slower retrieval of information. Thus, nurses and caregivers find that interventions such as reminiscence, memory photo books, and activities that draw on the client's long-practiced skills provide positive client outcomes.

Myth: Incontinence is an expected result of aging.
Reality: Incontinence is not an expected outcome of aging and, in most cases, can be reversed through assessment and treatment. Incontinence may be caused by infection, disease, injury, and certain types of medication. The challenge is that many people are embarrassed to discuss this problem with family or primary providers. Also, in long-term care settings, both the belief in this myth and the historically low staffing levels have served to dissuade clinical efforts at providing the needed nursing interventions (prompted voiding; consistent, nonhurried,

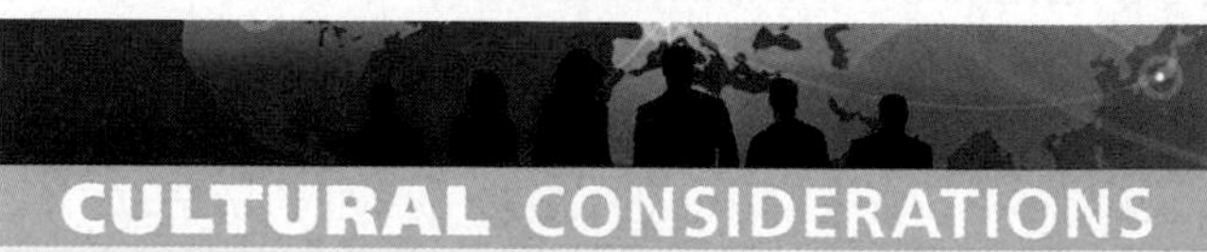

Aging

It is important to assess the older client's spiritual/religious beliefs, traditions, and culture because they can influence the client's health beliefs and health practices. When assessing a client of a different culture, show respect by using the client's full name.

TABLE 19-1 Theories of Aging

Biological Theories	
Title	**Major Premise**
Somatic mutation theory	Radiation or miscoding of enzymes causes changes in the DNA. Changes associated with aging are the result of decreased function and efficiency of the cells and organs.
Programmed aging theory	The life span is programmed within the cells. This genetic clock determines the speed at which the person ages and eventually dies.
Cross-linkage, or collagen theory	Collagen is the principal component of connective tissue and is also found in the skin, bones, muscles, lungs, and heart. Chemical reactions between collagen and cross-linking molecules cause loss of flexibility, resulting in diminished functional mobility.
Immunity theory	The thymus becomes smaller with age. The ability to produce T-cell differentiation decreases. This impairs immunologic functions and results in increased incidence of infections, neoplasms, and autoimmune disorders.
Stress theory	Stress throughout the lifetime causes structural and chemical changes in the body. These changes eventually cause irreversible tissue damage.
Psychosocial Theories	
Title	**Major Premise**
Activity theory	Roles and responsibilities change throughout the lifetime. Life satisfaction depends on maintaining an involvement with life by developing new interests, hobbies, roles, and relationships.
Disengagement theory	There is decreased interaction between the older person and others in his social system. The disengagement is inevitable, mutual, and acceptable to both the individual and society.
Continuity theory	Successful methods used throughout life for adjusting and adapting to life events are repeated. Characteristic traits, habits, values, associations, and goals remain stable throughout the lifetime, regardless of life changes.

timed voiding) to reverse urinary incontinence. In settings where care is provided to older adults, lack of funding, lack of policy support and education, and inconsistent enforcement of adequate staffing levels have often had a negative impact on client health outcomes. By developing urinary incontinence treatment programs, care facilities could improve clinical outcomes for clients and also reduce health-care costs.

Myth: Older adults are no longer interested in sexuality or sexual activity.
Reality: Sexuality is a lifelong need. Older adults can be and are sexually active, regardless of age. Although a slowing response time is a normal part of aging, many older adults want and lead a satisfying sex life, and persons of both genders are capable of orgasm into old age. Despite interest and desire, physiologic or psychological problems and medication side effects may present barriers to intercourse. In such situations, sexuality without coitus can provide older adults with love and intimacy. Just as small babies can fail to thrive without human touch (hugs, nurturing, companionship, valuing of the individual), so can older adults fail to thrive without these same human interactions and support (Figure 19-3).

A national survey by NCOA in 1998 revealed that half of those age 60 and older were sexually active. Approximately 72% of those were as satisfied or more satisfied with their sex lives compared to when they were in their forties (NCOA, 2001).

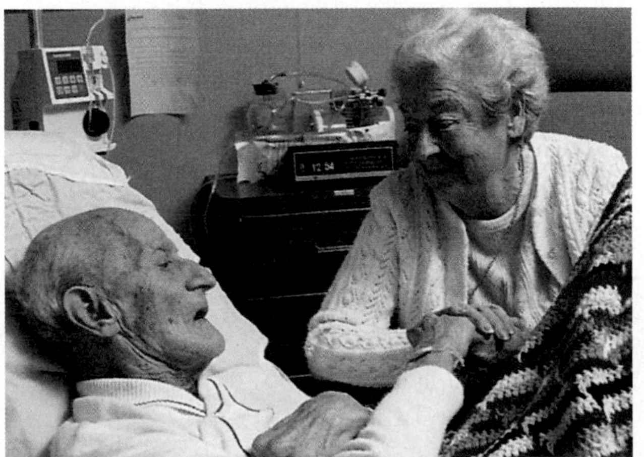

FIGURE 19-3 Individuals of all ages benefit from intimacy and companionship.

The medication sildenafil citrate (Viagra) has proven beneficial to many older couples as they work to meet their sexual health needs. The debate over the acceptance and funding of this medication for erectile dysfunction sheds light on just how far U.S. society still has to go in debunking this myth and replacing it with the truth that normal human sexuality needs continue throughout the life span.

Myth: Most people spend the last years of their lives in nursing homes.
Reality: According to NCOA (2002), in 2000, only 4.5% of those older than age 65 lived in nursing homes. The percentage rises steeply with age, however (1.1% of those 65 to 74 years of age, 4.7% of those 75 to 84 years of age, and 18% of those older than 85 years of age). For many, that stay will involve rehabilitation after surgery, a fracture, or stroke before returning home after a short hospital stay. The late 1990s saw a growing interest in the use of alternative care options for older adults (retirement communities, assisted-living centers, group homes, respite care, and partial hospitalization/adult day programs); however, most older adults continue to live in communities with varying levels of assistive services or support as they age. The projected trends in long-term care needs are for continued use of alternate settings that will support interventions to meet residents' physical, psychosocial, cultural, spiritual, cognitive, and mental health needs.

Traditionally, older adults in long-term care facilities have been taken from home environments where they have likely experienced the highest level of independence they have had in their lifetimes (to choose when to get up, eat, go to bed, and the like), and have been placed in settings where very few, if any, choices, including care decisions, are made based on their preferences. Gerontological nurses have an ongoing responsibility to help re-create the way care is provided and to advocate for older clients in long-term care facilities. Nurse leaders must learn to think in new ways about how to work with older clients and their families.

Myth: All older adults are financially impoverished.
Reality: Income range varies among those older than 65 years of age, just as it does among those in younger groups; however, the high costs of medications does disproportionately affect those older than age 65, who are more likely to have one or more chronic conditions that require management with medication. In the past, lack of reimbursement for preventive assessment, treatments, and medications led many older adults to go without medications or to delay care until they were too ill to wait any longer. This resulted in increased use of acute care services in hospitals.

In 2001, families headed by persons older than 65 years of age had a median income of $33,938 (AoA, 2002). The challenge for most older adults below the median (especially older women, who often have lower retirement incomes) is that most of their assets are tied up in the family home or in other nonliquid holdings. Thus, when an acute illness strikes, there is little financial reserve to help cover costs.

> **CRITICAL THINKING**
>
> **Myths/Stereotypes**
>
> A health team member makes an ageist remark to one of your older adult friends. How would you respond using a therapeutic communication technique?

HEALTH AND AGING

Like all age groups, older adults can do much to adopt a healthy lifestyle that will enhance their remaining years.

ACTIVITIES OF DAILY LIVING

Being well groomed enhances the self-esteem of all older adults. Adaptive devices and techniques are available for those who need assistance with the **activities of daily living** (ADLs), basic care activities that include mobility, bathing, hygiene, grooming, dressing, eating, and toileting.

Mobility

Many assistive devices are available to help the older client maintain mobility and independence. Handrails can decrease the risk of falls while the person is walking; they are also useful in the tub and, when used in conjunction with a plastic riser, can help the older adult get on and off the toilet safely.

Bathing

Skin dryness increases with aging; thus, it may be preferable for older adults to bathe or shower only two to three times per week and to take sponge baths in between. A gentle soap should be used sparingly for the bath, after which a moisturizing lotion should be applied. The individual or caregiver should be instructed to inspect the skin during bathing for any indication of skin breakdown, lumps, or changes in moles.

With aging, oil secretion decreases in the scalp, and hair can thus become dry. Shampooing one or two times per week is usually adequate for most older adults, and a simplified hairstyle may be helpful to those with limited mobility in the arms. The use of mild shampoos and conditioners can also enhance hair texture.

> **PROFESSIONALTIP**
>
> **Activities of Daily Living**
>
> Additional safety measures to consider during ADL include:
>
> - Filing nails instead of cutting because brittle nails may split
> - Avoiding perfumed bathing products due to their potential irritating effects
> - Showering (preferred) instead of taking a tub bath because it is easier to step into a shower stall than into a tub, the easier availability of shower chairs and hand bars that make it more accessable and safer than stepping into a tub, and clean water is constantly circulating over the client during the shower procedure

Hygiene

Fingernails may become more brittle with aging. Keeping the client's fingernails clean and short can prevent accidental injury or scratches to fragile older skin. Impaired circulation is common among older adults, so special attention should be given to care of the feet and lower extremities. Because toenails frequently become thick and tougher with aging, soaking the feet before trimming the toenails may ease the task. For clients with circulation or skin integrity problems of the feet and toes or for clients with diabetes, a referral to a podiatrist should be made for nail trimming. During bathing, monitor the client's feet for discomfort; inflammation; broken skin; color changes such as redness, pallor, or cyanosis (blue or purple discoloration resulting from lack of circulation); heat or coldness; cracking between toes; and corns or calluses.

The need for adequate oral care does not diminish with aging. Dental problems can result in poor eating habits and inadequate nutrition. Inadequate brushing and dental checkups can lead to gingivitis (bleeding and edematous gums), which, if left untreated, can progress to periodontal disease that can destroy connective tissue, alveolar bone, and periodontal ligaments. Monitor clients for proper oral care. Yoneyama et al. (2002) reports that nursing home residents who received oral hygiene after each meal and professional cleaning once a week were two times less likely to get pneumonia and two times less likely to die from it. For those clients with dentures, inspect the dentures for cleanliness and proper fit. Clients with dentures must brush the dentures and the gums regularly with a soft brush and a mild cleanser. It is helpful to label dentures with the client's name to facilitate identification of the dentures in the event that the client is admitted to a hospital or an assistive care setting.

Grooming

Good grooming is important in promoting the older client's self-esteem and confidence. Keeping the hair neat and tidy, choosing attractive clothing and jewelry, and making decisions about makeup and other personal care practices will all contribute to the older client's sense of well-being and independence (Figure 19-4).

Male clients may feel much better with a clean-shaven face. Infection-control principles demand that each razor (either electric or blade) be used for only one individual and that that razor be marked with the client's name. Women may also require attention to facial hair, as estrogen levels decrease after menopause. It is not uncommon for older women to notice hairs on the chin or upper lip that were not there in younger days. Also, both men and women are likely to notice graying and diminished hair on legs, underarms, and pubic areas as they age.

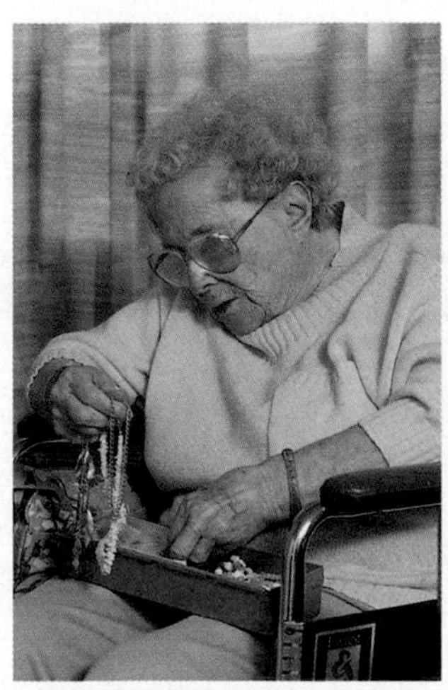
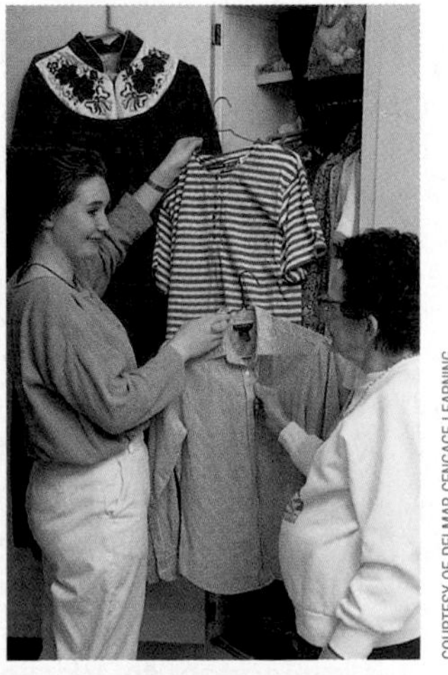

COURTESY OF DELMAR CENGAGE LEARNING

FIGURE 19-4 Good grooming for the older adult includes choosing personal items such as jewelry and clothing.

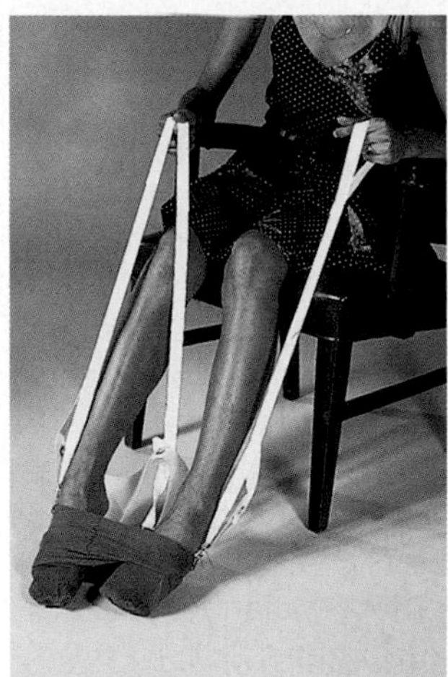
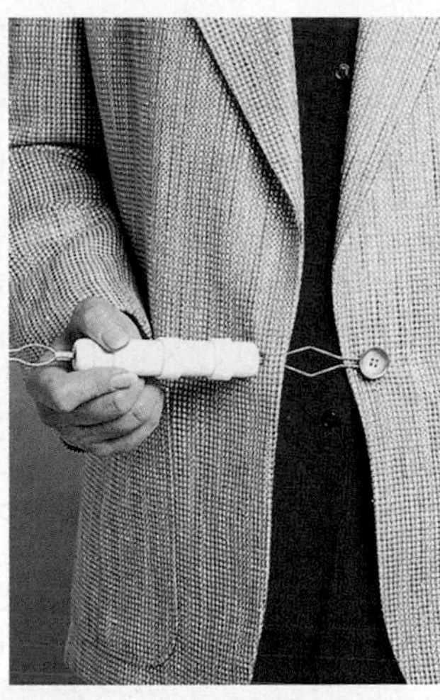

FIGURE 19-5 Assistive devices such as these for pantyhose and getting dressed are available to help older adults dress independently. (*Courtesy of Maddak, Inc.*)

Dressing

Dressing may be difficult for clients who have restricted joint movement, paralysis, or limited endurance because of health problems. Many choices are available to ease dressing, such as elastic waists, Velcro fasteners, and assistive reaching and dressing devices (Figure 19-5).

Eating

Many older adults are able to maintain the ability to self-feed, thereby promoting independence and self-esteem. Neurological and musculoskeletal alterations may, however, affect the ability to self-feed. Dysphagia, or difficulty swallowing, may place the older client at increased risk of choking. A mouth check is advisable until it is known that the client is safely swallowing. Diminished taste sensation affects the desire to eat. Adding seasonings and herbs to food may improve the taste. Encourage client to eat dessert after consuming nutrient dense foods.

Toileting

Toileting habits also change with aging. Bowel elimination problems can often be prevented as clients age by:

- Ensuring adequate fiber intake (whole grains, fresh fruit)
- Ensuring adequate fluid intake (minimum 1500 mL/day)
- Ensuring regular daily exercise (prescribed by physician)
- Developing regular elimination habits

For the client in the hospital or a long-term care facility, it is helpful to:

- Maintain previously effective habits such as drinking warm liquids upon arising
- Assist the client to the toilet approximately 30 minutes after eating, to take advantage of the gastrocolic reflex

PROFESSIONALTIP

Bowel Patterns in Older Adults

It is extremely important that caregivers of older adults monitor bowel patterns. Long periods of constipation (>2 to 3 days) should alert caregivers to the need for interventions to minimize the likelihood of bowel impaction, which can ultimately be life threatening if left untreated. Evacuation aids such as laxatives, lubricants, stool softeners, and enemas all have side effects and should thus be avoided if at all possible. Dietary changes or an exercise regimen should be introduced first.

As a result of the physical changes that occur with aging, increased frequency of urination may be noted in older adults of both genders. It is not uncommon for older adults to self-limit fluid intake because of a fear of incontinence. This habit is unhealthy and should be discouraged. Assess cases of incontinence to determine the cause and type, so that appropriate interventions and treatment can be implemented. Timing the use of prescribed diuretics in the morning rather than the evening can prevent the increased need for urination at night, which is especially helpful to older clients who are being treated for congestive heart failure (CHF).

EXERCISE

What was once accepted as the normal deterioration of old age is now considered the result of disuse through sitting and bed rest. Research indicates that high-intensity, progressive resistance training can improve muscle strength and muscle size in frail older adult clients. Walking and all other maneuvers required for ADLs are also beneficial. Individually plan exercise programs taking into consideration the older person's:

- General health status (Figure 19-6)
- Physiologic disorders (if present)
- Preference for solidarity or group activity
- Physical environment
- Financial status

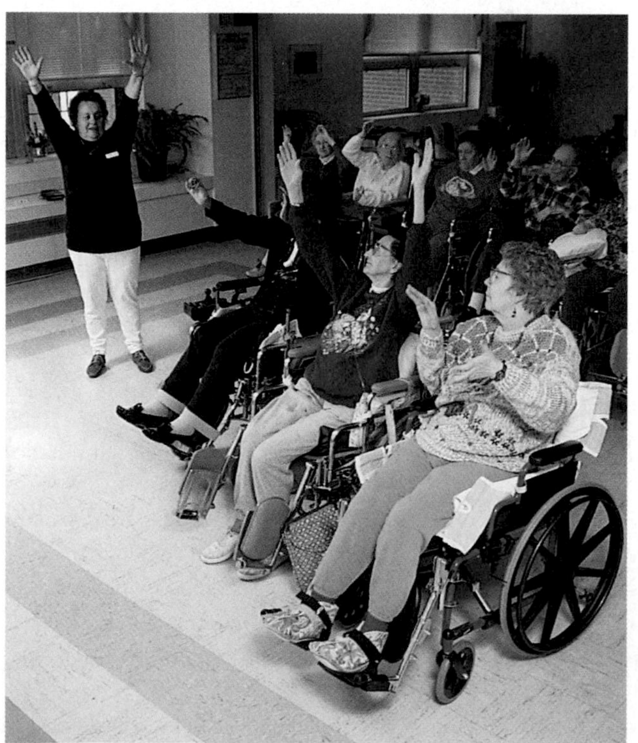

COURTESY OF DELMAR CENGAGE LEARNING

FIGURE 19-6 Exercise is important to all clients and should be tailored to interests and ability levels.

NUTRITION

For many older adults, cultural heritage, religious rites, ethnic practices, and family traditions are linked to food. The physiologic, psychological, sociological, and economic changes of aging may compromise nutritional status. Older adults must follow a balanced diet, often with lowered intakes of sugar, caffeine, and sodium. There are no universally accepted dietary guidelines specific to older adults. A dietitian can determine the needed food intake for a specific individual by taking into account the individual's height, ideal weight, activity level, and disease processes.

Older adults need 1,000 mg to 1,500 mg of calcium per day for both men and women. Calcium supplements should also contain vitamin D to provide for optimal metabolism by the body. Calcium supplements should not be taken at the same time as enteric coated medications because drugs containing calcium dissolve enteric coatings, thus leading to gastric irritation (Shepler, Grogan, & Pater, 2006). The need for additional supplements depends on the older individual's nutritional status and ability to maintain an adequate diet. Growing discussion supports the needs for adequate protein intake, to maintain both skin integrity and bone density, and moderate carbohydrate intake because carbohydrates metabolize to sugars.

It is important to know about community services designed to help older clients meet their nutritional needs. Such services include grocery transportation and delivery services, homebound meals (e.g., Meals On Wheels), group meals at senior food sites, and the Food Stamp program. Nurses and caregivers should also realize that socialization and companionship are necessary components of adequate dietary intake, and should ensure that these areas are addressed as part of any food-assistance intervention.

PSYCHOSOCIAL CONSIDERATIONS

Older adults, like all individuals, have psychosocial and cognitive needs for lifelong learning. Many colleges have

PROFESSIONALTIP

Iron

When iron is prescribed for an older adult, encourage taking with foods and fluids containing vitamin C to assist with iron absorption. A common side effect when taking iron is constipation. Clients may stop taking iron because of this problem. Therefore, it is important to ask clients about the constipating factor when reviewing their medications.

developed education program options for older adult students (often at no tuition), and employers are beginning to recruit older workers for part-time positions (recognizing their historically good work ethic and experience). Many older adults continue to volunteer countless hours each year, offering to help meet the social service needs of their communities. These efforts can result in feelings of productivity and self-worth for the older adult. Mental activity and emotional involvement are as necessary to the overall well-being as is physical activity. Older clients can benefit from building on their long-practiced skills to develop interesting and stimulating activities or hobbies. Such activities may be of an individual or group nature. Socialization with people of all age groups can help not only the older participants, but also the young and middle-aged participants, by illustrating that aging is not a disease but rather, a rich and natural part of the life process.

Strengths

Older adults generally have experienced many losses over the years. Some losses are slight and require only minor adaptation, whereas others may significantly affect the person. Physiologic changes or disease processes may result in losses, causing impairments in:

- Communication
- Vision and learning
- Mobility
- Cognition
- Psychosocial skills

If the impairment is severe, the individual could lose some degree of independence, and adaptations may be required. Furthermore, losses can cascade for the older client, as one loss contributes to another. For example, if an older adult with diabetes were to lose her driver's license because of impaired vision related to diabetic retinopathy, socialization might be restricted, which in turn might increase her feelings of loneliness and diminished self-esteem. If, however, her spouse provides caregiving and transportation, these adaptations might allow her to remain active socially while still living in her home. If her spouse later dies, and her health continues to decline, a move to an assisted-living facility may become necessary, if other community adaptations are unavailable. She would then be faced with adapting to the loss of both her home and her spouse.

Health-care professionals should remember that persons who have lived for many years are survivors and can adapt to life changes better if they are allowed to use their existing strengths. They are often much stronger and more ingenious and enterprising than they are given credit for. Identify the strengths of each individual (including past coping skills) and use them when planning care and assisting the older client to find new ways to adapt and maintain optimal independence in a new setting.

Health Promotion and Disease Prevention

Older adults must be alerted to ways of preventing disease and reducing risks. Being knowledgeable about self-care and participating in screening tests are important for health maintenance. For older men, an annual prostate examination and a prostate specific antigen (PSA) level lab test, which can detect prostate cancer in the early stages, are recommended every 1 to 2 years. For older women, the annual mammogram may be delayed by the physician depending on the client's risk factors. If a client's Pap smears have been negative (normal) for 5 consecutive years, they can be done less often. Men and women older than age 50 should have a yearly stool test for occult blood performed. A colonoscopy may be recommended to monitor for colon cancer. Teach clients habits for healthy living and inform them of signs and symptoms that require medical investigation. Older clients who have been exposed to environmental chemicals, tobacco, or extensive alcohol use over many years often experience serious health consequences as they reach older age. Older clients of any age can benefit from healthy lifestyles and from disease-prevention interventions, such as being inoculated yearly against influenza and every 5 years against pneumonia, assessment of tuberculosis (TB) status, and adequate safe food and clean water intake.

In many cases, by the time a person reaches 65 to 70 years of age, that person has been prescribed medication to address at least one ongoing (chronic) medical problem (e.g., hypertension, heart disease, diabetes, allergies, gastrointestinal disorders). The challenge many older adults face is that side effects from one medication are often treated with another prescription medication. If the client then goes to different doctors, these doctors may prescribe even more medications to address the same or other health concerns. This is called **polypharmacy**, or the problem of clients taking numerous prescription and over-the-counter medications for the same or various disease processes, with unknown consequences from the resulting combinations of chemical compounds and cumulative side effects. In many settings, primary care providers, nurses, clinical pharmacists, and social workers collaborate to assist the older client and the family to oversee the client's medication management and other health needs.

Among the biggest challenges facing older clients are shorter hospitalization stays and reduced time with physicians in the physician's offices. There is less time to ensure that the follow-up services the client will need are understood and in place and less time to educate client and family about medication regimens, including timing and possible interactions with other prescription and over-the-counter drugs or herbal remedies that the client may also be taking. The nurse, as part of the interdisciplinary team, plays a vital role as client advocate when ensuring that older clients have the teaching, services, and follow-up care they need. Figure 19-7 is a concept map that discusses safe nursing considerations when administering a medication to an older adult.

PHYSIOLOGIC CHANGES ASSOCIATED WITH AGING

Although the aging process brings with it many physiologic changes, it should be remembered that aging and disease are not synonymous. Whereas the physiologic changes of aging

CRITICAL THINKING

Polypharmacy

You are caring for a client who is suffering from the effects of polypharmacy. What interventions will you discuss with this client to prevent future polypharmacy problems?

PROFESSIONALTIP

Identifying Strengths of Older Adults as Part of Assessment

Assessment should include the identification of strengths as well as problems. Strengths are utilized to achieve or maintain optimal physical, mental, and emotional function. All of the following can be considered strengths:

- Cognitive health
- Freedom from or successful adaptation to deficits or impairments
- A history of healthy lifestyle with regard to diet, sleep, stress management, exercise, and chemical abuse (none)
- Adequate functional ability to carry out ADL
- Freedom from incapacitating physical discomfort and pain
- A physically safe living environment
- Feelings of security in present environment
- Realistic knowledge about capabilities
- Pattern of avoiding dangerous situations and unnecessary risks
- Compliance with health care regimen
- Capability with regard to managing own environment
- An intact support system
- Satisfying relationships with others
- Opportunities for sexual expression
- Access to transportation
- Adequate functional mobility
- Successful adaptation to life changes and crises
- History of relinquishing roles as phases of life require and replacing them with satisfying new roles
- A pattern of successful mourning for losses
- Participation in groups: religious, spiritual, community, hobbies
- Membership in family whose members respect each other and are willing to give and receive help when necessary
- Successful problem-solving skills
- Willingness to seek information to improve situation
- Evidence of initiative and self-confidence in abilities and judgment
- Participation in self-care by making decisions and accepting responsibility for decisions
- Acceptance of that which cannot be changed
- Successful use of assertive skills
- Ability to find comfort and strength in spiritual and religious practices
- Appreciation for aging, with demonstrative embrace of the positive aspects and adaptation to the negative aspects
- Participation in healthy reminiscing; evidence of few regrets about life past
- Appreciation for nature, art, music, hobbies, and activities
- A sense of humor

described in the following sections are normal for most people, the medical disorders described are not considered normal. Older adults age at different rates. The following aging changes for each system may not occur until late in the aging process.

Respiratory System

The following respiratory changes result from the aging process:

- Calcification of the rib cage and less flexible respiratory muscles may lead to a barrel chest and decreased vital capacity of the lungs.
- Decrease in functional capacity results in dyspnea on exertion or stress; usual activity does not affect breathing.
- Decreased ciliary action and a less effective cough mechanism increase the risk for lung infection.
- The alveoli thicken and decrease in number and size, causing less effective gas exchange (decreased oxygen saturation) and, in individuals who also have chronic lung disease, intensifying respiratory deficits.
- Structural changes in the skeleton, such as kyphosis (seen in clients with osteoporosis as an often asymmetrical convex curve of the spine) can decrease diaphragmatic expansion. Kyphosis in older clients can lead to a need for small, more frequent meals to balance nutritional requirements and respiratory function because of the restriction of adequate space for expansion and contraction of the diaphragm. It can also create skin integrity risks because the bony prominences of the client's back press against the backs of chairs.

Common respiratory disorders related to aging include the following:

- Respiratory tract infection (RTI)
- Chronic obstructive pulmonary disease (COPD)
- Pulmonary tuberculosis (TB)

Nursing Management: Respiratory Tract Infections

1. Encourage discussing the pneumovaccine with the primary care provider.
2. Encourage obtaining annual influenza vaccine.
3. Assist the client to assume a position of comfort and assist with medications and respiratory treatments, as ordered.

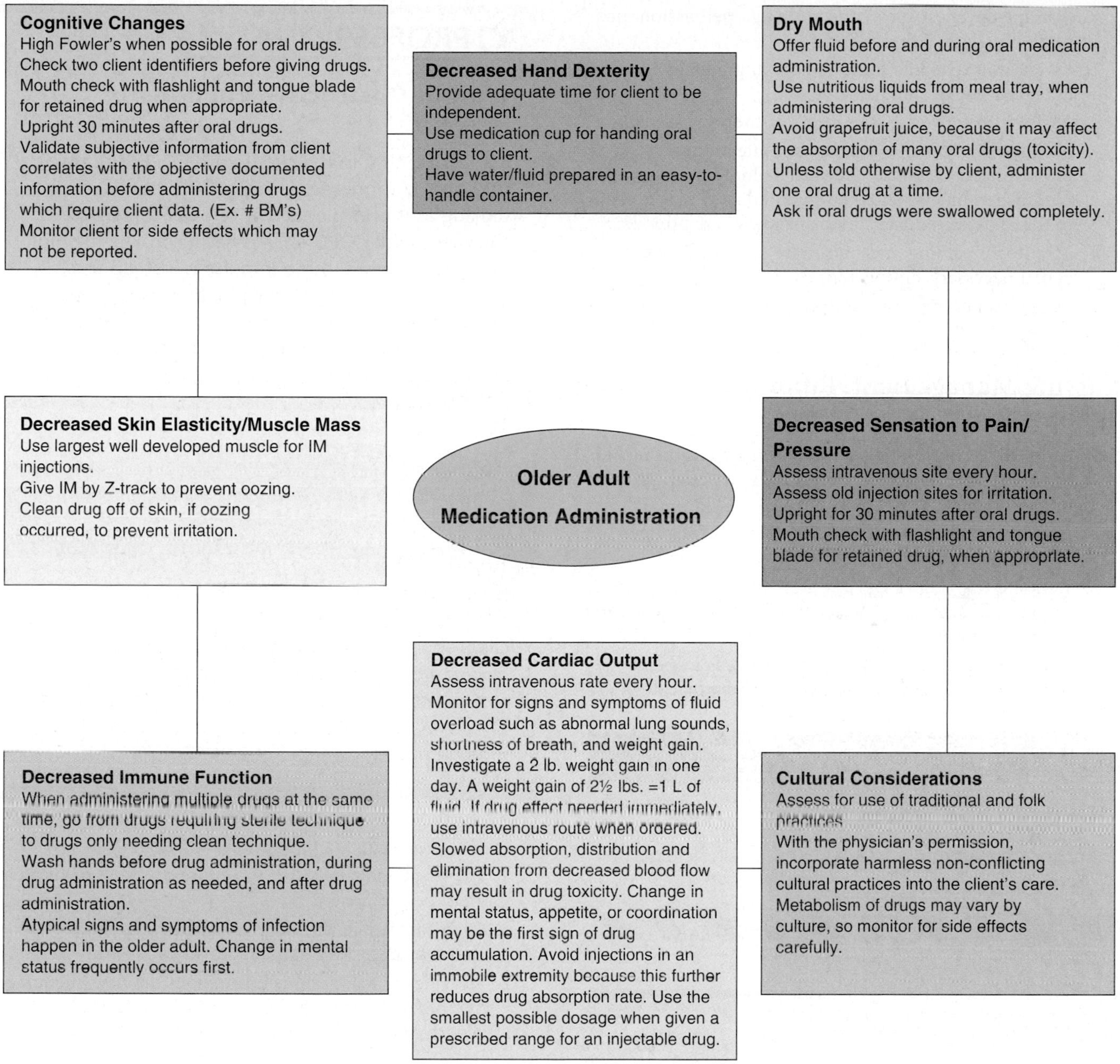

Cognitive Changes
High Fowler's when possible for oral drugs.
Check two client identifiers before giving drugs.
Mouth check with flashlight and tongue blade for retained drug when appropriate.
Upright 30 minutes after oral drugs.
Validate subjective information from client correlates with the objective documented information before administering drugs which require client data. (Ex. # BM's)
Monitor client for side effects which may not be reported.

Decreased Hand Dexterity
Provide adequate time for client to be independent.
Use medication cup for handing oral drugs to client.
Have water/fluid prepared in an easy-to-handle container.

Dry Mouth
Offer fluid before and during oral medication administration.
Use nutritious liquids from meal tray, when administering oral drugs.
Avoid grapefruit juice, because it may affect the absorption of many oral drugs (toxicity).
Unless told otherwise by client, administer one oral drug at a time.
Ask if oral drugs were swallowed completely.

Decreased Skin Elasticity/Muscle Mass
Use largest well developed muscle for IM injections.
Give IM by Z-track to prevent oozing.
Clean drug off of skin, if oozing occurred, to prevent irritation.

Older Adult
Medication Administration

Decreased Sensation to Pain/ Pressure
Assess intravenous site every hour.
Assess old injection sites for irritation.
Upright for 30 minutes after oral drugs.
Mouth check with flashlight and tongue blade for retained drug, when appropriate.

Decreased Immune Function
When administering multiple drugs at the same time, go from drugs requiring sterile technique to drugs only needing clean technique.
Wash hands before drug administration, during drug administration as needed, and after drug administration.
Atypical signs and symptoms of infection happen in the older adult. Change in mental status frequently occurs first.

Decreased Cardiac Output
Assess intravenous rate every hour.
Monitor for signs and symptoms of fluid overload such as abnormal lung sounds, shortness of breath, and weight gain.
Investigate a 2 lb. weight gain in one day. A weight gain of 2½ lbs. =1 L of fluid. If drug effect needed immediately, use intravenous route when ordered.
Slowed absorption, distribution and elimination from decreased blood flow may result in drug toxicity. Change in mental status, appetite, or coordination may be the first sign of drug accumulation. Avoid injections in an immobile extremity because this further reduces drug absorption rate. Use the smallest possible dosage when given a prescribed range for an injectable drug.

Cultural Considerations
Assess for use of traditional and folk practices.
With the physician's permission, incorporate harmless non-conflicting cultural practices into the client's care.
Metabolism of drugs may vary by culture, so monitor for side effects carefully.

FIGURE 19-7 **Concept Map: Safe Administration of Medication to an Older Adult**

4. Avoid distention of bowel, bladder, or stomach, any of which can increase breathing discomfort.
5. Allow adequate time for nursing care.
6. Administer humidified oxygen therapy, as prescribed.
7. Administer analgesics and antipyretics, as prescribed.
8. Assess for signs of dehydration and ensure that fluids are accessible to the client, unless contraindicated.
9. Review diagnostic data and monitor lung sounds and intake and output every 8 hours or as needed given changes in the client's condition. Weigh the client daily, assessing for fluid retention.
10. Monitor for any signs of respiratory distress (cyanosis of lips, mucous membranes, or nailbeds) and obtain pulse-oximetry readings, as needed.

Nursing Management: Chronic Obstructive Pulmonary Disease

1. Assist the client to a position of comfort.
2. Teach the client to use pursed-lip breathing to avoid hyperventilation when short of breath.
3. Teach the client diaphragmatic breathing for use when active.
4. Teach proper use of inhalers. Steroid inhalers should be used first, with a full 60-second wait between puffs; after waiting 5 minutes, any bronchodilator inhalers that are prescribed should then be used, also with a 60-second wait between puffs.
5. Teach the client to cough and clear the airway.

6. Administer chest physiotherapy (e.g., percussion, postural drainage), if prescribed.
7. Establish a schedule for ambulation, gradually increasing the distance ambulated.
8. Assist with active assistive range-of-motion exercises.
9. Monitor for signs and symptoms of infections (e.g., fever, blood-tinged or thick, greenish colored sputum, and diminished lung sounds) and immediately report same to the registered nurse and the primary care provider.
10. Monitor breathing and pulse rate and administer oxygen, if necessary, during periods of increased activity.
11. Suggest smoking cessation programs, if the client is a smoker.

Nursing Management: Pulmonary Tuberculosis

1. Monitor clients for TB status and for symptoms including fever, night sweats, weight loss, and cough producing blood-tinged sputum.
2. Inform the client, family, and caregivers of the need for adequate isolation techniques.
3. Evaluate the client's risk for infection with the human immunodeficiency virus (HIV) and related pneumocystic pneumonia.
4. Monitor that the client's psychosocial needs are being adequately met while the disease is being pharmacologically addressed with medications like isoniazid (Laniazid). Tell the client and family that the entire course of medication must be completed.
5. Monitor the client's nutrition intake and provide supplements as necessary to maintain adequate body weight.
6. Provide for rest periods throughout the day. Encourage the older client with TB to monitor activity level and length of visits by family so as not to become overtired.

SAFETY

Oxygen and Smoking

Ensure that no smoking is allowed around clients on oxygen therapy.

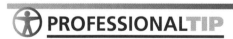

PROFESSIONALTIP

TB in the Older Adult

Older adults can be vulnerable to TB because of:

- An ineffective cough reflex and the resulting inability to clear the lungs.
- An altered immune system and a reduced response to extrinsic antigens. Not only are older adults at increased risk of infection via a new contagion, but older clients who contracted TB years ago and have been in remission since can experience reexacerbation. The risk of reexacerbation increases in cases where the initial infection was remote and healed (encapsulated) such that the immune system's memory of the T cells has been lost. Facilities where health care is provided to older clients and to immune-compromised clients thus must regularly assess the TB status of both their clients and their employees.

PROFESSIONALTIP

Chronic Obstructive Pulmonary Disease

Remember that in the client with COPD, breathing may not be triggered by a higher level of carbon dioxide as it is in clients without COPD, because the client with COPD always has a consistently high CO_2 level. The breathing impulse is instead triggered by a low level of oxygen. Increasing the oxygen level by more than 1 to 2 L/h in the client with COPD can shut down the trigger to breathe, and can put the client in respiratory failure.

CRITICAL THINKING

Chronic Obstructive Pulmonary Disease

A 69-year-old client with COPD was given some stressful news by a relative 1 hour ago. Now, the client reports that he can't breathe. He wants his nasal oxygen turned up. What physical respiratory assessment data will you collect? List the interventions that you will perform to assist the client to breathe easier.

CARDIOVASCULAR SYSTEM

The following cardiovascular changes result from the aging process:

- Left ventricle and heart valves become fibrotic leading to decreased cardiac output and slowed recovery time.

INFECTION CONTROL

TB

Remember that TB is spread through droplets when a client sneezes or coughs (direct and indirect contact). Consult the infection-control nurse on the client's interdisciplinary team and work to protect the client and others from transmission of *Mycobacterium tuberculosis* and other infections.

The heart requires more time to return to a normal rate after a rate increase in response to activity.

- The heart rate slows. Dysrhythmias are more common.
- Blood flow to all organs decreases. The brain and coronary arteries continue to receive a larger volume than do other organs.
- Arterial elasticity decreases (arteriosclerosis), causing increased peripheral resistance and, in turn, a rise in systolic blood pressure and a slight rise in diastolic blood pressure.
- Veins dilate, and superficial vessels become more prominent.

Common cardiovascular disorders related to aging include the following:

- Peripheral vascular disease (PVD)
- Hypertension
- Chronic CHF

Nursing Management: Peripheral Vascular Disease

1. Assess the lower extremities, including the peripheral pulses, for signs of arterial or venous insufficiency, such as cool pale skin and decreased sensation.
2. Evaluate lifestyle factors that may aggravate or advance atherosclerosis, such as a high-carbohydrate, high-fat diet and little exercise.
3. Teach the client about the disease, including treatment, medication actions and side effects, and signs of thrombosis.
4. Educate the client and caregivers about the care and inspection of the lower extremities.
5. Provide instructions on interventions specific to the client's type of PVD (arterial or venous).

Nursing Management: Hypertension

1. Evaluate food intake patterns, especially of cholesterol, fats, sodium, and carbohydrates. Make recommendations based on findings.
2. Evaluate for fluid retention. Weigh the client daily. Investigate a weight gain of 2 lbs. in one day.
3. Recommend a smoking-cessation program, if necessary.
4. Teach the client the importance of avoiding alcohol use.
5. Recommend and facilitate a consistent and appropriate exercise program.
6. Discuss the relationship of stress to hypertension and provide resources from which the client can learn relaxation techniques.
7. Provide information on medications and the importance of taking daily blood pressure medications as prescribed, regardless of health status on any given day.
8. Arrange for and encourage regular blood pressure checks and teach the client or significant others proper use of blood pressure equipment, if applicable.

Nursing Management: Chronic Congestive Heart Failure

1. Frequently monitor serum digitalis level and monitor for any signs of digoxin toxicity, for which older clients are at increased risk because of the decreased rate of renal clearance of the drug. Withhold the digoxin and immediately contact the registered nurse and the physician if abnormal serum level or signs and symptoms of toxicity are present.
2. Take the apical pulse for a full 1 minute before administering digoxin. Withhold the medication if the apical pulse is below 60, and consult the registered nurse and the physician if this or any other significant changes in vital signs are noted.
3. Monitor the client's blood pressure and lung sounds.
4. Monitor electrolyte levels, blood urea nitrogen (BUN), and creatinine level to observe system changes including decreased kidney efficiency.
5. Monitor for signs of fluid retention such as intake and output (output too small), weight gain, shortness of breath, coughing, and edema.
6. Encourage alternating periods of activity with periods of rest.
7. Encourage the client to maintain a level of exercise/physical activity appropriate to physical condition.
8. Teach the client and family about the safe use of the prescribed medications.
9. For clients on diuretics, which deplete potassium, monitor fluid intake and level of potassium, ensuring adequacy of each. Encourage administration of diuretics early in the day, unless contraindicated, to prevent increased urination at night.

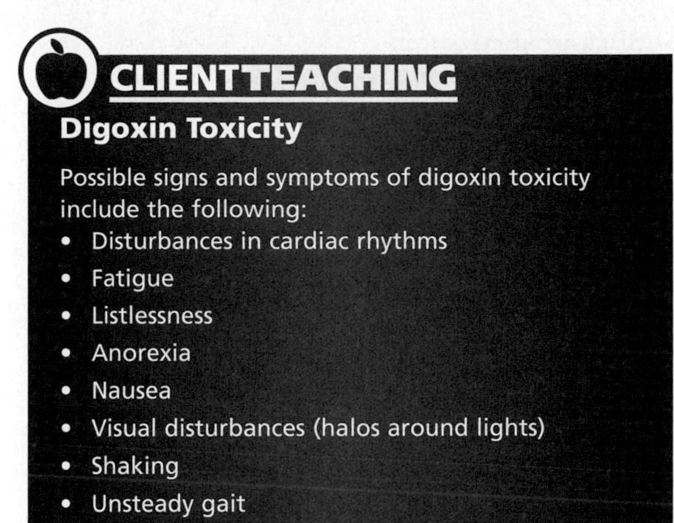

CLIENTTEACHING

Digoxin Toxicity

Possible signs and symptoms of digoxin toxicity include the following:

- Disturbances in cardiac rhythms
- Fatigue
- Listlessness
- Anorexia
- Nausea
- Visual disturbances (halos around lights)
- Shaking
- Unsteady gait
- Confusion

Gastrointestinal System

The following gastrointestinal changes result from the aging process:

- Tooth enamel thins.
- Periodontal disease rate increases.
- Taste buds decrease in number and sense of smell decreases. Saliva production diminishes leading to a dry mouth.
- Effectiveness of the gag reflex lessens, resulting in an increased risk of choking.
- Esophageal peristalsis slows, and the effectiveness of the esophageal sphincter lessens, causing delayed entry of food into the stomach and increasing the risk of aspiration.

- Hiatal hernia may occur.
- Gastric emptying slows. Food remains in the stomach longer, decreasing the capacity of the stomach.
- Peristalsis and nerve sensation of the large intestine decreases, contributing to constipation.
- The incidence of diverticulosis increases with age.
- Liver size decreases after age 70.
- Liver enzymes decrease, slowing drug metabolism and the detoxification process.
- Emptying of the gallbladder lessens in efficiency, resulting in thickened bile, increased cholesterol content, and increased incidence of gallstones.

Common gastrointestinal disorders related to aging include the following:

- Over-/undernutrition
- Constipation
- Dehydration
- Dental disorders

Nursing Management: Over-/ Undernutrition

1. Assess nutritional status.
2. Provide nutritional instruction based on assessment findings.
3. Recommend and discuss community nutrition programs (e.g., Meals On Wheels, senior center food sites, food pantries, and Food Stamp program).
4. Small, frequent meals may be more tolerable.
5. Maintain client in upright position for several hours after each meal to reduce the risk of aspiration.

Nursing Management: Constipation

1. Assess food and fluid intake.
2. Make recommendations based on assessment findings (e.g., increase fiber intake, increase fluid intake).
3. Discuss the relationship of exercise to bowel activity.
4. Discuss the importance of routine for regular bowel elimination.
5. Teach the importance of avoiding the overuse of laxatives. Frequent use leads to dependency.
6. Monitor adequate bowel elimination and provide interventions (e.g., prune juice, senna bars, milk of magnesia, as ordered) to assist the client in returning to a normal bowel elimination routine.

Nursing Management: Dehydration

1. Identify the reason for dehydration (e.g., inadequate fluid intake or excessive fluid output).
2. Identify the reason and corresponding interventions for inadequate fluid intake:
    - Fluids are inaccessible because of the client's physical limitations: offer fluids on a regular basis throughout the day.
    - The client dislikes water or other available fluids: identify fluid choices.
    - The client restricts fluids because of a fear of incontinence: explain the relationship of decreased fluid intake to bladder infections and arrange for assistance, as needed, for toileting.
3. Identify the reasons for any excessive fluid output and treat accordingly.

Nursing Management: Dental Disorders

1. Teach the oral hygiene procedures of brushing and flossing, and facilitate and encourage brushing of the teeth and gums and flossing of the teeth, as tolerated.
2. Inspect the mouth regularly for signs of dental disorders.
3. Encourage fluids to assist with salivary secretions and reduction of bacterial growth.
4. Advise regular dental checkups.

PROFESSIONALTIP

Determining Alterations in Nutrition

- Height and weight: Record actual body weight, usual body weight, and ideal body weight. If usual weight has varied significantly from the ideal for several years, the use of height/weight tables may be meaningless. Compare actual body weight to usual body weight to determine present status.
- Review laboratory values: hematocrit, hemoglobin, total iron-binding capacity, total protein, BUN.
- Determine whether client is on a weight-loss diet.
- Determine whether client was edematous when initially weighed and has lost weight with treatment.
- Evaluate cognitive status. Cognitively impaired clients may be unaware of hunger or be unable to attend to the task of eating.
- In clients with central nervous system damage, evaluate the presence of sensory–perceptual deficits that interfere with eating.
- Evaluate ability to pick up utensils and glasses and to get items from table to mouth.
- Evaluate dental/oral status: status of teeth/dentures, gums, presence of oral dryness (xerostomia).
- Determine presence of impaired swallowing.
- Determine whether client has distaste for certain food groups.
- Assess knowledge in regard to nutrition and food purchase and preparation.
- Determine whether client is taking medications that interfere with taste or food absorption.
- Determine whether financial status interferes with food purchasing.
- Evaluate for history of compulsive eating.

COMMUNITY/HOME HEALTH CARE

Nutritional Status

Evaluate the following when assessing a client's nutritional status in the home:

- Ability to shop for and prepare meals
- Mealtime environment, for unpleasant odors, noises, and visual stimuli
- Table setting, for appealing table cover, centerpiece, colorful dishes
- Appropriateness of food storage system (cabinets, refrigerator, freezer)

URINARY SYSTEM

The following urinary changes result from the aging process:

- Nephrons in the kidneys decrease in number and function, resulting in decreased filtration and gradual decrease in excretory and reabsorption functions of the renal tubules.
- Glomerular filtration rate decreases, resulting in decreased renal clearance of drugs. By age 75, renal blood flow typically diminishes by 40% (Shepler, Grogan, & Pater, 2006).
- Blood urea nitrogen increases. The creatinine clearance test is a better indicator than is BUN of renal function in older adults.
- Sodium-conserving ability diminishes.
- Bladder capacity decreases, causing increased frequency of urination, including nocturia.
- Renal function increases when the older client lies down, sometimes causing a need to void shortly after going to bed.
- Bladder and perineal muscles weaken, resulting in the inability to empty the bladder and predisposing the older client to cystitis.
- Incidence of stress incontinence increases in older females.
- The prostate may enlarge in older males, causing urinary frequency or dribbling.

Common urinary disorders related to aging include the following:

- Incontinence
- Urinary tract infections (UTIs)

Nursing Management: Incontinence

1. Complete an assessment for bladder management (Figure 19-8).
2. Identify the type of incontinence present (Table 19-2).
3. Implement an appropriate bladder management program (Table 19-3).
4. Frequently monitor for skin impairment.
5. Offer absorbent incontinent pads or briefs that draw the moisture away from the skin.
6. Teach all caregivers, the client, and the family the importance both of adequate cleansing of the genital area (proper retraction, cleansing, and replacement of the foreskin in the uncircumcised male and proper cleansing of the skin folds of the female), legs, and back and of the use of clean linens, to ensure that the client's skin is kept clean and dry. Apply a moisture barrier cream as needed to prevent skin maceration from excessive exposure to moisture.
7. Teach and employ effective infection-control techniques (e.g., wipe and clean [from front to back only] after toileting and when bathing).
8. Instruct client to avoid bladder irritants such as caffeine, spicy foods, and alcohol.

To be completed and reviewed every 90 days or as frequently as needed based on outcome and response.

CLIENT__________ Adm No. ________ Date__________ Diagnoses__________ Birthdate______

Bladder function: History of infection or other urinary problem.__________ Urinalysis: Date________

Protein___ Glucose__ Ketones__ RBC__ WBC__ Bacteria__ Crystals__ Sp.Gr.__ Culture: Date_____ Result______

Treatment________

BUN___ Ser.Creatinine___ Tot.Pro.___ FBS___ To be completed after 2-week assessment period.

Frequency of voiding______ Average amount______ Is client aware of need to void?____ Urgency?____ Dribbling?____

Incontinence preceded by laughing, sneezing_____

Medications affecting bladder function/continence__________

Mental status: Short-term memory_________ Orientation_________ Able to express self_________

Able to follow directions_________ Reaction to incontinence_________

Hydration baseline: Daily average fluid intake: Days______ Eve.______ Night______

Mobility/self-care skills: Ambulatory/self______ Cane______ Walker______ Requires assist of one or two______

Weight-bearing______ Propels self by w/c______ Transfers self______ Requires assistance______

Can manage clothing______ Cleanses self after toileting______ Washes hands______

FIGURE 19-8 Assessment for Bladder Management

Table 19-2 Types of Urinary Incontinence

TYPE	CHARACTERISTICS
Functional	Bladder emptying is unpredictable but complete. Incontinence is related to impairment of cognitive, physical, or psychological functioning or to environmental barriers.
Urge	Incontinence occurs immediately after the sensation to void is perceived.
Reflex	Incontinence is related to neurogenic bladder and central nervous system or spinal cord injury. Bladder fills, and uninhibited bladder contractions cause loss of urine.
Stress	Increased abdominal pressure is higher than urethral resistance. Stress associated with coughing or laughing causes incontinence.
Total	Unpredictable, unvoluntary, continuous loss of urine.

9. Encourage referral to discuss medical options (in addition to nursing interventions) for treatment of incontinence.
10. Allow the client to voice concerns over incontinence and assist to overcome any adverse effects on psychosocial functioning.

Nursing Management: Urinary Tract Infections

NOTE: Older persons frequently do not present with the usual signs and symptoms of urinary tract infections. Falling or signs of acute confusion (more than usual) often are the major clinical manifestations.

1. Monitor fluid intake and output. Increase intake unless contraindicated. Offer cranberry juice frequently, per ordered diet.
2. Teach and encourage client to empty the bladder every 3 to 4 hours.
3. Encourage the client to take all medication as prescribed.
4. Use proper infection-control techniques to minimize the risk of infection, including maintaining sterile technique for any urinary catheterization procedure (for urinalysis, assessment for bladder retention, or insertion of indwelling catheter), to prevent unnecessary introduction of bacteria into the bladder.
5. Teach female clients to wipe from front to back only; cleanse thoroughly after bowel movements; avoid bubble baths, colored toilet paper, douches, and vaginal sprays; and wear underwear made from cotton rather than synthetic fibers.
6. Teach the client and caregivers that hematuria (blood in the urine) and fever indicate the need for immediate assessment and intervention, as these signs and symptoms can signify a potentially serious infection or condition. Any signs and symptoms of bladder infection should be immediately reported to the registered nurse and the physician.

Musculoskeletal System

The following musculoskeletal changes result from the aging process:

- Muscle mass and elasticity diminish, resulting in decreased strength, endurance, coordination, and increased reaction time.
- Bone demineralization (osteoporosis) occurs, causing skeletal instability and shrinkage of intervertebral discs. The flexibility of the spine lessens, and spinal curvature

Table 19-3 Bladder Management Techniques

PROGRAM	DESCRIPTION
Kegel exercises	Used for stress incontinence in cognitively alert persons. Exercises strengthen pelvic floor musculature.
Scheduled toileting	Client is on a fixed schedule of toileting—usually every 2 hours. Technique can be used to facilitate voiding and emptying of the bladder.
Habit training	Client is toileted according to individual pattern of voiding. Several days must be spent assessing pattern.
Bladder retraining	Restores normal pattern of voiding/continence. Requires accurate assessment before establishing schedule with progressive shortening or lengthening of toileting intervals. Client must be cognitively alert.
Prompted voiding	Client is prompted to toilet at regular intervals and is given social reinforcement for appropriate toileting behavior.

(kyphosis) often occurs. Height may decrease 1 to 4 inches throughout the aging process.

- Joints undergo degenerative changes, resulting in pain, stiffness, and loss of range of motion.

Common musculoskeletal system disorders related to aging include the following:

- Osteoporosis
- Osteoarthritis
- Fractured hip

Nursing Management: Osteoporosis

1. Make dietary recommendations to ensure adequate intake of calcium, protein, and vitamin D.
2. Recommend a smoking cessation program, if necessary.
3. Teach the client the importance of avoiding alcohol.
4. Encourage the client to take a calcium supplement in conjunction with vitamin D, as ordered by the client's primary care provider.
5. Recommend consultation with the primary care provider regarding bone-density testing and to discuss estrogen replacement therapy (ERT) options for females or the use of medications like alendronate sodium (Fosamax) and ibandronate (Boniva) to address bone density loss associated with osteoporosis.
6. Teach the client, family, and caregivers about measures to reduce the risk of falling and sustaining fractures.
7. Recommend evaluation (x-ray) for the presence of stress, or compression, fractures of the spine in cases of severe back pain that occurs with or without a fall. In clients with osteoporosis, these fractures can occur more easily because the vertebrae are compacted by shrinkage of the intervertebral spaces as a consequence of aging.
8. Provide adequate pain control for back pain or other musculoskeletal discomfort.
9. Monitor for adequate dietary intake of calories and fluids and for effective elimination patterns.
10. Teach, encourage, and assist clients to establish exercise programs appropriate to their capabilities. Especially promote exercise programs that include walking or other weight-bearing activities, as tolerated.

Nursing Management: Osteoarthritis

1. Suggest a schedule for alternating periods of activity and rest.
2. Recommend a weight-reduction plan, if necessary, to eliminate extra strain on affected joints.
3. Teach, assist, and encourage the client to establish an exercise program that emphasizes gentle stretching and movement of all joints. For those clients who are more independent, exercise programs in warm water can have positive outcomes.
4. Provide adequate pain control. Teach clients and caregivers to monitor for gastrointestinal distress related to arthritis medications such as nonsteroidal anti-inflammatory drugs (NSAIDs) and to be aware that enteric-coated medications cannot be crushed because they are designed to protect the stomach by dissolving in the duodenum.
5. Encourage the client to seek ongoing evaluation by the physician, as new arthritis medications such as celecoxib (Celebrex) are continually being developed and trialed.

Nursing Management: Fractured Hip

NOTE: Nursing interventions may vary depending on whether the older client has an open reduction/internal fixation fracture (ORIF) or total hip arthroplasty (THA).

1. Maintain postoperative positioning as appropriate to the client's form of treatment.
2. Provide adequate pain control before physical therapy and on an ongoing basis throughout the recovery process.
3. Prevent complications, including skin breakdown, RTIs, infections at the surgical site, and dislocation of the prosthesis or internal fixation device.
4. Facilitate and monitor with the registered nurse the client's consistent use of antiembolism stockings as ordered and the administration of anticoagulant medications and the related monitoring of lab values, to decrease the risk of pulmonary embolism (which can be a significant risk to older clients after hip fracture and/or hip replacement).
5. Teach the client about fall prevention. Evaluate the client's environment (home, room, bathroom) for safety with regard to mobility and make recommendations for rectifying any threats to safety.

NEUROLOGICAL SYSTEM

The following neurological changes result from the aging process:

- Neurons in the brain decrease in number, resulting in decreased production of neurotransmitters and, thus, reduced synaptic transmission.

CRITICAL THINKING

Home Safety

Your 65-year-old grandmother tells you that she is planning to build a new home. She has been researching and gathering information about safety measures to include in her new home for people over age 60. She wants reassurance that her money is going to be well spent and asks you what are important safety measures to consider. Share pertinent information about the following along with rationale.

1. Location of home (country versus town)
2. One- versus two-story home
3. Paint colors to use
4. Gas versus electric appliances and heat
5. Type of door knobs for opening doors
6. Type and location of alarms
7. Location of lighting
8. Location for grab bars/railing
9. Type of flooring

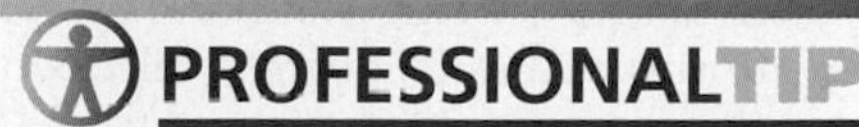

Neurological System in the Older Adult

In the absence of pathology, intellect and capacity for learning remain unchanged with aging.

- Cerebral blood flow and oxygen utilization decrease.
- Time required to carry out motor and sensory tasks requiring speed, coordination, balance, and fine-motor hand movements increases. Incidence of slight tremors is common.
- Short-term memory may somewhat diminish without much change in long-term memory.
- Night sleep disturbances occur because of more frequent and longer wakeful periods.
- Deep-tendon reflexes decrease, although reflexes at the knees remain fairly intact.

Many disorders that affect the neurological system are not unique to older adults; however, the risk of acquiring one of these disorders increases with age. One of the most common diagnoses among older adults in long-term care facilities is dementia, particularly one form of dementia called Alzheimer's disease (AD). **Dementia** is an organic brain pathology characterized by losses in intellectual functioning. The clinical manifestations associated with dementia are never considered normal aging changes.

It is important for care providers to assess the length of onset of confusion or cognitive changes in the client. Generally, dementia describes declines that have a slow onset of greater than 6 months, whereas **delirium** (or acute confusion) describes cognitive changes that have a shorter onset of 6 months or less. Acute confusion can occur independently or as an exacerbation of a current dementia-related disorder in the client. Acute confusion can result from many stresses such as infections, medication side effects, drug interactions, metabolic imbalances, dehydration, or injuries from falls (e.g., subdural hematomas). Elimination of the causative factor can often turn the acute confusion around in a relatively short period to the preexacerbation level of functioning, unless further pathology to the brain has occurred.

PROFESSIONALTIP

Mental Health in the Older Adult

Mood disorders including depression, bipolar disorder, anxiety disorders, late-onset psychosis, sleep disorders, substance abuse, schizophrenia (chronic and late-onset), and other psychiatric diseases certainly occur among older clients and often go unaddressed or are ineffectively treated. Appropriate assessment, treatment, and clinical management of these clients require effective interdisciplinary teams comprising a geriatric psychiatrist; a neurologist; a clinical nurse specialist specializing in gerontology and mental health; a licensed social worker; a clinical pharmacist; other multidisciplinary team members (including direct care nurses and staff and activity therapists); and the client's family and, whenever possible, the client.

Nursing Management: Alzheimer's Disease

1. Before diagnosis, encourage a medical and psychological diagnostic workup including a mental status examination.
2. Facilitate orientation in the early stages of the disease with calendars, lists, and consistent schedules.
3. Arrange an environment that is therapeutic, consistent, calm, and safe and that alternates rest with activities that require the use of long-practiced skills.
4. Encourage and facilitate access for the client and family to support groups where they can independently share their feelings and concerns and have questions addressed.
5. When assistance is needed with ADLs, implement consistent routines with consistent caregivers but allow for delay of care if needed because of client stress or irritability. Encourage independence of the client while assisting with ADLs (e.g., offer a warm washcloth for client to wash the face and assist with those ADLs that the client cannot complete without assistance).
6. Monitor general health status. Treat any underlying medical problems. Provide adequate pain control, as needed, and monitor for lack of sleep to minimize the risk of violent behavior. Observe for the client's better times of the day, and plan activities or interventions accordingly.
7. Build a trusting relationship with the client. Use clear, simple directions and treat clients with respect and as individuals, building on their strengths and their unique interests and histories. Doing so demonstrates appreciation for the individual and can help build the client's self-esteem.
8. Be aware that as much is communicated to the AD client through the caregiver's nonverbal behavior and tone and volume of voice as is communicated through actual words. A calm attitude allows the client time to process and retrieve information when spoken to or asked a question.
9. Support the client's mobility within a safe environment, recognizing that as the disease progresses, baseline wandering often increases as a coping skill, whereas verbal communication often decreases. Beanbag chairs, low mattresses, bed and chair alarms, positional (antisliding) wedges for chairs, merry walkers that support independent mobility, and assisted-ambulation programs to build leg strength are all therapeutic interventions for AD clients as the disease progresses and represent preferable alternatives to the use of restraints.

10. Monitor for changes in baseline behaviors and for intensity of wandering, pacing, and lethargy, as these often indicate underlying infections, metabolic imbalances, or stress. Encourage clients to alternate periods of activity and rest.

Nursing Management: Depression

1. Assess for signs of a physical basis for any fatigue (e.g., infection, pain, altered nutritional status, or shortness of breath upon exertion).
2. Administer treatment for underlying physiologic problems, if applicable.
3. If symptoms persist, encourage the client to have a medical diagnostic workup with a geriatric psychiatrist, if such a workup has not yet been done.
4. Monitor for verbal or nonverbal signs of suicidal thoughts/intent. Determine whether the client has a plan.
5. Provide one-on-one supervision of the client as needed and assure the client that the caregiver will keep him safe. If appropriate for the client, seek an agreement that he will not try to harm himself.
6. Administer antidepressant medication as ordered. Provide client and family education regarding medication, including length of time before therapeutic results should occur, and potential side effects. Report immediately to the registered nurse and primary care provider any extrapyramidal side effects (e.g., tremors, drooling, pin rolling of the fingers, shuffling gait) that are observed.
7. If the client is not assessed as being at risk for suicide but is isolating in his room, establish small goals with the client (e.g., coming out of the room and sitting safely in the hallway with the nurse for 5 minutes two times per day and for meals). Advance to more challenging goals as the client demonstrates increased tolerance for social interaction.
8. Facilitate the client's reintegration into a healthy support system and provide small community group time for the client to share his views.

Nursing Management: Transient Ischemic Attack

1. Assess for risk factors for stroke and for the existence of any previous carotid vascular tests for potential narrowing, stenosis, or blockage.
2. Provide client and family education explaining the relationship between risk factors and TIA and stroke.
3. Provide teaching to assist in reducing risk factors.
4. Monitor orthostatic blood pressure and encourage clients to change positions slowly to decrease the risk of falling.

SENSORY CHANGES

The following sensory changes in vision and hearing result from the aging process.

VISION

- With aging, the lens becomes less pliable and less able to increase its curvature in order to focus on near objects, causing presbyopia (trouble seeing objects up close) and decreased accommodation. The lens also yellows, causing distorted color perceptions, with greens and blues washing out and warm colors such as reds and oranges becoming more distinct. The incidence of cataracts also increases (Figure 19-9).

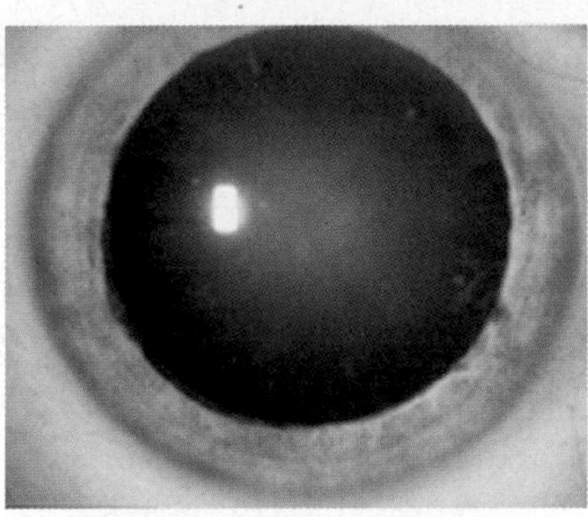

FIGURE 19-9 Cataract (*Courtesy of Salim L. Butrus, MD, Senior Attending, Department of Opthalmology, Washington Hospital Center, Washington, D.C., and Associate Clinical Professor, Georgetown University Medical Center, Washington, D.C.*)

- Accommodation of pupil size decreases, resulting in both decreased adjustment to changes in lighting and decreased ability to tolerate glare. For instance, high-gloss tile floors in hallways can appear like hills and valleys to older clients, especially those with perceptual deficits; this may increase anxiety and safety risks.
- Vitreous humor changes in consistency, causing blurred vision. Changes in the anterior chamber may increase the pressure of the aqueous humor, resulting in glaucoma.
- Lacrimal glands secrete less fluids, causing dryness and itching. Entropion or ectropion (turning of the eye inward) or ectropion (turning of the eye outward) occasionally occurs in older clients. These conditions can not only impact vision, but can also increase the risk of infection caused by dryness and ineffective blinking. In these conditions, obtaining an order for artificial tears, lacrilube, and eye drop treatments for dryness or infection may be necessary.
- Arcus senilus, a hazy grayish yellow ring around the cornea may develop, but it does not affect vision.

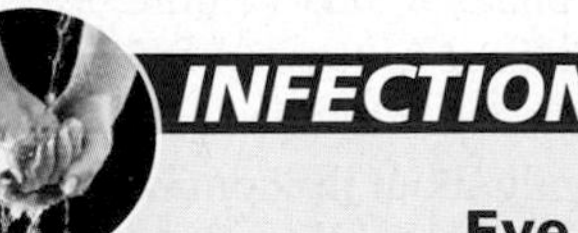

INFECTION CONTROL

Eye Care

To decrease infection risks, all caregivers should wash from the nose outward when washing clients' eyes.

Common vision disorders related to aging include the following:

- Presbyopia
- Cataract
- Glaucoma
- Age-related macular degeneration

Nursing Management: Visual Impairment

1. Teach visually impaired clients adaptive techniques for ADL, such as extra lighting.
2. Recommend regular examination by an ophthalmologist.
3. Provide preoperative and postoperative care and teaching to clients undergoing cataract surgery, including lifting and bending restrictions as well as measures to prevent infection.
4. Teach proper eye drop administration techniques to all clients who are prescribed eye drops, including holding the drop in the eye with the lid closed for 30 seconds after administration and lacrimal pressure for 1 minute when appropriate.
5. Ensure that older clients have their glasses on when needed to decrease perceptual and spatial deficits.

Teach clients that to have a better chance of keeping their vision they should not smoke, maintain a healthy weight, control blood pressure, and eat a healthy diet rich in fish and green leafy vegetables (Covell, Graziano, Rich, & Tobin, 2007).

HEARING

- As aging occurs, the pinna becomes less flexible, the hair cells in the inner ear stiffen and atrophy, and cerumen (earwax) increases.
- The number of neurons in the cochlea decrease, and the blood supply lessens, causing the cochlea and the ossicles to degenerate.
- Presbycusis, the impairment of hearing in older adults, is often accompanied by a loss of tone discrimination. High-frequency tones are lost first; thus, keeping the voice low and calm and decreasing any background noise can improve the client's comprehension of the caregiver's message.

Nursing Management: Hearing Impairment

1. Assess for ear pain, drainage, inflammation, abnormalities, surgeries, perforations, or impacted cerumen.
2. Evaluate medication regimen and assess for ototoxicity, if medication history reveals such a risk.
3. Recommend hearing testing by an audiologist, if the previous assessments are negative.
4. Monitor the care and use of a hearing aid by the older client with unilateral or bilateral aids (Figure 19-10). Provide teaching and assistance as needed for cleaning the hearing aid(s) and replacing batteries.
5. Instruct caregivers and family about the communication and socialization needs of the client. For some older clients, either the use of a small erasable board to augment verbal questions or communication with written text represents a therapeutic intervention for hearing impairment. If writing dexterity or ability is also impaired, a story board that has pictures indicating the client's needs (e.g., bathroom, food, rest) can assist the client to independently communicate needs to caregivers.
6. The consonants f, g, s, and t may become difficult to understand as the client ages. Rephrase sentences and questions when the client has difficulty with interpreting communication.

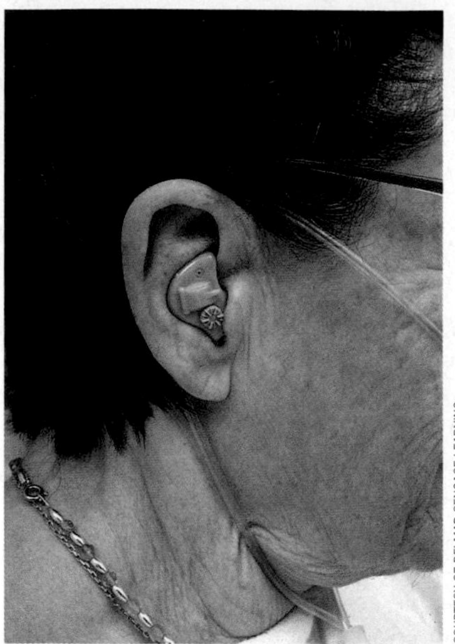

FIGURE 19-10 The use of hearing aids helps to compensate for hearing loss experienced by some clients.

CRITICAL THINKING

Driving Safety

An 80-year-old client is contemplating giving up automobile driving. What physical changes have occurred with aging that make it more difficult to drive safely? If the client decides to continue driving, what safety measures would you recommend?

PROFESSIONALTIP

New Technology for the Older Adult

Massachusetts Institute of Technology's (MIT) AgeLab designs new ideas to improve the quality of life for older adults and those who care for them. Health innovations that AgeLab is researching or has developed include: the Home Health Station, an intelligent cardiopulmonary decisions system that uses telemedicine at home to provide a "checkup a day" for managing chronic illnesses such as CHF and diabetes; the Smart Personal Advisor that uses the older adult's diet information to provide guidance when grocery shopping; Pill Pets, an electronic pill pet that uses emotions and play to remind the older adult to take their medication; Digital Danskins for older adults that integrate biosensors to monitor health conditions and chronic diseases; and the "Aware Car," a Volvo XC90 designed with cameras and sensors that provide the older adult driver with information to promote safe driving. To view additional technology being created by MIT for the aging population visit http://web.mit.edu/agelab/index.shtml (MIT, 2009).

SAMPLE NURSING CARE PLAN

The Client with Alzheimer's Disease (AD)

J.R., 64 years old, was admitted to the Alzheimer's unit of a long-term care facility. Last month, J.R. was visiting her daughter in another state and wandered away from the daughter's home. J.R. was found 60 miles away, unharmed but completely disoriented and agitated. J.R. had worked as a nursing assistant before she retired. She is a widow and has two children in the same community where the nursing home is located, in addition to the daughter who she was visiting in another state. Unless reminded, J.R. does not shower or change clothes. She awakens at least once each night and asks for breakfast.

NURSING DIAGNOSIS 1 *Disturbed Thought Processes* related to progressive dementia as evidenced by disorientation to time and place, loss of short-term memory, inability to concentrate, and periods of agitation

Nursing Outcomes Classification (NOC)
Memory
Cognitive Ability
Cognitive Orientation

Nursing Interventions Classification (NIC)
Dementia Management
Environmental Management

PLANNING/OUTCOMES	NURSING INTERVENTIONS	RATIONALE
J.R. will remain calm and will not experience agitation and anxiety as a result of her disorientation and memory loss.	Provide J.R. with clues for orientation: "Good morning, J.R. My name is Jean, and I will help you today." Avoid putting her on the spot.	Helps J.R. cope with her environment.
	Place a large sign on J.R.'s door with her name printed in large letters.	Helps her find her room.
	Have family bring in snapshots and photos taken in past years.	Stimulates reminiscing and allows her to recall happy times.
	Avoid changing J.R.'s room. Always put items back in the same place.	Consistency reduces frustration.
	Consult with activities staff in planning self-expressive, non-fail activities that require little concentration (e.g., painting with nontoxic paints, modeling with nontoxic clay).	Prevents boredom, which can lead to irritation.
	If J.R. is resistant to care, provide clear, simple, nonthreatening instructions and delay care as needed until she is calmer.	Often, delaying care for even 10 to 15 minutes when resistance is encountered improves client outcomes.

EVALUATION

J.R. remained calm and showed no signs of agitation or anxiety.

NURSING DIAGNOSIS 2 *Risk for Injury* related to risk factors of mode of transportation and cognitive and affective factors as evidenced by wandering behavior, impaired judgment, and disorientation

Nursing Outcomes Classification (NOC)
Safety Behavior: Personal
Safety Behavior: Home Physical Environment

Nursing Interventions Classification (NIC)
Pain Management
Dementia Management

(Continues)

SAMPLE NURSING CARE PLAN (Continued)

PLANNING/OUTCOMES	NURSING INTERVENTIONS	RATIONALE
J.R. will remain free of injury while retaining as much independence and freedom as possible.	Keep only nonpoisonous plants on the unit. Arrange furniture so that walkways are open. Pad sharp corners of tables and chests. Cover electrical outlets and hot radiators. Place electrical cords and telephone wires out of reach.	Does not recognize unsafe acts or conditions due to loss of impulse control and loss of judgment. Does not comprehend cause and effect.
	Provide assurance during fire drills.	Agitation increases especially when noise level is increased.

EVALUATION

J.R. has experienced no injury.

NURSING DIAGNOSIS 3 *Bathing/Hygiene and Dressing/Grooming **S**elf-Care Deficit* related to perceptual or cognitive impairment (memory loss and sensory–perceptual deficits) as evidenced by needing a reminder to shower and change clothes

Nursing Outcomes Classification (NOC)
Self-Care: Bathing
Self-Care: Hygiene
Self-Care: Dressing
Self-Care: Grooming

Nursing Interventions Classification (NIC)
Self-Care Assistance: Dressing/Grooming
Self-Care Assistance: Bathing/Hygiene

PLANNING/OUTCOMES	NURSING INTERVENTIONS	RATIONALE
J.R. will complete ADLs with minimal assistance now and with increasing assistance as the disease progresses.	Use verbal cues and hand-over-hand assistance with ADLs. Instruct staff to avoid doing tasks that J.R. can do by herself. Watch for signs of frustration and irritation and intervene when appropriate.	Minimizes the need for assistance, thereby increasing feelings of self-esteem.
	Ask family to bring in clothing that is easy to manipulate. Set clothing out in the order it is to be put on.	Allows J.R. to be more independent.
	Consider tub baths rather than showers. Provide privacy, check the temperature of the bathroom, and do not leave the client alone.	Showers may be threatening or confusing to persons with Alzheimer's disease. Tub baths are more relaxing.

EVALUATION

J.R. participates in ADLs.

NURSING DIAGNOSIS 4 *Disturbed **S**leep Pattern* related to disorientation as evidenced by wakefulness at night

Nursing Outcomes Classification (NOC)
Information Processing
Mood Equilibrium

Nursing Interventions Classification (NIC)
Sleep Enhancement
Simple Massage

SAMPLE NURSING CARE PLAN (Continued)

PLANNING/OUTCOMES	NURSING INTERVENTIONS	RATIONALE
J.R. will experience fewer periods of wakefulness during the night. If she awakens, she will remain calm and free of agitation.	Avoid stimulating activities prior to bedtime. Establish a consistent bedtime routine. Take J.R. to the bathroom and allow sufficient time for complete bladder emptying.	Overstimulation before bedtime may increase anxiety, preventing sleep. A consistent bedtime routine is helpful.
	Help J.R. with a sponge bath and with oral care; give her a back rub using warm lotion and slow, smooth strokes.	Provides relaxation.
	Provide a light snack of a warm, noncaffeinated beverage and a plain, easily digested cracker, cookie, or a piece of toast. Be patient and do not rush her.	Hunger or overeating can interfere with sleep.
	Question family concerning previous bedtime routines and sleeping habits.	Allows same routine to be followed.
	Repeat bedtime routine when J.R. awakens during night.	Makes J.R. think it is time to go to bed.
	Encourage a short nap early in the afternoon.	Sleep pattern disturbances may result from overfatigue.
	Avoid the use of sleeping medications.	Prevents confusion, disorientation, and restlessness.

EVALUATION

J.R. sleeps through the night several times a week.

Endocrine System

The following endocrine changes result from the aging process:

- Alterations occur in both the reception and the production of hormones.
- Release of insulin by the beta cells of the pancreas slows, causing an increase in blood sugar.
- Thyroid changes may lead to decreased T_4 and hypothyroidism.

The most common endocrine disorder related to aging is diabetes mellitus type 2.

Nursing Management: Diabetes Mellitus Type 2

1. Arrange for a consultation with a dietitian to assess nutritional status and to provide food-management instruction.
2. Teach the client, family members, or caregivers (as appropriate) the procedure for blood glucose monitoring specific to the equipment the client will be using.
3. Develop a personal exercise program with the client based on the client's physical condition, mental status, resources, and interests.
4. Provide information on prescribed oral hypoglycemic medications.
5. Teach the causes, signs, and treatment of hypoglycemia and hyperglycemia.
6. Educate on self-care and on careful monitoring of the extremities and of sores on the skin to minimize threats to skin integrity.
7. Encourage the client to wear shoes and to have nails trimmed by a podiatrist, if unable to safely perform self-care.

Reproductive System: Female

The following reproductive changes result from the aging process:

- Estrogen production decreases with the onset of menopause.
- Ovaries, uterus, and cervix decrease in size.

- The vagina shortens, narrows, and becomes less elastic, and the vaginal lining thins. Secretions decrease and become more alkaline, resulting in increased incidence of atrophic vaginitis. These changes may result in dyspareunia (discomfort during coitus), which can often be rectified with the use of a water-based lubricant. As at any age, protected intercourse (safe sex) through the use of a latex condom should be advised with new partners.
- Supporting musculature of the reproductive organs weakens, increasing the risk of uterine prolapse.
- Breast tissue diminishes and nipple erection lessens during sexual arousal.
- Libido and the need for intimacy and companionship in older women remain unchanged (Figure 19-11).

Common female reproductive system disorders related to aging include the following:

- Breast cancer (the risk of which increases with age)
- Altered sexuality patterns related to physiologic changes, medications, changes in body image, or psychosocial changes such as the loss of a significant other or a move to a setting that provides some level of assistive care (i.e., group home, assisted living center, or care facility)

Nursing Management: Female Reproductive System Disorders

1. Teach and encourage monthly breast self-exams and yearly mammograms for early detection and treatment of disorders.
2. Establish rapport and encourage the client to verbalize feelings and concerns related to sexuality, body image, and self-esteem.
3. Complete a sexual history and recommend interventions based on findings. Support the client's needs for companionship and intimacy throughout the life span.
4. Recommend that a bone density scan (Dexa-Scan) be discussed with the client's primary care provider to allow for early detection and treatment of osteoporosis.
5. Encourage annual gynecological examinations with the client's primary care provider.

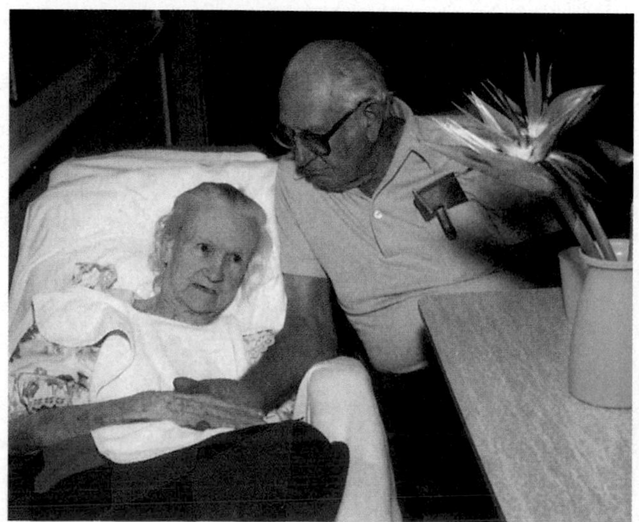

COURTESY OF DELMAR CENGAGE LEARNING

FIGURE 19-11 Sexuality and companionship remain important throughout the life span.

Reproductive System: Male

The following reproductive changes result from the aging process:

- Testosterone production decreases, resulting in decreased size of the testicles.
- Sperm count and viscosity of seminal fluid decrease.
- Although more time is required to obtain erection, the older man often finds that he and his partner can enjoy longer periods of lovemaking (greater control) before ejaculation. As at any age, protected intercourse (safe sex) through the use of a latex condom should be advised with new partners.
- The prostate gland may enlarge.
- Impotency may occur. Medications and other medical interventions have been successful in reversing impotency problems in many older males. A thorough evaluation by the primary care provider and a urologist can provide clients with available options given health status and current medication regimen.
- Libido and the need for intimacy and companionship remain unchanged in older males.

Common male reproductive disorders related to aging include the following:

- Altered sexuality patterns related to physiologic changes, medications, changes in body image, or psychosocial changes such as the loss of a significant other or a move to a setting that provides some level of assistive care (i.e., group home, assisted living center, or care facility)
- Benign prostatic hypertrophy (BPH)

Nursing Management: Male Reproductive System Disorders

1. Establish rapport and encourage the client to verbalize feelings and concerns related to sexuality, body image, and self-esteem.
2. Complete a sexual history and recommend interventions based on findings. Support the client's needs for companionship and intimacy throughout the life span.
3. Provide client and family education regarding the signs and symptoms of prostate disorders (e.g., difficulty in starting the urine stream, a smaller urine stream, frequent urination, frequent nighttime awakening for the purpose of urinating, or, in severe cases, the failure or inability to urinate).
4. Teach and encourage monthly testicular self-exam and yearly digital rectal examinations of the prostate gland by a primary care provider. The benefits of a PSA lab test performed every 1 to 2 years to facilitate early detection and treatment of prostate cancer are being researched and debated.

Integumentary System

The following integumentary changes result from the normal aging process:

- Subcutaneous tissue and elastin fibers diminish, causing the skin to become thinner, less elastic, and wrinkled.
- Ability of melanocytes to produce even pigmentation diminishes, resulting in hyperpigmentation or liver spots, typically on the hands and wrists (Figure 19-12).

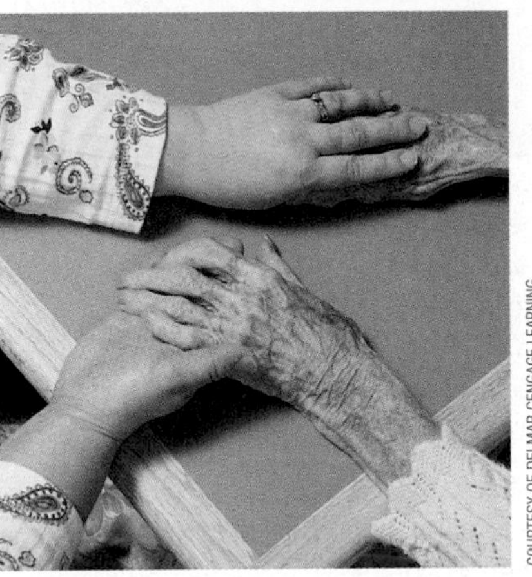

FIGURE 19-12 Hyperpigmentation is a normal result of the aging process.

- Eccrine, apocrine, and sebaceous glands decrease in size, number, and function, resulting in diminished secretions and moisturization and, thus, pruritis.
- Body temperature regulation diminishes because of decreased perspiration and, many times, decreased circulation, placing the older adult at risk for hypo- and hyperthermia.
- Capillary blood flow decreases, resulting in slower wound healing.
- Blood flow decreases, especially to lower extremities.
- Vascular fragility causes senile purpura
- Cutaneous sensitivity to pressure, touch, pain, and temperature decreases.
- Melanin production decreases, causing gray-white hair.
- Scalp, pubic, and axillary hair thin, and women display increased facial hair on the upper lip and chin.
- Nail growth slows, nails become more brittle, and longitudinal nail ridges form.

Common integumentary disorders related to aging include the following:

- Pressure ulcers (alteration in skin integrity)
- Herpes zoster (shingles)
- Skin cancer (included because the risk of skin cancer increases with age)

Nursing Management: Alteration in Skin Integrity

1. Perform a pressure ulcer risk assessment upon the client's admission to the health care setting (Figure 19-13).
2. Implement pressure ulcer prevention protocol for clients at risk for pressure ulcer formation. It is important to consider and document pressure-relieving interventions for all surfaces that the client will sit or lay on during the course of the day (Table 19-4).
3. Encourage adequate intake of protein and fluids to help ensure good skin integrity.
4. Dress clients in long sleeves and slacks, when appropriate, to protect fragile skin and provide warmth.
5. Assess skin turgor on sternum or forehead due to loss of skin elasticity.
6. Monitor client for exaggerated drug effects due to age related thinning of skin, potentially causing faster absorption of topical medications (Shepler, Grogan, & Pater, 2006).

Date of assessment: ____ Nurse: ________

Pressure ulcer present on admission: No ____ Yes ____ Stage ____

A score of 11 or more places a client at risk for pressure ulcer formation. Preventive protocol should be established.

Activity		**Total**	**Level of Consciousness**		**Total**
Ambulant without assistance	0		Alert	0	
Ambulant with assistance	2		Slow verbal response	1	
Chairfast	4		Responds to verbal or painful stimuli	2	
Bedfast	6	____	Absence of response to stimuli	3	____
Mobility—Range of Motion			**Nutritional Status**		
Full range of motion	0		Good (eats 75% or more of required intake)	0	
Moves with minimal assistance	2		Fair (eats less than 75% of required intake)	1	
Moves with moderate assistance	4		Poor (minimal intake, consistent weight loss)	2	
Immobile	6	____	Unable/refuses to eat/drink, emaciated	3	____
Skin Condition			**Incontinence—Bladder**		
Hydrated and intact	0		None	0	
Rashes or abrasions	2		Occasional (fewer than 2/24 hours)	1	
Decreased turgor, dry	4		Usually (more than 2/24 hours)	2	
Edema, erythema, pressure ulcers	6	____	Total (no control)	3	____
Predisposing Disease Process			**Incontinence—Bowel**		
No involvement	0		None	0	
Chronic, stable	1		Occasional (formed stool)	1	
Acute or chronic, unstable	2		Usually (semi-formed stool)	2	
Terminal	3	____	Total (no control, loose stool)	3	____

COURTESY OF DELMAR CENGAGE LEARNING

FIGURE 19-13 Pressure Ulcer Risk Assessment

Table 19-4 Protocol for Clients at Risk for Pressure Ulcers

OBJECTIVE	INTERVENTIONS
Relieve pressure	• Establish positioning schedule. • Place pressure relieving mattress on bed, cushions on chair. • Teach client wheelchair exercises. • Stand and/or ambulate client in chair frequently. • Use wheelchair for transporting only. • Allow client to sit on bedpan, commode, or toilet for only brief periods. • Check areas of pressure under casts, braces, splints, slings, prostheses.
Relieve friction and shearing	• Use turning sheet for positioning in bed and chair. • Keep head of bed lower than 30 degrees unless contraindicated. • Use supportive devices to prevent sliding in chairs. • Use appropriate transfer techniques. • Do not use powder on skin. • Place bed cradle under top covers.
Prevent moisture/maceration	• Implement scheduled toileting or bladder retraining program. • Use absorbent incontinent briefs or pads. • Check incontinent clients frequently. Wash and rinse thoroughly. Apply moisture barrier. • Avoid use of plastic/rubber sheets, protectors.
Prevent spasticity and contractures	• Avoid quick, rough movements. • Do range-of-motion exercises at least twice daily. • Assess for synergy patterns when positioning. • Administer oral antispasmodics if ordered.
Maintain hydration/nutritional status	• Assess nutritional status. • Investigate causes of anorexia. • Correct underlying nutritional deficits. • Encourage additional fluids, unless contraindicated. • Give high protein supplement, if necessary. • Monitor weight weekly.
Continue with routine skin care. Do skin checks with each position change.	

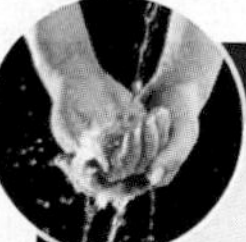

INFECTION CONTROL

Skin Integrity

It is a nursing responsibility to educate caregivers (including other staff members, as necessary) about the need to thoroughly wash and dry the client's perineal area and to keep linens and clothing clean and dry, especially when incontinence is a problem. Such education may also include instruction on maintaining client privacy; properly retracting, cleansing, and repositioning the foreskin of an uncircumcised older male client; and proper cleansing of the skin folds of female client's perineal area. Clients and caregivers should also be instructed to cleanse front to back only and to not rinse and reuse washcloths again or use them on other body areas. These simple hygiene and infection-control guidelines can help maintain the client's skin integrity and can also prevent unnecessary infections.

Nursing Management: Herpes Zoster

1. Treat the pain.
2. Treat the ulcer with medications (e.g., acyclovir [Zovirax] topical cream), as ordered, to reduce the length of time of the outbreak.
3. Develop a plan to ensure continuity in meeting the client's psychosocial needs, and allow the client time to share concerns.

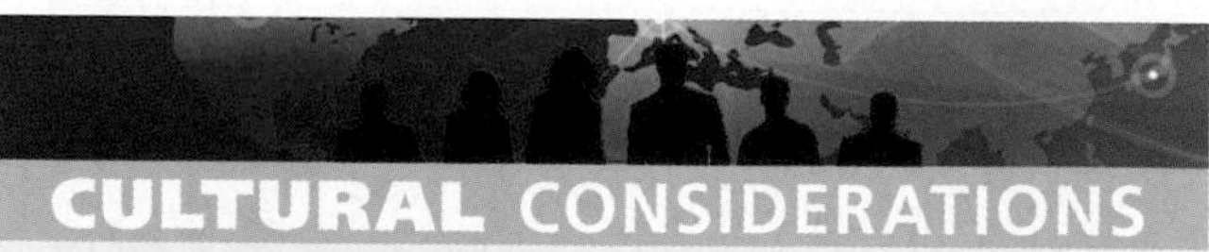

CULTURAL CONSIDERATIONS

Pain Assessment

Overt signs of pain may not be expressed by some cultures or sexes. Older adults may not sense pain until the condition has become severe. Therefore, a thorough pain assessment is crucial for effective pain management.

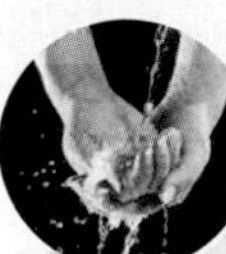

INFECTION CONTROL

Herpes Zoster

Prevent cross-infection from drainage from the vesicular eruptions by practicing proper hand hygiene and implementing appropriate isolation procedures, especially if the client is in the hospital or another health care facility.

Nursing Management: Skin Cancer

1. Teach clients and caregivers both cancer prevention methods and skin self-examination to detect lesions early. Early detection and treatment of skin cancers are essential to optimal client outcomes.
2. Provide information in both verbal and written form and in collaboration with the client's multidisciplinary team regarding treatment (surgery, chemotherapy, radiation, and other options).
3. Monitor for signs of infection at the lesion site.
4. Ensure that the client's psychological, psychosocial, spiritual, and dietary needs are also addressed.

FINANCING OLDER ADULT CARE

Since the 1960s, the U.S. Congress has developed and implemented a series of national entitlement programs to help ensure adequate income, housing, and access to medical care for older Americans. As the number of older clients (those older than age 65, particularly those older than age 85) continues to rise, caregivers and advocates for older-adult care should strive to understand the budgetary policies that have influenced and continue to influence the U.S. health care delivery system.

MEDICARE

Medicare (Title XVIII) is a nationwide health insurance program for Americans who are 65 years of age or older, for persons who are eligible for Social Security disability payments for longer than 2 years, and for certain workers and dependents who need kidney transplants or dialysis. The Health Care Financing Administration (HCFA) was the federal agency in charge of administering the Medicare program. Since July 2001, the HCFA is now the Centers for Medicare and Medicaid Services (CMS). More than the name has changed. Now there is an increased emphasis on responsiveness to beneficiaries and providers, and quality improvement (CMS, 2001).

The program was enacted as part of the Social Security Act of 1965 and became effective on June 1, 1966. It consists of two separate but coordinated programs: hospital insurance (called Part A) and medical insurance (called Part B), which covers physician's services, outpatient services, some medical supplies, and some skilled nursing and home health services. Medicare provides basic protection for the cost of health care but does not cover all expenses. Among the expenses *not* covered by Medicare for older Americans are those associated with the following:

- Acupuncture
- Chiropractic services (some exceptions)
- Cosmetic surgery
- Dental care and dentures (few exceptions)
- Eye exams (routine) and eye glasses
- Foot care (routine)
- Hearing aids
- Laboratory tests (screening)
- Long-term care
- Orthopedic shoes (few exceptions)
- Physical exams (routine)
- Prescription drugs (few exceptions)
- Travel (healthcare while traveling outside the United States) (Medicare, 2009a)

In the late 1990s, many insurance policies were available to supplement at varying levels the benefits paid by Medicare. This led many older clients to "stack" insurance policies or to buy numerous overlapping policies for fear of being underinsured. The insurance industry and Congress worked together to outlaw stacking of Medicare supplement policies.

Although there has been some improvement in insurance coverage for preventive screening tests such as mammograms, the lack of reimbursement for prescription drugs continues to significantly burden older Americans, many of whom must choose between costly medications and food.

On January 1, 2006, a new prescription drug coverage program began for persons older than 65 with Medicare regardless of income or health (CMS, 2009c). This program is referred to as Medicare Part D. This is insurance that should cover half of the cost of needed medications for the older adult. Medicare reports that 33% of persons covered by Medicare will meet the qualifying factors for extra help so that almost all of the medication costs for this group will be covered.

According to Kurtzman and Buerhaus (2008), the CMS, in an effect to refine Medicare's prospective payment system and improve quality care, implemented a new payment rule known as CMS-1533-FC to eliminate additional Medicare payments for eight preventable hospital-acquired conditions. The eight conditions include pressure ulcers, preventable injuries, catheter associated UTI's, vascular catheter associated infections, surgical site infections, air emboli, blood incompatibility reactions, and objects mistakenly left inside surgical clients.

In 2009, Medicare estimates coverage for items and services for more than 43 million beneficiaries (CMS, 2009b).

MEDICAID

The Medicaid program was also enacted as part of the Social Security Act of 1966 and is often referred to as Title XIX. This program, which is federally funded but state operated and administered, provides medical benefits to certain indigent, or low-income, Americans. Nursing home bills represent a staggering burden for many older Americans who require nursing care. In 1995, nursing home bills averaged $22,000 per person per year, and projections showed that two-thirds of older adults who lived alone would run out of savings after 13 weeks in a nursing home (Gallo, Paveza, Fulmer, 2003). Medicaid takes into account government-determined poverty levels when providing benefits, with coverage being extended to persons who are at certain percentages of the poverty level (e.g., 200% of poverty level, 150% of poverty level, and 100% of poverty level). Long-term care facilities serve both private-pay clients (those whose expenses are paid by themselves, their families, or their long-term care insurance policies) and Title XIX- (Medicaid-) funded clients. Medicaid coverage for long-term care is not available until a person's assets have been depleted to a certain set level. Older-adult care advocates continue their efforts to protect the assets of the spouse who is able to stay in the family home after the other spouse must be placed in a nursing home.

To some in the United States, the debate over Social Security, Medicare, and Medicaid financing is viewed as someone else's priority; however, the moral responsibility for providing access to quality services and care for our country's older adults is shared by all Americans. Older-adult care services should be developed to promote independence yet should provide assistance when needed.

Omnibus Budget Reconciliation Act

The Omnibus Budget Reconciliation Act (OBRA), first enacted in 1987 and reenacted in 1990, sought to ensure quality services for older Americans. The act included guidelines for services that were required to be made available to seniors and promoted the rights of seniors. As was the case with all health care costs, however, older-adult care costs continued to rise in the United States, and discussions and proposed legislation for financial reforms intensified.

Balanced Budget Act of 1997

Among the most significant influences on the financing of older-adult care is the Balanced Budget Act (BBA) of 1997. The BBA replaced cost-based reimbursement for care provided in skilled nursing facilities (SNFs) with a prospective payment system (PPS) based on client assessment within a resource utilization group system (RUGS). Reimbursement for home health services also shifted to a PPS.

The BBA also states that discharge from hospitals to SNFs or home care for 10 common but as yet unpublished diagnosis-related groups (DRGs) is to be considered as a transfer for payment purposes. Medicare's goal was to make a single blended payment that combined the traditional hospital DRG payment and the payment for postacute care services to be shared by the providers.

The intended implications for practice included reduced reimbursement to some SNFs, fewer discharges from hospitals to independent facilities for subacute care or home care, and, thus, encouraged the creation of integrated delivery systems and managed care. In reality, however, it has become more difficult to find placement in SNFs for clients with complex needs because the new reimbursement system simply does not fund all of their health care needs.

These reimbursement and regulatory changes surely represent only the beginning of such efforts to balance resources and need as the U.S. population continues to age. Certainly, significant work lies ahead for advocates of quality older-adult care in the United States and the world. Nurses will play a vital role in the ensuing debates, for they will see firsthand the positive and negative outcomes of their clients.

CRITICAL THINKING

Nurse Advocate

How can you, as a nurse, advocate for your older clients?

CASE STUDY

N.O., a 72-year-old man, was admitted to a skilled care facility for rehabilitation after an open reduction/internal fixation of the right hip. N.O. had fallen while going up the stairs of his home, suffering an intertrochanteric, comminuted fracture of the right femur. He has no recollection of what caused him to fall. He is married and, until his surgery, was working part time as a school-crossing guard. While in the hospital, N.O. exhibited mental status changes, including disorientation and confusion. His wife reports that he never had this problem before the surgery. He is continent of bowel and bladder. N.O. was in relatively good health until the fall. He and his wife agree that he should return home after rehabilitation is complete.

The following questions will guide your development of a nursing care plan for the case study.

1. Identify specific admission assessments that would be required for N.O. because of his age and condition.
2. Identify complications for which N.O. is at risk.
3. List interventions to prevent each complication.
4. Cite possible reasons for N.O.'s fall.
5. Describe methods for assessing N.O.'s mental status.
6. Describe possible reasons for his altered mental status.
7. Write three individualized nursing diagnoses and goals for N.O.
8. List nursing actions related to altered mental status.
9. List four successful outcomes for N.O.
10. Develop a teaching plan for N.O.
11. List the community resources N.O. may need after discharge.

SUMMARY

- The older adult population is rapidly growing.
- Although many stereotypes and myths are associated with aging, older adults are in fact very diverse in their characteristics.
- Health maintenance is as important for older adults as it is for younger persons. A healthy lifestyle can enhance the quality of life.
- Many changes are associated with aging. The disorders commonly seen among older adults are often the results of pathology and are thus not considered a normal part of aging; however, the risk of acquiring these disorders increases with age.
- Nurses knowledgeable about aging can plan interventions that will prevent complications for which older adults are at risk.
- Nurses have a responsibility to advocate for their older clients. Nurses should be active legislatively and should work collaboratively to develop older-adult care services that are affordable, provide equal access for all older Americans, and promote optimal wellness and independence.

REVIEW QUESTIONS

1. The senior citizens center has requested a nurse to speak to its members on the effects of aging. Which statement would be included in the presentation?
   1. All people eventually become senile if they live long enough.
   2. People lose interest in sex as they age.
   3. Most older adults are financially impoverished.
   4. Incontinence is not an expected or normal change of aging.
2. A student nurse is reading a book on the theories of aging. You know the student understands the programmed aging theory if the student states that:
   1. "Stress causes structural and chemical changes in the body, which, in turn, cause aging."
   2. "A genetic clock determines the speed at which people age."
   3. "Changes in collagen are the cause of aging."
   4. "The decreasing ability to produce T-cell differentiation causes aging."
3. The nurse is reviewing preventive respiratory tract infection care with an older adult client. A preventive instruction would include:
   1. obtaining an influenza vaccine each year.
   2. staying inside throughout the winter.
   3. avoiding exercise.
   4. limiting fluid intake.
4. The family of an older adult client is requesting information about the appropriate amount of exercise needed to maintain musculoskeletal function in their family member. As a nurse you would explain that:
   1. weight-bearing exercise is not recommended for older adults.
   2. high-intensity resistance training can improve muscle strength in older adults.
   3. muscle deterioration in older adults is to be expected.
   4. walking is the only healthy exercise for older adults.
5. While assisting an older client during bathing, the client asks "What is causing all of my skin problems?" How should the nurse respond?
   1. "The increased glandular secretions cause pruritus."
   2. "The increased capillary blood flow reduces body temperature."
   3. "The melanin production results in loss of hair."
   4. "The increased vascular fragility leads to ecchymosis."
6. The nurse assesses bilateral ectropion and presbycusis on an older client. As care is being planned, the nurse should:
   1. refer the client to a dermatologist and otologist for treatment.
   2. ask the nursing technician to obtain a walker for the client.
   3. provide additional fluids and extra protein in the client's diet.
   4. use a low-pitched voice to give the client directions while instilling artificial tears into his eyes.
7. The nurse is preparing medications for a newly admitted client. The medication sheet states the client is 95 years old. Which of the following age-related changes would the nurse expect to find which will increase the risk for drug toxicity?
   1. Faint pedal pulses and low body temperature.
   2. Loss of bone density and decreased blood flow.
   3. Urinary incontinence and thoracic rigidity.
   4. Dry skin and decreased heart conduction time.
8. An older adult nursing home client frequently repeats his World War II stories. The nursing assistant complains she is tired of hearing about his war stories. How should the nurse respond?
   1. "Yes, I'm tired of hearing about those war stories, too."
   2. "Reminiscing is good to help maintain long-term memory and self esteem."

3. "Whenever he starts to repeat another war story, change the subject."
4. "Just pretend you're listening to the war stories, so you won't hurt his feelings."

9. Your older adult client complains he feels bloated. Upon reading the chart, you note he has gained 2.5 pounds since yesterday. This 2.5 pounds would be equivalent to approximately how many milliliters of body fluid?
   1. 1000 mL
   2. 800 mL
   3. 600 mL
   4. 400 mL

10. A family member of a client with dementia asks the nurse the difference between delirium and dementia. The best response would be:
    1. dementia is a reversible confusion which is treatable.
    2. delirium is a chronic confusion with remissions and exacerbations.
    3. dementia is a slow progressive confusion which is irreversible.
    4. delirium is an acute confusion which is irreversible.

REFERENCES/SUGGESTED READING

Administration on Aging (AoA). (2001). The Administration on Aging and the Older American's Act. Retrieved from www.aoa.dhhs.gov/aoa/pages/aoafact.html

Administration on Aging (AoA). (2002). Income and poverty among the elderly. Retrieved from http://www.aoa.gov

Administration on Aging (AoA). (2009a). A profile of older Americans: 2008: Future growth. Retrieved August 4, 2009 from http://www.aoa.gov/AoARoot/Aging_Statistics/Profile/2008/4.aspx

Administration on Aging (AoA). (2009b). A profile of older Americans: 2008: The older population. Retrieved August 4, 2009 from http://www.aoa.gov/AoARoot/Aging_Statistics/Profile/2008/3.aspx

American Association of Retired Persons (AARP). (1998). *A profile of older Americans.* Washington, DC: Department of Health and Human Services.

Andersen, C. (1999). *Antecedents, correlates, and impact of violent behaviors in the elderly VA client.* Unpublished thesis, University of Iowa, Iowa City, IA.

Andersen, C. (1998). *Nursing student to nursing leader: The critical path to leadership development.* Clifton Park, NY: Delmar Cengage Learning.

Bendix, J. (2009). Exploiting the elderly. *RN,* 72(3), 42–46.

Bray, B., Van Sell, S., & Miller-Anderson, M. (2007). Stress incontinence: It's no laughing matter. *RN,* 70(4), 25–29.

Bulechek, G., Butcher, H., McCloskey, J., & Dochterman, J., eds. (2008). *Nursing Interventions Classification (NIC)* (5th ed.). St. Louis, MO: Mosby/Elsevier.

Covell, C., Graziano, J., Rich, D., & Tobin, K. (2007). New outlook for age-related macular degeneration. *Nursing2007,* 37(3), 22–24.

Centers for Medicare & Medicaid Services (CMS). (2002). Medicare aged and disabled enrollees by type of coverage. Retrieved from http://cms.hhs.gov/statistics/enrollment/natltrends/hi_smi.asp

Centers for Medicare & Medicaid Services (CMS). (2003). Medicare Part B physicians supplier data. Retrieved from http://cms.hhs.gov/data/betos/cy2001.asp

Centers for Medicare and Medicaid Services (CMS). (2009a). Medicare & you 2009. Retrieved August 7, 2009 from http://www.medicare.gov/Publications/Pubs/pdf/10050.pdf

Centers for Medicare and Medicaid Services (CMS). (2009b). Medicare coverage – general information overview. Retrieved August 7, 2009 from http://www.cms.hhs.gov/CoverageGenInfo/

Centers for Medicare and Medicaid Services (CMS). (2009c). Now Medicare covers more than ever. Retrieved August 7, 2009 from http://www.cms.hhs.gov/AIAN/Downloads/CMS-11142-N.pdf

Collins, J. (2002). Helping an older patient eat well to stay well. *Nursing2002, 32*(11), 32hn6–32hn8.

Dowling-Castronovo, A., & Specht, J. (2009). Assessment of transient urinary incontinence in older adults. *American Journal of Nursing, 109*(2), 62–71.

Estes, M. (2010). *Health assessment & physical examination* (4th ed.). Clifton Park, NY: Delmar Cengage Learning.

Flaherty, E. (2008). Using pain-rating scales with older adults. *American Journal of Nursing,* 108(6), 40–47.

Gallo, J., Paveza, G., & Fulmer, T. (2005). *Handbook of geriatric assessment.* Gaithersburg, MD: Jones & Bartlett.

Hamilton, S. (2001). Detecting dehydration & malnutrition in the elderly. *Nursing2001, 31*(12), 56–57.

Hogstel, M. (Ed.). (2001). *Gerontology: Nursing care of the older adult.* Clifton Park, NY: Delmar Cengage Learning.

Kimbell, S. (2001). Before the fall: Keeping your patient on his feet. *Nursing2001, 31*(8), 44–45.

Kurtzman, E., & Buerhaus, P. (2008). New Medicare payment rules: Danger or opportunity for nursing? *American Journal of Nursing, 108*(6), 30–35.

Logue, R. (2002). Self-medication and the elderly: How technology can help. *AJN, 102*(7), 51–55.

Manno, M., & Hayes, D. (2006). How medication reconciliation saves lives. *Nursing 2006, 36*(3), 63–64.

Massachusetts Institute of Technology (MIT). (2009). Innovations. Retrieved August 4, 2009 from http://web.mit.edu/agelab/index.shtml

Mezey, M., & Mitty, E. (2006). The teaching nursing home: Models for training clinicians in geriatrics. *American Journal of Nursing, 106*(10), 72.

Moorhead, S., Johnson, M., Maas, M., & Swanson, E. (2007). *Nursing Outcomes Classification (NOC)* (4th ed.). St. Louis, MO: Mosby.

Napoli, M. (2009). The marketing of osteoporosis. *American Journal of Nursing, 109*(4), 58–61.

National Council on Aging (NCOA) (2002). Facts about older Americans. Retrieved from http://www.ncoa.org/content.cfm5sectionID.106

National Institute on Aging. (2009). What's your aging IQ? Retrieved August 4, 2009 from http://www.niapublications.org/quiz/index.php

Peskin, B. (1999). *Beyond the zone.* Houston, TX: Noble.

Sharts-Hopko, N., & Glynn-Milley, C. (2009). Primary open-angle glaucoma. *American Journal of Nursing, 109*(2), 40–47.

Shepler, S., Grogan, T., & Pater, K. (2006). Keep your older patients out of medication trouble. *Nursing2006, 36*(9), 44–47.

Social Security Administration (SSA). (2000). The president signs the "Senior Citizens' Freedom to Work Act of 2000." Retrieved from www.ssa.gov/legislation/legis_bulletin_040700.html

Steffen, K. (2003). When your trauma patient is over 65. *Nursing2003, 33*(4), 53–56.

Stein, A. (2003). Aging is more than skin deep. *Nursing2003, 33*(2), 32hn7–32hn8.

Stockdell, R., & Amella, E. (2008). The Edinburgh feeding evaluation in dementia scale. *American Journal of Nursing, 108*(8), 46–53.

Victor, K. (2001). Properly assessing pain in the elderly. *RN*, 64(5), 45–49.

Wallhagen, M., Pettengill, E., & Whiteside, M. (2006). Sensory impairment in older adults: Part 1: Hearing loss. *American Journal of Nursing, 106*(10), 40–48.

Wilkinson, J. (1999). *A family caregiver's guide to planning and decision making for the elderly*. Minneapolis, MN: Fairview Press.

RESOURCES

Administration on Aging (AoA), http://www.aoa.gov

American Association for Geriatric Psychiatry, http://www.aagpgpa.org

American Association of Retired Persons (AARP), http://www.aarp.org

American Geriatrics Society, http://www.americangeriatrics.org

American Nurses Association (ANA), Council on Gerontological Nursing Practice, http://ww.nursingworld.org

National Council on Aging (NCOA), http://www.ncoa.org

UNIT 9 Nursing Care of the Client: Health Care in the Community

CHAPTER 20
Ambulatory, Restorative, and Palliative Care in Community Settings

MAKING THE CONNECTION

Refer to the following chapters to increase your understanding of nursing care within ambulatory/urgent, rehabilitative/restorative, home health, long-term, palliative, and hospice care settings:

Adult Health Nursing

- ***The Older Adult***

LEARNING OBJECTIVES

Upon completion of this chapter, you should be able to:

- Define key terms.
- List reasons for a significant change in the growth of nonacute care services.
- Describe the differences between Medicaid and Medicare.
- Explain the role of the licensed practical nurse/vocational nurse (LPN/VN) as a member of the interdisciplinary health care team in various health care settings.
- Discuss the types of clients that would benefit from participation in a rehabilitation/restorative care program.
- Explain the responsibilities of the LPN/VN in ambulatory care, rehabilitation/restorative care nursing, nursing in long-term care, in-home care, and hospice.

KEY TERMS

adult day care
age-appropriate care
ambulatory care
assisted living
disability
extended care facility (ECF)
handicap
hospice
impairment
long-term care
managed care
minimum data set (MDS)

TABLE 20-1 Interdisciplinary Health Care Team Roles

TEAM MEMBER	ROLE
Nurse	See text for description of roles
Physician or physiatrist	Prescribe medical and pharmacological treatment
Physical therapist	Muscle and joint training
Occupational therapist	Fine muscle training, self-care skills
Nutritionist	Assess for caloric intake
Speech therapist	Swallow evaluations, speech retraining
Psychologist	Test for cognitive, emotional, and psychological function; counseling for grief, loss, and depression
Social worker	Evaluate need for financial resources, community resources; counseling family issues
Visiting nurse	Evaluation of home setting; assess, teach, and coordinate home care
Vocational counselor	Vocational retraining, adaptation of work setting
Recreational therapist	Provides socialization opportunities; teaches how to adapt to community
Respiratory therapist	Treatment of respiratory or ventilatory equipment problems
Clergy	Spiritual counseling
Clinical nurse specialist	Case management

From *Nursing Fundamentals: Caring and Clinical Decision Making* (2nd ed.), by R. Daniels, R. Grendell, & F. Wilkins, 2010, Clifton Park, NY: Delmar Cengage Learning.

assesses individuals to regain or maintain their ADLs. Occupational therapy includes the use of assistive devices to reach a needed item, or pull up socks, or move a leg after a stroke or knee replacement. The speech therapist is the professional who assesses disabilities involving speech, communication whether spoken or written, and swallowing ability. All of these individuals are professionally trained to complete these tasks.

The social worker is a professionally trained individual who assists in the admissions process. Resident and family questions or concerns are usually addressed by a social worker in an extended care facility.

A pharmacist reviews the resident's medications monthly and oversees that the facility is meeting federal state regulations. If the resident's physician does not serve the facility, a medical director provides medical care to the resident and also to any residents in need of a physician while in the extended care facility. Depending on the facility, a dentist, podiatrist, and psychologist are available every month to every three months as needed.

Each discipline completes an assessment and pools this information at the care planning conference so that a consensus among members, including the client and family, are reached. The team process avoids both duplication of services and fragmented care. A holistic approach is used so that the client's physical, mental, and psychosocial needs are identified (Wenckus, 1995).

ROLE OF THE LPN/VN

Restorative nursing is a specialty practice and requires specialized knowledge, skills, and attitudes. A sound knowledge base in anatomy and physiology of the neurological, musculoskeletal, gastrointestinal, and urological systems is a prerequisite. The nurse has excellent clinical skills in the areas of therapeutic positioning, range of joint motion exercises, transfers, ambulation, and ADLs, as shown in Figure 20-6. The nurse is responsible for planning measures to prevent complications such as impaired skin integrity and contractures and to implement interventions for dysphagia, incontinence, and other identified problems.

The nurse is a member of the interdisciplinary team and functions as caregiver, counselor, coordinator of care, and client advocate (Mauk, 2007). The nurse seeks to understand the roles and responsibilities and to interrelate with each discipline. There is a steady demand for restorative nurses in all settings.

Nurses are advocates for the older adults and their families in the health care system. The nurse is aware of the residents needs and refers them to the appropriate health care service. The nurse continues to work alongside the health care services to reinforce the older adult's optimal health promotion and wellness.

FUNCTIONAL ASSESSMENT AND EVALUATION FOR REHABILITATION/RESTORATION

Terms such as disability, impairment, and handicap describe functional levels. **Disability** is an individual's lack of ability to complete an activity in the normal manner. **Impairment** refers to an abnormal psychological or physiologic behavior or an anatomic loss, such as a loss of a limb (Eliopoulos, 2005). According to the Self-identification of Handicap form, **handicap** means the physical or mental inability to complete a role in one or more major ADL (U.S. Office of Personnel Management, 1987).

Clients who need restorative care are screened before admission to a program. Assessments are completed by healthcare professionals whose services may be required by the client (Figure 20-7). The purpose of screening is to select the best setting for services. Criteria for admission to a program usually require that the client be:

- Medically stable
- Able to learn
- Able to sit supported for at least one hour a day and to actively participate in the program

Interdisciplinary programs may stipulate that the client has disabilities in 2 or more areas of function:

- Mobility
- Performance of ADL

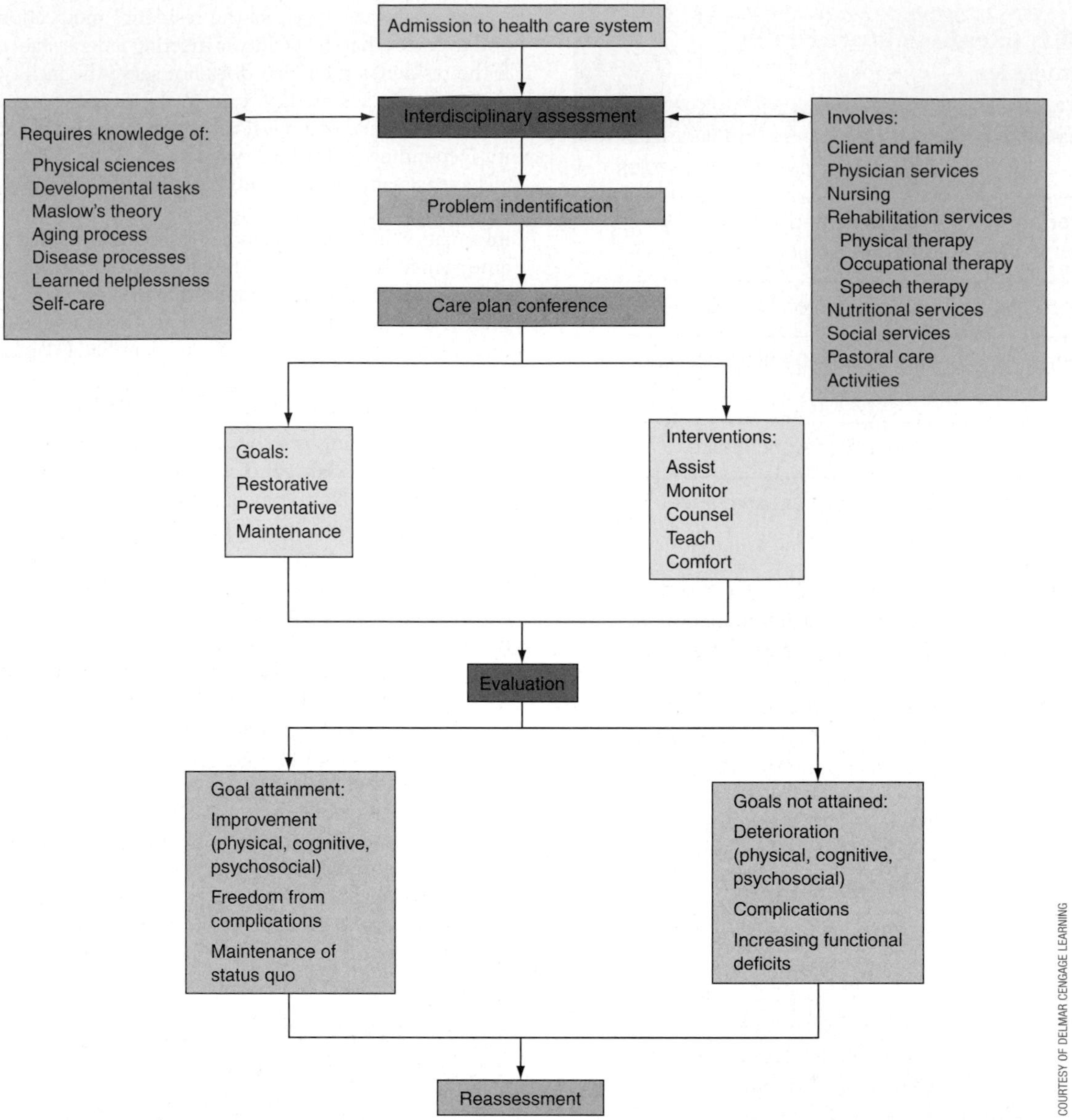

Admission to health care system

Interdisciplinary assessment

Requires knowledge of:
Physical sciences
Developmental tasks
Maslow's theory
Aging process
Disease processes
Learned helplessness
Self-care

Involves:
Client and family
Physician services
Nursing
Rehabilitation services
Physical therapy
Occupational therapy
Speech therapy
Nutritional services
Social services
Pastoral care
Activities

Problem indentification

Care plan conference

Goals:
Restorative
Preventative
Maintenance

Interventions:
Assist
Monitor
Counsel
Teach
Comfort

Evaluation

Goal attainment:
Improvement (physical, cognitive, psychosocial)
Freedom from complications
Maintenance of status quo

Goals not attained:
Deterioration (physical, cognitive, psychosocial)
Complications
Increasing functional deficits

Reassessment

FIGURE 20-4 The Interdisciplinary Health Care Team Process

- Bowel and bladder control
- Cognition
- Emotional function
- Pain management
- Swallowing
- Communication

There are a number of standardized assessment instruments that are designed to evaluate motor function, cognition, speech and language, mobility, and the client's performance of ADLs.

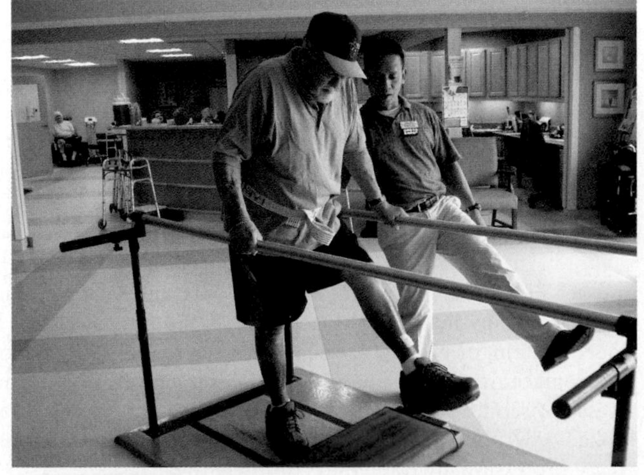

FIGURE 20-5 The physical therapist assists a client with a specific exercise program to improve or maintain physical mobility, function, and strength. (*Courtesy of Kingston Residence of Fort Wayne, Fort Wayne, IN.*)

ASSESSMENT OF ABILITIES

The Uniform Data System for Medical Rehabilitation (UDS) was developed by a grant from the U.S. Department of Education, National Institute on Disability and Rehabilitation Research. The UDS offers a uniform method to document a client's disability and medical rehabilitation, thereby providing a database of disability rehabilitation in more than 1,400

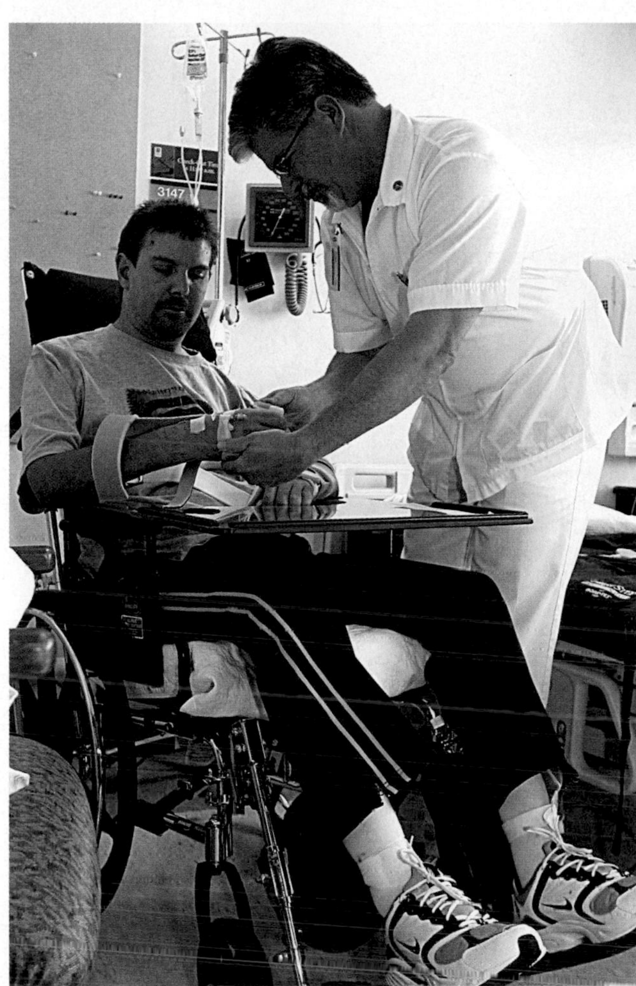

FIGURE 20-6 A nurse applies a splint to the arm of a rehabilitation client. (*Courtesy of Association of Rehabilitation Nurses.*)

facilities with more than 13 million clients for standardized rehabilitation comparison. The UDS measures impairment (function), disability (activity), and handicap (role).

There are several functional measurement tools to assess functional status. Three functional measurement tools are discussed in this chapter: Functional Independence Measure (FIM), Functional Assessment Measure (FAM), and the Barthel Index. The FIM and the FAM are more commonly used for the UDS.

Functional Independence Measure and Functional Assessment Measure

The FIM is an assessment tool that assesses cognitive and motor function status in relation to the amount of assistance needed to complete ADLs or IADL. Specific areas covered include independence in cognition problem solving, memory, communication, and social interaction. It also assesses physical independence in self care, control of bowel and bladder, transfers, and ambulation. The FIM is a widely used evaluation tool to review resident progress and rehabilitation/restorative outcomes.

The FAM assesses cognitive, behavioral, communication, and community functioning. The FAM is designed to use with the FIM (FIM+FAM) to provide a more comprehensive view of the rehabilitation client.

Barthel Index

The Barthel Index is a functional measurement tool that measures a person's level of independence in areas of self care and mobility. It is used in restorative care areas to predict length of stay and the amount of assisted care needed to complete ADL. The Barthel Index is included in the FIM and PULSES profile tools and only takes 5 minutes to complete.

These functional measurement tools assist in the objective documentation of changes that occur over time. With these tools, professionals recognize changes as they occur and promote optimal functional independence, which is the goal of restorative care.

REHABILITATION/RESTORATIVE CARE SETTINGS

Rehabilitation/restorative care settings are found in hospitals, extended care facilities with rehabilitation units, and rehabilitation hospitals as stand-alone facilities. Private rooms in hospitals and rehabilitation units are now the norm.

Special Beds

For residents with integumentary needs, whether they are the result of poor nutrition or poor circulation, there are special beds to aid in protecting the skin from breakdown. Pressure-relieving support surfaces, including special beds, mattresses, and mattress overlays, are available to support the body in bed. Special air-fluidized beds flow pressurized air through the oversized mattress to relieve pressure areas. A similar bed is a low-air-loss bed that works on the same principle of relieving pressure areas. Ring cushions (donuts) are not recommended because they cause fluid congestion and edema. None of these devices replace timely repositioning and assessing for skin breakdown on at risk residents. Repositioning the body decreases pressure point areas, and using positioning devices to raise vulnerable areas prone to pressure decreases skin breakdown. Pillows and foam wedges are placed between bony areas and under heels to relieve pressure points from the mattress. Avoid shearing force when moving residents in bed.

Urinary Devices

Incontinence causes skin tissue breakdown, and keeping the skin dry prevents skin breakdown. In the past, indwelling catheters were used. But years of research have proven that indwelling catheters cause urinary tract infections and are not used as frequently. For men, condom catheters are fit over the penis and drained into a leg bag. Other devices for men are urinary devices that act as an artificial sphincter for control of urinary incontinence. The male incontinence clamp attaches to the penis to restrict incontinence.

For women, there are medical devices to treat incontinence. One such device is a urethral insert, which is used in times of predictable incontinence, such as when taking part in an activity like running. The disposable device is a small tampon-like plug that inserts into the urethra to prevent leaking urine. These devices require a prescription and are not meant for everyday use. Another female urinary device is a pessary that is a stiff ring inserted into the vagina that holds up a prolapsed bladder or uterus to prevent leakage of urine. The device is worn all day and removed for cleaning on a regular basis.

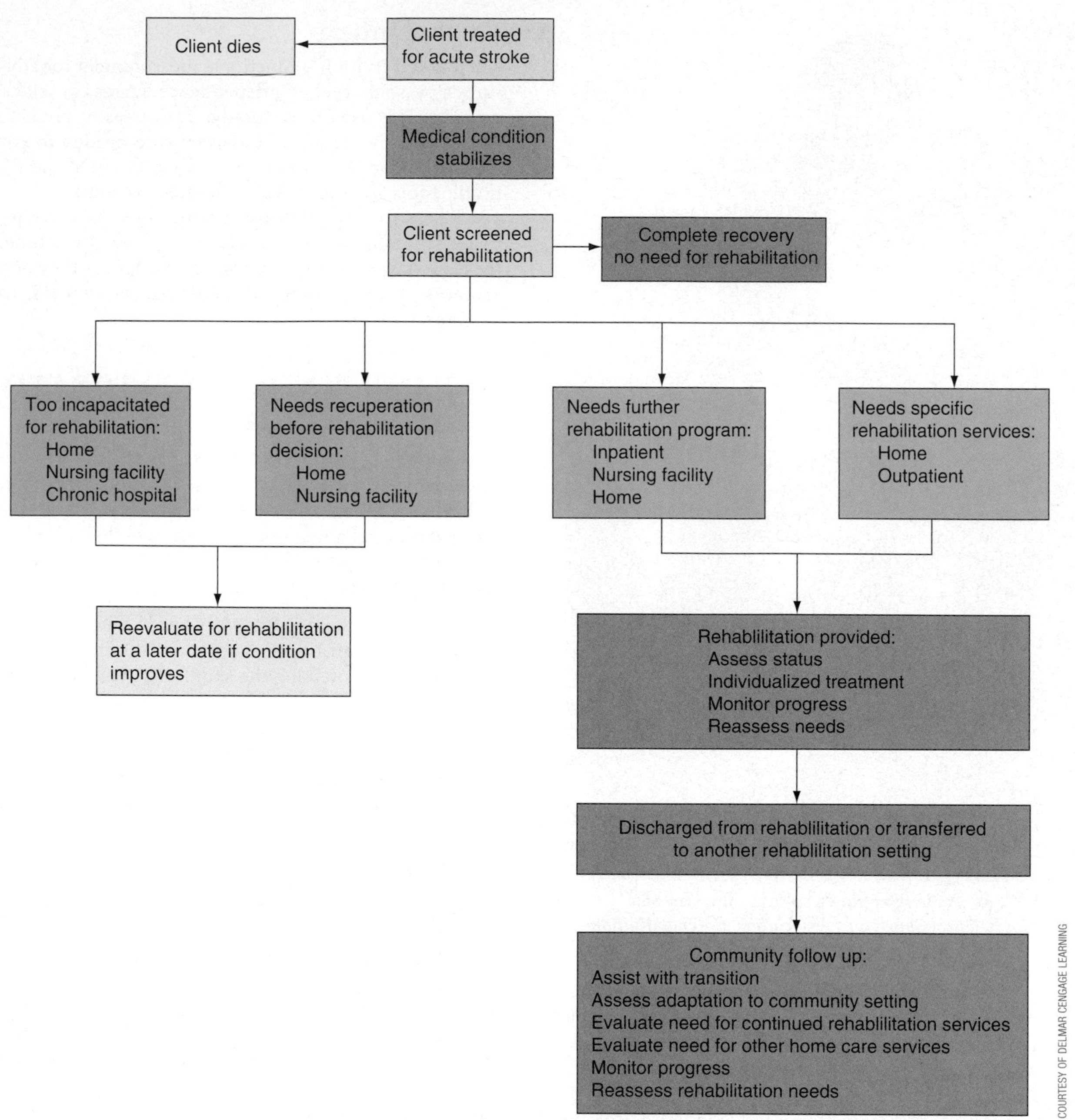

FIGURE 20-7 Assessing Potential Stroke Rehabilitation

HOME HEALTH CARE

Home care encompasses a number of services delivered to persons in their homes and is one of the fastest-growing segments of health care delivery. Clients are receiving intravenous therapy, ventilator care, parenteral nutrition, and chemotherapy at home. Many agencies have nurse specialists on staff for complicated cases involving care required for wounds, intravenous therapy, diabetes, and cardiac or respiratory problems.

Medicare-certified agencies provide intermittent care to persons meeting the criteria for care. A registered nurse calls on the client a specified number of times each week to assess the client's condition, supervise the work of LPN/VNs and nonlicensed staff, and deliver skilled nursing care. Nursing assistants are assigned to give personal care; check vital signs; and do positioning, transfers, and passive range-of-motion exercises. In addition to nursing staff, the agency provides therapists and social workers to serve their clients. These services are time-limited by Medicare and are not reimbursable if the client is not deemed to require skilled care.

CRITICAL THINKING

Choosing Housing for a Family Member

How could a nurse assist an individual in evaluating an extended care facility for a family member?

TYPES OF HOME-BASED CARE

There are two types of home-based care. One type is professional and the other is technical.

Professional

The professional division is based on scientific theory and principles bound by legal and professional standards and guidelines with licensed and certified employees. Employees offering skilled services are nurses, therapists, social workers, and nursing assistants. Other additional services offered are homemaker assistance, meal preparation, cleaning, sitter services, and transportation to physician offices. **Respite care** provides the caregiver with a short break from providing care. This short break may be a period of hours, days, or even weeks.

Technical

The technical division is driven by products sold for profit, following guidelines for reimbursement of payment. Included in the technical division would be the home medical equipment services or durable medical equipment that provides hospital beds, wheelchairs, scooters, walkers, oxygen, and related equipment. Also included in this division is the intravenous or home-infusion service that supplies the client with intravenous equipment. Personnel from the home-infusion service either teach the caregiver how to run the equipment or teach the client how to administer the infusion. Therapies include tube feedings, hyperalimentation, antibiotics, blood or blood products, analgesics, or antineoplastics. Reimbursement payment is determined by insurance companies, managed care companies, and Medicare.

Home Visit Outcomes

In 1999, that Medicare reimbursement requirements were mandated for home health agencies to validate client outcomes, quality improvement, and client satisfaction of care. An outcomes measurable tool called **Outcomes and Assessment Information Set (OASIS)** was developed and implemented to determine the care given and reimbursement required. OASIS data are reported to the Centers for Medicare and Medicaid Services. Each home health care agency uses this system to review the agencies' data results and compare their outcomes and client satisfaction to other similar agencies. Other home health care agencies, although not required by Medicare, use the Outcome Based Quality Improvement System to improve client outcomes.

Trends in Home Care

Home health care has evolved into a more technologic nursing care. Care within the home now includes apnea monitors, electrocardiographs, ventilators, parenteral nutrition, intravenous therapy, chemotherapy, chest tubes, and skeletal traction. Client x-rays are taken by mobile x-ray machines. The advanced technology provides client care without clients leaving their homes.

Telehealth

Telehealth is electronic information services that offer increased client and family participation. The nurse and client use interactive videos, telephone cardiac rate monitoring with EKG readout, digital subscriber lines, and internet transmission of data. Photos of client's wounds are viewed with an in-home computerized, two-way viewing screen. Home health care nurses use hand-held or laptop computers that hold the assessment and plan of care for each home care client. Most home health care facilities use an electronic clinical documentation system. The Centers for Medicare and Medicaid Services developed a computerized plan of care (Form 485) that is compatible with the home health care electronic system. Nurses electronically document their client assessments and delivery of nursing care on Form 485. The data are downloaded to the main frame computer in the main office for nurse managers to coordinate client care day or night. Through advanced technology, a nurse prioritizes the needs of the clients, implements a tighter control of nursing case management, and decreases the cost of health care.

Role of the Home Health Nurse

It is vital that the home health care nurse is experienced and knowledgeable in various disease processes seen in clients within the home setting. The nurse works alone, draws on previous experience, and knows when to call on or direct the client to community resources to meet the health needs of the client. The nurse has fine tuned assessment skills along with technological knowledge to use different equipment. The nurse manages home cases by using the federal government assessment and plan of care forms necessary for reimbursement. Communication techniques are crucial between all of the health team members.

Role of the LPN/VN

Although the role of the LPN is expanding, in 2006, 56,610 LPNs were working in home health care. This means that 7.5% of all employed LPNs worked in home care (Bureau of Labor Statistics, 2007). The responsibilities of the LPN/VN vary among agencies. All nurses working in home care must have excellent assessment skills and a keen ability to identify actual and potential problems. Teaching the client and family is a major responsibility for the home health nurse. Communication skills are essential as the nurse provides care to the client and meets the needs of the client's family (See Figure 20-8). The client with a chronic health problem will have ongoing needs after the home health care is discontinued. The home health nurse continually seeks out community resources to use in caring for clients. Clients and their family caregivers are taught the following:

The disease process

- Complications that may occur
- How to prevent the complications
- Signs and symptoms of the complications
- How to reduce risk factors such as dietary changes and exercise programs

Medications

- Actions of medications
- Special administration guidelines such as timing related to meals
- Side effects

Special skills

- Drawing up and administering insulin or other injectables
- Using a blood glucose monitor
- Changing dressings

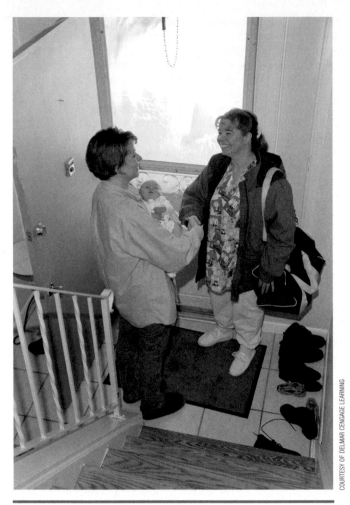

COURTESY OF DELMAR CENGAGE LEARNING

FIGURE 20-8 A home health nurse provides care to the client and meets the needs of the client's family.

- Monitoring vital signs
- Using special client care equipment, adaptive devices, and assistive devices

Documentation and communication

- How to keep records for nurse or physician visit; for example, blood glucose, blood pressure, and weight
- Communication with health care providers
- How and when to contact the home health nurse
- How and when to contact the physician
- How and when to contact emergency services

FUTURE OF HOME HEALTH CARE

Home health care has met the challenges of changes in the past with OASIS and reimbursement requirements of Medicare. It is imperative that home health care agencies and nurses continue to use evidence-based research to implement improvements to client care that is cost effective and ensures quality of healthcare.

ASSISTED LIVING

Assisted living combines housing and services for persons who require assistance with ADLs. Nursing care is usually provided for an additional fee. These are persons who cannot live alone but who do not need 24-hour care. It is a less restrictive environment than a long-term care facility and maintains the individual's independence and freedom of choice. This level of care may be offered in a freestanding facility or as a section of a long-term care facility. A monthly fee is charged and covers rent, utilities, housekeeping services, meals, transportation, health promotion, exercise programs, and assistance with ADL. There are an estimated 36,000 assisted living residences in the United States, with more than 1 million residents (Assisted Living Federation of America, 2009).

ADULT DAY CARE

Adult day care centers are located in a separate unit of a long-term care facility, in a private home, or are freestanding. They provide a variety of services in a protective setting for adults who are unable to stay alone but who do not need 24-hour care. The centers are generally open from 7:00 A.M. to 6:00 P.M., 5 days a week, and serve two or three meals in a day. A daily or hourly fee is charged with an additional charge for meals. Services are limited to socialization or may be comprehensive, offering modest restorative care services and nursing care. Adult day care is often used by working persons who have a spouse or a parent living with them who cannot be left alone.

RESPITE CARE

Respite care is offered by adult day care centers, long-term care facilities, or in private homes. It is intended to provide a break to caregivers and is used a few hours a week, for an occasional weekend, or for longer vacations. Planned activities, meals, and supervision are included in respite care services.

LONG-TERM CARE

Long-term care refers to a spectrum of services provided to individuals who have an ongoing need for health care. Long-term care has traditionally meant a community-based nursing home licensed for skilled or intermediate care. Although there is a great demand for this type of care, there is also a market for other levels of health care.

LONG-TERM CARE FACILITIES

Long-term care facilities provide services to individuals who are not acutely ill, have continuing health care needs, and cannot function independently at home. They are licensed for either intermediate care or skilled nursing care. Intermediate care facilities are not certified for reimbursement from Medicare but may be certified for Medicaid funding. Skilled nursing facilities are eligible for certification by both Medicare and Medicaid, but not all facilities choose to become certified. These facilities were formerly called nursing homes, rest homes, or convalescent centers. The term **extended care facility (ECF)** refers to any facility that provides care for a long period of time. It has no concrete definition and could refer to either an intermediate or skilled nursing facility. Facilities in every state that receive any government funds from any source are required by law to be in compliance with the Omnibus Budget Reconciliation Act of 1987 (OBRA) regulations. The Act requires that residents be free from all unneeded drugs and chemical restraints (psychotropic drugs).

A restorative philosophy of care provides direction for the interdisciplinary team. Emphasis is placed on assisting the client (usually called resident) to attain and maintain the highest level of physical, mental, and psychosocial function. A holistic approach is used, and families are important members of the care team. A large number of facilities have special units devoted to the care of residents with specific problems. These units care for persons with Alzheimer's disease, diabetes, respiratory disorders, wounds, and other conditions.

Long-term care or extended care facilities are available for older adults in need of nursing care 24 hours a day. The older adult receives assistance with ADLs, nursing supervision, and activities to keep the mind stimulated. Physical, speech, and occupational therapy are offered to assist the older adult. Also offered are three nutritious meals planned by a dietitian to meet the physician's orders, along with snacks for the older adult. The nursing staff includes registered nurses, LPNs, and certified nursing assistants 24 hours a day. Housekeeping services are available to keep the older adult's room and linens clean. An activity coordinator and social service personnel are included in the extended care facility staff. This could be one or two people based on the number of beds in the extended care facility. Added client expenses include medications, outside physician costs, various therapies, personal care items, and laundry services.

Reimbursement

Federal and state reimbursement is determined by the resident's functional abilities and services used while in the facility. The facility is reimbursed for a certain amount of money for expenses by Medicare and Medicaid. Each year, the Medicare/Medicaid facility is reviewed by state and/or federal personnel to ensure that the facility is meeting expected standards of care. If not, and if the infractions are severe enough, the facility is fined and/or loses Medicare/Medicaid funding. Facilities have closed their doors based on poor results. Every facility has to post these state/federal findings within the facility for the public.

Discharge

Client discharge planning begins at the time of admission and is included in the care plan. By placing the information on the care plan, all long-term care personnel know the same information and goals for a satisfactory outcome.

EXTENDED CARE FACILITIES

Extended care facilities are designed to provide different services to meet specific client needs. The basic extended care facility offers 24-hour supervised nursing care with a certified nursing aide to assist with ADLs. The next level is skilled nursing care. This level offers services of registered nurses and licensed practical nurses 24 hours a day that includes treatments, administration of medications, and procedures. Skilled care services include professionals in physical, speech, occupational, and respiratory therapies. Subacute care offers the same services as skilled care but is more focused on residents with acute or chronic illness or injury. Some extended care facilities are designed for special needs children and for older adults with special needs, such as Alzheimer's/dementia units. Senior communities offer living options to meet the older adults' needs such as totally independent apartments or condos, assisted-living areas, and skilled nursing care facilities.

Holistic Nursing in Extended Care

Holistic nursing reaches beyond treating diseases and meets the needs of the total person by nourishing the biological, psychological, social, and spiritual parts of a person. The holistic view promotes health and wellness.

As the body changes through the aging process and has acute and chronic health problems, the effect on the wellness of the body, mind, and spirit is diminished. Wellness develops from maintaining a positive purpose in life and an inner spiritual wholeness. Nurses change health outcomes as the result of their knowledge in the sciences and humanities. In caring for the older adult, nursing plays a significant role in assisting the older adult to find their balance of health promotion and wellness (See Figure 20-9).

Routines and Treatments

In an extended care facility, holistic gerontological nursing care goals are to: (1) enhance the older adult's growth to wholeness; (2) encourage improvement and learning from an acute or chronic disease; (3) optimize the quality of life during a terminal illness or disability; and (4) ensure comfort, peace, dignity and integrity in death (Eliopoulos 2005).

Activities

The enjoyment of life does not have to end when an older adult enters an extended care facility. An older adult can continue to find purpose in life. This time in life provides the individual with the freedom to reflect on life's work experiences, family life,

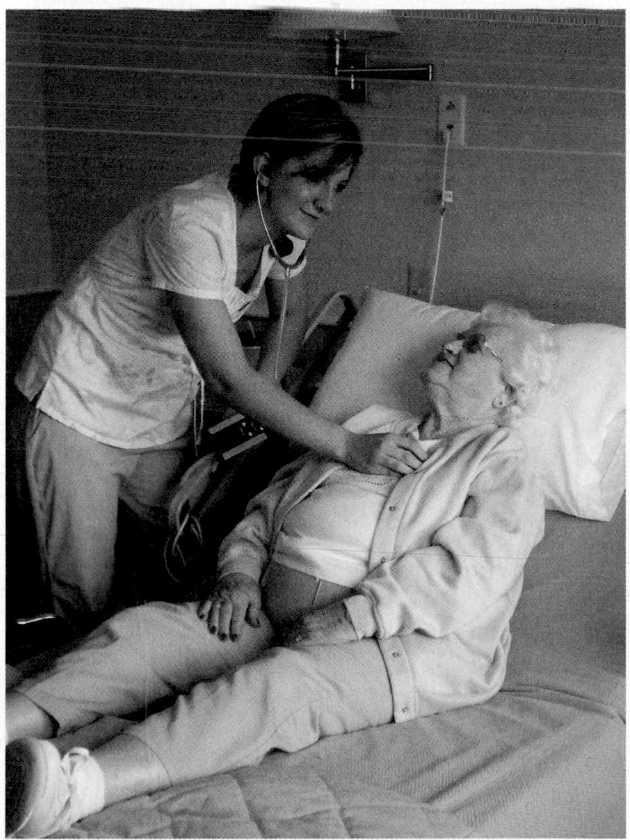

FIGURE 20-9 A nurse provides quality care to a client in an extended care facility. (*Courtesy of Kingston Residence of Fort Wayne, Fort Wayne, IN.*)

future goals, spiritual renewal, and social interactions. Taking part in extended care facility activities can assist in these pursuits.

The activity department is staffed with professionally trained personnel to create activities that meet the needs of each older adult. Some of the outside activities include trips to malls, picnics that include the family, gardening, shopping, and attending local concerts. Some of the indoor activities include musical activities; perhaps a local organ or piano talent, a choir, dances, or parties that may include a juke box. Christmas dinner with the resident's family, woodworking projects, pet therapy, craft making, exercise groups, bingo, Bible study, and cooking are other activities that are offered. Religious services of various beliefs are arranged by the activity department. The activity department can also assist in scheduling a visit to the beautician or barber. Individual activities such as the use of audio taped books are arranged when a resident is unable to leave the room. Monthly activities are posted so residents anticipate the event and participate as desired. Activities provide a social gathering and stimulation for the mind along with physical activity.

Dietary

There are several meals planned by a dietitian in an extended care facility. The dietitian consultant reviews each resident's intake of meals by percentage, fluid intake, and laboratory test values to avoid nutrition deficiencies and dehydration. The dietician then makes recommendations to the extended care facility's dietary manager and the director of nursing. Meal planning and dietary services are reviewed annually by the state government review board and, if necessary, the federal review board. It is the physician who determines and orders the diet for each resident. When a client is admitted, the dietary staff reviews personal food preferences.

Financial Issues

Private funds, Medicare, Medicaid, long-term care insurance, and supplemental security income cover the cost of extended care. Private funds are mostly used for independent and assistive living options. Assistive living facilities in some states accept Medicaid. Medicaid is a federal and state program that assists individuals and families who need financial assistance. Medicaid services vary from state to state; this is called a Medicaid waiver. The Medicaid rates are agreed on by the supplier of services and Medicaid and are accepted as full payment. Refer to Box 20-2 for expenses covered by Medicaid.

BOX 20-2 SERVICES COVERED FOR THE OLDER ADULT BY MEDICAID

Outpatient/inpatient hospital
Laboratory
Radiology
Medical expenses
Surgery expenses
Dental care exams
Home health care
Extended care facility
Physician expenses
Family nurse practitioner services

Medicare is a federal health insurance program for persons 65 years of age and older or disabled individuals, regardless of the income. There are two parts to Medicare: Part A and Part B. Part A is considered hospital insurance. Part A covers an extended care facility if the resident requires skilled care after a hospital stay of 3 days within a 30-day time limit for 100 days. Medicare covers home health and hospice care if the illness is terminal within 6 months. Medicare also covers hospital services such as laboratory, pharmacy, radiology, surgical operations, critical care, rehabilitation/restorative care, extended stays, and meals. Part B is a supplementary medical insurance plan and covers physician services, and non-physician services such as flu vaccinations and some therapies.

Long-term care insurance is paid monthly before the need of service to offset the cost of long-term care. Policies vary on what services are covered and type of facility.

Supplemental Security Income is not the same as social security but is similar in that the government supplies a monthly check to a disabled person or one with a financial need at age 65 and older. To receive Supplemental Security Income, a person has to have little or no income.

Veterans with a health condition can receive medical care or rehabilitation/restorative care in a veterans' affairs hospital or an extended care facility approved by the state to serve veterans. If the health condition is service related, the long-term care is provided as needed in an approved extended care facility.

CRITICAL THINKING

Social Isolation

Social isolation is a common psychological problem for clients who are admitted to rehabilitative or restorative facilities.

1. How can the nurse reduce the client's social isolation while in the rehabilitation/restorative care hospital?
2. What other disciplines within the rehabilitation/restorative care hospital reduce the client's social isolation?
3. In what ways can the nurse involve the family to resolve the client's social isolation?

PALLIATIVE CARE AND HOSPICE

Clients with chronic diseases or diseases that are not responsive to a cure are candidates for **palliative care**. Palliative care addresses the complications of the illness rather than the prognosis. Palliative care is separate from hospice care and is effective if started early in the disease process rather than at the end stages of the disease. Palliative care relieves symptoms of the disease and assists the family in setting and reaching goals, addressing and resolving conflict, and putting meaning to the dynamics of the illness and dying experience (Ferrell & Coyle, 2002). The illness affects the entire life of the client and family.

The interdisciplinary team works through multiple obstacles, such as client symptoms, family miscommunications, family members' grief, and cultural barriers to provide quality care. Nurses play a vital role as the client and family rely on them to meet their needs. Clients have countless emotions that nurses acknowledge and address such as anxiety, depression, sadness, loneliness, hopelessness, and anger (See

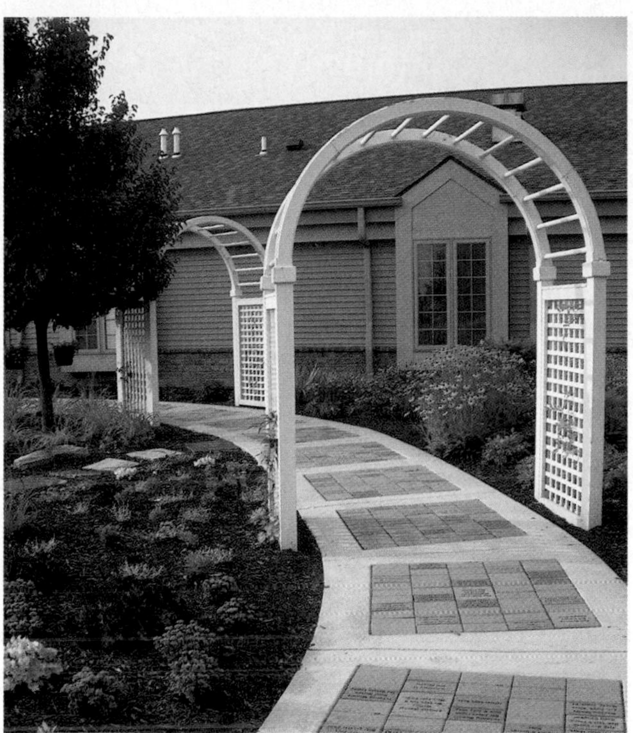

FIGURE 20-10 A garden is a place of solace for a hospice client and family. (*Courtesy of Visiting Nurse and Hospice Home, Fort Wayne, IN.*)

Figure 20-10). The palliative and hospice nurses not only attend to physical conditions but must be perceptive in handling psychological, psychosocial, and spiritual needs. The nurse acknowledges the client and family members' emotions and guides the client and family in gaining a sense of control and focusing on positive aspects of life.

Hospice provides care to the client and family through the dying process and assists the family in the grief process. Hospice provides pain relief for the client, focuses on the family during the loss of their loved one, and supports the family as they work through their grief (Ferrell & Coyle, 2002). End-of-life care is care provided in the last few weeks of life.

Medicare covers the cost of hospice if the client is eligible for Medicare Part A. The criteria for Medicare Part A is that the physician or hospice medical director states the client has 6 months or less to live, the client signs a paper choosing hospice care rather than curative care, and the client signs a paper to enter a Medicare-certified hospice program (Ferrell & Coyle, 2002).

BOX 20-3 HOSPICE SERVICES COVERED BY MEDICARE

Physician and nursing care
Home health aide care
House keeping services
Physical, occupational, and speech therapy
Counseling services
Pastoral services
Assistance with transportation, shopping, or other chores
Bereavement support
Medical equipment and supplies
Pain medication (no prescription costs more than $5)
Five days of respite care for caregiver

(Scala-Foley M, Caruso J, Archer D, & Reinhard S, 2004; Medicare.com, 2008)

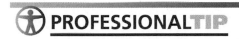

PROFESSIONALTIP

Questions about Medicare Hospice Benefits

The State Health Insurance Assistance Program (SHIP) answers question regarding Medicare coverage of Hospice benefits. The phone number is 800-MEDICARE or the website is www.medicare.gov (search for "Helpful Contacts"). Clients or nurses can call SHIP for any Medicare hospice benefit questions.

SAMPLE NURSING CARE PLAN

The Stroke Client

R.A. has had an altered state of wellness caused by a recede stroke and is living at the local restorative care hospital. She is distrustful of the new surroundings and is feeling socially isolated from her friends and family. She has left-sided paralysis and is scheduled for daily physical therapy to regain her strength and mobility. She walks with a cane.

NURSING DIAGNOSIS 1 *Impaired Physical Mobility* related to decreased strength and endurance as evidenced by paralysis of left arm and leg and inability to walk without a cane

Nursing Outcomes Classification (NOC)
Ambulation: Walking

Nursing Interventions Classification (NIC)
Exercise Therapy: Joint Mobility
Exercise Promotion: Strength Training
Exercise Therapy: Ambulation
Teaching: Prescribed Activity: Exercise
Teaching: Safety

SAMPLE NURSING CARE PLAN (Continued)

PLANNING/OUTCOMES	NURSING INTERVENTIONS	RATIONALE
R.A. will regain strength in left arm and leg and walk independently with a cane within 6 weeks.	Maintain the left arm and leg in natural alignment.	Prevents contractures and maintains proper alignment for future use.
	Place pillows to support left arm and leg in proper alignment.	Prevents pressure on body surfaces and maintains extremities in proper alignment for future use.
	Assist with ambulation frequently and gradually extend ambulation time frames.	Client gains strength in extremities and improves ambulation skills with cane.
	Teach safe crutch walking.	Teaches client correct use of cane when ambulating to prevent falls.
	Encourage use of left arm and leg for self-care activities.	Improves client's self esteem and improves self care.
	Encourage arm and leg exercises.	Client increases strength in affected arm and leg.

EVALUATION

At the end of 6 weeks, R.A. has full range of motion against gravity and flexes both arm and leg against resistance. R.A. walks independently with cane and relates ambulating safety precautions to the nurse.

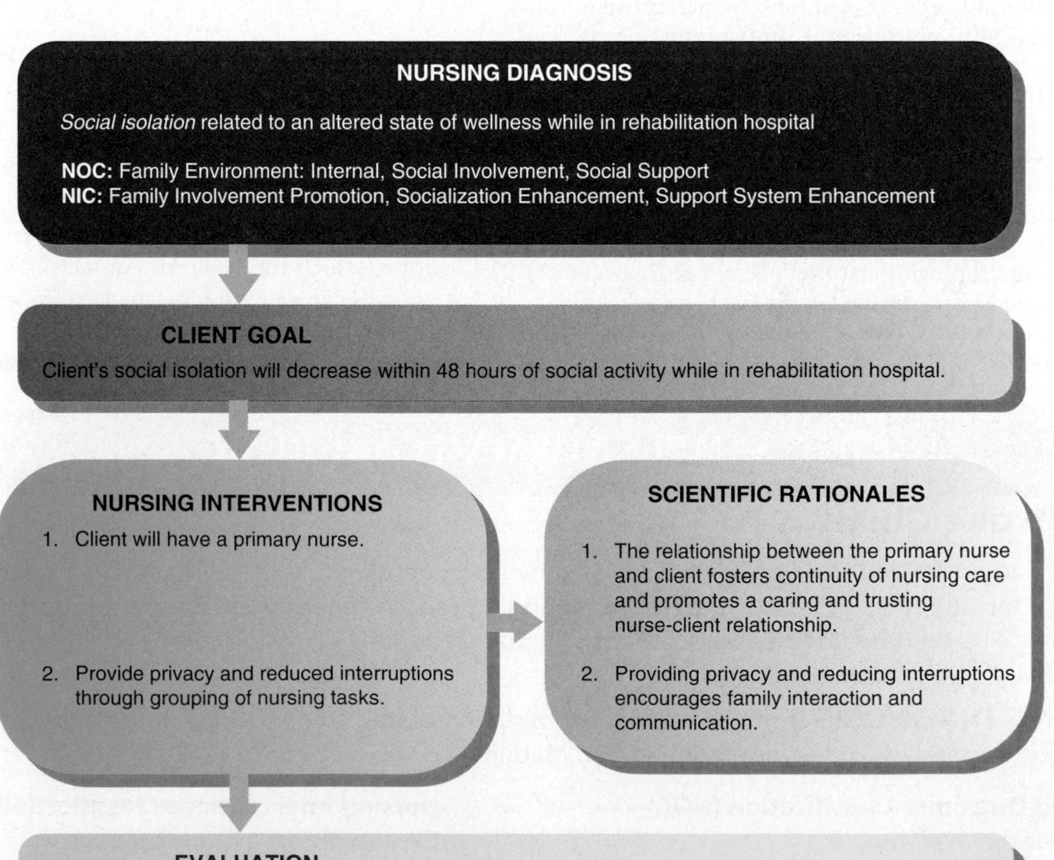

NURSING DIAGNOSIS
Social isolation related to an altered state of wellness while in rehabilitation hospital
NOC: Family Environment: Internal, Social Involvement, Social Support
NIC: Family Involvement Promotion, Socialization Enhancement, Support System Enhancement
CLIENT GOAL
Client's social isolation will decrease within 48 hours of social activity while in rehabilitation hospital.
NURSING INTERVENTIONS
1. Client will have a primary nurse.
2. Provide privacy and reduced interruptions through grouping of nursing tasks.
SCIENTIFIC RATIONALES
1. The relationship between the primary nurse and client fosters continuity of nursing care and promotes a caring and trusting nurse-client relationship.
2. Providing privacy and reducing interruptions encourages family interaction and communication.
EVALUATION
Is the client feeling less alone? Is the client content with social interactions?

CONCEPT CARE MAP 20-1

CASE STUDY

E.J., 72 years old, was admitted to Community Hospital for a left below-knee amputation. E.J. was an insulin-dependent diabetic for 35 years. The amputation followed a long and unsuccessful period of treatment for venous stasis ulcers. E.J. was transferred from the hospital to a rehabilitation hospital on her fourth postoperative day. After 2 weeks at the rehabilitation hospital, she was transferred to a skilled care facility near her home for additional restorative care and regulation of the diabetes. She is now ready to be discharged to her home. E.J. has a prosthesis and is able to ambulate with a walker. She performs her ADL with minimal assistance. She was on a sliding scale and blood glucose monitoring 4 times a day while in the long-term care facility. Her physician has now placed her on insulin twice a day with daily blood glucose checks. Her vision is somewhat impaired due to the diabetes. E.J. lives alone in a one-story home in a sage residential area. The discharge planner at the skilled care facility has arranged continuing care for E.J. through a local home health agency.

The following questions guide your development of a nursing care plan for the case study.

1. Identify the assessment factors that are most important in planning E.J.'s care.
2. List the nursing diagnoses that are applicable to E.J.'s assessment.
3. Describe the complications for which E.J. is at risk.
4. Describe nursing interventions for preventing the complications.
5. What specific actions would you take to prevent a recurrence of venous stasis ulcers?
6. What additional community services does E.J. need?
7. What nursing services (frequency of nurse visits, services from a nursing assistant, other home health services) would you plan to meet her needs? What services would each person provide?
8. Describe the outcomes you expect for E.J.?

SUMMARY

- Ambulatory care provides the nurse with opportunities to work with clients of all ages across the health continuum.
- Ambulatory care nurses require a high degree of skill in communication and client education.
- The goal of rehabilitation/restorative care is to assist individuals in reaching their optimal physical, mental, and psychosocial functioning level.
- The interdisciplinary health care team assesses, maintains, and evaluates the abilities of individuals in need of functional therapy.
- The minimum data set (MDS) is an assessment tool for assessing resident's physical, psychological, and psychosocial functioning in a Medicare and Medicaid-certified long term care facility.
- Long-term care facilities provide services to individuals who are not acutely ill, have continuing health care needs, and cannot function independently at home.
- Home Health Care requires the nurse to be technologically competent.
- The home health care nurse refers clients to community resources.
- The home health care nurse possesses knowledge of the various federal government forms and data systems necessary to carry out the position and ensure planned outcomes and quality of care to client.
- Palliative care relieves symptoms of the disease and assists the family in setting and reaching goals, addressing and resolving conflict, and putting meaning to the dynamics of the illness and dying experience.
- Hospice provides pain relief for the client, focuses on the family during the loss of their loved one, and supports the family as they work through their grief.

REVIEW QUESTIONS

1. A reason for the growth in nonacute health care services is: (Select all that apply.)
   1. the diminishing supply of physicians.
   2. an increase in the number of hospitals in the country.
   3. direct marketing of pharmaceuticals.
   4. the increase in Medicare reimbursement.
   5. the population shifts in the United States.
   6. the increased interest in alternative therapy.
2. Medicare is a reimbursement system for health care providers that:
   1. is based upon the client's personal financial resources.
   2. is available to persons 65 years of age and older or who have been disabled for 2 or more years.
   3. pays the full cost of all medical care.
   4. is managed by each state.

3. What client would be the most likely to benefit from rehabilitation/restorative care services?
   1. J.B., 64 years old, had a stroke, is responsive and stable.
   2. M.C., 89 years old, has Alzheimer's disease in the fourth stage.
   3. M.Z., 26 years old, is recovering from pneumonia.
   4. R. K., 56 years old, has terminal cancer of the lung.
4. As a member of the interdisciplinary health care team, the LPN/VN: (Select all that apply.)
   1. participates in the planning of client care.
   2. plans the appropriate diet for clients.
   3. teaches the new amputee how to walk with a prosthesis.
   4. advocates the needs of the client.
   5. provides alternative methods of communication for the client with recent stroke.
   6. understands the roles and responsibilities of each discipline.
5. In the home health care setting, it is essential that the LPN/VN possess skills in: (Select all that apply.)
   1. total parenteral nutrition.
   2. respiratory therapy treatments.
   3. data collection.
   4. planning and providing speech therapy.
   5. medication administration.
   6. client teaching.
6. In a long-term care facility, the LPN/VN serves as the:
   1. charge nurse of a unit.
   2. director of nursing.
   3. clinical nurse specialist.
   4. social worker.
7. The Minimum Data Set is a government tool to assess: (Select all that apply.)
   1. a functional need.
   2. psychosocial need.
   3. medical needs.
   4. discharge planning.
   5. psychological patterns.
   6. effect of medications.
8. What main factor determines the choice of housing for the older adult?
   1. The facility's floor plan.
   2. Dietary menu.
   3. Functional perimeters.
   4. Activity program.
9. The OASIS
   1. is used to assess a client's physical, psychological, and psychosocial functioning.
   2. is a computerized plan of care that is compatible with the home health care electronic system.
   3. provides a uniform method to document a client's disability and medical rehabilitation.
   4. is used to review the agencies' data results and measures home health care outcomes.
10. A client was just admitted to the rehabilitation unit. The nurse's restorative care goal for the client is to:
    1. restore health.
    2. assist in reaching optimal functional level.
    3. send residents home after two weeks of therapy.
    4. restore only ADLs.

REFERENCES/SUGGESTED READING

American Academy of Pediatrics. (2006). AAP Immunization Initiatives. Retrieved on October 10, 2007 from http://www.cispimmunize.org/aap/aap_main.html

Assisted Living Federation of America. (ALFA). (1999). What is assisted living? Retrieved from http://www.alfa.org

Assisted Living Federation of America (ALFA). (2009). About ALFA. Retrieved on May 31, 2009 from http://www.alfa.org/alfa/About_ALFA.asp?SnID=1173654858

Baker, L., Reifsteck, S., & Mann, W. (2003). Connected: Communication skills for nurses using the electronic medical record. *Nursing Economics, 21*(2), 85–88.

Bartz, K. (1999) The orientation experiences of urgent care nurses: Sources of learning. *Journal for Nurses in Staff Development, 15*(5), 210–216.

Bergman-Evans, B. (2004). Beyond the basics: Effects of the Eden alternative model on quality of life issues. *Journal of Gerontological Nursing, 30*(6), 27–34.

Brain Injury Resource Foundation. (2009). Bi assessment tools. Retrieved on May, 23, 2009 from http://www.birf.info/home/bi-tools/tests/fam.html

Bureau of Labor Statistics. (2007). National Employment Matrix, employment by industry, occupation, and percent distribution, 2006 and projected 2016. Retrieved on May 22, 2009 from ftp://ftp.bls.gov/pub/special.requests/ep/ind-occ.matrix/occ_pdf/occ_29-2061.pdf

Cameron, M. (2002). Older persons' ethical problems involving health. *Nursing Ethics, 9*(5), 537–556.

Castle, N. (2003). Searching for and selecting a nursing facility. *Medical Care Research and Review, 60*(2), 223–247.

Center for Disease Control. (2006). Clinical laboratory improvement amendments. Retrieved on October 10. 2007 from http://www.phppo.cdc.gov/clia/regs/subpart_a.aspx#493.15

Center for Disease Control. (2006). Healthy people—tracking the nation's health. Retrieved on October 12, 2007 from http://www.cdc.gov/nchs/hphome.htm#Healthy%20People%202010

Center to Improve Care of the Dying. (2006). Functional status. Retrieved on October 13, 2007 from http://www.gwu.edu/-cicd/toolkit/function.htm

Centers for Medicare and Medicaid Services. (2009). Long term care minimum data set (MDS). Retrieved on May 26, 2009 from http://www.cms.hhs.gov/IdentifiableDataFiles/10_LongTermCareMinimumDataSetMDS.asp

Cherlin, A. (1996) *Public and private families, and introduction*. New York, NY: McGraw Hill.

Cicatiello, J. (2000). A perspective of health care in the past insights and challenges for a health care system in the new millennium. *Nursing Administration Quarterly*, 25(1), 18–29.

Cusack, G., Jones-Wells, A., & Chisholm, L. (2004). Patient Intensity in an Ambulatory Oncology Research Center: A Step Forward for the Field of Ambulatory Care. *Nursing Economics*, 22(2), 58–63.

Department of Health and Human Services. (2006). HIPPA—general information. Retrieved on October 11, 2007 from http://www.cms.hhs.gov/HIPAAGenInfo/

Eliopoulos, C. (2005). *Gerontological nursing* (6th ed.). Philadelphia: Lippincott Williams & Wilkins.

Ferrell, B., & Coyle, N. (2002). An overview of palliative nursing care. *American Journal of Nursing*, 102(5), 26–31.

Futch, C., & Phillips, R. (2003) The mega issues of ambulatory care nursing. *Nursing Economics*, 21(3), 140–142.

Galarneau, L. (1993). An interdisciplinary approach to mobility and safety education for caregivers and stroke patients. *Rehabilitation Nursing*, 18(6), 395–398.

Glosner, G. (1995). How subacute care fills the gap. *Nursing95*, 25(3), 51.

Goldrick, B. (2005). Emerging infections: Infection in the older adult. *American Journal of Nursing*, 105(6), 31–34.

Hammons, T., Piland, N., Small, S., Hatlie, M., & Burstin, H. (2003) Ambulatory patient safety: What we know and need to know. *Journal of Ambulatory Care Management*, 26(1), 63–82.

Hawkins, D. (2001). *Migrant health issues: Introduction.* Buda, TX: National Center for Farmworker Health, Inc.

Health Resources and Services Administration (HSRA). (2009). Telehealth. Retrieved on May 24, 2009 from http://www.hrsa.gov/telehealth/

Hogstel, M. (2001). *Gerontology: Nursing Care of the Older Adult.* Albany, NY: Delmar Cengage Learning.

Hsu, C. (2006). The greening of aging. *US News & World Report*, 140(23), 48–52.

Illinois State University. (2006). Dr. William H. Thomas to Deliver Expanding Teaching Nursing Home Lecture on April 11. US Fed News Service, Including US State News. Washington, DC, March 28.

Indiana Health Facilities Rules. (1997). *Comprehensive care facilities. Resident's Rights.* 401 IAC 16.2-3.1.

Kimball, B., & O'Neil, E. (2002). Healthcare's human crisis: The American nursing shortage. The Robert Wood Johnson Foundation, Retrieved on October 14, 2007 from http://www.rwjf.org

Kolbe, L. (2005). A framework for school health programs in the 21st century. *Journal of School Health*, 75, 6.

Lasky, W. (1995). Assisted living: A brand new world. *Nursing Homes*, 44(7), 40–41.

Levac, K. (2002). Putting outcomes in practice in physician offices. *Journal of Nursing Care Quality*, 71(1), 51–62.

Lincoln Hospital. (2006). Long term care. Retrieved on October 10, 2007 from http://www.lincolnhospital.org/long_term_care.html

Lim, W., & Macfarlane, J. (2001). A prospective comparison of nursing home acquired pneumonia with community acquired pneumonia. *European Respiratory Journal*, 18(2), 362–368.

Male Incontinence Clamp. (2006). Retrieved from http://www.ppstop.com/

Mauk, K. (2007). *Specialty practice of rehabilitation nursing: A core curriculum* (5th ed.). Rehabilitation Nursing Foundation of the Association.

Maurer, F. & Smith, C. (2005). *Community/public health nursing practice: Health for families and populations* (3rd ed). St Louis, MO: Elsevier Saunders.

Mayo Clinic. (2006). Urinary incontinence: Treatment. Retrieved on November 10, 2007 from http://www.mayoclinic.com/health/urinary-incontinence/DS00404/DSECTION=8

Medicare.com. (2008). Hospice care. Retrieved August 5, 2009 from http://www.medicare.com/assisted-living/hospice-care.html?ht=

Meng, M. (1995). Starting an adult day care center. *Provider*, 21(12), 38–40.

National Center for Health Statistics. (2008). Americans make nearly four medical visits a year on average. Retrieved on May 24, 2009 from http://www.cdc.gov/nchs/pressroom/08newsreleases/visitstodoctor.htm

National Coalition for the Homeless: *How many people experience homelessness? Fact Sheet #3*, Washington DC, 1998a, NCH.

National Library of Medicare. (2006). AHCPR supported clinical practice guidelines: Treatment of pressure ulcers-managing tissue loads. Retrieved on November 11, 2007 from http://www.ncbi.nlm.nih.gov/book/bv.fcgi?rid=hstat2.section.5420

Nursing Homes and Senior Citizen Care. (1990). OBRA regulations and chemical restraints. (Omnibus budget Reconciliation Act of 1987). Retrieved on May 31, 2009 from http://www.accessmylibrary.com/comsite5/bin/aml_land_tt.pl?purchase_type=ITM&ite

O'Neill, P. (2002). *Caring for the older adult: A health promotion perspective.* Philadelphia: W.B. Saunders Company.

Parve, J. (2004) Remove vaccination barriers for children 12 to 24 months. *The Nurse Practitioner*, 29(4), 35–38.

Resnick, B., & Fleishell, A. (2002). Developing a restorative care program. *American Journal of Nursing*, 102(7), 91–95.

Saucier Lundy, K., & Janes, S. (2003). Essentials of community-based nursing. Jones and Bartlett Publishers. Retrieved on November 2, 2007 from http://communitynursing.jbpub.com/essentials/powerpoint.cfm

Scala-Foley, M., Caruso, J., Archer, D., & Reinhard, S. (2004). Making sense of Medicare: Medicare's hospice benefits. *American Journal of Nursing*, 104(9), 66–67.

Schim, S., Thornburg, P., & Kravutske, M. (2001). Time, task, and talents in ambulatory care nursing. *Journal of Nursing Administration*, 31(6), 311–315.

Senior Housing Net. (2006a). Assisted living. Retrieved on October 10, 2007 from http://www.seniorhousingnet.com/seniors/kyo/assisted_living.jhtml

Senior Housing Net. (2006b). Independent living. Retrieved on October 10, 2007 from http://www.seniorhousingnet.com/seniors/kyo/ind_living.jhtml

Senior Housing Net. (2006c). Nursing homes. Retrieved on October 10, 2007 from http://www.seniorhousingnet.com/seniors/kyo/nursing_home.jhtml

Senior Housing Net. (2006d). Payment options. Retrieved on October 10, 2007 from http://www.seniorhousingnet.com/seniors/finance_pay/plan/payment_options.jhtml

Smith, K. (2006). Appreciation of holistic nursing. *Journal of Holistic Nursing*, 24(2), 139.

Stanhope, M., & Lancaster, J. (2004). *Community & public health nursing* (6th ed). St Louis, MO: CV Mosby.

Symm, B., Averitt, M., Forjuoh, S., & Preece, C. (2006). Effects of using free sample medications on the prescribing practices of family physicians. *Journal of the American Board of Family Medicine*, 19, 443–449.

Swan, B., & Griffin, K. (2005). Measuring nursing workload in ambulatory care. *Nursing Economics*, 23(5), 253–260.

Uniform Data System for Medical Rehabilitation. (2009). The functional assessment specialists. Amherst, NY: Uniform Data System for Medical Rehabilitation. Retrieved on May 28, 2909 from http://www.udsmr.org/WebModules/UDSMR/Com_About.aspx

U.S. Office of Personnel Management. (1987). Self-identification of handicap. Retrieved May 23, 2009 from http://www.opm.gov/forms/pdfimage/sf256.pdf

Venes, D. (2005). *Taber's cyclopedic medical dictionary*. Philadelphia: F.A. Davis Company.

Walsh, G. (1995). How subacute care fills the gap. *Nursing95, 25*(3), 51.

Wellness Letter. (August 2006). Wellness guide to dietary supplements. Retrieved on October 15, 2007 from http://wellnessletter.com/html/ds/dsCalcium.php

Wenckus, E. (1995). Working for an interdisciplinary team. *The Nursing Spectrum, 8*(6), 11–12.

Wesley. (2006a). Assistive living. Retrieved on October 10, 2007 from http://www.wesleyhealth.com/Assistive-living-c29.html

Wesley. (2006b). Independent living. Retrieved on November 2, 2007 from http://www.wesleyhealth.com/Independent-living-c3.html

Wright, J. (2000). The Functional Assessment Measure. The Center for Outcome Measurement in Brain Injury. Retrieved on May 23, 2009 from http://www.birf.info/home/bi-tools/tests/fam.html

RESOURCES

Association of Rehabilitation Nurses, http://www.rehabnurse.org/

Brain Injury Resource Foundation, http://www.birf.info

City of Hope Pain/Palliative Care Resource Center, http://prc.coh.org

End-of-Life Nursing Education Consortium (ELNEC), http://www.aacn.nche.edu/elnec

Last Acts, http://www.lastacts.org

National Institute on Disability and Rehabilitation Research (NIDRR), http://www.ed.gov

American Association of Neuroscience Nurses (NNF), http://www.aann.org

UNIT 10 Applications

CHAPTER 21
Responding to Emergencies

MAKING THE CONNECTION

Refer to the following chapters to increase your understanding of emergency situations:

Adult Health Nursing

- ***Respiratory System***
- ***Cardiovascular System***
- ***Gastrointestinal System***
- ***Urinary System***
- ***Musculoskeletal System***
- ***Neurological System***
- ***Sensory System***
- ***Reproductive Systems***
- ***Integumentary System***
- ***Mental Illness***
- ***Substance Abuse***

LEARNING OBJECTIVES

Upon completion of this chapter, you should be able to:

- Define key terms.
- Describe the emergency medical services.
- Explain the role of the nurse in emergency situations.
- List personnel needed to respond to an in-hospital emergency.
- Discuss the steps in assessing an emergency client.
- Cite the different levels of triage.

KEY TERMS

chain of custody
disaster
emergency
emergency medical technician (EMT)
emergency nursing
Glasgow Coma Scale
paramedic
shock
trauma
triage

INTRODUCTION

An **emergency** can be defined as a medical or surgical condition requiring immediate or timely intervention to prevent permanent disability or death. Emergency nursing has developed rapidly over the years in response to the changing environment and expectations of the community. Many advancements in emergency care is attributed to the military. To manage vast numbers of injured soldiers, the military developed a systematic method of treating and responding to **trauma** (wound or injury). Casualties caused by wartime situations created the need for advancements in the care of large numbers of clients with injuries, wounds, and illness. Methods of caring for multiple clients were developed and implemented as a result of military influence.

In the United States, trauma is the number one killer of those younger than age 43 and the fourth leading cause of death overall (The American Association for the Surgery of Trauma, 2007). Motor vehicle collisions kill more than 43,000 people each year, with almost 5 million car crash victims cared for in emergency departments (EDs) (The American Association for the Surgery of Trauma, 2007; CDC, 2009).

Emergency nursing is the care of clients who require emergency intervention. The emergency nurse must be capable of rapid assessment and history taking and immediate intervention formulation and implementation utilizing the nursing process. This role carries great responsibility. Throughout the assessment and care of the client, the emergency nurse plans and teaches prevention and health promotion, as well as rapidly develops rapport with the client and family, including assisting with emotional needs. Clinical knowledge, communication, client teaching, and empathy skills are essential to effective emergency care. Although LP/VNs are seldom hired for EDs, they may float or help during emergency situations; therefore, a brief overview of emergency nursing is justified.

A **disaster** is a situation or event of greater magnitude than an emergency that has unforeseen, serious, or immediate threats to public health. They are *natural* events such as large fires, earthquakes, floods, hurricanes, or tornadoes; or *human-made* events such as war, terrorism, or overwhelming contamination of the environment (Gebbie & Qureshi, 2002).

EMERGENCY/DISASTER PREPAREDNESS

To prepare for emergencies or disasters, it is necessary to identify *who* needs to know *how* to do *what*. To this end, Gebbie and Qureshi (2002) have outlined the following core competencies for nurses that were modeled after the CDC's core emergency preparedness competencies for public health workers:

- *Describe* the agency's role in responding to a range of emergencies that might arise.
- *Describe* the chain of command in emergency response.
- *Identify* and locate the agency's emergency response plan (or the pertinent portion of it).
- *Describe* emergency response functions or roles and *demonstrate* them in regularly performed drills.
- *Demonstrate* the use of equipment (including personal protective equipment) and the skills required in emergency response during regular drills.
- *Demonstrate* the correct operation of all equipment used for emergency communication.
- *Describe* communication roles in emergency response within your agency, with news media, with the general public, and with personal contacts.
- *Identify* the limits of your own knowledge, skills, and authority and identify key system resources for referring matters that exceed these limits.
- *Apply* creative problem-solving skills and flexible thinking to the situation, within the confines of your role, and evaluate the effectiveness of all actions taken.
- *Recognize* deviations from the norm that might indicate an emergency and describe appropriate action.
- *Participate* in continuing education to maintain up-to-date knowledge in relevant areas.
- *Participate* in evaluating every drill or response and identify necessary changes to the plan.

CRITICAL THINKING

Stress

Describe factors that contribute to stress in an emergency room setting.

What can nurses do to effectively reduce stress when working in a stressful environment?

APPROACHES TO EMERGENCY CARE

There are three general approaches to emergency care: hospital triage, disaster triage, and the emergency medical services. To care for the emergent client, one first determines the severity of illness.

Hospital Triage

Each hospital with an ED has an established "triage" system in effect. **Triage** refers to classification of clients to determine priority of need and proper place of treatment. Triage is typically used in the ED to establish priorities and levels of care needed by the clients. Although clients and their families

PROFESSIONALTIP

Golden Rules of Emergency Care

1. Establish the safety of the scene.
2. Remove the client from danger.
3. Establish airway, breathing, and circulation.
4. Manage shock.
5. Attend to eye injuries.
6. Treat skin injuries.
7. Call for help.

INFECTION CONTROL

Mouth-to-Mouth Resuscitation

When delivering care to any client, the nurse is careful to practice Standard Precautions. Direct mouth-to-mouth breathing should not be administered; instead, use of a bag-valve-mask for resuscitation is more effective in both protecting the health care worker and the client from possible infection and in administering respirations.

define emergency according to their perceptions, it is the triage nurse's responsibility to sort and prioritize the clients as they arrive in the ED.

The simplest method of triaging clients is to use the American Heart Association's basic life support principles: Airway, Breathing, and Circulation (ABCs). By using this method, clients with airway problems are immediately assessed and become a top priority of care. If any of the ABCs are not functioning, either the Heimlich maneuver or cardiopulmonary resuscitation (CPR) is initiated.

Most hospitals have a triage system established to provide expedient care to those requiring it first. Although the term *emergency department* implies emergency care, the client using this department does not always require immediate care. In 2000, there were 108 million visits to hospital EDs (McMahon, 2003). The most commonly used triage classifications are emergent, urgent, and nonurgent and are recognized by the Emergency Nurses Association (McMahon, 2003) (Table 21-1). Emergent clients require immediate care in order to sustain life or limb. Examples of emergent conditions include foreign bodies in the eye, shortness of breath, impending birth, and cardiopulmonary arrest. Urgent clients require care within 1 to 2 hours to prevent worsening of their conditions. Examples of urgent situations include acute abdominal pain and compound fractures. For nonurgent clients, care can be delayed without the risk of permanent consequences. Contusions and sprains are examples of nonurgent complaints.

Table 21-1 Triage Categories

CATEGORY/ PRIORITY	CLIENT NEEDS	EXAMPLES
Emergent	Immediate intervention is required to sustain life or limb.	Cardiac arrest Multiple trauma
Urgent	Care is required within 1 to 2 hours to prevent deterioration of condition.	Compound fractures Persistent vomiting and diarrhea
Nonurgent	Care may be delayed without risk of permanent sequelae.	Contusions Minor sprains and fractures

Developed from Military Standard Operating Procedure (SOP) for General Hospitals.

COURTESY OF DELMAR CENGAGE LEARNING

Disaster Triage and Mass Casualty Incidents

Disaster or mass casualty incident triage systems represent a second approach to emergency care. In the event of a mass casualty incident (MCI), where there are more victims than care providers, these systems are used. The disaster may be a natural occurrence like a tornado, hurricane, or flood, or human-made, such as a train accident, chemical spill, or terrorism. In the event of an MCI, an Incident Command System is established to provide safe and orderly management. Given the possibility of large numbers of casualties as a result of disasters, different approaches to triaging from that of the hospital system may be used. Another similar system developed for pre-hospital providers is the START (Simple Triage and Rapid Treatment) system, where the victims are rapidly color coded based on respirations, perfusion, and mental status (Figure 21-1). A victim is given a red tag if immediate treatment is needed, such as shock or a severe head injury, and is at risk for death. Yellow tags are given to victims who have serious injuries but their respirations are <30 per minute, the capillary refill is <2 seconds, and they can follow simple commands. A yellow tag indicates the victim can receive delayed treatment. Green tags are given to victims with minor injuries. The treatment for these victims is reassurance and transportation to a facility when other clients with more urgent needs have been transferred. A navy tag is given to victims who are dead or whose injuries are so severe they will die soon (BCEMS Web, 2009).

Most communities have disaster/mass casualty committees or an emergency management agency (EMA) director. These committees include all hospitals, the emergency medical services (EMS) system, and citizens needed to alert the community of an impending or real disaster.

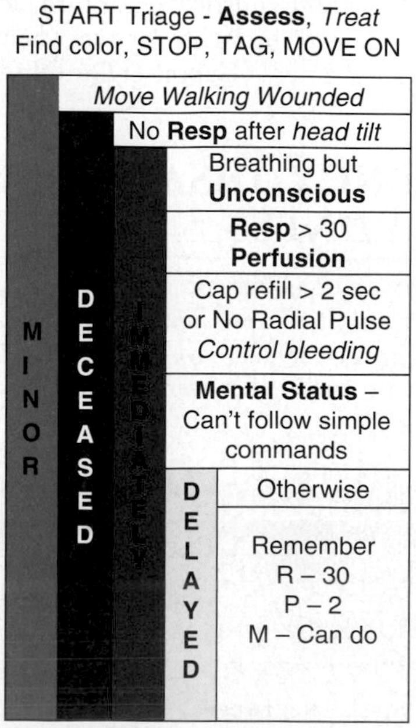

START Triage - **Assess**, *Treat*
Find color, STOP, TAG, MOVE ON

MINOR: *Move Walking Wounded*
DECEASED: No **Resp** after *head tilt*
IMMEDIATELY: Breathing but **Unconscious**
Resp > 30
Perfusion
Cap refill > 2 sec or No Radial Pulse
Control bleeding
Mental Status – Can't follow simple commands
DELAYED: Otherwise
Remember
R – 30
P – 2
M – Can do

Figure 21-1 START Triage (*Courtesy of Critical Illness and Trauma Foundation, Inc.*)

Emergency Medical Services

Before admission to the ED, the client usually is cared for by a first responder or an **emergency medical technician (EMT)**. An EMT-B (Basic) is a health care professional trained to provide basic lifesaving measures before arrival at the hospital. An EMT-P (**Paramedic**) is a more specialized health care professional educated to provide advance life support to the client requiring emergency interventions (Figure 21-2). Both are part of the EMS and are essential to prehospital care of the emergency client.

Principles of first aid, developed for emergency medicine, are part of the triage process and include what are referred to as the golden rules of emergency care. The first of these rules cautions the health care worker to assess the physical environment for self-protection. That is, safety at the scene must be established before rescue is attempted (Figure 21-3). The next rule is to remove the client from danger, such as that presented by passing vehicles. These first two rules typically apply to emergencies occurring outside of an institutional setting.

Once the safety at the emergency scene and of the client have been established, assessment turns to the ABCDs of emergency care—airway, breathing, circulation, and disability. Obtain and maintain an open *airway*. Assess *breathing* and provide resuscitative breathing as needed. *Circulation* includes starting CPR to restore cardiac output, assessing and controlling bleeding, and assessing and treating possible shock. Care for a potential central nervous system *disability* by assessing neurological status using the Glasgow Coma Scale and apply a neck collar for any head or neck injury (Integrated Publishing: Medical, 2009). Eye and skin injuries are evaluated next.

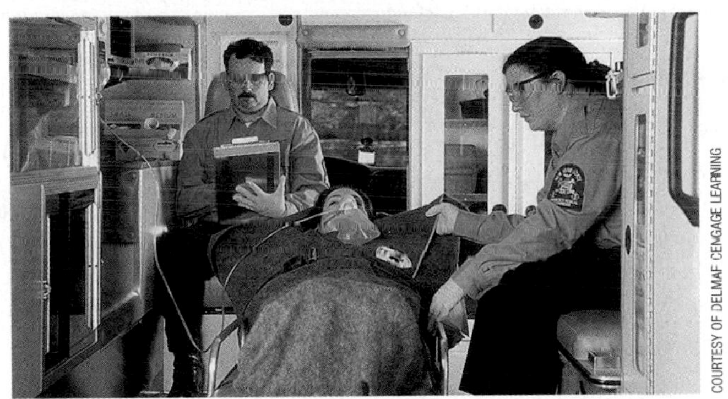

COURTESY OF DELMAR CENGAGE LEARNING

FIGURE 21-2 EMTs and paramedics are often the first to arrive at an emergency scene.

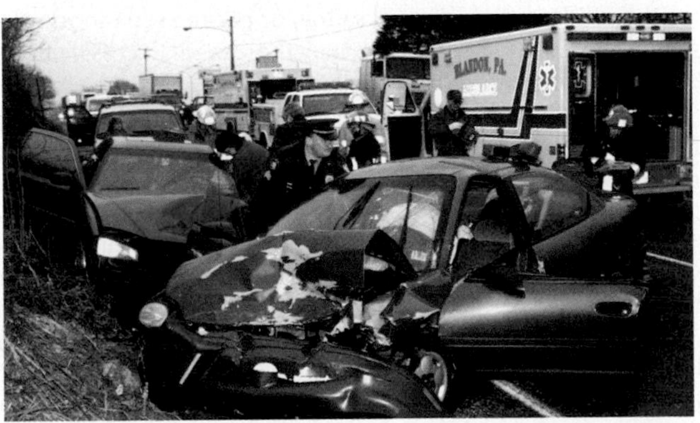

FIGURE 21-3 Establishing the safety of the scene is the first priority in emergency care, as in this scene of a motor vehicle accident, where rescue workers may be in danger from oncoming vehicles. (*Courtesy of David J. Reimer, Sr.*)

MEMORY**TRICK**

Use the **ABCDs** of emergency care when assessing a client in a prehospital setting:

- **A** = Airway – Establish a patent airway.
- **B** = Breathing – Provide ventilation; use resuscitation measures as needed.
- **C** = Circulation – Restore and maintain circulation by restoring cardiac output, controlling bleeding, and providing adequate fluid volume.
- **D** = Disability – Assess for and prevent neurological disability by using the Glasgow Coma Scale.

SHOCK

Shock is a condition of profound hemodynamic and metabolic disturbance characterized by inadequate tissue perfusion (the body's inability to meet tissue demand for oxygen) (Table 21-2). Shock can result from trauma, injury, or insult. Recognizing and immediately treating shock are critical to the client's survival. There are four major types of shock: hypovolemic shock, cardiogenic shock, distributive shock, and obstructive shock (Chavez & Brewer, 2002).

Hypovolemic shock is usually easily recognized. It results from severe fluid volume depletion through vomiting, dehydration, diarrhea, or blood loss. Severe external bleeding may be obvious, but internal bleeding, such as that from a gastric ulcer, is not readily observable.

Cardiogenic shock may be caused by several different heart conditions that result in loss of the contractile property of the heart muscle. The most common of these is acute myocardial infarction (heart attack). Severe heart failure and certain arrhythmias may also cause shock.

There are three types of distributive shock: septic, anaphylactic, and neurogenic. In all of these, shock results from vasodilation and an abnormal fluid distribution within the circulatory system.

Septic shock is usually caused by overwhelming infection. Certain organisms may cause severe reactions, resulting in collapse of the circulatory system. Toxic shock syndrome, gram-negative shock, and urogenic shock are types of septic shock.

Anaphylactic shock is a severe allergic reaction to a toxin to which a client has been exposed. Causes of anaphylactic reaction include insect bites and certain medications.

Neurogenic shock is the body's response to extreme pain or trauma to the spinal cord. As with the other forms of shock, it results in inadequate supply of oxygen, electrolytes, and other essential chemicals to the tissues.

Obstructive shock is the result of indirect pump failure that leads to decreased cardiac function and reduced circulation. Conditions causing obstructive shock include pulmonary

TABLE 21-2 Types of Shock

TYPE	CAUSES	SIGNS AND SYMPTOMS	TREATMENT
Hypovolemic	Hemorrhage,* burns	Increased heart rate; hypotension, cold, clammy skin; profound thirst	Replace fluids
Cardiogenic	Myocardial infarction*	Increased heart rate; hypotension; cold, clammy skin	Initiate drug therapy for myocardial infarction; replace fluids; consider possible emergency coronary bypass surgery
Septic	Overwhelming infection	Hot, dry, flushed skin; hypotension; increased heart rate	Locate source of infection and treat with broad-spectrum antibiotic; replace fluids
Anaphylactic	Medications,* insect bites or stings, foods	Throat edema in conjunction with increasing difficulty breathing; hypotension; increased heart rate	Manage ABCs; administer epinephrine (Adrenalin); administer diphenhydramine hydrochloride (Benadryl)
Neurogenic	Spinal cord injury, head trauma	Slowed heart rate; hypotension	Replace fluids, administer drugs to increase blood pressure and heart rate
Obstructive	Arterial stenosis, pulmonary embolism, pulmonary hypertension, cardiac tamponade	Increased heart rate, dyspnea	Treat underlying cause

*Most common cause

embolism, pulmonary hypertension, arterial stenosis, and cardiac tamponade.

In all types of shock, diminished blood flow causes the signs and symptoms. There is usually no clinical evidence of shock in the *early stage*. There may be an increase in heart rate (above client's baseline), restlessness, and the client may have a sense of impending doom. In the *compensatory stage*, respirations and heart rate increase; pulses may be weak; urinary output decreases; skin is cold and clammy, mottled, and pale; pupils dilate; bowel sounds are hypoactive, and there is hyperglycemia. Interventions at this stage reduce the possibility of permanent damage. If shock advances to the *progressive stage*, the client's condition noticeably deteriorates. The pulse may be too rapid to count, blood pressure falls below 80 mm Hg, peripheral pulses disappear, there is metabolic acidosis, peripheral edema, pulmonary crackles and wheezes are heard, and the client may be unresponsive. In the *refractory stage*, there is too much cell death and tissue damage from inadequate oxygenation. The client does not respond to treatment. Multiple organ failure occurs, which generally results in death.

MEDICAL–SURGICAL MANAGEMENT

Medical

Management of shock is supportive in nature during initial resuscitation. The immediate priority is maintenance of the ABCs. Active bleeding should then be stopped. Blood is administered in the event of major blood loss. After the client is stabilized, the underlying cause of shock is identified and treated.

Pharmacological

Initial treatment involves the administration of oxygen and the insertion of two large-bore intravenous (IV) lines. Intravenous lines are instituted to establish lifelines through which life saving drugs and fluids are administered. Fluid resuscitation and oxygen delivery are critical to management of the client in shock. Medications, including epinephrine, are administered to improve circulation.

NURSING MANAGEMENT

The focus is to identify the type of shock and initiate interventions as soon as possible. For hypovolemic shock, the treatment goal is to restore volume. Administer IV solutions such as Ringer's lactate or normal saline, or packed red blood cells, serum albumin, plasma, or dextran as ordered. Excessive fluids dilute clotting factors and worsen bleeding.

For cardiogenic shock, treatment focuses on improving myocardial function. Medications for hypotension are frequently ordered. Provide oxygen. Monitor the client's respiratory and cardiac status.

Septic shock is the most common type of distributive shock. Administer IV antibiotics and fluids as ordered. Monitor vital signs.

Clients in neurogenic shock generally have hypotension, bradycardia, hypothermia, and dry warm skin. Administer medications as ordered for hypotension and bradycardia. Monitor vital signs. Provide warmth.

For clients in anaphylactic shock, talk with family (or client if able) to identify the cause. After assessing ABCs, administer IV fluids, epinephrine, and antihistamines as ordered. Monitor vital signs.

Obstructive shock is managed by identifying the source of the obstruction and treating it. Administer fluids cautiously. Seldom are diuretics used.

NURSING PROCESS

ASSESSMENT

Subjective Data

Determine whether the client is responsive and able to respond to questions or is unconscious. When the client is alert and stabilized, assessment includes obtaining a history of the events leading to the injury or illness, including any food consumed or medication taken and any unusual event (such as a bee sting) that precipitated the shock state. Ask the client to describe any pain with regard to intensity, location, and duration.

Objective Data

Immediate assessment involves evaluating the ABCs. Take vital signs, because many clients in shock will present with hypotension, tachycardia, tachypnea, and pale, diaphoretic, clammy skin.

Nursing diagnoses for a client in shock include the following:

NURSING DIAGNOSES	PLANNING/OUTCOMES	NURSING INTERVENTIONS
*Risk for Deficient **Fluid** Volume* related to acute blood loss/vomiting/diarrhea	The client will maintain adequate fluid balance.	Initiate and maintain fluid replacement with two large-bore IV access lines. Administer blood as ordered.
*Ineffective **Tissue** Perfusion* related to decreased oxygen-carrying hemoglobin secondary to blood loss and fluid depletion	The client will maintain adequate tissue perfusion as manifested by stable vital signs.	Assess vital signs at least every 30 minutes. Administer oxygen per physician order.
*Anticipatory **Grieving*** related to grave nature of illness/injury	The client will cope with illness/injury by cooperating with care provided by health care workers and will discuss outcomes with nurse and family.	Communicate with client and family. Explain all interventions as they occur, to decrease acute anxiety. Allow client and family to express their fears and worries about the situation. Answer questions about care.

Evaluation: Evaluate each outcome to determine how it has been met by the client.

CARDIOPULMONARY EMERGENCIES

Cardiopulmonary emergencies are those emergencies that jeopardize the function of the heart and lungs. These emergencies can result from trauma or illness. Cardiopulmonary emergencies such as drowning, foreign body obstruction of the airway, chest trauma, and chest pain are grouped together, because the effects, medical management, and nursing priorities are similar.

Near-drowning episodes occur most frequently in the summer. Many clients will suffer other related injuries associated with drowning, such as head and spinal cord injuries (Table 21-3).

Foreign-body obstruction of the airway most commonly occurs in the larger, right main bronchus. The most common source of airway obstruction is the tongue. Other sources of airway obstruction include hot dogs, candy, steak, and coins (especially in children).

Penetrating or blunt trauma to the chest can cause multiple injuries. Penetrating injuries are insults that puncture the chest, such as gunshot or knife wounds. Blunt trauma is more likely caused by falls or by forceful contact with a blunt object, such as a baseball bat or steering wheel. Injuries associated with pneumothorax include cardiac tamponade, fractured ribs, fractured sternum, and flail chest.

TABLE 21-3 Freshwater versus Saltwater Near-Drowning

TYPE	CLIENT SYMPTOMS	PATHOPHYSIOLOGY	SIGNS
Freshwater	Fatigue, anxiety, difficulty breathing, fear	Water in lungs causes changes in surfactant, which in turn causes alveolar collapse.	Hypoxia, collapsed alveoli
Saltwater	Fatigue, anxiety, difficulty breathing, fear, rales, rhonchi	Hypertonic salt water pulls fluid into the alveoli.	Hypoxia, pulmonary edema

One of the most common complaints evaluated in the ED is chest pain. Those clients presenting with the symptom of chest pain must be clearly and carefully evaluated. Chest pain has a multitude of potential causes and can be frightening to the client until the cause is confirmed.

Medical–Surgical Management

Medical

Management of all cardiopulmonary emergencies is directed at maintaining the ABCs. If indicated, intubation is part of resuscitation in cardiopulmonary emergencies. Establishment of an IV line is essential for medical management, because the line provides access for administration of lifesaving medications.

After resuscitation is achieved, other treatment modalities are instituted. Obtain chest x-rays, electrocardiograms (EKGs), and blood tests. Initiate pain control. Morphine sulfate is the drug of choice for clients with these types of emergencies, because morphine decreases both pain and anxiety in the client, which, in turn, leads to improved breathing.

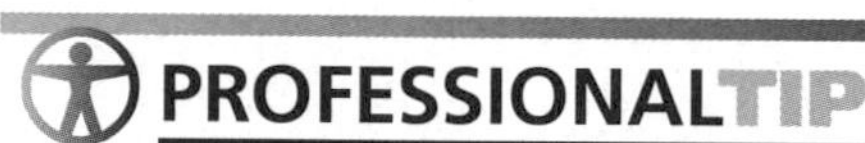

Flail Chest

A flail chest is defined as instability in the chest wall. This condition is caused by fracture of three or more ribs in two or more places. With a flail chest, breathing is unique: The flail segment moves inward during inspiration and outward during expiration. This is called paradoxical breathing.

Pharmacological

With the near-drowning client, mannitol (Osmitrol) and furosemide (Lasix) are occasionally indicated in the event of fluid overload. Pain medication is essential for the client with chest injury, because hypoventilation may occur as a result of the pain associated with deep breathing. Pain control is also essential for the client experiencing chest pain. Pain medications vary from sublingual nitroglycerine to IV morphine sulfate.

Activity

Most clients with cardiopulmonary emergencies are initially confined to bed and must frequently be rolled from side to side. Encourage deep breathing and coughing to prevent stasis of fluid and development of pneumonia.

Nursing Management

Initiate CPR if indicated. Remain with the client to reduce anxiety. Administer pain medication as ordered. Suction as necessary to keep airway patent. Monitor vital signs and lung sounds. Encourage turning and deep breathing.

NURSING PROCESS

Assessment

Subjective Data

Evaluate for restlessness, an early sign of hypoxia. Note pain description. Other areas to include in assessment are fatigue, anxiety, and level of consciousness. Ability to give a brief history of events before the cardiopulmonary emergency is evaluated.

Objective Data

Immediately assess airway and breathing. Note any cough, stridor, cyanosis, or inability to talk. Initial vital signs are essential for a baseline.

Nursing diagnoses for a client with a cardiopulmonary emergency include the following:

NURSING DIAGNOSES	PLANNING/OUTCOMES	NURSING INTERVENTIONS
*Ineffective **A**irway Clearance* related to accumulation of fluid and blood in the airway and to the client's inability to cough	Client's lungs will be clear bilaterally to auscultation.	Maintain airway and breathing with suctioning, if secretions accumulate. Turn client frequently to mobilize secretions. Encourage deep breathing and coughing. Listen to lungs hourly, or more frequently, to evaluate secretions and suctioning.
*Ineffective **B**reathing Pattern* related to injury to the chest and inability to fully expand the lungs	Client will regain spontaneous respiration within normal rate range and pattern.	Initiate CPR, if indicated. Administer pain medications as ordered to ease the work of breathing. Note response to pain medications. Remain with the client during episodes of respiratory distress, because being left alone at these times escalates both the anxiety and breathing problems. Explain all procedures.

Evaluation: Evaluate each outcome to determine how it has been met by the client.

NEUROLOGICAL/ NEUROSURGICAL EMERGENCIES

Head injuries are the most common type of neurological trauma. Spinal cord trauma can also occur as a result of injuries sustained in a head injury. Head trauma most often results from motor vehicle collisions (MVCs) (Figure 21-4). Head injuries vary from very minor contusions to major head trauma.

Clients experiencing any altered level of consciousness (LOC) are admitted to the health care system for prompt evaluation and care. Cerebrovascular accidents (CVA), also called strokes or "brain attacks," occur in different areas of the brain when it becomes starved for oxygen or hypoxic. These events are caused by a blood clot (ischemic stroke) or a bleeding blood vessel (hemorrhagic stroke), which causes symptoms ranging from mild confusion or a slight lip droop to total unresponsiveness. Establishing the exact time of onset, if possible, is extremely important for prompt and effective treatment. CVAs, or "brain attacks," require the same initial consideration given to myocardial infarctions, or "heart attacks."

Another common event causing an altered LOC is low blood sugar (hypoglycemia). The client appears lethargic, intoxicated and combative, or comatose. Prompt restoration of adequate blood glucose levels and supplemental oxygen support are critical to protect the brain from further insult. Other medical emergencies that cause an altered LOC include carbon monoxide poisoning, drug overdose, severe infections, and electrolyte imbalances.

MEDICAL–SURGICAL MANAGEMENT

Medical

As with all trauma, management is aimed at maintaining the ABCs. In addition, if head, neck, or spinal cord trauma is suspected, the client is placed on a backboard, with the head and neck immobilized. Blood alcohol level is determined. Intravenous access is initiated early in the resuscitation phase. Radiological examination is necessary to determine the extent of damage. If the client does not have spontaneous respirations, the injury has probably occurred at C-4 or above, meaning that the client will not be able to independently maintain respirations. The client is continuously monitored for increased intracranial pressure. Early signs of increased intracranial pressure include a headache; later signs include widened pulse pressure, dilated pupils, and spontaneous emesis without warning. Hiccups are an ominous sign and thus are reported immediately. Use of the **Glasgow Coma Scale**, a neurological screening test that measures a client's best verbal, motor, and eye response to stimuli, is indicated (Figure 21-5).

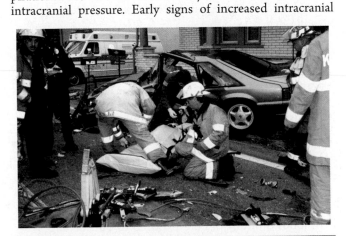

FIGURE 21-4 MVCs are the most common cause of head trauma. (*Courtesy of David J. Reimer, Sr.*)

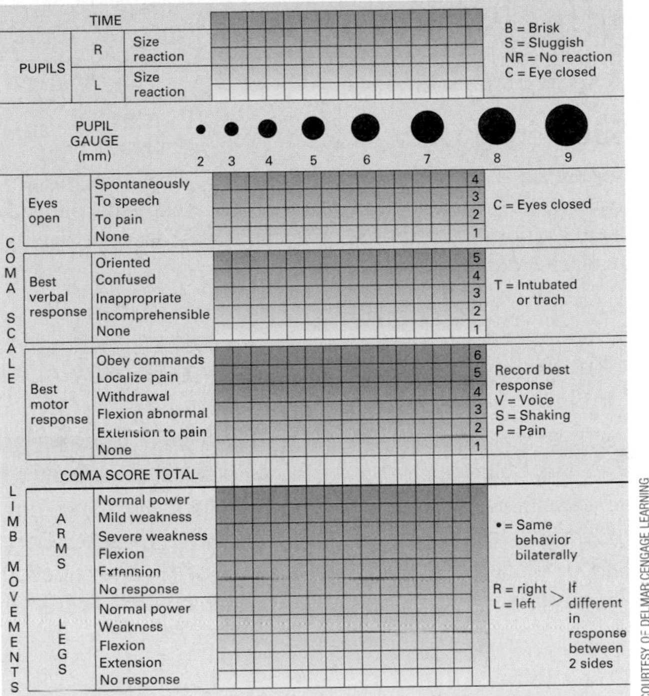

FIGURE 21-5 Neurological Flow Sheet, Including Glasgow Coma Scale

Pharmacological

Increased cranial pressure and buildup of carbon dioxide complicate the client's condition, oxygen most often alleviates the resultant complications. Thus, administer oxygen immediately. Pain management is accomplished through IV access.

Activity

Clients with head injuries are placed in semi-Fowler's position to decrease edema and intracranial pressure.

NURSING MANAGEMENT

Immediately administer oxygen as ordered. Monitor vital signs. Assess Glasgow Coma Scale score. Maintain the client in a semi-Fowler's position or as ordered. Orient to date and time as needed.

CRITICAL THINKING

Motor Vehicle Crash

You come upon an MVC involving several vehicles and no emergency response vehicles have yet arrived. What steps can you take to secure the accident site and aid the victims until emergency services arrive?

NURSING PROCESS

Assessment

Subjective Data

Obtain a history of the accident and the mechanism of injury. Evaluate the client's perception of what happened and the client's emotional response. The client may describe having a headache and difficulty seeing.

Objective Data

Assess the client's vital signs and Glasgow Coma Scale level. Note cerebrospinal fluid leaks, such as clear fluid coming from the nares or ear. Document the client's unequal pupillary response, trouble making self understood, or difficulty swallowing.

Nursing diagnoses for the client with a neurological/neurosurgical emergency include the following:

NURSING DIAGNOSES	PLANNING/OUTCOMES	NURSING INTERVENTIONS
*Excess **Fluid** Volume (Cerebral)* related to accumulation of fluid/blood in cranium	The client will remain conscious, maintain a Glasgow Coma Scale score of 15, and experience no further increase in cranial fluid volume.	Monitor intracranial pressure. Maintain the client in semi-Fowler's position. Document vital signs hourly. Assess Glasgow Coma Scale level and record hourly. Administer oxygen.
*Impaired Verbal **Communication*** related to injury to speech center	The client will be able to communicate with the nurse and family.	Orient the client frequently to date and time. Explain all nursing interventions. Modify communication methods, such as use of a message board, depending on the client needs. Encourage client to verbalize feelings about condition; offer support.

Evaluation: Evaluate each outcome to determine how it has been met by the client.

ABDOMINAL EMERGENCIES

Abdominal emergencies are diverse in nature. Trauma to the upper body and torso can result in multiple abdominal injuries, from a simple contusion and bruising to a ruptured spleen. Clients presenting to the ED with complaints of abdominal pain require careful evaluation. Illnesses causing abdominal pain range from gastroenteritis to gastrointestinal bleeding.

Abdominal injuries can result from blunt or penetrating trauma. It is important to determine the mechanism of injury, because certain causes, such as MVCs, often result in multisystem trauma. Blunt trauma, for instance from falling on the abdomen, usually results in injury to internal organs, such as the kidneys or spleen. Penetrating injuries such as gunshot wounds can affect any internal organ. Hemorrhage is a potential complication of both types of trauma.

Medical–Surgical Management

Medical

Initial management of abdominal emergencies is IV access with large-bore catheters. Oxygen is administered immediately, and standard protocol calls for managing the ABCs. Blood products or plasma expanders are administered in the event of large-volume blood loss. Insertion of a nasogastric tube decompresses the stomach. A peritoneal lavage may be performed to check for blood in the abdominal cavity of clients with abdominal trauma. Presence of blood indicates a need for immediate surgical intervention. A computed tomography (CT) scan of the abdomen may be indicated as well. Blood work is drawn, and a urinalysis is done. Hematuria is evaluated, and x-rays may be indicated.

Pharmacological

If the client is in severe pain and has been evaluated, narcotics are indicated.

Nursing Management

Administer oxygen and follow agency protocol for managing ABCs. Initiate IV access. Administer analgesics as ordered. Monitor vital signs, bowel sounds, and abdominal girth. Administer medications and ambulate as allowed.

PROFESSIONALTIP

Open Abdominal Wound

If loops of intestines are exposed to outside air, cover with sterile saline-soaked gauze.

NURSING PROCESS

ASSESSMENT

Subjective Data

Ask about the location, duration, severity, and radiation of pain. Obtain history of nausea, vomiting, and diarrhea. Note the times of the client's last meal, bowel movement, and urination.

Objective Data

Assess vital signs, active bleeding, abdominal girth, and weight. Inspect the abdomen for bruises, edema, and wounds.

Nursing diagnoses for the client with an abdominal emergency include the following:

NURSING DIAGNOSES	PLANNING/OUTCOMES	NURSING INTERVENTIONS
*Deficient **F**luid Volume* related to active bleeding	The client will stabilize, and vital signs and fluid balance will return to normal.	Establish IV access with at least two large-bore catheters. Monitor vital signs frequently, at least hourly. Evaluate abdominal girth and bowel sounds hourly.
*Risk for **I**nfection* related to penetrating injury	The client will not experience an elevated temperature or show signs and symptoms of infection.	Administer antibiotics as ordered to reduce the risk of infection. Monitor temperature at least every 2 hours. Change saturated dressings as needed. Note amount and quality of any drainage.
Activity Intolerance related to pain and bleeding	The client will ambulate with assistance the evening of or 1 day after surgical correction.	Turn client hourly from side to side. Assist client to ambulate when able to prevent stasis of fluid and to diminish the risk of infection.

Evaluation: Evaluate each outcome to determine how it has been met by the client.

GENITOURINARY EMERGENCIES

Rape is a legal term and is not considered a medical condition. It is defined as sexual penetration of a forceful and threatening nature with a nonconsenting person. Included under this legal term is penetration of persons who are unable to consent because of intoxication or mental illness. *Alleged sexual assault* is the terminology used by most centers for rape survivors. Because of the many legal implications and the fact that there are not only physical symptoms, but also long-lasting psychological consequences of sexual assault, accurate and methodical care must be given to the survivors of sexual assault. Most communities have hospitals designated to care for rape survivors. These facilities are staffed with registered nurses and doctors familiar with the medical, psychological, and legal issues particular to caring for the client who has experienced a sexual assault. Many facilities now have a Sexual Assault Nurse Examiner (SANE). These nurses are trained in collecting and accurately documenting the forensic evidence needed to protect the rights of the victim.

Straddle injuries are another type of genitourinary emergency. These injuries occur when a client falls while straddling an object, such as a fence or metal bar, thereby injuring the perineum. Though not a very common injury, it is imperative to assess the client and promptly initiate treatment. These injuries can occur with multiple traumas or as a single injury.

MEDICAL–SURGICAL MANAGEMENT

Medical

As with all emergencies, the ABCs must be managed first. Intravenous access is established, and blood and urine specimens are obtained. Rape crisis intervention is essential for the sexual assault victim. Those with straddle injuries are evaluated for fractures. If blood is seen at the external urethral meatus, a urethral tear is suspected, and catheterization is avoided because it will further damage the urethra. Radiological examination is done to confirm injury.

Surgical

Certain injuries such as urethral or vaginal tears may require surgical repair.

Pharmacological

Douching and bathing for the sexual assault survivor is delayed until all specimens are collected and all examinations are performed. For the sexual assault client, antibiotics are usually prescribed for possible sexually transmitted infection. Blood tests for baseline human immunodeficiency virus (HIV) and acquired immunodeficiency syndrome (AIDS) and a pregnancy test are usually part of the protocol. In addition, a "morning after" pill, such as diethylstilbestrol diphosphate (DES), may be prescribed in the event of a possible pregnancy.

PROFESSIONAL TIP

Chain of Custody

Care is taken in handling the clothing and belongings of a survivor of sexual assault, as these items may become valuable in legal proceedings. For purposes of potential future litigation, it is thus imperative to maintain a strict **chain of custody** of evidence. The chain of custody is the documentation of the transfer of evidence from one worker to the next in a secure fashion. This means that to follow the rape protocol, each person handling the client's clothing or lab work must sign the document used by the facility to indicate receipt and release of items. The fewer the names on the chain, the more secure the integrity of evidence.

Diet

The client is designated nothing by mouth (NPO) in case of the need to go to immediate surgery. Fluids can be given intravenously.

Activity

The sexual assault survivor returns to full activity as soon as able, although counseling may be needed before the client regains the desire to resume activities of daily living. Those with straddle injuries need bed rest and careful observation until testing is complete. Clients are taught to resume sexual activities only when they feel physically and emotionally ready.

Nursing Management

Manage the ABCs and establish IV access. Obtain blood and urine specimens. Monitor output and test urine for blood. Make a list of the client's clothing worn during the assault and keep the clothing for evidence in case of legal proceedings. Instruct client to delay bathing or douching until all examinations are completed and all specimens are collected.

NURSING PROCESS

Assessment

Subjective Data

Obtain a description of the rape or assault. A history of menstrual cycles, including date of last menstrual period, is vital in determining the potential for pregnancy.

Objective Data

Assess all bruises, scrapes, or abrasions caused by the assault. Make a list of the client's clothing worn during the assault, and keep the clothing for evidence in case of legal proceedings.

Nursing diagnoses for the client with genitourinary emergencies include the following:

NURSING DIAGNOSES	PLANNING/OUTCOMES	NURSING INTERVENTIONS
*Impaired **U**rinary Elimination* related to break in urethra	Client will void clear urine before discharge and will regain normal pre-injury elimination patterns.	Closely monitor output. Test urine for blood using dipstick. Note and report hematuria. Offer bladder retraining and encourage client to resume pre-assault elimination patterns.
*Risk for **I**nfection (Sexually Transmitted Infection)* related to alleged sexual assault	Client will have negative outcomes on all lab specimens obtained.	Obtain all specimens as ordered. Teach the client how and when to obtain further specimens, as needed. Keep the client informed about all test results.
***R**ape-Trauma Syndrome* related to alleged sexual assault and violence of event	Client will state awareness of help groups for therapy and follow-up care.	Maintain open and nonjudgmental communication with the client. Call rape crisis center for immediate referral and assistance for the client. Refer the client to crisis help per community offerings. Teach the client that the trauma does not resolve overnight and that help is available at all times.

Evaluation: Evaluate each outcome to determine how it has been met by the client.

OCULAR EMERGENCIES

Most eye emergencies are urgent to emergent in nature. Foreign bodies can cause damage to vision very rapidly, and thus they require immediate attention. Clients with objects impaled in the eye must be immediately evaluated by an ophthalmologist. An eyeball may be avulsed, or forcibly torn out of its socket, either by blunt or penetrating trauma; such an injury requires immediate referral to and treatment by an ophthalmologist. Retinal detachment is a surgical emergency, as it is one of the leading causes of accidental blindness.

Medical–Surgical Management

Medical

The primary goal of care is restoring the health of the eye. The foreign body or impaled object is removed as soon as the client's condition allows and the effects on the eye of removal of the object have been determined. The client's eye is protected until definitive treatment is provided. Protective dressings are needed. In the event of ocular avulsion, the eyeball is protected with a warm saline dressing. Because both eyes move together, patching of the opposite eye decreases movement of the affected eye, allowing it to heal more quickly.

Surgical

Immediate surgical intervention is needed for retinal detachment.

Pharmacological

As a prophylactic measure, all eye trauma is treated with an antibiotic eye medication.

Diet

There are no modifications to the diet of the client with a foreign body in the eye. Clients with avulsed eyes are kept NPO in case immediate surgical intervention is needed.

Activity

Because sensory and depth perceptions may be altered when one eye is patched, activity is limited initially. Clients are maintained in semi-Fowler's position to prevent or alleviate intraocular edema.

Nursing Management

Maintain the client in semi-Fowler's position. Instill eye medications and apply an eye patch (sometimes both eyes are patched to decrease eye movement). Assist the client to ambulate while wearing an eye patch.

NURSING PROCESS

Assessment

Subjective Data

Obtain both the client's perception of what happened to the eye and a history of the accident, including the time it occurred. Document care given to an avulsed eye, such as placement in a plastic bag with water.

Objective Data

Assessment includes visual acuity testing and observation of tearing and/or redness of the eye.

Nursing diagnoses for the client with an ocular emergency include the following:

NURSING DIAGNOSES	PLANNING/OUTCOMES	NURSING INTERVENTIONS
*Disturbed **S**ensory Perception (Visual)* related to impaired vision	The client will regain partial preinjury vision.	Maintain the client in semi-Fowler's position in cases of ocular avulsion or retinal detachment. Assist the client to walk while wearing an eye patch and discuss problems that may be encountered and ways to accommodate decreased vision. Ask the client to name one resource person to assist with decreased vision at home.
*Risk for **I**nfection* related to trauma caused by foreign body	The client will not develop ocular infection.	Instill initial eye medication and apply initial eye patch for the client. Teach the client to instill eye medication and apply eye patch. Instruct the client to immediately report any visual changes or drainage. Be alert and listen to the client's concerns.

Evaluation: Evaluate each outcome to determine how it has been met by the client.

MUSCULOSKELETAL EMERGENCIES

Musculoskeletal emergencies can vary from simple muscle strains to major trauma. A muscle strain is the overstretching of a muscle. A sprain is defined as a twisting of the joint with partial rupture of ligaments, which can cause injury to surrounding tissue. Sprains often occur in the wrist and ankle. A dislocation is the displacement of a bone from its joint. The most common sites of dislocation are the fingers and toes. A fracture is a break in the continuity of a bone. In the event of a long-bone fracture, care also is given to the cardiopulmonary system: Fat emboli from the fracture site can develop and cause severe respiratory problems if they settle in the pulmonary system.

Medical–Surgical Management

Medical

Initial treatment of simple strains and sprains are managed by use of the "RICE" formula, meaning rest, ice, compression, and elevation. Fractures are immediately immobilized, with attention to body areas proximal to the fracture. Radiological examination is indicated to validate the diagnosis. Dislocations are immediately reduced. Many fractures and dislocations are reduced in the ED by the use of procedural sedation. Tetanus toxoid is given to any client with an open injury.

Surgical

Some fractures require immediate surgical intervention. Most open, compound fractures fall into this category. Debridement is often indicated, because most fractures are trauma related, and dirt and other matter imbed in the wound.

Pharmacological

Pain control is a major consideration in relation to musculoskeletal system injuries. Reduction and immobilization often significantly decrease pain. Those clients with minor sprains and strains respond well to anti-inflammatory medications such as ibuprofen (Advil, Motrin) and other nonsteroidal anti-inflammatory drugs (NSAIDs). Those with major or multiple fractures initially require narcotic relief.

Diet

Clients with sprains, strains, and simple fractures do not need special diets. Those with major fractures and trauma are kept NPO pending surgical intervention.

Activity

Depending on the site of the fracture, activity may be limited because of casting or immobilization. To help strengthen the muscles and minimize atrophy in cases of immobilization, teach the client to contract and release those muscles immobilized in the casting.

MEMORYTRICK

Treatment for Strains and Sprains

Remember **RICE** when treating a strain or sprain:

R = Rest

I = Ice

C = Compression

E = Elevation

Nursing Management

Immobilize the affected part. Administer analgesic as ordered. Elevate the injured area. Apply ice packs, as ordered. Assess pulse, skin color, capillary refill, ability to move fingers or toes, and sensation in the injured area.

NURSING PROCESS

Assessment

Subjective Data

The client will initially verbalize intense pain, tingling, and loss of use of the injured part.

Objective Data

Obvious deformities, edema, cool skin, and decreased capillary refill are present on the affected part. Note breaks in the skin and visual bone fragments.

Nursing diagnoses for the client with a musculoskeletal emergency include the following:

NURSING DIAGNOSES	PLANNING/OUTCOMES	NURSING INTERVENTIONS
*Acute **Pain** related to traumatic fracture/dislocation*	The client's pain will decrease with immobilization and pain medications.	Administer pain medications as ordered. Immobilize affected body part. Elevate injured extremity. Apply ice packs as directed. Listen attentively to the client's concerns and verbalizations of pain.
*Ineffective Tissue **Perfusion** related to edema and fracture/dislocation*	The client's pulses will be equal bilaterally, and capillary refill will be less than 2 seconds at the affected site.	Assess the client's pulse, skin color, capillary refill, and ability to move the fingers and toes every 30 minutes. Ask the client about sensation in the injured body part. Instruct the client to move the toes and fingers. Apply an elastic bandage for compression in cases of a sprain.
*Impaired Physical **Mobility** related to limitations of pain and immobilization of fracture/dislocation*	The client will demonstrate the ability to mobilize with cast or other assistive devices.	Teach the client to care for the cast. Teach the client exercises to minimize muscle atrophy and crutch walking, if needed.

Evaluation: Evaluate each outcome to determine how it has been met by the client.

SOFT-TISSUE EMERGENCIES

Minor abrasions, lacerations, puncture wounds, contusions, bites of all varieties (human, insect, animal, and snake), and burn injuries fall into the category of soft-tissue injuries. Although most such injuries do not require emergency care, some are more severe than others, and some are potentially fatal. Clients will seek medical attention for these injuries because of fear.

MEDICAL–SURGICAL MANAGEMENT

Medical

Skin emergencies require prompt intervention. All injuries must be cleansed or debrided. Infection is a major consideration, and prophylactic treatment must therefore be initiated immediately. If a laceration is large, suturing is necessary. Bites, unless extremely large, are usually not sutured because of the increased risk of infection presented by suturing these lacerations, which provide an excellent growth medium for bacteria. Burns sometimes are treated in an ED, with follow-up care provided at home. The application of cool water decreases the pain associated with minor burns. The burn is carefully debrided with the use of running cool water and then an antiseptic solution is applied. Because burns are painful, debridement is performed after administration of pain medication. A silver sulfadiazine (Silvadene) dressing is usually applied after debridement.

Major burns may require client resuscitation with rapid EMS transport to a burn center. Initially, the ABCs are established. "Packaging" the client for transport to a burn unit usually involves insertion of at least two large-bore IV lines, insertion of a nasogastric tube, intubation, Foley catheterization, sterile wrapping, and temperature regulation/monitoring.

Snakebites do not always result in envenomation (poisoning). A rubber band (not a tourniquet) above the site is the best intervention to control rapid spreading of the venom. Most snakebites occur in the foot, so a rubber band is easy to apply. In managing snakebites, it is best to establish the ABCs and, once the type of snake is identified, start antivenom treatment as necessary.

> **PROFESSIONAL TIP**
>
> **Animal Bites**
>
> Many states require that all instances of clients seeking treatment in an ED for animal bites be reported to animal control officials. Know your state reporting rules and regulations.

Pharmacological

All clients with soft-tissue injuries, including those with burns, must be current with regard to immunizations, especially the diphtheria and tetanus (Td) immunizations. Pain medication is given to alleviate pain related to lacerations, bites, and burns. Topical antibiotic agents are applied to all injuries. Silver sulfadiazine (Silvadene) is the most widely used topical agent for burn injuries. Systemic antibiotics are often included in the treatment regimen.

Activity

Movement may be somewhat limited depending on the location of injury. Because muscle weakness and atrophy occur rapidly, physical therapy is initiated immediately for immobilized clients.

NURSING MANAGEMENT

Determine the client's immunization status. Use aseptic technique when cleansing soft-tissue injuries. Administer analgesic, immunization(s), and antibiotic as ordered. Encourage the client to keep the wound and dressing dry and clean, but instruct how to remove and change the dressing when dirty or wet.

NURSING PROCESS

ASSESSMENT

Subjective Data

Elicit the client's report of the injury. Evaluate and document the client's level of pain.

Objective Data

Obtain vital signs. Assess the wound or damaged area with regard to depth, location, and size (in centimeters). In the event of a bite, note the location and source of the bite.

> **PROFESSIONAL TIP**
>
> **Snakebites**
>
> In the event of snakebite, it is essential to note the location of the fang marks and the distance (in centimeters) between the marks. Doing so helps determine the size of the snake and, thus, the likelihood of envenomation, as smaller, younger snakes typically have not yet learned to control the amount of venom released.

Nursing diagnoses for the client with a soft-tissue injury include the following:

NURSING DIAGNOSES	PLANNING/OUTCOMES	NURSING INTERVENTIONS
Impaired Skin Integrity related to break/wound in skin	The client's wound will heal.	Prepare client for cleansing and possible suturing of wound. Assist with possible suturing.
Risk for Infection related to imbedded dirt/bacteria in the wound	The client's wound will heal without evidence of infection.	Cleanse wound thoroughly with soap and water. Administer tetanus intramuscularly (IM) if ordered. Teach the client to keep the wound and sutures dry and clean. Apply a topical antibiotic and clean dressing, if indicated. Teach the client to remove and change the dressing if it becomes dirty or wet. Tell the client to return for additional care if wound becomes red, edematous, or painful or exhibits purulent discharge.

Evaluation: Evaluate each outcome to determine how it has been met by the client.

SAMPLE NURSING CARE PLAN

The Client with a Soft-Tissue Injury

E.H., a 23-year-old Hispanic rancher, was brought to the ED after an accident at his ranch. He was riding his horse and fixing fences. The horse threw E.H. over its head and stomped E.H.'s left upper abdomen with its right forefoot. E.H., who states that he has never been hurt or previously admitted in the hospital, presents with a large, 6-centimeter-by-3-centimeter and 2-centimeter in depth, jagged laceration imbedded with dirt and other foreign material. There are no other associated injuries. A large pressure bandage that is saturated with bright-red blood is controlling the bleeding.

NURSING DIAGNOSIS 1 *Deficient Fluid Volume* related to active bleeding from traumatic abdominal laceration as evidenced by a large, jagged laceration measuring 6 centimeters by 3 centimeters and a large, bulky, saturated dressing

Nursing Outcomes Classification (NOC)
Fluid Balance
Hydration

Nursing Interventions Classification (NIC)
Wound Care
Fluid Monitoring

PLANNING/OUTCOMES	NURSING INTERVENTIONS	RATIONALE
E.H. will lose no more blood.	Apply clean pressure dressing.	Controls amount of bleeding.
	Prepare E.H. for suturing of the laceration.	Provides E.H. with knowledge of what is to happen.
	Monitor vital signs.	Identifies the client is going into shock from blood loss. Increased pulse and respiration and hypotension require immediate attention and intervention.

EVALUATION

E.H.'s wound was sutured. The dressing applied after suturing is clean and dry and showed no further evidence of bleeding at discharge.

SAMPLE NURSING CARE PLAN (Continued)

NURSING DIAGNOSIS 2 *Impaired Skin Integrity* related to abdominal injury as evidenced by a jagged laceration measuring 6 centimeters by 3 centimeters and 2 centimeters in depth

Nursing Outcomes Classification (NOC)
Tissue Integrity: Skin and Mucous Membranes
Wound Healing: Primary Intention

Nursing Interventions Classification (NIC)
Wound Care
Infection Protection

PLANNING/OUTCOMES	NURSING INTERVENTIONS	RATIONALE
E.H. will have regained skin integrity with sutures.	Prepare sterile environment for suturing.	Prevents additional bacteria from contaminating the wound.
	Assist physician with suturing of E.H.'s wound.	The nurse is responsible for assisting the physician, who is suturing.

EVALUATION

E.H. had intact skin integrity, with 22 sutures in place.

NURSING DIAGNOSIS 3 *Risk for Infection* related to laceration as evidenced by dirt and other foreign material imbedded in abdominal wound

Nursing Outcomes Classification (NOC)
Treatment Behavior: Illness or Injury
Immune Status

Nursing Interventions Classification (NIC)
Immunization/Vaccination Management
Infection Protection

PLANNING/OUTCOMES	NURSING INTERVENTIONS	RATIONALE
E.H.'s wound will not become infected.	Administer tetanus booster.	All wounds require that the client be current with regard to tetanus booster.
	Cleanse E.H.'s wound thoroughly after local anesthesia has been administered.	Wound is cleansed with the least discomfort to E.H.
	Remove as much dirt and foreign material as possible.	Prevents inflammation and infection at the wound site.
	Cleanse sutured wound and demonstrate care to E.H.	Removes old blood and other debris from the suturing. Teaches E.H. how to cleanse wound at home.
	Give E.H. explicit directions regarding taking oral antibiotics after discharge.	It is imperative that E.H. takes the full course of the antibiotics to prevent infection.
	Teach E.H. to care for wound.	Provides E.H. with knowledge to remove the dressing when it becomes wet or dirty and apply a new and clean dressing.
	Teach E.H. the signs and symptoms that require a return visit to the doctor (redness, inflammation, increased pain, purulent drainage).	Provides E.H. with knowledge to identify if the wound becomes infected.

(Continues)

SAMPLE NURSING CARE PLAN (Continued)

EVALUATION

E.H. was given a tetanus booster because he remembered having received his last at the age of 15. He verbalized the need to take the complete course of antibiotics when he went home.

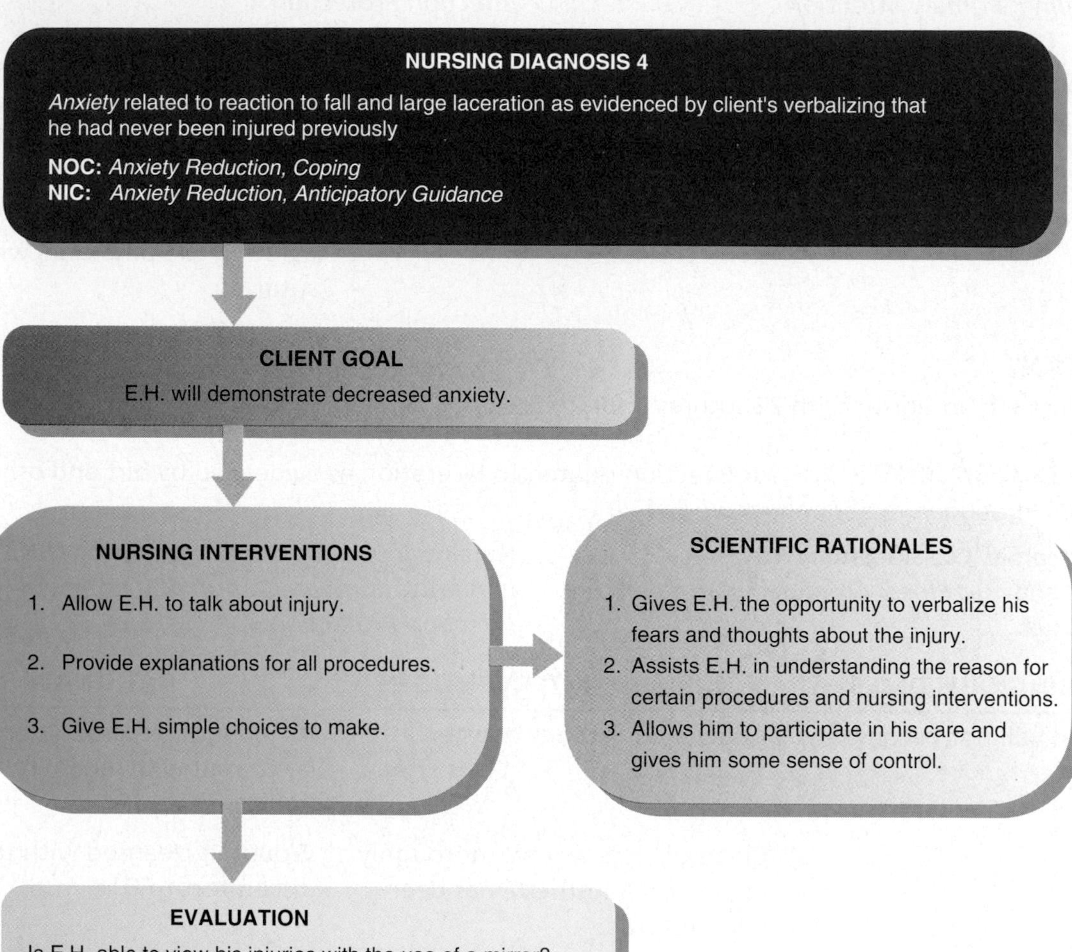

NURSING DIAGNOSIS 4
Anxiety related to reaction to fall and large laceration as evidenced by client's verbalizing that he had never been injured previously
NOC: *Anxiety Reduction, Coping*
NIC: *Anxiety Reduction, Anticipatory Guidance*
CLIENT GOAL
E.H. will demonstrate decreased anxiety.
NURSING INTERVENTIONS
1. Allow E.H. to talk about injury.
2. Provide explanations for all procedures.
3. Give E.H. simple choices to make.
SCIENTIFIC RATIONALES
1. Gives E.H. the opportunity to verbalize his fears and thoughts about the injury.
2. Assists E.H. in understanding the reason for certain procedures and nursing interventions.
3. Allows him to participate in his care and gives him some sense of control.
EVALUATION
Is E.H. able to view his injuries with the use of a mirror?
How is E.H. coping with the injuries?
Is E.H. able to assist with the care of his sutures?

POISONING AND DRUG OVERDOSES

Poisoning or drug overdose, whether accidental or intentional, is treated as an emergency. Poison is defined as any substance that causes harm to the body and may be tasteless, odorless, or colorless. There are many types of poisonings and drug overdoses with several different entry routes. Ingested poisonings are most common. The nurse obtains a clear history of the route of entry: inhalation, ingestion, topical, or injection. Poison exposure is difficult to diagnose and accurate identification of the substance is the most important aspect of safe and effective treatment. Poison control centers are the best source of antidote information for the client suffering from poisoning or drug overdose. The nationwide Poison Help Hotline (1-800-222-1222) is staffed 24 hours a day, 7 days a week, in the event of a poison related emergency, to help identify potential poisons and serve as a resource for medical treatment. In addition to treating for poisoning or drug overdose, evaluate the client for any associated injuries, such as lacerations from a fall.

MEDICAL–SURGICAL MANAGEMENT

Medical

The ABCs are still the number one client priority. Oxygen is immediately initiated and IV access established. In addition, institute cardiac monitoring and obtain blood and urine samples for toxicology screening. Once the client is stabilized with adequate breathing, a protected airway, and sufficient perfusion of the brain and organs, try to identify the substance to minimize or reverse the effects. Treatments for ingestion include client monitoring and gastric lavage. Treatments for exposure include flushing the affected area or treating as a soft tissue injury.

Pharmacological

If the substance has been ingested, and institutional protocol dictates, administer activated charcoal. Give clients who have ingested caustic products copious amounts of water to dilute the substance. Sometimes the health care provider orders reversal agents, antidotes, and medications with complex nomograms and regimens of multiple labs to track blood concentrations.

In the event of accidental ingestion of pills or medication, the client may not be aware that over the counter (OTC) drugs, herbs or vitamins can cause serious side effects in combination with prescription drugs. When interviewing the client, review all forms of oral medication and supplements. Elderly clients sometimes see multiple physicians and receive medications of which other prescribing physicians are unaware. The nurse utilizes resources and teaches the clients to identify and eliminate these safety hazards.

Diet

The client who has overdosed is typically kept NPO until cleared by the health-care provider.

NURSING MANAGEMENT

Assess ABCs, initiate IV access, and administer oxygen. Begin cardiac monitoring. Obtain blood and urine samples. Keep client NPO. Obtain a history of the entire incident. Maintain a calm, supportive, nonjudgmental environment with the client and family while administering the prescribed treatment regimen. Continually monitor the client for changes in mental status or vital signs. Insure that the client and/or family receive adequate instruction regarding the use of OTC medications or supplements.

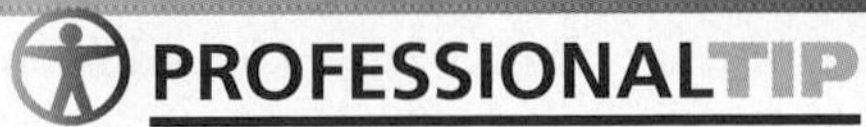

Interviewing a Client of Intentional Drug Overdose

The nurse requests additional family members to leave the room during the interview so the client is more free to answer questions. A client of intentional drug overdose may be reluctant to reveal what was taken. Ask the client or family to see the pill bottles if they are available. Look at the date the prescription was filled and then calculate how many pills should be in the bottle. If an excessive number of pills are missing from a bottle, it is considered suspect for intentional drug overdose. Admission to taking any form of pill or drug is recorded and evaluated.

NURSING PROCESS

ASSESSMENT

Subjective Data

Ask about the timing and the route of overdose. Evaluate mental status to establish whether the exposure was intentional. Document other incidences related to an overdose, such as an altercation with a loved one.

Objective Data

The client's vital signs are critical for baseline data. Try to identify the substance involved, as well as the amount.

Nursing diagnoses for the client with an overdose include the following:

NURSING DIAGNOSES	PLANNING/OUTCOMES	NURSING INTERVENTIONS
*Risk for **Poisoning*** related to ingestion of toxin	The client will recover with no residual effects of poisoning.	Manage the ABCs and stabilize the client. Monitor baseline laboratory work and ECG. Administer antidotes to toxins. Document the client's response.
*Risk for Self-Directed **Violence*** related to harmful ingestion of toxic substance	The client will not harm self and will participate in help groups to work through issues.	Encourage the client to share reasons for overdose. Maintain a supportive, calm, reassuring environment for the client. If overdose was accidental, discuss exposure to toxin and ways to avoid exposure in the future. Teach varying methods of coping. Refer to help groups.

(*Continues*)

Nursing diagnoses for the client with an overdose include the following: (Continued)

NURSING DIAGNOSES	PLANNING/OUTCOMES	NURSING INTERVENTIONS
*Interrupted **Family** Processes* related to ingestion of harmful toxin	Client will begin to discuss problems with family.	Encourage client and family to discuss their problems openly and supportively and assist them in identifying different methods of coping. Encourage family counseling.

Evaluation: Evaluate each outcome to determine how it has been met by the client.

ENVIRONMENTAL/TEMPERATURE EMERGENCIES

Exposure to extremes of heat and cold can be potentially life threatening. Severe cold, or hypothermia, occurs in very cold weather and from prolonged submersion in cold water. Heart rate and metabolic rate fall, and cardiac arrest may follow. Frostbite is another potentially dangerous result of exposure to cold (Table 21-4). The most common sites of frostbite are the fingers, toes, ears, and nose. Initially, frostbite causes paleness and numbness to the affected areas. If exposure continues, frostbite can progress to blistering and loss of feeling. The client may lose voluntary control over the affected body part. Rewarming in an emergency setting is imperative.

Extreme heat also causes potentially serious problems, especially in very young or elderly clients. As temperature rises, the body's ability to cool lessens. Table 21-5 compares heat injuries.

TABLE 21-4 Degrees of Frostbite Severity

DEGREE	SYMPTOMS	TREATMENT
Mild	Skin is cold to touch, pale, tingling, and numb, with a prickly sensation	Use blankets, warm clothing to warm cold flesh
Moderate	Affects deeper body tissue; skin appears waxy and is puffy to touch and itchy and burning with pain	Use gloves, blankets, warm clothing to warm cold flesh, observe closely for deeper injuries
Severe	Blistering, damage to all layers of soft tissue; flesh appears lifeless and is hard to the touch; no pain sensation in or ability to move frozen area	Initiate emergency rewarming in an ED using warm-water baths at 40.6°C (105°F); observe carefully for increased edema

TABLE 21-5 Comparison of Heat Injuries

TYPE	SYMPTOMS	TREATMENT
Heat cramps	Muscle cramps in arms, legs, and abdomen	Move client to cool, shady area. Slowly administer copious amounts of water. Reevaluate.
Heat exhaustion	Diaphoresis, with pale, moist, cool skin, headache, weakness, dizziness; muscle cramps, nausea, chills, tachypnea, confusion, tingling of hands and feet	Move client to cool, shady area. Loosen/remove constrictive clothing. Pour water over client; place client near fan. Encourage client to slowly drink water. Elevate client's legs. Reevaluate.
Heat stroke (a medical emergency)	Red, flushed, hot, dry skin; no diaphoresis	Reduce client's body temperature by removing client's clothing and pouring cool water over client. Start two large-bore IV lines. Use fan to cool client. Place client on cardiac monitor. Elevate client's legs. Assess client's vital signs, especially core (rectal) temperature. Check for neurological signs (confused, combative, disoriented). Check client's core (rectal) temperature frequently.

Developed from U.S. Army Training Support Command Protocols.

Medical–Surgical Management

Medical

For those exposed to extreme cold, rewarming is essential to resuscitation. The body's core (rectal) temperature is taken. Gradual warming is initiated using warm blankets, warmed oxygen, warmed IV fluids, warmed nasogastric tubes, and, in extreme instances, warmed enemas. Resuscitation should continue until the body has reached a core temperature of at least 34.4°C (94°F).

For frostbite, rewarming of the exposed body part is indicated. If the frostbite is severe, rapid rewarming is essential. This involves placing the frozen area in warm-water baths not exceeding 40.6°C (105°F). Tetanus is administered. Acute pain is treated with analgesics.

For heat injuries, rapidly reducing the body's temperature is vital. Supplemental oxygen may be administered. Pouring cool water over the client, chilling IV fluids, and fanning the client accelerates the cooling process.

Pharmacological

For heat and cold injuries, establishment of at least two large-bore IV lines is essential. Supplemental oxygen should be administered. Replacement of fluid and electrolytes is essential.

Diet

In the event of heat injuries, fluids, especially water, should be encouraged, if the client is able.

Nursing Management

Initiate CPR if needed. Monitor vital signs. Establish IV access. Provide oxygen and administer fluid and electrolytes as ordered. Warm or cool body as indicated. Monitor cardiac response.

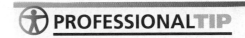

Frostbite

Do not massage or rub frostbite injuries because doing so can increase the severity of damage to tissue. Caffeine, alcohol, and smoking are avoided because they decrease circulation to the damaged tissue.

NURSING PROCESS

Assessment

Subjective Data

Ask the client to give a history of the heat/cold injury, if able, and any current medications taken.

Objective Data

Measure and document core (rectal) body temperature and vital signs. Record the client's skin color and temperature. Initiate cardiac monitoring to track any cardiac response to the heat or cold stress to the body. Evaluate pupillary response because neurological problems may result from the heat/cold injury.

Nursing diagnoses for the client with a temperature/environmental injury include the following:

NURSING DIAGNOSES	PLANNING/OUTCOMES	NURSING INTERVENTIONS
***H**ypothermia* related to exposure to cold environment/long submersion in cold water	The client will regain normal core body temperature.	Administer supplemental oxygen. Monitor cardiac response carefully. If CPR is in progress, continue until the client's core temperature reaches 94°F and cardiac status is evaluated. Administer warmed IV fluids. Place warmed blankets on the client.
***H**yperthermia* related to environmental exposure to heat	The client will regain normal core body temperature.	Remove the client's clothing. Pour cool water over the client. Use large fan to cool the client. Administer chilled IV fluids and supplemental oxygen. Initiate cardiac monitoring. Evaluate client's neurological status with reference to orientation to time, person, and place. Measure core temperature every 30 minutes to assess progress.

Evaluation: Evaluate each outcome to determine how it has been met by the client.

MULTIPLE-SYSTEM TRAUMA

Multiple-system trauma is injury sustained in more than one body system. During the initial care of the emergent client, the mechanism of injury is determined. Blunt injuries and penetrating trauma are most likely to result in multiple-system involvement.

Medical–Surgical Management

Medical

Immediate management of the ABCs is imperative. Bleeding is stopped by the use of pressure applied to the wound. Two to four large-bore IV lines are started. Remove all clothing for visualization of bleeding and injuries. Obtain blood and urine specimens. Radiographic studies are performed. A tetanus booster also is administered.

Nursing Management

Assess and manage ABCs. Establish IV access. Remove the client's clothing for visualization of injuries. Obtain blood and urine specimens. Assess level of consciousness. Monitor vital signs and neurological status.

CRITICAL THINKING

Multiple-System Trauma

Under what circumstances might a client present with multiple-system trauma? How would you proceed with the assessment of such a client? What immediate actions would the nurse take to maintain the stability of this client?

NURSING PROCESS

Assessment

Subjective Data

Assess for level of consciousness and orientation to time, person, and place. Evaluate verbalizations of pain. Ask the client for an account of the accident.

Objective Data

Airway, breathing, and circulation are immediately assessed. Assess vital signs and neurological status by use of the Glasgow Coma Scale. Assess and control active bleeding.

Nursing diagnoses for the client with multiple-system trauma include the following:

NURSING DIAGNOSES	PLANNING/OUTCOMES	NURSING INTERVENTIONS
Impaired Spontaneous Ventilation related to major trauma and severe hypotension	The client will breathe without assistive devices.	Maintain open airway. Initiate rescue breathing. Ventilate per CPR protocol. Assist with insertion of endotracheal tube. Maintain pulse oximetry reading at 94% to 99%. Start multiple large-bore IV lines.
Powerlessness related to the inability to sustain life without emergency interventions	The client will survive the emergency and within several hours be able to indicate simple choices about care.	Explain all nursing/medical interventions to client. Provide emotional and physiological support to client and family as much as possible throughout resuscitation. Allow the client to make simple choices about care.

Evaluation: Evaluate each outcome to determine how it has been met by the client.

TERRORISM

Terrorist acts can appear in many forms; the events of September 11, 2001, is one example. Nuclear, chemical, and biological terrorism are other forms.

NUCLEAR TERRORISM

According to Kilpatrick (2002), the threat of nuclear terrorism is real. One example is the use of a radiation dispersal device (RDD), a so-called dirty bomb, which has nuclear waste in a conventional bomb. Another example is an attack on a domestic nuclear weapon facility. The effects of either example would be severe and widespread.

The source of radiation on contaminated clients is on the body or clothing, or has been ingested, or absorbed through a skin opening. The amount of radiation absorbed determines the effects on the client. Absorbed radiation, now measured by the gray (Gy), is equal to 100 Rads (old measurement) (Kilpatrick, 2002). When less than 0.75 Gy are absorbed, clients are not likely to have any symptoms, clients with 8 Gy would die, and 30 Gy is always fatal. The Occupational Safety and Health Administration (OSHA) requires that hospitals have an emergency plan for treating clients contaminated with radioactive substances. A decontamination area is set up in or near the ED.

The client who absorbs more than 0.75 Gy can develop acute radiation syndrome (ARS). Symptoms of ARS depend on the dose of radiation and include:

- *Hematopoietic.* Deficiency of WBCs and platelets leading to bleeding, anemia, infections, impaired wound healing, and immunodeficiency
- *Gastrointestinal.* Loss of mucosal barrier and cells lining intestines leading to fluid and electrolyte loss, vomiting, diarrhea, loss of normal flora, and sepsis
- *Cerebrovascular/CNS.* Cerebral edema, hyperpyrexia, hypotension, confusion, and disorientation
- *Skin.* Loss of epidermis and possibly dermis

Signs and symptoms in one or more of these areas appear immediately after exposure. This is the *prodromal phase*. In a day or so, all symptoms generally disappear for a few days to a few weeks. This is the *latent phase*. Next is the *illness phase*, in which the signs and symptoms reappear and intensify. After the peak of the illness phase, the client either begins to recover or dies from infection or other complications.

CHEMICAL TERRORISM

Several types of agents can be used in chemical terrorism, including nerve agents, pulmonary agents, cyanide agents, vesicant agents, and incapacitating agents. All clients exposed to chemical agents must be decontaminated.

Nerve Agents

Nerve agents include taubin (GA), sarin (GB), sonan, cyclosarin (GF), and one called VX (Armstrong, 2003; Yergler, 2002; Reilly & Deason, 2003). These are the most toxic of chemical agents and cause death within minutes. Clinical effects depend on dose and route of exposure, i.e., inhalation, skin contact, or ingestion. Inhalation is the most dangerous. These agents cause acetylcholine to accumulate either by preventing its breakdown or by desensitizing the receptor sites.

Symptoms range from increased saliva production, chest pressure, rhinorrhea, and vomiting to muscle weakness, incontinence, and convulsions. Symptoms may take up to 18 hours to appear with low exposure.

The antidotes are atropine and pralidoxime (2-PAM). Seizures are treated with diazepam (Valium).

Pulmonary Agents

Pulmonary agents include chlorine (CL), phosgene (CG), diphosgene (DP), and chloropicrin (PS). These agents, when inhaled, destroy the alveoli and capillary bed, resulting in pulmonary edema. There may be a 2- to 24-hour latent period before pulmonary edema occurs. The fluid in the lungs leads to hypovolemia and hypotension (Armstrong, 2002; Reilly & Deason, 2003).

Cyanide Agents

Hydrogen cyanide (AC) and cyanogen chloride (CR), which forms cyanide when metabolized, can be either ingested or inhaled. Cyanide prevents the transfer of oxygen from the blood to tissues. A client in severe respiratory distress but not cyanotic probably was exposed to cyanide. It has a pungent odor like bitter almonds or peaches. Death occurs in 5 to 10 minutes when exposed to a high concentration. Amyl nitrite is the antidote (Reilly & Deason, 2003).

Vesicant Agents

Sulfur mustard (HD), lewisite (L), and phosgene oxime (CX) are in the vesicant group. Phosgene oxime causes skin lesions not vesicles, as do the other two. These agents are more lethal than pulmonary agents and cyanide agents because they can remain in the environment for weeks, providing a continuing source of exposure to populations. Sulfur mustard smells like mustard or garlic, lewisite smells like geraniums, and phosgene oxime has a peppery smell.

All three agents affect the skin, eyes, and airway. Sulfur mustard, in large quantities, damages the bone marrow. Lewisite is immediately irritating, causing vesicles that progress to severe tissue necrosis and sloughing. Symptoms from sulfur mustard exposure appear in 4 to 8 hours, but cellular damage begins in 2 minutes (Reilly & Deason, 2003; Armstrong, 2002). Supportive care is primary treatment.

Incapacitating Agents

BZ, a glycolate anticholinergic compound, and Agent 15, a BZ "copy" made by Iraq, impair rather than kill or seriously injure victims (Armstrong, 2002). The effects are understimulation of organs similar to those of high doses of atropine. Hyperthermia, hallucinations, illusions, and erratic behavior are the greatest risks. The antidote is physostigmine sulfate (Eserine sulfate) or physostigmine salicylate (Antilirium).

BIOTERRORISM

Bioterrorism is deliberate releasing of pathogenic microorganisms such as viruses, bacteria, fungi, or toxins into a community. Many biologic agents are easily made and disseminated and can potentially injure or kill many people. The CDC has categorized these agents into three categories (Persell et al., 2002).

- *Category A* agents are easily disseminated or transmitted, have a high mortality, cause public panic, and require special public health management.
- *Category B* agents usually spread through water and food, have moderate morbidity and low mortality.
- *Category C* agents have not yet been weaponized (put into a form for mass destruction) but cause high morbidity and mortality.

The category A agents are the ones considered most likely to be used in a bioterrorism attack. Included are anthrax, smallpox, plague, botulism, viral hemorrhagic fevers (VHF), and tularemia. Many of these diseases begin with flu-like symptoms and are difficult to identify early. Knowledge about these diseases, careful observation for the sudden appearance of a disease or symptoms occurring at an unusual time, and some critical thinking may help identify a bioterrorist attack. An example is if many people suddenly have flu symptoms in the middle of summer (Steinhauer, 2002).

Anthrax

Anthrax is caused by *Bacillus anthracis*. It may manifest as a cutaneous, inhalation, or gastrointestinal disease. Cutaneous anthrax develops when spores enter a break in the skin. A pruritic macule or papule becomes vesicular and then forms a black, depressed scab. It is completely curable with treatment. Inhalation anthrax has an incubation period of up to 60 days. Mild flulike symptoms improve for 1 to 2 days and are followed by acute, severe dyspnea; stridor; and cyanosis. Gastrointestinal anthrax is unlikely because aerosolizing anthrax is easier than sabotaging food supplies.

Use Standard Precautions. No isolation is necessary. Treatment recommendations include ciprofloxacin (Cipro) or doxycycline calcium (Vibramycin, Monodox) given orally for cutaneous anthrax. These two drugs are initially given IV for inhalation anthrax along with one or two other antimicrobials, such as rifamin (Rifadin), vancomycin HCl (Vancocin), imipenem (Primaxin), penicillin, ampicillin, clindomycin HCl (Clocin), or clarithromycin (Biaxin) (Steinhauer, 2002). Later, clients are given the medications orally.

Smallpox

Smallpox, caused by variola virus, is easily transmitted from person to person by direct contact or inhalation of respiratory droplets. It has an incubation period of 7 to 19 days and is most contagious during the first week. This disease produces lesions in a body area in the same level of development. They progress from macules to vesicles to pustules and then scabs. Smallpox can be transmitted until all scabs fall off. This is unlike chicken pox, which has some lesions at each level of development in a body area at the same time.

Vaccination after exposure may decrease disease severity if given within 3 to 4 days of exposure. Standard Precautions, as well as isolation, airborne, and contact precautions, must be observed. Treatment is supportive with adequate hydration. All laundry and wastes must be autoclaved before washing or incinerating (Persell et al., 2002).

Plague

Plague, also called "black death," is caused by *Yersinia pastis*. When it is transmitted from an infected rodent to humans by an infected flea bite, it is called bubonic plague. Transmission from an infected individual to an uninfected individual by inhalation of respiratory droplets is called pneumonic plague. Terrorists would probably aerosolize the bacteria to cause pneumonic plague. Respiratory symptoms are the main manifestation.

The incubation period for pneumonic plague is 1 to 6 days. Clients must be treated with antibiotics within 24 hours of the first symptoms. Recommended antibiotics are streptomycin IM or gentamicin sulfate (Garamycin). For postexposure prophylaxis, doxycycline calcium (Vibramycin), ciprofloxacin (Cipro), or tetracycline HCl (Sumycin, Tetracyn) may be used.

Standard Precautions including gown, gloves, mask, and eye protection are used. Droplet precautions are followed for the first 48 hours of antibiotic therapy and until clinical improvement occurs.

Botulism

Botulism is caused by a toxin made by *Clostridium botulinum*, which paralyzes muscles. The toxin, one of the most poisonous substances known, is usually food borne. Terrorists would probably aerosolize the toxin for inhalation. The absorbed toxin irreversibly blocks cholinergic synapses, resulting in bilateral descending paralysis. There is no elevation of temperature, and clients retain complete cognitive functioning, although they may appear comatose.

Standard Precautions are used. Passive immunization with botulinum antitoxin may be used if botulism is recognized early. Care is supportive and may involve intensive care.

Viral Hemorrhagic Fevers

VHF includes Ebola, Lassa, Marburg, Crimean-Congo, Argentine, Yellow fever, and Dengue fever. Fever onset is sudden with signs and symptoms of circulatory compromise. All are infectious by aerosol except for Dengue fever. Ebola, Marburg, Lassa, and Crimean-Congo can be spread from person to person, especially during later stages of the disease.

Isolation in a negative-pressure room is recommended. Caregivers use a personal respirator, gown, gloves, face shield, and shoe and head covers. Care is supportive. There is no treatment or proven cure.

Tularemia

Tularemia, caused by *Francisella tularensis*, is not nearly as deadly as anthrax or plague. Inhalation of the bacteria is the likely route used in bioterrorist acts. Terrorists are believed to have developed antibiotic-resistant strains, so the number of fatalities could be high (Persell et al., 2002). There are currently no methods of rapid identification.

Standard Precautions are followed. For small outbreaks, parenteral therapy with either streptomycin or gentamicin sulfate (Garamycin) is recommended. When there are large outbreaks or for postexposure prophylaxis, oral doxycycline calcium (Vibramycin) or ciprofloxacin (Cipro) are the drugs of choice. Refer to Table 21-6 for isolation guidelines for biological agents.

LEGAL ISSUES

Emergency medicine allows medical personnel to care for clients without obtaining informed consent. In life-threatening and emergency situations, consent is implied. In addition, the Good Samaritan Law, one of the laws and regulations enforced for the benefit of both the caregiver and the client, provides protection against malpractice to persons who stop at the scene of an accident and render care. It should be noted, however, that the Good Samaritan Law offers protection only to those who provide safe and appropriate care; it does not protect those charged with gross negligence or willful misconduct.

There are other legal issues specific to emergency care. Several injuries/illnesses are reported to proper authorities. For instance, most states require that police be notified of MVCs, assaults, or rape. Likewise, animal control authorities require that animal bite reports be filed to facilitate follow-up on the possibility of rabies.

DEATH IN THE EMERGENCY DEPARTMENT

Death can occur in the ED at any time as a result of trauma, sudden illness, or even extended illness. This creates a delicate situation, because the death is usually unexpected. Family members may have a difficult time dealing with sudden death. If their loved one is being resuscitated in the ED, there is little time for health care personnel to comfort the family because the personnel are very busy providing care to the client. In the event of sudden death, the family is usually in a state of shock and will need further assistance to cope with the death of their loved one. Special support groups are available for this assistance and are contacted for the family.

TABLE 21-6 Isolation Guidelines for Biological Agents

	Bacterial Agents	Anthrax	Brucellosis	Cholera	Glanders	Bubonic plague	Pneumonic plague	Tularemia	Q fever	***Viruses***	Smallpox	Venez, equine encephalitis	Viral hemorrhagic fever	***Biological Toxins***	Botulism	Ricin
Isolation Precautions																
Standard precautions for all aspects of patient care		X	X	X	X	X	X	X	X		X	X	X		X	X
Contact precautions (gown and gloves; wash hands after each patient encounter)			X[c]	X[a]	X[a]						X		X			
Airborne precautions (negative pressure room and N-95 masks for all individuals entering the room)											X		X[b]			
Droplet precautions (surgical mask)							X									
Patient Placement																
No restrictions		X	X	X	X			X	X			X			X	X
Cohort like patients when private room unavailable				X[c]	X[a]	X	X				X		X			
Private room				X[c]	X[a]	X[a]	X				X		X			
Negative pressure											X		X[b]			
Door closed at all times											X		X[b]			
Patient Transport																
No restrictions		X	X	X	X	X		X	X			X			X	X
Limit movement to essential medical purposes only				X[c]	X[a]	X[a]	X[a]				X[a]		X			
Place mask on patient to minimize dispersal of droplets							X[a]				X[a]		X[b]			
Discontinuation of Isolation																
48 hours of appropriate antibiotic and clinical improvement							X									
Until all scabs separate											X					
Until skin decontamination completed (1 hour contact time)																
Duration of illness				X[c]	X[a]	X[a]							X			

[a] Contact precautions needed only if the patient has skin involvement (bubonic plague: draining bubo) or until decontamination of skin is complete.

[b] A surgical mask and eye protection should be worn if you come within three feet of patient. Airborne precautions are needed if patient has cough, vomiting, diarrhea, or hemorrhage.

[c] Contact precautions needed only if the patient is diapered or incontinent.

Adapted by R. Daniels, L. H. Nicoll, & L. J. Nosek, 2007, from Biological weapons and emergency preparedness, Part I, by R. Stilp, 2004. Retrieved June 27, 2006, from nsweb.nursingspectrum.com

CASE STUDY

J.D. fell from a fishing boat into deep, cold water. He was wearing a life vest and was rescued within 10 minutes, at which time he was immediately dried, placed in a blanket, and brought to the ED. He is alert and oriented to person, time, and place, but is shivering uncontrollably and pale in color. His core temperature is 93°F.

The following questions will guide your development of a nursing care plan for the case study.

1. List the assessments according to the priority of performance.
2. Identify the priority nursing diagnoses for J.D.
3. List nursing interventions according to the priority of performance.
4. Identify the treatment outcomes for J.D.

SUMMARY

- Clients in shock need immediate assessment and intervention.
- Rapid assessment and observation of ABCs is essential in treating all cardiovascular emergencies.
- Evaluation of abdominal emergencies include taking a history of the onset of pain because this is critical to outcome and survival.
- Ocular emergencies can be a threat to vision and thus require immediate assessment and treatment.
- Musculoskeletal and soft-tissue injuries are painful but manageable with rapid assessment and treatment.
- In cases of poisoning or drug overdoses, the ABCs are first established, then the agent to which the client was exposed is immediately identified so that prompt treatment is initiated.
- Major trauma is a life-threatening and unexpected occurrence for both client and loved ones.
- Terrorism is a viable threat and emergency nurses need to be knowledgeable about possible biological, chemical and nuclear exposure agents, symptoms of exposed victims, and nursing interventions for each situation.
- Nurses must be aware of the legal issues related to emergency care, such as Good Samaritan Laws and mandated reporting.

REVIEW QUESTIONS

1. Triage is a system of:
   1. identifying clients by disease.
   2. prioritizing client care.
   3. counting clients waiting for care.
   4. medical diagnosing.

2. A client with a small branch sticking out of the right midchest arrives at the ED during a hurricane. There is bubbling and oozing at the site. Medical personnel should first:
   1. remove the branch and save it.
   2. administer pain medication to the client.
   3. start the ABCs of CPR.
   4. stop the bleeding and take vital signs.

3. An example of a nonurgent client is one with:
   1. CPR in progress.
   2. fractures of both legs.
   3. heat stroke.
   4. a sprained ankle.

4. The ambulance brings a client with a large, bleeding laceration of the upper leg to the ED. Vital signs are as follows: blood pressure 78/62 mm Hg, pulse 112 beats/min, and respirations 26 breaths/min. A priority nursing diagnosis is:
   1. *Deficient **F**luid Volume.*
   2. *Risk for **A**spiration.*
   3. *Risk for **I**nfection.*
   4. *Disturbed **B**ody Image.*

5. Interventions for a client in shock include:
   1. pain control and assessment of vital signs.
   2. administration of oxygen and IV fluids.
   3. insertion of a nasogastric tube.
   4. calling the physician.

6. For which client should the nurse provide care first?
   1. A client who needs her dressing changed.
   2. A client who needs to be suctioned.
   3. A client who needs to be medicated for incisional pain.
   4. A client who is incontinent and needs to be cleaned.

7. An adult suffered a diving accident and is brought in by an ambulance intubated and on a backboard with a cervical collar. What is the nurse's first action when the client arrives at the hospital?
   1. Take the client's vital signs.
   2. Check the lungs for equal breath sounds bilaterally.

3. Insert a large bore IV line according to physician orders.
4. Perform a neurologic check using the Glasgow Coma Scale.

8. An adult is brought in by ambulance after a motor vehicle crash. He is unconscious and on a backboard, with his neck immobilized. He is bleeding profusely from a large gash on his right thigh. What is the nurse's second priority action in caring for the client?
   1. Stop the bleeding.
   2. Check the airway.
   3. Connect the client to a cardiac monitor.
   4. Cleanse the wound.
9. A client is brought to the emergency room after taking an overdose of several different types of pills. What choice is the last priority for the nurse?
   1. Check the airway.
   2. Connect the client to the cardiac monitor.
   3. Identify the pills the client swallowed.
   4. Lavage the stomach contents according to physician orders.
10. What symptoms are third in the sequence of signs and symptoms of nuclear exposure?
   1. Signs and symptoms reappear and intensify.
   2. After the peak of the symptoms, the client begins to recover.
   3. Signs and symptoms appear immediately after exposure.
   4. Symptoms disappear for a few day or weeks.

REFERENCES/SUGGESTED READINGS

American Heart Association. (1997). *Advanced cardiac life support.* Dallas, TX: Author.

Arbour, R. (1998). Aggressive management of intracranial dynamics. *Critical Care Nurse, 18*, 30–40.

Armstrong, J. (1998). Bombs and other blasts. *RN, 61*(11), 26–29.

Armstrong, J. (2002). Chemical warfare. *RN, 65*(4), 32–39.

BCEMS Web. (2009). START. Retrieved July 24, 2009 from http://emsstaff.buncombecounty.org/inhousetraining/start/start_overview2.htm

Blank-Reid, C. (1999). Strangulation. *RN, 62*(2), 32–35.

Bowen, T., & Bellamy, R. (Eds.). (1998). *Emergency war surgery*. United States Department of Defense. Washington, DC: United States Government Printing Office.

Bulechek, G., Butcher, H., McCloskey, J., & Dochterman, J., eds. (2008). *Nursing Interventions Classification (NIC)* (5th ed.). St. Louis, MO: Mosby/Elsevier.

Carroll, P. (1999). Chest injuries. *RN, 62*(1), 36–43.

Centers for Disease Control and Prevention (CDC). (2009). Motor vehicle safety. Retrieved July 24, 2009 from http://www.cdc.gov/Motorvehiclesafety/index.html

Chavez, J., & Brewer, C. (2002). Stopping the shock slide. *RN, 65*(9), 30–34.

Coleman, E. (2001). Anthrax. *AJN, 101*(12), 48–52.

Coleman, E. (2002). Tularemia. *AJN, 102*(6), 65–69.

Coleman, E., & Yergler, M. (2002). Botulism. *AJN, 102*(9), 44–47.

Critical Illness and Trauma Foundation, Inc. (2001). START. Retrieved July 24, 2009 from http://www.citmt.org/start/flowchart.htm#Simplified

Daniels R., Nosek, L., & Nicoll, L. (2007). *Contemporary medical-surgical nursing*. Clifton Park, NY: Delmar Cengage Learning.

Easter, A. (2002). Ebola. *AJN,* 102(12), 49–52.

Estes, M. (2010). *Health assessment & physical examination* (4th ed.). Clifton Park, NY: Delmar Cengage Learning.

Gebbie, K., & Qureshi, K. (2002). Emergency and disaster preparedness: Core competencies for nurses. *AJN, 102*(1), 46–51.

Harrison, T., Gustafson, E., & Dixon, J. (2003). Radiologic emergency: Protecting schoolchildren & the public. *AJN, 103*(5), 41–48.

Hayes, L. (2000). Poison emergency. *Nursing2000, 30*(9), 34–39.

Huston, C. (2001). Dog bite. *Nursing2001, 31*(7), 88.

Integrated Publishing: Medical. (2009). Primary survery. Retrieved July 27, 2009 from http://www.tpub.com/content/medical/14295/css/14295_144.htm

Kilpatrick, J. (2002). Nuclear attacks. *RN, 65*(5), 46–51.

Laskowski-Jones, L. (2000a). Responding to summer emergencies. *Nursing2000, 30*(5), 34–39.

Laskowski-Jones, L. (2000b). Responding to winter emergencies. *Nursing2000, 30*(1), 34–39.

Laskowski-Jones, L. (2002). Responding to an out-of-hospital emergency. *Nursing2002, 32*(9), 36–42.

Lewis, A. (1999). Neurologic emergency. *Nursing99, 29*(10), 54–56.

McMahon, M. (2003). ED triage. *AJN, 102*(3), 61–63.

Moorhead, S., Johnson, M., Maas, M., & Swanson, E. (2007). *Nursing Outcomes Classification (NOC)* (4th ed). St. Louis, MO. Mosby.

National Association of Emergency Medical Technicians. (2006). PHTLS. Basic and advanced pre-hospital trauma life-support (6th ed.). St. Louis, MO: Mosby/JEMS.

North American Nursing Diagnosis Association International. (2010). *NANDA-I nursing diagnoses: Definitions and classification 2009–2011*. Ames, IA: Wiley-Blackwell.

Persell, D., Arangie, P., Young, C., Stokes, E., Payne, W., Skorga, P., & Gilbert-Palmer, D. (2002). Preparing for bioterrorism. *Nursing2002, 32*(2), 36–43.

Pettinicchi, T. (1998). Lightning strike. *Nursing98, 28*(7), 33.

Quinn, S. (1998). ED triage. *RN, 61*(9), 53–60.

Ramponi, D. (2000). Go with the flow during an eye emergency. *Nursing2000, 30*(8), 54–56.

Rebmann, T., Carrico, R., & English, J. (2002). Are you prepared for a bioterrorist attack? *Nursing2002, 32*(9), 32hn1–32hn6.

Reilly, C., & Deason, D. (2002). Plague: A naturally occurring bacterial species can be weaponized *AJN, 102*(11), 47–50.

Reilly, C., & Deason, D. (2002). Smallpox: Eradicated more than 20 years ago, this killer is again causing concern. Will you know it when you see it? *AJN, 102*(2), 51–55.

Reilly, C., & Deason, D. (2003). How would you respond to a chemical release? *Nursing2003, 33*(1), 36–42.

Ruffolo, D. (2002). Hypothermia in trauma. *RN, 65*(2), 46–51.

Schulmerich, S. (1999). When nature turns up the heat. *RN, 62*(8), 35–38.

Sibley, C. (2002). Smallpox: Vaccination revisited. *AJN, 102*(9), 26–32.

Siwula, C. (2003). Managing pediatric emergencies. *Nursing2003, 33*(2), 48–51.

Sommers, M. (1998). Missed injuries. *RN, 61*(10), 28–31.

Spratto, G., & Woods, A. (2009). *2009 PDR nurses' drug handbook*. Clifton Park, NY: Delmar Cengage Learning.

Stacy, P. (1998). On-scene care. *RN, 61*(9), 50–52.

Steffen, K. (2003). When your trauma patient is over 65. *Nursing2003, 33*(4), 53–56.

Steinhauer, R. (2002). Bioterrorism. *RN, 65*(3), 48–54.

Talbert, S., & Talbert, P. (1998). Flight nursing: Summary of strategies for managing severe traumatic brain injury during early posttraumatic phase. *Journal of Emergency Nursing, 24*, 254–257.

The American Association for the Surgery of Trauma. (2007). Introduction. Retrieved July 24, 2009 from http://www.aast.org/TraumaFacts/dynamic.aspx?id=964

TRAUMA! (1998). *RN, 61*(9), 49.

Veenema, T. (2002). The smallpox vaccine debate. *AJN, 102*(9), 33–38.

Veenema, T., & Daram, P. (2003). Radiation. *AJN 103*(5), 32–40.

Wiebelhaus, P., & Hansen, S. (2001). Burn emergencies. *Nursing2001, 31*(1), 36-41.

Woods, A. (2002). New threat from an ancient microbe: Anthrax. *Nursing2002, 32*(1), 44–45.

Yergler, M. (2002). Nerve gas attack. *AJN, 102*(7), 57–60.

RESOURCES

Agency for Toxic Substances and Disease Registry, http://www.atsdr.cdc.gov

American Association of Critical Care Nurses (AACN), http://www.aacn.org

American Association of Poison Control Centers, http://www.aapcc.org/DNN/

American Red Cross, http://www.redcross.org

Centers for Disease Control and Prevention, http://www.cdc.gov

Emergency Nurses Association (ENA), http://www.ena.org

International Nursing Coalition for Mass Casualty Education, http://www.nursing.vanderbilt.edu

Johns Hopkins University, Center for Civilian Biodefense Strategies, http://www.jhu.edu/

Oak Ridge Institute for Science and Education, Radiation Emergency Assistance Center/Training Site, http://www.orau.gov/reacts

Salvation Army USA National Headquarters, http://www.salvationarmyusa.org

U. S. Food and Drug Administration, http://www.fda.gov

CHAPTER 22
Integration

MAKING THE CONNECTION

Through careful study of Adult Health Nursing, a knowledge base is developed in preparation for the critical thinking exercises in this chapter. Each critical thinking exercise begins with an index of the body systems relevant to the case study. Refer back to these chapters as needed while working through the case study.

LEARNING OBJECTIVES

Upon completion of this chapter, you should be able to:

- Integrate how a condition affects several body systems and causes multiple clinical problems.

INTRODUCTION

The format of this chapter is different than previous chapters. Multiple system disease processes are presented in a case study format. Answering the case study questions enhances problem-solving techniques and critical thinking skills. Information learned in previous chapters is integrated into the case studies to develop a holistic view of the disease as it affects multiple systems. The student examines the interweaving of pathophysiology causing the disease process and develops the nursing process for the disease. An example is diabetes that affects other body systems such as the integumentary, nervous, musculoskeletal, cardiac, vascular, blood, gastrointestinal, urinary, and reproductive.

Read the case study, and then analyze how the condition affects other body systems. It may be helpful to first outline the condition presented in the case study by making a grid of the signs and symptoms, pathophysiology, diagnostic studies, and nursing interventions. Refer to the grid when answering the questions (see Table 22-1).

The case study questions can be completed alone, in a study group, or in a classroom setting. When completed, share the answers and charts with the entire group to enhance everyone's learning experience. Remember, each student or group of students arrives at the answers or present the answers in a different manner. The process followed is less important than the opportunity to integrate all aspects of the

TABLE 22-1 Grid for Reviewing the Case Study Disease

DISEASE	
Pathophysiology	
Incidence/Risk factors	
Diagnostic tests	
Signs and symptoms	
Nursing interventions	

condition and use critical thinking skills, as long as sound, logical nursing judgment is utilized in obtaining an appropriate answer. This is an opportunity to think creatively and freely.

SYSTEMS REVIEWED IN DIABETES MELLITUS MULTISYSTEM CASE STUDY

- Cardiovascular system
- Urinary system
- Neurological system
- Sensory system
- Endocrine system
- Reproductive systems
- Integumentary system

DIABETES MELLITUS CASE STUDY

M.B., a 46-year-old insurance salesman, is admitted to the hospital with the diagnosis of diabetes type 1.

- List the etiological risk factors for diabetes type 1.
- Brainstorm subjective and objective data that would be included in the assessment of M.B.
- Develop a patho-flow diagram identifying the symptoms M.B. may have been experiencing on admission and relate the pathophysiology of diabetes to the symptoms (see the examples of a patho-flow diagram in Figure 22-1 and an interrelationship chart in Figure 22-2).
- What diagnostic tests could the physician have ordered to confirm the diagnosis of diabetes?
- Relate the possible results of the diagnostic tests to the pathophysiological cause of the results on the patho-flow diagram.
- If M.B. had been diagnosed with diabetes type 2, how would the pathophysiology and nursing care vary?

A couple of days after M.B. was diagnosed with diabetes, he said to the nurse, "One of my friends at work said there are a lot of future problems with diabetes. I am concerned about this. What are some of the problems? What can I do to keep these problems from occurring?"

- What would be appropriate responses of the nurse?
- List local resources or support groups where M.B. and his family could be referred.

The discharge teaching included insulin administration, diet, exercise, foot care, and eye exams.

- What is important to include in the discharge teaching regarding:
  - insulin administration
  - diet
  - exercise
  - foot care
  - eye exams
- Develop a care plan for M.B.

Eight years after M.B. was diagnosed with diabetes, he had a routine physical examination. At that time his blood pressure (BP) was 174/96. The physician monitored the

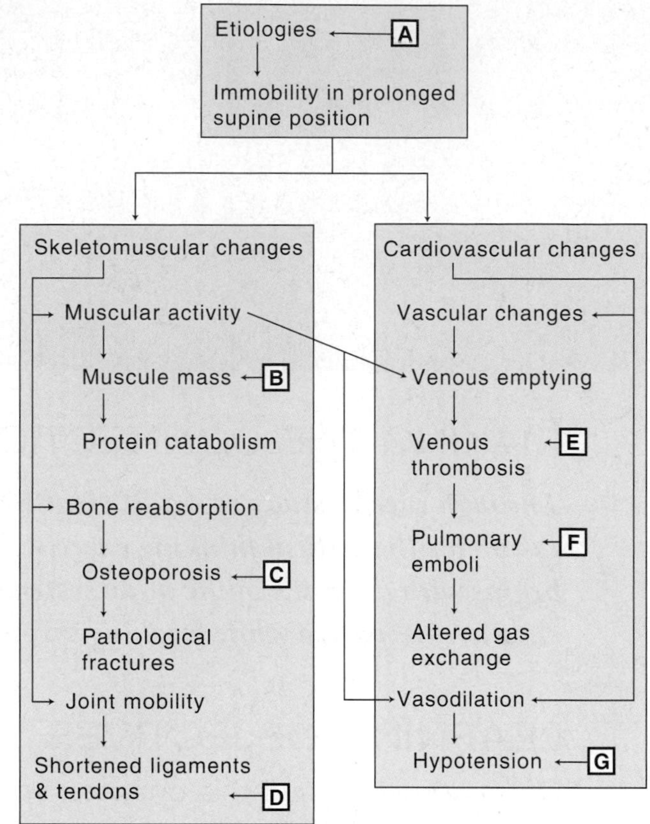

FIGURE 22-1 An example of a patho-flow diagram of skeletomuscular and cardiovascular changes caused by immobility. Complete the following instructions corresponding to the letters located at specific points along the pathophysiologic sequence of events. *A,* List the risk conditions that may lead to immobility. *B,* Name the assessment data at this point. *C,* List the interventions that would minimize calcium loss. *D,* Name the outcome criteria associated with effective nursing interventions at this point. *E,* State the assessment data at this point. *F,* List the interventions that may prevent the development of this complication. *G,* List the nursing interventions to minimize this consequence. (*Courtesy of the* Journal of Nursing Education.)

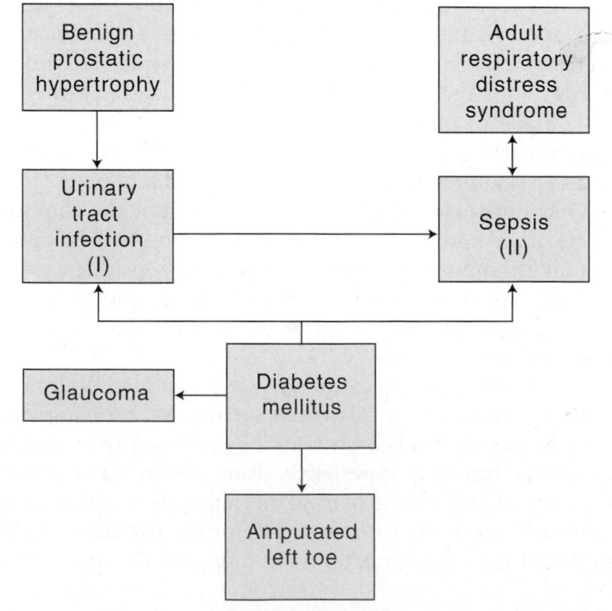

FIGURE 22-2 Interrelationships of Conditions and Symptoms (*Courtesy of the* Journal of Nursing Education.)

BP for 3 weeks and then placed M.B. on enalapril maleate (Vasotec). His urine had a trace of albumin.

- What common complication of diabetes could be occurring to cause M.B. to have hypertension? Explain the pathophysiology of the complication.
- What is the action of Vasotec in lowering BP?
- What is the rationale for placing M.B. on enalapril maleate (Vasotec) rather than propranolol hydrochloride (Inderal), verapamil (Calan), or clonidine hydrochloride (Catapres)?
- What other complications could have a circulatory etiology?
- What could be the possible long-term renal complication from diabetes mellitus?
- Explain the pathophysiology of renal complications as they relate to diabetes. Relate these to the patho-flow diagram previously developed.

One evening, M.B. was massaging his foot while watching television. He noticed an ulcerated area between his third and fourth toe.

- State possible reasons M.B. may not have felt pain from the ulcerated area. Relate these to the patho-flow diagram previously developed.

During a yearly physical, M.B. relates difficulty obtaining an erection.

- Explain the rationale for this complication.
- What nursing interventions are appropriate at this time?

In later years, M.B. may experience some symptoms from autonomic neuropathies.

- List symptoms that may occur and relate the symptoms to the pathophysiological etiology.

SYSTEMS REVIEWED IN CIRRHOSIS MULTISYSTEM CASE STUDY

- Respiratory system
- Cardiovascular system
- Hematologic and lymphatic systems
- Gastrointestinal system
- Urinary system
- Musculoskeletal system
- Neurological system
- Endocrine system
- Integumentary system

CIRRHOSIS CASE STUDY

B.W., a 60-year-old male client, is admitted to the hospital with hematemesis. He has a history of alcohol abuse. B.W.'s wife and two daughters accompany him. B.W. is 5'10" tall and weighs 140 lbs. His vital signs are temperature (T) 98.2°F, apical pulse (AP) 98 and slightly irregular, respiration (R) 24 breaths/min, and BP 152/88. He is lethargic, confused, and jaundiced. When the nurse assesses his lung sounds, she hears pulmonary crackles in all lobes. His abdominal girth measures 44 inches. His wife states he has not gone to the bathroom all morning. He has +3 edema in his feet and ankles. B.W.'s primary diagnosis is hematemesis with a secondary diagnosis of cirrhosis.

- Brainstorm other subjective and objective data that are important to include in the assessment of B.W.
- Relate the pathophysiology of cirrhosis to the assessed symptoms and other symptoms B.W. may have experienced. Develop a patho-flow chart relating the symptoms to the pathological cause.
- List diagnostic tests that would be appropriate for the health care provider to order for B.W. What abnormal laboratory results would be typical of cirrhosis?
- Relate the possible results of the diagnostic tests to the developed patho-flow chart.
- Besides alcohol abuse, what are some other causes of cirrhosis?
- List complications of cirrhosis caused by chronic alcohol abuse.
- Explain the pathophysiology of portal hypertension as it relates to cirrhosis. Relate these to the patho-flow chart previously developed.
- List diuretics that may be ordered for B.W. to decrease the ascites.
- How does the action of lactulose (Cephulac) lower the level of ammonia in the blood?
- What other complications result from portal hypertension?
- Explain the rationale for the complication of pleural effusion.
- Identify possible nursing diagnoses for B.W.
- What nursing interventions would be appropriate at this time?
- Develop a care plan for B.W.
- If B.W.'s condition improved and he was scheduled for discharge, what is important to include in the discharge teaching regarding:
  - bleeding tendencies
  - exercise
  - nutrition
  - skin care
- Develop diet instructions for B.W. according to various cultural influences.
- List local resources/support groups where B.W. and his family could be referred.

B.W.'s daughter says, "I wish Dad would have quit drinking years ago. I was always embarrassed by his behavior when he had too much to drink. His life could have had so much potential."

- What would be appropriate therapeutic responses of the nurse?

SYSTEMS REVIEWED IN HYPERTENSION, CONGESTIVE HEART FAILURE, AND CHRONIC RENAL FAILURE MULTISYSTEM CASE STUDY

- Respiratory system
- Cardiovascular system
- Hematologic and lymphatic systems

- Gastrointestinal system
- Urinary system
- Musculoskeletal system
- Neurological system
- Endocrine system
- Reproductive systems
- Integumentary system
- Immune system

HYPERTENSION, CONGESTIVE HEART FAILURE, AND CHRONIC RENAL FAILURE CASE STUDY

M.B has a 20-year history of hypertension. She has been noncompliant in taking her antihypertensive medications that were prescribed by her physician. She recently developed symptoms of congestive heart failure and renal failure.

- Brainstorm some reasons for M.B.'s noncompliance.
- Name some medications that may have been prescribed to treat M.B.'s hypertension. List the advantage and disadvantage of each medication.
- Using Table 8-4, Effects of Chronic Renal Failure by Body System, develop a concept map showing the relationship of hypertension to the effects of renal failure on each listed system.
- What is the relationship between hypertension, increased peripheral resistance, cardiac hypertrophy, and congestive heart failure?
- What is the relationship of blood pressure (hypotension and hypertension) and renal failure?
- What is the relationship between the heart's decreasing ability to pump blood through the blood vessels and pulmonary edema?
- Explain the relationship between fluid in the alveoli and dyspnea.
- Physiologically, what is occurring in M.B.'s body to cause an increased rate of respiration?
- List laboratory results that would indicate that M.B. is developing chronic renal failure.
- List symptoms that would indicate M.B. is developing chronic renal failure.
- List subjective and objective data for which the nurse would assess for symptoms of chronic renal failure.
- List laboratory results that would indicate that M.B. is developing congestive heart failure.
- List symptoms that would indicate M.B. is developing congestive heart failure. Give the cause/etiology for each symptom.
- List subjective and objective data for which the nurse would assess for symptoms of congestive heart failure.
- Identify possible nursing diagnoses for M.B.
- List nursing interventions and give rationale for each intervention.

M.B.'s abdomen is distended, and she has lost her appetite for the last 2 days. She has had hiccups constantly for 2 hours. She says, "I am so tired of these hiccups. Why am I having them?"

- Explain to M.B. the cause for her hiccups.
- What are some medical and nursing interventions to relieve the distress of constant hiccups?

SYSTEMS REVIEWED IN PARKINSON DISEASE CASE STUDY

- Respiratory system
- Gastrointestinal system
- Urinary system
- Musculoskeletal system
- Neurological system
- Sensory system
- Integumentary system

PARKINSON DISEASE CASE STUDY

P.K. is a 76-year-old man who was exposed to several chemicals during his farming career. For the last 7 years, he has walked with his arms flexed, leaning forward with his head bowed. Recently, he has had difficulty rising from a chair and balancing himself when he walks. He fell twice when doing odd jobs around the house. He started making a "to-do list" because he has difficulty remembering. He goes to the store for three items but returns with only two. His wife noticed that he has a slight tremor in his hand when he eats and often rolls his forefinger and thumb together in a circular motion.

- Use deductive reasoning and identify P.K.'s possible diagnosis.
- With these symptoms, what diagnostic tests may the doctor order?

P.K. shared his symptoms with his family physician. After some tests were completed and results of referrals to specialists were returned, the physician told P.K. he was suspecting Parkinson disease. P.K. said, "Tell me about Parkinson disease."

- Relate what a nurse could teach P.K. about Parkinson disease.
- List objective and subjective data needed to make an appropriate and thorough assessment on P.K.
- List etiological causes of Parkinson disease. What possible etiological factors does P.K. have?
- Explain the function of dopamine, a neurotransmitter, to the symptoms displayed in a client with Parkinson disease.
- List drugs that interfere in the synthesis and storage of dopamine.
- List the signs and symptoms of Parkinson disease. Think of a client with Parkinson disease, and relate his or her symptoms to the textbook symptoms.
- Develop a patho-flow map or concept map relating the pathophysiology of Parkinson disease to the systems that could be affected and the typical symptoms of that system.
- List drugs that P.K. may receive to control symptoms of Parkinson disease. List the symptoms and side effects that need monitoring with each of the drugs listed.

P.K. is becoming more rigid, having difficulty swallowing food, falling frequently, reaching for items to assist in ambulating, experiencing frequent incontinence, complaining of his eyes itching, and having severe memory loss. His voice has become soft, and his speech is slurred.

- List P.K.'s autonomic symptoms.
- Develop diet instructions for P.K. and his wife.
- What possible surgical procedures could be done to relieve P.K.'s symptoms.
- Develop a nursing care plan for P.K. listing nursing diagnoses, goals, and nursing interventions to address each symptom.
- Using the Internet, research new therapies for Parkinson disease, and share them with other students.

After a year, P.K. is unable to walk and is lifted from his bed to his wheelchair. He is unable to verbally communicate. He no longer has bladder control. When he was fed his lunch, he started coughing and perhaps aspirated some food.

- List appropriate subjective and objective data needed in a nursing assessment.
- Reevaluate the previously developed nursing care plan and revise appropriately.

SYSTEMS REVIEWED IN HEMATOLOGIC DISORDER MULTISYSTEM CASE STUDY

- Respiratory system
- Cardiovascular system
- Hematologic system
- Lymphatic system
- Gastrointestinal system
- Urinary system
- Musculoskeletal system
- Neurological system
- Integumentary system

HEMATOLOGIC DISORDER CASE STUDY

J.D., a 69-year-old man, visits the health care clinic. When seen by the health-care provider, he states he has had a cold for 4 weeks and cannot seem to get over it. He also mentions that the bones in his legs are "hurting." The nurse notes on his chart that he has a productive cough and nasal drainage. He states he is tired all the time and cannot seem to get rested. His skin is pale, and he became short of breath walking from the waiting room to the exam room. His vital signs are T 100.2°F, P 92 beats/min, R 22 breaths/min, SaO_2 90, and weight is 140 lbs, a decrease of 10 pounds since his last visit 3 months ago. During his physical exam the health care provider notes two open sores in J. D's mouth, petechiae on his lower extremities, an ecchymosed spot on his right lower arm, and swollen lymph nodes in his neck and groin.

- From the listed symptoms, what do you suspect is J.D.'s diagnosis?
- What diagnostic tests are appropriate for the health care provider to order for J.D.?

The health care provider ordered a complete blood count (CBC), fibrin degradation fragment, and activated partial thromboplastin time (APTT) for J.D. The results of the CBC are hemoglobin (Hgb) 13.0 g/dL, hematocrit (HCT) 40%, white blood cells (WBCs) 75,000, red blood cells (RBCs) 3.5 M/mL, platelets 130 K/mL. The fibrin degradation fragment is 25 mg/mL, and the APTT is 45 sec.

- Complete the lab values chart and compare normal lab values with J.D.'s results.

CBC TEST	NORMAL VALUES	J.D.'S RESULTS
Hgb		13.0 g/dL
HCT		40%
WBC		75 K/mL
RBC		3.5 M/mL
Platelet count		130 K/mL
Fibrin degradation fragment		25 mg/mL
APTT		45 sec

- What hematologic diagnosis does J.D.'s lab results suggest?
- What lab results, either ones ordered or not ordered, rule out thrombocytopenia, myeloma, Hodgkin disease, and non-Hodgkin's lymphoma?
- According to your data-gathering skills, what is the next confirmative diagnostic test the health care provider would order?

The health-care provider orders a chest x-ray and a skeletal bone x-ray. With J.D.'s potential diagnosis, what do you think the x-rays will reveal?

The health-care provider completes a bone biopsy on J.D. and the results confirm the diagnosis of leukemia. The health care provider determines that J.D. has AML.

- What other symptoms could J.D. have with AML?
- Normally increased WBCs fight off an infection. Explain the reason the increased WBCs are not able to fight the bacteria causing J.D.'s infection.
- J.D. has bone pain. Explain the pathophysiology of the bone pain.
- J.D. has dyspnea with slight exertion. Explain the pathophysiology of the dyspnea.
- The health-care provider places J.D. on a bland, high-protein, high-carbohydrate diet. Following the health care provider's orders, develop a nutritious diet for J.D. for 3 days.
- What are the treatment options for J.D.?
- What type of chemotherapy is used for AML?
- Explain the steps of bone marrow transplantation.
- J.D.'s gums are bleeding. What nursing assessments and nursing interventions are appropriate at this time?
- What nursing interventions are taken when starting or removing J.D.'s IV?

After the chemotherapy treatments, J.D.'s condition goes into remission for 3 months. Then, he starts having headaches, and blurred vision. He recently fell when rising from a chair.

- What do these symptoms indicate?
- What safety precautions should the nurse take since these symptoms occurred?

- What nursing assessment and nursing interventions are appropriate at this time?
- J.D. states "I know the leukemia is active again. Are there any other treatments I can have?"
- What other treatment options does J.D. have?
- What are some possible therapeutic responses from the nurse?
- Develop a concept map relating the different body systems to the possible symptoms and to the pathophysiology causing the symptoms. Then map nursing interventions for each symptom.

SUMMARY

This may be the first time anatomy and physiology were related to a disease process, or understanding was gained as to why clients have particular symptoms with a specific disease or condition. Ill clients rarely have only one problem but several inter-related problems. These exercises provide an opportunity to think through situations before they are encountered in a clinical situation. The case studies asked pertinent questions, evaluated clinical situations, and allowed the student to make clinical decisions, much the way it is done in the clinical environment. Analyzing and synthesizing skills were used to work through these questions. Perhaps a renewed interest and amazement at the complexity of the body was gained while discovering the inter-relatedness of the body systems. Hopefully, these integration exercises and the critical thinking experience are catalysts to becoming a proficient, critical thinking nurse.

APPENDIX A
NANDA-I Nursing Diagnoses 2009–2011

Domain 1
Health Promotion
Ineffective **Health** Maintenance
Ineffective Self **Health** Management
Impaired **Home** Maintenance
Readiness for Enhanced **Immunization** Status
Self **Neglect**
Readiness for Enhanced **Nutrition**
Ineffective Family **Therapeutic** Regimen Management
Readiness for Enhanced **Self Health** Management

Domain 2
Nutrition
Ineffective Infant **Feeding** Pattern
Imbalanced **Nutrition**: Less Than Body Requirements
Imbalanced **Nutrition**: More Than Body Requirements
Risk for Imbalanced **Nutrition**: More Than Body Requirements
Impaired **Swallowing**
Risk for Unstable Blood **Glucose** Level
Neonatal **Jaundice**
Risk for Impaired **Liver** Function
Risk for **Electrolyte** Imbalance
Readiness for Enhanced **Fluid** Balance
Deficient **Fluid** Volume
Excess **Fluid** Volume
Risk for Deficient **Fluid** Volume
Risk for Imbalanced **Fluid** Volume

Domain 3
Elimination and Exchange
Functional Urinary **Incontinence**
Overflow Urinary **Incontinence**
Reflex Urinary **Incontinence**
Stress Urinary **Incontinence**
Urge Urinary **Incontinence**
Risk for Urge urinary **Incontinence**
Impaired **Urinary** Elimination
Readiness for Enhanced **Urinary** Elimination
Urinary Retention
Bowel Incontinence
Constipation
Perceived **Constipation**
Risk for **Constipation**
Diarrhea
Dysfunctional Gastrointenstinal **Motility**
Risk for Dysfunctional Gastrointestinal **Motility**
Impaired **Gas** Exchange

Domain 4
Activity Rest
Insomnia
Disturbed **Sleep** Pattern
Sleep Deprivation
Readiness for Enhanced **Sleep**
Risk for **Disuse** Syndrome
Deficient **Diversional** Activity
Sedentary **Lifestyle**
Impaired Bed **Mobility**
Impaired Physical **Mobility**
Impaired Wheelchair **Mobility**
Delayed **Surgical** Recovery
Impaired **Transfer** Ability
Impaired **Walking**
Disturbed **Energy** Field
Fatigue
Activity Intolerance
Risk for **Activity** Intolerance
Risk for **Bleeding**
Ineffective **Breathing** Pattern
Decreased **Cardiac** Output
Ineffective Peripheral Tissue **Perfusion**
Risk for Decreased Cardiac Tissue **Perfusion**
Risk for Ineffective Cerebral Tissue **Perfusion**
Risk for Ineffective Gastrointestinal

Perfusion
Risk for **Ineffective Renal Perfusion**
Risk for **Shock**
Impaired Spontaneous **Ventilation**
Dysfunctional **Ventilatory** Weaning Response
Readiness for Enhanced **Self-Care**
Bathing **Self-Care** Deficit
Dressing **Self-Care** Deficit
Feeding **Self-Care** Deficit
Toileting **Self-Care** Deficit

Domain 5
Perception/Cognition
Unilateral **Neglect**
Impaired **Environmental** Interpretation Syndrome
Wandering
Disturbed **Sensory** Perception (Specify: Visual, Auditory, Kinesthetic, Gustatory, Tactile, Olfactory)
Acute **Confusion**
Chronic **Confusion**
Risk for Acute **Confusion**
Deficient **Knowledge**
Readiness for Enhanced **Knowledge**
Impaired **Memory**
Readiness for Enhanced **Decision-Making**
Ineffective **Activity** Planning
Impaired Verbal **Communication**
Readiness for Enhanced **Communication**

Domain 6
Self-Perception
Risk for Compromised Human **Dignity**
Hopelessness
Disturbed Personal **Identity**
Risk for **Loneliness**
Readiness for Enhanced **Power**
Powerlessness
Risk for **Powerlessness**
Readiness for Enhanced **Self-Concept**
Situational Low **Self-Esteem**
Chronic Low **Self-Esteem**
Risk for Situational Low **Self-Esteem**
Disturbed **Body** Image

Domain 7
Role Relationships
Caregiver Role Strain
Risk for **Caregiver** Role Strain
Impaired **Parenting**
Readiness for Enhanced **Parenting**
Risk for Impaired **Parenting**
Risk for Impaired **Attachment**
Dysfunctional **Family** Processes
Interrupted **Family** Processes
Readiness for Enhanced **Family** Processes
Effective **Breastfeeding**
Ineffective **Breastfeeding**
Interrupted **Breastfeeding**
Parental Role **Conflict**
Readiness for Enhanced **Relationship**
Ineffective **Role** Performance
Impaired **Social** Interaction

Domain 8
Sexuality
Sexual Dysfunction
Ineffective **Sexuality** Pattern
Readiness for Enhanced **Childbearing** Process
Risk for Disturbed **Maternal/Fetal** Dyad

Domain 9
Coping/Stress Tolerance
Post-Trauma Syndrome
Risk for **Post-Trauma** Syndrome
Rape-Trauma Syndrome
Relocation Stress Syndrome
Risk for **Relocation** Stress Syndrome
Anxiety
Death **Anxiety**
Risk-Prone Health **Behavior**
Compromised Family **Coping**
Defensive **Coping**
Disabled Family **Coping**
Ineffective **Coping**
Ineffective Community **Coping**
Readiness for Enhanced **Coping**
Readiness for Enhanced Community **Coping**
Readiness for Enhanced Family **Coping**
Ineffective **Denial**
Fear
Grieving
Complicated **Grieving**
Risk for Complicated **Grieving**
Impaired Individual **Resilience**
Readiness for Enhanced **Resilience**
Risk for Compromised **Resilience**
Chronic **Sorrow**
Stress Overload

Autonomic Dysreflexia
Risk for **Autonomic** Dysreflexia
Disorganized **Infant** Behavior
Risk for Disorganized **Infant** Behavior
Readiness for Enhanced Organized **Infant** Behavior
Decreased **Intracranial** Adaptive Capacity

Domain 10
Life Principles
Readiness for Enhanced **Hope**
Readiness for Enhanced **Spiritual** Well-Being
Decisional **Conflict**
Moral **Distress**
Noncompliance
Impaired **Religiosity**
Readiness for Enhanced **Religiosity**
Risk for Impaired **Religiosity**
Spiritual Distress
Risk for **Spiritual** Distress

Domain 11
Safety/Protection
Risk for **Infection**
Ineffective **Airway** Clearance
Risk for **Aspiration**
Risk for Sudden Infant **Death** Syndrome
Impaired **Dentition**
Risk for **Falls**
Risk for **Injury**
Risk for Perioperative-Positioning **Injury**
Impaired **Oral** Mucous Membrane
Risk for **Peripheral** Neurovascular Dysfunction
Ineffective **Protection**
Impaired **Skin** Integrity
Risk for Impaired **Skin** Integrity
Risk for **Suffocation**
Impaired **Tissue** Integrity
Risk for **Trauma**
Risk for Vascular **Trauma**
Self-Mutilation
Risk for **Suicide**
Risk for Other-Directed **Violence**
Risk for Self-Directed **Violence**
Contamination
Risk for **Contamination**
Risk for **Poisoning**
Latex **Allergy** Response
Risk for Latex **Allergy** Response
Risk for Imbalanced **Body** Temperature
Hyperthermia
Hypothermia
Ineffective **Thermoregulation**

Domain 12
Comfort
Readiness for Enhanced **Comfort**
Impaired **Comfort**
Nausea
Acute **Pain**
Chronic **Pain**
Social Isolation

Domain 13
Growth/Development
Adult **Failure** to Thrive
Delayed **Growth** and Development
Risk for Disproportionate **Growth**
Risk for Delayed **Development**

APPENDIX B
Recommended Immunization Schedules

Recommended Immunization Schedule for Persons Aged 0 Through 6 Years—United States • 2009

For those who fall behind or start late, see the catch-up schedule

Vaccine ▼ Age ►	Birth	1 month	2 months	4 months	6 months	12 months	15 months	18 months	19–23 months	2–3 years	4–6 years
Hepatitis B[1]	HepB	HepB		*see footnote 1*	HepB						
Rotavirus[2]			RV	RV	*RV*[2]						
Diphtheria, Tetanus, Pertussis[3]			DTaP	DTaP	DTaP	*see footnote 3*	DTaP				DTaP
Haemophilus influenzae type b[4]			Hib	Hib	*Hib*[4]	Hib					
Pneumococcal[5]			PCV	PCV	PCV	PCV				PPSV	
Inactivated Poliovirus			IPV	IPV	IPV						IPV
Influenza[6]					Influenza (Yearly)						
Measles, Mumps, Rubella[7]						MMR		*see footnote 7*			MMR
Varicella[8]						Varicella		*see footnote 8*			Varicella
Hepatitis A[9]						HepA (2 doses)				HepA Series	
Meningococcal[10]										MCV	

Legend: Range of recommended ages (shaded); Certain high-risk groups (black)

This schedule indicates the recommended ages for routine administration of currently licensed vaccines, as of December 1, 2008, for children aged 0 through 6 years. Any dose not administered at the recommended age should be administered at a subsequent visit, when indicated and feasible. Licensed combination vaccines may be used whenever any component of the combination is indicated and other components are not contraindicated and if approved by the Food and Drug Administration for that dose of the series. Providers should consult the relevant Advisory Committee on Immunization Practices statement for detailed recommendations, including high-risk conditions: http://www.cdc.gov/vaccines/pubs/acip-list.htm. Clinically significant adverse events that follow immunization should be reported to the Vaccine Adverse Event Reporting System (VAERS). Guidance about how to obtain and complete a VAERS form is available at http://www.vaers.hhs.gov or by telephone, 800-822-7967.

1. **Hepatitis B vaccine (HepB).** ***(Minimum age: birth)***
   At birth:
   - Administer monovalent HepB to all newborns before hospital discharge.
   - If mother is hepatitis B surface antigen (HBsAg)-positive, administer HepB and 0.5 mL of hepatitis B immune globulin (HBIG) within 12 hours of birth.
   - If mother's HBsAg status is unknown, administer HepB within 12 hours of birth. Determine mother's HBsAg status as soon as possible and, if HBsAg-positive, administer HBIG (no later than age 1 week).

   After the birth dose:
   - The HepB series should be completed with either monovalent HepB or a combination vaccine containing HepB. The second dose should be administered at age 1 or 2 months. The final dose should be administered no earlier than age 24 weeks.
   - Infants born to HBsAg-positive mothers should be tested for HBsAg and antibody to HBsAg (anti-HBs) after completion of at least 3 doses of the HepB series, at age 9 through 18 months (generally at the next well-child visit).

   4-month dose:
   - Administration of 4 doses of HepB to infants is permissible when combination vaccines containing HepB are administered after the birth dose.
2. **Rotavirus vaccine (RV).** ***(Minimum age: 6 weeks)***
   - Administer the first dose at age 6 through 14 weeks (maximum age: 14 weeks 6 days). Vaccination should not be initiated for infants aged 15 weeks or older (i.e., 15 weeks 0 days or older).
   - Administer the final dose in the series by age 8 months 0 days.
   - If Rotarix® is administered at ages 2 and 4 months, a dose at 6 months is not indicated.
3. **Diphtheria and tetanus toxoids and acellular pertussis vaccine (DTaP).** ***(Minimum age: 6 weeks)***
   - The fourth dose may be administered as early as age 12 months, provided at least 6 months have elapsed since the third dose.
   - Administer the final dose in the series at age 4 through 6 years.
4. ***Haemophilus influenzae*** **type b conjugate vaccine (Hib).** ***(Minimum age: 6 weeks)***
   - If PRP-OMP (PedvaxHIB® or Comvax® [HepB-Hib]) is administered at ages 2 and 4 months, a dose at age 6 months is not indicated.
   - TriHiBit® (DTaP/Hib) should not be used for doses at ages 2, 4, or 6 months but can be used as the final dose in children aged 12 months or older.
5. **Pneumococcal vaccine.** ***(Minimum age: 6 weeks for pneumococcal conjugate vaccine [PCV]; 2 years for pneumococcal polysaccharide vaccine [PPSV])***
   - PCV is recommended for all children aged younger than 5 years. Administer 1 dose of PCV to all healthy children aged 24 through 59 months who are not completely vaccinated for their age.
   - Administer PPSV to children aged 2 years or older with certain underlying medical conditions (see *MMWR* 2000;49[No. RR-9]), including a cochlear implant.
6. **Influenza vaccine.** ***(Minimum age: 6 months for trivalent inactivated influenza vaccine [TIV]; 2 years for live, attenuated influenza vaccine [LAIV])***
   - Administer annually to children aged 6 months through 18 years.
   - For healthy nonpregnant persons (i.e., those who do not have underlying medical conditions that predispose them to influenza complications) aged 2 through 49 years, either LAIV or TIV may be used.
   - Children receiving TIV should receive 0.25 mL if aged 6 through 35 months or 0.5 mL if aged 3 years or older.
   - Administer 2 doses (separated by at least 4 weeks) to children aged younger than 9 years who are receiving influenza vaccine for the first time or who were vaccinated for the first time during the previous influenza season but only received 1 dose.
7. **Measles, mumps, and rubella vaccine (MMR).** ***(Minimum age: 12 months)***
   - Administer the second dose at age 4 through 6 years. However, the second dose may be administered before age 4, provided at least 28 days have elapsed since the first dose.
8. **Varicella vaccine.** ***(Minimum age: 12 months)***
   - Administer the second dose at age 4 through 6 years. However, the second dose may be administered before age 4, provided at least 3 months have elapsed since the first dose.
   - For children aged 12 months through 12 years the minimum interval between doses is 3 months. However, if the second dose was administered at least 28 days after the first dose, it can be accepted as valid.
9. **Hepatitis A vaccine (HepA).** ***(Minimum age: 12 months)***
   - Administer to all children aged 1 year (i.e., aged 12 through 23 months). Administer 2 doses at least 6 months apart.
   - Children not fully vaccinated by age 2 years can be vaccinated at subsequent visits.
   - HepA also is recommended for children older than 1 year who live in areas where vaccination programs target older children or who are at increased risk of infection. See *MMWR* 2006;55(No. RR-7).
10. **Meningococcal vaccine.** ***(Minimum age: 2 years for meningococcal conjugate vaccine [MCV] and for meningococcal polysaccharide vaccine [MPSV])***
    - Administer MCV to children aged 2 through 10 years with terminal complement component deficiency, anatomic or functional asplenia, and certain other high-risk groups. See *MMWR* 2005;54(No. RR-7).
    - Persons who received MPSV 3 or more years previously and who remain at increased risk for meningococcal disease should be revaccinated with MCV.

The Recommended Immunization Schedules for Persons Aged 0 Through 18 Years are approved by the Advisory Committee on Immunization Practices (www.cdc.gov/vaccines/recs/acip), the American Academy of Pediatrics (http://www.aap.org), and the American Academy of Family Physicians (http://www.aafp.org).

DEPARTMENT OF HEALTH AND HUMAN SERVICES • CENTERS FOR DISEASE CONTROL AND PREVENTION

Recommended Immunization Schedule for Persons Aged 7 Through 18 Years—United States • 2009

For those who fall behind or start late, see the schedule below and the catch-up schedule

Vaccine ▼ Age ►	7–10 years	11–12 years	13–18 years
Tetanus, Diphtheria, Pertussis[1]	*see footnote 1*	Tdap	Tdap
Human Papillomavirus[2]	*see footnote 2*	HPV (3 doses)	HPV Series
Meningococcal[3]	MCV	MCV	MCV
Influenza[4]	Influenza (Yearly)		
Pneumococcal[5]	PPSV		
Hepatitis A[6]	HepA Series		
Hepatitis B[7]	HepB Series		
Inactivated Poliovirus[8]	IPV Series		
Measles, Mumps, Rubella[9]	MMR Series		
Varicella[10]	Varicella Series		

Range of recommended ages

Catch-up immunization

Certain high-risk groups

This schedule indicates the recommended ages for routine administration of currently licensed vaccines, as of December 1, 2008, for children aged 7 through 18 years. Any dose not administered at the recommended age should be administered at a subsequent visit, when indicated and feasible. Licensed combination vaccines may be used whenever any component of the combination is indicated and other components are not contraindicated and if approved by the Food and Drug Administration for that dose of the series. Providers should consult the relevant Advisory Committee on Immunization Practices statement for detailed recommendations, including high-risk conditions: http://www.cdc.gov/vaccines/pubs/acip-list.htm. Clinically significant adverse events that follow immunization should be reported to the Vaccine Adverse Event Reporting System (VAERS). Guidance about how to obtain and complete a VAERS form is available at http://www.vaers.hhs.gov or by telephone, 800-822-7967.

1. Tetanus and diphtheria toxoids and acellular pertussis vaccine (Tdap). ***(Minimum age: 10 years for BOOSTRIX® and 11 years for ADACEL®)***
- Administer at age 11 or 12 years for those who have completed the recommended childhood DTP/DTaP vaccination series and have not received a tetanus and diphtheria toxoid (Td) booster dose.
- Persons aged 13 through 18 years who have not received Tdap should receive a dose.
- A 5-year interval from the last Td dose is encouraged when Tdap is used as a booster dose; however, a shorter interval may be used if pertussis immunity is needed.

2. Human papillomavirus vaccine (HPV). ***(Minimum age: 9 years)***
- Administer the first dose to females at age 11 or 12 years.
- Administer the second dose 2 months after the first dose and the third dose 6 months after the first dose (at least 24 weeks after the first dose).
- Administer the series to females at age 13 through 18 years if not previously vaccinated.

3. Meningococcal conjugate vaccine (MCV).
- Administer at age 11 or 12 years, or at age 13 through 18 years if not previously vaccinated.
- Administer to previously unvaccinated college freshmen living in a dormitory.
- MCV is recommended for children aged 2 through 10 years with terminal complement component deficiency, anatomic or functional asplenia, and certain other groups at high risk. See *MMWR* 2005;54(No. RR-7).
- Persons who received MPSV 5 or more years previously and remain at increased risk for meningococcal disease should be revaccinated with MCV.

4. Influenza vaccine.
- Administer annually to children aged 6 months through 18 years.
- For healthy nonpregnant persons (i.e., those who do not have underlying medical conditions that predispose them to influenza complications) aged 2 through 49 years, either LAIV or TIV may be used.
- Administer 2 doses (separated by at least 4 weeks) to children aged younger than 9 years who are receiving influenza vaccine for the first time or who were vaccinated for the first time during the previous influenza season but only received 1 dose.

5. Pneumococcal polysaccharide vaccine (PPSV).
- Administer to children with certain underlying medical conditions (see *MMWR* 1997;46[No. RR-8]), including a cochlear implant. A single revaccination should be administered to children with functional or anatomic asplenia or other immunocompromising condition after 5 years.

6. Hepatitis A vaccine (HepA).
- Administer 2 doses at least 6 months apart.
- HepA is recommended for children older than 1 year who live in areas where vaccination programs target older children or who are at increased risk of infection. See *MMWR* 2006;55(No. RR-7).

7. Hepatitis B vaccine (HepB).
- Administer the 3-dose series to those not previously vaccinated.
- A 2-dose series (separated by at least 4 months) of adult formulation Recombivax HB® is licensed for children aged 11 through 15 years.

8. Inactivated poliovirus vaccine (IPV).
- For children who received an all-IPV or all-oral poliovirus (OPV) series, a fourth dose is not necessary if the third dose was administered at age 4 years or older.
- If both OPV and IPV were administered as part of a series, a total of 4 doses should be administered, regardless of the child's current age.

9. Measles, mumps, and rubella vaccine (MMR).
- If not previously vaccinated, administer 2 doses or the second dose for those who have received only 1 dose, with at least 28 days between doses.

10. Varicella vaccine.
- For persons aged 7 through 18 years without evidence of immunity (see *MMWR* 2007;56[No. RR-4]), administer 2 doses if not previously vaccinated or the second dose if they have received only 1 dose.
- For persons aged 7 through 12 years, the minimum interval between doses is 3 months. However, if the second dose was administered at least 28 days after the first dose, it can be accepted as valid.
- For persons aged 13 years and older, the minimum interval between doses is 28 days.

The Recommended Immunization Schedules for Persons Aged 0 Through 18 Years are approved by the Advisory Committee on Immunization Practices (www.cdc.gov/vaccines/recs/acip), the American Academy of Pediatrics (http://www.aap.org), and the American Academy of Family Physicians (http://www.aafp.org).

DEPARTMENT OF HEALTH AND HUMAN SERVICES • CENTERS FOR DISEASE CONTROL AND PREVENTION

Recommended Adult Immunization Schedule

UNITED STATES · 2009

Note: These recommendations *must* be read with the footnotes that follow containing number of doses, intervals between doses, and other important information.

Figure 1. Recommended adult immunization schedule, by vaccine and age group

<table>
<tr><th>VACCINE ▼ AGE GROUP ▶</th><th>19–26 years</th><th>27–49 years</th><th>50–59 years</th><th>60–64 years</th><th>≥65 years</th></tr>
<tr><td>Tetanus, diphtheria, pertussis (Td/Tdap)[1,*]</td><td colspan="4">Substitute 1-time dose of Tdap for Td booster; then boost with Td every 10 yrs</td><td>Td booster every 10 yrs</td></tr>
<tr><td>Human papillomavirus (HPV)[2,*]</td><td>3 doses (females)</td><td></td><td></td><td></td><td></td></tr>
<tr><td>Varicella[3,*]</td><td colspan="5">2 doses</td></tr>
<tr><td>Zoster[4]</td><td></td><td></td><td></td><td colspan="2">1 dose</td></tr>
<tr><td>Measles, mumps, rubella (MMR)[5,*]</td><td colspan="2">1 or 2 doses</td><td colspan="3">1 dose</td></tr>
<tr><td>Influenza[6,*]</td><td colspan="5">1 dose annually</td></tr>
<tr><td>Pneumococcal (polysaccharide)[7,8]</td><td colspan="4">1 or 2 doses</td><td>1 dose</td></tr>
<tr><td>Hepatitis A[9,*]</td><td colspan="5">2 doses</td></tr>
<tr><td>Hepatitis B[10,*]</td><td colspan="5">3 doses</td></tr>
<tr><td>Meningococcal[11,*]</td><td colspan="5">1 or more doses</td></tr>
</table>

*Covered by the Vaccine Injury Compensation Program.

- (Light shading) For all persons in this category who meet the age requirements and who lack evidence of immunity (e.g., lack documentation of vaccination or have no evidence of prior infection)
- (Dark shading) Recommended if some other risk factor is present (e.g., on the basis of medical, occupational, lifestyle, or other indications)
- (Blank) No recommendation

Report all clinically significant postvaccination reactions to the Vaccine Adverse Event Reporting System (VAERS). Reporting forms and instructions on filing a VAERS report are available at www.vaers.hhs.gov or by telephone, 800-822-7967.

Information on how to file a Vaccine Injury Compensation Program claim is available at www.hrsa.gov/vaccinecompensation or by telephone, 800-338-2382. To file a claim for vaccine injury, contact the U.S. Court of Federal Claims, 717 Madison Place, N.W., Washington, D.C. 20005; telephone, 202-357-6400.

Additional information about the vaccines in this schedule, extent of available data, and contraindications for vaccination is also available at www.cdc.gov/vaccines or from the CDC-INFO Contact Center at 800-CDC-INFO (800-232-4636) in English and Spanish, 24 hours a day, 7 days a week.

Use of trade names and commercial sources is for identification only and does not imply endorsement by the U.S. Department of Health and Human Services.

Figure 2. Vaccines that might be indicated for adults based on medical and other indications

VACCINE ▼ / INDICATION ▶	Pregnancy	Immuno-compromising conditions (excluding human immunodeficiency virus [HIV])[13]	HIV infection[3,12,13] CD4+ T lymphocyte count <200 cells/µL	HIV infection[3,12,13] CD4+ T lymphocyte count ≥200 cells/µL	Diabetes, heart disease, chronic lung disease, chronic alcoholism	Asplenia[12] (including elective splenectomy and terminal complement component deficiencies)	Chronic liver disease	Kidney failure, end-stage renal disease, receipt of hemodialysis	Health-care personnel
Tetanus, diphtheria, pertussis (Td/Tdap)[1,*]	Td	Substitute 1-time dose of Tdap for Td booster; then boost with Td every 10 yrs							
Human papillomavirus (HPV)[2,*]		3 doses for females through age 26 yrs							
Varicella[3,*]	Contraindicated			2 doses					
Zoster[4]	Contraindicated				1 dose				
Measles, mumps, rubella (MMR)[5,*]	Contraindicated			1 or 2 doses					
Influenza[6,*]	1 dose TIV annually								1 dose TIV or LAIV annually
Pneumococcal (polysaccharide)[7,8]	1 or 2 doses								
Hepatitis A[9,*]	2 doses								
Hepatitis B[10,*]	3 doses								
Meningococcal[11,*]	1 or more doses								

*Covered by the Vaccine Injury Compensation Program.

For all persons in this category who meet the age requirements and who lack evidence of immunity (e.g., lack documentation of vaccination or have no evidence of prior infection)

Recommended if some other risk factor is present (e.g., on the basis of medical, occupational, lifestyle, or other indications)

No recommendation

These schedules indicate the recommended age groups and medical indications for which administration of currently licensed vaccines is commonly indicated for adults ages 19 years and older, as of January 1, 2009. Licensed combination vaccines may be used whenever any components of the combination are indicated and when the vaccine's other components are not contraindicated. For detailed recommendations on all vaccines, including those used primarily for travelers or that are issued during the year, consult the manufacturers' package inserts and the complete statements from the Advisory Committee on Immunization Practices (www.cdc.gov/vaccines/pubs/acip-list.htm).

The recommendations in this schedule were approved by the Centers for Disease Control and Prevention's (CDC) Advisory Committee on Immunization Practices (ACIP), the American Academy of Family Physicians (AAFP), the American College of Obstetricians and Gynecologists (ACOG), and the American College of Physicians (ACP).

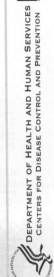

DEPARTMENT OF HEALTH AND HUMAN SERVICES
CENTERS FOR DISEASE CONTROL AND PREVENTION
CDC

CS200484-A

Footnotes

Recommended Adult Immunization Schedule—UNITED STATES - 2009

For complete statements by the Advisory Committee on Immunization Practices (ACIP), visit www.cdc.gov/vaccines/pubs/ACIP-list.htm.

1. Tetanus, diphtheria, and acellular pertussis (Td/Tdap) vaccination

Tdap should replace a single dose of Td for adults aged 19 through 64 years who have not received a dose of Tdap previously.

Adults with uncertain or incomplete history of primary vaccination series with tetanus and diphtheria toxoid-containing vaccines should begin or complete a primary vaccination series. A primary series for adults is 3 doses of tetanus and diphtheria toxoid-containing vaccines; administer the first 2 doses at least 4 weeks apart and the third dose 6–12 months after the second. However, Tdap can substitute for any one of the doses of Td in the 3-dose primary series. The booster dose of tetanus and diphtheria toxoid-containing vaccine should be administered to adults who have completed a primary series and if the last vaccination was received 10 or more years previously. Tdap or Td vaccine may be used, as indicated.

If a woman is pregnant and received the last Td vaccination 10 or more years previously, administer Td during the second or third trimester. If the woman received the last Td vaccination less than 10 years previously, administer Tdap during the immediate postpartum period. A dose of Tdap is recommended for postpartum women, close contacts of infants aged less than 12 months, and all health-care personnel with direct patient contact if they have not previously received Tdap. An interval as short as 2 years from the last Td is suggested; shorter intervals can be used. Td may be deferred during pregnancy and Tdap substituted in the immediate postpartum period, or Tdap may be administered instead of Td to a pregnant woman after an informed discussion with the woman.

Consult the ACIP statement for recommendations for administering Td as prophylaxis in wound management.

2. Human papillomavirus (HPV) vaccination

HPV vaccination is recommended for all females aged 11 through 26 years (and may begin at 9 years) who have not completed the vaccine series. History of genital warts, abnormal Papanicolaou test, or positive HPV DNA test is not evidence of prior infection with all vaccine HPV types; HPV vaccination is recommended for persons with such histories.

Ideally, vaccine should be administered before potential exposure to HPV through sexual activity; however, females who are sexually active should still be vaccinated consistent with age-based recommendations. Sexually active females who have not been infected with any of the four HPV vaccine types receive the full benefit of the vaccination. Vaccination is less beneficial for females who have already been infected with one or more of the HPV vaccine types.

A complete series consists of 3 doses. The second dose should be administered 2 months after the first dose; the third dose should be administered 6 months after the first dose.

HPV vaccination is not specifically recommended for females with the medical indications described in Figure 2, "Vaccines that might be indicated for adults based on medical and other indications." Because HPV vaccine is not a live-virus vaccine, it may be administered to persons with the medical indications described in Figure 2. However, the immune response and vaccine efficacy might be less for persons with the medical indications described in Figure 2 than in persons who do not have the medical indications described or who are immunocompetent. Health-care personnel are not at increased risk because of occupational exposure, and should be vaccinated consistent with age-based recommendations.

3. Varicella vaccination

All adults without evidence of immunity to varicella should receive 2 doses of single-antigen varicella vaccine if not previously vaccinated or the second dose if they have received only one dose unless they have a medical contraindication. Special consideration should be given to those who 1) have close contact with persons at high risk for severe disease (e.g., health-care personnel and family contacts of persons with immunocompromising conditions) or 2) are at high risk for exposure or transmission (e.g., teachers; child care employees; residents and staff members of institutional settings, including correctional institutions; college students; military personnel; adolescents and adults living in households with children; nonpregnant women of childbearing age; and international travelers).

Evidence of immunity to varicella in adults includes any of the following: 1) documentation of 2 doses of varicella vaccine at least 4 weeks apart; 2) U.S.-born before 1980 (although for health-care personnel and pregnant women, birth before 1980 should not be considered evidence of immunity); 3) history of varicella based on diagnosis or verification of varicella by a health-care provider (for a patient reporting a history of or presenting with an atypical case, a mild case, or both, health-care providers should seek either an epidemiologic link with a typical varicella case or to a laboratory-confirmed case or evidence of laboratory confirmation, if it was performed at the time of acute disease); 4) history of herpes zoster based on health-care provider diagnosis or verification of herpes zoster by a health-care provider; or 5) laboratory evidence of immunity or laboratory confirmation of disease.

Pregnant women should be assessed for evidence of varicella immunity. Women who do not have evidence of immunity should receive the first dose of varicella vaccine upon completion or termination of pregnancy and before discharge from the health-care facility. The second dose should be administered 4–8 weeks after the first dose.

4. Herpes zoster vaccination

A single dose of zoster vaccine is recommended for adults aged 60 years and older regardless of whether they report a prior episode of herpes zoster. Persons with chronic medical conditions may be vaccinated unless their condition constitutes a contraindication.

5. Measles, mumps, rubella (MMR) vaccination

Measles component: Adults born before 1957 generally are considered immune to measles. Adults born during or after 1957 should receive 1 or more doses of MMR unless they have a medical contraindication, documentation of 1 or more doses, history of measles based on health-care provider diagnosis, or laboratory evidence of immunity.

A second dose of MMR is recommended for adults who 1) have been recently exposed to measles or are in an outbreak setting; 2) have been vaccinated previously with killed measles vaccine; 3) have been vaccinated with an unknown type of measles vaccine during 1963–1967; 4) are students in postsecondary educational institutions; 5) work in a health-care facility; or 6) plan to travel internationally.

Mumps component: Adults born before 1957 generally are considered immune to mumps. Adults born during or after 1957 should receive 1 dose of MMR unless they have a medical contraindication, history of mumps based on health-care provider diagnosis, or laboratory evidence of immunity.

A second dose of MMR is recommended for adults who 1) live in a community experiencing a mumps outbreak and are in an affected age group; 2) are students in postsecondary educational institutions; 3) work in a health-care facility; or 4) plan to travel internationally. For unvaccinated health-care personnel born before 1957 who do not have other evidence of mumps immunity, administering 1 dose on a routine basis should be considered and administering a second dose during an outbreak should be strongly considered.

Rubella component: 1 dose of MMR vaccine is recommended for women whose rubella vaccination history is unreliable or who lack laboratory evidence of immunity. For women of childbearing age, regardless of birth year, rubella immunity should be determined and women should be counseled regarding congenital rubella syndrome. Women who do not have evidence of immunity should receive MMR upon completion or termination of pregnancy and before discharge from the health-care facility.

6. Influenza vaccination

Medical indications: Chronic disorders of the cardiovascular or pulmonary systems, including asthma; chronic metabolic diseases, including diabetes mellitus, renal or hepatic dysfunction, hemoglobinopathies, or immunocompromising conditions (including immunocompromising conditions caused by medications or human immunodeficiency virus [HIV]); any condition that compromises respiratory function or the handling of respiratory secretions or that can increase the risk of aspiration (e.g., cognitive dysfunction, spinal cord injury, or seizure disorder or other neuromuscular disorder); and pregnancy during the influenza season. No data exist on the risk for severe or complicated influenza disease among persons with asplenia; however, influenza is a risk factor for secondary bacterial infections that can cause severe disease among persons with asplenia.

Occupational indications: All health-care personnel, including those employed by long-term care and assisted-living facilities, and caregivers of children less than 5 years old.

Other indications: Residents of nursing homes and other long-term care and assisted-living facilities; persons likely to transmit influenza to persons at high risk (e.g., in-home household contacts and caregivers of children aged less than 5 years old, persons 65 years old and older and persons of all ages with high-risk condition[s]); and anyone who would like to decrease their risk of getting influenza. Healthy, nonpregnant adults aged less than 50 years without high-risk medical conditions who are not contacts of severely immunocompromised persons in special care units can receive either intranasally administered live, attenuated influenza vaccine (FluMist®) or inactivated vaccine. Other persons should receive the inactivated vaccine.

7. Pneumococcal polysaccharide (PPSV) vaccination

Medical indications: Chronic lung disease (including asthma); chronic cardiovascular diseases; diabetes mellitus; chronic liver diseases, cirrhosis; chronic alcoholism, chronic renal failure or nephrotic syndrome; functional or anatomic asplenia (e.g., sickle cell disease or splenectomy [if elective splenectomy is planned, vaccinate at least 2 weeks before surgery]); immunocompromising conditions; and cochlear implants and cerebrospinal fluid leaks. Vaccinate as close to HIV diagnosis as possible.

Other indications: Residents of nursing homes or long-term care facilities and persons who smoke cigarettes. Routine use of PPSV is not recommended for Alaska Native or American Indian persons younger than 65 years unless they have underlying medical conditions that are PPSV indications. However, public health authorities may consider recommending PPSV for Alaska Natives and American Indians aged 50 through 64 years who are living in areas in which the risk of invasive pneumococcal disease is increased.

8. Revaccination with PPSV

One-time revaccination after 5 years for persons with chronic renal failure or nephrotic syndrome; functional or anatomic asplenia (e.g., sickle cell disease or splenectomy); and for persons with immunocompromising conditions. For persons aged 65 years and older, one-time revaccination if they were vaccinated 5 or more years previously and were aged less than 65 years at the time of primary vaccination.

9. Hepatitis A vaccination

Medical indications: Persons with chronic liver disease and persons who receive clotting factor concentrates.

Behavioral indications: Men who have sex with men and persons who use illegal drugs.

Occupational indications: Persons working with hepatitis A virus (HAV)-infected primates or with HAV in a research laboratory setting.

Other indications: Persons traveling to or working in countries that have high or intermediate endemicity of hepatitis A (a list of countries is available at wwwn.cdc.gov/travel/contentdiseases.aspx) and any person seeking protection from HAV infection.

Single-antigen vaccine formulations should be administered in a 2-dose schedule at either 0 and 6–12 months (Havrix®), or 0 and 6–18 months (Vaqta®). If the combined hepatitis A and hepatitis B vaccine (Twinrix®) is used, administer 3 doses at 0, 1, and 6 months; alternatively, a 4-dose schedule, administered on days 0, 7 and 21 to 30 followed by a booster dose at month 12 may be used.

10. Hepatitis B vaccination

Medical indications: Persons with end-stage renal disease, including patients receiving hemodialysis; persons with HIV infection; and persons with chronic liver disease.

Occupational indications: Health-care personnel and public-safety workers who are exposed to blood or other potentially infectious body fluids.

Behavioral indications: Sexually active persons who are not in a long-term, mutually monogamous relationship (e.g., persons with more than 1 sex partner during the previous 6 months); persons seeking evaluation or treatment for a sexually transmitted disease (STD); current or recent injection-drug users; and men who have sex with men.

Other indications: Household contacts and sex partners of persons with chronic hepatitis B virus (HBV) infection; clients and staff members of institutions for persons with developmental disabilities; international travelers to countries with high or intermediate prevalence of chronic HBV infection (a list of countries is available at wwwn.cdc.gov/travel/contentdiseases.aspx); and any adult seeking protection from HBV infection.

Hepatitis B vaccination is recommended for all adults in the following settings: STD treatment facilities; HIV testing and treatment facilities; facilities providing drug-abuse treatment and prevention services; health-care settings targeting services to injection-drug users or men who have sex with men; correctional facilities; end-stage renal disease programs and facilities for chronic hemodialysis patients; and institutions and nonresidential daycare facilities for persons with developmental disabilities.

If the combined hepatitis A and hepatitis B vaccine (Twinrix®) is used, administer 3 doses at

0, 1, and 6 months; alternatively, a 4-dose schedule, administered on days 0, 7 and 21 to 30 followed by a booster dose at month 12 may be used.

Special formulation indications: For adult patients receiving hemodialysis or with other immunocompromising conditions, 1 dose of 40 µg/mL (Recombivax HB®) administered on a 3-dose schedule or 2 doses of 20 µg/mL (Engerix-B®) administered simultaneously on a 4-dose schedule at
0, 1, 2 and 6 months.

11. Meningococcal vaccination

Medical indications: Adults with anatomic or functional asplenia, or terminal complement component deficiencies.

Other indications: First-year college students living in dormitories; microbiologists who are routinely exposed to isolates of *Neisseria meningitidis*; military recruits; and persons who travel to or live in countries in which meningococcal disease is hyperendemic or epidemic (e.g., the "meningitis belt" of sub-Saharan Africa during the dry season [December–June]), particularly if their contact with local populations will be prolonged. Vaccination is required by the government of Saudi Arabia for all travelers to Mecca during the annual Hajj.

Meningococcal conjugate (MCV) vaccine is preferred for adults with any of the preceding indications who are aged 55 years or younger, although meningococcal polysaccharide vaccine (MPSV) is an acceptable alternative. Revaccination with MCV after 5 years might be indicated for adults previously vaccinated with MPSV who remain at increased risk for infection (e.g., persons residing in areas in which disease is epidemic).

12. Selected conditions for which *Haemophilus influenzae* type b (Hib) vaccine may be used

Hib vaccine generally is not recommended for persons aged 5 years and older. No efficacy data are available on which to base a recommendation concerning use of Hib vaccine for older children and adults. However, studies suggest good immunogenicity in persons who have sickle cell disease, leukemia, or HIV infection or who have had a splenectomy; administering 1 dose of vaccine to these persons is not contraindicated.

13. Immunocompromising conditions

Inactivated vaccines generally are acceptable (e.g., pneumococcal, meningococcal, and influenza [trivalent inactivated influenza vaccine]), and live vaccines generally are avoided in persons with immune deficiencies or immunocompromising conditions. Information on specific conditions is available at www.cdc.gov/vaccines/pubs/acip-list.htm.

APPENDIX C
Abbreviations, Acronyms, and Symbols

$>$	greater than
$<$	less than
ʒ	dram
℥	ounce
♏	minum
ā	before
AAPB	Association of Applied Psychophysiology and Biofeedback
AARP	American Association of Retired Persons
AASM	American Academy of Sleep Medicine
AAT	animal-assisted therapy
AATH	American Association for Therapeutic Humor
ABC	airway, breathing, circulation
ABD	abdominal
ABG	arterial blood gases
ABO	blood types
a.c.	before meals
ACIP	Advisory Committee on Immunization Practices
ACS	American Cancer Society
ACTH	adrenocorticotropic hormone
AD	Alzheimer's disease
AD	right ear
ad lib	freely, as desired
ADA	Americans with Disabilities Act
ADH	antidiuretic hormone
ADLs	activities of daily living
ADN	associate degree nurse (nursing)
AEB	as evidenced by
AFP	alpha-fetoprotein
AHA	American Hospital Association
AHCA	American Health Care Association
AHCPR	Agency for Health Care Policy and Research
AHNA	American Holistic Nurses' Association
AHRQ	Agency for Healthcare Research and Quality
AI	adequate intake
AIDS	acquired immunodeficiency syndrome
AJN	*American Journal of Nursing*
ALFA	Assisted Living Federation of America
ALT	alanine aminotransferase
AMA	against medical advice
AMA	American Medical Association
ANA	American Nurses Association
ANA	antinuclear antibody
AoA	Administration on Aging
AP	anterior/posterior
AP	apical pulse
APIC	Association for Practitioners in Infection Control and Epidemiology
APRN	advance practice registered nurse
APS	Adult Protective Services
APS	American Pain Society
APTT	activated partial thromboplastin time
AROM	active range of motion
AS	left ear
ASA	acetylsalicylic acid
ASO	antireptolysin-O
AST	aspartate aminotransferase
AT	axillary temperature
ATC	around the clock
ATP	adenosine triphosphatase
AU	both ears
B_1	thiamine
B_2	riboflavin
B_6	pyridoxine
B_{12}	cobolomine
BBA	Balanced Budget Act
BE	base excess
bid	twice a day
BMD	bone mineral density
BMI	body mass index
BMR	basal metabolic rate

BP blood pressure
BPH benign prostatic hypertrophy
BPM beats per minute
BSA body surface area
BSE breast self-examination
BSI body substance isolation
BSN bachelor of science in nursing
BUN blood urea nitrogen
c cup
c̄ with
C Celsius
Ca calcium
Ca^{++} calcium ion
$CaCl_2$ calcium chloride
C/A complementary/alternative
CAD coronary artery disease
CAI computer-assisted instruction
CAM complementary/alternative medicine
C & S culture and sensitivity
cap capsule
CARF Commission on Accreditation of Rehabilitation Facilities
CAT computed axial tomography
CAT computerized adaptive testing
CBC complete blood count
CBD common bile duct
CBE charting by exception
cc cubic centimeter
CCRC continuing care retirement community
CCU coronary care unit
CDC Centers for Disease Control and Prevention
CEA carcinoembryonic antigen
CEPN-LTC™ Certification Examination for Practical and Vocational Nurses in Long-Term Care
CEU continuing education unit
CHAP Community Health Accreditation Program
CHD coronary heart disease
CHF congestive heart failure
CHIP Children's Health Insurance Program
CHO carbohydrate (carbon, hydrogen, oxygen)
CHON protein (carbon, hydrogen, oxygen, nitrogen)
CK or CPK creatine kinase or creatine phosphokinase
Cl chlorine, chloride
Cl^- chloride ion
CLTC certified in long-term care
cm centimeter
CMS Centers for Medicare and Medicaid Services
CN cranial nerve
CNA certified nursing assistant
CNM certified nurse midwife
CNO community nursing organization
CNS central nervous system
CNS clinical nurse specialist
Co cobalt
CO_2 carbon dioxide
CO_2^- carbon dioxide ion
COBRA Comprehensive Omnibus Budget Reconciliation Act
COOH carboxyl group
COPD chronic obstructive pulmonary disease
CPAP continuous positive airway pressure
CPNP Council of Practical Nursing Programs
CPR cardiopulmonary resuscitation
CPR computerized patient record
Cr chromium
CRNA Certified Registered Nurse Anesthetist
CRP C-reactive protein
C&S culture and sensitivity
CSF cerebrospinal fluid
CSM circulation, sensation, motion
CT computed tomography
Cu copper
CVA cerebrovascular accident
CVC central venous catheter
D_5W dextrose 5% in water
D & C dilatation and curettage
DAR document, action, response
dc discontinue
DDB Disciplinary Data Bank
DDS doctor of dental surgery
DEA Drug Enforcement Agency
DHHS Department of Health and Human Services
DIC disseminated intravascular coagulation
DICC dynamic infusion cavernosometry and cavernosography
dL deciliter
DMD doctor of dental medicine
DNA deoxyribonucleic acid
DNR do not resuscitate
DO doctor of osteopathy
DPAHC durable power of attorney for health care
dr dram, or ʒ
DRG diagnosis-related group
DRI dietary reference intake
DSM-IV *Diagnostic and Statistical Manual of Mental Disorders,* 4th edition
DST dexamethasone suppression test
DT delirium tremens
DTaP diphtheria, tetanus, acellular pertussis
DTP diphtheria, tetanus, pertussis
DVT deep vein thrombosis
EAR estimated average requirement
ECF extended care facility
ECF extracellular fluid
ED emergency department
EDTA ethylenediaminetetraacetic acid
EEG electroencephalograph
EGD esophagogastroduodenoscopy
EKG (ECG) electrocardiogram
ELISA enzyme-linked immunosorbent assay
elix elixir
EMG electromyogram
EMLA eutectic (cream) mixture of local anesthetics
EMS emergency medical services

EMT emergency medical technician
EMT-P emergency medical technician-paramedic
EPA Environmental Protection Agency
EPO exclusive provider organization
ER emergency room
ERCP endoscopic retrograde cholangiopancreatogram
ERG electroretinogram
ERT estrogen replacement therapy
ESR erythrocyte sedimentation rate
ET ear (tympanic) temperature
EVAD explantable venous access device
F fahrenheit
FAS fetal alcohol syndrome
FBS fasting blood sugar
FCA False Claims Act
FDA Food and Drug Administration
Fe iron
$FeSO_4$ iron sulfate
fl fluid
Fl fluorine
FOBT fecal occult blood test
FSH follicle-stimulating hormone
ft foot or feet
FVD fluid volume deficit
g gram
GAO General Accounting Office
GAS general adaptation syndrome
GCS Glasgow Coma Scale
g/dL grams per deciliter
GED general education development
GER gastroesophageal reflux
GFR glomerular filtration rate
GGT (GGTP) gammaglutamy transpeptidase
GH growth hormone
GHB glycosylated hemoglobin
GI gastrointestinal
gr grain
gtt drop
GTT glucose tolerance test
gtt/min drops per minute
GU genitourinary
h hour(s)
H^+ hydrogen ion
H_2CO_3 carbonic acid
H_2O water
H&H hemoglobin and hematocrit
HB_sAG hepatitis B surface antigen
HBV hepatitis B virus
HCFA Health Care Financing Administration
hCG human chorionic gonadotropin
HCl hydrochloric acid, hydrochloride
HCO_3^- bicarbonate ion
Hct hematocrit
HCV hepatitis C virus
HDL high density lipoprotein
HDV hepatitis D virus
Hep B hepatitis B
HFA Hospice Foundation of America
Hg mercury
Hgb hemoglobin
Hgbs hemoglobins
HICPAC Hospital Infection Control Practices Advisory Committee
HIS hospital information system
HIV human immunodeficiency virus
HLA human leukocyte antigen
HMO health maintenance organization
HPO_4 phosphate
HR heart rate
HRSA Health Resources and Services Administration
h.s. hour of sleep
I iodine
IADLs instrumental activities of daily living
I&O intake and output
IASP International Association for the Study of Pain
ICF intermediate care facility
ICF intracellular fluid
ICN International Council of Nurses
ICU intensive care unit
ID identification
ID intradermal
IgG immunoglobulin G
IgM immunoglobulin M
IHCT interdisciplinary health care team
IM intramuscular
in inch
INR International Normalized Ratio
I&O intake and output
IOL intraocular lens
IOM Institute of Medicine
ITT insulin tolerance test
IV intravenous
IVAD implantable vascular access device
IVP intravenous push, intravenous pyelogram
IVPB intravenous piggyback
JCAHO Joint Commission on Accreditation of Healthcare Organizations
K potassium
K^+ potassium ion
kcal kilocalorie
KCl potassium chloride
kg kilogram
KS ketosteroids
KUB kidneys/ureters/bladder
KVO keep vein open
L liter
LAS local adaptation syndrome
lb pound
LDH lactic dehydrogenase
LDL low density lipoprotein
LE lupus erythematosus
LES lower esophageal sphincter
LFT liver function test

LH	luteinizing hormone
LLQ	left lower quadrant
LMP	last menstrual period
L/min	liters per minute
LOC	level of consciousness
LP	lumbar puncture
LP/VN	licensed practical/vocational nurse
LPN	licensed practical nurse
LUQ	left upper quadrant
LVN	licensed vocational nurse
m	meter
m^2	square meter
MAO	monoamine oxidase
MAOI	monoamine oxidase inhibitor
MAR	medication administration record
mcg (or μg)	microgram
MD	doctor of medicine
MDI	metered-dose inhaler
MDR	multidrug-resistant
MDR-TB	multidrug-resistant tuberculosis
MDS	minimum data set
mEq	milliequivalent
mEq/L	milliequivalents per liter
mg	milligram
mg/dL	milligrams per deciliter
Mg	magnesium
Mg^{++}	magnesium ion
MgCl	magnesium chloride
$MgSO_4$	magnesium sulfate
MI	myocardial infarction
min	minute
mL	milliliter
mm^3	cubic millimeter
mm Hg	millimeters of mercury
mmol/L	millimoles per liter
MMR	measles, mumps, rubella
Mn	manganese
Mo	molybdenum
MOM	Milk of Magnesia
mOsm/kg	milliosmoles/kilogram
MRI	magnetic resonance imaging
MRSA	methicillin-resistant *staphylococcus aureus*
MS	morphine sulfate
MSDS	material safety data sheet
MUGA	multi-gated acquisition
N_2	nitrogen
Na	sodium
Na^+	sodium ion
Na_2SO_4	sodium sulfate
NaCl	sodium chloride
NA	not applicable
NADSA	National Adult Day Services Associations
NaH_2PO_4	sodium dihydrogen phosphate
Na_2HPO_4	disodium phosphate
NAHC	National Association for Home Care
$NaHCO_3$	sodium bicarbonate
$NaHPO_4$	sodium monohydrogen phosphate
NANDA	North American Nursing Diagnosis Association
NaOH	sodium hydroxide
NAPNE	Natonal Association of Practical Nurse Education
NAPNES	National Association for Practical Nurse Education and Services
NCCAM	National Center for Complementary and Alternative Medicine
NCHS	National Center for Health Statistics
NCLEX®	National Council Licensure Examination
NCLEX-PN®	National Council Licensure Examination—Practical Nurse
NCLEX-RN®	National Council Licensure Examination—Registered Nurse
NCLD	National Center for Learning Disabilities
NCOA	National Council on Aging
NCSBN	National Council of State Boards of Nursing
NCVHS	National Committee on Vital and Health Statistics
NF	*National Formulary*
NFLPN	National Federation of Licensed Practical Nurses, Inc.
NG	nasogastric
NH_2	amino group
NHO	National Hospice Organization
NIA	National Institute on Aging
NIC	Nursing Interventions Classification
NIH	National Institutes of Health
NIOSH	National Institute of Occupational Safety and Health
NIS	nursing information system
NLEA	Nutrition, Labeling, and Education Act
NLN	National League for Nursing
NLNAC	National League for Nursing Accrediting Commission
NMDS	nursing minimum data set
NOC	Nursing Outcomes Classification
NP	nurse practitioner
NPDB	National Practitioner Data Bank
NPO	*nil per os*, Latin for "nothing by mouth"
NREM	non-rapid eye movement
NS	normal saline
NSAID	nonsteroidal anti-inflammatory drug
NSF	National Sleep Foundation
O_2	oxygen
OAM	Office of Alternative Medicine
O&P	ova and parasite
OBRA	Omnibus Budget Reconciliation Act
OD	right eye
OH^-	hydroxyl
OR	operating room
ORIF	open reduction/internal fixation
OS	left eye
OSHA	Occupational Safety and Health Administration
OT	occupational therapist
OT	oral temperature

OTC over-the-counter
OU both eyes
oz ounce
p̄ after
P phosphorus
P pulse
PA physician's assistant
PA posterioanterior
$PaCO_2$ partial pressure of carbon dioxide
PaO_2 partial pressure of oxygen
Pap Papanicolaou test
p.c. after meals
PCA patient-controlled analgesia
PCO_2 ($PaCO_2$) partial pressure of carbon dioxide
PCP primary care provider
PCR polymerase chain reaction
PCV pneumococcal conjugate vaccine
PDPH postdural puncture headache
PEG percutaneous endoscopic gastrostomy
PERRLA pupils equal, round, reactive to light and accommodation
PET positron emission tomography
PFT pulmonary function test
pH potential hydrogen
PICC peripherally inserted central catheter
PIE problem, implementation, evaluation
PKU phenylketonuria
PLMS periodic limb movements in sleep
PMI point of maximum intensity
PMR progressive muscle relaxation
PMS premenstrual syndrome
PNI psychoneuroimmunology
PNS peripheral nervous system
po *per os,* Latin for "by mouth"
PO_2 (PaO_2) partial pressure of oxygen
PO_4^{--} phosphate ion
POMR problem-oriented medical record
POR problem-oriented record
PPBS post prandial blood sugar
PPE personal protective equipment
PPG post prandial glucose
PPO preferred provider organization
PPS prospective payment system
PRA plama renin activity
PRL prolactin level
PRN *pro re nata,* Latin for "as required"
PRO peer review organization
PROM passive range of motion
PSA prostate specific antigen
PSDA Patient Self-Determination Act
PSP phenolsulfonphtalein
pt pint
PT physical therapist
PT prothrombin time
PTH parathyroid hormone
PTSD post-traumatic stress disorder
PTT partial thromboplastin time
PVD peripheral vascular disease
q *quaque,* Latin for "every"
qd every day
qh every hour
qid four times a day
qod every other day
qs quantity sufficient
q2h every 2 hours
qt quart
R (Resp) respiration
RAIU radioactive iodine uptake
RAST radio allergosorbent test
RBC red blood count, red blood cell
RD registered dietician
RDA recommended dietary allowance
REM rapid eye movement
RF rheumatoid factor
RLQ right lower quadrant
RLS restless leg syndrome
RN registered nurse
RNA ribonucleic acid
RNFA registered nurse first assistant
ROM range of motion
ROS review of systems
RPCH rural primary care hospital
RPh registered pharmacist
RPR rapid plasma reagin
RR recovery room
RSV respiratory syncytial virus
R/T related to
RT rectal temperature
RT respiratory therapist
RTI respiratory tract infection
RUGS resource utilization group system
RUQ right upper quadrant
RWJF Robert Wood Johnson Foundation
s̄ without
S sulfur
SAMe S-adenosylmethionine
SaO_2 oxygen saturation
SBC school-based clinic
SC/SQ subcutaneous
SCHIP State Children's Health Insurance Program
Se selenium
SGOT serum glutamate oxaloacetate transaminase
SGPT serum glutamic pyruvic transaminase
SL sublingual
SNF skilled nursing facility
SOAP subjective data, objective data, assessment, plan
SOAPIE subjective data, objective data, assessment, plan, implementation, evaluation
SOAPIER subjective data, objective data, assessment, plan, implementation, evaluation, revision
SPF sun protection factor
s̄s̄ one half
SSA Social Security Administration
STAT *statim,* Latin for "immediately"
STD sexually transmitted disease

supp suppository
susp suspension
SW social worker
T temperature
T_3 triiodothyronine
T_4 thyroxine
tab tablet
TAC tetracaine, adrenaline, cocaine
TB tuberculosis
Tbsp tablespoon
Td tetanus/diphtheria
TDD telecommunication device for the deaf
TEFRA Tax Equity Fiscal Responsibility Act
TENS transcutaneous electrical nerve stimulation
TF tube feeding
THA total hip arthroplasty
TIA transient ischemic attack
TIBC total iron binding capacity
t.i.d. three times a day
TMJ temporomandibular joint
t.o. telephone order
TPN total parenteral nutrition
TPR temperature, pulse, respirations
Tr or tinct tincture
TRH thyrotropin-releasing hormone
TSE testicular self examination
TSH thyroid-stimulating hormone
tsp teaspoon
U unit
U/L unit per liter
UA routine urinalysis
UAP unlicensed assistive personnel
UIS Universal Intellectual Standards
UL upper intake level
UMLS Universal Medical Language System
UNOS United Network for Organ Sharing
U-100 100 units insulin per cc
UPP urethra pressure profile
URQ upper right quadrant
USDHHS United States Department of Health and Human Services
USP *United States Pharmacopeia*
USPHS United States Public Health Service
UTI urinary tract infection
VA Veterans Administration, Veterans Affairs
VAD ventricular assist device, vascular access device
VAS Visual Analog Scale
VDRL venereal disease research laboratory
VLDL very low-density lipoprotein
VMA vanilymandelic acid
VRE vancomycin-resistant enterococci
VS vital signs
WASP white, Anglo-Saxon, Protestant
WBC white blood cell, white blood count
WHO World Health Organization
WNL within normal limits
WPM words per minute
wt weight
YWCA Young Women's Christian Association
Zn Zinc

APPENDIX D
English/Spanish Words and Phrases

Being able to say a few words or phrases in the client's language is one way to show that you care. It lets the client know that you as a nurse are interested in the individual. There are three rules to keep in mind regarding the pronunciation of Spanish words.

- If a word ends in a vowel, or in *n* or *s,* the accent is on the next to the last syllable.
- If the word ends in a consonant other than *n* or *s,* the accent is on the last syllable.
- If the word does not follow these rules, it has a written accent over the vowel of the accented syllable.

Courtesy phrases, names of body parts, and expressions of time and numbers are included in this section for quick reference. The English version will appear first, followed by the Spanish translation and Spanish pronunciation.

Courtesy Phrases

Please	Por favor	Por fah-**vor**
Thank-you	Grácias	**Grah**-the-as
Good morning	Buénos dias	Boo-**ay**-nos **dee**-as
Good afternoon	Buénas tardes	Boo-**ay** nas **tar**-days
Good evening	Buénas noches	Boo-**ay**-nas **no**-chays
Yes/No	Si/no	See/no
Good	Bien	Be-en
Bad	Mal	Mahl
How many?	¿Cuántos?	¿Coo-**ahn**-tos?
Where?	¿Dónde?	¿**Don**-day?
When?	¿Cuándo?	¿Coo**ahn**-do?

Body Parts

abdomen	el abdomen	el ab-doh-men
ankle	el tobillo	el to-**beel**-lyo
anus	el ano	el **ah**-no
anvil (incus)	el yunque	el **yoon**-kay
appendix	el apéndice	el ah-**pen**-de-thay
aqueous humor	el humor acuoso	el oo-**mor** ah-coo-**o**-so
bladder	la vejiga	lah vay-**nee**-gah
brain	el cerebro	el thay-**ray**-bro
breast	el pecho	el **pay**-cho
buttock	la nalga	lah **nahl**-gah
calf	la pantorrilla	lah pan-tor-**reel**-lyah
cervix	la cerviz	lah ther-**veth**
cheek	la mejilla	lah may-**heel**-lyah

chin	la barbilla	lah bar-**beel**-lyah
choroid	la coroidea	lah co-ro-e-**day**-ah
ciliary body	el cuerpo ciliar	el coo-**err**-po the-le-**ar**
clitoris	el clítoris	el **clee**-to-ris
coccyx	el coxis	el **coc**-sees
conjunctiva	la conjuntiva	lah con-hoon-**tee**vah
cornea	la córnea	lah **cor**-nay-ah
penis	el pene	el **pay**-nay
prostate gland	la próstata	lah **pros**-ta-tah
pupil	la pupila	lah poo-**pee**-lah
rectum	el recto	el **rec**-to
retina	la retina	lah ray-**tee**-nah
sclera	la esclerótica	lah es-clay-**ro**-te-cah
scrotum	el escroto	el es-**cro**-to
seminal vesicle	la vesícula seminal	lah vay-**see**-coo-lah say-me-**nahl**
shoulder	el hombro	el **om**-bro
small intestine	el intestino delgado	el in-tes-**tee**-no del-**gah**-do
spinal cord	la médula espinal	lah **may**-doo-lah es-pe-**nahl**
spleen	el bazo	el **bah**-tho
stirrup (stapes)	el estribo	el es-**tree**-bo
stomach	el estómago	el es-**toh**-mah-go
temple	la sien	lah se-**ayn**
testis	el testículo	el tes-**tee**-coo-lo
thigh	el muslo	el **moos**-lo
thorax	el tórax	el **to**-rax
tongue	la lengua	lah **len**-goo-ah
trachea	la tráquea	lah **trah**-kay-ah
upper extremities	las extremidades superiores	las ex-tray-me-**dahd**-es soo-pay-re-**or**-es
ureter	el uréter	el oo-**ray**-ter
uterus	el útero	el **oo**-tay-ro
vagina	el vagina	lah vah-**hee**-nah
vitreous humor	el humor vítreo	el oo-**mor vee**-tray-o
wrist	la muñeca	lah moo-**nyay**-cah

Expressions of Time, Calendar, and Numbers

after meals	después de comer	des-poo-**es** day co-**merr**
at bedtime	al acostarse	al ah-cos-**tar**-say
before meals	antes de comer	**ahn**-tes day co-**merr**
daily	el diario	el de-**ah**-re-o
date	la fecha	lah **fay**-chah
day	el dia	el **dee**-ah
every hour	a cada hora	ah **cah**-dah **o**-rah
hour (time)	la hora	lah **o**-rah
how often	cada cuánto tiempo	**cah**-dah coo-**ahn**-to te-**em**-po
noon	el mediodia	el may-de-o-**dee**-ah
now	ahora	ah-**o**-rah
once	una vez	**oo**-nah veth
today	hoy	**oh**-e
tomorrow	mañana	mah-**nyah**-nah
tonight	esta noche	**es**-tah **no**-chay
week	la semana	lah say-**mah**-nah
year	año	**a**-nyo
Sunday	el domingo	el do-**meen**-go
Monday	el lunes	el **loo**-nes
Tuesday	el martes	el **mar**-tes
Wednesday	el miércoles	el me-**err**-co-les
Thursday	el jueves	el hoo-**ay**ves
Friday	el viernes	el ve-**err**-nes

Saturday	el sábado	el **sah**-bah-do
zero	cero	**thay**-ro
one	uno	**oo**-no
two	dos	dose
three	tres	trays
four	cuatro	coo-**ah**-tro
five	cinco	**theen**-co
six	seis	**say**-ees
seven	siete	se-**ay**-tay
eight	ocho	**o**-cho
nine	nueve	noo-**ay**-vay
ten	diez	de-**eth**

Nursing Care Sentences and Questions

What is your name?
¿Como se llama usted?
¿**Co**-mo say **lyah**-mah oos-**ted?**

I am a student nurse.
Soy estudiente enfermera(o).
Soy es-too-de-**ahn**-tay en-fer-**may**-ra(o).

My name is . . .
Mi nombre es . . .
Mee **nom**-bray es . . .

Do you need a wheelchair?
¿Necesita usted una silla de rueda?
¿Nay-thay-**se**-ta oos-**ted oo**-nah **seel**-lyah day roo-**ay**-dah?

How do you feel?
¿Como se siente?
¿**Co**-mo say se-**ayn**-tah?

When is your family coming?
¿Cuándo viene su familia?
¿Coo-**ahn**-do vee-**en**-nah soo fah-**mee**-le-ah?

This is the call light.
Esta es la luz para llamar a la enfermera.
Es-tah es lah looth **pah**-ra lyah-**mar** a lah en-fer-**may**-ra.

If you need anything, press the button.
Si usted necesita algo, oprima el botón.
See oos-**ted** nay-thay-**se**-ta **ahl**-go o-pre-**ma** el bo-**tone.**

Do not turn without calling the nurse.
No se voltee sin llamar a la enfermera.
No say **vol**-tay seen lyah-**mar** a lah en-fer-**may**-ra.

The side rails on your bed are for your protection.
Los rieles del costado están para su protección.
Los re-**el**-es del cos-**tah**-do es-**tahn pah**-ra soo pro-tec-the-**on.**

Please do not try to lower or climb over the side rail.
Por favor no pretenda bajarlos (barjarlas) o treparse sobre ellos.
Por fah-**vor** no pray-**ten**-dah ba-**har**-los o tray-**par**-say **so**-bray **ayl**-lyos.

The head nurse is . . .
La jefa de enfermeras es . . .
La **hay**-fay day en-fer-**may**-ras es . . .

Do you need more blankets or another pillow?
¿Necesita usted más frazadas u orta almohada?
¿Nay-thay-**si**-ta oos-**ted** mahs frah-**thad**-dahs oo **o** trah al mo **ah**-dah?

You may not smoke in the room.
No se puede fumar en el cuarto.
No say poo-**ay**-day foo-**mar** en el coo-**ar**-to.

Do you want me to turn on (turn off) the lights?
¿Quiere usted que encienda (apague) la luz?
¿Ke-**ay**-ray oos-**ted** day en-the-**en**-dah (a-**pah**-gay) lah looth?

Are you thirsty?
¿Tiene usted sed?
¿Tee-**en**-nah oos-**ted** sayd?

Are you allergic to any medication?
¿Es usted alérgico(a) a alguna medicina?
¿Es oos-**ted** ah-**lehr**-hee-co(a) ah ah-**goo**-nah nay-de-**thee**-nah?

You may take a bath.
Usted puede bañarse.
Oos-**ted** poo-**ay**-day bah-**nyar**-say.

Do not lock the door, please.
No cierre usted la puerta con llave, por favor.
No the-**err**-ray oos-**ted** lah poo-**err**-tah con **lyah**-vay por fah-**vor.**

Call if you feel faint or in need of help.
Llame si usted se siente débil o si necesita ayuda.
Lyah-mah see oos-**ted** say se-**ayn**-tah **day**-bil o see nay-thay-**se**-ta ah-**yoo**-dah.

Call when you have to go to the toilet.
Llame cuando tenga que ir al inodoro.
Lyah-mah coo-**ahn**-do **ten**-gah kay eer al in-o-**do**-ro.

I will give you an enema.
Le pondré una enema.
Lay pon-**dray oo**-nah ay-**nay**-mah.

Turn on your left (right) side.
Voltese a su lado izquierdo (derecho).
Vol-**tay**-say ah soo **lah**-do ith-ke-**er**-do(dah) (day-**ray**-cho[cha]).

Here is an appointment card.
Aqui tiene usted una tarjeta con la información escrito.
Ah-**kee** tee-**en**-nah oos-**ted oo**-nah tar-**hay**-tah con lah in-for-mah-the-**on** es-**cree**-to.

You are going to be discharged (released) today.
A usted le van a dar de alta hoy.
Ah oos-**ted** lay vahn ah dar day **ahl**-tah **oh**-e.

How did this illness begin?
¿Como empezó esta enfermedad?
¿**Co**-mo em-pa-**tho es**-tah en-fer-may-**dahd**?

Is the pain better after the medicine?
¿Siente usted alivio depués de tomar la medicina?
¿Se-**ayn**-tah oos-**ted** al-**lee**-ve-o des-poo-**es** day to-**mar** lah may-de-**thee**-nah?

Where is the pain?
¿Que la duele? (or) Dónde le duele?
¿Kay lah doo-**ay**-le? (or) **Don**-day lay doo-**ay**-le?

Do you have pains in your chest?
¿Tiene usted dolores in el pecho?
¿Tee-**en**-nah oos-**ted** do-**lor**-es en el **pay**-cho?

Are you in pain now?
¿Tiene usted dolores ahora?
¿Tee-**en**-nah oos-**ted** do-**lor**-es ah-**o**-rah?

Is it constant pain or does it come and go?
¿Es un dolor constante o va y vuelve?
¿Es oon do-**lor** cons-**tahn**-tay o vah ee voo-**el**-vah?

Is there anything that makes the pain better?
¿Hay algo que lo alivie?
¿**Ah**-ee **ahl**-go kay lo al-**le**-ve?

Is there anything that makes the pain worse?
¿Hay algo que lo aumente?
¿**Ah**-ee **ahl**-go kay lo ah-oo-**men**-tay?

Where do you feel the pain?
¿Dónde siente usted el dolor?
¿**Don**-day se-**ayn**-tah oos-**ted** el do-**lor**?

Point to where it hurts.
Apunte usted por favor, adonde le duele.
Ah-**poon**-tay oos-**ted** por fah-**vor** ah-**don**-day lay doo-**ay**-le.

Show me where it hurts.
Enséñeme usted donde le duele.
En-**say**-nah-may oos-**ted don**-day lay doo-**ay**-le.

Is the pain sharp or dull?
¿Es agudo o sordo el dolor?
¿Es ah-**goo**-do o **sor**-do el do-**lor**?

Do you know where you are?
¿Sabe usted donde esta?
¿Sah-**bay** oos-**ted don**-day es-**tah**?

You are in the hospital.
Usted está en el hospital.
Oos-**ted** es-**tah** en el os-pee-**tahl**.

You will be okay.
Usted va a estar bien.
Oos-**ted** vah a es-**tar be**-en.

Do you have any drug reactions?
¿Tiene usted alguna sensibilidad a productos químicos?
¿Te-**en**-nah oos-**ted** al-**goo**-nah sen-se-be-le-**dahd** a pro-**dooc**-tos **kee**-me-cos?

Have you seen another doctor or native healer for this problem?
¿Ha visto usted a otro médico o curandero tocante a este problema?
¿Ah **vees**-to oos-**ted** a **o**-tro **may**-de-co o coo-ran-**day**-ro to-**cahn**-tay a **es**-ah pro-**blay**-mah?

Have you vomited?
¿Ha vomitado usted?
¿Ah vo-me-**tah**-do oos-**ted**?

Do you have any difficulty in breathing?
¿Tiene usted alguna dificultad para respirar?
¿Te-**en**-nah oos-**ted** ah-**goo**-nah de-fe-cool-**tahd pah**-ra res-pe-**rar**?

Do you smoke?
¿Fuma usted?
¿Foo-**mar** oos-**ted**?

How many per day?
¿Cuántos al dia?
¿Coo-**ahn**-tos al **dee**-ah?

For how many years?
¿Por cuántos años?
¿por coo-**ahn**-tos **a**-nyos?

Do you awaken in the night because of shortness of breath?
¿Se despierta usted por la noche por falta de respiración?
¿Say des-pee-**err**-tah oos-**ted** por lah **no**-chay por **fahl**-tah day res-pe-rah-the-**on**?

Is any part of your body swollen?
¿Tiene usted alguna parte del cuerpo hinchada?
¿Te-**en**-nah oos-**ted** ah-**goo**-nah **par**-tay del coo-**err**-po in-**chah**-da?

How much water do you drink daily?
¿Cuántos vasos de agua bebe usted diariamente?
¿Coo-**ahn**-tos **vah**-sos day **ah**-goo-ah **bay**-be oos-**ted** de-ah-re-ah-**men**-tay?

Are you nauseated?
¿Tiene náusea?
¿Te-**en**-nah **nah**-oo-say-ah?

Are you going to vomit?
¿Va a vomitar?
¿Vah a vo-me-**tar**?

When was your last bowel movement?
¿Cuánto tiempo hace que evacúa usted?
¿Coo-**ahn**-to te-**em**-po **ah**-the kay ay-vah-**coo**-ah oos-**ted**?

Do you have diarrhea?
¿Tiene usted diarrea?
¿Te-**en**-nah oos-**ted** der-ar-**ray**-ah?

How much do you urinate?
¿Cuánto orina usted?
¿Coo-**ahn**-to o-**re**-nah oos-**ted**?

Did you urinate?
¿Orinó usted?
¿O-re-**no** oos-**ted**?

What color is your urine?
¿De qué color es la orina?
¿Day kay co-**lor** es lah o-**re**-nah?

Call when you have to go to the toilet.
Llame usted cuando tenga que ir al inodoro.
Lyah-mah oos-**ted** coo-**ahn**-do **ten**-gah kay eer al in-o-**do**-ro.

I need a urine specimen from you.
Necesito una muestra de orina de usted.
Nay-thay-**se**-to **oo**-nah moo-**ays**-trah day o-**re**-nah day oos-**ted**.

We will put a tube in your bladder so that you can urinate.
Le pondremos un tubo en la vejiga para que puede orinar.
Lay pon-**dray**-mos un **too**-be en lah vay-**hee**-gah **pah**-rah kay poo-**ay**-day o-re **nar.**

When was your last menstrual period?
¿Cuándo fue se última menstruación?
¿Coo-**ahn**-do foo-**ay** soo **ool**-te-mah mens-troo-ah-the-**on?**

Are you bleeding heavily?
¿Está sangrando mucho?
¿Es-**tah** san-**grahn**-do **moo**-cho?

Take off your clothes, please
Desvístase usted, por favor.
Des-**ves**-tah-say oos-**ted** por-fah-**vor.**

Just relax.
Relaje usted el cuerpo.
Ray-**lah**-he oos-**ted** el coo-**err**-po.

I am going to listen to your chest.
Voy a escucharle el pecho.
Voye a es-coo-**char**-lay el **pay**-cho.

Let me feel your pulse.
Déjeme tomarle el pulso.
Day-ha-me to-**bar**-lay el **pool**-so.

I am going to take your temperature.
Voy a tomarle la temperatura.
Voye a to-**mar**-lay lah tem-pay-rah-**too**-rah.

Lie down, please.
Acuéstese, por favor.
Ah-coo-**es**-tah-say por fah-**vor.**

Do you understand?
¿Me comprende usted?
¿May com-**pren**-day oos-**ted?**

That's right.
Así. Bien.
Ah-**see. Be**-en.

You are doing very well.
Usted va muy bien.
Oos-**ted** vah **moo**-e **be**-en.

Do not take any medicine from home.
No tome usted ninguna medicina traída de su casa.
No **to**-may oos-**ted** nin-**goon**-ay may-de-**thee**-nah trah-**ee**-dah day soo **cah**-sah.

I am going to give you an injection.
Voy a ponerle ana inyección.
Voye a po-**nerr**-lay **oo**-nah in-yec-the-**on.**

Take a sip of water.
Tome usted un traguito de agua.
To-may oos-**ted** un trah-**gee**-to day **ah**-goo-ah.

Very good. That was fine.
Muy bien. Excelente.
Moo-e **be**-en. Ex-thay-**len**-tay.

Don't be nervous.
No se ponga nervioso(a).
No say **pon**-gah ner-ve-**o**-so(ah).

Do you feel dizzy?
¿Se siente vertigo?
¿Say see-**ayn**-tah **verr**-to-go?

Please lie still.
Quédese inmóvil, por favor.
Kay-day-say in-**mo**-veel por fah-**vor.**

You must drink lots of liquids.
Usted debe tomar muchos líquidos.
Oos-**ted day**-bay to-**mar moo**-chos **lee**-ke-dos.

References

Kelz, R. K. (1982.) *Conversational Spanish for Medical Personnel.* Clifton Park, NY: Delmar Cengage Learning.

Velazquez de la Cadena, M., Gray, E., & Iribas, J. (1985). *New Revised Velazquez Spanish and English Dictionary.* Clinton, NJ: New Win Publishing, Inc.

GLOSSARY

A

abduction Lateral movement away from the body

ability Competence in an activity

abortion Termination of pregnancy before the age of fetal viability, usually 24 weeks

abruptio placenta Premature separation, from the wall of the uterus, of normally implanted placenta

absorption Passage of a drug from the site of administration into the bloodstream; process whereby the end products of digestion pass through the epithelial membranes in the small and large intestines and into the blood or lymph system

abuse Incident involving some type of violation to the client; misuse, excessive, or improper use of a substance, the absence of which does not cause withdrawal symptoms

acanthosis nigricans A velvety hyperpigmented patch on the back of neck, in axilla, or anticubital area found in children with type 2 diabetes

accreditation Process by which a voluntary, nongovernmental agency or organization appraises and grants accredited status to institutions, programs, services, or any combination of these that meet predetermined structure, process, and outcome criteria

acculturation Process of learning beliefs, norms, and behavioral expectations of a group

acid Any substance that in a solution yields hydrogen ions bearing a positive charge

acidosis Condition characterized by an excessive number of hydrogen ions in a solution

acme Peak of a contraction

acquired immunity Formation of antibodies (memory B cells) to protect against future invasions of an already experienced antigen

acquired immunodeficiency syndrome (AIDS) Progressively fatal disease that destroys the immune system and the body's ability to fight infection; caused by the human immunodeficiency virus (HIV)

acrocyanosis Blue coloring of hands and feet

actively suicidal Descriptor of an individual intent upon hurting or killing him- or herself and who is in imminent danger of doing so

activities of daily living Basic care activities that include mobility, bathing, hygiene, grooming, dressing, eating, and toileting

acupressure Technique of releasing blocked energy within an individual when specific points (tsubas) along the meridians are pressed or massaged by the practitioner's fingers, thumbs, and heel of the hands

acupuncture Technique of application of needles and heat to various points on the body to alter the energy flow

acute pain Has a sudden onset, relatively short duration, mild to severe intensity, with a steady decrease in intensity over several days or weeks

adaptation Ongoing process whereby individuals use various responses to adjust to stressors and change; change resulting from assimilation and accommodation

adaptive energy Inner forces that an individual uses to adapt to stress (phrase coined by Selye)

adaptive measure Measure for coping with stress that requires a minimal amount of energy

addiction Overwhelming preoccupation with obtaining and using a drug for its psychic effects; used interchangeably with dependence

adhesion Internal scar tissue from previous surgeries or disease processes

adjuvant medication Drug used to enhance the analgesic efficacy of opioids, treat concurrent symptoms that exacerbate pain, and provide independent analgesia for specific types of pain

adult day care Centers that provide a variety of services in a protective setting for adults who are unable to stay alone but who do not need 24-hour care; the centers are located in a separate unit of a long-term care facility, in a private home, or are freestanding

adventitious breath sound Abnormal sound, including sibilant wheezes (formerly wheezes), sonorous wheezes (formerly rhonchi), fine and course crackles (formerly rales), pleural friction rubs, and stridor

affect Outward expression of mood or emotions

affective domain Area of learning that involves attitudes, beliefs, and emotions

afferent nerve pathway Ascending spinal cord pathway that transmits sensory impulses to the brain

afferent pain pathway Ascending spinal cord

afterpains Discomfort caused by the contracting uterus after the infant's birth

age appropriate care Nursing care that takes into consideration the client's physical, mental, emotional, and spiritual developmental levels

age of viability Gestational age at which a fetus could live outside the uterus, generally considered to be 24 weeks

agent Entity capable of causing disease

agglutination Clumping together of red blood cells

agglutinin Specific kind of antibody whose interaction with antigens is manifested as agglutination

agglutinogen Any antigenic substance that causes agglutination by the production of agglutinin

agnosia Inability to recognize, either by sight or sound, familiar objects such as a hairbrush

agnostic Individual who believes that the existence of God cannot be proved or disproved

agranulocytosis Acute condition causing a severe reduction in the number of granulocytes (basophils, eosinophils, and neutrophils)

Airborne Precautions Measures taken in addition to Standard Precautions and for clients known to have or suspected of having illnesses spread by airborne droplet nuclei

airborne transmission Transfer of an agent to a susceptible host through droplet nuclei or dust particles suspended in the air

Aldrete Score Scoring system for objectively assessing the physical status of clients recovering from anesthesia; serves as a basis for dismissal from the postanesthesia care unit (PACU) and ambulatory surgery; also known as the postanesthetic recovery score

algor mortis Decrease in body temperature after death, resulting in lack of skin elasticity

alkalosis Condition characterized by an excessive loss of hydrogen ions from a solution

allergen Type of antigen commonly found in the environment

allogeneic From a donor of the same species

alopecia Partial or complete baldness or loss of hair

alternative therapy Therapy used instead of conventional or mainstream medical practices

ambulatory care A facility that provides clients diagnostic treatment, medical treatment, preventive care, and rehabilitative care on an outpatient basis

ambulatory surgery Surgical operation performed under general, regional, or local anesthesia, involving less than 24 hours of hospitalization

amenorrhea Absence of menstruation

amnesia Inability to remember things

amniocentesis Withdrawal of amniotic fluid to obtain a sample for specimen examination

amnion Inner fetal membrane originating in the blastocyst

amniotomy Artificial rupture of the membranes

amphiarthrosis Articulation of slightly movable joints such as the vertebrae

amputation Removal of all or part of an extremity

anabolism Constructive process of metabolism whereby new molecules are synthesized and new tissues are formed, as in growth and repair

analgesia Pain relief without producing anesthesia

analgesic Substance that relieves pain

analyte Substance that is measured

anaphylaxis Type I systemic reaction to allergens

anasarca Generalized edema

anesthesia Absence of normal sensation

anesthesiologist Licensed physician educated and skilled in the delivery of anesthesia who also adds to the knowledge of anesthesia through research or other scholarly pursuits

anesthetist Qualified RN, dentist, or medical doctor who administers anesthetics

aneurysm Weakness in the wall of a blood vessel

anger control assistance Nursing intervention aimed at facilitating the expression of anger in an adaptive and nonviolent manner

angina pectoris Chest pain caused by a narrowing of the coronary arteries

angiocatheter Intracatheter with a metal stylet

angioedema Allergic reaction consisting of edema of subcutaneous tissue, mucous membranes, or viscera

angiogenesis Formation of new blood vessels

angiography Visualization of the vascular structures through the use of fluoroscopy with a contrast medium

angioma Benign vascular tumor involving skin and subcutaneous tissue; most are congenital

anion Ion bearing a negative charge

annulus Valvular ring in the heart
anorexia Loss of appetite
anosognosia Lack of awareness of own neurological deficits
anthrax An acute, infectious disease caused by the bacterium Bacillus anthracis, which has an incubation period of 2-60 days; it is an Important potential agent for bioterrorism
anthropometric measurements Measurements of the size, weight, and proportions of the body
antibody Immunoglobulin produced by the body in response to bacteria, viruses, or other antigenic substances; destroys antigens
anticipatory grief Occurrence of grief before an expected loss actually occurs
anticipatory guidance Information, teaching, and guidance given to a client in anticipation of an expected event
antigen Any substance identified by the body as nonself
antineoplastic Agent that inhibits the growth and reproduction of malignant cells
antioxidant Substance that prevents or inhibits oxidation, a chemical process wherein a substance is joined to oxygen
antipyretic Drug used to reduce an abnormally high temperature
anxiety Subjective response that occurs when a person experiences a real or perceived threat to well-being; a diverse feeling of dread or apprehension
anxiolytic Antianxiety medication
aphasia Absence of speech; often the result of a brain lesion
apheresis Removal of unwanted blood components
appendicitis Inflammation of the vermiform appendix
appropriate for gestational age Infant's weight falls between the 90th and 10th percentile for gestational age
areflexia Absence of reflexes
aromatherapy Therapeutic use of concentrated essences or essential oils extracted from plants and flowers
arousal State of wakefulness and alertness
arterial blood gases Measurement of levels of oxygen, carbon dioxide, pH, partial pressure of oxygen (PO2 or PaO2), partial pressure of carbon dioxide (PCO2 or PaCO2), saturation of oxygen (SaO2), and bicarbonate (HCO3) in arterial blood
arteriography Radiographic study of the vascular system following the injection of a radiopaque dye through a catheter
arteriosclerosis Cardiovascular disease wherein plaque forms on the inside of artery walls, reducing the space for blood flow
arthroplasty Replacement of both articular surfaces within a joint capsule
ascites Abnormal accumulation of fluid in the peritoneal cavity
asepsis Absence of pathogenic microorganisms
aseptic technique Collection of principles used to control and/or prevent the transfer of pathogenic microorganisms from sources within (endogenous) and outside (exogenous) the client
aspiration Procedure performed to withdraw fluid that has abnormally collected or to obtain a specimen; also inhalation of secretion or fluids into the pulmonary system
assent Voluntary agreement to participate in a research project or to accept treatment
assisted living A facility that combines housing and services for persons who require assistance with activities of daily living
asthma Condition characterized by intermittent airway obstruction due to antigen antibody reaction
astigmatism Asymmetric focus of light rays on the retina
ataxia Inability to coordinate voluntary muscle action
atelectasis Collapse of a lung or a portion of a lung
atheist Individual who does not believe in God or any other deity
atherosclerosis Cardiovascular disease of fatty deposits on the inner lining, the tunica intima, of vessel walls
atom Smallest unit of an element that still retains the properties of that element and that cannot be altered by any chemical change
atresia Absence or closure of a body orifice
attachment Long-term process that begins during pregnancy and intensifies during the postpartum period, which establishes an enduring bond between parent and child, and develops through reciprocal (parent-to-child and child-to-parent) behaviors
attitude Manner, feeling, or position toward a person or thing
attribute Characteristic that belongs to an individual
audible wheeze Wheeze that can be heard without the aid of a stethoscope
auditory hallucination Perception by an individual that someone is talking when no one in fact is there
auditory learner Person who learns by processing information through hearing
augmentation of labor Stimulation of uterine contractions after spontaneously beginning but having unsatisfactory progress of labor
aura Peculiar sensation preceding a seizure or migraine; may be a taste, smell, sight, sound, dizziness, or just a "funny feeling"

auscultation Physical examination technique that involves listening to sounds in the body that are created by movement of air or fluid
autoimmune disorder Disease wherein the body identifies its own cells as foreign and activates mechanisms to destroy them
autologous From the same organism (person)
automatism Mechanical, repetitive motor behavior performed unconsciously
autonomic nervous system That part of the peripheral nervous system consisting of the sympathetic and parasympathetic nervous systems and controlling unconscious activities
autonomy Self-direction; ethical principle based on the individual's right to choose and the individual's ability to act on that choice
autopsy Examination of a body after death by a pathologist to determine cause of death
autosomal Pertaining to a condition transmitted by a nonsex chromosome
awareness Capacity to perceive sensory impressions through thoughts and actions
azotemia Nitrogenous wastes present in the blood

B

bacteremia Condition of bacteria in the blood
bactericide Bacteria-killing chemicals; found in tears
ballottement Rebounding of the floating fetus when pushed upward through the vagina or abdomen
bands Immature neutrophils
barium Chalky-white contrast medium
Barrier Precautions Use of personal protective equipment, such as masks, gowns, and gloves, to create a barrier between the person and the microorganisms and thus prevent transmission of the microorganism
basal metabolism Energy needed to maintain essential physiologic functions when a person is at complete rest; the lowest level of energy expenditure
base Substance that when dissociated produces ions that will combine with hydrogen ions
baseline level Lab value that serves as a reference point for future value levels
behavioral tolerance Compensatory adjustments of behavior made under the influence of a particular substance
benign Not progressive; favorable for recovery
bereavement Period of grief that follows the death of a loved one
bioavailability Readiness to produce a drug effect
biofeedback Measures physiologic responses that assist individuals to improve their health by using signals from their own bodies
biologic response modifier Agent that destroys malignant cells by stimulating the body's immune system
biological agent Living organism that invades a host, causing disease
biological clock Internal mechanism in a living organism capable of measuring time
biopsy Excision of a small amount of tissue
bioterrorism the purposeful use of a biological preparation for the purposes of harming, killing large numbers of people, and/or instilling fear in large numbers of people
blanching White color of the skin when pressure is applied
blastic phase Intensified phase of leukemia that resembles an acute phase in which there is an increased production of white blood cells
blastocyst Cluster of cells that will develop into the embryo
bloody show Expulsion of cervical secretions, blood-tinged mucus, and the mucus plug that blocked the cervix during pregnancy
body image Individual's perception of physical self, including appearance, function, and ability
body mass index Measurement used to ascertain whether a person's weight is appropriate for height; calculated by dividing the weight in kilograms by the height in meters squared
body mechanics Use of the body to safely and efficiently move or lift objects
bodymind Inseparable connection and operation of thoughts, feelings, and physiologic functions
bonding Rapid process of attachment, parent to infant, that takes place during the sensitive period, the first 30 to 60 minutes after birth
borborygmi High-pitched, loud, rushing sounds produced by the movement of gas in the liquid contents of the intestine
bradycardia Heart rate less than 60 beats per minute in an adult
bradykinesia Slowness of voluntary movement and speech
bradypnea Respiratory rate of 10 or fewer breaths per minute
Braxton-Hicks contractions Irregular, intermittent contractions felt by the pregnant woman toward the end of pregnancy
breakthrough pain Sudden, acute, temporary pain that is usually precipitated by a treatment, a procedure, or unusual activity of the client
brief dynamic therapy Short-term psychotherapy that focuses on resolving core conflicts deriving from personality and living situations

bronchial sound Loud, high-pitched, hollow-sounding breath sound normally heard over the sternum; longer on expiration than inspiration
bronchiectasis Lung disorder characterized by chronic dilation of the bronchi
bronchitis Inflammation of the bronchial tree accompanied by hypersecretion of mucus
bronchovesicular sound Breath sound normally heard in the area of the scapula and near the sternum; medium in pitched blowing sound, with inspiratory and expiratory phases of equal length
bruxism Grinding of teeth during sleep
buffer Substance that attempts to maintain pH range, or hydrogen ion concentration, in the presence of added acids or bases
burnout State of physical and emotional exhaustion occurring when caregivers use up their adaptive energy
butterfly needle Wing tipped needle

C

cachectic Being in a state of malnutrition and wasting
cachexia State of malnutrition and protein wasting
calculus Concentration of mineral salts in the body leading to the formation of stone
calorie Amount of heat required to raise the temperature of 1 gram of water 1 degree Celsius
cancer Disease resulting from the uncontrolled growth of cells, which causes malignant cellular tumors
capitated rate Preset fee based on membership rather than services provided; payment system used in managed care
caput succedaneum Edema of the newborn's scalp which is present at birth, may cross suture lines, and is caused by head compression against the cervix
carcinogen Substance that initiates or promotes the development of cancer
carcinoma Cancer occurring in epithelial tissue
cardiac cycle Cycle of an impulse going completely through the conduction system of the heart, and the ventricles contracting
cardiac output Volume of blood pumped per minute by the left ventricle
cardiac tamponade Collection of fluid in the pericardial sac hindering the functioning of the heart
carrier Person who harbors an infectious agent but has no symptoms of disease
caseation Process whereby the center of the primary tubercle formed in the lungs as a result of tuberculosis becomes soft and cheese-like due to decreased perfusion
catabolism Destructive process of metabolism whereby tissues or substances are broken into their component parts
cataplexy Sudden loss of muscle control
catharsis Process of talking out one's feelings; "getting things off the chest" through verbalization
cation Ion bearing a positive charge
cavitation Process whereby a cavity is created in the lung tissue through the liquefaction and rupture of a primary tubercle
ceiling effect Medication dosage beyond which no further analgesia occurs
cellular immunity Type of acquired immunity involving T-cell lymphocytes
Centers for Disease Control & Prevention (CDC) An agency of the federal government that provides for the investigation, identification, prevention, and control of diseases; it plays an important role in preparing for, and disseminating information about, possible terrorist attacks
central line Venous catheter inserted into the superior vena cava through the subclavian or internal or external jugular vein
central nervous system System of the brain and spinal cord
cephalalgia Headache; also known as cephalgia
cephalhematoma Collection of blood between the periosteum and the skull of a newborn; appears several hours to a day after birth, does not cross suture lines, and is caused by the rupturing of the periosteal bridging veins due to friction and pressure during labor and delivery
cephalopelvic disproportion Condition in which the fetal head will not fit through the mother's pelvis
certification Voluntary process that establishes and evaluates standards of care; mandatory for any health care services receiving federal funds
cerumen Earwax
cervical dilatation Enlargement of the cervical opening (os) from 0 to 10 cm (complete dilatation)
cesarean birth Birth of an infant through an incision in the abdomen and uterus
Chadwick's sign Purplish-blue color of the cervix and vagina noted about the eighth week of pregnancy
chain of custody Documentation of the transfer of evidence (of a crime) from one worker to the next in a secure fashion
chain of infection Describes the development of an infectious process
chalazion Cyst of the meibomian glands
chancre Clean, painless, syphilitic primary ulcer appearing 2 to 6 weeks after infection at the site of body contact
change Dynamic process whereby an individual's response to a stressor leads to an alteration in behavior
change agent Person who intentionally creates and implements change

chemical agent Substance that interacts with a host, causing disease
chemical name Precise description of the drug's chemical formula
chemical restraint Medication used to control client behavior
chemical warfare agents Poisonous chemicals and gases that are used to harm or kill a large number of persons; examples of chemical agents include nerve agents, blood agents, choking or vomiting agents, and blister or vesicant agents
Chemical, Biological, Radiological/Nuclear, and Explosive Enhanced Response Force Package A program of the National Guard that responds rapidly, following a call by the governor, and can be at the scene of a disaster, ready to function in 6 hours; it can also include a surgical suite, if needed
chemoreceptor Receptor that monitors the levels of carbon dioxide, oxygen, and pH in the blood
chemotherapy Use of drugs to treat illness, especially cancer
Cheyne-Stokes respirations Breathing characterized by periods of apnea alternating with periods of dyspnea
child abuse Any intentional act of physical, emotional, or sexual abuse or neglect committed by a person responsible for the care of a child
child life specialist Health care professional with extensive knowledge of psychology and early childhood development
chloasma Darkening of the skin of the forehead and around the eyes during pregnancy; also called the "mask of pregnancy"
cholecystitis Inflammation of the gallbladder
cholelithiasis Presence of gallstones or calculi in the gallbladder
cholesterol Sterol produced by the body and used in the synthesis of steroid hormones
chorea Condition characterized by abnormal, involuntary, purposeless movements of all musculature of the body
chorion Outer fetal membrane formed from the trophoblast
chronic acute pain Discomfort that occurs almost daily over a long period, months or years, and may never stop; also known as progressive pain
chronic nonmalignant pain Discomfort that occurs almost daily, has been present for at least 6 months, and ranges from mild to severe in intensity; also known as chronic benign pain
chronic pain Discomfort usually defined as long term (lasting 6 months or longer), persistent, nearly constant, or recurrent pain producing significant negative changes in a person's life
chronobiology Science of studying biorhythms
Chvostek's sign Abnormal spasm of the facial muscles in response to a light tapping of the facial nerve
chyme Acidic, semi-fluid paste found in the gastrointestinal tract
circadian rhythm Biorhythm that cycles on a daily basis
circulating nurse RN responsible and accountable for management of personnel, equipment, supplies, the environment, and communication throughout a surgical procedure
circumcision Surgical removal of the prepuce (foreskin), which covers the glans penis
circumoral cyanosis Bluish discoloration surrounding the mouth
cirrhosis Chronic degenerative changes in the liver cells and thickening of surrounding tissue
claiming process Process whereby a family identifies the infant's "likeness to" and the "differences from" family members, and the infant's unique qualities
clean object Object on which there are microorganisms that are usually not pathogenic
cleansing Removal of soil or organic material from instruments and equipment used in providing client care
client behavior accident Mishap resulting from the client's behavior or actions
clinical Observing and caring for living clients
closed reduction Repair of a fracture done without surgical intervention
coarse crackle Moist, low-pitched crackling and gurgling lung sound of long duration
codependent Description for persons who live based on what others think of them
cognition Intellectual ability to think
cognitive behavior therapy Treatment approach aimed at helping a client identify stimuli that cause the client's anxiety, develop plans to respond to those stimuli in a nonanxious manner, and problem-solve when unanticipated anxiety-provoking situations arise
cognitive domain Area of learning that involves intellectual understanding
cognitive reframing Stress-management technique whereby the individual changes a negative perception of a situation or event to a more positive, less threatening perception
coitus (copulation) Sexual act that delivers sperm to the cervix by ejaculation of the erect penis
cold stress Excessive heat loss
colic Condition of acute abdominal pain
colonization Multiplication of microorganisms on or within a host that does not result in cellular injury
colostomy Opening created anywhere along the large intestine

colostrum Antibody-rich yellow fluid secreted by the breasts during the last trimester of pregnancy and the first 2–3 days after birth; gradually changes to milk
comedone Whitehead or blackhead
command hallucination Perception by an individual of a voice or voices telling the individual to do something, usually to himself and/or someone else
communicable agent Infectious agent transmitted to a client by direct or indirect contact, via vehicle, vector, or airborne route
communicable disease Disease caused by a communicable agent
comorbidity Simultaneous existence of more than one disease process within an individual
complementary therapy Therapy used in conjunction with conventional medical therapies
complete protein Protein containing all nine essential amino acids
complicated grief Grief associated with traumatic death such as death by accident, violence, or homicide; survivors often have more intense emotions than those associated with normal grief
compound Combination of atoms of two or more elements
compromised host Person whose normal body defenses are impaired and is therefore susceptible to infection
computed tomography Radiological scanning of the body with x-ray beams and radiation detectors to transmit data to a computer that transcribes the data into quantitative measurement and multidimensional images of the internal structures
conditioning Teaching a person a behavior until it becomes an automatic response; method of conserving adaptive energy
conduction Loss of heat by direct contact with a cooler object
conductive hearing loss Condition characterized by the inability of sound waves to reach the inner ear
confabulation The making up of information to fill in memory gaps
congruence Agreement between two things
conjunctivitis Inflammation of the conjunctiva
consciousness State of awareness of self, others, and surrounding environment
constipation Condition characterized by hard, infrequent stools that are difficult or painful to pass
Contact Precautions Measures taken in addition to Standard Precautions for clients known to have or suspected of having illnesses easily spread by direct client contact or by contact with fomites
contact transmission Transfer of an agent from an infected person to a host by direct contact with that person, indirect contact with an infected person through a fomite, or close contact with contaminated secretions
contraception Measure taken to prevent pregnancy
contracture Permanent shortening of a muscle
contrast medium Radiopaque substance that facilitates roentgen (x-ray) imaging of the body's internal structures
convalescent stage Time period in which acute symptoms of an infection begin to disappear until the client returns to the previous state of health
convection Loss of heat by the movement of air
copulation Sexual act that delivers sperm to the cervix by ejaculation of the erect penis
cotyledon Subdivision of the maternal side of the placenta
couvade Development of physical symptoms by the expectant father such as fatigue, depression, headache, backache, and nausea
crackle Abnormal breath sound that resembles a popping sound, heard on inhalation and exhalation; not cleared by coughing
crenation Condition wherein cells decrease in size, shrivel and wrinkle, and are no longer functional when in a hypertonic solution
crepitus Grating or crackling sensation or sound
cretinism Congenital lack of thyroid hormones causing defective physical development and mental retardation
crisis Acute state of disorganization that occurs when usual coping mechanisms are no longer adequate; stressor that forces an individual to respond and/or adapt in some way
crisis intervention Specific technique used to help a person regain equilibrium
critical thinking The disciplined intellectual process of applying skillful reasoning, imposing intellectual standards and self-reflective thinking as a guide to a belief or action
cross-tolerance Decreased sensitivity to other substances in the same category
crowning When the largest diameter of the fetal head is past the vulva
cryotherapy Use of cold applications to reduce swelling
cryptorchidism Failure of one or both testes to descend
cultural assimilation Process whereby members of a minority group are absorbed by the dominant culture, taking on characteristics of the dominant culture
cultural diversity Differences among people resulting from ethnic, racial, and cultural variations
culture Integrated, dynamic structure of knowledge, attitudes, behaviors, beliefs, ideas, habits, customs, languages, values, symbols, rituals, and ceremonies that

are unique to a particular group of people; growing of microorganisms to identify a pathogen
curative To heal or restore health
curing Ridding one of disease
cutaneous pain Discomfort caused by stimulating the cutaneous nerve endings in the skin
cyanosis Bluish discoloration of the skin and mucous membranes observed in lips, nail beds, and earlobes
cycling Alteration in mood between depression and mania
cystitis Inflammation of the urinary bladder
cystocele Downward displacement of the bladder into the anterior vaginal wall
cytology Study of cells

D

dawn phenomenon Early morning glucose elevation produced by the release of growth hormone
death rattle Noisy respirations in the period preceding death caused by a collection of secretions in the larynx
debride To remove dead or damaged tissue or foreign material from a wound
decerebration Severing of the spinal cord
decidua The endometrium after implantation
decomposition Chemical reaction wherein the bonding between atoms in a molecule is broken and simpler products are formed
decrement Decreasing intensity of a contraction
defense mechanism Unconscious functions protecting the mind from anxiety
deglutition Swallowing of food
dehiscence Complication of wound healing wherein the wound edges separate
dehydration Condition wherein more water is lost from the body than is being replaced
delirium Cognitive changes or acute confusion of rapid onset (less than 6 months)
delusion False belief that misrepresents reality
dementia Organic brain pathology characterized by losses in intellectual functioning and a slow onset (longer than 6 months)
dental caries Cavities
dependence Reliance on a substance to such a degree that abstinence causes functional impairment, physical withdrawal symptoms, and/or psychological craving for the substance; see also addiction
depersonalization Treating an individual as an object rather than as a person
depolarization Contraction of the heart
depression State wherein an individual experiences feelings of extreme sadness, hopelessness, and helplessness
detoxification Elimination of a substance from the body
development Behavioral changes in skills and functional abilities
dialysate Solution used in dialysis, designed to approximate the normal electrolyte structure of plasma and extracellular fluid
dialysis Mechanical means of removing nitrogenous waste from the blood by imitating the function of the nephrons; involves filtration and diffusion of wastes, drugs, and excess electrolytes and/or osmosis of water across a semipermeable membrane into a dialysate solution
diarthrosis Freely movable joint
didactic Systematic presentation of information
diet therapy Treating disease or disorder with special diet
dietary prescription/order Order written by the physician for food, including liquids
differentiation Acquisition of characteristics or functions different from those of the original
diffusion Process whereby a substance moves from an area of higher concentration to an area of lower concentration
digestion Mechanical and chemical processes that convert nutrients into a physically absorbable state
diplopia Double vision
dirty object Object on which there is a high number of microorganisms, some that are potentially pathogenic
disability An individual's lack of ability to complete an activity in the normal manner
disaster A situation or event of greater magnitude than an emergency and that has unforeseen, serious, or immediate threats to public health
disciplined Trained by instruction and exercise
disenfranchised grief Grief not openly acknowledged, socially sanctioned, or publicly shared
disinfectant Chemical solution used to clean inanimate objects
disinfection Elimination of pathogens, with the exception of spores, from inanimate objects
dislocation Injury in which the articular surfaces of a joint are no longer in contact
disorientation State of mental confusion in which awareness of time, place, self, and/or situation is impaired
disseminated intravascular coagulation Abnormal stimulation of the clotting mechanism causing small clots throughout the vascular system and widespread bleeding internally, externally, or both
distraction Technique of focusing attention on stimuli other than pain
distress Subjective experience that occurs when stressors evoke an ineffective response
distribution Movement of drugs from the blood into various tissues and body fluids
diverticula Sac-like protrusion of the intestinal wall that results when the mucosa herniates through the bowel wall

diverticulitis Inflammation of one or more diverticula
diverticulosis Condition in which multiple diverticula are present in the colon
domestic violence Aggression and violence involving family members
dominant culture The group whose values prevail within a given society
Down syndrome Congenital chromosomal abnormality; also called trisomy 21
Droplet Precautions Measures taken in addition to Standard Precautions for clients known to have or suspected of having serious illnesses spread by large particle droplets
drug allergy Hypersensitivity to a drug
drug incompatibility Undesired chemical or physical reaction between a drug and a solution, between a drug and the container or tubing, or between two drugs
drug interaction Effect one drug can have on another drug
drug tolerance Reaction that occurs when the body is accustomed to a specific drug that larger doses are needed to produce the desired therapeutic effects
ductus arteriosus Fetal vessel connecting the pulmonay artery to the aorta
ductus venosus Branch of the umbilical vein that enters the inferior vena cava
duration Length of one contraction, from the beginning of the increment to the conclusion of the decrement
dysarthria Difficult and defective speech due to a dysfunction of the muscles used for speech
dysfunctional grief Persistent pattern of intense grief that does not result in reconciliation of feelings
dysfunctional labor Labor with problems of the contractions or of maternal bearing down
dysmenorrhea Painful menstruation
dyspareunia Painful intercourse
dysphagia Difficulty in swallowing
dysplasia Abnormal development
dyspnea Difficulty breathing as observed by labored or forced respirations through the use of accessory muscles in the chest and neck
dysrhythmia Irregularity in the rate, rhythm, or conduction of the electrical system of the heart
dystocia Long, difficult, or abnormal labor caused by any of the four major variables (4 Ps) that affect labor
dysuria Difficult or painful urination

E

early deceleration Reduction in fetal heart rate that begins early in the contraction and virtually mirrors the uterine contraction
ecchymosis Large, irregular hemorrhagic area on the skin; also called a bruise
eclampsia Convulsion occurring in pregnancy-induced hypertension
ectopic pregnancy Pregnancy in which the fertilized ovum is implanted outside the uterine cavity
edema Detectable accumulation of increased interstitial fluid
effacement Thinning of the cervix
efferent nerve pain pathway Descending spinal cord pathway that transmits sensory impulses from the brain
effluent Liquid output from an ileostomy
electrocardiogram Graphic recording of the heart's electrical activity
electroconvulsive therapy Procedure whereby clients are treated with pulses of electrical energy sufficient to cause brief convulsions or seizures
electroencephalogram Graphic recording of the brain's electrical activity
electrolyte Compound that, when dissolved in water or another solvent, dissociates (separates) into ions (electrically charged particles)
element Basic substance of matter
emancipated minor Child who has the legal competency of an adult because of cicumstances involving marriage, divorce, parenting of a child, living independently without parents, or enlistment in the armed services
embolus Mass, such as a blood clot or an air bubble, that circulates in the bloodstream
embryonic phase Development occuring during the first 2 to 8 weeks after fertilization of a human egg
emergency Medical or surgical condition requiring immediate or timely intervention to prevent permanent disability or death
emergency medical technician (EMT) Health care professional trained to provide basic lifesaving measures prior to arrival at the hospital
emergency nursing Care of clients who require emergency interventions
emotional lability Loss of emotional control
empathy Capacity to understand another person's feelings or perception of a situation
emphysema Lung disease wherein air accumulates in the tissues of the lungs
empowerment A process through which an individual is enabled to change situations, and uses resources, skills, and opportunities to do so
empty calories Calories that provide few nutrients
encephalitis Inflammation of the brain
encoding Laying down tracks in areas of the brain to enhance the ability to recall and use information
encopresis Passage of watery colonic contents around a hard fecal mass

endemic Occurring continuously in a particular population and having low mortality
endocrine Group of cells secreting substances directly into the blood or lymph circulation and affecting another part of the body
endometriosis Growth of endometrial tissue on structures outside of the uterus, within the pelvic cavity
endorphins Group of opiate-like substances produced naturally by the brain that raise the pain threshold, produce sedation and euphoria, and promote a sense of well-being
endoscopy Visualization of a body organ or cavity through a scope
energetic-touch therapy Technique of using the hands to direct or redirect the flow of the body's energy fields and enhance balance within those fields
engagement Condition of the widest diameter of the fetal presenting part (head) entering the inlet to the true pelvis
engorgement Distentions and swelling of the breasts in the first few days following delivery
engrossment Parents' intense interest in and preoccupation with the newborn
enriched Descriptor for food in which nutrients that were removed during processing are added back in
enteral instillation Administration of drugs through a gastrointestinal tube
enteral nutrition Feeding method meaning both the ingestion of food orally and the delivery of nutrients through a gastrointestinal tube, but generally meaning the latter
entrainment Infant's ability to move in rhythm to the parent's voice
enzyme Globular protein produced in the body that catalyzes chemical reactions within the cells
enzyme-linked immunosorbent assay Basic screening test currently used to detect antibodies to HIV
epidemic Infecting many people at the same time and in the same geographic area
epidural analgesia Analgesics administered via a catheter that terminates in the epidural space
episiotomy Incision in the perineum to facilitate passage of the baby
epispadias Placement of the urinary meatus on the top of the penis
epistaxis Hemorrhage of the nares or nostrils; also known as nosebleed
Epstein's pearls Small, whitish-yellow epithelial cysts found on the hard palate
equipment accident Accident resulting from the malfunction or improper use of medical equipment
erythema Redness of the skin due to increased blood flow to the area
erythema toxicum neonatorum Pink rash with firm, yellow-white papules or pustules found on the chest, abdomen, back, and/or buttocks of a newborn
erythematous Characterized by redness of the skin
erythrocytapheresis Procedure that removes abnormal red blood cells and replaces them with healthy ones
erythropoiesis Production of red blood cells and their release by the red bone marrow
eschar Dry, dark, leathery scab composed of denatured protein
ethnicity Cultural group's perception of itself or a group identity
ethnocentrism Assumption of cultural superiority and inability to accept another culture's ways
euglycemia Normal blood glucose level
euphoric Characterized by elation out of context to the situation
eupnea Easy respirations with a rate that is age-appropriate
eustress Stress that results in positive outcomes
evaporation Loss of heat when water is changed to a vapor
evisceration Complication of wound healing characterized by a complete separation of wound edges, accompanied by visceral protrusion
exacerbation Increase in the symptoms of a disease
exclusive provider organization Organization wherein care must be delivered by providers in the plan in order for clients to receive any reimbursement
excretion Elimination of drugs or waste products from the body
Expeditionary Medical Support A total package that includes everything necessary to screen, treat, and release clients to other facilities for longer-term care
exposure Contact with an infected person or agent
extended care facility The term refers to any facility that provides care for a long period of time. It has no concrete definition and could refer to either an intermediate or skilled nursing facility
external respiration Exchange of gases between the atmosphere and the lungs
external version Manipulation of the fetus through the mother's abdomen to a presentation facilitating birth
extracellular fluid Fluid outside of the cells; includes interstitial, intravascular, synovial, cerebrospinal, and serous fluids; aqueous and vitreous humor; and endolymph and perilymph
extravasation Escape of fluid into the surrounding tissue

F

faith Confident belief in the truth, value, or trustworthiness of a person, idea, or thing
false labor Contractions that do not cause the cervix to dilate

family-centered care A philosophy of caring recognizing the centrality of the family in the child's life and including the family's contribution and involvement in the plan of care and its delivery (Potts & Mandleco, 2000)
fasciculation Involuntary twitching of muscle fibers
fat-soluble vitamin Vitamin requiring the presence of fats for its absorption from the gastrointestinal tract into the lymphatic system and for cellular metabolism: vitamins A, D, E, and K
fee for service System in which the health care recipient directly pays the provider for services as they are provided
feedback Response from the receiver of a message so that the sender can verify the message
Ferguson's reflex Spontaneous, involutary urge to bear down during labor
fertilization Union of an ovum and a sperm
fetal attitude Relationship of fetal body parts to one another, either flexion or extension
fetal biophysical profile Assessment of five variables: fetal breathing movement, fetal movements of body or limbs, fetal tone (flexion/extension of extremities), amniotic fluid volume, and reactive NST
fetal lie Relationship of the cephalocaudal axis of the fetus to the cephalocaudal axis of the mother, either longitudinal or transverse
fetal phase Intrauterine development from 8 weeks to birth
fetal position Relationship of the identified landmark on the presenting part to the four quadrants of the mother's pelvis
fetal presentation Determined by the fetal lie and the part of the fetus that enters the pelvis first
fibrinolysis Process of breaking fibrin apart
fight-or-flight response State wherein the body becomes physiologically ready to defend itself by either fighting or fleeing from the stressor
filtration Process of fluids and the substances dissolved in them being forced through the cell membrane by hydrostatic pressure
fine crackle Dry, high-pitched crackling and popping lung sounds of short duration
first assistant Physician or RN who assists the surgeon to retract tissue, aids in the removal of blood and fluids at the operative site, and assists with homeostasis and wound closure
first responders Persons who have been identified as the first ones to appear at the scene of a disaster or accident; designated first responders include health care workers, emergency medical personnel, police, and firepersons
flashback Rushing of blood back into intravenous tubing when a negative pressure is created on the tubing; reliving of an original trauma as if the individual were currently experiencing it
flora Microorganisms that occur or have adapted to live in a specific environment, such as intestinal, skin, vaginal, or oral flora
flow rate Volume of fluid to infuse over a set period of time
fluoroscopy Immediate, serial images of the body's structure or function
fomite Object contaminated with an infectious agent
fontanelle Membranous area where sutures meet on the fetal skull
foramen ovale Flap opening in the atrial septum that allows only right-to-left movement of blood
forceps Metal instruments used on the fetal head to provide traction or to provide a method of rotating the fetal head to an occiput-anterior position
foremilk Watery first milk from the breast, high in lactose, like skim milk, and effective in quenching thirst
formal teaching Teaching that takes place at a specific time, in a specific place, and on a specific topic
fortified Descriptor for food in which nutrients not naturally occurring in the food are added to it
fracture Break in the continuity of a bone
free radical Unstable molecule that alters genetic codes and triggers the development of cancer growth in cells
frequency Time for the beginning of one contraction to the beginning of the next contraction
friction Force of two surfaces moving against one another
fulguration Procedure to destroy tissue with long, high-frequency electric sparks
fundus Top of the uterus
funic souffle Sound of the blood pulsating through the umbilical cord; rate the same as the fetal heartbeat

G

gastric ulcer Erosion in the stomach
gastritis Inflammation of the stomach mucosa
gate control pain theory Theory that proposes that the cognitive, sensory, emotional, and physiologic components of the body can act together to block an individual's perception of pain
general adaptation syndrome Physiologic response that occurs when a person experiences a stressor
general anesthesia Method of producing unconsciousness; amnesia, motionlessness, muscle relaxation, and complete insensibility to pain
generic name Name assigned by the U.S. Adopted Names Council to the manufacturer who first develops a drug
genogram A way to visualize family members, their birth and death dates, or ages and specific health problems
genuineness Sincerity

germicide Chemical that can be applied to both animate and inanimate objects for the purpose of eliminating pathogens

germinal phase Development beginning with conception and lasting approximately 10 to 14 days

gerontological nursing Specialty within nursing that addresses and advocates for the special care needs of older adults

gerontologist Specialist in gerontology in advanced practice nursing, geriatric psychiatry, medicine, and social services

gerontology Study of the effects of normal aging and age-related diseases on human beings

gingivitis Inflammation of the gums

Glasgow Coma Scale Neurological screening test that measures a client's best verbal, motor, and eye response to stimuli

glucagon Hormone secreted by the alpha cells of the pancreas, which stimulate release of glucose by the liver

gluconeogenesis Conversion of amino acids into glucose

glycogenesis Conversion of glucose into glycogen

glycogenolysis Conversion of glycogen into glucose

glycosuria Presence of excessive glucose in the urine

goiter Enlargement of the thyroid gland

Goodell's sign Softening of the cervix noted about the 8th week of pregnancy

Gower's sign Walking the hands up the legs to get from sitting to standing position (as in Duchenne muscular dystrophy)

granulation tissue Delicate connective tissue consisting of fibroblasts, collagen, and capillaries

graphesthesia Ability to identify letters, numbers, or shapes drawn on the skin

gravida Pregnancy, regardless of duration, including present pregnancy

grief Series of intense psychological and physical responses occuring after a loss; these responses are necessary, normal, natural, and adaptive responses to the loss

growth Measurable changes in the physical size of the body and its parts

gynecomastia Abnormal enlargement of one or both breasts in males

H

half-life Time it takes the body to eliminate half of the blood concentration level of the original dose of medication

halitosis Bad breath

hallucination Sensory perception that occurs in the absence of external stimuli and that is not based on reality

hallux varus Placement of the great toe farther from the other toes

hand hygiene Rubbing together of all surfaces and crevices of the hands using a soap or chemical and water, followed by rinsing in a flowing stream of water

handicap The physical or mental inability to complete a role in one or more major ADL (U.S. Office of Personnel Management, 1987)

healing Process that activates the individual's recovery forces from within; to make whole

healing touch Energy therapy using the hands to clear, energize, and balance the energy field

health According to the World Health Organization, the state of complete physical, mental, and social well-being, not merely the absence of disease or infirmity

health care delivery system Method for providing services to meet the health needs of individuals

health care surrogate law Law enacted by some states that provides a legal means for decision making in the absence of advance directives

health continuum Range of an individual's health, from highest health potential to death

health history Review of the client's functional health patterns prior to the current contact with a health care agency

health maintenance organization Prepaid health plan that provides primary health care services for a preset fee and focuses on cost-effective treatment methods

hearing Act or power of receiving sounds

heart sound Sound heard by auscultating the heart

Heberden's nodes Enlargement and characteristic hypertrophic spurs in the terminal interphalangeal finger joints

Hegar's sign Softening of the uterine isthmus about the 6th week of pregnancy

HELLP syndrome Pregnancy-induced hypertension with liver damage characterized by hemolysis, elevated liver enzymes, and low platelet count

hemarthrosis Bleeding into the joints

hematemesis Vomiting of blood

hematocrit Percentage of red blood cells in a given volume of blood

hematopoiesis Process of blood cell production and development

hematuria Blood in the urine

hemiparesis Weakness of one side of the body

hemiplegia Paralysis of one side of the body

hemolysis Breakdown of red blood cells and the release of hemoglobin

hemopneumothorax Presence of blood and air within the pleural space

hemorrhagic exudate Discharge that has a large component of red blood cells

hemorrhoid Swollen vascular tissue in the rectal area

hemostasis Cessation of bleeding

hemothorax Condition wherein blood accumulates in the pleural space of the lungs

hepatitis Chronic or acute inflammation of the liver
hesitancy Difficulty initiating the urinary stream
hindmilk Follows foremilk, is higher in fat content, leads to weight gain, and is more satisfying
hirsutism Excessive body hair in a masculine distribution
histamine Substance released during allergic reactions
holistic Whole; includes physical, intellectual, sociocultural, psychological, and spiritual aspects as an integrated whole
Homans' sign Test to check for the presence of clots in the leg
homeostasis Balance or equilibrium among the physiologic, psychological, sociocultural, intellectual, and spiritual needs of the body; maintenance of internal environment
homonymous hemianopia Loss of vision in half of the visual field on the same side of both eyes
hope To look forward to with confidence or expectation; a resource clients can use to promote physical, psychological, and spiritual wellness
hormone Substance that initiates or regulates activity of another organ, system, or gland in another part of the body
hospice Humane, compassionate care provided to clients who can no longer benefit from curative treatment and have 6 months or less to live; allows individuals to die with dignity
host Organism that can be affected by an agent
human immunodeficiency virus (HIV) Retrovirus that causes AIDS
human leukocyte antigen Antigen present in human blood
humoral immunity Type of immunity dominated by antibodies
hydatidiform mole Abnormality of the placenta wherein the chorionic villi become fluid filled, grape-like clusters; the trophoblastic tissue proliferates; and there is no viable fetus
hydramnios (polyhydramnios) Excess amount of amniotic fluid
hydrocele Fluid around the testes in the scrotum
hydrostatic pressure Pressure that a fluid exerts against a membrane; also called filtration force
hygiene Study of health and ways of preserving health
hyperbilirubinemia Excess of bilirubin in the blood
hyperemesis gravidarum Excessive vomiting during pregnancy
hypergylcemia Condition wherein the blood glucose level becomes too high as a result of the absence of insulin
hyperopia Farsightedness
hypersensitivity Excessive reaction to a stimulus
hypersomnia Alteration in sleep pattern characterized by excessive sleep, especially in the daytime
hyperthermia Condition in which the core body temperature rises above 106°F
hypertonic solution Solution that has a higher molecular concentration than the cell; also called a hyperosmolar solution
hypertrophy Increase in muscle mass
hyperuricemia Increased uric acid blood level
hyperventilation Breathing characterized by deep, rapid respirations
hypervigilant Condition of constantly scanning the environment for potentially dangerous situations
hypervolemia Increased circulating fluid volume
hypnosis Altered state of consciousness or awareness resembling sleep and during which a person is more receptive to suggestion
hypoglycemia Condition wherein the blood glucose level is exceedingly low
hypomania Mild form of mania without significant impairment
hypospadias Placement of the urinary meatus on the underside of the penis
hypothermia Condition in which the core body temperature drops below 95°F
hypotonia Lax muscle tone
hypotonic solution Solution that has a lower molecular concentration than the cell; also called hypo-osmolar solution
hypoventilation Breathing characterized by shallow respirations
hypovolemia Abnormally low circulatory blood volume
hypoxemia Decreased oxygen level in the blood

I

iatrogenic Caused by treatment or diagnostic procedures
ideal self The person whom the individual would like to be
identity An individual's conscious description of who he or she is
idiopathic Occurring without a known cause
idiosyncratic reaction Very unpredictable response that may be an overresponse, an underresponse, or an atypical response
ileal conduit Implantation of the ureters into a piece of ileum, which is attached to the abdominal wall as a stoma so urine can be removed from the body
ileostomy Opening created in the small intestine at the ileum
illness stage Time period when the client is manifesting specific signs and symptoms of an infectious agent

illusion Inaccurate perception or misinterpretation of sensory stimuli
imagery Relaxation technique of using the imagination to visualize a pleasant, soothing image
immune response Body's reaction to substances identified as nonself
immunity Body's ability to protect itself from foreign agents or organisms
immunization Process of creating immunity or resistance to infection in an individual
immunotherapy Treatment to suppress or enhance immunologic functioning
implantable cardioverter-defibrillator (ICD) Implantable device that senses a dysrythmia and automatically sends an electrical shock directly to the heart to defibrillate it
implantable port Device made of a radiopaque silicone catheter and a plastic or stainless steel injection port with a self-sealing silicone-rubber septum
implantation Embedding of a fertilized egg into the uterine lining
impotence Inability of an adult male to have an erection firm enough or to maintain it long enough to complete sexual intercourse
incidence Frequency of disease occurrence
incompetent cervix Descriptor for when the cervix begins to dilate, usually during the second trimester
incomplete protein Protein with one or more of the essential amino acids missing
increment Increasing intensity of a contraction
incubation period Time between entry of an infectious agent in the host and the onset of symptoms
independent nursing intervention Nursing action initiated by the nurse and do not require direction or an order from another health care professional
induction of labor Stimulation of uterine contractions before contractions begin spontaneously for the purpose of birthing an infant
infancy Development from the end of the first month to the end of the first year of life
infection Invasion and multiplication of pathogenic microorganims in body tissue that results in cellular injury
infectious agent Microorganism that causes cellular injury
infertility Inability or diminished ability to produce offspring
infiltration Seepage of foreign substances into the interstitial tissue, causing swelling and discomfort at the IV site
inflammation Nonspecific cellular response to tissue injury
informal teaching Teaching that takes place anytime, anyplace, and whenever a learning need is identified
informed consent Legal form signed by a competent client and witnessed by another person that grants permission to the client's physician to perform the procedure described by the physician and that demonstrates the client's understanding of the benefits, risks, and possible complications of the procedure, as well as alternate treatment options
ingestion The taking of food into the digestive tract, generally through the mouth
initial planning Development of a preliminary plan of care by the nurse who performs the admission assessment and gathers the comprehensive admission assessment data
insensible water loss Water loss of which the person is not generally aware
insomnia Difficulty in falling asleep initially or in returning to sleep once awakened
inspection Physical examination technique that involves thorough visual observation
insulin Pancreatic hormone that aids in both the diffusion of glucose into the liver and muscle cells, and the synthesis of glycogen
intellectual wellness Ability to function as an independent person capable of making sound decisions
intensity Strength of the contraction at the acme
interdependent nursing intervention Nursing action that is implemented in a collaborative manner with other health care professionals
internal respiration Exchange of oxygen and carbon dioxide at the cellular level
interstitial fluid Fluid in tissue spaces around each cell
interval Resting period between two contractions
intoxication Reversible effect on the central nervous system soon after the use of a substance
intracath Plastic tube for insertion into a vein
intracellular fluid Fluid within the cells
intradermal Injection into the dermis
intramuscular Injection into the muscle
intraoperative phase Time during the surgical experience that begins when the client is transferred to the operating room table and ends when the client is admitted to the postanesthesia care unit
intrathecal analgesia Administration of analgesics into the subarachnoid space
intravascular fluid Fluid consisting of the plasma in the blood vessels and the lymph in the lymphatic system
intravenous Injection into a vein
intravenous therapy Administration of fluids, electrolytes, nutrients, or medications by the venous route
intravesical Within the urinary bladder
intussusception Telescoping of one part of the intestine into another

invasive Accessing the body tissues, organs, or cavities through some type of instrumentation procedure
involution Return of the reproductive organs, especially the uterus, to their pre-pregnancy size and condition
ion Atom bearing an electrical charge
ischemia Oxygen deprivation, usually due to poor perfusion
ischemic pain Discomfort resulting when the blood supply to an area is restricted or cut off completely
isolation Separation from other persons, especially those with infectious diseases
isotonic solution Solution that has the same molecular concentration as does the cell; also called an isosmolar solution
isotopes Atom of the same element that has a different atomic weight (i.e., different numbers of neutrons in the nucleus)
iv push (bolus) The administration of a large dose of medication in a relatively short time, usually 1–30 minutes

J

jaundice Yellow discoloration of the skin, sclera, mucous membranes, and body fluids that occurs when the liver is unable to fully remove bilirubin from the blood
Johnsonian intervention Confrontational approach to a client with a substance problem that lessens the chance of denial and encourages treatment before the client "hits bottom"
judgment Conclusion based on sound reasoning and supported by evidence

K

Kardex A brief worksheet with basic client care information
keloid Abnormal growth of scar tissue that is elevated, rounded, and firm with irregular, clawlike margins
keratin Tough, fibrous protein produced by cells in the epidermis called keratinocytes
keratitis Inflammation of the cornea
kernicterus Severe neurological damage resulting from a high level of bilirubin (jaundice)
Kernig's sign Diagnostic test for inflammation in the nerve roots; the inability to extend the leg when the thigh is flexed against the abdomen
ketone Acidic by-product of fat metabolism
ketonuria Presence of ketones in the urine
ketosis Condition wherein acids called ketones accumulate in the blood and urine, upsetting the acid–base balance
kilocalorie Equivalent to 1,000 calories
kinesthetic learner Person who learns by processing information through touching, feeling, and doing
kwashiorkor Condition resulting when there is a sudden or recent lack of protein-containing foods
kyphosis Increased roundness of the thoracic spinal curve

L

lanugo Fine hair covering the fetus's body
large for gestational age Infant's weight falls above the 90th percentile for gestational age
late deceleration Reduction in fetal heart rate that begins after the uterus has begun contracting and increases to the baseline level after the uterine contraction has ceased
learning Act or process of acquiring knowledge, skill, or both in a particular subject; process of assimilating knowledge resulting in behavior changes
learning disability Heterogenous group of disorders manifested by significant difficulties in the acquisition and use of listening, speaking, reading, writing, reasoning, or mathematical abilities
learning plateau Peak in the effectiveness of teaching and depth of learning
learning style Individual preference for receiving, processing, and assimilating information about a particular subject
lecithin Major component of surfactant
Leopold's maneuvers Series of specific palpations of the pregnant uterus to determine fetal position and presentation
let-down reflex Neurohormonal reflex that causes milk to be expressed from the alveoli into the lactiferous ducts
leukocytosis Increased number of white blood cells
leukopenia Decreased number of white blood cells
licensure Mandatory system of granting licenses according to specified standards
life review Form of reminiscence wherein a client attempts to come to terms with conflict or to gain meaning from life and die peacefully
ligation Application of a band or tie around a structure
lightening Descent of the fetus into the pelvis, causing the uterus to tip forward, relieving pressure on the diaphragm
linea nigra Dark line on the abdomen from umbilicus to symphysis during the pregnancy
lipid Organic compound that is insoluble in water but soluble in organic solvents such as ether and alcohol; also known as fats
lipodystrophy Atrophy or hypertrophy of subcutaneous fat
lipoma Benign tumor consisting of mature fat cells
lipoprotein Blood lipid bound to protein

liquefaction necrosis Death and subsequent change of tissue to a liquid or semi-liquid state; often descriptive of a primary tubercle

listening Interpreting the sounds heard and attaching meaning to them

litholapaxy Procedure involving crushing of a bladder stone and immediate washing out of the fragments through a catheter

lithotripsy Method of crushing a calculus anyplace in the urinary system with ultrasonic waves

liver mortis Bluish-purple discoloration of the skin that is a by-product of red blood cell destruction; it begins within 20 minutes of death

living will Legal document that allows a person to state preferences about the use of life-sustaining measures should he or she be unable to make his or her wishes known

local adaptation syndrome Physiologic response to a stressor (e.g., trauma, illness) affecting a specific part of the body

localized infection Infection limited to a defined area or single organ

lochia Uterine/vaginal discharge after childbirth; initially bright red, then changing to a pink or pinkish brown, then to a yellowish white

locomotor Pertaining to movement or the ability to move

long-term care facility Health care facility that provides services to individuals who are not acutely ill, have continuing health care needs, and cannot function independently at home

long-term care managed care Care that refers to a spectrum of services provided to individuals who have an ongoing need for health care; traditionally a community-based nursing home licensed for skilled or intermediate care

long-term goal Statement that profiles the desired resolution of the nursing diagnosis over a long period of time, usually weeks or months

lordosis Exaggeration of the curvature of the lumbar spine

loss Any situation, either potential, actual, or perceived, wherein a valued object or person is changed or is not accessible to the individual

lumbar puncture Aspiration of cerebrospinal fluid from the subarachnoid space

lung stretch receptor Receptor that monitors the patterns of breathing and prevents overexpansion of the lungs

lymphokine Chemical substance released by sensitized lymphocytes (T cells) and that assists in antigen destruction

lymphoma Tumor of the lymphatic system

M

macrosomia Excessive fetal growth characterized by a fetus weighing more than 4,000 g (8.8 lb.)

magnetic resonance imaging Imaging technique that uses radiowaves and a strong magnetic field to make continuous cross-sectional images of the body

maladaptive measure Measure used to avoid conflict or stress

malignant Becoming progessively worse and often resulting in death

malpractice Negligent acts on the part of a professional; relates to the conduct of a person who is acting in a professional capacity

managed care A cost-saving system where a case management, individual, or team control what specialists the client sees, as well as the frequency or duration of that specialty care

mania Extremely elevated mood with accompanying agitated behavior

marasmus Condition resulting from severe malnutrition; afflicts very young children who lack both energy and protein foods as well as vitamins and minerals

Maslow's hierarchy of needs Theory of behavioral motivation based on needs; includes physiologic, safety and security, love and belonging, self-esteem, and self-actualization needs

mastication Chewing food into fine particles and mixing the food with enzymes in saliva

mastitis Inflammation of the breast, generally during breastfeeding

material principle of justice Rationale for determining those times when there can be unequal allocation of scarce resources

matter Anything that occupies space and possesses mass

maturation Process of becoming fully grown and developed; involves physiologic and behavioral aspects

maturational loss Loss that occurs as a person moves from one developmental stage to another

mechanism of labor Series of movements of the fetus as it passes through the pelvis and birth canal

meconium Fecal material stored in the fetal intestines

meconium ileus Impacted feces in the newborn, causing intestinal obstruction

Medicaid Government title program (XIX) that pays for health services for people who are older, poor, or disabled, and for low-income families with dependent children

medical asepsis Practices that reduce the number, growth, and spread of microorganisms

medical diagnosis Clinical judgment by the physician that identifies or determines a specific disease, condition, or pathological state

medical model Traditional approach to health care wherein the focus is on treatment and cure of disease not prevention

Medicare Amendment (Title XVIII) to the Social Security Act that helps finance the health care of persons over 65 years old and younger persons who are permanently disabled to receive Social Security disability benefits

Medigap insurance Insurance plan for persons with Medicare that pays for health care costs not covered by Medicare

meditation An activity that brings the mind and spirit in focus on the present and provokes a sense of peace and relaxation

melanin Pigment that gives skin its color

melena Stool containing partially broken down blood usually black, sticky, and tar-like

menarche Onset of the first menstrual period

meningitis Inflammation of the meninges

meningocele Saclike protrusion along the vertebral column filled with cerebrospinal fluid and meninges

menopause Cessation of menstruation

menorrhagia Excessively heavy menstrual flow

mental disorder Clinically significant behavior or psychological syndrome or pattern that occurs in an individual and is associated with present distress or disability or with a significantly increased risk of suffering, death, pain, disability, or an important loss of freedom (APA, 1994)

mental illness Condition wherein an individual has a distorted view of self, is unable to maintain satisfying personal relationships, and is unable to adapt to the environment

mentation Ability to concentrate, remember, or think abstractly

metabolic rate Rate of energy utilization in the body

metabolism Sum total of all the biological and chemical processes in the body

metastasis Spread of cancer cells to distant areas of the body by way of the lymph system or bloodstream

metritis Inflammation of the uterus including the endometrium and parametrium

metrorrhagia Vaginal bleeding between menstrual periods

micturition Process of expelling urine from the urinary bladder; also called urination or voiding

middle adulthood Development from the ages of 40 years to 65 years

milia Pearly white cysts on the face

minimum data set An assessment tool for assessing a resident's physical, psychological, and psychosocial functioning in a Medicare and Medicaid-certified long-term care facility

minority group Group of people constituting less than a numerical majority of the population and are often labeled and treated differently from others in the society

miscarriage Spontaneous abortion

misdemeanor Offense that is less serious than a felony and may be punished by a fine or by sentence to a local prison for less than 1 year

misuse Use of a legal substance for which it was not intended, or exceeding the recommended dosage of a drug

mixed agonist-antagonist Compound that blocks opioid effects on one receptor type while producing opioid effects on a second receptor type

mixture Substances combined in no specific way

mnemonic Method to aid in association and recall; a memorable sentence created from the first letters of a list of items to be used to recall the items later

mode of transmission Process of the infectious agent moving from the reservoir or source through the portal of exit to the portal of entry of the susceptible "new" host

modulation Central nervous system pathway that selectively inhibits pain transmission by sending signals back down to the dorsal horn of the spinal cord

molding Shaping of the fetal head to adapt to the mother's pelvis during labor

molecule Atoms of the same element that unite with each other

Mongolian spots Large patches of bluish skin on the buttocks of dark-skinned infants

monounsaturated fatty acid Forms a glycerol ester with a double or triple bond; nuts, fowl, and olive oil

mood Subjective report of the way an individual is feeling

moral maturity Ability to decide for oneself what is "right"

morbidity Illness

mortality Death

morula Mass of cells resembling a mulberry

mourning Period during which grief is expressed and integration and resolution of the loss occur

multigravida Condition of being pregnant two or more times

multipara Condition of having delivered twice or more after 24 weeks' gestation

myelomeningocele Saclike protrusion along the vertebral column that is filled with spinal fluid, meninges, nerve roots, and spinal cord

myocardial infarction Necrosis (death) of the myocardium caused by an obstruction in a coronary artery; commonly known as heart attack

myocarditis Inflammation of the myocardium of the heart

myofascial pain syndrome Group of muscle disorders characterized by pain, muscle spasm, tenderness, stiffness, and limited motion
myopia Nearsightedness
myringotomy Surgical incision of the eardrum
myxedema Severe hypothyroidism in adults

N

narcolepsy Sleep alteration manifested as sudden uncontrollable urges to fall asleep during the daytime
narrative charting Chronological account written in paragraphs describes the client's status, the interventions and treatments, and the client's response to treatments
necrosis Tissue death as the result of disease or injury
neglect Situation wherein a basic need of the client is not being provided
negligence General term referring to careless acts on the part of an individual who is not exercising reasonable or prudent judgment
neonatal stage First 28 days of life following birth
neonatal transition First few hours after birth wherein the newborn makes changes to and stabilizes respiratory and circulatory functions
neonate Newborn from birth to 28 days of life
neoplasm Any abnormal growth of new tissue
nephrotoxic Quality of a substance that causes kidney tissue damage
nerve agents Powerful acetylcholinesterase inhibitors that alter cholinergic synaptic transmission at neuroeffector junctions, at skeletal myoneural junctions and autonomic ganglia, and in the central nervous system
nesting Surge of energy late in pregnancy when the pregnant woman organizes and cleans the house
neuralgia Paroxysmal pain that extends along the course of one or more nerves
neurogenic shock Hypotensive situation resulting from the loss of sympathetic control of vital functions from the brain
neuropeptide Amino acid produced in the brain and other sites in the body that acts as a chemical communicator
neurotransmitter Chemical substance produced by the body that facilitates or inhibits nerve-impulse transmission
neutral thermal environment Environment in which the newborn can maintain internal body temperature with minimal oxygen consumption and metabolism
nevi Pigmented areas in the skin; commonly known as birthmarks or moles
nevus flammeus Large, reddish-purple birthmark usually found on the face or neck and does not blanch with pressure
nevus vascularis Birthmark of enlarged superficial blood vessels, elevated and red in color
nociceptor Receptive neuron for painful sensations
nocturia Awakening at night to void
nocturnal enuresis Incontinence that occurs during sleep
noninvasive Descriptor for procedure wherein the body is not entered with any type of instrument
nonmaleficence Ethical principle based on the obligation to cause no harm to others
nonshivering thermogenesis Metabolism of brown fat; process unique to the newborn
nonverbal communication Body language or a method of sending a message without words
nosocomial infection Infection acquired in the hospital or other health care facility that was not present or incubating at the time of the client's admission
noxious stimulus Underlying pathology that causes pain
nuchal cord Condition of the umbilical cord being wrapped around the baby's neck
nuchal rigidity Pain and rigidity in the neck
nulligravida Condition of never having been pregnant
nullipara Condition of never having delivered an infant after 24 weeks' gestation
nursing The art and science of assisting individuals in learning to care for themselves whenever possible and of caring for them when they are unable to meet their own needs
nursing audit Method of evaluating the quality of care provided to clients
nursing care plan Written guide of strategies to be implemented to help the client achieve optimal health
nursing diagnosis Second step in the nursing process; a clinical judgment about individual, family, or community (aggregate) responses to actual or potential health problems/life processes
nursing intervention Action performed by a nurse that helps the client achieve the results specified by the goals and expected outcomes
nursing interventions classification Standardized language for nursing interventions
nursing minimum data set Elements that should be in clinical records and abstracted for studies on the effectiveness and costs of nursing care
nursing outcomes classification Standardized language for nursing outcomes
nursing practice act Statute that is enacted by the legislature of a state and that outlines the scope of nursing practice in that state

nursing process Systematic method for providing care to clients, consisting of five steps: assessment, diagnosis, outcome identification and planning, implementation, and evaluation
nutrition All of the processes (ingestion, digestion, absorption, metabolism, and elimination) involved in consuming and using food for energy, maintenance, and growth
nystagmus Constant, involuntary movement of the eye in various directions

O

obesity Weight that is 20% or more above the ideal body weight
objective data Observable and measurable data that are obtained through standard assessment techniques performed during the physical examination and through laboratory and diagnostic tests
occult blood Blood in the stool that can be detected only through a microscope or by chemical means
occult blood test (guaiac) Test for microscopic blood done on stool
older adulthood Development occurring from age 65 years until death
oligomenorrhea Decreased menstrual flow
oliguria Diminished production of urine
oncology Study of tumors
ongoing assessment Type of assessment that includes systematic monitoring of specific problems
ongoing planning Updates the client's plan of care
onset of action Time for the body to respond to a drug after administration
oophoritis Inflammation of the ovary
open reduction Surgical procedure that enables the surgeon to reduce (repair) a fracture under direct visualization
ophthalmia neonatorum Inflammation of a newborn's eyes that results from passing through the birth canal when a gonorrheal or chlamydial infection is present
opinion Subjective belief
opisthotonos Complete arching of the body with only the head and feet on the bed
opportunistic infection Infection in persons with a defective immune system that rarely causes harm in healthy individuals
oppression Condition wherein the rules, values, and ideals of one group are imposed on another group
orchiectomy Removal of a testis
orientation Person's awareness of self in relation to person, place, time, and in some cases, situation
orthopedics (orthopaedics) Branch of medicine that deals with the prevention or correction of the disorders and diseases of the musculoskeletal system
orthopnea Difficulty breathing while lying down
orthostatic hypotension Significant decrease in blood pressure that results when a person moves from a lying or sitting (supine) position to a standing position
osmolality Measurement of the total concentration of dissolved particles (solutes) per kilogram of water
osmolarity Concentration of solutes per liter of cellular fluid
osmosis Movement of a solvent, usually water, through a semipermeable membrane, from a region of higher concentration to a region of lower concentration
osmotic pressure Pressure exerted against the cell membrane by the water inside a cell
osteoporosis Increase in the porosity of bone
Outcomes and Assessment Information Set An outcomes measurable tool developed and implemented to determine the care given and reimbursement required; Outcomes and Assessment Information Set (OASIS) data is reported to the Centers for Medicare and Medicaid Services (CMS)
overflow incontinence Leaking of urine when the bladder becomes very full and distended
oxidation Chemical process of combining with oxygen
oxidized Joined with oxygen

P

pain Unpleasant sensory and emotional experience associated with actual or potential tissue damage or described in terms of such
pain threshold Level of intensity at which pain becomes appreciable or perceptible
pain tolerance Level of intensity or duration of pain that a person is willing to endure
palliative care Care that relieves symptoms, such as pain, but does not alter the course of disease
pallor Abnormal paleness of the skin, seen especially in the face, conjunctiva, nail beds, and oral mucous membranes
palpation Physical examination technique that uses the sense of touch to assess texture, temperature, moisture, organ location and size, vibrations and pulsations, swelling, masses, and tenderness
pancreatitis Acute or chronic inflammation of the pancreas
Papanicolaou test Smear method of examining stained exfoliative cells
paracentesis Aspiration of fluid from the abdominal cavity
paradoxical reaction Opposite effect of that which would normally be expected
paramedic Specialized health care professional trained to provide advanced life support to the client requiring emergency interventions

paraplegia Paralysis of lower extremities

parasomnia Disorders that intrude on sleep in very active ways

parenteral Any route other than the oral-gastrointestinal tract

parenteral nutrition Feeding method whereby nutrients bypass the small intestine and enter the blood directly

paresthesia Abnormal sensation such as burning, prickling, or tingling

paroxysmal Descriptor for a symptom that begins and ends abruptly

paroxysmal nocturnal dyspnea Condition of suddenly awakening, sweating, and having difficulty breathing

passive euthanasia Process of working with the client's dying process

patency Being freely opened

pathogen Microorganism that causes disease

pathogenicity Ability of a microorganism to produce disease

patient-controlled analgesia Device that allows the client to control the delivery of intravenous or subcutaneous pain medication in a safe, effective manner through a programmable pump

peak plasma level Highest blood concentration of a single dose of a drug until the elimination rate equals the rate of absorption

peer assistance program Rehabilitation program that provides an impaired nurse with referrals, professional and peer counseling support groups, and assistance and monitoring back into nursing

peptic ulcer Erosion formed in the esophagus, stomach, or duodenum resulting from acid/pepsin imbalance

perception Ability to experience, recognize, organize, and interpret sensory stimuli

percussion Physical examination technique that uses short, tapping strokes on the surface of the skin to create vibrations of underlying organs

perfectionism Overwhelming expectation of being able to get everything done in a flawless manner

perfusion Blood flow through an organ or body part

pericardial friction rub Short, high-pitched squeak heard as two inflamed pericardial surfaces rub together

pericardiocentesis Removal of fluid from the pericardial sac

pericarditis Inflammation of the membrane sac surrounding the heart

perineal care Cleansing of the external genitalia, perineum, and the surrounding area

perioperative Period of time encompassing the preoperative, intraoperative, and postoperative phases of surgery

peripheral nervous system System of the cranial nerves, spinal nerves, and the autonomic nervous system

peripheral resistance Pressure within a vessel that resists the flow of blood such as plaque buildup or vasoconstriction

peristalsis Rhythmic, coordinated, serial contraction of the smooth muscles of the gastrointestinal tract

peritonitis Inflammation of the peritoneum, the membranous covering of the abdomen

permeability Ability of a membrane to permit substances to pass through it

petechiae Pinpoint hemorrhagic spots on the skin

phantom limb pain Neuropathic pain that occurs after amputation with pain sensations referred to an area in the missing portion of the limb

pharmacokinetics Study of the absorption, distribution, metabolism, and excretion of drugs to determine the relationship between the dose of a drug and the drug's concentration in biological fluids

phimosis Condition wherein the opening in the foreskin is so small that it cannot be pulled back over the glans

phlebitis Inflammation in the wall of a vein without clot formation

phlebothrombosis Formation of a clot because of blood pooling in the vessel, trauma to the vessel's endothelial lining, or a coagulation problem with little or no inflammation in the vessel

phlebotomist Individual who performs venipuncture

phlebotomy Removal of blood from a vein

phospholipid Lipid composed of glycerol, fatty acids, and phosphorus; the structural component of cells

physical agent Factor in the environment capable of causing disease in a host

physical restraint Equipment that reduces the client's movement

physical wellness Healthy body that functions at an optimal level

physically aggressive Descriptor of an individual who threatens or actually harms someone

physiologic anemia of pregnancy Condition of having delivered after 24 weeks' gestation, whether infant is born alive or dead or number of infants born

phytochemical Physiologically active compound present in plants in very small amounts that gives plants flavor, odor, and color

pica Practice of eating substances not considered edible and that have no nutritive value, such as laundry starch, dirt, clay, and freezer frost

pie charting Documentation method using the problem, intervention, evaluation (PIE) format

piggyback Addition of an intravenous solution to infuse concurrently with another infusion

placenta Membranous vascular organ connecting the fetus to the mother, which produces hormones to sustain a pregnancy, supplies the fetus with oxygena and food, and transports waste products out of the fetal system

placenta previa Condition in which the placenta forms over or very near the internal cervical os

plague An infectious disease transmitted by a bite of a flea from a rodent (usually a rat) infected with the bacillus Yersinia pestis; plague is a potential agent of bioterrorism

planning Third step of the nursing process; includes both the establishing of guidelines for the proposed course of nursing action to resolve the nursing diagnoses and developing the client's plan of care

plateau Level at which a drug's blood concentration is maintained

pleural effusion Collection of fluid within the pleural cavity

pleural friction rub Abnormal breath sound that is creaky and grating in nature and is heard on inspiration and expiration

pleurisy Condition arising from inflammation of the pleura, or sac, that encases the lung

pneumonia Inflammation of the bronchioles and alveoli accompanied by consolidation, or solidification of exudate, in the lungs

pneumothorax Condition wherein air or gas accumulates in the pleural space of the lungs, causing the lungs to collapse

point-of-care charting Documentation system that allows health care providers to gain immediate access to client information at the bedside

poison Any substance that when taken into the body interferes with normal physiologic functioning; may be inhaled, injected, ingested, or absorbed by the body

polydipsia Excessive thirst

polymenorrhea Menstrual periods that are abnormally frequent, generally less than every 21 days

polyp Abnormal growth of tissue

polyphagia Increased hunger

polypharmacy Problem of clients taking numerous prescription and over-the-counter medications for the same or various disease processes, with unknown consequences from the resulting combinations of chemical compounds and cumulative side-effects

polyunsaturated fatty acid Forms a glycerol ester with many carbons unbonded to hydrogen atoms; fish, corn, sunflower seeds, soybeans, cotton seeds, and safflower oil

polyuria Increased urination

Port-a-Cath Port that has been implanted under the skin with a catheter inserted into the superior vena cava or right atrium through the subclavian or internal jugular vein

portal of entry Route by which an infectious agent enters the host

portal of exit Route by which an infectious agent leaves the reservoir

postictal After a seizure

post-mortem care Care given immediately after death before the body is moved to the mortuary

postoperative phase Time during the surgical experience that begins at the end of the surgical procedure and ends when the client is discharged, not just from the hospital or institution, but from medical care by the surgeon

postpartum blues Mild transient condition of emotional lability and crying for no apparent reason, which affects up to 80% of women who have just given birth, and lasts about 2 weeks

postpartum depression Condition similar to postpartum blues but is more serious, intense, and persistent

postpartum hemorrhage Blood loss of more than 500 mL after the third stage of labor or 1,000 mL following a cesarean birth

postpartum psychosis Condition more severe than postpartum depression and characterized by delusions and thoughts of self-harm or infant harm

postprandial After eating

postterm Delivery after 42 weeks' gestation

post-void residual Urine that remains in the bladder after urination

prayer A type of communication between an individual and spiritual entities

preadolescence Development from the ages of approximately 10 years to 12 years

precipitate birth Birth occurring suddenly and unexpectantly without a CNM/physician present to assist

precipitate labor Labor lasting less than 3 hours from the onset of contractions to the birth of the infant

preeclampsia Phase of pregnancy-induced hypertension prior to convulsions

preferred provider organization Type of managed care model wherein member choice is limited to providers within the system for full reimbursement and other providers for less reimbursement

prenatal care Care of a woman during pregnancy, before labor

prenatal stage Development beginning with conception and ending with birth

preoperative phase Time during the surgical experience that begins when the client decides to have surgery and ends when the client is transferred to the operating table

presbycusis Sensorineural hearing loss associated with aging

presbyopia Inability of the lens of the eye to change curvature to focus near objects
preschool stage Development from the ages of 3 years to 6 years
prescriptive authority Legal recognition of the ability to prescribe medications
presenting part Part of the fetus in contact with the cervix
pressured speech Rapid, intense style of speech
preterm Delivery after 24 weeks' gestation but before 38 weeks (full term)
preterm birth Birth that takes place before the end of the 37th week of gestation
preterm labor Onset of regular contractions of the uterus that cause cervical changes between 20 and 37 weeks' gestation
prevention Obstructing, thwarting, or hindering a disease or illness
priapism Prolonged erection that does not occur in response to sexual stimulation
primary care provider Health care provider whom a client sees first for health care, typically a family practitioner (physician/nurse), internist, or pediatrician
primary health care Client's point of entry into the health care system; includes assessment, diagnosis, treatment, coordination of care, education, prevention services, and surveillance
primary hypertension High blood pressure, the cause of which is unknown; also known as essential hypertension
primary prevention All practices designed to keep health problems from developing
primary source Major provider of information about a client
primary tubercle Nodule that contains tubercle bacilli and forms within lung tissue
primigravida Condition of being pregnant for the first time
primipara Condition of having delivered once after 24 weeks' gestation
privacy The right to be left alone, to choose care based on personal beliefs, to govern body integrity, and to choose when and how sensitive information is shared (Badzek & Gross, 1999)
problem-oriented medical record Documentation method employs a structured, logical format and focuses on the client's problem
process Series of steps or acts that leads to accomplishing some goal or purpose
procrastination Intentionally putting off or delaying something that should be done
prodromal stage Time interval from the onset of nonspecific symptoms until specific symptoms of the infectious process begin to manifest
professional boundaries Limits of the professional relationship that allow for a safe, therapeutic connection between the professional and the client
progressive muscle relaxation Stress-management strategy in which muscles are alternately tensed and relaxed
projectile vomiting Forceful ejection (up to 3 feet) of the contents of the stomach
prolapsed cord Condition in which the umbilical cord lies below the presenting part of the fetus
prolapsed uterus Downward displacement of the uterus into the vagina
prospective payment Predetermined rate paid for each episode of hospitalization based on the client's age and principal diagnosis and the presence or absence of surgery or comorbidity
protocol Series of standing orders or procedures that should be followed under certain specific conditions
proxemics Study of the space between people and its effect on interpersonal behavior
pruritus Severe itching
pseudocyesis False pregnancy
pseudomenstruation Blood-tinged mucus discharge from the vagina of a newborn caused by the withdrawal of maternal hormones
psychoanalysis Therapy focused on uncovering unconscious memories and processes
psychological wellness Enjoyment of creativity, satisfaction of the basic need to love and be loved, understanding of emotions, and ability to maintain control over emotions
psychomotor domain Area of learning that involves performance of motor skills
psychoneuroimmunology Study of the complex relationship among the physical, cognitive, and affective aspects of humans
psychoprophylaxis Mental and physical preparation for childbirth; synonymous with Lamaze
psychosis State wherein an individual has lost the ability to recognize reality
psychotherapy Treatment of mental and emotional disorders through psychological rather than physical methods
ptosis Drooping upper eyelid
puberty Emergence of secondary sex characteristics that signal the beginning of adolescence
public law Law that deals with an individual's relationship to the state
public self What the client thinks others think of him or her
pudendal block Injection of a local anesthetic into the pudendal nerve to provide perineal, external genitalia, and lower vaginal anesthesia

puerperal (postpartum) infection Infection following childbirth occurring between the birth and 6 weeks postpartum
puerperium Term for the first 6 weeks after the birth of an infant
pulse amplitude Measurement of the strength or force exerted by the ejected blood against the arterial wall with each heart contraction
pulse deficit Condition in which the apical pulse rate is greater than the radial pulse rate
pulse rate Indirect measurement of cardiac output obtained by counting the number of peripheral pulse waves over a pulse point
pulse rhythm Regularity of the heartbeat
purpura Reddish-purple patches on the skin indicative of hemorrhage
purulent exudate Discharge resulting from infection; also called pus
pyelonephritis Bacteral infection of the renal pelvis, tubules, and interstitial tissue of one or both kidneys
pyorrhea Periodontal disease
pyuria Pus in the urine

Q

quadriplegia Dysfunction or paralysis of both arms, both legs, and bowel and bladder
quickening Descriptor for when the mother first feels the fetus move, about 16 to 20 weeks' gestation

R

race A group of people with biological similarities
radiation Loss of heat by transfer to cooler near objects, but not through direct contact
radiation sickness An abnormal condition resulting from exposure to ionizing radiation, either purposefully or by accident
radiography Study of x-rays or gamma-ray-exposed film through the action of ionizing radiation
radiotherapy Treatment of cancer with high-energy radiation
rapport Mutual trust established between two people
readiness for learning Evidence of willingness to learn
real self How the individual really thinks about him- or herself
reasoning Use of the elements of thought to solve a problem or settle a question
reconstructive To rebuild or reestablish
rectocele Anterior displacement of the rectum into the posterior vaginal wall
recurrent acute pain Identified by repetitive painful episodes that recur over a prolonged period or throughout a client's lifetime
referred pain Discomfort from the internal organs that is felt in another area of the body
reframing Technique of monitoring negative thoughts and replacing them with positive ones
regional anesthesia Method of temporarily rendering a region of the body insensible to pain
rehabilitation Process or therapy designed to assist individuals to reach their optimal level of physical, mental, and psychosocial functioning
relapse Return to a previous behavior or condition
relaxation technique Method used to decrease anxiety and muscle tension
religion A system of organized beliefs, rituals, and practices with which a person identifies and wishes to be associated
religious support system Group of ministers, priests, nuns, rabbis, shamans, mullahs, or laypersons who are able to meet clients' spiritual needs
REM movement disorder Condition wherein the normal paralysis of REM sleep is absent or incomplete and the sleeper acts out the dream
remission Decrease or absence of symptoms of a disease
renal colic Severe pain in the kidney that radiates to the groin
repolarization Recovery phase of the cardiac muscle
reportable conditions Diseases or injuries that the government requires be reported to the appropriate authority or agency; include suspected abuse and/or neglect, sexually transmitted diseases (STDs), and certain other contagious illnesses that could threaten the health of the general public
reservoir Place where the agent can survive
resident flora Microorganisms that are always present, usually without altering the client's health
residual urine Urine remaining in the bladder after the individual has urinated
respect Acceptance of an individual as is and in a nonjudgmental manner
respiration Process of exchanging oxygen and carbon dioxide
respite care Care and service that provides a break to caregivers and is used for a few hours a week, for an occasional weekend, or for longer periods of time
rest State of mental and physical relaxation and calmness
restitution Rotation of the fetal head back to normal alignment with the shoulders after delivery of the fetal head
restless leg syndrome Condition characterized by uncomfortable sensations of tingling or crawling in the muscles, and twitching, burning, prickling, or deep aching in the foot, calf, or upper leg when at rest

restraint Protective device used to limit the physical activity of a client or to immobilize a client or extremity
resuscitation Support measures implemented to restore consciousness and life
reticulocyte Immature red blood cell
retroperitoneal Behind the peritoneum outside the peritoneal cavity
reverse isolation Barrier protection designed to prevent infection in clients who are severely compromised and highly susceptible to infection; also known as protective isolation
reverse tolerance Phenomenon whereby a smaller amount of substance will elicit the desired psychic effects
review of systems Brief account of any recent signs or symptoms related to any body system
rhinorrhea Watery nasal discharge
Ricin A poison made from the waste products of castor bean processing; a potential agent of bioterrorism because of its ease of dissemination
rigor mortis Natural stiffening of muscles after death; begins about 4 hours after death
risk nursing diagnosis Nursing diagnosis indicating that a problem does not yet exist but that specific risk factors are present; composed of "Risk for" followed by the diagnostic label and a list of the risk factors
role An ascribed or assumed expected behavior in a social position or group
role performance Specific behaviors a person exhibits within each role
rooming-in Practice of staying with the client 24 hours a day to provide care and comfort

S

salpingitis Inflammation of the fallopian tube
salt Product formed when an acid and a base react with each other
sanguineous Bloody drainage from a wound or surgical drain
sarcoma Cancer occurring in connective tissue
Sarin A dangerous man-made nerve agent, first developed as an insecticide that is a potential agent for bioterrorism
satiety Feeling of adequate fullness from food
school-age stage Development from the ages of 6 years to 10 years
sclerotherapy Treatment that involves injecting a chemical into the vein, causing the vein to become sclerosed (hardened) so blood no longer flows through it
sclerotic Hardened tissue
scoliosis Lateral curvature of the spine
scrub nurse RN, LP/VN, or surgical technologist who provides services under the direction of the circulating nurse and who is qualified by training or experience to prepare and maintain the integrity, safety, and efficiency of the sterile field throughout an operation
sebaceous cyst Sebaceous gland filled with sebum
sebum Oily substance secreted by the sebaceous glands of the skin
secondary care Care focused on diagnosis and treatment after the client exhibits symptoms of illness
secondary hypertension High blood pressure occurring as a sequel to a pre-existing disease or injury
secondary prevention Early detection, screening, diagnosis, and intervention, to reduce the consequences of a health problem
sedation Reduction of stress, excitement, or irritability via some central nervous system depression
self-awareness Consciously knowing how the self thinks, feels, believes, and behaves at any specific time
self-care deficit State wherein an individual is not able to perform one or more activities of daily living
self-concept Individual's perception of self; includes self-esteem, body image, and ideal self
self-efficacy Belief in one's ability to succeed in attempts to change behavior
self-esteem A personal opinion of oneself
semipermeable membrane Membrane that allows passage of only certain substances
sensation Ability to receive and process stimuli received through the sensory organs
sensible water loss Water loss of which the person is aware
sensitivity Susceptibility of a pathogen to an antibiotic
sensorineural hearing loss Condition in which the inner ear or cochlear portion of cranial nerve VIII is abnormal or diseased
sensory deficit Change in the perception of sensory stimuli; can affect any of the senses
sensory deprivation State of reduced sensory input from the internal or external environment, manifested by alterations in sensory perception
sensory overload State of excessive and sustained multisensory stimulation manifested by behavior change and perceptual distortion
sensory perception Ability to receive sensory impressions and, through cortical association, relate the stimuli to past experiences and form an impression of the nature of the stimulus
seroconversion Evidence of antibody formation in response to disease or vaccine
serosanguineous exudate Discharge that is clear with some blood tinge; seen with surgical incisions
serous exudate Discharge composed primarily of serum; is watery in appearance and has a low protein level.

serum lithium level Laboratory test done to determine whether the client's lithium level is within a therapeutic range

shaman Folk healer-priest who uses natural and supernatural forces to help others

shearing Force exerted against the skin by movement or repositioning

shift report Report about each client between shifts

shock Condition of profound hemodynamic and metabolic disturbance characterized by inadequate tissue perfusion and inadequate circulation to the vital organs

shroud Covering for the body after death

sibilant wheeze Abnormal breath sound that is high pitched and musical in nature and is heard on inhalation and exhalation

sickle When red blood cells become crescent-shaped and elongated

single point of entry Common feature of HMOs wherein the client is required to enter the health care system through a point designated by the plan

single-payer system Health care delivery model wherein the government is the only entity to reimburse health care costs

situational loss Loss that takes place in response to external events generally beyond the individual's control

slander Words that are communicated verbally to a third party and that harm or injure the personal or professional reputation of another

sleep State of altered consciousness during which a person has minimal physical activity, changes in levels of consciousness, and a slowing of physiologic processes

sleep apnea A period during sleep of not breathing; often associated with heavy snoring

sleep cycle Sequence of sleep beginning with the four stages of NREM sleep, a return to stage 3 and then stage 2 (first phase), followed by the first REM sleep (second phase)

sleep deprivation Prolonged inadequate quality and quantity of sleep

small for gestational age Infant's weight falls below the 10th percentile for gestational age

smallpox (variola) A highly contagious and frequently fatal viral disease, which is a potential agent for a bioterroristic attack; there are two varieties, known as variola major and variola minor

Snellen Chart Chart containing various-sized letters with standardized numbers at the end of each line of letters

sociocultural wellness Ability to appreciate the needs of others and to care about one's environment and the inhabitants of it

somatic nervous system Nerves that connect the central nervous system to the skin and skeletal muscles and control conscious activities

somatic pain Nonlocalized discomfort originating in tendons, ligaments, and nerves

somnambulism Sleepwalking

Somogyi phenomenon In response to hypoglycemia, the release of glucose-elevating hormones (epinephrine, cortisol, glucose), which produces a hyperglycemic state

sonorous wheeze Abnormal breath sound that is low pitched and snoring in nature and is louder on expiration

spermatogenesis Production of sperm

spina bifida occulta Failure of the vertebral arch to close

spinal shock Cessation of motor, sensory, autonomic, and reflex impulses below the level of injury; characterized by flaccid paralysis of all skeletal muscles, loss of spinal reflexes, loss of sensation, and absence of autonomic function below the level of injury

spiritual care Recognition of and assistance toward meeting spiritual needs

spiritual distress A client in this situation may have a troubled, fragmented, or possibly disintegrating spirit

spiritual needs Individual's desire to find purpose and meaning in life, pain, and death

spiritual wellness Inner strength and peace

spirituality The core of a person's being, a higher experience or transcendence of oneself

spore Bacteria in a resistant stage that can withstand unfavorable environments

sprain Injury to ligaments surrounding a joint caused by a sudden twist, wrench, or fall

stable Alert with vital signs within the client's normal range

staff development Delivery of instruction to assist nurses achieve the goals of the employer

standard Level or degree of quality

Standard Precautions Preventive practices to be used in the care of all clients in hospitals regardless of their diagnosis or presumed infection status

standards of practice Guidelines established to direct nursing care

startle response Overreaction to minor sounds or noises

stasis dermatitis Inflammation of the skin due to decreased circulation

station Relationship of the fetal presenting part to the ischial spines

status asthmaticus Persistent, intractable asthma attack

status epilepticus Acute, prolonged episode of seizure activity that lasts at least 30 minutes and may or may not involve loss of consciousness

statutory law Law enacted by legislative bodies

steatorrhea Fatty stool

stent Tiny metal tube with holes in it that prevents a vessel from collapsing and keeps the atherosclerotic plaque pressed against the vessel wall; any material used to hold tissue in place or provide support
stereognosis Ability to recognize an object by feel
stereotyping Belief that all people within the same ethnic, racial, or cultural group act the same way, sharing the same beliefs and attitudes
sterile Without microorganisms
sterile conscience Individual's personal sense of honesty and integrity with regard to adherence to the principles of aseptic technique, including prompt admission and correction of any errors and omissions
sterile field Area surrounding the client and the surgical site that is free from all microorganisms; created by draping of the work area and the client with sterile drape
sterilization Destroying all microorganisms, including spores
stock supply Medications dispensed and labeled in large quantities for storage in the medication room or nursing unit
stoma Surgical opening between a cavity and the surface of the body
stomatitis Inflammation of the oral mucosa
strabismus Inability of the eyes to focus in the same direction
strain Injury to a muscle or tendon due to overuse or overstretching
stress Nonspecific response to any demand made on the body (Selye, 1974)
stress incontinence Leakage of urine when a person does anything that strains the abdomen, such as coughing, laughing, jogging, dancing, sneezing, lifting, making a quick movement, or even walking
stress test Measure of a client's cardiovascular response to exercise
stressor Any situation, event, or agent that produces stress
striae gravidarum Reddish streaks frequently found on the abdomen, thighs, buttocks, and breasts; also called "stretch marks"
stridor High-pitched, harsh sound heard on inspiration when the trachea or larynx is obstructed
stroke volume Volume of blood pumped by the ventricle with each contraction
stye Pustular inflammation of an eyelash follicle or sebaceous gland on the eyelid margin
subacute care Short-term, aggressive care for clients who are out of the acute stage of illness but who still require skilled nursing, monitoring, and ongoing treatment
subcutaneous Injection into the subcutaneous tissue
subinvolution Incomplete return of the uterus to its prepregnant size and consistency
subluxation Partial separation of an articular surface
substance A drug, legal or illegal, that may cause physical or mental impairment
suicidal ideations Thoughts of hurting or killing oneself
supine hypotensive syndrome Lowering of blood pressure in a pregnant woman when lying supine due to compression of the vena cava by the enlarged, heavy uterus
surfactant Phospholipids that are present in the lungs and lower surface tension to prevent collapse of the airways
surgery Treatment of injury, disease, or deformity through invasive operative methods
suture Thin, fibrous, membrane-covered space between skull bones
synarthrosis Immovable joint
syndactyly Fusion of two or more fingers or toes
synergism Result of two or more agents working together to achieve a greater effect than either could produce alone
synthesiasis Hearing colors and seeing sounds
synthesis Chemical reaction when two or more atoms, called reactants, bond and form a more complex molecular product; putting data together in a new way

T

tachycardia Heart rate in excess of 100 beats per minute in an adult
tachypnea Respiratory rate greater than 24 beats per minute
talipes equinovarus A congenital deformity in which the foot and ankle are twisted inward and cannot be moved to a midline position; also known as clubfoot
teaching Active process wherein one individual shares information with another as a means to facilitate learning and thereby promote behavioral changes
teaching strategy Technique to promote learning
teaching–learning process Planned interaction that promotes a behavioral change that is not a result of maturation or coincidence
telangiectasic nevi Birthmarks of dilated capillaries that blanch with pressure; also called stork-bites
telangiestasia Permanent dilation of groups of superficial capillaries and venules; commonly known as "spider veins"
telehealth An electronic information services that offer increased client and family participation; for example, nurse and client use interactive videos, telephone

cardiac rate monitoring with EKG readout, digital subscriber lines, and Internet transmission of data

telemedicine An element of telehealth permitting physicians to provide care through a telecommunication system

teleology Ethical theory that states that the value of a situation is determined by its consequences

tenesmus Spasmodic contradiction of the anal or bladder sphincter, causing pain and a persistent urge to empty the bowel or bladder

teratogen Agent such as radiation, drugs, viruses, and other microorganisms capable of causing abnormal fetal development

teratogenic Causing abnormal development of the embryo

teratogenic substance Substance that crosses the placenta and impairs normal growth and development

term Descriptor for a pregnancy between 38 and 42 weeks' gestation

terrorism Instilling fear in large groups of persons by using any product, weapon, or the threat of using a harmful act or substance to kill or injure people

tertiary care Care focused on restoring the client to the state of health that existed before the development of an illness; if unattainable, then care is directed to attaining the optimal level of health possible

tertiary prevention Treatment of an illness or disease after symptoms have appeared, so as to prevent further progression

tetany Sharp flexion of the wrist and ankle joints, involving muscle twitching or cramps

therapeutic communication Communication that is purposeful and goal directed, creating a beneficial outcome for the client

therapeutic massage Application of hand pressure and motion to improve the recipient's well-being

therapeutic procedure accident Accident that occurs during the delivery of medical or nursing interventions

therapeutic touch Technique of assessing alterations in a person's energy fields and using the hands to direct energy to achieve a balanced state

thermogenesis Production of heat

thermoregulation Maintenance of body temperature

thoracentesis Aspiration of fluid from the pleural cavity

thrombocytopenia Decrease in the number of platelets in the blood

thrombophlebitis Formation of a clot due to an inflammation in the wall of the vessel

thrombosis Formation of a clot due to an inflammation in the wall of the vessel

thrombus Formed clot that remains at the site where it formed

time management System to help meet goals through problem solving

tinnitus Ringing sound in the ear

tocolysis Process of stopping labor with medications

tocolytic agent Medication that inhibits uterine contractions

toddler stage Development begins at approximately 12 to 18 months of age, when a child begins to walk, and ends at approximately 3 years of age

tolerance Decreased sensitivity to subsequent doses of the same substance; an increased dose of the substance is needed to produce the same desired effect

tophi Subcutaneous nodules of sodium urate crystals

tort Civil wrong committed by a person against another person or property

tort law Enforcement of duties and rights among individuals and independent of contractual agreements

touch Means of perceiving or experiencing through tactile sensation

toxic effect Reaction that occurs when the body cannot metabolize a drug and the drug accumulates in the blood

trade (brand) name Name assigned to a drug by the pharmaceutical company; always capitalized

transcendence A state of being or existence above and beyond the limits of material experience

transcutaneous electrical nerve stimulation Process of applying a low-voltage electrical current to the skin through cutaneous electrodes

transducer Instrument that converts electrical energy to sound waves

transduction Noxious stimulus that triggers electrical activity in the endings of afferent nerve fibers (nociceptors)

transmission Process whereby the pain impulse travels from the receiving nociceptors to the spinal cord

Transmission-based Precautions Practices designed for clients documented as, or suspected of, being infected with highly transmissible or epidemiologically important pathogens for which additional precautions beyond Standard Precautions are required to interrupt transmission in hospitals

trauma Wound or injury

traumatic imagery Imagining the feelings of horror felt by the victim or reliving the horror of the incident

triage Classification of clients to determine priority of need and proper place of treatment

triglyceride Lipid compound consisting of three fatty acids and a glycerol molecule

trocar Sharply pointed surgical instrument contained in a cannula

Trousseau's sign Carpal spasm caused by inflating a blood pressure cuff above the client's systolic pressure and leaving it in place for 3 minutes

trust Ability to rely on an individual's character and ability

tumor marker Substance found in the serum that indicates the possible presence of malignancy

turgor Normal resiliency of the skin

type and cross-match Laboratory test that identifies the client's blood type (e.g., A or B) and determines the compatibility of the blood between potential donor and recipient

U

ultrasound Use of high-frequency sound waves to visualize deep body structures; also called an echogram or sonogram

umbilical cord Structure that connects the fetus to the placenta

uncomplicated grief Grief reaction normally following a significant loss

unilateral neglect Failure to recognize or care for one side of the body

unit dose form System of packaging and labeling each dose of medication by the pharmacy, usually for a 24-hour period

urethrocele Downward displacement of the urethra into the vagina

urethrostomy Formation of a permanent fistula opening into the urethra

urge incontinence Inability to suppress the sudden urge or need to urinate

urgent care center A facility designed for the effective and efficient treatment of acute illnesses and injuries; clients do not require an appointment, do not see the same provider consistently, and are usually seen in the order of arrival or the order of acuity

urobilinogen Colorless derivative of bilirubin formed by the normal bacterial action of intestinal flora on bilirubin

urticaria Allergic reaction causing raised pruritic, red, nontender wheals on the skin; also called hives

uterine retraction Unique ability of the muscle fibers of the uterus to remain shortened to a small degree after each contraction

uterine souffle Sound of blood pulsating through the uterus and placenta

utility Ethical principle that states that an act must result in the greatest positive benefit for the greatest number of people involved

V

value system Individual's collection of inner beliefs that guides the way the person acts and helps determine the choices the person makes

values Influences on the development of beliefs and attitudes rather than behaviors; a principle, standard, or quality considered worthwhile or desirable

values clarification Process of analyzing one's own values to better understand those things that are truly important

variable deceleration Reduction in fetal heart rate that has no relationship to contractions of the uterus

vasectomy Surgical resection of the vas deferens

venipuncture Puncturing of a vein with a needle to aspirate blood

ventilation Movement of gases into and out of the lungs

veracity Ethical principle based on truthfulness (neither lying nor deceiving others)

verbal communication Using words, either spoken or written, to send a message

verbally aggressive Descriptor of an individual who says things in a loud and/or intimidating manner

vernix caseosa White, creamy substance covering a fetus's body

vertigo Dizziness

vesicant Agent that may produce blisters and tissue necrosis

vesicular sound Soft, breezy, low-pitched sound heard longer on inspiration than expiration resulting from air moving through the smaller airways over the lung periphery, with the exception of the scapular area

villi Finger-like projections that line the small intestine

viral load test Test that measures copies of HIV RNA

visceral pain Discomfort felt in the internal organs

visual hallucination Perception by an individual that something is present when nothing in fact is

visual learner Person who learns by processing information through seeing

vitamin Organic compounds essential to life and health

vitiligo Depigmentation of the skin caused by destruction of melanocytes; appears as milk-white patches on the skin

void Process of urine elimination

volvulus Twisting of a bowel on itself

W

water-soluble vitamin Vitamin that must be ingested daily in normal quantities because it is not stored in the body: vitamins C and B-complex

wellness State of optimal health wherein an individual maximizes human potential, moves toward integration of human functioning, has greater self-awareness and self-satisfaction, and takes responsibility for health
Western blot test Confirmatory test used to detect HIV infection
Wharton's jelly Thick substance surrounding and protecting the vessels of the umbilical cord
whistleblowing Calling public attention to unethical, illegal, or incompetent actions of others
windowing Cutting a hole in a plaster cast to relieve pressure on the skin or a bony area and to permit visualization of the underlying body part
witch's milk A whitish fluid secreted by a newborn's nipples
withdrawal Symptoms produced when a substance on which an individual has dependence is no longer used by that individual
word salad Nonsensical combination of words that is meaningless to others
wound Disruption in the integrity of body tissue

Y

yin and yang Opposing forces that yield health when in balance
young adulthood Development from the ages of 21 years through approximately 40 years

Z

zoonotic disease A disease of animals that is directly transmissible to humans from the primary animal host
zygote Fertilized ovum

INDEX

Page numbers followed by "f" denote figures, "t" denote tables, and "b" denote boxes.

A

B

C

D

E

F

G

H

I

J

K

L

M

N

O

P

Q

R

S

U

V

W

X

Y

Z